Difficult Medical Management

Difficult Medical Management

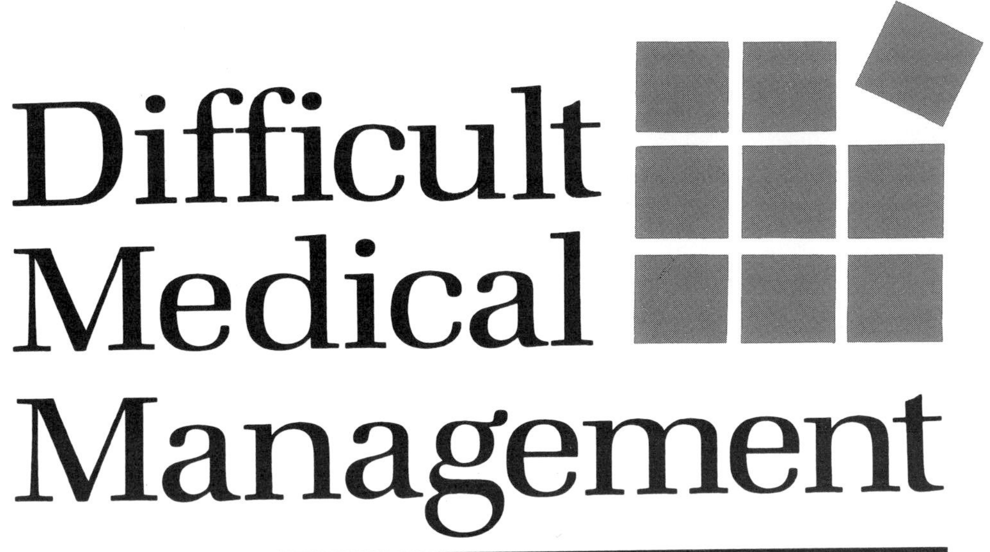

Robert B. Taylor, M.D.

Professor and Chairman, Department of Family Medicine
Oregon Health Sciences, University School of Medicine
Portland, Oregon

1991

W. B. SAUNDERS COMPANY

Harcourt Brace Jovanovich, Inc.

Philadelphia ○ London ○ Toronto ○ Montreal ○ Sydney ○ Tokyo

W. B. SAUNDERS COMPANY

Harcourt Brace Jovanovich, Inc.
The Curtis Center
Independence Square West
Philadelphia, PA 19106

Library of Congress Cataloging-in-Publication Data

Difficult medical management / (edited by) Robert B. Taylor.
    p. cm.
    Includes index.
    ISBN 0-7216-8768-7
    1. Clinical medicine. I. Taylor, Robert B.
    (DNLM: 1. Clinical Medicine. WB 100 D569)
RC48.D54 1991
616—dc20
DNLM/DLC
for Library of Congress
                                                    90-8706
                                                       CIP

Editor: John Dyson
Designer: Karen O'Keefe
Production Manager: Linda R. Turner
Manuscript Editor: Wynette Kommer
Illustration Coordinator: Cecelia Kunkle
Indexer: Julie Schwager
Cover Designer: Kim Jones

Difficult Medical Management   ISBN 0-7216-8768-7

Printed in the United States of America

Last digit is the print number: 9   8   7   6   5   4   3   2   1

Contributors

RICHARD F. AFABLE, M.D.
Assistant Professor of Clinical Medicine, Northwestern University Medical School; St. Joseph's Hospital, Chicago, Illinois.
Hypertension, Refractory

BRUCE D. AGINS, M.D.
Assistant Professor of Medicine, Cornell University College of Medicine; Director of AIDS Program, Division of Infectious Diseases and Immunology, North Shore University Hospital, Manhasset, New York.
Infections in the Acquired Immunodeficiency Syndrome Patient

MICHAEL W. ANDERSON, M.D.
Staff, Orlando Regional Medical Center and Arnold Palmer Children's and Women's Hospitals, Orlando, Florida.
Anaphylaxis and Anaphylactoid Reactions

PENG-TIAM ANG, M.D., M.R.C.P. (U.K.)
Fellow in Medical Oncology, University of Texas Medical School at Houston; M. D. Anderson Cancer Center, Houston, Texas.
Breast Cancer

DAVID M. ARBESFELD, M.D.
Clinical Instructor of Dermatology, New Jersey Medical School, Newark, New Jersey.
Herpes Simplex Virus Infections

MICHAEL E. ASSEY, M.D.
Associate Professor of Medicine and Director, Adult Cardiac Catheterization Laboratories, Medical University of South Carolina, Charleston, South Carolina.
Endocarditis, Infective

LUIS A. BALART, M.D.
Clinical Assistant Professor of Medicine, Tulane University School of Medicine; Director, Gastroenterology Training, Department of Internal Medicine, Ochsner Clinic, New Orleans, Louisiana.
Transplantation Patient, Medical Care of the

LES L. BARRICKMAN, D.O.
Associate in Child Psychiatry, University of Iowa College of Medicine, Iowa City, Iowa.
Attention-Deficit Hyperactivity Disorder

RALPH E. BENNETT, M.D.
Arthritis Center, Ltd., Phoenix, Arizona.
Rheumatoid Arthritis

ELLEN BERKOWITZ, M.D.
Faculty, Family Practice Residency Program, Tallahassee Memorial Regional Medical Center, Tallahassee, Florida.
Borderline Personality Disorder

ALICE N. BESSMAN, M.D.
Professor of Medicine, University of Southern California School of Medicine, Los Angeles; Co-Chief, Ortho/Diabetes Services, Rancho los Amigos Medical Center, Downey, California.
Infections in the Diabetic Patient

FREDERICK C. BITTIKOFER, M.D.
Senior Physician and Assistant Chief, Department of Psychiatry, Kaiser Permanente Medical Group, Santa Clara, California.
Panic Disorder and Agoraphobia

JOSEF BLANKSTEIN, M.D.
Staff Physician, Section of Reproductive Endocrinology and Infertility, Department of Gynecology, The Cleveland Clinic Foundation, Cleveland, Ohio.
Anovulation

ALVIN S. BLAUSTEIN, M.D.
Associate Professor of Medicine, Division of Cardiology, University of Cincinnati College of Medicine; Chief of Cardiovascular Noninvasive Diagnostic Laboratory, and Associate Chief, Medical Intensive Care Unit, Veterans Administration Medical Center, Cincinnati, Ohio.
Angina Pectoris, Unstable

PETER J. BOOSALIS, B.A.
American Heart Association Medical Student Research Fellow, University of Minnesota School of Medicine, Minneapolis, Minnesota.
Congestive Heart Failure

V. ALIN BOTOMAN, M.D.
Assistant Clinical Professor of Medicine, University of Washington School of Medicine; Attending Gastroenterologist, Virginia Mason Clinic and Hospital, Seattle, Washington.
Inflammatory Bowel Disease

ALEX H. BRUCKSTEIN, M.D.
Clinical Associate Professor of Medicine, New York Medical College, Valhalla; Assistant Attending, Department of Medicine, Division of Gastroenterology, St. Vincent's Medical Center of Richmond, Staten Island, New York.
Ascites
Peptic Ulcer Disease in Elderly Patients

RUTH DOWLING BRUUN, M.D.
Clinical Associate Professor of Psychiatry, Cornell University Medical College; Attending Psychiatrist, New York Hospital–Cornell Medical Center, New York, New York.
Tourette's Syndrome

ROBERT BURAKOFF, M.D.
Associate Professor of Medicine, State University of New York at Stony Brook, School of Medicine, Stony Brook; Chief, Division of Gastroenterology, Winthrop-University Hospital, Mineola, New York.
Cirrhosis of the Liver in the Alcoholic Patient

SIDNEY N. BUSIS, M.D.
Clinical Professor of Otolaryngology, University of Pittsburgh School of Medicine; Senior Staffs, Eye and Ear Hospital, Children's Hospital, and Montefiore Hospital, Pittsburgh, Pennsylvania.
Meniere's Disease

AMAN U. BUZDAR, M.D.
Professor of Medicine, Department of Medical Oncology, University of Texas Medical School at Houston; M. D. Anderson Cancer Center, Houston, Texas.
Breast Cancer

PAUL H. CALDRON, D.O.
Arthritis Center, Ltd.; Staff Physician, Humana-Phoenix Center, Phoenix, Arizona.
Rheumatoid Arthritis

STEPHEN M. CAMPBELL, M.D.
Associate Professor of Medicine, Division of Arthritis and Rheumatic Disease, Oregon Health Sciences University School of Medicine; Chief, Rheumatology Section, Veterans Administration Medical Center; Portland, Oregon.
Reflex Sympathetic Dystrophy Syndrome

LOUIS A. CANNON, M.D.
Instructor, Emergency Medicine, University of Cincinnati College of Medicine; Research Fellow, Ohio Affiliate A.H.A., University of Cincinnati Medical Center, Cincinnati, Ohio.
Angina Pectoris, Unstable

JOHN B. CHAWLUK, M.D.
Clinical Associate Professor of Neurology, Medical College of Pennsylvania; Clinical Assistant Professor of Neurology, University of Pennsylvania School of Medicine, Philadelphia, Pennsylvania; Staff Neurologist, Episcopal Hospital, Philadelphia, and Good Samaritan Hospital, Pottsville, Pennsylvania.
Transient Ischemic Attacks

ANTHONY W. CHOW, M.D., F.A.C.P., F.R.C.P.C.
Professor of Medicine, University of British Columbia; Head, Division of Infectious Diseases, Vancouver General Hospital, Vancouver, British Columbia.
Antimicrobial Use During Pregnancy and Lactation

IRA SETH COHEN, M.D.
Director, Noninvasive Laboratory, Sinai Hospital of Detroit, Detroit, Michigan.
Atrial Fibrillation

JOHN D. CONGER, M.D.
Professor of Medicine, Division of Renal Diseases, University of Colorado School of Medicine; Director, Hemodialysis Unit, Veterans Administration Medical Center, Denver, Colorado.
Renal Failure, Acute

DONALD R. COUSTAN, M.D.
Professor of Obstetrics and Gynecology, Brown University Program in Medicine; Director of Obstetrics and Maternal-Fetal Medicine, Women and Infants Hospital of Rhode Island, Providence, Rhode Island.
Diabetes Mellitus in Pregnancy

GARY WALTER CROOKS, M.D.
Assistant Professor of Medicine, University of Pennsylvania School of Medicine; Staff Physician, Section of General Internal Medicine, Hospital of the University of Pennsylvania, Philadelphia, Pennsylvania.
Hypercholesterolemia

GERALD M. CROSS, M.D.
Lieutenant Colonel, United States Army Medical Corps; Director, Residential Treatment Facility, William Beaumont Army Medical Center, El Paso, Texas.
Alcohol Withdrawal Syndromes

KENT CROSSLEY, M.D.
Professor of Medicine, University of Minnesota School of Medicine, Minneapolis; Chief, Infectious Disease Section, St. Paul-Ramsey Medical Center, St. Paul, Minnesota.
Meningitis and Encephalitis

DAVID C. CUMMING, M.B., Ch.B., F.R.C.O.G., F.R.C.S.C.
Associate Professor, Department of Obstetrics and Gynaecology and Division of Endocrinology, Department of Medicine, University of Alberta; Active Staff, Obstetrics and Gynaecology and Consultant Staff, Endocrinology, University of Alberta Hospital, Edmonton, Alberta, Canada.
Polycystic Ovarian Disease

JEFFREY L. CUMMINGS, M.D.
Associate Professor of Neurology and Psychiatry and Biobehavioral Sciences, University of California, Los Angeles School of Medicine; Director, Neurobehavior Unit, West Los Angeles Veterans Administration Medical Center, Los Angeles, California.
Alzheimer's Disease

RICHARD D. deSHAZO, M.D.
Professor of Medicine and Pediatrics; Chairman, Department of Internal Medicine, University of South Alabama College of Medicine; University of South Alabama Medical Center, Mobile, Alabama.
Anaphylaxis and Anaphylactoid Reactions

ADRIAN S. DOBS, M.D.
Assistant Professor of Medicine, Department of Internal Medicine, Division of Endocrinology and Metabolism, Johns Hopkins University School of Medicine; Staff, Johns Hopkins Hospital, Baltimore, Maryland.
Obesity in the Diabetic Patient

MICHAEL DONAHOE, M.D.
Assistant Professor of Medicine, Division of Pulmonary/Critical Care Medicine, University of Pittsburgh School of Medicine; Director, Medical Intensive Care Unit, Presbyterian University Hospital, Pittsburgh, Pennsylvania.
Sleep Apnea

PAUL M. DORINSKY, M.D.
Associate Professor of Medicine, Division of Pulmonary and Critical Care Medicine, The Ohio State University College of Medicine; Director, Medical Intensive Care Unit, Ohio State University Hospital, Columbus, Ohio.
Adult Respiratory Distress Syndrome

BRUNO ESCALER, M.D.
Fellow in Cardiovascular Diseases, Wayne State University School of Medicine; Sinai Hospital of Detroit, Detroit, Michigan.
Atrial Fibrillation

STANLEY FAHN, M.D.
H. Houston Merritt Professor of Neurology, Columbia University College of Physicians and Surgeons; Attending Neurologist, Columbia-Presbyterian Medical Center, New York, New York.
Parkinson's Disease

SEBASTIAN FARO, M.D., Ph.D.
Professor of Obstetrics and Gynecology, Section of Infectious Diseases, Baylor College of Medicine; Attending, St. Luke's Episcopal Hospital, Methodist Hospital, Ben Taub Hospital, Lyndon B. Johnson County Hospital, Houston, Texas.
Vaginitis, Recurrent

JAMES V. FELICETTA, M.D.
Associate Clinical Professor of Internal Medicine, University of Arizona College of Medicine, Tucson; Chief of Medical Service, Carl T. Hayden Veterans Administration Medical Center, Phoenix, Arizona.
Thyroid Disease in the Elderly Patient

ROBERT B. FICK, Jr., M.D.
Associate Professor of Medicine and Chair, Senior Curriculum in Medicine, University of Iowa College of Medicine; Division of Pulmonary and Critical Care Medicine, University of Iowa Hospitals and Clinics, Iowa City, Iowa.
Cystic Fibrosis

JULIO E. FIGUEROA, M.D.
Head, Section on Nephrology, Department of Internal Medicine, Ochsner Clinic, New Orleans, Louisiana.
Transplantation Patient, Medical Care of the

MORRIS A. FLAUM, M.D.
Staff Physician, Section on Hematology, Department of Internal Medicine, Ochsner Clinic and Alton Ochsner Medical Foundation, New Orleans, Louisiana.
Transplantation Patient, Medical Care of the

KATHLEEN A. FLETCHER
Assistant Director, The Center for Research in Sleep Disorders, Mercy Hospital, Hamilton/Fairfield, Ohio.
Narcolepsy

GARY S. FRANCIS, M.D.
Professor of Medicine, University of Minnesota School of Medicine; Director, Acute Cardiac Care, University of Minnesota Hospital, Minneapolis, Minnesota.
Congestive Heart Failure

HOWARD FRUMIN, M.D.
Assistant Professor of Medicine, Wayne State University School of Medicine; Director, Electrophysiology and Pacing Laboratory, Sinai Hospital of Detroit, Detroit, Michigan.
Atrial Fibrillation

DAVID L. GARBOWIT, M.D.
Attending, Memorial Hospital, Burlington County, New Jersey.
Hypertensive Crisis

JUDITH G. GEARHART, M.D.
Assistant Professor of Family Medicine, University of Mississippi School of Medicine; Staff Physician, University Hospital, Mississippi Baptist Medical Center, and St. Dominic Memorial Hospital, Jackson, Mississippi.
Pelvic Infections

BIMAL C. GHOSH, M.D., F.A.C.S.
Professor of Surgery, Uniformed Services University of the Health Sciences; Chairman, Division of Surgical Oncology, National Naval Medical Center, Bethesda, Maryland.
Malignant Melanoma

A. JAMES GIANNINI, M.D.
Clinical Professor of Psychiatry, Ohio State University; Medical Director, A. James Giannini, Inc.; Medical Director, Chemical Abuse Centers, Inc., Youngstown, Ohio.
Anorexia Nervosa and Bulimia

AARON E. GLATT, M.D.
Assistant Professor of Medicine, State University of New York at Stony Brook School of Medicine, Stony Brook; Assistant Chief of Infectious Diseases, Nassau County Medical Center, East Meadow, New York.
Infections in the Acquired Immunodeficiency Syndrome Patient

IRWIN GOLDSTEIN, M.D.
Associate Professor of Urology, Boston University School of Medicine, Boston, Massachusetts.
Impotence

MARC B. GOLDSTEIN, M.D.
Professor of Medicine, University of Toronto; Medical Director, Hemodialysis Program, St. Michael's Hospital, Toronto, Ontario, Canada
Hyponatremia

REX L. GOMEZ, M.D.
Attending Physician, South West Florida Regional Medical Center and Lee County Memorial Hospital, Fort Myers, Florida. Formerly: Senior Fellow in Gastroenterology, Medical College of Georgia, Augusta, Georgia.
Esophageal Motility Disorders

JOSEPH W. GRIFFIN, Jr., M.D.
Professor of Medicine, Medical College of Georgia Hospital and Clinics, Augusta, Georgia.
Esophageal Motility Disorders

TROY H. GUTHRIE, Jr., M.D.
Associate Professor of Medicine, Section of Hematology/Medical Oncology, Medical College of Georgia, and Medical College of Georgia Hospital and Clinics, Augusta, Georgia.
Prostate Cancer

NANCY K. HANSEL, Dr.P.H.
Associate Professor, Department of Family Practice and Community Medicine, The University of Texas Medical School at Houston and Health Science Center, Houston, Texas.
Near-Drowning

RICHARD L. HARRIS, M.D.
Associate Professor of Clinical Medicine, Baylor College of Medicine; Medical Epidemiologist, The Methodist Hospital, Houston, Texas.
Bacteremia and Sepsis

DANIEL H. HAYES, M.D.
Clinical Instructor of Surgery, Louisiana State University Medical Center; Director, Liver Transplant Program, Ochsner Foundation Hospital, New Orleans, Louisiana.
Transplantation Patient, Medical Care of the

KEITH HENRY, M.D.
Assistant Professor of Medicine, University of Minnesota School of Medicine, Minneapolis; Staff Physician and Director, HIV Clinic, St. Paul–Ramsey Medical Center, St. Paul, Minnesota.
Meningitis and Encephalitis

HAROLD HOROWITZ, M.D.
Assistant Professor of Medicine, Division of Infectious Diseases, New York Medical College; Westchester County Medical Center, Valhalla, New York.
Human Immunodeficiency Virus (HIV)–Infected Patient
Human Immunodeficiency Virus–Related Disease

RANDY L. HOWARD, M.D.
Fellow in Renal Diseases, Department of Internal Medicine, University of Colorado School of Medicine, Denver, Colorado.
Renal Failure, Acute

MICHAEL F. HOYT, Ph.D.
Associate Clinical Professor, Langley Porter Psychiatric Institute, University of California, San Francisco, School of Medicine; Chief Consultant, Veterans Administration Medical Center, San Francisco; Staff Psychologist and Director of Adult Services, Department of Psychiatry, Kaiser Permanente Medical Center, Hayward, California.
Panic Disorder and Agoraphobia

JOHN L. HUSSEY, M.D.
Section Head, Division of Transplantation, Department of Surgery, Ochsner Clinic; Attending, Ochsner Foundation Hospital, New Orleans, Louisiana.
Transplantation Patient, Medical Care of the

THOMAS J. IBERTI, M.D.
Associate Professor of Surgery and Anesthesiology, Mount Sinai School of Medicine of the City University of New York; Associate Attending, Departments of Anesthesiology and Surgery, and Director, Surgical Intensive Care Unit, Mount Sinai Medical Center, New York, New York.
Smoke Inhalation

STEPHEN W. JENNINGS, M.D., A.C.P.
Director of Sleep Disorders Centers, St. Luke Hospital, Fort Thomas, Florence, Kentucky.
Narcolepsy

LARRY W. JOHNSON, M.D.
Associate Professor of Family Medicine and Residency Director, Medical College of Ohio and St. Vincent Medical Center, Toledo, Ohio.
Urinary Tract Infections, Recurrent

THOMAS H. JOHNSON, M.D.
Fellow in Cardiology, University of Minnesota School of Medicine, Minneapolis, Minnesota.
Congestive Heart Failure

D. M. KAJI, M.D.
Associate Professor of Medicine, Renal Section, Mt. Sinai School of Medicine, New York; Assistant Chief, Renal Section, Veterans Administration Medical Center, Bronx, New York.
Dialysis Patient, Medical Management of the

MARY KENNEDY, R.N., M.S.N.
Program Coordinator, Continuing Care Hospice Program, University of California, Davis, Sacramento Medical Center, Sacramento, California.
Pain Management in the Terminally Ill Patient

NICHOLAS Z. KERIN, M.D.
Associate Professor of Medicine, Wayne State University School of Medicine; Associate Chief, Section of Cardiovascular Diseases, Sinai Hospital of Detroit, Detroit, Michigan.
Atrial Fibrillation

GEORGE KIHICZAK, M.D.
Clinical Assistant Professor of Dermatology, New Jersey Medical School; Attending Physician, UMDNJ University Hospital, Newark, New Jersey.
Herpes Simplex Virus Infections

RICHARD A. KOZAREK, M.D.
Associate Clinical Professor of Medicine, University of Washington School of Medicine; Chief of Gastroenterology, Virginia Mason Medical Center, Seattle, Washington.
Inflammatory Bowel Disease

GREGORY A. KOZENY, M.D.
Associate Professor of Medicine, Section of Nephrology, Loyola University Medical Center/Stritch School of Medicine, Maywood, Illinois.
Hypertension, Refractory

LAWRENCE R. KRAKOFF, M.D.
Professor of Medicine, Chief of the Division of Hypertension, Mount Sinai School of Medicine; Attending Physician, Mount Sinai Hospital, New York, New York.
Hypertensive Crisis

SUBHASH C. KUKREJA, M.D.
Professor of Medicine, University of Illinois College of Medicine; Chief, Nuclear Medicine Service and Endocrinology Section, Veterans Administration West Side Medical Center; Acting Chief, Section of Endocrinology, University of Illinois Hospital, Chicago, Illinois.
Endocrine Manifestations of Cancer

DANIEL L. KULICK, M.D.
Assistant Professor of Medicine, University of Southern California School of Medicine; Director, Cardiac Catheterization Laboratory, Los Angeles County–University of Southern California Medical Center, Los Angeles, California.
Myocardial Infarction, Acute

STEVEN P. KUTALEK, M.D.
Assistant Professor of Medicine and Clinical Pharmacology, Division of Cardiac Electrophysiology, Hahnemann University School of Medicine; Director, Clinical Cardiac Electrophysiology, Hahnemann University Hospital, Philadelphia, Pennsylvania.
Ventricular Arrhythmias

THOMAS E. LAD, M.D.
Associate Professor of Clinical Medicine, University of Illinois College of Medicine; Chief, Oncology Section, West Side Veterans Administration Hospital; Interim Chief, Medical Oncology Section, University of Illinois Hospital, Chicago, Illinois.
Endocrine Manifestations of Cancer

LAWRENCE B. LEHMAN, M.D.
Assistant Professor of Clinical Neurosurgery and Acting Vice Chairman, Department of Neurosurgery, State University of New York (Brooklyn); Assistant to the Director, Department of Surgery, Maimonides Medical Center; Chief, Division of Neurosurgery, Coney Island Hospital; Attending Neurosurgeon, State University Hospital and King's County Hospital, New York, New York.
Cervical Spine Injury

CAMILO A. LESLIE, M.D.
Associate Professor of Clinical Medicine, University of Miami School of Medicine; Staff, Department of Medicine, Diabetes and Metabolism Unit, Jackson Memorial Hospital, Miami, Florida.
Infections in the Diabetic Patient

ANGELO A. LICATA, M.D., Ph.D.
Assistant Clinical Professor of Medicine, Case Western Reserve University School of Medicine; Cleveland Clinic Foundation, Cleveland, Ohio.
Osteoporosis

ALAN E. LICHTIN, M.D.
Staff Physician, Department of Hematology/Medical Oncology; Cleveland Clinic Foundation, Cleveland, Ohio. Formerly: Assistant Professor of Internal Medicine, University of Missouri–Kansas City School of Medicine, Kansas City, Missouri.
Sickle Cell Disease

L. KEITH LLOYD, M.D.
Professor of Surgery, Division of Urology, University of Alabama School of Medicine; Director, Urological Rehabilitation and Research Center, Spain Rehabilitation Center, Birmingham, Alabama.
Urinary Incontinence

JOHN T. MacDONALD, M.D.
Department of Pediatric Neurology, Minneapolis Children's Medical Center, Minneapolis, Minnesota.
Seizures During Childhood

DOUGALD C. MacGILLIVRAY, M.D., F.A.C.S.
Assistant Professor of Surgery, Uniformed Services University of the Health Sciences; Surgeon, National Naval Medical Center, Bethesda, Maryland.
Malignant Melanoma

MICHAEL K. MAGILL, M.D.
Director, Family Practice Residency Program, Tallahassee Memorial Regional Medical Center, Tallahassee; Clinical Assistant Professor of Family Practice, University of Florida College of Medicine, Gainesville, Florida.
Borderline Personality Disorder

A. MALIK, M.D.
Fellow, Renal Section, Department of Medicine, Mount Sinai School of Medicine, City University of New York, New York, New York; currently Attending/Consulting Physician in Nephrology, St. Augustine General Hospital and Flagler Hospital, St. Augustine, Florida.
Dialysis Patient, Medical Management of the

ROBERT T. MANNING, M.D.
Professor of Internal Medicine, University of Kansas School of Medicine; Director, Internal Medicine Education, HCA–Wesley Medical Center, Wichita, Kansas.
Hepatitis, Chronic Active

RAYMOND A. MARTIN, M.D.
Clinical Assistant Professor, Department of Neurology and Department of Family Practice and Community Medicine, University of Texas School of Medicine; Chief, Department of Neurology, Memorial Southwest Hospital, Houston, Texas.
Peripheral Neuropathy

RICHARD W. McCALLUM, M.D., F.A.C.P., F.R.A.C.P. (Aust.), F.A.C.S.
Paul Janssen Professor of Internal Medicine; Chief, Division of Gastroenterology; Director, Gastrointestinal Fellowship Program, University of Virginia, School of Medicine, Charlottesville, Virginia.
Toxic Megacolon in Inflammatory Bowel Disease

KAY F. McFARLAND, M.D.
Professor of Medicine, University of South Carolina School of Medicine, Columbia, South Carolina.
Diabetes Mellitus, Type I

DEAN McGINTY, M.D.
Clinical Assistant Professor of Family Medicine, Oregon Health Sciences University School of Medicine, Portland, Oregon.
Hypertension in Pregnancy

LARRY G. McLAIN, M.D.
Director, Ambulatory Pediatrics, Division of Pediatrics, Lutheran General Hospital, Park Ridge, Illinois.
Laryngotracheobronchitis, Bacterial Tracheitis and Epiglottitis in Children

RICHARD E. MELCHER, M.D.
Clinical Assistant Professor of Family Medicine, Medical College of Georgia; Active Staff, Departments of Family Practice–Internal Medicine, Humana Hospital and St. Joseph's Hospital; Consulting Medical Staff, University Hospital, Augusta, Georgia.
Pressure Sores

ROBERT L. MELLMAN, M.D.
Senior Fellow in Gastroenterology and Clinical Assistant Instructor, Department of Internal Medicine, Winthrop University Hospital/State University of New York at Stony Brook School of Medicine, Stony Brook, New York.
Cirrhosis of the Liver in the Alcoholic Patient

FREDERICK H. MEYERS, M.D.
Professor, Department of Pharmacology, University of California at Davis, School of Medicine, Sacramento, California.
Pain Management in the Terminally Ill Patient

FREDERICK J. MEYERS, M.D.
Associate Professor of Medicine and Pathology, Division of Hematology/Oncology, University of California at Davis; Medical Director, University of California-Davis Medical Center Hospice Program, Sacramento, California.
Pain Management in the Terminally Ill Patient

JOEL MORGANROTH, M.D.
Clinical Professor of Medicine, University of Pennsylvania School of Medicine; Director, Center of Excellence for Cardiovascular Studies, The Graduate Health System, Philadelphia, Pennsylvania.
Ventricular Arrhythmias

ODDVAR A. MYHRE, M.D.
Assistant Clinical Professor of Surgery, University of California, Los Angeles, School of Medicine and Medical Center, Los Angeles; Active Staff, Memorial Medical Center of Long Beach, California, Long Beach, California.
Coronary Artery Disease in the Surgical Patient

DAVID B. NASH, M.D., M.B.A.
Assistant Professor of Medicine, Thomas Jefferson University Medical College; Director of Health Policy and Clinical Outcomes, Thomas Jefferson University Hospital, Philadelphia, Pennsylvania.
Hypercholesterolemia

HAROLD G. OLSON, M.D.
Associate Professor of Medicine, Department of Cardiology, University of California School of Medicine, Irvine; Director, Coronary Care Unit, Long Beach Veterans Administration Medical Center, Long Beach, California.
Coronary Artery Disease in the Surgical Patient

PETER J. PAPADAKOS, M.D.
Senior Instructor, Department of Anesthesiology, University of Rochester, School of Medicine and Dentistry; Clinical Director, Surgical Intensive Care Unit, University of Rochester Medical Center, Rochester, New York.
Smoke Inhalation

LAIRD PATTERSON, M.D.
Associate Clinical Professor of Medicine, Section of Neurology, University of Washington School of Medicine; Virginia Mason Hospital, Harborview Hospital, and Seattle Veterans Administration Medical Center, Seattle, Washington.
Myasthenia Gravis

D. MELESSA PHILLIPS, M.D.
Professor and Chairman, Department of Family Medicine, University of Mississippi School of Medicine and Medical Center; Staff Physician, University Hospital, Mississippi Baptist Medical Center, Hinds General Hospital, St. Dominic Memorial Hospital, Jackson, Mississippi.
Pelvic Infections

ROBERT A. PHILLIPS, M.D., Ph.D.
Assistant Professor of Medicine, Division of Hypertension and Cardiology, Mount Sinai School of Medicine; Assistant Attending Physician, Mount Sinai Hospital, New York, New York.
Hypertensive Crisis

FRANK M. PRICE, M.D.
Department of Internal Medicine, Carl T. Hayden Veterans Administration Medical Center, Phoenix, Arizona.
Thyroid Disease in the Elderly Patient

E. EDWARD PROCTOR, M.D.
Senior Fellow in Cardiology, Medical University of South Carolina, Charleston, South Carolina.
Endocarditis, Infective

HAROLD T. PRUESSNER, M.D.
Professor and Chairman, Department of Family Practice and Community Medicine, The University of Texas Medical School at Houston; Medical Staff, St. Luke's Episcopal Hospital, Memorial Southwest Hospital, and Hermann Hospital, Houston, Texas.
Near-Drowning

MARTIN M. QUIGLEY, M.D.
Head, Section of Reproductive Endocrinology and Infertility, Department of Gynecology, Cleveland Clinic Foundation, Cleveland, Ohio.
Anovulation

SHAHBUDIN H. RAHIMTOOLA, M.B., F.R.C.P.
George C. Griffith Professor of Cardiology and Professor of Medicine, University of Southern California School of Medicine; Chief, Division of Cardiology, Los Angeles County–University of Southern California Medical Center, Los Angeles, California.
Myocardial Infarction, Acute

JOHN RAVITS, M.D.
Assistant Clinical Professor, Department of Medicine, University of Washington School of Medicine; Virginia Mason Medical Center, Harborview Hospital, Seattle Veterans Administration Medical Center, Seattle, Washington.
Myasthenia Gravis

MARY L. REICHARDT-FICK, R.N., M.S.
Graduate Research Assistant, College of Education, University of Iowa, Iowa City, Iowa.
Cystic Fibrosis

INGRAM M. ROBERTS, M.D.
Associate Professor of Medicine, George Washington University School of Medicine; Attending Physician in Gastroenterology and Internal Medicine, George Washington University Hospital and Medical Center, Washington, D.C.
Malabsorption

TIMOTHY M. RODDY, M.D.
Northwest Hospital, Seattle, Washington. Formerly Fellow, Department of Urology, Boston University School of Medicine, Boston, Massachusetts.
Impotence

THOMAS J. ROMANO, M.D., Ph.D., F.A.C.P.
Clinical Assistant Professor of Medicine, Rheumatology Division, West Virginia University School of Medicine; Staff, Ohio Valley Medical Center and Wheeling Hospital, Wheeling, West Virginia.
Fibromyalgia Syndrome

SANFORD H. ROTH, M.D.
Professor and Director, Aging and Arthritis Program, Arizona State University, Tempe, Arizona; Medical Director, Arthritis Center, Ltd., and Medical Director, Arthritis and Orthopedic Center for Excellence, Humana-Phoenix, Phoenix, Arizona.
Rheumatoid Arthritis

REBECCA A. ROUBENOFF, M.P.H., R.D.
Metabolic Support Dietitian, Department of Nutrition, The Johns Hopkins Hospital, Baltimore, Maryland.
Nutritional Support of the Acutely and Chronically Ill Patient

RONENN ROUBENOFF, M.D., M.H.S.
Fellow, Divisions of Molecular and Clinical Rheumatology and Clinical Epidemiology, Johns Hopkins University Schools of Medicine and of Public Health and Hygiene; Fellow, The Johns Hopkins Hospital, Baltimore, Maryland.
Nutritional Support of the Acutely and Chronically Ill Patient

MELVYN RUBENFIRE, M.D.
Professor of Medicine, Wayne State University School of Medicine; Chairman, Department of Medicine, Sinai Hospital of Detroit, Michigan.
Atrial Fibrillation

MICHAEL SALCMAN, M.D.
Professor and Head, Division of Neurological Surgery, University of Maryland School of Medicine; Chief of Neurological Surgery, University of Maryland Hospital and the Maryland Institute for Emergency Medical Services Systems (Shock Trauma), Baltimore, Maryland.
Head Injury

MARK H. SANDERS, M.D., F.C.C.P.
Associate Professor of Medicine, Division of Pulmonary/Critical Care Medicine, University of Pittsburgh School of Medicine; Director, Pulmonary Sleep Evaluation and Control of Breathing Laboratories, Presbyterian–University Hospital, Pittsburgh, Pennsylvania.
Sleep Apnea

FRANCISCO L. SAPICO, M.D., F.A.C.P.
Professor of Medicine, University of Southern California School of Medicine, Los Angeles; Associate Chief, Division of Infectious Diseases, and Physician Specialist, Rancho Los Amigos Medical Center, Downey, California.
Infections in the Diabetic Patient

CHRISTOPHER D. SAUDEK, M.D.
Associate Professor of Medicine, Division of Endocrinology and Metabolism, Johns Hopkins University School of Medicine; Director, Johns Hopkins Diabetes Center, Johns Hopkins Hospital, Baltimore, Maryland.
Obesity in the Diabetic Patient

JOHN W. SAULTZ, M.D.
Associate Professor of Family Medicine, Oregon Health Sciences University School of Medicine, Portland, Oregon.
Hypertension in Pregnancy

DAVID S. SCHADE, M.D.
Professor of Medicine, Division of Endocrinology and Metabolism, The University of New Mexico School of Medicine; Staff Physician, University of New Mexico Hospital, Albuquerque, New Mexico.
Diabetes Mellitus in the Surgical Patient

MARTIN B. SCHARF, Ph.D., A.C.P.
Clinical Associate Professor of Psychiatry, University of Cincinnati College of Medicine; Director, The Center for Research in Sleep Disorders, Mercy Hospital, Hamilton/Fairfield, Ohio.
Narcolepsy

ROBERT W. SCHRIER, M.D.
Professor and Chairman, Department of Medicine, Division of Renal Diseases, University of Colorado School of Medicine, Denver, Colorado.
Renal Failure, Acute

TERRY K. SCHULTZ, M.D.
Director of Addiction Medicine, Department of Psychiatry, Walter Reed Army Medical Center, Washington, D.C.
Alcohol Withdrawal Syndromes

ROBERT A. SCHWARTZ, M.D., M.P.H.
Professor and Chairman, Division of Dermatology, New Jersey Medical School; Chief of Dermatology, UMDNJ University Hospital, Newark, New Jersey.
Herpes Simplex Virus Infections

STEPHEN D. SHAFRAN, M.D., F.R.C.P.C.
Assistant Professor of Medicine, Division of Infectious Diseases, University of Alberta; Active Staff, University of Alberta Hospitals, Edmonton, Alberta, Canada.
Antimicrobial Use During Pregnancy and Lactation

HEIDI M. SHALE, M.D.
Associate in Clinical Neurology, Columbia–Presbyterian Medical Center; Associate in Neurology, Division of Neurology, St. Lukes–Roosevelt Hospital, New York, New York.
Parkinson's Disease

JUDD SHELLITO, M.D.
Associate Professor of Medicine, Section of Pulmonary/Critical Care, Louisiana State University School of Medicine in New Orleans, Louisiana.
Asthma, Refractory

I. DAVID SHOCKET, M.D.
Assistant Professor of Medicine, Boston University School of Medicine; Staff Physician, Boston Veterans Administration Medical Center, Boston, Massachusetts.
Pancreatitis, Chronic

JACK C. SIPE, M.D.
Clinical Professor of Neurosciences, University of California, San Diego, School of Medicine, San Diego; Consultant in Neurology, Scripps Clinic and Research Foundation, La Jolla, California.
Multiple Sclerosis

DAVID L. SMITH, M.D.
Assistant Professor of Medicine, Division of General Medicine, Ambulatory Care and Medical Service, Section of Arthritis and Rheumatic Disease, Oregon Health Sciences University School of Medicine; Portland Veterans Administration Medical Center, Portland, Oregon.
Reflex Sympathetic Dystrophy Syndrome

DOUGLAS R. SMUCKER, M.D.
Assistant Professor of Family Medicine, Medical College of Ohio; Assistant Director, MCO/St. Vincent Family Practice Residency, Toledo, Ohio.
Urinary Tract Infections, Recurrent

CLIFFORD C. SNYDER, M.D.
Professor Emeritus of Surgery; Distinguished Honors Professor; Associate Dean, University of Utah School of Medicine; Professor of Surgery, University Medical Center, Salt Lake City, Utah.
Snakebite

STUART JON SPECHLER, M.D.
Associate Professor of Medicine, Boston University School of Medicine; Associate Chief, Gastroenterology, Boston Veterans Administration Medical Center, Boston, Massachusetts.
Pancreatitis, Chronic

RONALD C. STRICKLER, M.D.
Professor of Obstetrics and Gynecology, Washington University School of Medicine; Active Staff, Jewish Hospital and Barnes Hospital, St. Louis, Missouri.
Endometriosis

DAVID L. SULTZER, M.D.
Neurobehavior Fellow, Department of Neurology and Department of Psychiatry and Biobehavioral Sciences, University of California, Los Angeles, School of Medicine, Los Angeles, California.
Alzheimer's Disease

ROBERT B. TAYLOR, M.D.
Professor and Chairman, Department of Family Medicine, Oregon Health Sciences University School of Medicine, Portland, Oregon.
Cluster Headache

JOCELYNE TESSIER, M.D.
Fellow in Urology, Boston University School of Medicine, Boston, Massachusetts.
Impotence

JOSEPH THURN, M.D.
Graduate Student, School of Public Health, University of Minnesota; Staff Physician, St. Paul–Ramsey Medical Center; Director, Human Immunodeficiency Virus Clinic of Minnesota Correctional Facilities, St. Paul, Minnesota.
Meningitis and Encephalitis

JANET RUTH TODORCZUK, M.D.
Division of Digestive Diseases, Barnes Hospital, St. Louis, Missouri. Formerly: Fellow, Division of Gastroenterology, University of Virginia School of Medicine, Charlottesville, Virginia.
Toxic Megacolon in Inflammatory Bowel Disease

WILLIAM L. TOFFLER, M.D.
Assistant Professor of Family Medicine, Oregon Health Sciences University School of Medicine, Portland, Oregon.
Recreational Athlete, Medical Care of the

E. P. TRULOCK, M.D.
Assistant Professor of Medicine, Division of Respiratory and Critical Care, Washington University School of Medicine; Assistant Physician, Barnes Hospital, St. Louis, Missouri.
Pulmonary Embolic Disease

CHRISTOPHER D. TRUSS, M.D.
Associate Professor of Medicine, University of Alabama School of Medicine, Birmingham, Alabama.
Diarrhea, Infectious

EDWARD TSOU, M.D.
Associate Professor of Medicine, Division of Pulmonary and Critical Care Medicine, Georgetown University School of Medicine and Medical Center, Washington, D.C.
Pneumonia, Nosocomial

CLIFFORD H. VAN METER, Jr., M.D.
Department of Surgery, Ochsner Clinic, New Orleans, Louisiana.
Transplantation Patient, Medical Care of the

HECTOR O. VENTURA, M.D.
Section on Cardiology, Department of Internal Medicine, Ochsner Clinic, New Orleans, Louisiana.
Transplantation Patient, Medical Care of the

WILLIAM WAGNER, M.D.
Department of Allergy and Immunology, Cleveland Clinic Foundation, Cleveland, Ohio.
Urticaria and Angioedema

ANNE D. WALLING, M.B., Ch.B.
Associate Professor of Family and Community Medicine, University of Kansas School of Medicine; Active Staff, HCA/Wesley Medical Center and St. Joseph's Medical Center, Wichita, Kansas.
Premenstrual Syndromes

JEFFREY E. WEILAND, M.D.
Assistant Professor of Medicine, The Ohio State University College of Medicine, Columbus, Ohio.
Adult Respiratory Distress Syndrome

NANETTE KASS WENGER, M.D.
Professor of Medicine (Cardiology), Emory University School of Medicine; Director, Cardiac Clinic, Grady Memorial Hospital, Atlanta, Georgia.
Cardiomyopathy

AIZIK L. WOLF, M.D.
Assistant Professor of Neurological Surgery, University of Maryland School of Medicine; Attending Neurological Surgeon, University of Maryland Hospital and Maryland Institute for Emergency Medical Services Systems (Shock Trauma), and Maryland Epilepsy Center, Baltimore, Maryland.
Head Injury

GARY P. WORMSER, M.D.
Professor of Medicine and Pharmacology and Chief, Division of Infectious Diseases, New York Medical College; Chief, Section of Infectious Diseases, Westchester County Medical Center, Valhalla, New York.
Human Immunodeficiency Virus (HIV)–Infected Patient
Human Immunodeficiency Virus–Related Disease

xviii Contributors

WILLIAM R. YATES, M.D.
Assistant Professor of Psychiatry, University of Iowa College of Medicine; Director, Adult Psychiatric Outpatient Clinic and Consultation Service, University of Iowa Hospitals and Clinic, Iowa City, Iowa.
Attention-Deficit Hyperactivity Disorder

JOHN E. YOUNT, M.D.
Assistant Professor of Pediatrics, Oregon Health Sciences University School of Medicine; Doernbecher Memorial Children's Hospital, Portland, Oregon.
Apnea and Apparent Life-Threatening Events in Infancy

H. MICHAEL ZAL, D.O., F.A.C.N.
Clinical Professor of Psychiatry, Philadelphia College of Osteopathic Medicine; Chairman, Psychiatric Service, Metropolitan Hospital—Central Division, Philadelphia, Pennsylvania.
Depression in the Elderly Patient

Preface

Difficult Medical Management is intended to be a multidisciplinary reference source describing the therapy of selected complicated clinical problems. These problems include diseases that offer various therapeutic options (e.g., reflex sympathetic dystrophy), involve several diagnoses (e.g., diabetes in pregnancy), or require therapy that is complex or hazardous (e.g., alcohol withdrawal syndromes). The problems may be especially disabling, recurrent, or communicable—such as osteoporosis, cluster headache, or acquired immunodeficiency syndrome.

Many of these clinical problems, such as medical care of the recreational athlete, transcend traditional specialty lines. They are not necessarily rare or serious, and some, such as pressure sores, may be encountered frequently. They share in common that they are difficult to manage.

The book's articles cover the full spectrum of clinical medicine from obstetrics and neonatology to geriatrics. The selection of topics reflects my own experience as a family physician, first as a rural practitioner and currently as an academician.

The intended reader is the practicing clinician—the primary care provider as well as the specialist who encounters therapeutic problems outside his or her field of expertise. The book should also be helpful for resident physicians and medical students during their clinical years. I hope that Difficult Medical Management will prove to be a useful resource in day-to-day practice.

The idea for the book came when I realized that I use only a small part of my large reference textbooks. The parts I use describe problems that are especially difficult to treat. These topics, such as breast cancer, AIDS, and transient ischemic attacks, I seem to look up over and over. What's new in therapy? What do I do when usual recommendations don't work? What therapeutic innovations are on the horizon? Most physicians do not need to have valuable book pages devoted to the treatment of viral upper respiratory infections, otitis media, gastritis, contraception, and essential hypertension. What we clinicians need is a book that focuses on the tough problems.

This book is intended as a companion to Difficult Diagnosis, also published by the W. B. Saunders Company. The emphasis of the current book is on therapy, whereas Difficult Diagnosis emphasizes evaluation. The topics are almost entirely different; topics that are difficult to diagnose are not necessarily difficult to treat. This book begins each article with diagnosis and devotes most space to therapeutic management.

As editor, I wish to thank the contributing authors responsible for the 93 articles in this book. Among those in our department who provided help and guidance, special thanks are due to Coelleda Koches, Sherri Johnson, and Richard Bernard, M.D. The editors at W. B. Saunders Company provided vital encouragement and support during the preparation of this work. I also thank my family and the families and colleagues of all the book's contributors.

ROBERT B. TAYLOR

Adult respiratory distress syndrome

Jeffrey E. Weiland ■ *Paul M. Dorinsky*

In the adult, severe failure of the lung to exchange oxygen has been termed the adult respiratory distress syndrome (ARDS). As the name suggests, rather than a discrete entity, ARDS is a constellation of clinical findings, the most prominent of which are refractory hypoxemia and noncardiogenic (high permeability) pulmonary edema. ARDS usually develops 18 to 24 hours after a catastrophic medical or surgical insult. Although the pathogenesis of the syndrome remains controversial, there is nearly always a well-defined inciting event (Table 1). Approximately 250,000 cases of ARDS occur each year, with a mortality that approaches 50 per cent. There is no age predilection, and ARDS frequently occurs in otherwise healthy young adults. Most important, since specific therapy for ARDS has not been developed as yet, the judicious use of supportive care remains the mainstay of treatment.

■ Background

This disease was initially described in 1967. Nearly 90 per cent of the patients who developed ARDS died with respiratory failure.[1] Advances in supportive care have improved our ability to manage the respiratory failure, yet nearly 50 per cent of patients who develop ARDS continue to succumb, mainly from multiple organ failure.[2] This shift in the cause of death has major implications for the management of ARDS, as will be discussed in subsequent sections.

ARDS can arise from insults either systemically (e.g., sepsis) or from direct injury to the lung (e.g., gastric aspiration). In this regard, the clinical scenarios in which ARDS occurs are multiple and varied. However, regardless of the etiology, four physiologic disturbances are common: (1) shunting of blood through collapsed, atelectatic, or fluid-filled alveoli, resulting in refractory hypoxemia; (2) decreased lung compliance, resulting in high peak inspiratory pressures; (3) increased dead space ventilation, resulting in high minute ventilatory requirements; and (4) increased pulmonary vascular resistance, resulting in elevated pulmonary arterial pressures. While the last phenomenon is a consequence of vascular obstruction by platelet, granulocyte, and fibrin thrombi, the first three disturbances are a direct result of edema formation and inflammatory cell infiltrate into the lung parenchyma.

Edema formation occurs as a direct result of increased permeability of the alveolar capillary membrane. The forces governing fluid flux from the vascular space into the lung parenchyma are defined by the Starling equation (Figure 1A). In the setting of ARDS, diffuse injury to the alveolar capillary membrane results in a dramatic increase in the permeability constant (Figure 1B). As a result, the barrier to movement of plasma proteins into the lung parenchyma is effaced, and plasma proteins are no longer restricted to the vascular space.[3] In this context, the

TABLE 1. Frequent Causes of the Adult Respiratory Distress Syndrome

Infections
Bacterial sepsis
Pneumocystis pneumonia

Inhalation
Gastric aspiration
Smoke inhalation
Oxygen toxicity

Drugs
Narcotics
Salicylates

Trauma
Near drowning
Fat embolism
Hypertransfusion
Lung contusion

A.

$$\text{Fluid Flux} = K \, (\Delta P_{hyd} - \Delta P_{onc})$$

B.

$$\text{Fluid Flux} = \uparrow K \, (\Delta P_{hyd} - \Delta \cancel{P_{onc}})$$

Figure 1. The forces governing fluid flux from the vascular to the interstitial and alveolar spaces on the lung. K = permeability coefficient of the alveolar capillary membrane, P_{hyd} = the difference in hydrostatic pressures (vascular to interstitium), P_{onc} = the difference in oncotic pressures (plasma to interstitium). Panel *A* depicts the normal relationship. Panel *B* depicts the relationship in the presence of injury to the alveolar capillary membrane. Fluid flux becomes directly related to hydrostatic pressure.

oncotic pressure gradient, which normally favors retention of fluid in the vascular space, is lost and fluid flux becomes directly related to hydrostatic pressure (i.e., fluid flux occurs at all levels of pulmonary capillary hydrostatic pressure). In contrast, fluid flux occurs in hydrostatic (cardiogenic) pulmonary edema only when the pulmonary capillary wedge pressure (PCWP) exceeds 15 mm Hg. This observation has major implications in the management of patients with ARDS.

The pathogenesis of the injury to the alveolar capillary membrane remains controversial.[4] Nonetheless, it is clear that the injury stems from a derangement in the host's inflammatory response. Multiple factors, including complement activation,[5] prostaglandins,[6] interleukin-1,[7] and tumor necrosis factor[8] have been proposed as potential initiators or amplifiers of this inflammatory response. Although the pathogenesis of the capillary injury is undoubtedly complex, most investigators agree that the neutrophil plays a significant role.[9] The putative importance of the neutrophil in acute lung injury arose from the clinical observations that hemodialysis often induced neutropenia and pulmonary dysfunction[10] and that white cell transfusions in neutropenic, septic patients receiving amphotericin[11] caused catastrophic lung injury. Further support for this hypothesis came from clinical investigations that documented the tremendous influx of neutrophils into the lungs of patients with ARDS, as well as the observation that the magnitude of the neutrophil influx correlated with the degree of hypoxemia and the permeability defects in the lung.[12,13] Moreover, studies describing the occurrence of ARDS in neutropenic patients are infrequent and suggest that non-neutrophil–mediated lung injury is the exception rather than the rule in this syndrome.[14,15]

The neutrophil is well equipped for its putative role in acute lung injury. Upon stimulation, the neutrophil is a potent producer of oxidant species, and oxidized products have been recovered from the lungs of patients with ARDS.[16] In addition, the neutrophil can release several connective tissue proteases that may injure lung parenchymal cells and degrade the connective tissue matrix of the lung. Foremost among these is elastase, which has been shown to cause injury in isolated perfused lungs and is immunologically present in the lungs of most patients with ARDS.[12,13] However, the recovery of free elastolytic activity from the lungs of ARDS patients has been more difficult to document.[13,17] This finding probably relates to the increased presence of the elastase inhibitor α-1 antitrypsin in the lungs of patients with ARDS.[18] In this context it may be reasonable to question the role of elastase in ARDS. However, recent studies have elegantly demonstrated that in the microenvironment of the cell-substrate interface, the large molecular weight protein α-1 antitrypsin may be unable to inhibit the function of elastase secreted by the neutrophil.[19]

In summary, ARDS is a syndrome of hypoxemic respiratory failure resulting from diffuse injury to the alveolar capillary membrane. The capillary injury alters the normal membrane characteristics in such a way that there is a linear relationship between fluid flux and intravascular pressure at *all* hydrostatic pressures. The injury is due to a nonfocused activation of the host's inflammatory response, and the neutrophil appears to play an important role.

■ Management

The first objective in managing a patient with ARDS is to diagnose and treat the underlying disease that precipitated the syndrome. In most cases, the underlying disease is readily apparent. When an obvious etiology is lacking, bronchoscopy and bronchoalveolar lavage should be performed to look for a primary lung infection. Thoracotomy and lung biopsy are rarely indicated, given the very low yield in negative bronchoalveolar lavages.[20] One clinical caveat that has gained attention is that miliary tuberculosis should be considered in the alcoholic or diabetic patient with ARDS in the setting of a subacute (2- 3-month) illness with no clear precipitating factor.[21] In addition, in the current era, patients who have ARDS without an apparent cause should be expediently evaluated for the acquired immunodeficiency syndrome (AIDS) and *Pneumocystis* infection.[22]

In discussing the management of ARDS, it is useful to divide therapeutic interventions into specific and nonspecific management strategies. Discussion of the former is largely theoretic at the present time; therefore, nonspecific interventions represent the mainstay of current therapy for ARDS.

■ NONSPECIFIC MANAGEMENT

The therapeutic goal of supportive care in ARDS is the maintenance of adequate tissue delivery of substrate (oxygen). Oxygen delivery is the product of cardiac output (CO) and oxygen content of the blood. Since the oxygen content of blood is determined by the hemoglobin concentration (Hgb) and the per cent saturation of hemoglobin with oxygen (% SAT), three variables (i.e., CO, Hgb, % SAT) emerge that can be manipulated to improve oxygen delivery. Thus, supportive care in ARDS can be simplified into those interventions that improve the oxygen content of the blood and those that improve cardiac output (Table 2).

Oxygen Content

The first therapeutic intervention employed in the management of ARDS is the administration of supplemental oxygen. Improvement in arterial saturation occurs by elimination of the contribution of ventilation-perfusion (v/Q) mismatch to the hypoxemia. Unfortunately, this improvement is usually inadequate since the majority of the hypoxemia in ARDS is due to the shunting of blood through collapsed or very poorly ventilated alveoli.[23] In addition, the potential injurious effects to the lung of high concentrations of oxygen are a constant source of concern. In the setting of an injured lung, the absolute "safe" level of oxygen supplementation is unknown. However, most cli-

TABLE 2. Therapeutic Interventions in ARDS

Intervention	Benefit	Risk
Improve Oxygen Content		
$\uparrow$ F_1O_2	Overcome v/Q mismatch	O_2 toxicity
PEEP	$\downarrow$ Shunt	$\downarrow$ Cardiac output
Transfusion	$\uparrow$ O_2 = carrying capacity	$\uparrow$ PCWP
Improve Cardiac Output		
Increase preload	$\uparrow$ Cardiac output	$\uparrow$ PCWP
Reduce afterload	$\uparrow$ Cardiac output	$\uparrow$ Shunt
Inotropic agents	$\uparrow$ Cardiac output	Arrhythmias ? Organ blood flow

nicians agree that supplemental oxygen of less than 55 per cent is a reasonable therapeutic goal.

Positive end expiratory pressure (PEEP) has become an extremely useful adjunct to mechanical ventilation in patients with ARDS. However, as with many beneficial interventions, the use of PEEP has spread to clinical situations (e.g., prophylactic PEEP, "super" PEEP) in which data to support its use are nonexistent, and the risks clearly outweigh the benefits. PEEP improves arterial oxygenation by re-expanding atelectatic alveoli and increasing the functional residual capacity of the lung. Although this results in a decrease in shunt fraction in most patients with ARDS, a subpopulation fails to receive benefit from the use of PEEP. Presumably, rather than displaying atelectatic alveoli, the lung parenchyma in this subgroup is completely effaced by edema and inflammatory cell infiltrate. PEEP also exerts greatest therapeutic benefit in patients with reduced lung compliance from diffuse alveolar injury rather than in patients with severe obstructive lung disease or focal pneumonias. The main adverse consequences of PEEP are decreased cardiac output and pneumothorax. These complications are directly related to mean airway pressure and become clinically significant when levels of PEEP exceed 10 cm H_2O.

The therapeutic endpoint in using PEEP has evolved drastically over the years. Initially, the optimal level of PEEP was defined in terms of improvement in lung compliance and maximal oxygen delivery.[24] Subsequently, the concept of "goal-directed" PEEP evolved, in which the "best PEEP" was defined as the level of PEEP at which the pulmonary shunt fraction was minimized.[25] However, numerous studies have delineated the adverse consequences of high levels of PEEP, not only in regard to overdistention of normal alveoli with subsequent pulmonary barotrauma but also in the context of cardiovascular barotrauma and alterations in regional organ blood flow.[26] Consequently, the use of PEEP in ARDS patients has been refined to reflect a balance between its salutory effects on gas exchange and its adverse effects on cardiopulmonary function. "Best PEEP" is defined clinically as the lowest level of PEEP necessary to maintain adequate arterial oxygen tension (i.e., $PaO_2 > 60$ mm Hg) at a "safe" level of inspired oxygen concentration[27] (i.e., $F_IO_2 < 0.55$).

The final intervention to improve oxygen content of the blood is the transfusion of packed red blood cells. From the equation for oxygen delivery cited earlier, transfusion of packed cells has obvious merit but is frequently overlooked. The major adverse effect of red blood cell transfusions is the potential to increase pulmonary vascular hydrostatic pressure and cause deterioration in gas exchange. However, in contrast to crystalloids and colloids, red cells are more likely to be retained within the vascular space. In this regard, red cell transfusions are particularly useful for hemodynamic support when there is evidence of significant intravascular volume depletion.

Hemodynamic Interventions

Efforts to improve cardiac output can be divided into interventions that increase preload, decrease afterload, or directly stimulate myocardial contractility. Intravascular volume expansion, albeit an effective measure for increasing preload and cardiac output, also increases pulmonary vascular hydrostatic pressure. Therefore, since pulmonary capillary permeability is markedly increased in ARDS, this intervention should be avoided if at all possible. When volume expansion is necessary to maintain adequate blood pressure, this should be accomplished by the transfusion of packed red cells. Afterload reduction by means of arterial vasodilators also can improve cardiac output.

However, vasodilators must be employed with caution in ARDS, since vasodilation also occurs in the pulmonary vascular bed, ablating hypoxic vasoconstriction. This may lead to an increase of blood flow into nonventilated alveoli and an elevation of the shunt fraction. Finally, positive inotropic agents are frequently employed in the management of patients with ARDS. Both dobutamine and dopamine possess relative merit. Theoretically, dobutamine would be the drug of choice for increasing cardiac output in ARDS patients with elevated left ventricular filling pressures.[28] However, in practice, PEEP and the aggressive use of diuretics usually lower preload to such an extent that hypotension ensues, and dopamine is required for its effects on the systemic vasculature.

■ SPECIFIC MANAGEMENT

Currently, major investigative efforts have focused on interventions that may have an impact on the inflammatory processes occurring in the lung during ARDS. The design of these trials has been hindered by the difficulty in predicting which patients at risk for lung injury will proceed to develop ARDS. Therefore, specific interventions frequently are not implemented until the inflammatory processes underlying ARDS are well established. In this context, infusions of corticosteroids have failed to improve survival in ARDS.[29] Future trials using specific inhibitors of neutrophil elastase, as well as scavengers of oxygen radicals, are being considered. However, it is reasonable to speculate that any hope of improving survival in ARDS will depend on early detection and intervention before the clinical syndrome of ARDS becomes manifest.

■ Issues and Risks

■ VOLUME MANAGEMENT

The aggressive use of diuretics in the management of ARDS remains controversial. Recent studies have shown improvement in mortality when management strategies are employed to reduce intravascular volume.[30]

However, these promising findings need to be interpreted with caution, since diuretics also may hasten the development of azotemia, which is a grave prognostic sign in ARDS. In addition, although reducing pulmonary hydrostatic pressure may improve gas exchange, it may also decrease delivery of substrate to vital organs via reductions in cardiac output, and it may contribute to the multiorgan failure of ARDS. Although this issue remains to be clarified, current evidence supports the use of diuretics, especially in those patients whose gas exchange defect is critical—namely, those patients requiring high levels of supplemental oxygen and PEEP.

■ MULTIPLE ORGAN FAILURE

At present, evidence suggests that mortality in most ARDS patients is not due to progressive pulmonary failure. Rather, mortality in ARDS is frequently due to the development of multiple nonpulmonary organ failure. In this regard, patients with ARDS not only manifest the hallmark gas exchange abnormalities attendant to the lung injury in this syndrome but also develop systemic gas exchange abnormalities, which present clinically as altered relationships between oxygen uptake and delivery, as well as defects in oxygen extraction.[31,32] Moreover, increasing evidence suggests that nonpulmonary organs are directly injured in ARDS, and that this injury occurs through mechanisms similar to those responsible for the lung injury in this syndrome (i.e., activation of inflammatory cells and their mediators). Consequently, the rationale described earlier for edema reduction in the management of the lung injury may also apply directly to the management of nonpulmonary organ failure in ARDS.

An additional contributing factor to multiple organ failure in ARDS is the development of secondary bacterial infection.[33] This is probably not surprising, given the need for prolonged mechanical ventilation, central venous access, and parenteral or enteral feeding in these patients. In addition, the systemic nature of the injury in ARDS may result in alterations in local host defenses owing to liver injury or intestinal mucosal injury or both, resulting in an increased susceptibility to bacterial infection. In this con-

text, attention should be given to meticulous sterile techniques during the insertion and maintenance of central lines. Furthermore, Gram stains of endotracheal secretions should be obtained daily. Although positive cultures from these secretions usually are not helpful, a significant change in the morphology of endotracheal bacteria, coupled with fever or new infiltrates, may herald the development of superinfection and help guide the selection of appropriate antibiotics.

■ INVASIVE MONITORING

Currently, controversy exists regarding the utility of Swan-Ganz catheterization in the management of patients with ARDS. The advantages of central hemodynamic monitoring are that it provides access to a variety of parameters (e.g., mixed venous oxygen tension, cardiac output, oxygen delivery, shunt fraction) that are not readily attainable by other methods. In addition, central hemodynamic monitoring often is the only means available to distinguish cardiogenic from noncardiogenic pulmonary edema. This is not a trivial distinction, since numerous studies have emphasized the inaccuracies in differentiating these entities on clinical grounds. By contrast, opponents of Swan-Ganz catheterization have enumerated the often life-threatening complications attendant on the use of these devices.[34] More important, the use of these catheters has never clearly been shown to improve outcome. Nonetheless, given the uncertainties in accurate diagnosis/classification of the ARDS patients, it seems prudent to employ central hemodynamic monitoring in those patients in whom volume status, cardiovascular function, or diagnosis are in question.

■ PROGNOSIS AFTER SURVIVAL

Despite the catastrophic nature of this syndrome, multiple studies have shown that the prognosis of patients who survive the acute lung injury is excellent: lung function in survivors, measured 1 year after discharge, is essentially normal.[35] Thus, regardless of the severity of the gas exchange defect or the duration of mechanical ventilation, diligent efforts should be maintained to support these patients through to the resolution of this syndrome.

REFERENCES

1. Ashbaugh DG, Bigelow DB, Petty TL, Levine BE. Acute respiratory distress in adults. Lancet 1967; 2:319–323.
2. Bell RC, Coalson J, Smith JD, Johanson WG. Multiple organ system failure and infection in adult respiratory distress syndrome. Ann Intern Med 1983; 99(3):293–298.
3. Holter JF, Weiland JE, Pacht ER, Gadek JE, Davis WB. Protein permeability in the adult respiratory distress syndrome: loss of size selective of the alveolar epithelium. J Clin Invest 1986; 78:1513–1522.
4. Rinaldo JE, Rogers RM. Adult respiratory distress syndrome: changing concepts of lung injury and repair. N Engl J Med 1982; 300:900–909.
5. Hammerschmidt DE, Weaver LJ, Hudson LD, Craddock PR, Jacob HS. Association of complement activation and elevated plasma-C5a with adult respiratory distress syndrome. Lancet 1980; 1:947–949.
6. Brigham KL, Ogletree ML. Effects of prostaglandins and related compounds on lung vascular permeability. Bull Euro Physiopathol Respir 1981; 17:703–722.
7. Goldblum SE, Jay M, Yoneda K, Cohen DA, McClain CJ, Gillespie MN. Monokine-induced acute lung injury in rabbits. J Appl Physiol 1987; 63(5):2093–2100.
8. Tracey KJ, Beutler B, Lowry SF, Merryweather J, Wolpe S, Milsark IW, Hariri RJ, Fahey TJ, Zentella A, Albert JD, Shires GT, Cerami A. Shock and tissue injury induced by recombinant human cachectin. Science 1986; 234:470–474.
9. Tate RM, Repine JE. Neutrophils and the adult respiratory distress syndrome. Am Rev Respir Dis 1983; 128:552–559.
10. Craddock PR, Fehr J, Brigham KL, Kronenberg RS, Jacob HS. Complement and leukocyte-mediated pulmonary dysfunction in hemodialysis. N Engl J Med 1977; 296:769–774.
11. Wright DG, Robichaud KJ, Pizzo PA, Deisseroth AB. Lethal pulmonary reactions associated with the combined use of amphotericin B and leukocyte transfusions. N Engl J Med 1981; 304(20):1185–1189.
12. Lee CT, Fein AM, Lippman M, Holtzman H, Kimbel P, Wienbaum G. Elastolytic activity in pulmonary lavage fluid from patients with adult respiratory distress syndrome. N Engl J Med 1981; 304:192–196.
13. Weiland JE, Davis WB, Holter JF, Mohammed JR, Dorinsky PJ, Gadek JE. Lung neutrophils in the adult respiratory distress syndrome. Am Rev Respir Dis 1986; 133:218–225.
14. Laufe MD, Simon RH, Flint A, Keller JB. Adult respiratory distress syndrome in neutropenic patients. Am J Med 1986; 80:1022–1026.
15. Ognibene FP, Martin SE, Parker MM, Schlesinger T, Roach P, Burch C, Shelhamer JH, Parillo JE. Adult respiratory distress syndrome in patients with severe neutropenia. N Engl J Med 1986; 315:547–551.
16. Cochrane CG, Spragg R, Revak SD. Pathogenesis of the adult respiratory distress syndrome: evidence of oxidant activity in bronchoalveolar lavage fluid. J Clin Invest 1983; 71:754–761.
17. Fowler AA, Walchak S, Giclas PC, Henson PA, Hyers TM. Characterization of antiprotease activity in the adult respiratory distress syndrome. Chest 1982; 81:50S–51S.
18. Wewers MD, Herzyk DJ, Gadek JE. Alveolar fluid neutrophil elastase activity in the adult respiratory distress syndrome is complexed to alpha-2 macroglobulin. J Clin Invest 1988; 82:1260–1267.
19. Campbell EJ, Senior RM, McDonald JA, Cox DL. Proteolysis by neutrophils: relative importance of cell-substrate contact and oxidative inactivation of proteinase inhibitors in vitro. J Clin Invest 1982; 70:845–852.
20. Poe RH, Utell MJ, Israel RH, Hall WJ, Eshleman JD. Sensitivity and specificity of the nonspecific transbronchial lung biopsy. Am Rev Respir Dis 1979; 119:25–31.
21. Piqueras AR, Marruecos L, Artigas A, Rodriguez C. Miliary tuberculosis and adult respiratory distress syndrome. Intensive Care Med 1987; 13:175–182.
22. Baumann WR, Jung RC, Koss M, Boylen T, Navarroh J, Sharma OP. Incidence and mortality of adult respiratory distress syndrome: a prospective analysis from a large metropolitan hospital. Crit Care Med 1986; 14(1):1–4.
23. Dantzker DR, Brook CJ, Dehart P, Lynch JP, Weg JG. Ventilation-perfusion distributions in the adult respiratory distress syndrome. Am Rev Respir Dis 1979; 120:1039–1052.
24. Suter PM, Fairley HB, Isenberg MD. Optimum end-expiratory airway pressure in patients with acute pulmonary failure. N Engl J Med 1975; 292:284–289.
25. Gallagher TJ, Civetta JM, Kirby RR. Terminology update: optimal PEEP. Crit Care Med 1978; 6:323–326.
26. Dorinsky PM, Hamlin RL, Gadek JE. Alterations in regional blood flow during positive end-expiratory pressure. Crit Care Med 1987; 15:106–113.
27. Weisman IM, Rinaldo JE, Rogers RM. Positive end-expiratory pressure in adult respiratory failure. N Engl J Med 1982; 307:1381–1384.
28. Regnier B, Safran D, Carlet J, et al. Comparative hemodynamic effects of dopamine and dobutamine in septic shock. Intensive Care Med 1979; 5:115–120.
29. Bernard GR, Luce JM, Sprung CL, Rinaldo JE, Tate RM, Sibbald WJ, Kariman K, Higgins S, Bradley R, Metz CA, Harris TR, Brigham KL. High dose corticosteroids in patients with adult respiratory distress syndrome. N Engl J Med 1987; 317:1565–1570.
30. Simmons RS, Berdine GG, Seidenfeld JJ, Prihoda TJ, Harris GD, Smith JD, Gilbert TJ, Mota E, Johanson WG. Fluid balance and the adult respiratory distress syndrome. Am Rev Respir Dis 1987; 135:924–929.
31. Danek SJ, Lynch JP, Weg JG, Dantzker DR. The dependence of oxygen uptake on oxygen delivery in the adult respiratory distress syndrome. Am Rev Respir Dis 1980; 122:387–395.
32. Kariman K, Burns SR. Regulation of tissue oxygen extraction is disturbed in adult respiratory distress syndrome. Am Rev Respir Dis 1985; 132:109–114.
33. Seidenfeld JJ, Pohl DF, Bell RC, Harris GD, Johanson WG. Incidence, site, and outcome of infections in patients with the adult respiratory distress syndrome. Am Rev Respir Dis 1986; 134:12–16.
34. Wiedemann HP, Matthay MA, Matthay RA. Cardiovascular-pulmonary monitoring in the intensive care unit (part 2). Chest 1984; 85:656–668.
35. Lakshminarayan S, Stanford RE, Petty TL. Prognosis after recovery from adult respiratory distress syndrome. Am Rev Respir Dis 1976; 113:7–16.

Alcohol withdrawal syndromes

Gerald M. Cross ■ *Terry K. Schultz*

Until 1955, it was believed that alcohol* withdrawal played no role in precipitating delirium tremens. In that year, Isbell and associates published an experiment demonstrating that stopping heavy alcohol consumption did produce rum fits and delirium tremens.[1] Today, our understanding of detoxification allows us to bring most patients through withdrawal comfortably and safely. The physician's ultimate goal, however, is to guide the alcoholic patient into a successful recovery.

The number of patients who may need detoxification is substantial. Conservatively, 7 per cent of adults are alcohol dependent. In general hospitals, the percentage is much higher. One study at Johns Hopkins Hospital, for example, found that 25 per cent of adult patients admitted were diagnosable as alcoholic.[2] The prevalence by hospital department was: 24 per cent were medical patients; 30 per cent, psychiatric; and 43 per cent, ear, nose, and throat patients. This chapter offers our best advice for treating patients in detoxification.

■ Background

■ PHYSIOLOGY OF WITHDRAWAL

The pathophysiology of alcohol dependence and withdrawal is extremely complex, and no comprehensive understanding is yet possible. Nevertheless, rapid developments in cell biology have provided new insights into alcohol-induced changes at the cellular and subcellular levels.[3] Understanding these alterations, as summarized in the following pages, has important clinical implications for handling detoxification. This understanding is reflected in current treatment protocols and the promising novel treatment approaches now under development.[4]

Neurophysiology

Alcohol disorders the structure of cell membranes by increasing their fluidity. Membranes become more rigid with chronic alcohol use and retain the rigidity into withdrawal, with functional consequences. Cell membrane rigidity alterations include newly discovered bilipid membrane changes,[5] with increases in cholesterol, decreases in gangliosides, and changes in specific acidic phospholipids.

GABA-Benzodiazepine-Chloride

The gamma-aminobutyric acid (GABA)–benzodiazepine-chloride receptor complex is the major inhibitory pathway in the brain. Alcohol potentiates the GABA receptor complex,[6] but during withdrawal its sensitivity is decreased, which may underlie the withdrawal symptoms from alcohol, as well as other drugs, since this receptor complex is the primary site of action for the sedative-hypnotic drugs. These drugs are cross-tolerant with alcohol and can be used to maintain GABA receptor functioning during alcohol withdrawal. The commonly used GABA receptor complex agonist drugs are barbiturates and benzodiazepines.

The Hyperadrenergic State

Alcohol withdrawal may be viewed as a hyperactive noradrenergic state[7] in which the patient's central nervous system is suddenly relieved of the chronic suppression produced by alcohol and rebounds with a pro-

---

The opinions presented in this paper are those of the authors and no endorsement or approval by the Federal Government is intended or implied.

*The term *alcohol* will be used interchangeably with the term *ethanol*. The term *alcoholism* will be used interchangeably with the term *alcohol dependence*.

longed surge of activity. The level of breakdown products from norepinephrine increases during alcohol withdrawal and then declines. Increased noradrenergic release correlates with peripheral symptoms, such as hypertension, tachycardia, and general autonomic reactivity.

As alcoholic persons undergo repeated cycles of intoxication and withdrawal, their withdrawal neuroexcitation becomes progressively worse. This phenomenon is called *kindling*.[8] Norepinephrine breakdown products and diastolic blood pressure provide a measure of this progressive change. These measures correlate with the patient's lifetime withdrawal experience. A second phenomenon related to kindling is *reinstatement*. As cycles of intoxication and withdrawal continue, the duration of each drinking episode tends to be shorter. In other words, the duration of drinking necessary to produce tolerance and withdrawal tends to decrease.

Adenosine

Adenosine is an inhibitory neuromodulator with anticonvulsant properties. Adenosine may mediate the effects of alcohol in the brain. Chronic alcohol exposure causes a significant down-regulation of adenosine function, perhaps through an alteration in gene expression and regulation of adenosine-dependent cAMP in neural cells.[9] These changes could play a role in generating alcohol withdrawal seizures or contribute to kindling effects. Since xanthine substances, including theophylline and caffeine, are known adenosine antagonists, use of these drugs may increase the risk of withdrawal seizures; therefore they should be used with caution or avoided during detoxification.

Calcium Channels

Calcium channels play a central role in both alcohol intoxification and withdrawal, with likely implications for kindling. Alcohol acutely inhibits N-methyl-D-aspartate (NMDA)–activated calcium channels[10] and chronically up-regulates neuronal dihydropyridine-sensitive calcium channels that contribute to withdrawal neuroexcitation and convulsions.[11] These findings have opened up the possibility that calcium channel inhibitors, shown to be beneficial in animal models of withdrawal, may also have clinical usefulness in human detoxification.

Physiology

The release of vasopressin (antidiuretic hormone) is inhibited while the patient's alcohol level is rising. This effect is less apparent in patients over the age of 50 years. The release of vasopressin is increased while the alcohol level is declining. The general effect is that chronic alcohol use causes increased total body water. Serum electrolytes in alcoholic persons may not reflect these changes. For this reason, unless other complications exist, alcoholic withdrawal should not be treated with intravenous fluids.

Chronic alcohol use increases the urinary loss of magnesium. Hypomagnesemia, as measured in cerebrospinal fluid (CSF), is associated with the development of withdrawal seizures. Serum and CSF levels of magnesium are not correlated, so blood levels of magnesium are unreliable for deciding for or against magnesium supplementation. The evidence for the routine use of magnesium to treat alcohol withdrawal is controversial. In a study of 100 patients treated for alcohol withdrawal, the use of magnesium did not alter the patient's outcome.[12] Later studies, including one with 781 patients,[13] found that magnesium was an effective addition to sedative therapy for preventing seizures. Along with these changes, acid-base disorders may occur. Alkalosis is the most frequent acid-base disorder seen in these patients. Usually it is a simple respiratory alkalosis or a mixed respiratory and metabolic alkalosis.[14] Hypokalemia is another common occurrence in chronic alcoholic patients during withdrawal. It does not necessarily reflect a true total body potassium depletion. Potassium supplementation is usually not necessary.

Inadequate diet and the effects of alcohol combine to produce vitamin deficiencies in alcoholism. Alcoholic patients may be deficient in thiamine without clinical signs of the deficiency. Thiamine is effective in preventing paresis of the sixth cranial nerve. Prophylactic use of thiamine should be given prior to the administration of glucose to prevent an acute Wernicke-Korsakoff syndrome. If the patient's magnesium level is low, resistance to thiamine therapy may occur. In addition to thiamine, supplementation with other vitamins, especially pyridoxine hydrochloride (B₆) and folate, is appropriate.

■ DIAGNOSIS

Initial Examination

Physicians called to the emergency room to examine a possible alcohol withdrawal patient should initially focus on several basic questions. Is the patient obtunded or agitated? If the patient is obtunded, is the blood alcohol concentration (BAC) high enough to explain it? Drunkenness generally produces the maximum level of obtundation within about 90 minutes of the last drink, but obtundation should improve noticeably 1 or 2 hours after that peak.[15] Is there any evidence of trauma, hypoglycemia, or drug overdose? If the patient is agitated, consider the possibility of other drug reactions—especially that of a psycho-stimulant or PCP. Also rule out primary seizure disorders and thyrotoxicosis. Obtain corroborative information from the patient's family to verify alcohol and other drug use. The BAC, urine drug screen, prothrombin time, and measurement of mean cell volume (MCV) and transaminase levels can be helpful in diagnosing alcohol dependence.

The aspartate aminotransferase (AST): alanine aminotransferase (ALT) ratio has been shown to be greater than 1 in alcoholic patients. The reliability of the ratio may be age specific, since the youthful military alcoholic population is more likely to have an AST:ALT ration of less than 1. The elevation of either of these liver enzymes does not correlate with the severity of alcoholic liver disease found at biopsy.[16] Any elevation of liver enzymes should raise the possibility of alcoholism as the cause. An increase in prothrombin time seems to correlate best with alcohol-induced liver disease.

Measurement of carbohydrate-deficient transferrin (CDT) can confirm a history of heavy alcohol consumption. A CDT of 80 mg/liter is found in more than 80 per cent of alcoholics who had consumed 50 grams (approximately four regular beers) or more of alcohol per day during the previous month or longer.[17] A definitive Diagnostic and Statistical Manual (DSM-III-R) alcohol diagnosis can wait until after the patient is

TABLE 1. The CAGE Questions

C	Have you ever felt you ought to Cut down on your drinking?
A	Have people ever Annoyed you by criticizing your drinking?
G	Have you ever felt Guilty about your drinking?
E	Have you ever had a drink first thing in the morning to steady your nerves or to get rid of a hangover? (Eye opener)

(From Ewing JA: Detecting alcoholism: the CAGE questionnaire. JAMA 1984; 1905–1907. Copyright 1984, American Medical Association.)

alert and coherent. At that time, a paper and pencil test such as the Michigan Alcoholism Screening Test (MAST) is helpful, but for a screening interview the CAGE questions are simple and quick. CAGE is an acronym for the key words in four questions (Table 1).[18] Two or three positive responses highly suggest alcohol dependency and should lead to further investigation.

■ Withdrawal

Stages of Withdrawal

Alcohol withdrawal can be divided into four clinically recognizable stages. Although more complex models have been proposed, this four-stage model is commonly used because of its simplicity for clinical use. The time of onset and the duration for each stage are variable. Occasionally, patients may seem to skip stages and develop a severe withdrawal quite rapidly.

Stage 1 usually begins 6 to 8 hours after the last drink. The symptoms are commonly described as a "hangover." Patients typically experience nausea, insomnia, vivid dreaming, anxiety, tachycardia, and the "shakes."

If the patient progresses, stage 2 begins about 24 hours after stopping or reducing alcohol intake. In this stage, the patient has continued stage 1 signs, tremor, and autonomic hyperactivity. Visual hallucinations may occur, especially at night, but when auditory hallucinations occur, they are more frightening to the patient. These hallucinations can be distinguished from those that occur during delirium tremens, since in stage 2 the patient remains oriented to reality.

Seizures herald the onset of stage 3. Seizures occur in as few as 2.5 per cent of patients,[19] usually within 48 hours of the last drink. Withdrawal seizures are typically grand mal in type, with no bowel or bladder loss of control. One third of these stage 3 patients may go on to delirium tremens if not treated. The percentage of patients who develop severe withdrawal symptoms depends on the population served.

Delirium tremens (DTs)—stage 4—usually occurs within 3 to 5 days after the last drink. Delirium tremens includes hallucinations accompanied by autonomic hyperactivity, disorientation, global confusion, fever, hypertension, and tachycardia. Electrolyte imbalance and vascular collapse may lead to death. Failure to recognize and treat withdrawal in its early stages increases the patient's morbidity. Even with currently available treatment, mortality may be 5 per cent or more, depending on the population served.

A protracted alcohol withdrawal syndrome may exist in some recovering alcoholics. Sleep electroencephalographic studies have shown ongoing disturbances for more than 30 days, and animal studies have shown central nervous system hyperexcitability for up to 8 weeks after drinking was stopped. An intermediate duration (subacute) mental disorder also has been described based on brain imaging and neuropsychologic testing.[20] During this period there is an increased risk of relapse. Cumulative alcohol damage to the brain was further demonstrated in an autopsy series in which nondemented alcoholic patients were compared with age-matched controls.[21] The alcoholic patients had a 40 per cent decrease in the density of cholinergic muscarinic receptors in the frontal cortex. This diminished synaptic function produces a clinical spectrum of impaired cognition that precedes brain atrophy and dementia and supports the concept of a protracted withdrawal syndrome.

Withdrawal from Alcohol and a Second Drug

The course of withdrawal from alcohol and a cross-tolerant sedative depends on the half-life of the sedative. If the sedative has a relatively short half-life, such as that of alprazolam, the course of withdrawal for both drugs may be almost simultaneous but more severe than for alcohol alone. The combination of alcohol and a longer-acting sedative may result in prolongation of withdrawal. If a patient is addicted to both alcohol and a noncross-tolerant drug, withdraw the more medically dangerous drug first while maintaining the less dangerous drug.

■ RISK ASSESSMENT FOR WITHDRAWAL

Certain patient characteristics should serve as a warning that alcohol withdrawal will be severe. The total amount of alcohol consumed and the length of exposure to alcohol is related to withdrawal severity. Patients over the age of 45 years and those with poor health or a history of prior difficult withdrawal are at higher risk. While these predictive factors are helpful, a more objective and standardized measure is the revised version of the Clinical Institute Withdrawal Assessment for Alcohol (CIWA-A).[22] This scale requires only about 5 minutes to use. Scores greater than 15 suggest a more severe withdrawal. Trauma, such as a fractured femur, may mask the severity of withdrawal and may result in an artificially low score.

■ Management

■ SUPPORTIVE CARE

Carry out admission procedures rapidly so that therapy is not delayed. Supportive care may be all that is required for patients with minimal risk for a difficult withdrawal. After the preliminary history and physical and laboratory data are obtained, place the patient in an environment that minimizes photic stimulation while avoiding sensory deprivation. A quiet room with even lighting is best. If the patient shows signs of severe withdrawal, the presence of an attendant may help avoid the rare necessity of restraints. Stable sleep is the therapeutic goal at this point. If the patient is too agitated for sleep, sedative medication is appropriate. Intravenous fluids are rarely necessary, and oral fluids can be provided when the patient is thirsty. Psychostimulants such as caffeine are to be avoided because of the possibility of lowering the seizure threshold.

Metabolic changes in elderly patients allow blood alcohol levels to remain higher for longer periods of time. Intoxicated behavior persists longer, and recovery from intoxication is slower. During their detoxification, elderly patients are more likely to have sleep disturbances, neuropathy, and memory impairment. Instructions to elderly patients should be repeated several times to insure understanding, and environmental changes should be minimized to avoid disorientation.

The physician's role during this period extends far beyond the physical examination. The physician can play a key role in penetrating the patient's denial, as well as in responding to medical complications. The patient's interaction with the physician reinforces the disease concept and can help avoid discharges against medical advice. Throughout this period, patients may have many minor physical complaints. Reassurance is an adequate response to minor complaints that will resolve spontaneously after detoxification.

■ STANDARD MEDICATIONS

Protocols for detoxification should not be rigid formulas. The protocols that follow are general guidelines that can be adapted to an individual patient's needs. Alcohol withdrawal is usually treated by discontinuing alcohol and substituting a cross-tolerant sedative medication, which is then gradually withdrawn. There is an ongoing and lively debate about which medication offers the most effective and safe detoxification. We feel that our guidelines are appropriate for most patients. The issues in the debate over the best protocol are presented later.

Generic Protocol Recommendations

The frequency with which vital signs are measured depends on the patient's stability. Oral liquids are usually adequate for hydration during alcohol withdrawal. Thiamine should be given immediately, 100 mg IM. If the patient is at risk for the Wernicke-Korsakoff syndrome, thiamine should be continued IM at this dose for 3 days, then orally at the same dose for up to 2 months. Otherwise, a daily dose of oral vitamins, including thiamine, pyridoxine hydrochloride, and folate, is adequate. Finally, magnesium sulfate ($MgSO_4$) (50 per cent), 2 ml IM every 6 to 8 hours for up to six doses, is appropriate for patients who are at risk for a difficult withdrawal or who have a magnesium deficiency that would interfere with thiamine replacement. Magnesium supplementation provides the additional benefit of inhibiting NMDA calcium channel function, which helps to reduce withdrawal neuroexcitation.

Phenobarbital Sample Protocol

For mild withdrawal, phenobarbital is given orally on a tapering schedule: 30 mg QID for 3 days, then 15 mg QID for 2 days, and finally 15 mg BID for 1 day. The keys to success in using this protocol are the staff's attentiveness in frequently monitoring changes in the patient's withdrawal state and the administration of intramuscular phenobarbital (240 mg IM as needed, up to approximately 500 mg in 1 day) early in the treatment of patients at risk for a severe withdrawal. An alternative oral loading dose protocol may be used. In this method, 120 mg of phenobarbital is given every 1 to 2 hours until withdrawal symptoms are controlled or until side effects occur—including ataxia, nystagmus, or drowsiness.

Benzodiazepine Sample Protocol

If benzodiazepines are used, the oral loading technique is effective[23] and is preferred by coauthor TKS. Patients at risk for withdrawal are given 20 mg of diazepam PO every 1 to 2 hours until a minimum cumulative dose of 60 mg is reached, the patient's CIWA-A score is 10 or less, or the patient becomes drowsy. Because of diazepam's long half-life, usually no additional doses are necessary beyond that point. The Project Cork Institute of Dartmouth College Medical School recommends a variation of this protocol in which oxazepam, with its shorter half-life, is titrated to an objective scale of withdrawal signs.

When prescribing any sedative, physicians should be careful to avoid causing excessive drowsiness, ataxia, or aspiration. Nevertheless, the most common mistake of physicians is the failure to provide the adequate dosages of medication necessary to treat severe withdrawal.

Chlormethiazole (Heminevrin)

This sedative-hypnotic is popular in some other countries due to its wide spectrum of effects in severe withdrawal. Studies have compared chlormethiazole favorably with chlordiazepoxide, neuroleptics, and, most recently, clonidine.[24] This medication has not been approved for use in the United States.

■ ADJUNCTIVE MEDICATIONS

Beta-Blockers

Since withdrawal involves a surge in the sympathetic nervous system's activity, beta-blockers should be an appropriate treatment. The actual treatment results have been mixed. Propranolol has produced a high level of psychotoxic reactions when used during alcohol withdrawal. Propranolol failed to prevent or reduce the symptoms of hangover, although a slight improvement in hand tremor was noted.[25] Atenolol seemed to avoid the psychotoxic problems of propranolol, and when used as an addition to standard sedative therapy, vital signs returned to normal more rapidly.[26] Beta-blockers may prove to be a useful adjunct to standard therapy when withdrawal symptoms are mild and consist primarily of tremor and tachycardia.

Clonidine

Clonidine is a centrally acting alpha-2 adrenoceptor agonist that has been useful both in the treatment of hypertension and for attenuating opiate withdrawal. It has also been used for the treatment of alcohol withdrawal. Clonidine, as with the beta-blockers, improves diaphoresis, tremor, tachycardia, and hypertension. Severe withdrawal states, including hallucinations, seizures, or delirium, are not prevented. Sympatholytic drugs may have an adjunctive role, but their use as a sole therapy in patients at risk for withdrawal is inappropriate.[24]

Antiepileptic Drugs

Phenytoin or carbamazepine has been combined with sedatives for detoxification. The addition of phenytoin to treatment protocols has not reduced the incidence of seizures. A double-blind randomized study revealed that phenytoin is no better than placebo in alcohol withdrawal.[27] On the other hand, carbamazepine has been shown to have an antikindling effect and to be effective for alcohol withdrawal seizures.[28] For patients suspected of dual dependence on alcohol and benzodiazepines, carbamazepine may prove to be especially useful.[29]

Amino Acid Loading

Neurotransmitter precursor loading using amino acids[4] has been reported to ease withdrawal craving and to reduce treatment drop-out rates. A variety of amino acid compounds is being tried. An example is tyrosine loading in the morning to reduce anxiety. Precursor loading improves dysfunctional serotonergic, catecholaminergic, enkephalinergic, and GABAergic mechanisms. Such treatments are currently considered investigational.

Other Medications

If hallucinosis is a prominent feature of withdrawal, haloperidol may be given as an adjunct to a standard sedative medication in a dose ranging from 0.5 to 5.0 mg IM every 1 to 2 hours for up to five doses.[30] An interesting but unconfirmed report is that dexamethasone will reverse delirium tremens that is resistant to benzodiazepine therapy. Dexamethasone was given IV, 3 mg every 12 hours. The mechanism of action may be corticosteroid's ability to stabilize cell membranes.[31]

■ ASPECTS OF COMPLICATED WITHDRAWAL

Wernicke-Korsakoff Syndrome

This is a neurologic disorder caused by thiamine deficiency. Wernicke's encephalopathy is the acute phase and Korsakoff's psychosis is the chronic phase of this syndrome.

Although it is usually associated with alcoholism, it also can occur in other conditions associated with poor thiamine intake or inadequate absorption. The onset of the syndrome may be abrupt and includes the triad of mental confusion, cerebellar ataxia, and oculomotor disturbances. The ocular findings vary but may include a range of signs from nystagmus to total ophthalmoplegia. The ataxia is a broad-based, lurching gait. Disorientation and drowsiness are characteristic of the mental state, but coma may also occur. It is emphasized that thiamine should be given before glucose in any patient at risk for Wernicke's encephalopathy.

Korsakoff's psychosis is characterized by memory defects and confabulation, with preservation of other intellectual function. Whereas Korsakoff's psychosis might be prevented by prompt treatment of Wernicke's encephalopathy, many cases progress to a chronic condition that, in the end, requires institutionalization.

Coma

Naloxone was once viewed as a promising treatment for coma secondary to alcohol intoxication. Later experience with this treatment has been disappointing, except in those cases in which other depressants had been ingested.[19] The treatment for combined alcohol and benzodiazepine coma is the newly released benzodiazepine antagonist RO 15-1788 (Flumazenil). This drug has been shown to be effective in reversing CNS depression because of benzodiazepine overdose, in overdose with benzodiazepines and other drugs, and in one patient who had only ethanol intoxication. The dosage recommended was 3 to 5 mg given at a rate of 1 mg/min IV. If long-acting benzodiazepines are present, a continuous infusion may be necessary to prevent a relapse of coma.[32]

Hepatic Encephalopathy

Hepatic encephalopathy (HE) is a complex neuropsychiatric disorder that complicates hepatocellular failure, regardless of its cause. The earliest signs of HE are subtle changes in behavior and intellectual function, which reflect bilateral forebrain dysfunction. Progression results in ataxia, motor impairment, and eventually the loss of consciousness. The differential diagnosis between delirium tremens and hepatic encephalopathy is important, although both conditions may coexist. Patients with delirium tremens are typically more anxious, with a tremor that is fine and fast. HE patients are more obtunded, with asterixis and a slow tremor. If the diagnosis is not clear, an EEG will be helpful. Patients in withdrawal have EEGs with hyperactivity, whereas with encephalopathy the EEG shows slowing of electrical activity. An elevated ammonia level also supports the diagnosis of HE.

These patients pose an especially difficult problem during detoxification if they need treatment for agitation. Encephalopathy may be worsened by central nervous system depressants, especially if the drug requires hepatic metabolism. Benzodiazepines may intensify the confusion associated with HE, whereas haloperidol may reduce confusion and agitation. A promising new treatment for hepatic encephalopathy is the benzodiazepine antagonist RO 15-1788 (Flumazenil), the use of which has demonstrated improvement in both gross behavior and EEG visual evoked response in patients with hepatic encephalopathy.[33] This observation supports the possibility that the GABA-benzodiazepine receptor complex is a mediator for HE. When there appears to be a paradoxic response to benzodiazepines, suspect hepatic encephalopathy.

Seizures

If seizures that occur before admission are included, the percentage of seizures during withdrawal increases to 10 per cent.[34] These seizures typically occur in one or two episodes and are generalized and nonfocal. The key to preventing seizures is early treatment with sedative medication. One study found that a single IV loading dose of phenobarbital successfully prevented withdrawal seizures.[27] Patients who have withdrawal seizures but no prior history of seizures should be evaluated to rule out metabolic, infectious, or neurologic causes. If withdrawal seizures do occur, they may be managed in the acute stage with diazepam, 5 mg as an IV push over 2 minutes, followed by additional smaller doses every 5 to 10 minutes if appropriate. Remember that withdrawal seizures indicate a greater risk that the patient will develop delirium tremens.

Muscle Deterioration

Skeletal and cardiac muscular function deteriorates in alcoholic patients.[35] This is due to the effect of alcohol on muscle tissue, instead of a nutritional deficiency. Cardiac ejection fraction, which may be the earliest diagnostic marker for alcoholic cardiomyopathy, declines as the total lifetime dose of ethanol increases. Atrial fibrillation is the most common dysrhythmia associated with binge drinking in alcoholics, but other dysrhythmias may also occur, especially in withdrawal. There is evidence in animals that changes in muscular function can be reversed with abstinence.

■ PSYCHOLOGIC INTERVENTION

Early interactions with alcoholic patients will bring the physician face to face with denial. Harsh, forceful attempts to break through denial should be discouraged. Instead, provide a warm, supportive atmosphere in which the patient feels comfortable. Honest, caring, and direct confrontation can be the foundation of good counseling. The medical staff can promote the patient's long-term recovery by focusing attention on the need for rehabilitation and by introducing the patient to Alcoholics Anonymous. Craving is another problem that should be explicitly discussed with the patient and family. The best ally for overcoming craving and supporting continued treatment is a prepared family that understands enabling behavior and is educated about rehabilitation.

Acute alcohol intoxication and withdrawal symptoms may mistakenly be interpreted as a variety of psychiatric disorders. Psychiatric diagnoses should be made cautiously during acute and extended withdrawal. Depression, for instance, resolves spontaneously during withdrawal and early rehabilitation in the great majority of alcoholic patients. In general, wait 4 to 6 weeks at least, before an in-depth neuropsychologic assessment is requested.

Clinicians should be aware that age can be an important factor in withdrawal states. Adolescents experience alcohol withdrawal differently than do older patients. Adolescents externalize discomfort and have less somatization. More often, they may complain about the hospital, parents, and so on. These complaints may be evidence of withdrawal and require medication. Failure to recognize this may result in a patient leaving treatment prematurely. Adolescents usually do better in a clearly structured environment, since peer pressure, or autonomous strivings, may drive them to test limits. In this situation, controls act as a face-saving mechanism for adolescents. Respectful, firm interaction with adolescents opens the way for a therapeutic relationship that will promote education and rehabilitation.

■ Issues and Risks

■ THE IDEAL MEDICATION FOR DETOXIFICATION

Few studies comprehensively compare the effectiveness of various drugs for alcohol withdrawal. Although a review of 81 studies published since 1954 found no conclusive evidence that one drug was superior to others for alcohol withdrawal,[36] several of the studies are worth review. Phenobarbital has been compared with several medications, including carbamazepine and diazepam. In each case, phenobarbital was found to be equal or superior in effectiveness. The comparison with carbamazepine showed both drugs to be equally effective for mild or moderate withdrawal symptoms, although the carbamazepine-treated group had more side effects, especially dizziness.[28] In a double-blind study, diazepam was compared with phenobarbital and found to be equivalent, except in severe withdrawal, when phenobarbital was superior in relieving delirium tremens.[37] Phenobarbital has the advantages of a long half-life, an excellent anticonvulsant effect, and predictable IM absorption. In addition, phenobarbital is a prudent choice for pregnant patients who require seizure prophylaxis.[38] Although phenobarbital has been effectively used in alcohol withdrawal for decades, it has the advantage that today's patients are less likely to recognize it. Patient recognition of tranquilizers like diazepam (Valium) resulted in inappropriate requests for the medication.[39] Philosophically, some physicians prefer to use phenobarbital during detoxification, since currently it is less commonly abused than are the benzodiazepines.

The various benzodiazepines are therapeutically equivalent,[19] although a patient's specific characteristics may argue for one agent over another in cases of liver disease or when an IM medication is desired. Lorazepam is the only benzodiazepine recommended for IM use. Whichever medication is selected, it should have a half-life that is longer than the abused medication. Approximate doses equivalent to 20 mg of diazepam are chlordiazepoxide, 100 mg; lorazepam, 4 mg; and oxazepam, 120 mg. Benzodiazepines are most commonly used because of their cross-tolerant sedative, anxiolytic, and anticonvulsant effects combined with their superior safety to toxicity ratio, as compared with other sedative-hypnotics.

In the final analysis, it is unlikely that medication selection will be the most critical factor in a patient's recovery. The therapeutic environment, the familiarity of the staff with a specific protocol, and their commitment to the patient's rehabilitation are the critical factors.

■ MEDICAL VERSUS SOCIAL DETOXIFICATION

Evidence concerning kindling and reinstatement after repeated cycles of withdrawal suggests that progressive changes occur in the brain. These changes include alterations in neuronal cell membranes, adrenal hyperplasia, and autonomic reactivity. While rehabilitation is the best defense against this progression, the contributory role of withdrawal neuroexcitation and kindling has been highlighted during the past decade, raising new concerns about detoxification methods.[7] As the mystery of the cellular mechanism of alcoholism has unfolded, it is clear that pharmacotherapy has an essential role in the prophylaxis of the diseases's progression. Research validation of this approach has called into question the clinical role of social detoxification. As this information has been confirmed, it has further strengthened the rationale for medical treatment of alcohol withdrawal, in addition to the usual reasons such as patient comfort, seizure prophylaxis, and treatment of other medical complications.

Allowing alcoholic patients to go "cold turkey" through withdrawal is losing credibility, especially because of the imprecision of predicting which patients will have a difficult withdrawal. Nevertheless, the nurturing aspects of social detoxification—especially the promotion of respect, reality, and reassurance—should be combined with medical therapy based on our current understanding of the cellular and subcellular changes that alcohol withdrawal produces in the central nervous system.

REFERENCES

1. Isbell H, Fraser H, Wikler A, Belleville M, Eisenman A. An experimental study of the etiology of "Rum Fits" and delirium tremens. Q J Studies Alcoholism 1955; 16:1–33.
2. Moore R, Bone L, Geller G, Mamon J, Stokes E, Levine D. Prevalence, detection, and treatment of alcoholism in hospitalized patients. JAMA 1989; 261:403–407.
3. Rubin E (ed). Alcohol and the cell. Ann NY Acad Sci 1987; 492:1–412.
4. Wallace J. The relevance to clinical care of recent research in neurobiology. J Subst Abuse Treat 1988; 5:207–217.
5. Goldstein D. Ethanol-induced adaptation in biological membranes. Ann NY Acad Sci 1987; 492:103–111.
6. Ticku MK, Burch TP, Davis WC. Interactions of ethanol with the benzodiazepine-GABA ionophore complex. Pharm Bio Behav 1983; 18(Suppl 1):15–18.
7. Linnoila M, Mefford I, Nutt D, Adinoff B. Alcohol withdrawal and noradrenergic function. Ann Intern Med 1987; 108:875–889.
8. Ballenger JC, Post RM: Kindling as a model for the alcohol withdrawal syndromes. Br J Psychiatry 1978; 133:1–14.
9. Mochly-Rosen D, Chang F, Cheever L, et al. Chronic ethanol causes heterologous desensitization of receptors by reducing alpha subunits of messenger RNA. Nature 1988; 333:848–850.
10. Lovinger DM, White G, Weight FF. Ethanol inhibits NMDA-activated ion currents in hippocampal neurons. Science 1989; 243:1721–1724.
11. Carlen PL, Wu PH. Calcium and sedative hypnotics drug action. Int Rev Neurobiol 1988; 29:161–189.
12. Wilson A, Vulcano B. A double-blind, placebo-controlled trial of magnesium sulfate in the ethanol withdrawal syndrome. Alcoholism Clin Exp Res 1984; 8:542–545.
13. Daus A, Freeman W, Wilson J, Aponte C. Clinical experience with 781 cases of alcoholism evaluated and treated on an inpatient basis by various methods. Int J Addict 1985; 20:643–650.
14. Pitts T, Van Thiel D. Disorders of the serum electrolytes, acid-base balance, and renal function. In Gallante M (ed). Recent Developments in Alcoholism. Vol 4. New York: Plenum Press, 1986:315–321.
15. Baum R, Iber F. Initial treatment of the alcoholic patient. In Gitlow S, Peyser H (eds). Alcoholism: A Practical Treatment Guide. Philadelphia: Grune & Stratton, 1988:55.

16. Marshall J, Burnett D, Zetterman R, Sorrell M. Clinical and biochemical course of alcoholic liver disease following sudden discontinuation of alcoholic consumption. Alcoholism Clin Exp Res 1983; 7:312–315.
17. Behrens U, Worner T, Braly L, Schaffner F, Lieber C. Carbohydrate-deficient transferrin, a marker for chronic alcohol consumption in different ethnic populations. Alcoholism Clin Exp Res 1988; 12:427–432.
18. Ewing JA. Detecting alcoholism: the CAGE questionnaire. JAMA 1984; 252:1905–1907.
19. Liskow B, Goodwin D. Pharmacological treatment of alcohol intoxication, withdrawal and dependence: a critical review. J Stud Alcohol 1987; 48:356–370.
20. Grant I, Adams KM, Reed R. Intermediate duration (subacute) organic mental disorder of alcoholism. In Neuropsychiatric Correlates of Alcoholism. Washington, DC: American Psychiatric Press Inc., 1986.
21. Freund G, Ballinger WE. Loss of cholinergic muscarinic receptors in the frontal cortex of alcohol abusers. Alcoholism Clin Exp Res 1988; 12:630–638.
22. Foy A, March S, Drinkwater V. Use of an objective clinical scale in the assessment and management of alcohol withdrawal in a large general hospital. Alcoholism Clin Exp Res 1988; 12:360–364.
23. Naranjo CA, Sellers EM. Clinical assessment and pharmacotherapy of the alcohol withdrawal syndrome. In Gallanter M (ed). Recent Developments in Alcoholism. Vol 4. New York: Plenum Press, 1986:265–281.
24. Robinson BJ, Robinson GM, Maling TJB, et al. Is clonidine useful in the treatment of alcohol withdrawal? Alcoholism Clin Exp Res 1989; 13:95–98.
25. Bogin TM, Nostrant TT, Young MJ. Propranolol for the treatment of the alcoholic hangover. Am J Drug Alcohol Abuse 1987; 13:175–180.
26. Kraus M, Gottlieb L, Horwitz R, Anscher M. Randomized clinical trial of atenolol in patients with alcohol withdrawal. N Engl J Med 1985; 313:905–909.
27. Simon RP. Alcohol and seizures. N Engl J Med 1988; 319:715–716.
28. Flygenring HJ, Hoist B, Petersen E, Sorensen A. Treatment of alcohol withdrawal symptoms in hospitalized patients. Acta Psychiatr Scand 1984; 69:398–408.
29. Ries R, Roy-Byrne P, Ward N, Neppe V, Cullison S. Carbamazepine treatment for benzodiazepine withdrawal. Am J Psychiatr 1989; 146:536–537.
30. Rosenbloom AJ. Emerging treatment options in the alcohol withdrawal syndrome. J Clin Psychiatr 1988; 49 (12):28–31.
31. Fischer D, Simpson R, Smith F, Mattox K. Efficacy of dexamethasone in benzodiazepine-resistant delirium tremens. Lancet 1988; 1 (8598):1340–1341.
32. Lheureux P, Askenasi R. Specific treatment of benzodiazepine overdose. Hum Toxicol 1988; 7:165–170.
33. Basile AS, Gammal SH, Mullen KD, et al. Differential responsiveness of cerebellar Purkinje neurons to GABA and benzodiazepine receptor ligands in an animal model of hepatic encephalopathy. J Neurosci 1988; 8:2414–2421.
34. Hillbom ME, Hjelm-Jäger M. Should alcohol withdrawal seizures be treated with anti-epileptic drugs? Acta Neurol Scand 1984; 69:39–42.
35. Urbano-Marquez A, Estruch R, Navarro-Lopez F, Grau J, Mont L, Rubin E. The effects of alcoholism on skeletal and cardiac muscle. N Engl J Med 1989; 320:409–415.
36. Moskowitz G, Chalmers T, Sacks H, Fagerstrom R, Smith H. Deficiencies of clinical trials of alcohol withdrawal. Alcoholism Clin Exp Res 1983; 7:42–46.
37. Kramp P, Rafaelsen O. Delirium tremens: a double-blind comparison of diazepam and barbital treatment. Acta Psychiatr Scand 1978; 58:174–190.
38. Aminoff M. Maternal neurologic disorders. In Creasy R, Resnik R (eds). Maternal-Fetal Medicine. Philadelphia: WB Saunders, 1984;1005–1010.
39. Francis DA, Nelson AA. Effect of patient recognition of tranquilizers on their use in alcohol detoxification. Am J Hosp Pharm 1984;41:488–492.

Alzheimer's disease

David L. Sultzer ■ *Jeffrey L. Cummings*

Dementia of the Alzheimer type (DAT) is a common illness with significant medical, behavioral, and social morbidity. The reported prevalence of clinically diagnosed DAT varies between 1.9 and 5.8 cases per 100 persons over the age of 65 years,[1] and the prevalence rate doubles every 4.5 years after age 65 years.[2] As the elderly population of the United States expands, the number of patients with DAT progressively increases, making DAT a major health care concern.

DAT presents difficult medical management challenges because of the complexity and uncertainty of clinical diagnosis, the lack of definitive treatment for the underlying illness, the occurrence of disabling behaviors, the comorbid conditions of aging, the vulnerability to secondary complications, and the magnitude of family stress. Although DAT is an irreversible illness, treatment options are available for many aspects of the disorder.

This chapter reviews the clinical features of DAT, provides strategies for managing behavioral and medical conditions in patients with DAT, and discusses family and ethical issues associated with management.

■ Background

■ CLINICAL IDENTIFICATION AND DIFFERENTIAL DIAGNOSIS

Dementia is defined as an acquired, persistent impairment in intellectual function, with deterioration in at least three of five domains: memory, language, visuospatial skills, personality, and cognition (calculation, abstraction, and so on).[3] Dementia must be distinguished from delirium (acute confusional state), mental retardation, and illnesses with more restricted areas of dysfunction, such as amnesia or aphasia.

The differential diagnosis of dementia is broad (Table 1), and patients suspected of having a dementing illness require a thorough evaluation, including clinical history (specific areas of disability, extent of disability, time course of illness, exposure to toxins or alcohol), review of medical and psychiatric history, review of medications, mental status examination, general physical and neurologic examinations, laboratory evaluation (electrolytes, blood sugar, blood urea nitrogen, liver enzyme and thyroid hormone assays, serum calcium and phosphorus levels, VDRL, B_{12} and folate levels, complete blood count, erythrocyte sedimentation rate, urinalysis), and an imaging study of the brain (computed tomography [CT] or magnetic resonance imaging [MRI]). Many patients require additional evaluation, including electroencephalogram (EEG), cerebrospinal fluid evaluation, supplemental laboratory tests (e.g., serum human immunodeficiency virus [HIV] antibody testing), or extended neuropsychologic testing.

Clinical Features

DAT accounts for approximately 40 per cent of all cases of dementia.[3] The clinical diag-

TABLE 1. Common Causes of Dementia

Degenerative conditions
  Cortical dementia
    Alzheimer's disease
    Pick's disease
  Extrapyramidal syndromes with dementia
    Huntington's disease
    Parkinson's disease
    Wilson's disease
    Progressive supranuclear palsy

Metabolic conditions
  Systemic illnesses
  Electrolyte disorders
  Endocrine imbalance
  Vitamin deficiencies

Toxic conditions
  Alcoholic dementia
  Heavy metal toxicity
  Medication toxicity

Dementia syndrome of depression

Multi-infarct dementia

Dementia secondary to infection
  HIV dementia
  Jakob-Creutzfeldt disease
  Syphilis

Dementia secondary to structural neurologic conditions
  Trauma
  Neoplasm

nosis of DAT is complex; it requires excluding alternative causes of dementia and identification of a characteristic clinical syndrome. The most widely accepted diagnostic criteria are those proposed in 1984 by the Work Group on the Diagnosis of Alzheimer's Disease established by the National Institute of Neurological and Communicative Disorders and Stroke and the Alzheimer's Disease and Related Disorders Association (NINCDS-ADRDA criteria).[4] Criteria for diagnosis of Probable Alzheimer's Disease include:

- dementia established by clinical examination and documented by cognitive rating scale assessment and neuropsychologic testing,
- deficits in two or more areas of cognition, including memory,
- progressive worsening of cognitive dysfunction,
- no disturbance of consciousness,
- onset between ages 40 and 90 years,
- and absence of other illnesses that could account for the cognitive decline.

Use of both the clinical and laboratory portions of these criteria results in diagnostic accuracy rates of approximately 90 per cent.[5]

Patients with DAT develop the insidious onset and gradual deterioration of cognitive functions, usually beginning after age 55 years. Death usually occurs 6 to 12 years after the onset of illness. In approximately 20 per cent of families, DAT is inherited in an autosomal dominant pattern, and there is a tendency for familial clustering of DAT in families, without clear dominant inheritance.[6]

Early in the course of illness, patients may exhibit impaired calculations, memory, or concentration; they may have difficulty adapting to new situations or finding their way in previously familiar environments. On mental status testing, there is a deficit in learning new information, impaired copying of three-dimensional figures, poor word list generation, and anomia. There may be subtle personality changes. The motor system, electroencephalogram (EEG), and brain imaging studies are usually normal in the initial phases of the illness.

During the middle stage of disease, patients have more difficulty with remembering and get lost easily. Family members may report personality changes, irritability, or indifference. Examination reveals impairment of recent and remote memory, spatial disorientation, poor constructional ability, acalculia, and aphasia with fluent language output, low information content ("empty speech"), poor comprehension, and paraphasias. There may be motor restlessness with excessive pacing. The electroencephalogram often shows diffuse slowing of background rhythms; brain imaging studies are normal or demonstrate diffuse atrophy.

In the final stage of illness, patients depend on others for self-care. There is severe impairment of nearly all cognitive functions. Urinary or fecal incontinence occur and limb rigidity or flexion supervenes. The EEG is diffusely slow, and brain imaging reveals diffuse atrophy.

In addition to the cognitive impairments of DAT, a number of personality and psychiatric changes occur. Early in the disorder, personality changes such as indifference are most striking, and depressive symptoms may occur. As the illness progresses, there may be inappropriate laughing, paranoid delusions, or agitation.

■ LABORATORY FINDINGS

No specific biologic markers for DAT have been identified. Diagnosis is based on clinical findings and results of cognitive testing. Neuropsychologic testing can quantify and further characterize the mental status abnormalities noted on clinical examination. CT, MRI, and EEG evaluations show characteristic but nonspecific findings. Single-photon emission computed tomography (SPECT) scan or positron emission tomography (PET) scan may identify characteristic patterns of reduced blood flow or metabolic changes in the temporal and parietal regions of the brain.

■ NEUROPATHOLOGY

On gross examination, the brain is atrophic with reduced brain weight. Histologically, the hallmarks of DAT are the presence of neurofibrillary tangles, senile plaques, granulovacuolar degeneration, and neuronal loss. These changes are most severe in the hippocampus, amygdala, and association areas of the cortex, particularly in the temporoparieto-occipital junction.[6] Neurochemical studies reveal depletion of acetylcholine. Alterations in levels of other neurotransmitters, including norepinephrine, serotonin, somatostatin, neuropeptide Y, and corticotropin-releasing factor (CRF), may also occur.

■ Management

There is no "cure" for DAT, but many symptoms are treatable. Treatment of the underlying neurodegenerative process has been unsuccessful; management emphasizes control of the psychiatric and behavioral syndromes of DAT and optimizing long-term care.

■ TREATMENT OF THE PRIMARY CONDITION

Cholinergic Agents

The use of cholinergic agents in the treatment of DAT was stimulated by the finding of decreased acetylcholine and choline acetyltransferase in the brains of patients with DAT. The loss of cholinergic neurons or diminished cerebral cholinergic activity or both was hypothesized to be important in the pathogenesis of cognitive deficits. Three approaches to enhancing cholinergic activity have been pursued: (1) precursor therapy (choline, lecithin), (2) treatment with inhibitors of acetylcholinesterase (physostigmine, tetrahydroaminoacridine), and (3) treatment with cholinergic receptor agonists (arecholine, bethanechol). None of these approaches has resulted in consistent clinically significant improvement.

Agents That Enhance Neuronal Metabolism

Several agents whose mechanism of action is related to the ability to enhance cerebral metabolism have been used in the treatment of patients with DAT.

Dihydroergotoxine (Hydergine), a compound containing several dihydrogenated alkaloids of ergot, has been used in the treatment of dementia for more than 30 years and is the most commonly used agent for the treatment of memory loss. Clinical trials generally have demonstrated significant improvement or amelioration of cognitive decline in treated patients,[7,8] but the improvements have been small. The dosage used in most clinical trials has been 3 mg per day, although more recent studies have used higher doses.[9] A dosage of 6 mg per day (in three divided doses) for a minimum period of 6 months is recommended in order to accurately assess amelioration of cognitive decline. Side effects include bradycardia and hypotension, although these problems are generally minimal. The cost for a 6-month trial has been estimated to be $260.[10]

None of the other metabolism-enhancing agents has been sufficiently useful to gain clinical endorsement.

■ TREATMENT OF BEHAVIORAL DISTURBANCES IN PATIENTS WITH DAT
(Table 2)

Psychosis

The prevalence of paranoid delusions in patients with DAT has been reported to be between 10 and 75 per cent.[11] The most common delusions are those of paranoia ("people are stealing things"), misidentification of familiar places, abandonment, and Capgras' syndrome.[12,13] Auditory and visual hallucinations occur, but are generally less common than delusions.[11]

Neuroleptic agents can be useful in the treatment of psychotic symptoms. Consideration of side effects is paramount in drug choice. The following side effects should be monitored:

1. *Sedation* can occur with all neuroleptic agents. Although sedation may be therapeutically beneficial in some cases, it may also lead to falls and fractures.
2. *Anticholinergic effects* include peripheral actions, such as dry mouth, blurred vision, constipation, and urinary retention. Central actions include anticholinergic delirium and exacerbation of the underlying cognitive impairment. These effects are most common with high doses of low-potency neuroleptics like chlorpromazine (Thorazine) and thioridazine (Mellaril).
3. *Extrapyramidal symptoms* include parkinsonism, dystonia, and akathisia (a subjective sense of restlessness, associated with increased motor activity such as pacing). These symptoms are more common with high-potency neuroleptics such as haloperidol (Haldol), fluphenazine (Prolixin), trifluoperazine (Stelazine), and thiothixene (Navane). The side effects may be treated with amantadine (Symmetrel) if reduction of the neuroleptic dosage is impossible. The addition of anticholinergic agents such as benztropine (Cogentin) or trihexyphenidyl (Artane) also may help ameliorate extrapyramidal symptoms, but elderly patients with dementia are particulary vulnerable to the adverse peripheral and central effects of anticholinergics. Treatment with neuroleptic agents also may cause tardive dyskinesia.
4. *Cardiovascular effects* include hypotension secondary to alpha-adrenergic blockade, tachycardia, and arrhythmias.
5. *Other side effects* include hepatotoxicity and agranulocytosis.

The recommended approach to treating psychosis in patients with DAT is to administer a low dose of a high-potency neurolep-

TABLE 2. Common Drugs for Psychiatric and Behavioral Disturbances in DAT

Class	Indications	Side Effects	Agents	Initial Dose (Mg) (PO)	Routine Daily Dose (Mg) (PO)*
Antidepressant	Major depression	Hypotension Anticholinergic symptoms Cardiac conduction disturbance Cardiac arrhythmia Confusion	Desipramine (Norpramin, Pertofrane) Nortriptyline (Pamelor) Doxepin (Adapin, Sinequan)	25 10 25	50–150 20–75 50–150
Neuroleptic	Psychosis Agitation Hostility	Sedation Anticholinergic symptoms Extrapyramidal symptoms Tardive dyskinesia Hypotension Hepatotoxicity Confusion	Haloperidol (Haldol) Fluphenazine (Prolixin) Molindone (Moban) Chlorpromazine (Thorazine) Thioridazine (Mellaril)	0.5 0.5 5 10 10	0.5–5 0.5–5 5–50 10–200 10–200
Benzodiazepine	Anxiety Insomnia Agitation	Sedation Ataxia Confusion Increased agitation	Oxazepam (Serax) Lorazepam (Ativan)	10 0.5	10–30 0.5–2

Beta-
  adrenergic
  antagonist
	Restlessness
	Agitation
	Hostility
		Bradycardia
		Hypotension
		Depression
			Propranolol
			(Inderal)
				20	60–600

*Severe or persistent symptoms may require higher dose; side effect frequency and severity may increase with higher dose.

tic (e.g., haloperidol, 0.25 to 1.0 mg, or trifluoperazine, 1 to 2 mg) once or twice daily. If extrapyramidal side effects develop, consider decreasing the neuroleptic dose or switching to a less potent neuroleptic. If the psychotic symptoms do not improve, consider increasing the neuroleptic dose. Extreme caution is advised when neuroleptic doses exceed 200 chlorpromazine milligram-equivalents per day (e.g., haloperidol, 5 mg per day).

Depression

Estimates of the prevalence of depression in patients with DAT have varied considerably. A recent study found a frequency of 17 per cent in a sample of 144 patients.[14] Recognition of depression may be difficult in patients with DAT owing to the disability in activities of daily living, coexistent medical problems, and considerable concern for the failing cognition and changing social roles that appear early in the dementing illness.

Some studies have demonstrated significant improvement in mood, neurovegetative symptoms, and activities of daily living in depressed patients with heterocyclic antidepressant treatment. There is no clear evidence of increased efficacy with any specific agent. Treatment can be initiated with a relatively low dose of drug with minimal anticholinergic toxicity, such as doxepin (Adapin, Sinequan), 25 mg; desipramine (Norpramin, Pertofrane), 25 mg; or nortriptyline (Pamelor), 10 mg daily. Dosage should be increased slowly to a moderate level (e.g., 100 to 150 mg of desipramine or doxepin daily, or 50 to 75 mg of nortriptyline daily), with careful monitoring for side effects (hypotension, anticholinergic effects, cardiac conduction disturbance and arrhythmia, and increasing confusion). Alternative antidepressant agents include fluoxetine (Prozac), monoamine oxidase inhibitors, or electroconvulsive treatment (ECT), although there are fewer clinical data supporting their efficacy.

Anxiety

Anxiety can occur in patients in any stage of DAT.[12] Benzodiazepines may be effective for treatment of anxiety in patients with mild dementia. Side effects of treatment include sedation, ataxia, confusion, and exacerbation of memory disturbance. Untoward effects are more prominent in patients with moderate or severe dementia,[15] and the use of benzodiazepines in these patients is not usually recommended. Short-acting agents like oxazepam (Serax) or lorazepam (Ativan) are recommended to minimize the potential for drug accumulation.

Agitation

Agitation is a nonspecific term, generally used to describe inappropriate verbal or motor behaviors. It is common in patients with DAT[12] and a frequent source of distress for caregivers. It is important to identify the determinants of agitation, including medical abnormalities (pain, hypoxia, urinary retention, metabolic changes, medication toxicity), psychiatric disturbances such as psychosis or depression, or difficulty adjusting to environmental changes.[16] The initial treatment approach to agitation includes minimizing environmental stresses, identifying factors that precipitate agitation, providing reassurance, minimizing frustration, instituting behavior modification strategies when possible, and appropriate treatment of underlying medical or psychiatric conditions.

The use of neuroleptic medications to help control agitation in demented patients is controversial. In many cases, neuroleptic agents have been prescribed too frequently and without clear indications. Most investigators, however, have found that neuroleptic agents can be helpful in managing agitation when they are prescribed appropriately and the response is monitored closely. Salzman concluded from a review of 68 studies involving over 5000 patients[17] that (1) Neuroleptic agents are superior to placebo and are therapeutically useful in the control of agitation, restlessness, and hostility in elderly patients. (2) There is no clear therapeutic difference among neuroleptic agents. (3) The therapeutic efficacy of neuroleptic agents is modest. (4) Some agitated patients do not improve with neuroleptic treatment, and frank behavioral deterioration may occur.

The choice of the neuroleptic drug and dosage to control agitation is similar to that described earlier in treating psychosis. Long-term use of neuroleptic agents should be avoided. After stabilization of agitation or psychosis for several months, the clinician should attempt to discontinue the neuroleptic agent or determine the lowest dose that controls the symptoms.

Agents other than neuroleptic drugs have been successfully used to control agitation in demented elderly patients.[18] Oxazepam, a short-acting benzodiazepine, has been shown to reduce psychomotor agitation and aggressiveness in some patients, although it may aggravate aggression in others. Propranolol and trazodone also have been reported effective. Propranolol treatment should be initiated at a low dose and the dose increased slowly, with attention to development of side effects (bradycardia, hypotension, depression). A clinical response may require 4 to 6 weeks of treatment. The effective dose for a particular patient can vary between 60 and 600 mg/day.

Wandering

Wandering is common in patients with DAT. Wandering may result from a number of factors, including attempts by the patient to minimize anxiety or to increase visuospatial cues. Getting lost is also common, caused by wandering, impaired integration of visuospatial cues, inability to recognize familiar places, and memory loss. Wandering should not be viewed as a behavior that must necessarily be stopped, but strategies should be devised to minimize the extent of wandering and to ensure safety. Interventions include identifying provocations that stimulate wandering, increasing observation of mobile demented patients, increasing ambient lighting, physically limiting access to exits, redirecting the wandering patient in a supportive way, providing positive feedback for nonwandering behavior, providing more structured activities, or having the patients wear an identification bracelet bearing the phone number of a contact person. Physical restraints should be avoided, as they can increase the risk of injury. Practical, ethical, and legal issues should be considered in the determination of institutional policy regarding the use of restraints, and institutional restraint policies should be discussed with patients' family members.

Insomnia

Nighttime insomnia and alteration of the diurnal sleep-wake cycle are common in patients with DAT. These symptoms may also reflect the presence of depression or delirium. It may not be necessary to treat insomnia in DAT; maximizing the patient's safety and avoiding the disturbance of others' sleep is more useful. Medications such as chloral hydrate, or a short-acting benzodiazepine (e.g., lorazepam, oxazepam) may help induce sleep but are not recommended for long-term use. These medications may cause oversedation, exacerbate confusion, and produce paradoxic excitation. If the patient is receiving neuroleptic agents, shifting the dose to bedtime may help normalize sleep patterns.

■ LONG-TERM CARE OF THE PATIENT WITH DAT

Medical Care

Patients with DAT have a lower survival rate than do nondemented elderly persons.[19] The increased mortality is largely due to coexistent medical illnesses. The clinician should be involved in prevention, early detection, and prompt treatment of medical illnesses in demented patients. Demented patients are particularly vulnerable to malnutrition, dehydration, aspiration pneumonia, urinary tract infection, decubitus ulcers, psychotropic medication side effects, and falls. Preventive measures are extremely important: providing adequate nutrition, hydration, and skin care; avoiding catheterization; avoiding unnecessary medications; using gastrostomy feeding tubes when there are chronic swallowing difficulties; and providing regular physical and laboratory examinations.

Delirium is common in medically ill demented patients, and the mortality rate of delirium is high. Recognition of delirium in DAT is complicated by the presence of chronic cognitive dysfunction in demented patients, but fluctuating alterations in attention or level of alertness, hallucinations, increased agitation, or exaggerated sleep-wake cycle disturbances may reflect a superimposed encephalopathy. Common etiologies are infections, metabolic disturbances, or psychotropic medication toxicity.

Community Resources and Residential Choice

Medical care should be directed by a physician who is involved with both the patient and the family. The physician can provide liaison with nurses and social workers and can coordinate subspecialty consultation when appropriate. Early in the course, specific diagnosis of the dementing illness can be complex, and referral to a specialized center may be appropriate.

The choice of living situation is generally determined by the needs of the patient and of the family. Early in the course of the illness, the patient may need to make adjustments in work activities, financial arrangements, and transportation. As the dementia progresses, assistance with daily domestic activities becomes more important. Interventions in the home may be useful: limit access to exits, provide outdoor fencing, remove low-lying obstructions, render gas ranges and automobiles inoperable, and place toilet facilities in direct view of the patient. Adult day care programs, in which the patient attends structured activities for several hours per day, may provide additional assistance for patients and valuable relief for caregivers. Respite care, in which the patient is admitted to a hospital or nursing home for a limited time period, may also provide an important rest for caregivers.

If behavioral disturbances become unmanageable, or if care needs exceed the level that can be provided at home by caregivers, nursing home placement may be indicated. The decision of *when* placement is appropriate varies considerably among different patients and their families. The most important aspect is balancing the patient's physical and emotional needs with those of the family and other caregivers. A wide variety of facilities exist. Assistance with the choice of facility can be provided by the health care team or other families who have made previous residential decisions.

A number of organizations can help provide essential information and assist with decision-making. These include the Alzheimer's Association, the National Institute on Aging, and many local community social service programs and support groups.

■ Issues and Risks

■ FAMILY CARE

Family members of patients with DAT experience considerable stress: the physical needs of patients are overwhelming; the lack of certainty regarding diagnosis and lack of definitive treatment can be perplexing; the behaviors exhibited by patients can be embarrassing to caregivers and physically dangerous to patients. In addition, a number of psychologic factors may contribute to the caregiver's burden. Patients with DAT can undergo significant changes in personality and can be perceived as no longer "acting like themselves." There is a considerable shift in family roles: in the past, the patient may have been perceived as independent and a source of strength within the family but now may be dependent and childlike. The shift in family roles may bring to the surface prior intrafamily conflicts. There may be feelings of guilt, anger, and abandonment associated with caring for a demented relative. As the illness progresses, there is usually a feeling of loss and grieving among family members. Finally, at the time of death family members often feel a distressing mixture of guilt due to their inability to "save" the patient and relief that their caretaking job is over.

Family members may respond to the stress with denial, anger, anxiety, or depression. Physicians should be aware of the high likelihood of distress among family members. Useful interventions may include

- talking with families about their sources of stress,
- allowing families to ventilate feelings of sadness, anger, and frustration,
- supporting coping strategies by providing sources of information or outside help (*The 36-Hour Day* is a useful, informative book[20]),
- referral to community support groups, or
- referral for additional evaluation or treatment.

■ LEGAL ISSUES

DAT involves a progressive decline in cognitive ability, and the physician and family members should be aware of the potential need for surrogate decision-making. Legal counsel should be sought and a decision-maker appointed in anticipation of future needs.

Potential medical and financial decisions should be discussed with the patient early in the illness so that his or her needs and wishes are understood by decision-makers later on. This can relieve the family of some of the emotional conflict generated by these decisions. Common issues that arise include the desirability of life-sustaining technology, preferences toward research and autopsy, and disposition of financial assets. The financial burden of caring for patients with DAT can be enormous. Family members should consider obtaining financial advice, including criteria for eligibility for governmental benefits, to help minimize erosion of the family's financial resources.

■ ETHICAL ISSUES

Ethical questions frequently arise during the course of treating patients with DAT, particularly during the later stages of illness. Common ethical questions include (1) When should surrogate decisions be made for the demented patient? (2) Who should make particular surrogate decisions? and (3) How extensive should medical interventions be during the final stage of illness? As with all such dilemmas, there is no "right answer" for all patients at all times. The family should be involved in these decisions. The physician should not adopt a sense of therapeutic nihilism but should recognize that there is no ethical obligation to treat if the treatment will not benefit the patient. Discussing the treatment options and goals with the patient's family will usually elicit a consensus approach. Preserving the dignity of the patient and maintaining as much of the quality of the patient's life as possible should receive the highest priorities.

REFERENCES

1. Rocca WA, Amaducci LA, Schoenberg BS. Epidemiology of clinically diagnosed Alzheimer's disease. Ann Neurol 1986; 19:415–424.
2. Jorm AF, Korten AE, Henderson AS. The prevalence of dementia: a quantitative integration of the literature. Acta Psychiatr Scand 1987; 76:465–479.
3. Cummings JL, Benson DF. Dementia: definition, prevalence, classification, and approach to diagnosis. *In* Cummings JL, Benson DF (eds.). Dementia: A Clinical Approach. Boston: Butterworth, 1983:1–14.
4. McKhann G, Drachman D, Folstein M, Katzman R, Price D, Stadlan E. Clinical diagnosis of Alzheimer's disease: Report of the NINCDS-ADRDA Work Group under the auspices of the Department of Health and Human Services Task Force on Alzheimer's Disease. Neurology 1984; 34:939–944.
5. Katzman R. Alzheimer's disease. N Engl J Med 1986; 314:964–973.
6. Cummings JL, Benson DF. Cortical dementias: Alzheimer and Pick diseases. *In* Cummings JL, Benson

DF (eds). Dementia: A Clinical Approach. Boston: Butterworth, 1983:35–72.

7. Yesavage JA, Tinklenberg JR, Hollister LE, Berger PA. Vasodilators in senile dementias. A review of the literature. Arch Gen Psychiatr 1979; 36:220–223.

8. Fanchamps A. Dihydroergotoxine in senile cerebral insufficiency. *In* Agnoli A, Crepaldi G, Spano PF, Trabucchi M (eds). Aging Brain and Ergot Alkaloids. New York: Raven Press, 1983:311–322.

9. Thienhaus OJ, Wheeler BG, Simon S, Zemlan FP, Hartford JT. A controlled double-blind study of high-dose dihydroergotoxine mesylate (Hydergine) in mild dementia. J Am Geriatr Soc 1987; 35:219–223.

10. Hollister LE, Yesavage J. Ergoloid mesylates for senile dementias: unanswered questions. Ann Intern Med 1984; 100:894–898.

11. Wragg RE, Jeste DV. Neuroleptics and alternative treatments. Management of behavioral symptoms and psychosis in Alzheimer's disease and related conditions. Psychiatr Clin North Am 1988; 11:195–213.

12. Reisberg B, Borenstein J, Salob SP, Ferris SH, Franssen E, Georgotas A. Behavioral symptoms in Alzheimer's disease: phenomenology and treatment. J Clin Psychiatr 1987; 48(Suppl 5):9–15.

13. Merriam AE, Aronson MK, Gaston P, Wey S-L, Katz I. The psychiatric symptoms of Alzheimer's disease. J Am Geriatr Soc 1988; 36:7–12.

14. Rovner BW, Broadhead J, Spencer M, Carson K, Folstein MF. Depression and Alzheimer's disease. Am J Psychiatr 1989; 146:350–356.

15. Salzman C. Treatment of agitation, anxiety, and depression in dementia. Psychopharm Bull 1988; 24:39–42.

16. Leibovici A, Tariot P. Agitation associated with dementia: a systematic approach to treatment. Psychopharm Bull 1988; 24:49–53.

17. Salzman C. Treatment of agitation in the elderly. *In* Meltzer HY (ed). Psychopharmacology: The Third Generation of Progress. New York: Raven Press, 1987:1167–1176.

18. Salzman C. Treatment of the elderly agitated patient. J Clin Psychiatr 1987; 48(Suppl 5):19–22.

19. Chandra V, Philipose V, Bell PA, Lazaroff A, Schoenberg BS. Case-control study of late onset "probable Alzheimer's disease." Neurology 1987; 37:1295–1300.

20. Mace NL, Rabins PV. The 36-hour day: a family guide to caring for persons with Alzheimer's disease. Baltimore: Johns Hopkins Press, 1981.

Anaphylaxis and anaphylactoid reactions

Michael W. Anderson ■ *Richard D. deShazo*

■ Background

■ EPIDEMIOLOGY AND MECHANISMS OF ANAPHYLAXIS

Anaphylaxis and anaphylactoid reactions represent a potentially life-threatening symptom complex resulting from the sudden release of mast cell– and basophil-derived mediators into the circulatory system. Such reactions are not uncommon. One in every 2700 hospitalized patients experiences drug-induced anaphylaxis, and between 400 and 800 patients die each year from allergic reactions to beta-lactam antibiotics alone.[1]

The chemical mediators that cause anaphylaxis are released from preformed mast cell and basophil granules (histamine, tryptase, glycosidases, and granulocyte chemotactic factors) or are generated from membrane lipids by the activated cell (prostaglandin D_2, leukotrienes, and platelet-activating factor).[2] These mediators may be released by immunologic means (anaphylactic) or by nonimmunologic mechanisms (anaphylactoid reactions). Immunologic mediator release results from the interaction of specific IgE antibody to the responsible agent and subsequent IgE-triggered mast cell degranulation. Nonimmunologic mediator release results from direct activation of the mast cell or basophil membrane by the agent, independent of IgE. The distinction between anaphylaxis and anaphylactoid reactions has little clinical meaning, however, as the symptom complex and treatment are the same.

■ AGENTS THAT CAUSE ANAPHYLAXIS

At least 11 classes of agents have been reported to cause anaphylaxis (Table 1). Although drugs, especially antibiotics, continue to be the most common culprits, the list of reported agents continues to grow. Recent additions include anaphylaxis associated with murine monoclonal antibodies used for diagnostic purposes or in cancer therapy, reactions to chymopapain used for chemonucleolysis, anaphylaxis to the venom of the imported fire ant (a growing problem in the southern United States), reactions to streptokinase used in the therapy of ischemic heart disease, and reactions occurring during dialysis to ethylene oxide gas used in the sterilization of dialysis tubing.

A similarly diverse group of agents has been associated with anaphylactoid reactions (Table 2). Included in the table are several agents with which IgE antibody has been implicated in a few reports, but these appear to be nonimmunologic in the majority of cases. Anaphylactoid reactions to iodinated contrast media have been studied extensively.[3] These agents not only cause direct release of mediators from mast cells and basophils but also activate the complement and coagulation systems.[4,5] Nonsteroidal anti-inflammatory agents and bisulfite preservatives may cause acute anaphylactoid reactions in individuals with no previous history of asthma or, more commonly, in a subpopulation of patients with chronic asthma. Physical stimuli, including cold and exercise, also can cause anaphylactoid reactions in some individuals.

■ NEWLY RECOGNIZED SYNDROMES OF ANAPHYLAXIS TO CONSIDER

A number of newly recognized syndromes of anaphylaxis have been reported (Table 3). *Exercise-induced anaphylaxis* occurs with prolonged strenuous exercise, frequently in conditioned runners, and is usually preceded by a short prodrome of generalized

TABLE 1. Classes and Examples of Agents That Cause Anaphylaxis

Hormones: ACTH, insulin, hydrocortisone
Animal or human proteins: horse serum (snake antivenin), seminal fluid, factor VIII, protamine sulfate, monoclonal antibodies
Enzymes: chymotrypsin, chymopapain, streptokinase
Venoms: fire ants, wasps, hornets, etc.
Animal danders: cat, horse, etc.
Allergen extracts: pollen, mold, dust, food extracts
Foods: eggs, milk, shellfish, nuts, chocolate, etc.
Drugs: penicillin, cephalosporin, insulin, etc.
Ethylene oxide gas on dialysis tubing
Polysaccharides: dextran, iron dextran
Hydatid cyst rupture

pruritus.[6] In some cases, exercise-induced anaphylaxis occurs only after the ingestion of certain foods, such as lettuce or celery, or drugs such as aspirin.[7] *Progesterone-associated anaphylaxis* has been described in women previously thought to have idiopathic anaphylaxis.[8] Induction or change in the pattern of anaphylactic episodes associated with pregnancy, lactation, or other hormonal flux has been associated with progesterone hypersensitivity. Positive intradermal challenges with medroxyprogesterone and *resolution* of symptoms with the administration of a luteinizing hormone–releasing hormone (LHRH) analog to suppress gonadotropin release has been reported to confirm this diagnosis.[9] A syndrome of repeated episodes of anaphylaxis for which no etiology can be determined despite extensive evaluation has been termed *idiopathic anaphylaxis*.[10] Individuals on *beta-blockers*

TABLE 2. Representative Agents That Cause Anaphylactoid Reactions

Nonsteroidal anti-inflammatory agents: aspirin, indomethacin, ibuprofen, etc.
Diagnostic agents: iodinated contrast media*
Opiates
Muscle relaxants: D-curare, succinylcholine
Preservatives: bisulfites
Cold: cold urticaria
Exercise
Intravenous gamma globulin

*The incidence of repeat reactions decreased to less than 5 per cent by pretreatment with prednisone, 50 mg PO at 6-hour intervals for three doses, with the last dose 1 hour before the procedure, plus diphenhydramine (50 mg PO or IM) and ephedrine (25 mg PO) 1 hour before administration.

TABLE 3. Newly Recognized Syndromes of Anaphylaxis

Exercise-induced anaphylaxis
Food-associated, exercise-induced anaphylaxis
Recurrent idiopathic anaphylaxis
Protracted anaphylaxis associated with beta-adrenergic blockade
Biphasic anaphylaxis

are more likely to experience anaphylaxis and to have reactions that are more severe and resistant to treatment.[11] Patients with underlying medical conditions, such as asthma and coronary artery disease, are also at a higher risk for dying from anaphylaxis.[2] Moreover, myocardial dysfunction and infarction during anaphylaxis probably occur more commonly than previously recognized.[2]

Life-threatening manifestations of anaphylaxis recur in up to 20 per cent of patients treated for an initial episode of anaphylaxis. These second-wave reactions can appear up to 8 hours after apparent remission of the syndrome and have been labeled *biphasic anaphylactic* reactions.[2] They are distinguishable from *persistent anaphylaxis*, a form of anaphylaxis that may last from 5 to 32 hours and occurs in up to 28 per cent of patients. Isolated acute anaphylaxis appears to be the predominant pattern in only about half of patients with severe anaphylaxis.

■ CLINICAL MANIFESTATIONS

In addition to the three temporal patterns of anaphylaxis (acute, biphasic, and persistent) discussed earlier, clinical manifestations of anaphylaxis may involve multiple organ systems or be confined to a single organ system, such as the skin. Anaphylactic reactions are commonly preceded by a short prodrome of nasal, eye, and genital itching or burning, followed by generalized erythema and itching, and then by urticaria and angioedema. In cases of massive mediator release, laryngospasm, bronchospasm, hypotension, diarrhea, and syncope may ensue. These reactions usually occur within 20 to 30 minutes after exposure to the responsible agent but may be delayed for hours with some agents, especially foods.

■ DIFFERENTIAL DIAGNOSIS

Vasovagal reactions that occur under stress, for instance during dental surgery, must be distinguished from anaphylactic reactions. In vasovagal reactions (as compared with anaphylaxis), the pulse rate is slow rather than rapid, the blood pressure is normal or elevated rather than decreased, and the skin is cool (rather than warm) from vasodilation. Patients with systemic mastocytosis have recurrent episodes of flushing, tachycardia, pruritus, headache, abdominal pain, diarrhea, or syncope. Pseudoanaphylactic reactions have been described after intramuscular injection of procaine penicillin and are thought to be caused by the release of free procaine. Symptoms include visual hallucinations, unusual tastes, fright, combativeness, twitching, and seizures. Patients with hereditary angioneurotic edema have episodes of laryngeal edema and painless nonpruritic swelling of the extremities, frequently associated with abdominal pain. Factitious anaphylaxis is defined as repeated, self-induced episodes of anaphylaxis. The diagnosis of anaphylaxis can be confirmed by elevated serum levels of mast cell tryptase or elevated serum or urine levels of histamine or prostaglandin D-2 (PGD_2).[12]

■ Management

A step-by-step approach to the management of anaphylaxis is outlined in Figure 1. If exposure to the causative agent is ongoing, such exposure obviously should be discontinued. This includes stopping infusions of culprit agents or putting a tourniquet proximal to the site of a therapeutic injection. The treatment of anaphylaxis depends on the severity of the reaction. Basic life support is the initial strategy in the management of life-threatening anaphylaxis. The use of aqueous epinephrine is central in both mild and severe anaphylaxis, as epinephrine prevents further mediator release from mast cells and basophils and restores vasomotor tone.[13] Overtreatment can be just as hazardous as the reaction itself. Therefore, treatment modalities must be carefully considered and must be continuously monitored, so that complications of therapy can be detected early on.

The deaths that occur during witnessed anaphylaxis usually result from delay in administration of epinephrine and severe respiratory involvement. In life-threatening anaphylaxis, early intubation is required to facilitate the management of shock, as well as to avoid the difficulty of intubation once laryngeal edema has become severe. If there is difficulty in obtaining IV access, epinephrine and atropine can be given via the endotracheal tube. Once IV access is obtained, H_1 and H_2 blockers, as well as steroids, can be infused along with volume expanders. Subsequent measures depend on the response to the initial epinephrine.

■ HOW TO USE EPINEPHRINE

Epinephrine remains the drug of choice in treatment of systemic anaphylactic shock. The route and dosage remain a variable, depending on the clinical situation and the patient history.[14] Epinephrine has potent alpha, beta-1, and beta-2 activity. The alpha-agonist action of epinephrine increases blood pressure and reverses peripheral vasodilation and systemic hypotension. In addition, the peripheral vasoconstriction decreases angioedema and urticaria.[15] The beta-agonist properties of epinephrine cause bronchodilation, increase the force and volume of cardiac contraction, and prevent further mediator release from mast cells and basophils. Actions of epinephrine that are beneficial are also potentially dangerous. Excessive alpha-agonist activity can precipitate a hypertensive crisis or an intracranial bleed. This can be compounded by beta-stimulation causing increased cardiac oxygen consumption, possibly leading to myocardial ischemia with arrhythmias and infarction.[14]

For mild anaphylaxis, without cardiovascular compromise, the recommended dose of epinephrine in adults is 300 to 500 μg, which is 0.3 to 0.5 ml of a 1:1000 dilution. This is administered subcutaneously and repeated every 15 to 20 minutes. In **children,** the dose suggested is 0.01 ml/kg of a 1:1000 dilution, subcutaneously, every 15 to 30 minutes.[14]

For the patient with persistent or prolonged hypotension or frank cardiovascular

Inject Aqueous Epinephrine 1:1000 (0.01 ml per kg up to 0.3 ml) intramuscularly into the upper arm and massage site. This may be repeated every 5 to 10 minutes while carefully monitoring blood pressure, pulse, respiration, and cardiac rhythm.

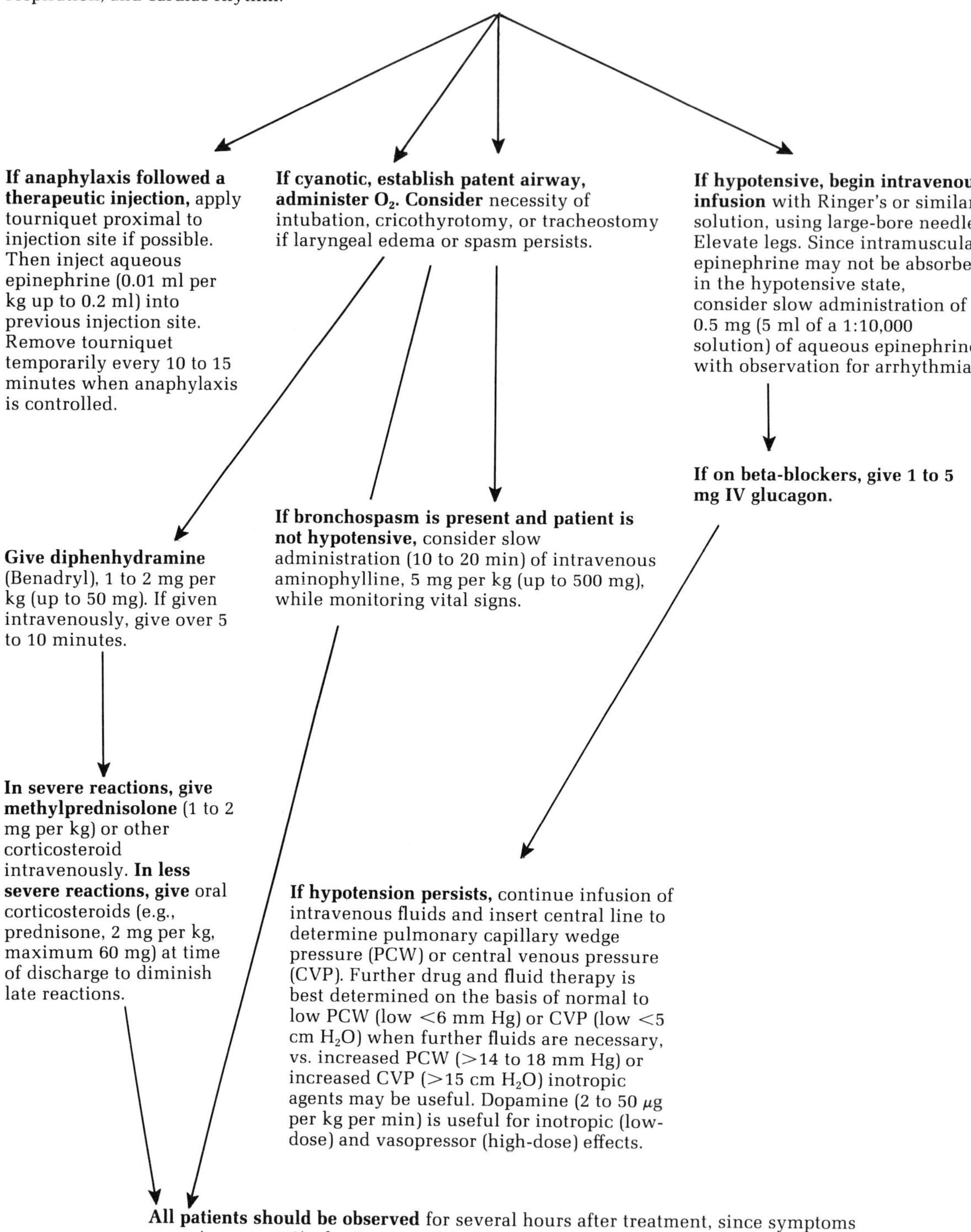

All patients should be observed for several hours after treatment, since symptoms recur in up to 20% of patients within 8 hours of the resolution of the first episode.

Figure 1. Treatment of anaphylaxis.

collapse, diluted IV epinephrine is indicated. Because there are neither definitive studies nor consensus regarding the use of IV epinephrine, and because adverse reactions have been reported with dilutions of 1:10,000, it seems prudent to begin with small doses and observe the clinical effects before increasing the dose. Intravenous bolus therapy should not be used, because of the risk of inducing dangerous cardiac arrhythmias. An initial dose of 0.1 mg (0.1 ml) of a 1:1000 dilution of aqueous epinephrine, mixed with 10 ml of normal saline and infused over 5 to 10 minutes, is a good starting point in adults.[16,17] If response to this is inadequate, a continuous infusion should be prepared. The Advanced Cardiac Life Support protocol for adults recommends that 1.0 mg (1.0 ml) of a 1:1000 dilution of epinephrine be added to 250 ml of D5W to give a concentration of 4.0 μg/ml. This is infused at a rate of 1.0 μg/min (15 drops/min using a microdrop apparatus), increasing to a maximum of 4.0 μg/min.[18] The slower the rate of infusion, the greater the beta-receptor stimulation, compared with the alpha-receptor stimulation.[19] This is desired because of the extreme danger of excessive alpha stimulation. In **children,** a rate of 0.1 μg/kg/min is recommended, increasing by 0.1 mg/kg/min to sustain a systolic blood pressure of 80 mm Hg. This infusion is prepared by adding 0.5 mg (0.5 ml) of a 1:1000 solution of epinephrine to 100 ml of normal saline, producing a solution with a concentration of 5.0 μg/ml.[20]

At all times during epinephrine infusion, the patient's cardiovascular status (i.e., blood pressure, rate, and rhythm) should be continuously monitored.

■ HOW TO USE ANCILLARY MEDICATIONS

In our opinion, whether the reaction is life threatening or mild, the standard treatment of all episodes of anaphylaxis should include antihistamines and corticosteroids in addition to epinephrine. Even at their maximum dosage, antihistamines (H_1 blockers) are unable to induce remission of anaphylaxis when massive amounts of histamine already occupy their receptors. It appears, however, that angioedema, urticaria, and pruritus can be reduced with H_1 blockers and that relapse may be prevented with these agents.

For these reasons, it is appropriate to give 50 mg of diphenhydramine (1 mg/kg IV) following cardiovascular and respiratory stabilization. The role of H_2 blockers such as cimetidine and ranitidine is more controversial. There are case reports of persistent hypotension responding to intravenous use of these agents.[21] However, efficacy in anaphylaxis has been shown only when these agents are given before the release of histamine. Since untoward reactions to these agents are uncommon, their use after initial stabilization is recommended. Because there are both in vitro data that cimetidine may inhibit the metabolism of beta antagonists and in vivo data that cimetidine inhibits theophylline metabolism, we use ranitidine, 50 mg, infused over 10 to 15 minutes.

Corticosteroids may not have any immediate effect on anaphylaxis, but their use may attenuate the course of the immediate reaction and prevent late reactions. Because of this, corticosteroids should be given intravenously early in the attack, at a dose equivalent to 1.0 mg/kg of methylprednisolone every 6 hours for a sustained attack. Oxygen should be routinely administered to patients whose symptoms require multiple doses of epinephrine, to those with pre-existing hypoxemia or cardiac dysfunction, or when the course of anaphylaxis is protracted. Therapy is best directed by measurement of arterial blood gases.

If there is a persistent bronchospastic component, inhaled B_2 agonists or IV aminophylline may also be cautiously administered. Because the mechanism by which aminophylline produces bronchodilation is different from that of sympathomimetics, its effect may be additive to beta-agonistic bronchodilation effects. In this light, aminophylline may be lifesaving in those patients with bronchoconstriction on beta-blocker therapy. A loading dose of 5.0 mg/kg, with 0.9 mg/kg/hour as a maintenance dose, with serum levels monitored, is recommended. The use of this drug in the face of hypoxemia or cardiac dysfunction, which frequently accompanies severe anaphylaxis, may induce life-threatening cardiac arrhythmias. Therefore, the initial infusion should be given slowly (over 20 to 30 minutes, preferably with cardiac monitoring). If nausea, vomiting, or arrhythmias occur, the infusion should be stopped and a theophylline level obtained.

MANAGEMENT OF COMPLICATED ANAPHYLAXIS

Several unique circumstances should be appreciated when treating anaphylaxis. These include coexisting diseases, such as asthma and coronary artery disease, and concurrent drug therapy with beta-blockers.

Patients with asthma are twice as likely to die if anaphylaxis occurs.[2] This is due not only to their hyper-responsive airways but also to the intrinsic beta-unresponsiveness that these patients exhibit. These patients are less likely to respond to the usual doses of epinephrine and may require larger doses in addition to other therapy, such as supplemental oxygen, inhaled beta-agonists, H_1 and H_2 blockers, and aminophylline.

Patients with coronary artery disease are obviously at increased risk when epinephrine is used. Their already compromised circulation may be further reduced by the alpha-agonist effects of epinephrine.

The *patient on beta-blockers* may not respond to the normal doses of epinephrine, and higher doses may cause predominant alpha-agonist effects, which may be especially undesirable in this group. For this reason, attempts to overcome beta-blockade with massive doses of epinephrine are not recommended. In these situations, we recommend volume expansion with isotonic fluids and the use of glucagon, 1.0 to 5.0 mg given by IV infusion. This provides an alternative pathway to raise intracellular cAMP levels via bypass of the blocked beta-receptors.

MANAGEMENT OF PERSISTENT HYPOTENSION

In the patient with persistent hypotension, despite subcutaneous epinephrine, a solution should be prepared as described previously for IV infusion of epinephrine. The patient's airway should be double-checked to insure adequate ventilation. Oxygen supplementation should be added to counteract possible hypoxemic cardiac dysfunction. With the patient in the Trendelenburg position, central venous access (preferably with placement of a Swan-Ganz catheter) should be attempted for the rapid administration of fluids and continuous assessment of intravascular fluid status. If possible, a

history should be obtained to be certain there are no other factors such as concomitant beta-blocker therapy, asthma, or cardiac disease before proceeding with IV epinephrine therapy. Refractory hypotension may be the result of myocardial infarction caused by prolonged hypoxemia or hypotension during the initial anaphylactic reaction.

The proper choice of vasopressor drug therapy for persistent hypotension is unclear. Some investigators suggest that *norepinephrine* is optimal.[2] Four ml of a 1 mg/ml solution in 1000 ml of D5W provides a 4 μg/ml solution to be infused at 2 to 3 ml/min (8 to 12 μg/min) to sustain a systolic blood pressure of 80 to 90 mm Hg. Care must be taken to prevent extravasation of this solution. Other options include continuous *epinephrine* therapy infused at 1 μg/min[18] or *dopamine* used as described in Figure 1. Again, assessment of left atrial pressure is optimal in this setting via Swan-Ganz catheterization. Some patients with intractable hypotension will require aortic balloon placement. This should be considered early so that a cardiologist can be notified to assist and the apparatus obtained.

MANAGEMENT OF PERSISTENT AIRWAY OBSTRUCTION

Persistent Upper Airway Obstruction

Severe laryngospasm may occur so quickly that intubation is impossible. Therefore, the rule is, when in doubt, intubate early. An endotracheal tube with a 4- to 5-mm internal diameter is more likely to be placed than larger sizes and is adequate to ventilate adults. If subcutaneous epinephrine does nothing to facilitate aborted attempts at intubation, aerosolized epinephrine, along with supplemental oxygen, extension of the neck, and insertion of an oropharyngeal airway may be helpful.

Under these circumstances, a cricothyrotomy is the next step. This procedure is accomplished much easier in the emergency setting than is a tracheostomy. Briefly, the patient's neck is hyperextended, and the area of the cricothyroid membrane is located below the thyroid cartilage and above the cricoid cartilage. A small incision is made, the membrane is punctured, and the opening is enlarged with a blunt instrument, such as a scalpel handle. Finally, a small-diameter endotracheal tube (internal diameter of 4 to 5 mm) is inserted. Alternatively, if the situation does not permit endotracheal tube, an 11-gauge needle or polyethylene catheter will suffice for a short term with high O_2 delivery. Complications of this procedure include vocal cord injury, bleeding, and subcutaneous emphysema.

Persistent Lower Airway Obstruction

Once the upper airway has been managed, attention is directed toward the pulmonary reaction. Often epinephrine will reduce the severe bronchospasm associated with anaphylaxis; however, despite a good airway, ventilation and oxygenation may remain a problem. This situation resembles status asthmaticus and should be treated similarly. Measurements of blood gases are essential in guiding therapy and assessing results of interventions. Inhaled beta-2 agonists such as albuterol (0.5 ml or 2.5 mg of a 5 per cent solution), delivered by nebulization with oxygen, are often effective. If further treatment is necessary, intravenous aminophylline should be used. The precautions concerning the use of aminophylline in this situation are reviewed in the earlier section on Ancillary Medications. Aminophylline should be administered to obtain therapeutic levels (10 to 20 μg/ml). This may be achieved with a loading dose of 5.0 mg/kg of aminophylline given over 20 minutes with cardiac monitoring. If the patient is already on theophylline, dosage selection is based on the prior dosage and current levels. Usually, no more than half the calculated loading dose is given. Therapeutic blood levels are maintained by giving a maintenance dose in the range of 0.9 mg/kg/hr, but monitoring of blood levels is essential.

Some patients on mechanical ventilation will continue to deteriorate. Unfortunately, morbidity and mortality in these situations are still high, largely because of the treatment itself. Pulmonary barotrauma and cardiocirculatory failure resulting from the extremely high pressures needed to overcome airway obstruction are frequent complications. In those patients with persistent hypotension despite adequate ventilation, one must consider the effects of the mechanical ventilation. High inspiratory pressure can be responsible for right heart failure by de-

creasing venous return and increasing right ventricular afterload. In this situation, inadequate oxygen delivery may lead to arrhythmia and cardiac arrest.

One study from Switzerland reported a large series of patients treated with a new approach to mechanical ventilation.[22] Once intubated, these patients were maintained with tidal volumes and inspiratory rates such that insufflation pressures were maintained below 50 cm H_2O, regardless of the pCO$_2$. Adequate oxygenation was maintained by increasing the FiO$_2$. In this way, the patients tolerated the mechanical ventilation with relatively few complications, while oxygen levels were maintained in the normal range. This approach decreased the incidence of barotrauma, circulatory failure, and hypoxic encephalopathy often associated with high-pressure mechanical ventilation in status asthmaticus, while maintaining adequate oxygenation to sustain life.

If this approach is undesirable, other alternatives are available. Some investigators suggest the induction of general anesthesia with specific anesthetics possessing bronchodilating properties. Specifically, there are case reports of halothane, ketamine, and ether relieving severe bronchospasm unresponsive to conventional agents.[23-25]

Adult respiratory distress syndrome (ARDS) does occur in the setting of profound anaphylaxis. The treatment of ARDS is discussed in the first chapter in this book.

■ MANAGEMENT OF ANAPHYLAXIS IN PREGNANCY

Although rare, anaphylaxis does occur in pregnancy. Inadequate data are available to make firm recommendations on the treatment of anaphylaxis in the pregnant patient. Because the uteroplacental arteries are extremely responsive to alpha-adrenergic stimulation, the use of agents with alpha-adrenergic effects must be carefully considered.[26] Obstetric anesthesiologists commonly use ephedrine, in doses ranging from 25 to 50 mg IV, to support the blood pressure of pregnant patients. Ephedrine primarily supports blood pressure as a beta-agonist by increasing cardiac output. At high doses, ephedrine will stimulate alpha-receptors, causing contraction of the uteroplacental arteries and possibly jeopardizing fetal circulation. Therefore this drug, as any adrenergic drug, should be used with extreme caution in the pregnant patient.

■ MANAGEMENT FOLLOWING RESUSCITATION

Following the stabilization of the patient with anaphylaxis, several matters should be considered. Most patients will require a minimum of overnight observation, depending on the severity of their reaction. The possibility of recurrence of anaphylaxis after 6 to 12 hours (late-phase anaphylaxis) should be anticipated. Treatment is similar to that for the early phase of anaphylaxis. In addition, it may be important to measure coagulation values, as severe reactions have been associated with intravascular coagulation and consumption of clotting factors.[27] Prior to discharge, the patient should be educated regarding the cause of the reaction and the likelihood of recurrence. Depending on the situation, most patients should be given an automated epinephrine delivery device (for instance, Epi-Pen), with instructions for its use, and a Medic-Alert bracelet in the event of future anaphylaxis.

■ Summary

Prevention of anaphylaxis is preferred to treatment. In those situations of increased risk, such as the necessary re-exposure to an agent like iodinated contrast dye that previously caused anaphylaxis, pretreatment with H_1 and H_2 blockers, as well as systemic steroids, is indicated.[28] Once anaphylaxis has occurred, successful management requires rapid diagnosis and initiation of therapy. Epinephrine remains the mainstay of treatment. Frequent and critical assessment of therapy, and consideration of other variables such as underlying medical conditions, will insure the best possible outcome.

REFERENCES

1. Wasserman SI. Anaphylaxis. *In* Middleton E Jr (ed). Allergy: Principles and Practice. St. Louis: CV Mosby, 1983:689–700.
2. Sullivan TJ. Systemic anaphylaxis. *In* Lichtenstein LM, Fauci AS (eds). Current Therapy in Allergy, Immunology, and Rheumatology—3. Philadelphia: BC Decker, 1988:91–98.
3. Greenberger PA. Contrast media reactions. J Allergy Clin Immunol 1984; 74:600–605.
4. Lieberman P, Siegle PL, Taylor WW. Anaphylactoid reactions to iodinated contrast material. J Allergy Clin Immunol 1978; 62:174–180
5. Lasser EC, Slivka J, Lang JM, et al. Complement and coagulation: causative considerations in contrast catastrophes. Am J Radiol 1979; 132:171–176.
6. Sheffer AL, Austin KF. Exercise induced anaphylaxis. J Allergy Clin Immunol 1984; 73:699–703.
7. Kidd J, Cohen S, Sussman A, Fink S. Food dependent exercise-induced anaphylaxis (abstract). J Allergy Clin Immunol 1982; 69:103.
8. Meggs WJ, Pesconitz OM, Metcalfe D, Loriaux DL, Cutler G Jr, Kaliner M. Progesterone sensitivity as a cause of recurrent anaphylaxis. N Engl J Med 1984; 311(19):1236–1238.
9. Slater JE, Raphael G, Cutler GB Jr, Loraux DL, Meggs WJ, Kaliner M. Recurrent anaphylaxis in menstruating women: treatment with a luteinizing hormone–releasing hormone agonist—a preliminary report. Obstet Gynecol 1987; 70(4):542–546.
10. Lieberman P, Taylor WW Jr. Recurrent idiopathic anaphylaxis. Arch Intern Med 1979; 139:1032–1034.
11. Toogood JH. Beta-blocker therapy and the risk of anaphylaxis. Can Med Assoc J 1987; 136(9):929–933.
12. Schwartz LB, Metcalfe DD, Sullivan TJ. Tryptase levels as an indicator of mast-cell activation in systemic anaphylaxis and mastocytosis. N Engl J Med 1987; 316:1622–1626.
13. Austen KF. Systemic anaphylaxis in the human being. N Engl J Med 1974; 291(13):661–664.
14. Barach EM, Nowak RM, Lee TG, Tomanovich MC. Epinephrine for treatment of anaphylactic shock. JAMA 1984; 251(16):2118–2122.
15. Harvey SC. Sympathomimetic drugs. *In* Osol A (ed). Remington's Pharmaceutical Sciences. Easton, PA: Mack Publishing Company, 1980:815–824.
16. Lockey RF, Fox RW. Allergic emergencies. Hosp Med 1979: 15:64–68.
17. Chatton MJ. Anaphylactic reactions. *In* Krupp MA, Chatton MJ (eds). Current Medical Diagnosis and Treatment. Los Altos, CA: Lange Medical Publications, 1983:15.
18. White RD. Cardiovascular pharmacology: Part 1. *In* McIntyre KM, Lewis AJ (eds). Textbook of Advanced Cardiac Life Support. Dallas: American Heart Association, 1981:VIII-8.
19. Modell W, Schild HO, Wilson A. Applied Pharmacology. Philadelphia: WB Saunders, 1976:272–273.
20. Chameides L, Melker R, Raye JR, et al. Resuscitation of infants and children. *In* McIntyre KM, Lewis AJ (eds). Textbook of Advanced Cardiac Life Support. Dallas: American Heart Association, 1981: XVII-11.
21. Mayumi N, Kimura S, Asano M, Shimokawa T, Au-Yong T, Yagama T. Intravenous cimetidine as an effective treatment for systemic anaphylaxis and acute allergic skin reactions. Ann Allergy 1987; 58:447–450.
22. Darioli R, Perret C. Mechanical controlled hypoventilation in status asthmaticus. Am Rev Respir Dis 1984; 129:385–387.
23. Fisher MM. Ketamine hydrochloride in severe bronchospasm. Anaesthesia 1977; 32:771–772.
24. Schwartz S. Treatment of status asthmaticus with halothane. JAMA 1984; 251:2688–2689.

25. Robertson CE, Steedman D, Sinclair CJ, Brown D, Malcolm-Smith N. Use of ether in life-threatening acute severe asthma. Lancet 1985; 2:187–188.
26. Entman SS, Moise KJ. Anaphylaxis in pregnancy. South Med J 1984; 77(3):402.
27. Watkins, J. Immunologic problems in anaesthesia. Br J Hosp Med 1980; 23:583–590.
28. Lasser EC, Berry CC, Alner LB, et al. Pretreatment with corticosteroids to alleviate reactions to intravenous contrast material. N Engl J Med 1987; 317:845–849.

Angina pectoris, unstable

Alvin S. Blaustein ■ *Louis A. Cannon*

■ Background

The patient with *unstable angina pectoris* (UAP) may present to the physician in several ways: new-onset, accelerating, or post-infarction angina, or acute coronary insufficiency. All these share in common that they arise de novo or from a plateau of stable exertional symptoms, and they include pain at rest that is often poorly responsive to sublingual nitroglycerin. A decrease of variability in exertional threshold progressing over 1 to 3 months also may be classified as UAP, but it is unusual for rest symptoms to be absent. Finally, a change in the accompanying features of stable angina (diaphoresis, dyspnea, palpitations) or radiation to a new site may herald UAP.

The clinical syndrome of unstable angina pectoris identifies an abrupt, critical change in the course of chronic coronary artery disease (CAD). Often, it marks the end of a previously stable or even asymptomatic stage. In either situation, the patient has entered a period in which risk for significant cardiac events (uncontrollable symptoms, nonfatal myocardial infarction, or sudden cardiac death) rises far above that for stable or asymptomatic CAD. In classic studies, the 1-year mortality ranged from 12 to 25 per cent and the morbidity/mortality from 17 to 35 per cent, with the majority of events occurring in the first 4 months. Even more recent trials report a comparable incidence of cardiac events.

The acute change in symptoms reflects the pathophysiology. During the asymptomatic phase or period of stable symptoms, the atherosclerotic plaque grows slowly, producing a smooth, endothelialized protrusion into the vascular lumen. Eventually the reduction in cross-sectional area exceeds the capacity to increase flow by available regulatory mechanisms (vasomotion, collateral vessels, gradient for coronary perfusion). Symptoms are first manifested under conditions of increased myocardial oxygen demand (e.g., exercise). Other factors, such as emotional or mental stress, or eating large meals, also may precipitate symptoms. The usual nature of atherosclerotic lesions is to evolve slowly, but on occasion radical changes in a plaque may occur and reduce the vascular cross-sectional area.

The exact sequence of events is not yet known, but some important components have been established. Plaque fissuring and intraintimal hemorrhage seem to be initiating factors, exposing subendocardial collagen, the fatty content of the plaque, and perhaps even deeper layers of the vessel wall to the thrombogenic components of blood. Following this, there is platelet activation and aggregation, with concomitant production of potent vasoconstrictor substances. Recruitment of the clotting cascade may also occur. The platelet and fibrin clot appears to be the most important factor in narrowing the residual lumen and producing a primary reduction in coronary blood flow and ischemia. The intermittent symptoms may reflect cycles of clot lysis, or fragmentation and reconstitution, or inappropriate vasoconstriction. With further flow reduction, the clot may become more adherent, may enlarge, and may occlude the vessel, resulting in myocardial infarction. A close association between plaque fissuring and sudden cardiac death has been observed.[3] This working hypothesis, proposed and reviewed by Fuster, accounts for the dynamic clinical presentation and predicts our most effective therapies.[4]

■ Management

■ DIAGNOSIS AND EVALUATION

Correct identification and appropriate assignment to a appropriate coronary care unit rely almost exclusively on obtaining the history. As with other coronary syndromes, the patient may not experience pain but rather heaviness, squeezing, fullness, burning, or shortness of breath. The symptoms may not be confined to, or even involve, the thorax but may be present in the arms, neck, jaw, back or epigastrium. The symptoms may be nocturnal or emotionally provoked but almost always are recognized as disturbing.

In some instances the alarming change in symptoms is not a result of the pathophysiology just described. These other precipitants (Table 1) must be sought and corrected. Some heart diseases are associated with angina even though there is no coronary artery disease. Patients with dilated or hypertrophic cardiomyopathies, aortic stenosis, and syndrome X (angina associated with normal heart function and presumed small vessel abnormalities) all may have classic symptoms with normal epicardial vessels. In these disorders, abnormal regulation of blood flow or anatomic inadequacy of intramyocardial vessels may contribute to ischemia. Extramyocardial disorders may mimic UAP. Esophageal spasm or reflux, thoracic outlet or chest wall syndromes, pulmonary embolism, pericarditis, and mitral prolapse are some of the more common.

History and Physical Examination. Since intercurrent noncardiac disorders can trigger UAP, the physician should perform a comprehensive history and physical examination. The physical examination may be helpful in two ways. First, examination during pain may reveal transient pulmonary congestion, gallop sounds or murmurs, or a

TABLE 1. Precipitants of Unstable Angina

Cardiovascular Disorders
  Aortic stenosis
  Cardiomyopathies
  Congestive heart failure
  Tachyarrhythmias
  Uncontrolled hypertension
Extracardiac Disorders
  Anemia
  Fever, sepsis
  Hemodialysis
  Hypoxemia
  Hyperviscosity
  Thrombocytosis
  Thyrotoxicosis
Medication and Drugs
  Amphetamines
  Beta-agonists
  Cocaine
  Ergot derivatives
  Theophylline toxicity
  Thyroid hormone

visible ectopic impulse supporting the diagnosis of ischemia. Second, signs of heart failure, severe aortic stenosis, or acute pericarditis may modify the physician's thinking regarding the proximate cause of the current episode. One patient admitted recently for UAP had an examination during pain with ST depression; a spiking temperature to 39.4°C (103°F) and right upper quadrant tenderness were revealed. Treatment with antibiotics and, later, cholecystectomy led to complete resolution of the UAP syndrome.

Electrocardiogram. The electrocardiogram (ECG) is important in evaluating patients suspected of having UAP. In particular, a reference ECG during a prior quiescent or stable period must be compared with those obtained during symptoms and upon their resolution. The refence ECG should be examined for evidence of CAD (old scar, localized primary ST and T wave abnormalities). It also will establish the stable baseline for the patient. The ECG obtained with the patient pain-free will disclose interval events—new Q waves or loss of R waves compatible with infarction, new conduction disturbances or hypertrophy indicating progressive myocardial disease, or new global or localized ST elevation demonstrating evolving infarction or pericarditis. Forty per cent of patients with a convincing story will have a nondiagnostic or stable ECG. Therefore, the absence of ECG changes should not exclude the diagnosis of UAP. When changes are present, they usually include transient ST depressions or elevations or T wave inversions. Prior T wave inversions may normalize transiently ("pseudonormalization"). A rapid supraventricular or even ventricular tachycardia may be recorded, providing insight into the source of the symptoms. Resolution of ECG changes may coincide with or lag slightly behind spontaneous or pharmaceutic pain relief. However, persistent new ST or T wave changes, even in the absence of Q waves or ST elevation, should be regarded as myocardial infarction.

Serum Enzymes. Evaluation of serum enzymes may provide useful information. Most sensitive and specific are the MB fraction of creatine kinase (CKMB) and the fastest electrophoretic component of lactate dehydrogenase (LDH-1). While it is not certain that small increases (2 to 3 times baseline) in these enzymes represent cell death, it is generally felt that such changes reflect at least reversible myocardial injury. Measured elevations may clarify equivocal symptoms or ECG changes and provide useful prognostic information. It is important to remember that enzyme elevations will not occur, even with profound ischemia, if there is neither cell injury nor death. Enzyme tests should be made when the patient is first seen, then every 6 to 8 hours for the first 24 hours, to maximize diagnostic utility. Enzyme analysis should be performed in patients whose symptoms persist for more than 20 minutes and who are unresponsive to nitroglycerin, or whose ECG changes persist despite pain relief.

Cardiac Catheterization. Cardiac catheterization should be performed on virtually every patient with a convincing or confirmed history for UAP, generally early in the hospital admission. A few patients are unsuitable for or unwilling to undergo revascularization, and these patients may be managed without catheterization. In general, both hemodynamic and angiographic data assist the clinician to select among therapeutic options. Clinically inapparent elevations in diastolic chamber pressures or unsuspectedly severe valvular or muscle disease can lead to alternative or adjunctive therapy. The hemodynamic information also may be helpful in guiding the surgeon or interventional cardiologist to identify patients at unusually high risk.

Coronary arteriography provides the most important information gained from the catheterization. It defines the severity of the CAD and reveals qualitative information useful in deciding which therapy—medical, surgical bypass, or angioplasty—is most appropriate. Ambrose and colleagues have demonstrated that eccentric lesions with irregular borders and those with identifiable thrombus are most commonly associated with UAP and are likely to progress over the next few months; sometimes an intraluminal thrombus is discovered. In contrast these findings are rare in patients with chronic stable angina.[5] Angiography may not be sufficient to select the vessel responsible for the pain syndrome. In rare instances, provocative testing may be indicated (e.g., to induce angina or vasospasm in patients with Prinzmetal's variant angina). More often, thallium or positron imaging may identify the ischemic zone and implicate a specific vessel.

The timing of cardiac catheterization depends on the patient's clinical course. A rapid resolution of symptoms and a stable clinical course permit angiography to be carried out electively. If medications and rest fail to induce a prompt remission in symptoms, or if episodes of pain are associated with pulmonary edema or hypotension, it should be performed urgently. Under these circumstances, an intra-aortic balloon pump that augments coronary flow and reduces systolic load may quiet symptoms and permit angiography to be safely completed.

Dangers inherent to cardiac catheterization may be amplified in certain patients. A careful cardiologist will "design" the appropriate protocol based on the clinical assessment and evaluation of the risks. The administration of radiopaque contrast material may be more hazardous in patients who are hypovolemic or diabetic or who have prior renal disease. Some patients may have iodine or contrast sensitivity and will have to be pretreated to prevent dangerous reactions. Patients with peripheral vascular disease may alter the cardiologist's choice of catheters and anatomic approach, whereas those who are hemodynamically unstable or who have disease of the left main coronary artery may require intra-aortic balloon pump for mechanical support. Despite these risks, cardiac catheterization can be safely performed with a very low incidence of death, threatening arrhythmia, cerebral ischemia, or myocardial infarction. Postcatheterization, the clinician should provide adequate hydration, assure that medications have been continued, and watch for local bleeding, vascular occlusion, and recurrent chest pain.

■ THERAPY

With the patient now admitted to a monitored setting, certain measures should be initiated immediately. A secure intravenous line should be inserted and orders written to keep the patient at bed rest. An anxiolytic such as lorazepam should be administered, and the objectives of therapy should be explained reassuringly to the patient. In line with general stress reduction, the frequency and duration of visits by family and friends should be carefully restricted. Once the patient is stable, a diet of 1200 to 1800 calories in small portions is reasonable. The therapeutic value of oxygen is unknown, but oxygen should certainly be administered to correct even baseline hypoxemia and given to patients with metabolic stress or anemia. There are several approaches to the management of pain and ischemia: anticoagulation and lytic therapy to alter the cascade of endothelial injury, thrombosis, and occlusion: heparin, platelet inhibitors, streptokinase, and tissue plasminogen activator; medical treatment altering myocardial oxygen delivery and demand: nitrates, calcium channel blockers, and beta-blockers; invasive interventional techniques: intra-aortic balloon counterpulsation and angioplasty; and surgery.

Early Management (The First 48 Hours)

The most important change in the early medical treatment of UAP is routine use of aspirin or heparin. Each has been shown to reduce the incidence of death and nonfatal infarction. In the VA Cooperative Study, a single buffered aspirin lowered the cumulative event rate in 1200 men from 10.1 per cent to 5 per cent over the 3-month follow-up.[6] A smaller but equally impressive study conducted by Theroux and associates showed that heparin or aspirin were effective, reducing the event rate from 11.9 per cent to 0.8 per cent and 3.3. per cent, respectively.[7] Whereas each drug had similar effects on the incidence of infarction, heparin decreased mortality more than aspirin did. Moreover, heparin's benefit persisted beyond the period of infusion. Combination therapy increased the risk of bleeding without additional benefit.

In the absence of strong contraindications, heparin should be given first by administering an intravenous bolus of 5000 to 10,000 units and then initiating a maintenance drip of 10 to 15 units/kg/hour. Routinely, 40,000 units are placed in 1 liter of normal saline and maintained at 25 ml/hour (1000 units per hour). When fluids need to be restricted, a double concentrated mixture may be used. To reduce bleeding complications, the partial thromboplastin time should be monitored and maintained approximately twice control. Platelet count and blood pressure also should be closely observed. After a minimum of 5 to 7 days of heparin therapy (or in patients unable to tolerate heparin), 325 mg/day of buffered or enteric-coated aspirin should be prescribed and heparin discontin-

ued. These treatments will not interfere with catheterization, angioplasty, or surgery.

Typical angina reflects myocardial ischemia, and, therefore, some therapy is initially directed toward pain control. Short-acting nitrates administered sublingually are usually effective in relieving pain and reversing ECG changes. In patients with new-onset angina or in those whose systolic blood pressure is 90 to 100 mm Hg, use the smallest dosage (200 μg) to minimize the risk of a hypotensive response, then increase as tolerated. Sublingual nitroglycerin may be repeated every 5 minutes if hemodynamics permit. For recurring pain, it is best to begin an intravenous continuous infusion of nitroglycerin beginning at 10 to 25 μg/min and escalating as necessary. When the dosage is increased in response to symptoms, it is advisable to use a sublingual nitroglycerin to elevate the serum level rapidly at the same time the infusion rate is advanced. Persistent pain may require the use of morphine, an excellent anxiolytic with beneficial effects on pulmonary artery pressure.

In patients with tachycardia and hypertension, early administration of beta-adrenergic blockers is warranted. Beta-blockers pose a special risk only to patients with reduced heart function or bronchospastic lung disease. In such cases, esmolol, an utrashort-acting intravenous drug, can produce an effect rapidly. Infusions from 50 to 200 μg/kg/min are safe even in patients with moderate elevations of pulmonary capillary wedge pressures.[8] The infusion can be used until a short-acting oral preparation—for example, propranolol—has produced desirable effects. Therapy should maintain a heart rate below 70 beats per minute, a systolic blood pressure between 110 and 130 mm Hg, and relief of chest pain. In patients exhibiting inferior wall ST segment changes during periods of ischemia, beta-blocker therapy should also be used cautiously, as these individuals are prone to develop bradycardia and second-degree Mobitz Type I block (Wenckebach). The choice of a specific agent is largely based on selectivity, half-life, and relative contraindications. Table 2 reviews some of these considerations.

The calcium channel blockers are a heterogeneous group of compounds with varied effects on the peripheral circulation, contractility and conduction. These factors should always be considered in choosing

TABLE 2. Pharmacologic Properties of the Beta-Blockers

| Generic (Trade) | Half-Life Elimination | | Dosages |
	Hours	Hepatic/Renal	
Propranolol (Inderal)	3–6	hepatic	10–20 mg QID
Timolol (Blocadren)	3–4	80%/20%	10–20 mg BID
Nadolol (Corgard)	14–24	renal	40–80 mg QD
Metoprolol* (Lopressor)	3–4	hepatic	100–200 mg BID
Acebutolol*† (Sectral)	3–4†	60%/40%	200–600 mg BID
Atenolol* (Tenormin)	6–9	renal	50–100 mg QD
Esmolol* (Brevibloc)	9 min	RBC esterase	50–200 μg/kg/min

*Cardioselective.
†Diacetolol, active metabolite present for 8 to 13 hours.

these agents. In patients with low ejection fractions and a history of congestive heart failure, a calcium channel blocker that is a strong negative inotrope may precipitate heart failure and worsen symptoms; however, patients with underlying tachycardia and hypercontractility, such as those with hypertrophic cardiomyopathy, may benefit from this effect.

Although calcium blockers are used extensively for stable angina in which their effectiveness is unquestioned, surprisingly few studies have examined their use in UAP. The most extensively studied is nifedipine, which effectively controls pain and ECG evidence of ischemia only in patients previously treated with nitrates and beta-blockers. It has not reduced mortality or nonfatal infarction, even in this setting. Verapamil, nicardipine, and diltiazem simply have not been carefully studied in UAP

Early use of calcium blockers is probably most beneficial in patients already taking nitrates and beta-blockers, when there are clear contraindications to beta-blockade (see Table 3), and when rest pain is accompanied by evidence of coronary spasm, such as ST elevation. Use extra caution when combining beta- and calcium blockers (especially verapamil and diltiazem), because of additive effects on cardiac function and conduction. Table 4 reviews the commonly prescribed calcium channel blockers and their effects on heart rate and contractility.

Intermediate Management (48–96 Hours)

When the patient is pain-free and hemodynamically stable, longer-acting medications should be substituted for intravenous, cutaneous, or short-acting antianginals. Nitrate

TABLE 3. Recommended Therapy for Unstable Angina: Relative Indications for Calcium Channel Blockers or Beta Blockade

Calcium Blocker	Beta-Blocker
Sinus bradycardia*	Sinus tachycardia
Supraventricular tachycardia†‡	Supraventricular tachycardia
Hypertrophic cardiomyopathy	Mitral stenosis
Congestive heart failure	Ventricular arrhythmias
Asthma/COPD	Hyperthyroidism
Raynaud's phenomenon§	Anxiety/hyperadrenergic state
IDDM§	Hypertrophic cardiomyopathy‡
Arterial insufficiency§	Sustained hypertension
Prior beta-blocker therapy*†	
ST elevation with pain*†	

*Nifedipine.
†Diltiazem.
‡Verapamil.
§ Cardioselective beta-blocker. Metoprolol, atenolol, and esmolol also may be used.

TABLE 4. Cardiovascular Effects and Dosages of the Calcium Channel Blockers

Generic (Trade)	Dosages	HR	Contractility
Verapamil* (Calan)	80–120 mg q 6–8 hr	decrease	Negative effects, avoid if congestive heart failure
Diltiazem* (Cardizem)	30–90 mg q 6–8 hr	decrease	Minor negative effects, usually unimportant except in those with ejection fraction < 40%
Nifedipine (Procardia)	10–30 mg q 6–8 hr	increase	Offset by sympathetic activation and arterial dilation

*May slow A-V conduction and should be used cautiously with first-degree A-V block or inferior wall ischemia. Contraindicated with second-degree block unless prophylactic pacemaker is present.

tolerance complicates not only the use of intravenous nitroglycerin, which must be escalated over 24 to 48 hours to maintain effectiveness, but also cutaneous and oral preparations. Continuous nitrate levels deplete cyclic guanidine-monophosphate (GMP), and there is inadequate time for cells to regenerate the compound. Patients will respond less to the same preparations after 24 hours, and many completely lose the beneficial hemodynamic and vascular effects.

A nitrate schedule should include a nitrate-free interval of 8 to 12 hours. Commonly used preparations and dosages are outlined in Table 5, with the nitrate "holiday" included. The drug-free period should coincide with a period in which other antianginals are active and when the likelihood of symptoms is minimal.

As the switch is being made to a chronic drug regimen, the patient's activities may be liberalized. The patient may take meals while sitting in a chair and use a bedside commode. These two measures simplify care while providing an opportunity to observe changes in heart rate and blood pressure. In asymptomatic patients, an inhospital cardiac rehabilitation team may begin daily visits and instruction, as in the postinfarction patients.

Revascularization

With the anatomic data available from coronary angiography, the physician has the information to make a rational therapeutic plan, including revascularization. Two options for revascularization are now widely available—percutaneous transluminal coronary angioplasty (PTCA) and coronary artery bypass surgery (CABS). A number of other options are under investigation, including thrombolysis, vascular stenting, and atherectomy.

There has been no systematic randomized trial of acute PTCA in the treatment of UAP. The largest published series is from the Netherlands. Procedures were performed between 1983 and 1985.[9] No patients with a significant left main coronary artery lesion underwent PTCA. Major complications (death, infarction, or urgent coronary artery bypass graft) occurred in 10.5 per cent of patients at the time of the procedure; risk factors were ST elevation with pain, persistent T wave inversion and stenosis of over 65 per cent. Of the remainder, 4 per cent suffered either myocardial infarction (MI) or death, and 26 per cent had stable angina after 1 year. Results were similar in single-vessel disease, and in multivessel disease with dilation of the offending lesion only. Tech-

TABLE 5. Nitrates Used in Management of Angina

Medication	Dosage	Onset	Interval
Intravenous	10–500 μg/min	1–2 min	Continuous infusion
Sublingual	300–600 μg	2–5 min	5 to 20 min
Oral isosorbide	5–40 mg	15–30 min	6 to 8 hr; 8–12 off
Isosorbide (SR)	40 mg	20–60 min	8 to 12 hr; 8–12 off
Ointment, 2%	0.5–2 inches	20–60 min	6 to 8 hr; 8–12 off
Transdermal	5–10 mg	30–60 min	12 hr on; 12 hr off

niques for PTCA are evolving rapidly and newer studies must be scrutinized. If early complications can be avoided, PTCA is a promising treatment.

The results of a Veterans Administration Cooperative randomized trial comparing medicine and surgery have recently been published.[10] This study supersedes those of the National Cooperative Study Group published in the late 1970s, which found that surgery was superior to medical management in preventing recurrent angina but not in reducing the incidence of myocardial infarction or cardiovascular death.[11] The Veterans Administration Cooperative Study included 468 patients under age 70 years, with complete follow-up of at least 24 months. Surgical therapy was compared with use of nitrates and beta- and/or calcium blockers. Surgical treatment was statistically advantageous in patients with multivessel disease and abnormal left ventricular function—that is, an ejection fraction of less than 55 per cent. As the ejection fraction approached 30 per cent (the lower limit acceptable for entry into the study), the difference became quite large: that is, the 2-year mortality was 5 per cent for surgically treated and 15 per cent for medically treated patients. In addition, 34 per cent of the medical patients had symptoms sufficient to require cross-over from medical to surgical therapy, a factor that biased results in favor of medicine.

In summary, surgery is clearly beneficial for the relief of symptoms and reduced mortality (but not necessarily nonfatal MI) for patients in high-risk groups of UAP, including those with multivessel disease and an ejection fraction of less than 45 to 50 per cent. However, it is unknown whether surgery is superior to medical management that includes heparin or aspirin or both. Clearly, randomized trials are essential to answer these complex questions and to clarify the evolving role of PTCA. Given the published data, our strategy is to treat all patients with heparin, nitroglycerin, and/or beta blockers, initially. Those found to have multivessel disease, reduced ejection fraction, or risk factors for acute occlusion postPTCA (including visible intraluminal thrombi) should be revascularized surgically if suitable. The remainder should be treated with aspirin and antianginals and considered for PTCA. As technology and therapy for re-stenosis evolve, PTCA may be used more ex-

tensively. The physician also should consider the expertise of the surgical and angioplasty teams when selecting the option for revascularization.

■ Issues and Risks

■ RISK STRATIFICATION

As indicated in the beginning of this article, the morbidity and mortality of UAP are unacceptably high even when only the most optimistic figures are chosen. It is clear that the control of symptoms acutely does not necessarily predict a favorable outcome. A number of factors have been identified that may assist the physician in identifying patients at highest risk for cardiovascular events. It is convenient to divide these factors into the following categories: clinical course, electrocardiogram, and stress testing.

Two clinical syndromes identify patients at particularly high risk: episodes of rest angina persisting more than 48 hours after CCU admission despite aggressive treatment, and ischemic pain following myocardial infarction. Patients in whom pain persists may have a 1-month morbidity and mortality rate as high as 40 per cent, while in those with postinfarction angina, the 6-month mortality may be even higher.[12,13] Patients with these syndromes have more extensive CAD, and often a history of stable angina precedes their admission.

Several electrocardiographic findings identify patients who are more likely to die or have a nonfatal cardiovascular event. Recurrent episodes of ST elevation during pain are associated with a high risk of early, acute myocardial infarction and should be interpreted as impending infarction. These patients may have small elevations of CK-MB and lactic dehydrogenase (LDH), even in the absence of new Q waves or loss of R waves. In some patients, T wave inversions occur but do not resolve with the pain.[14] Coronary arteriography in these patients often discloses a significant stenosis corresponding to the region identified by the inverted T waves.

ST segment depression on a continuously recorded (Holter) ECG, even in the absence of symptoms (silent ischemia), identifies patients who are likely to have recurrent symptoms or infarctions, most commonly in the first month.[15] In one survey, ischemia totaling more than 60 minutes in a 24-hour period predicted cardiovascular events in 17 of 18 patients, whereas only 4 of 31 with fewer than 60 minutes of ischemia had events.[16] However, it is not clear whether such monitoring is necessary in light of the aggressive approach generally taken and the reduced morbidity/mortality with newer therapies.

The incidence of coronary events in the "low"-risk groups whose symptoms are easily controlled and who have little evidence of injury or silent ischemia is 10 to 20 per cent. It is appropriate to ask who among these patients is most likely to have a complication. In these patients a symptom-limited graded exercise test with or without thallium imaging may be helpful. Unfortunately, few data have been systematically collected, but those that have indicate that an ischemic ECG response, limiting angina, or low maximal cardiac work were all predictive of events.[17] There are insufficient data to evaluate the additional impact of a reversible thallium defect, but extrapolation from post-MI studies implies its potential usefulness.

■ THROMBOLYSIS

The early use of thrombolysis in the treatment of acute myocardial infarction, while still under intense scrutiny, clearly increases the overall rate of infarct vessel patency (which may be important for reasons other than myocyte salvage) and reduces mortality. Despite the general acceptance that thrombus formation is an important element in the pathophysiology of UAP, similar support for thrombolysis is lacking. Several studies in unstable angina have shown successful clot lysis and decreased severity of stenosis; some have shown relief of symptoms after thrombolytic therapy. However, the number of patients requiring revascularization is high. In addition, an unacceptably large number of patients require blood transfusions or discontinuance of therapy because of bleeding from puncture sites. Thrombolytic therapy cannot be recommended on a routine basis for those patients presenting with unstable angina, although it may be useful when a clot has been visualized angiographically. At this time, however, there is no indication for thrombolysis in the routine management of UAP.

■ SUMMARY CASES

(1) JD is a 65 year old white man with chronic exertional angina who has been followed in the office for years. His last catheterization was 5 years ago, and he underwent three-vessel bypass with saphenous grafts to his right coronary artery (RCA) and proximal circumflex artery and an internal mammary graft to his left anterior descending artery. His medications include propranolol 40 mg per day, and isosorbide dinitrate at breakfast, lunch, and dinner to avoid nitrate tolerance. He also takes one enteric-coated aspirin per day.

JD is awakened from sleep with a burning substernal chest pressure associated with burping and hiccoughs. The pain is different from his usual angina in that it lasts somewhat longer, radiates into his epigastric area, and is associated with a feeling of stomach distress. His pain subsides after he takes an antacid mix and three new nitroglycerin sublingual tablets, but it returns in the emergency care unit. Physical examination reveals a blood pressure of 154/92, a heart rate of 50 beats per minute, and a normal heart and lung examination with the exception of an S4. His electrocardiogram reveals 1 to 2 mm of ST segment depression in leads II, III, and AVF with pain.

JD's rest pain syndrome is different from his previous exertional angina, and in light of his electrocardiogram, his gastrointestinal symptoms are probably related to inferior wall myocardial ischemia and unstable angina. He should be admitted to the coronary care unit. Considering his hypertension, he should probably be started on a nitroglycerin drip or aggressive oral nitrate management. In addition, heparin should be started intravenously to decrease the likelihood of further clot propagation. He is already taking aspirin, so you may elect to discontinue it while administering heparin. If a calcium channel blocker is chosen, nifedipine or nicardipine would be the most reasonable choice, since resting bradycardia is already present.

If the patient becomes stable, you may elect to continue medical management over the short term, before proceeding to catheterization. An exercise test with thallium will help determine whether there has been a reduction in exercise tolerance and will assess the region of reversible ischemia. Depending on whether there has been graft closure or stenosis, or progression of atherosclerosis in the native coronary circulation, PTCA or medical management would be most desirable, because the risk of a second CABS exceeds that of the first (especially when an internal mammary graft is in place).

(2) DM is a 58 year old man who presents for the first time with a complaint of increasing chest pressure occurring with exertion. The pressure lasts for 15 to 20 minutes, is substernal without radiation, and is associated with a feeling of light-headedness that subsides with rest. In the examining room, he once again had pain. He also relates a 6-month decline in exercise tolerance. He is on no medications, and his physical examination is remarkable for a resting heart rate of 92 beats per minute, a blood pressure of 160/84, and a harsh midsystolic murmur along the left sternal border and base. His electrocardiogram when pain is not present shows Q waves in the anterior leads, a slight left axis deviation, and left ventricular hypertrophy.

The recent onset and progressive nature of the symptoms, as well as the very abnormal electrocardiogram are cause for aggressive management. On your physical examination, you should characterize the carotid pulses to assess whether aortic valvular or subvalvular disease is likely and perform bedside maneuvers to characterize the murmur. Admission to a monitored unit is indicated. There the patient should be evaluated for impending or ongoing infarction. However, before initiating nitrate therapy, an urgent echocardiogram and cardiology consultation should be obtained. Nitrate therapy may be hazardous in valvular aortic stenosis or hypertrophic obstructive cardiomyopathy. Therefore, if initial management is required before a definitive answer is available, heparin or aspirin and diltiazem or verapamil might be best. These would have beneficial effects on heart rate and the inotropic state and would be effective antianginals even in the absence of epicardial coronary disease. The patient's syndrome may still reflect atherosclerotic CAD, a fact which only cardiac catheterization will clarify.

REFERENCES

1. Gazes PC, Mobley EM, Faris HM, Duncan RC, Humphries GB. Preinfarction (unstable) angina; a prospective study—ten year follow-up. Circulation 1983; 48:331–337.
2. Scanlon PJ, Nemioicas R, Moran JF, Talano JV, Amirparviz F, Pifarre R. Accelerated angina pectoris: clinical and hemodynamic arteriographic and therapeutic experience in 85 patients. Circulation 1973; 47:19–26.
3. Davies MJ, Thomas A. Thrombosis and acute coronary-artery lesions in sudden cardiac ischemic death. N Engl J Med 1984; 310:1137–1140.
4. Fuster V, Badimon L, Cohen M, Ambrose J, Badimon JJ, Chesebro J. Insights into the pathogenesis of acute ischemic syndromes. Circulation 1988; 77:1213–1220.
5. Ambrose JA, Hjamdahl-Monsen CE. Arteriographic anatomy and mechanisms of myocardial ischemia in unstable angina. J Am Coll Cardiol 1987; 7:1397–1402.
6. Lewis HD, Davies JW, Archibald DG, et al. Protective effect of aspirin against acute myocardial infarction and death in men with unstable angina: results of V.A. Cooperative Trial. N Engl J Med 1983; 309:396–403.
7. Theroux P, Ouimet H, McCans J, et al. Aspirin, heparin or both to treat acute unstable angina. N Engl J Med 1988; 319:1105–1111.
8. Kirshenbaum JM, Kloner RF, McGowan N, Antman EH. Use of an ultrashort-acting beta-receptor blocker (Esmolol) in patients with acute myocardial ischemia and relative contraindications to beta-blockade therapy. J Am Coll Cardiol 1988; 12:773–780.
9. De Feyter PJ, Suryapranata H, Serruys P, et al. Coronary angioplasty for unstable angina: immediate and late results in 200 consecutive patients with identification of risk factors for unfavorable early and late outcomes. J Am Coll Cardiol 1988; 12:324–333.
10. Luchi RJ, Scott SM, Deupree RH, and the principal investigators and their associates of Veterans Administration Cooperative Study No. 28. Comparison of medical and surgical treatment for unstable angina pectoris. N Engl J Med 1987; 316:977–984.
11. Russell RD, Moraski RE, Kouchoukos N, et al. Unstable angina pectoris: National Cooperative Study Group to compare surgical and medical therapy. Am J Cardiol 1978; 42:837–848.
12. Olson HG, Lyons KP, Aronow WS, Sanson PJ, Kuperus J, Waters HJ. The high risk angina patient: identification by clinical features, electrocardiography and technetium-99m stannous pyrophosphate scintigraphy. Circulation 1981; 64:674–684.
13. Schuster EH, Bulkley BH. Ischemia at a distance after acute myocardial infarction: a cause of early postinfarction angina. Circulation 1980; 62:509–515.
14. Haines DE, Raabe DS, Gundel WD, Wackers FJ. Anatomic and prognostic significance of new T wave inversions in unstable angina. Am J Cardiol 1983; 52:14–18.
15. Gottlieb SO, Weisfeldt ML, Ouyang P, Mellits ED, Gerstenblith G. Silent ischemia as a marker for unfavorable outcomes in patients with unstable angina. N Engl J Med 1986; 314:1214–1219.
16. Nademanee K, Intarachot V, Josephson MA, Reiders D, Mody FV, Singh BN. Prognostic significance of silent myocardial ischemia in patients with unstable angina. J Am Coll Cardiol 1987; 10:1–9.
17. Swahn E, Arestog M, Wallention L. Prognostic importance of early exercise testing in men with suspected unstable coronary artery disease. Eur Heart J 1987; 8:861–869.

Anorexia nervosa and bulimia

A. James Giannini

■ Background

Anorexia nervosa and its companion disease, bulimia nervosa, have been a part of the social and medical fabric of Western civilization for at least 2000 years. Titus Petronius Arbiter described the socially accepted practice of bingeing and purging in his contemporaries in Neronian Rome. A phenomenon of middle and upper class Romans, the forced emesis was a social ritual following each course of a banquet. Large households invariably contained a "vomitarium" attached to the dining area. In the fifteenth century, Giovanni Bocaccio described anorexia in literate Italian men. Certainly, anorectic men and women populate the paintings of his near-contemporaries, Piero della Francesca and Sandro Botticelli. In both periods, Imperial Rome and Renaissance Italy, feeding disturbances were reported in an educated elite.[1] In both cases, a lithe figure was a sign of success.

In 1668, Thomas Hobbes made the first clinical description of anorexia, and 36 years later Richard Morton described it as a clinical entity.[2] The term *anorexia nervosa* was coined by Sir William Gull at Guy's Hospital in 1874. Bulimia has also threaded through Western history but under much less intense scrutiny.

Though anorexia is popularly connected with the image of a middle class adolescent girl, the stereotype is incorrect. Young men have been reported with the symptom anorexia, as have elderly men and women. First-time anorectic episodes have been reported to occur in adults in their 70s. In addition, a variety of conditions, including lung cancer, Alzheimer's disease, major depression, Addison's disease, Crohn's disease, superior mesenteric artery syndrome, and ischemic heart disease can mimic anorexia and sometimes bulimia.[3]

Studies have placed the prevalence of anorexia at about 2 per cent among English schoolgirls. The incidence has been reported at approximately 5 per cent in areas as disparate as Aberdeen, Scotland; Zurich, Switzerland; Groningen, Holland; and Rochester, Minnesota.[4,5]

■ PRESENTATION

The presentation of anorexia and bulimia may occur in combination or separately. The symptoms of anorexia are listed in Table 1.

Bulimia, while having some characteristics of anorexia, presents the symptoms shown in Table 2.

The patient may be any age or of either sex; however, the typical anorectic patient is young, middle class, upwardly mobile, and female. There is stress either to present a svelte image or to suppress menses. The personal image is distorted. When emaciated, a girl will see herself as obese, even though her observation of the physiognomy of others is unremarkable. Typically, drawings by the patient show accurate representations of family members while she herself is drawn as a grotesquely obese figure. Contradictions abound. She will feel satiated when fasting; conversely, she experiences hunger when eating or overeating.

She may continue to eat to the point of painful abdominal distention. As the extreme dieting continues, the patient becomes increasingly obsessed with her weight. Her behavior may become secretive, hoarding food or surreptitiously disposing of it. Compulsive cleansing rituals such as handwashing, bathing, douching, or enemas, may occur with a high level of frequency.

TABLE 1. Symptoms of Anorexia

amenorrhea	hypotension
bradycardia	lanugo
cold sensitivity	MAO platelet level
compulsive behavior	decreased
constipation	mortality rate of 15 to 20%
distorted body image	overactivity
edema	reversal of nocturnal
emesis	luteinizing hormone
hoarding of food	(LH) curve
hypercarotenemia	reverse satiety
	weight loss of 25%

■ Management

Treatment of anorexia is difficult since no definitive etiology has been discovered. Recently, elevated levels of serum cholecystokinin (CCK) have been associated with bulimic behavior. In spite of a variety of sophisticated biochemical, behavioral, and psychotherapeutic modalities, the mortality rate for anorexia hovers at 15 to 20 per cent. Unlike most illnesses, these feeding disorders provide positive reinforcement. Therein lies the physician's dilemma. The anorexia provides a means to a desirable body image. Also, during times of starvation, a near-transcendental euphoria may ensue. Bulimia allows the patient to keep both the mouth of a glutton and the body of a god(dess). The major difficulty in treatment is that the patient does not really wish to be cured.

In addition to poor motivation, a plethora of poorly understood biochemical processes increases the difficulty of treatment. The major biogenic amines all appear to play a role. Norepinephrine seems to increase appetite. Serotonin, which controls norepi-

TABLE 2. Symptoms of Bulimia

abdominal distention relieved by emesis
abuse of diuretics
abuse of laxatives
bingeing associated with abdominal distention
bingeing terminated by abdominal pain
bingeing terminated by sleep
bingeing terminated by social intervention
bingeing without control
bolting of food
electrolyte imbalances
elevated cholecystokinin (CCK) serum levels
parotid enlargement
postbinge depression
postbinge emesis
weight fluctuation of 10 or more pounds

nephrine release, both increases and decreases feeding behavior, depending upon which serotonergic receptor is activated. Dopamine, a precursor of norepinephrine, may inhibit appetite. Beta-endorphin inhibits release of norepinephrine in the brain. However, in elderly people, low β-endorphin is associated with a "natural" decline in appetite.[6]

Seemingly controlling all these mechanisms is corticotropin-releasing factor (CRF). In itself, it is a powerful anorexogenic agent. Secondarily, it inhibits norepinephrine-induced hunger by hypothalamic action. It also assists in the breakup of the precursor macromolecule β-lipotropin to form β-endorphin.[6,7]

Using these fundamental neurotransmitter principles, pharmacologic intervention may be made. It is emphasized, however, that medication therapy is not at all effective as a primary treatment intervention. Nevertheless, it can serve as a useful treatment adjunct. In both young and old patients, a reversal of the primary biochemical imbalance is the key. In elderly anorectic patients, flavor enhancement and zinc repletion also may be useful.

■ THERAPEUTIC OPTIONS

The tricyclic antidepressants that block deaminative reuptake of the biogenic amines may reverse somewhat the symptoms of anorexia. In more limited fashion, bulimia also can be diminished. The noradrenergic antidepressant desipramine (Norpramin) can be useful in daily dosages of 3.26 mg/kg to a maximum of 100 mg for patients in early adolescence and 200 mg for those in late adolescence and adulthood. Amitriptyline (Elavil), a predominately serotonergic antidepressant, is also useful at similar dosages.[7]

Neither of these medications is without risks. Both have been reported to cause death at a dosage of only 1800 mg in adults. A far smaller dosage can be lethal in children. The toxicity is due to the anticholinergic activity shared by all tricyclic antidepressants. It also seems true, however, that anticholinergic activity is also counteranorectic. The tetracyclic and bicyclic antidepressants that have little or no anticholinergic activity are not useful for this purpose.

If a tricyclic agent is begun, it should be

titrated slowly upward. Dosage should begin at 25 to 50 mg QD. Increments of another 25 to 50 mg can be added every second or third day until optimal daily dosage levels are achieved. The physician should not expect to observe improvements until 3 to 4 weeks after initiation of optimal dosage. This dosage should then be maintained for a period of 6 to 8 months.

Cyproheptadine (Periactin) is used chiefly in the treatment of rhinitis and allergic reactions. It is a serotonin antagonist with antihistaminic and anticholinergic properties. It is also moderately effective as an appetite stimulant. It comes in both tablet and syrup forms. Dosage for preteens is 4 mg BID to TID. Adult and adolescent dosage is 12 to 20 mg QD. It is recommended that syrup of cyproheptadine be given in the initial stages of treatment, with an optional conversion to tablet form in the latter stages of therapy. Compliance issues are vastly simplified with liquids.[8]

Bulimia is sometimes responsive to low-to-moderate doses of carbamazepine (Tegretol). Carbamazepine usually brings quick initial results, but most patients relapse within 2 to 3 weeks. If a clinical trial seems warranted, 100 mg QD to TID should be maintained until the medication becomes ineffective. Since carbamazepine therapy is associated with bone marrow depression, frequent blood cell counts should be conducted throughout the treatment period of this drug. Also, weekly serum levels of carbamazepine can assist in dosage titration.[9]

Chlorpromazine (Thorazine), a dopamine antagonist, has been used to achieve weight gain in anorectics.[18] However, much of this increase occurs through fluid retention, reversible hypothalamic changes, and lethargy. It is therefore not recommended. Also, long-term use of chlorpromazine can produce irreversible tardive dyskinesia in over 5 per cent of patients.

Levodopa has been used with encouraging results. In addition to stimulating appetite and weight gain, it has been reported to diminish the obsessive-compulsive rituals associated with eating in these patients. The recommended dosage in adult and late adolescent patients is 200 to 300 mg QD. Effects continue throughout administration and may persist for several months after discontinuance. Hair loss over the scalp has been the only troublesome side effect thus far reported.[9]

Chemical intervention in anorexia and bulimia is not limited to pharmacologic treatment of the patient. In some cases, the food itself can be treated. Flavor enhancement is especially useful in middle-aged and elderly anorectic patients. In these latter phases of the life cycle, general taste losses are commonly reported. In fact, olfactory-gustatory thresholds can be 12 times higher than those in the young. Also, the capacity to discriminate among a variety of odors and tastes is much diminished.

Substance P is a neurotransmitter that can increase appetite. It also produces the taste sensations we associate with highly spiced food. The flavor-inducing antianorectic effects of these spices occurs because of the presence of capsaicin, which inhibits the breakdown of substance P. Some capsaicin-rich spices include black pepper, chili, curry powder, coriander, savory, oregano, cumin, and basil. Meals prepared for the anorectic patient should include these whenever possible.[10]

In addition to spices, flavor enhancers can offset the chemosensory losses that contribute to adult anorexia.[11] Commercially available enhancers can be used to fortify the taste of nearly every basic food in the North American diet. For example, beef flavoring can be added to roast beef and broccoli flavor to broccoli. This is a variation on the cook's trick of using fish stock in fish dishes and chicken bouillon cubes in chicken dishes. Gravies and sauces also serve this function.

Minimal fluctuations in zinc levels can also decrease both appetite and flavor perception. Zinc is thought to act by decreased activity of the opioid feeding system.[12] Multivitamins containing zinc should be provided. One such commercial preparation is Vicon-C, which should be prescribed at a dosage of 1 to 2 capsules per day. However, since dietary copper antagonizes zinc, the clinician should avoid vitamin preparations containing copper.

■ MANAGEMENT OF COMPLICATIONS

Management of anorexia and bulimia is quite difficult. The total long-term mortality rate approaches 20 per cent, with anorexia accounting for nearly all deaths. In addition to specific weight loss, cardiovascular, electrolyte and renal pathologies are the grim companions of induced starvation. Most deaths by starvation are presumed to be cardiovascular. Approximately 60 per cent of anorectic patients and 80 per cent of bulimic patients have postural hypotension. About 90 per cent of both groups manifest bradycardia. Electrocardiographic changes show atrial flutter and fibrillation, premature ventricular contractions, ventricular escape, and right bundle branch block. Occasionally, congestive heart failure is seen.[13]

Acute and life-threatening cardiac arrhythmias should be treated with intravenous lidocaine. In adults, give 50 to 100 mg, with an electrocardiographic monitor. The dosage rate should range between 0.35 and 0.70 mg/kg/min. If a therapeutic response is absent, the dose may be repeated after 5 minutes. For children, this dose should be adjusted to 1 mg/kg.

A continuous lidocaine infusion can be prepared by mixing 1 to 2 gm of lidocaine with 1 liter of D5W. This 0.2 per cent lidocaine solution can thus be diluted according to charts found in the *Physicians Desk Reference* and other sources. This preparation is stable for 24 hours. Treatment usually is not needed past this time. For children, the infusion should run at 20 to 30 μg/kg/min. In adults, the recommended rate is 0.014 to 0.057 mg/kg/min.

The usual electrolyte imbalances include sodium, potassium, calcium,[27] chloride, and phosphate. Of these, potassium is the most critical. Whereas hypokalemia is seen only in endstage anorexia nervosa, 25 per cent of all bulimic patients manifest this imbalance.[28] It can be treated by giving potassium chloride IV at a rate of 5 mEq/hr. The cardiac activity should be monitored by ECG during this time. After potassium is brought to a therapeutic level, it should be maintained by the oral route. A powder, such as K-Lor, rather than a tablet, is preferred. The adult dosage, 20 to 80 mEq QD, is recommended. It should be given in doses of 20 mEq each dissolved in 4 ounces of juice or water. Never give it with milk or milk products. In the initial phases of oral therapy, compliance should be observed by staff members.[14]

Chloride deficiencies can lead to hypochloremic alkalosis. This can be treated with potassium therapy plus volume expansion. Calcium deficiency is rare and usually is not life threatening.[29] If necessary, commercial calcium tablets can be given. Recent studies demonstrated that dietary boron (available in broccoli and plums) may be useful in stabilizing intracellular calcium. Phosphate and sodium imbalances are rarely a problem and can be treated simply with a commercial electrolyte drink, such as Gatorade. A 0.9 N sodium chloride IV drip can be used for the rare cases of clinical hyponatremia.[15]

Renal status is often impaired but should be treated with very conservative management. BUN levels are elevated in 20 per cent of anorectic patients and in 10 per cent of bulimic patients. This evaluation responds to nutritional therapy. Serum creatinine is rarely altered. Pyuria is found in 50 per cent of both anorectic and bulimic patients.[16] Occasionally, this is accompanied by hematuria or proteinuria or both. All these conditions will respond to rehydration and refeeding. Since resolution does not occur until well into the refeeding process, however, the physician should resist the impulse to intervene unless these conditions absolutely warrant such a move.[16]

Endocrine abnormalities usually involve the female gonadotropins. Low levels of follicle-stimulating hormone (FSH) and luteinizing hormone (LH) are commonly seen. Lowered levels of these hormones are associated with amenorrhea. Nearly a third of all anorectic patients do not achieve menstruation until their twenties, if at all. These may respond to refeeding but not in all cases. Hormonal therapy is never indicated. Thyroid studies may reveal marginal or low-normal levels. Again, treatment with thyroid hormone is not warranted.[17]

■ NONPHARMACOLOGIC THERAPY

Interventions may take forms other than pharmacologic. Nutritional therapy is one such useful form. A proper nutritional therapy/dietary intervention can avoid such extreme measures as parenteral or nasogastric feeding. Eating is influenced by its social environment. The family and primary caregivers (i.e., primary physicians, psychiatrists, nurses, psychologists) should not be responsible for monitoring and altering food intake and eating behavior. Enlisting a registered dietitian as part of the treatment team can reduce much staff and patient frustration.[18]

Rigid meal plans are to be avoided. They

are usually unrealistic and tend to reinforce the patient's previous ritualization of eating. Food intake patterns should be only gradually modified. A number of small meals and variable times should replace the traditional "three meals a day" regimen. This should reduce abdominal distention and further decrease the ritualization of eating. To divorce eating from weight, the patient should not be allowed to know her or his weight. High carbohydrate/high protein foods should predominate. Foods with high fat content or cooked with fats or oils may provoke nausea and bingeing.[19,20]

Specific nutritional deficiencies are best treated through diet. High-calcium foods can be given for patients with low bone density (e.g., milk, milk products). Hypokalemic patients can be given such foods as oranges, tomatoes, plums, and bananas. The patient should be encouraged to participate in this part of the nutritional treatment process. A positive view toward food can be developed when food is seen as maintaining body integrity rather than body size.

Intake and output should be monitored. Bathroom privileges should not be unsupervised during the initial phases of therapy. Anorectic patients generally need 6000 to 10,000 Kcal of food to gain 1 pound of body weight. This is opposed to about 3200 Kcal for the nonanorectic adult. Therefore, exercise should be carefully monitored to prevent sabotage of the treatment program.[21]

■ Comprehensive Approach to Management

The staff should be organized as a treatment team. Assignment of specific goals can help prevent staff subversion of therapy. Generally, subversion occurs when personnel do not view the patients as "sick" in the traditional sense. Therefore, they will not give anorectic and bulimic patients the care normally due those "entitled" to a "sick role." While lectures and in-service programs are helpful, these interventions alone will only drive the problem underground with a false patina of understanding.[22]

Generally, the structure of the treatment unit needs attention. A true treatment team can be developed to deal with anorectic and

bulimic patients.[23] The therapeutic-administrative split is a useful and easily adapted strategy. Some team members, such as the physician, dietitian, and some nurses, should adopt administrative roles in which medication and dietary orders are given and compliance checked. Other personnel should be engaged in talking and listening to patients in structured and unstructured therapy sessions, activity sessions, or in physical therapy. These latter personnel could include house physicians, nonadministrative nurses, and activity, occupational, and physical therapists.

Psychotherapy and counseling should focus initially on themes of responsibility and adaptation. Later, patient-identified issues and reintegration into family and work or school milieu can be stressed. Relaxation techniques are to be stressed. While this is occurring, a normal eating pattern should be developed as meals become deritualized.

Family therapy involves de-emphasis of eating as a control issue.[20] As a spin-off of control, weight loss is perceived by the patient as part of the achievement process, especially in upwardly mobile families. The conscious and unconscious signals given by parents need to be semiotically translated and examined. The possible pathology of the family needs to be identified and modified in the context of the patient's treatment program.

The discharge from acute treatment involves reintegration. Staff and family members should encourage passes to purchase clothing and to eat outside the hospital confines. Socialization skills, including assertiveness training, should be practiced.

Outpatient therapy should focus on family and individual therapy or counseling. Weight and food intake should not be subjected to intense monitoring. Since it is imperative that feeding rituals do not re-emerge, intake should not be a control issue. Weight should be monitored at specific times by the physician, not the parent. Again, remove control as an issue.

The patient should be encouraged to develop peer support from self-help groups. Addresses of local groups can be obtained by writing to these national organizations:

1. American Anorexia
   Nervosa Association (AANA)
   Teaneck, NJ 07666

2. Anorexia Nervosa and Related Eating Disorders (ANRED)
   P.O. Box 1012
   Grover City, CA 93433
3. Bulimia and Anorexia Self-Help Foundation (BASH)
   % Deaconess Hospital
   6150 Oakland Avenue
   St. Louis, MO 63139
4. National Anorexia Aid Society (NAAS)
   P.O. Box 29461
   Columbus, OH 43229

In addition, the Bulimia and Anorexia Self-Help Foundation maintains a 24-hour crisis hot line for anorectic and bulimic people and those who live with one. Their toll-free number is (800) 762-3334. (Call [314] 768-3838 in Missouri.)

REFERENCES

1. Giannini AJ. Anorexia nervosa—a retrospective view. Int J Psychiatr Med 1982; 11:199–202.
2. Morton R. Phthisiologia: A Treatise of Consumptions. London: Smith & Walford, 1694.
3. Giannini AJ, Telew F. Anorexia nervosa in geriatric patients. Geriatr Psychiatr 1987; 6(12):76–78.
4. Szmukler GI. The epidemiology of anorexia and bulimia. J Psychiatr Res 1985; 19:143–154.
5. Hoek HW, Brook FG. Patterns of care of anorexia nervosa. J Psychiatr Res 1985; 19:155–160.
6. Giannini AJ. Drug abuse and depression: possible models for geriatric anorexia. Neurobiol Aging 1988; 9:26–27.
7. Morley JE, Silver AJ. Anorexia in the elderly. Neurobiol Aging 1988; 9:9–16.
8. Halmi KA, Eckert E, LaDu TJ, Cohen J. Anorexia nervosa: treatment efficacy with cyproheptadine and amitriptyline. Arch Gen Psychiatr 1988; 2:177–181.
9. Johansson AJ, Knorr NJ. Treatment of anorexia nervosa by levodopa. Lancet 1974; 2:591.
10. Nishimoto T, Akai M, Inagaki S, Shissaka Y, Shimizo K. On the distribution and origin of substance P in the papillae of rat tongue. J Comp Neurol 1982; 207:85–92.
11. Essatara MD, Morley JE, Levine, AJ. The role of endogenous opiates in zinc deficiency anorexia. Physiol Behav 1984; 32:475–478.
12. Essatara MB, Morley JE, McClain CJ: The role of endogenous opiates in zinc deficiency anorexia. Physiol Behav 1984; 32:475–478.
13. Kalager T, Brubak O, Bassoe HH. Cardiac performance in patients with anorexia nervosa. Cardiology 1978; 63:1–4.
14. Fonseca GA, Howard CWH. Electrolyte disturbances and cardiac failure with hypomagnesemia in anorexia nervosa. Br Med J 1985; 291:1680–1682.
15. Fonseca VA, De Souza V, Houlder S, Thomas M, Dundona P. Vitamin D deficiency and low osteocalcitonin in anorexia nervosa. J Clin Pathol 1988; 41:195–197.
16. Palla B, Litt IF. Medical complications of eating disorders in adolescents. Pediatrics 1988; 81:613–623.
17. Jeuniewic N, Brown GB, Garfinkel PE, Moldafsky H. Hypothalamic function as related to body weight and body fat in anorexia nervosa. Psychosom Med 1978; 40(3):187–198.
18. Storey M. Nutrition management and the dietary treatment of bulimia. J Am Diet Assoc 1986; 86:4–9.
19. Bayer L, Bauers C. Psychosocial aspects of nutritional support. Nurs Clin North Am 1983; 1:1–5.
20. Omizo SA, Oda EA. Anorexia nervosa: psychological consideration for nutritional counseling. J Am Diet Assoc 1988; 88:49–51.
21. Kage WH, Gwirtsman HV, Orazzanek E, George DT. Relative importance of calorie intake to gain weight and level of physical activity in anorexia nervosa. Am J Clin Nutr 1988; 47:989–994.
22. Herzog DB, Copeland PM. Eating disorders. N Engl J Med 1985; 313:295–298.
23. DoCouto J, Reiff D, Steward E, Lampson-Reiff K. Nutrition intervention in the treatment of anorexia nervosa and bulimia nervosa. J Am Diet Assoc 1988; 88:68–71.

Anovulation

Josef Blankstein ■ *Martin M. Quigley*

Infertility is a descriptive term rather than a diagnosis. It refers to the inability of a couple to achieve parenthood. For practical purposes, a couple can be considered infertile if pregnancy has not been achieved after a year of unprotected intercourse. Infertility affects approximately 10 to 15 per cent of couples,[1] and roughly one third of infertile women seeking treatment present with ovulation failure. To manage ovulatory dysfunction, several cycle-regulating and ovulation-inducing drugs are available, and each of them may be used at various dosages and in different treatment schemes.

To manage an anovulatory patient properly, a decision must be made initially on the type of therapy each patient should receive. The treatment will be reasonably successful and safe only if the decision is correct. In other words, proper diagnosis and classification of patients are essential for effective and safe therapy. In this chapter, we first review ways to document ovulation. Only then is attention focused on the proper usage of conventional ovulation-inducing agents. Finally, we describe the application of recently released pharmaceutical agents that may be employed in patients with anovulation who do not respond to conventional therapy. In addition, we review the major risks and concerns associated with ovulation induction.

■ Background

■ DOCUMENTATION OF OVULATION

Women with regular menstrual cycles are probably ovulating, but this should be documented in the infertile woman by one or more of the following tests:

- basal body temperature,
- serum progesterone,
- endometrial biopsy,
- ultrasound.

Basal Temperature Charting

The basal body temperature shows a mean increase of 0.2 to 0.5 degrees C following ovulation owing to secretion of progesterone during the luteal phase of the cycle; the length of the luteal phase (from the temperature nadir to next menses) should be at least 12 days. The patient should be instructed to take her temperature each morning prior to getting out of bed.

Temperature charts are often difficult to interpret, are *not* useful in timing intercourse to facilitate conception, and should never be used as the single diagnostic parameter. The prolonged use of basal body temperature charts may encourage the development of an unhealthy obsession in some couples.

Serum Progesterone

Serum progesterone measurements should be made 5 to 8 days after the temperature rise shown by the basal body temperature chart. This will usually coincide with the midluteal phase (days 22 to 24 of a 30-day cycle) and can indicate whether ovulation has occurred and can give an estimate of its normality. The main problem with single progesterone levels is that progesterone secretion in women is pulsatile,[2,3] and a single estimation might provide insufficient data to judge the adequacy of the luteal phase.

Endometrial Biopsy

The endometrium demonstrates a predictable pattern of histologic changes over the menstrual cycle, especially in the luteal phase. Endometrial sampling is the most reliable test to assess ovulation and luteal phase adequacy. This procedure is performed in the week preceding the next menstruation and should reveal the typical secretory changes of the endometrial glands that are consistent with an ovulatory cycle. It is important to interpret the endometrial biopsy in accordance with the date of onset of the *subsequent* menstrual period.

Ultrasound Determinations

Although ultrasonography is important in the study of follicular growth, it is less precise in the detection of ovulation. Ultrasonic criteria for ovulation are the disappearance or collapse of the follicle after the LH surge or decrease of follicular size, appearance of fluid in the cul-de-sac, and/or opacification within the follicular structure.[4]

Other "ovulation" tests, such as home kits for urinary LH determination, recently have become available. In experienced hands, these tests can predict the time of ovulation accurately.

■ MINIMAL ENDOCRINE TESTING IN THE ANOVULATORY PATIENT

After the initial evaluation, further assessment of endocrine causes of anovulation requires consideration of three factors:

- prolactin,
- gonadotropins (especially follicle-stimulating hormone), and
- androgens (ovarian or adrenal).

Prolactin. Excess secretion of prolactin can cause anovulation in the female. Hyperprolactinemia has many underlying causes, of which the most important one is a possible pituitary tumor.

Follicle-Stimulating Hormone (FSH). In hypoestrogenic, anovulatory women, FSH determinations should be performed. Elevated levels indicate gonadal failure, whereas low or normal levels suggest hypothalamic or pituitary insufficiency.

Endogenous Androgens. When adrenal or ovarian androgens are secreted in excess, they may interfere with the complex feedback mechanism regulating the ovarian cycle. Polycystic ovarian disease (PCOD) is the most common clinical condition in which ovulatory dysfunction and elevated androgen secretion are combined. Patients with this disease present a variety of men-

strual cycle disturbances; usually they have some clinical signs of androgenization, such as hirsutism, and often, a tendency toward obesity. Proper management of these patients requires that the source of androgens be determined.[5]

■ Management

Women who have anovulatory cycles but spontaneous uterine bleeding and amenorrheic patients with endogenous estrogen activity (who exhibit withdrawal bleeding to progestogen administration) are classified as having hypothalamic-pituitary dysfunction. For these women, the first treatment of choice is clomiphene citrate (Clomid; Serophene).

Women with low endogenous gonadotropins and estrogens may require gonadotropin treatment. In the United States, the only suitable gonadotropin preparations are human menopausal gonadotropins (hMG, Pergonal), a 1:1 mixture of luteinizing hormone (LH) and FSH, and "pure" FSH (Metrodin). An alternative treatment for these women is gonadotropin hormone–releasing hormone (GnRH). The pulsatile administration of GnRH (Factryl), using portable minipumps that give a bolus of the hormone subcutaneously or intravenously every 60 to 90 minutes, may be successful in these patients, except for those with absent gonadotroph cells in the anterior pituitary.

Hyperprolactinemia is usually treated medically with the use of bromocriptine (Parlodel).

■ CLOMIPHENE CITRATE

Clomiphene citrate (CC) has been used as the first line of therapy for induction of ovulation in the anovulatory patient. At the recommended doses in humans, CC is an antiestrogen. Although the exact mechanism of action of an antiestrogen is not yet clear, it is thought that CC acts in estrogen target organs through the estrogen receptor machinery (that is, competes for the receptor-binding sites with endogenous estrogens). The stereoscopic configuration of CC is sufficiently similar to that of estradiol to compete with it for available estrogen receptor sites in all estrogen-dependent target cells in the hypothalamus, pituitary, ovary, uterus, and cervical glands.

The mode of action of clomiphene in the induction of ovulation may be tentatively described as follows: "Blinded" by clomiphene molecules occupying the estrogen receptor sites, the hypothalamus and pituitary are unable to perceive correctly the real level of estrogens in the blood. A false message of insufficient estrogen concentration is registered and acted upon, resulting in exaggerated secretion of FSH and LH. The occupation of hypothalamic estrogen receptors by clomiphene is a time-limited process of rather short duration. A fair chance exists that, by the time ovarian follicles that are stimulated by the clomiphene-induced gonadotropin elevation reach the preovulatory stage, the hypothalamus is already free of clomiphene influence and ready to perceive the correct steroid signal. From this moment on, the events are regulated and controlled by the endogenous feedback mechanism within the hypothalamic-pituitary-ovarian axis.

Antiestrogenic Effects on the Cervix and Endometrium. The antiestrogenic effect of CC may exert an adverse effect on the uterine cervix and its mucus. This detrimental effect, owing to the drug's competiton for estrogen receptors on the cervical epithelium, is claimed to be one factor responsible for the discrepancy between the ovulation rate (85 per cent) and the pregnancy rate (43 per cent) of women receiving CC treatment.[6]

Selection of Patients. Considering its mode of action, an antiestrogen such as clomiphene should be effective in anovulatory patients who have a hypothalamus capable of producing GnRH, a pituitary gland capable of response to GnRH, and an ovary containing normal follicles at various stages of development. Clomiphene should be used in patients with hypothalamic-pituitary dysfunction who lack the proper regulation within the hypothalamic-pituitary-ovarian axis. These infertile women probably have irregularities in the pulsatile secretion of GnRH, even though they do have fluctuating, detectable levels of gonadotropins and estrogens. They have various types of menstrual disorders and anovulatory cycles, such as oligomenorrhea, regular or irregular cycles with absent or infrequent ovulation, luteal phase deficiencies, and amenorrhea with endogenous estrogenic activity (positive progesterone withdrawal).

Treatment Scheme. Clomiphene citrate should be begun at a dosage of 50 mg (1 tablet) daily from cycle day 5 through 9 after induced or spontaneous menstrual bleeding. The patient should be instructed to keep a basal body temperature chart and return in about 4 weeks. At that time, the presence or absence of spontaneous menstrual bleeding, changes in cervical mucus, and the pattern of temperature changes will suggest whether ovulation has been successfully induced. If ovulation has not occurred, another withdrawal period is induced and the clomiphene is increased to 100 mg a day, days 5 through 9. The dosage of clomiphene is increased by 50 mg per month each month until ovulation appears to be occurring, based on the temperature chart and spontaneous menstrual bleeding. If ovulation has occurred, the clomiphene dose should be repeated and should *not* be increased. In each cycle prior to reinstitution of clomiphene, whether or not ovulation is occurring, a bimanual pelvic examination must be done to exclude ovarian cyst formation. Clomiphene-induced ovarian cysts resolve spontaneously as long as additional clomiphene is not administered during the subsequent cycle.

Once ovulation appears to be occurring, a premenstrual endometrial biopsy must be done to ensure that there is an adequate luteal phase with a receptive endometrium. In addition, a postcoital test (generally scheduled on cycle day 15 or 16) is performed to ensure that the antiestrogenic effect of clomiphene has not adversely affected the quantity and quality of the cervical mucus. If the mucus has been adversely affected, then ethinyl estradiol, 20 μg, is added from days 9 through 16.

■ HUMAN MENOPAUSAL GONADOTROPINS

Both follicle-stimulating hormone (FSH) and luteinizing hormone (LH) are required to stimulate follicular maturation. The FSH is necessary for the recruitment of follicles and is probably responsible for the selection of the dominant follicle. The LH stimulates theca cells to produce androgens, which are aromatized to estrogens by granulosa cells under FSH stimulation. Most gonadotropic preparations used for therapeutic purposes contain both FSH and LH in various proportions. Final maturation of the follicles is brought about by the combination of FSH and LH, and the subsequent ovulation is induced by a surge of LH secretion by administration of LH or the LH-like material, human chorionic gonadotropin (hCG).

Selection of Patients

Ovulation induction with human menopausal gonadotropin (hMG) is effective in patients who lack endogenous gonadotropins but have ovaries capable of responding normally to gonadotropic stimuli. In this latter group, a 60 to 80 per cent pregnancy rate can be expected.[7] Moreover, patients who fail to ovulate or conceive within a reasonable time during clomiphene therapy are considered "clomiphene failures" and can be considered for hMG therapy, although their pregnancy rate is lower than that of the hypogonadotropic patients.

The difference in pregnancy rates between hypothalamic-pituitary amenorrhea and clomiphene failure may be explained by the fact that the patients belonging to the latter group are negatively selected; that is, many of these patients failed to conceive following clomiphene therapy, despite the fact that many of them did ovulate. It is possible that additional factors may contribute to the lower pregnancy rate.

Monitoring of hMG Therapy

The monitoring of treatment serves to assess the effective dose to evoke an ovarian response, the length of time required for follicular maturation, and the appropriate time for induction of ovulation with hCG. Furthermore, it should aim to prevent the ovarian hyperstimulation syndrome, especially in patients with polycystic ovarian disease, since high rates of multiple births and ovarian hyperstimulation have been observed frequently in these patients.

In practice, hMG is generally administered beginning between cycle days 2 and 5 of a spontaneous or induced menstrual period. Patients are monitored every 1 to 4 days by clinical examination of the cervical mucus; ultrasound study of follicular number, diameter, and growth rate; and serum estradiol determinations. The dosage of hMG is adjusted on the basis of these parameters. When sufficient follicular maturation has been achieved, as shown by follicular size and estradiol levels, the ovulatory dose of hCG (10,000 IU) is administered. In general, hCG should be administered when estradiol levels are between 900 and 1200 pg per ml, and mean follicular diameters of 16 to 18 mm have been reached.

In case of multifollicular development, much higher levels of estrogens will be obtained. In this case, the decision to inject hCG should be carefullly weighed against the risk of hyperstimulation or multiple pregnancies. When multifollicular development occurs and estrogen levels rise above 2500 pg per ml, hCG definitely should be withheld, because our experience shows that hyperstimulation is likely to complicate the treatment, especially if pregnancy occurs.

■ "PURE" FSH

Patients with polycystic ovarian disease (PCOD), who have a tonically elevated level of LH, theoretically should respond better to ovulation induction with pure FSH than with hMG. It has been shown that pure FSH is capable of inducing ovulation in PCOD patients. In general, pure FSH is administered and monitored the same way as hMG is. Some researchers have postulated that treatment with pure FSH should be associated with a better pregnancy rate than treatment with hMG.

At present, the few patients treated with FSH do not permit a final conclusion about the optimal gonadotropin therapy for PCOD patients. More studies are needed to determine the most effective form of gonadotropin therapy for these patients.

■ GONADOTROPIN-RELEASING HORMONE

GnRH is a linear decapeptide that binds to specific receptors in the extracellular surface on the plasma membrane of the pituitary gonadotrophs. It has been shown that only the pulsatile discharge of GnRH will activate the pituitary to synthesize and secrete FSH and LH. It is now well documented that GnRH can be used to induce follicular development and ovarian estradiol secretion as long as GnRH is given in a pulsatile fashion.

GnRH is administered by a computerized minipump via a chronic indwelling intravenous or subcutaneous catheter. Several commercial infusion pumps are now available that allow delivery of measured amounts of the hormone in a pulsatile fashion.

■ BROMOCRIPTINE

Bromocriptine is an ergot derivative whose structure resembles that of dopamine. Bromocriptine acts directly as a potent dopamine agonist, thus decreasing prolactin secretion. The initial dosage is 2.5 mg daily, taken with dinner for 1 week. (If nausea occurs, the dosage can be decreased to 1.25 mg daily for 1 week, followed by 2.5 mg daily for 1 week). The dosage then should be increased to 2.5 mg twice a day for 1 week, after which prolactin levels are measured. When a serum prolactin level of between 5 and 15 ng/ml is reached, the patient is asked to begin charting basal body temperature. If spontaneous ovulation and menses do not begin within 6 to 8 weeks, bromocriptine therapy is continued, and clomiphene is added to the regimen.

■ Concerns and Risks

■ COMPLICATIONS FOLLOWING GONADOTROPIC THERAPY

Ovarian Hyperstimulation Syndrome (OHSS)

The ovarian hyperstimulation syndrome is one of the most severe complications associated with the use of hMG for ovulation induction. Death and severe morbidity have been reported with this syndrome. This reaction occurs when ovaries respond to exogenous gonadotropins by forming too many follicles and, after the administration of hCG, develop massive ovarian follicular and corpus luteum cysts. A comprehensive classification of the OHSS into three grades has been suggested:[8]

Grade I includes patients with variable ovarian enlargement and small cysts. Laboratory findings in Grade I hyperstimulation cases include serum E2 levels above 2000 pg per ml and serum progesterone above 30 ng per ml. While treatment is not necessary, it is important that patients report back immediately if additional symptoms appear, since severe complications may develop from initially innocent-looking disturbances.

Grade II includes patients with distinct ovarian cysts, accompanied by various additional symptoms such as abdominal distention, nausea, vomiting, diarrhea, and weight gain. In cases of rapid weight gain associated with vomiting and diarrhea, hospitalization for symptomatic treatment may be advisable.

Grade III (severe hyperstimulation) includes patients with large ovarian cysts, ascites, and sometimes hydrothorax.

The clinical symptoms of OHSS usually appear 5 to 10 days following hCG administration. Hyperstimulation apparently leads to capillary damage and permeability, with loss of fluid from the intravascular compartment, which leads to hypovolemia, hemoconcentration, and decreased renal perfusion, together with increased blood viscosity and coagulation abnormalities. Aldosterone production also increases salt retention. The elevation of aldosterone and antidiuretic hormone can be considered as secondary to the intravascular volume deficit produced by the loss of fluid and protein into the peritoneal and pleural cavities as plasma renin is elevated.[9]

If not promptly recognized and vigorously treated, the syndrome may be complicated by the occurrence of dangerous thromboembolic phenomena. Ovarian hyperstimulation can be alleviated by indomethacin, a blocker of prostaglandins. Shenker has postulated that the increased capillary permeability might be due to an excess of prostaglandins secreted by the ovary after gonadotropin stimulation.[10]

The treatment of severe OHSS is directed primarily toward correction of the disturbed fluid and electrolyte balance. A careful intake/output record should be kept, and 5 per cent glucose in water may be administered initially. Diuretic agents should be used with caution, if at all, because the artificially induced diuresis may further diminish the intravascular volume but will be unable to reduce the ascites or hydrothorax. Plasma expanders seem to be a much more logical treatment and should be used early.

Abdominal and pulmonary symptoms may be alleviated or at least diminished by puncture and drainage of fluid from the abdominal and/or pleural cavities. Anticoagulant therapy is usually unnecessary if the aforementioned steps are employed promptly. Except for torsion or rupture of cysts and internal hemorrhage, there is no reason for contemplating laparotomy. Because the cysts are so large and so extremely brittle, ultrasound examination for monitoring should be performed in a very gentle manner; moreover, for the same reasons one should try to avoid pelvic examinations.

The close observation of patient response, as monitored by serum estradiol levels and ovarian follicular ultrasound, is useful in preventing, or at least reducing, the incidence of clinical hyperstimulation. The most important hint is the slope of ascent of blood estrogens. A steep increase of estrogens—that is, 2 or 3 consecutive days during which serum estrogen more than doubles—should be regarded as a serious warning sign. The decision whether, when, and at what dosage hCG should be administered must be carefully evaluated. It has been recommended that whenever estrogen levels exceed 1500 pg per ml, the administration of hCG to induce ovulation should be withheld in that treatment cycle. A recent prospective study was undertaken to correlate preovulatory sonographic findings in the ovaries on the day of hCG administration and the occurrence of OHSS following hMG therapy.[11] It was found that patients with OHSS had significantly more follicles at the time of hCG, emphasizing the value of ovarian ultrasonography in predicting OHSS.

Multiple Ovulation

A high multiple pregnancy rate is also a complication of gonadotropin therapy and has contributed much to the high pregnancy wastage. It has been shown that the multiple pregnancy rate and the inherent complications may be reduced by adhering to a "ceiling limit" of estrogens at which hCG may be administered. In regard to preovulatory ultrasonic assessment, it has been shown recently that during hMG therapy no differences in the number or distribution of ovarian follicles could be found in cycles that subsequently resulted in single or multiple pregnancies.[12]

■ Summary

Ovulatory dysfunction is a leading cause of female infertility. Fortunately, ovulatory dysfunction is often amenable to treatment. Thorough testing is necessary to identify the exact cause of anovulation before conventional ovulation-inducing therapy is started. Careful patient monitoring is essential to avoid risks, such as hyperstimulation and multiple gestation.

REFERENCES

1. Pratt WF, Mosher WED, Bachrach C, Horn MC. Infertility—United States, 1982. MMWR 1985; 34:197–200.
2. Filicori M, Buler JP, Crowley WF. Neuroendocrine regulation of the corpus luteum in the human: evidence for pulsatile progesterone secretion. J. Clin Invest 1984; 73:1638–1647.
3. Soules MR, Clifton DK, Steiner RA, Cohen NL, Bremner WJ. The corpus luteum: determinants of progesterone secretion in normal menstrual cycle. Obstet Gynecol 1988; 71:659–666.
4. de Crespigny LC, O'Herlihy C, Robinson HP. Ultrasonic observation of the mechanism of human ovulation. Am J Obstet Gynecol 1981; 139:636–639.
5. Blankstein J, Mashiach S, Lunenfeld B. Ovulation Induction and in Vitro Fertilization. Chicago: Year Book Medical Publishers, 1986;61–76.
6. Gysler M, March CM, Mishell DR, Bailey EJ. A decade's experience with an individualized clomiphene treatment regimen, including its effect on the post-coital test. Fertil Steril 1982; 37:161–167.
7. Lunenfeld B, Insler V, Rabau E. Induction de l'ovulation par les gonadotropines. In Moricard R, Ferin J (eds): L'Ovulation. Paris: Masson et Cie, 1969;291–300.
8. WHO Scientific Group. Agents stimulating gonadal function in the human. WHO Tech Rep Ser 1973; 5:4.
9. Haning RV, Strawn EY, Nolten WE. Pathophysiology of the ovarian hyperstimulation syndrome. Obstet Gynecol 1985; 66:220–224.
10. Shenker JY. Ovarian hyperstimulation syndrome. In Hafez ESE (ed): Human Ovulation: Mechanisms, Prediction, Detection and Induction. Amsterdam: North Holland Publishing Company, 1978;32–40.
11. Blankstein J, Shalev J, Saadon T, Kukia E, Rabinovici J, Pariente C, Lunenfeld B, Serr DM, Mashiach S. Ovarian hyperstimulation syndrome: prediction by number and size of preovulatory ovarian follicles. Fertil Steril 1987; 47:597–602.
12. Goldenberg M, Rabinovici J, Shalev J, Bider D, Mashiach S, Blankstein J: Association of the occurrence of multiple pregnancies in menotropin cycles with follicular size and number. Submitted to Fertil Steril, 1989.

Antimicrobial use during pregnancy and lactation

Stephen D. Shafran ■ *Anthony W. Chow*

■ Background

It is frequently necessary to administer antimicrobial agents to pregnant or lactating women. According to previous studies, 25 per cent to 40 per cent of pregnant women are exposed to these agents.[1]

Drug usage during pregnancy is complicated by two critical considerations. First, maternal physiologic changes of pregnancy can alter drug absorption, distribution, metabolism, and excretion. Second, virtually any drug administered to a pregnant woman is also administered to her fetus via the placenta, thereby exposing the fetus to potential adverse drug reactions, some of which are teratogenic.

Drug use in lactating women is somewhat less complicated than in pregnant women, as teratogenicity is not a consideration. Nevertheless, many drugs are excreted in breast milk and may cause adverse effects in breast-fed infants.

In this chapter, we review both maternal and fetal considerations and then discuss specific antimicrobial agents. Diagnosis and specific treatment regimens will not be discussed here.

■ MATERNAL PHYSIOLOGIC AND PHARMACOKINETIC CONSIDERATIONS

The critical maternal considerations in the pharmacokinetics of antimicrobial agents are absorption, distribution, metabolism and elimination. These are depicted in Figure 1.

Absorption. The tone and motility of the maternal gastrointestinal tract are reduced during pregnancy, resulting in delayed gastric emptying and prolonged intestinal transport.[2] In addition, gastric acid secretion is reduced. Drugs administered orally will be in contact with gastric acid for longer periods of time, and this will reduce the bioavailability of acid-labile drugs, such as erythromycin base. On the other hand, once active drug traverses the pylorus, the delayed transit time within the small intestine generally will result in increased absorption.

Distribution. During pregnancy, there is a marked increase in both the intravascular and extravascular fluid volumes. Consequently, the volume of drug distribution increases, and the serum drug levels fall. Additionally, serum albumin levels fall substantially during pregnancy, resulting in a decreased ratio of bound to unbound drug.[3] This latter effect will partially offset the effects of increased volume of distribution for highly protein-bound drugs, such as the isoxazolyl penicillins, but not for those agents like the aminoglycosides, which are poorly bound to proteins.

Metabolism. The hormonal changes of pregnancy stimulate hepatic microsomal enzyme activity, which may result in increased metabolism of certain drugs.[4]

Elimination. During pregnancy, renal blood flow and glomerular filtration increase by up to 50 per cent.[5] Since the majority of antimicrobial agents are eliminated via the kidney, the result of the increased glomerular filtration rate is more rapid clearance of these drugs.

■ PLACENTAL TRANSFER

The maternal and fetal circulations are separate, with no direct mixing. Within the placenta, however, the two circulations are separated only by the placental membrane. Until about 20 weeks' gestation, this membrane consists of four layers: the syncytiotrophoblast, the cytotrophoblast, the connective tissue core, and the endothelium of

"

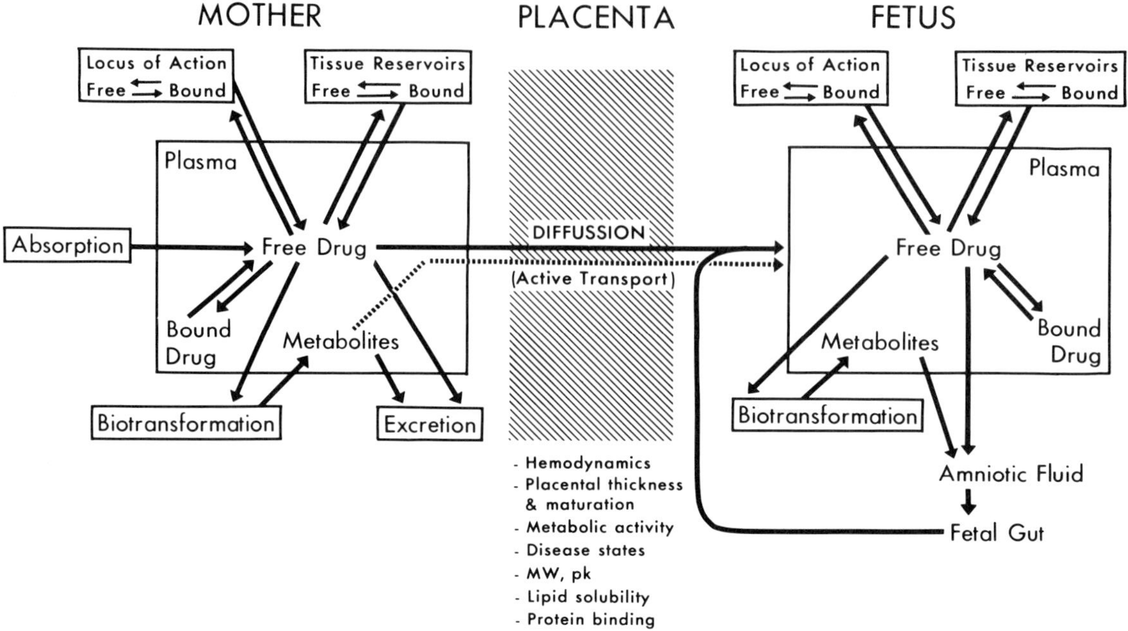

Figure 1. Major pathways and interrelations of drug pharmacokinetics in the mother, the fetus, and the placenta. (Reproduced with permission of the University of Chicago from Chow AW, Jewesson PJ. Pharmacokinetics and safety of antimicrobial agents during pregnancy. Rev Infect Dis 1985; 7:287–311.)

the fetal capillary.[6] After about 20 weeks, the cytotrophoblast no longer forms a continuous layer, the relative amount of connective tissue is reduced, and the number and size of fetal capillaries increase. Therefore, as pregnancy advances, the placental membranes become progressively thinner.

The mechanisms that regulate the transfer of pharmacologically active molecules across biologic membranes in other body sites also operate in the placenta. Transfer of antimicrobial agents across the placenta occurs by simple diffusion, and the rate of diffusion may be expressed by the equation $KA(Cm - Cf)/X$, where A represents the surface area available for transfer, Cm represents the concentration of unbound drug in maternal blood, Cf represents the concentration of unbound drug in fetal blood, X represents the thickness of the placental membranes, and K represents the diffusion constant of the drug.[7] The diffusion constant, in turn, is increased by lower molecular weight, lower degree of ionization, and higher lipid solubility and also can be influenced by the spatial configuration of the molecule.

Since the placental membrane becomes thinner and its surface area increases during gestation, placental transfer of drugs will be greater toward the end of pregnancy than in the first trimester.

Placental homogenates have been shown to possess metabolic activity in vitro.[8] It is conceivable, therefore, that the placenta could play a small role in drug metabolism, but this theory remains unproved.

■ FETAL PHARMACOKINETIC CONSIDERATIONS

Drugs are able to reach the fetus by two mechanisms: parenterally via the umbilical vein and orally via the swallowing of amniotic fluid. After placental transfer, drugs are carried to the fetal liver via the umbilical vein. Some of the drug will then be diverted via the ductus venosus into the inferior vena cava and the systemic circulation, while the remainder will perfuse the fetal liver where, depending on the agent, it may be subject to metabolism, since the fetal liver possesses many of the metabolic activities of the adult liver.

Amniotic fluid is derived primarily from the maternal blood.[6,9] Once the fetal urinary system is established, fetal urine also contributes significantly to the amniotic fluid. Since many antimicrobial agents are excreted unchanged by the kidney, these can be recirculated through ingestion of amniotic fluid by the fetus, provided they are absorbed enterally.

■ THERAPEUTIC EFFICACY CONSIDERATIONS

Antibiotics may be used during pregnancy to treat infections in the mother, the fetus, or the amniotic fluid (amnionitis). Most frequently, they are given to treat maternal infections.

The majority of antimicrobial agents attain lower serum levels and are eliminated more rapidly in pregnancy. Therefore, it is frequently necessary to increase the dosage or the frequency of administration of these drugs or both for optimal efficacy.

Treating fetal infections is more difficult. Some drugs cannot cross the placenta in therapeutic concentrations. The majority of antimicrobial agents will cross the placenta to the fetus, but there are two therapeutic obstacles. First, fetal serum levels are generally lower than maternal levels, and sometimes profoundly so. Second, there is a delay between the administration of drug to the mother and the achievement of therapeutic levels in the fetus. Frequently, the most prudent course of action is to deliver the infected fetus and then treat the neonate, thus improving the chances for successful treatment while sparing the mother from drug toxicity.

Treating amnionitis presents the same two problems as treating fetal infections, except that the delay in achieving therapeutic levels in the amniotic fluid is more significant, since by the late stage in pregnancy when this infection may occur, fetal urine is the major contributor to the composition of amniotic fluid. Again, early delivery of the infant is an important component of therapy of this infection.

■ ADVERSE EFFECTS

Maternal Adverse Effects. There is no evidence that pregnant women experience adverse effects of antimicrobial agents with greater frequency or severity than nonpregnant individuals, with the possible exception of tetracycline, which will be discussed later. Indeed, adverse effects that are dose dependent theoretically should be observed less frequently during pregnancy because of lower serum levels of most drugs.

Fetal Adverse Effects. Fetal development can be divided into three periods: (1) the fertilization and implantation period (usually days 0 to 17), (2) the embryonic period (usually days 18 to 55), and (3) the fetal period (beyond 8 weeks). The first period is characterized by rapid replication of totipotent cells, and it is believed that drugs exert an all-or-nothing effect when administered at this time.[10] The embryonic period is characterized by organogenesis; during this period teratogenic effects are most likely to occur. During the fetal period, by which time the major organ systems have already formed, the potential for major congenital malformation is considerably diminished.

Major congenital malformations occur in 2 per cent to 3 per cent of neonates, and minor defects occur in up to 9 percent.[1] Given this background rate of congenital malformations, it is inappropriate to label a drug teratogenic merely because a defective infant was born to a mother who received that drug during pregnancy. Teratogenicity is evaluated by comparing the incidence of congenital malformations in drug-exposed women to unexposed women who are matched by age, parity, and exposure to other potential toxins. In recent years, most newer drugs have been tested for possible teratogenicity in animals. This method is imperfect, since teratogenicity is sometimes restricted to certain species. Nevertheless, when a drug is found to be teratogenic in animals, prudence dictates that it be avoided in human pregnancy.

■ LACTATION

Breast-feeding is considered the optimal way to feed infants and is currently practiced by a majority of mothers. As breast-feeding may continue for many months, a significant number of breast-feeding women may require drug therapy during this time.

Drug Excretion in Breast Milk. Studies of drug excretion in breast milk are complicated by the fact that breast milk is not a homogeneous fluid. For example, the fat content of hind (or after-) milk contains four- to fivefold the amount of fore-milk, and this will affect the amount of lipophilic drug contained.[11] In addition, the timing of the sampling of milk relative to drug administration will affect the concentration of drug measured in the milk. In general, drugs are transferred from blood into breast milk by simple diffusion, and the rate of diffusion is enhanced by higher concentration gradients (only unbound, nonionized drug will diffuse), lower molecular weight, and higher lipid solubility.[11] Most drugs studied have been detected in breast milk, generally in concentrations below that of maternal plasma; however, data are not available for many drugs.[11,12] The extent of excretion of a drug into breast milk is commonly expressed at the M/P (milk/plasma) ratio.

Absorption of Drugs by Breast-Fed Infants. It is not enough to know whether a given drug is present in breast milk; it is also necessary to know whether the drug is absorbed, and to what extent. Drugs which are acid labile and thus used only parenterally, such as aminoglycosides, will not be absorbed by the nursing infant even if present in breast milk. It is possible, however, that such drugs can be absorbed in trace amounts to sensitize the child or to result in allergic reaction, but this remains to be established. Data regarding absorption of most drugs from breast milk are scant; however, it is presumed that drugs that are absorbed through the alimentary tract are also absorbed when administered via breast milk.

Adverse Effects in Breast-Fed Infants. Only drugs that are excreted in breast milk in an absorbable form are capable of causing dose-related adverse effects. However, the majority of such drugs are present in low concentrations and are unlikely to cause such effects. Dose-unrelated adverse effects conceivably could occur with such drugs, although some of these effects may require a minimal duration of therapy. It is likely that all breast-fed infants of mothers receiving antibiotics will undergo changes in their intestinal flora, especially when the agents utilized are poorly absorbed from the alimentary tract. Whether such effects are clinically evident is uncertain.

Adverse effects of drugs administered via breast milk have been reported very infrequently and have been similar to the known adverse effects of these drugs.[12] Unlike the case in pregnancy, in which maternally administered drugs are invariably also administered to the fetus, during lactation there is the option of formula feeding the infant, either transiently during short-term maternal drug therapy or longer if drug therapy is likely to be prolonged. This strategy is frequently used, especially for drugs contraindicated in young children.[13]

Specific Antimicrobial Agents in Pregnancy and Lactation

Current information regarding the pharmacokinetics and safety of many antimicrobial drugs in pregnancy is summarized in Table 1. Specific agents are discussed next.

BETA-LACTAMS

Penicillin and ampicillin have been used for many years for pregnant women. It is clear that these agents are not associated with an increased rate of adverse effects, and they are considered among the safest drugs to administer during pregnancy.[1,12] Fewer data are available regarding antistaphylococcal and antipseudomonal penicillins, but these appear to be as safe.

All penicillins cross the placenta, but since these agents have a low degree of lipid solubility, and some such as the isoxazolyl penicillins are highly protein bound, fetal levels are considerably lower than maternal levels.

Less is known about cephalosporins in pregnancy, but these drugs have pharmacokinetics and mechanisms of action similar to those of penicillins, with less frequent allergic reactions in nonpregnant patients. Experience with first-generation cephalosporins in pregnancy supports the belief that these agents are safe during pregnancy. Experience during pregnancy with second- and third-generation cephalosporins, monobactams, and carbapenems is much more limited but is also favorable, and there are no reasons to believe that these agents will be more toxic than their ancestors.

Most beta-lactam antibiotics that have been studied have been detected in very low concentrations in breast milk.[11–13] Many of these agents are acid labile and would not be absorbed by the infant (e.g., antipseudomonal penicillins and third-generation cephalosporins). Even absorbable drugs, such as

TABLE 1. Pharmacokinetic and Toxicologic Characteristics of Selected Antimicrobial Agents During Pregnancy and Lactation

Group, Agent	Approx. % Protein-Bound (Maternal)	Degree of Placental Transfer	Fetal/ Maternal Serum Level Ratio	Milk/ Maternal Plasma (M/P) Ratio	Pharmacokinetics		Potential Toxicity	
					Maternal	Fetal/ Neonatal	Maternal	Fetal/Neonatal
Penicillins	Variable	Moderate to high	0.1–0.7	Variable	↓ Serum level; ↑ excretion; ↑ VD; ↓ t½	Probably un-changed	Allergic reactions; safe	Allergic reactions; safe
Benzathine	50	—	0.1–0.7	0.13	—	—	As above	As above
Phenoxymethyl	80	—	—	—	—	—	As above	As above
Oxacillin	94	—	—	—	↑ Excretion; ↑ VD	—	As above	As above
Dicloxacillin	98	—	Low (0.1–0.3)	—	—	—	As above	As above
Methicillin	37	High	High (0.8–1.4)	—*	↓ Serum level	—	As above	As above
Nafcillin	90	—	—	—	—	68% protein-bound	As above	As above
Carbenicillin	50	—	—	—*	—	—	As above	As above
Ampicillin	22	High	High (0.3–0.9)	0.2	—	10% protein-bound	As above	Diarrhea, candidiasis
Cephalosporins	Variable	Moderate to high	0.2–1.0	0–0.5	↓ Serum level; ↑ excretion; ↑ VD; ↓ t½	Probably unchanged	Cross-hypersensitivity with penicillin; safe	Allergic reactions; safe
Cephalothin	72	Moderate	0.1	0.5*	↓ Serum level	—	—	Probably safe
Cefazolin	80	Moderate	0.3	.02*	↓ Serum level; ↓ t½	—	—	Probably safe
Cephradine	10	High	0.1–0.4	0.2	↓ Serum level; ↑ excretion; ↑ VD; ↓ t½	—	—	Probably safe
Cephalexin	12	Moderate	—	0.14	↓ Serum level	—	—	Probably safe
Cefoxitin	70	High	0.6	0.05*	↓ Serum level	—	—	Probably safe
Cefuroxime	33	High	0.3	— *	↓ Serum level; ↑ excretion; ↑ VD; ↓ t½	—	—	Probably safe
Moxalactam	40	High	0.4	0.1*	↓ t½	—	—	Probably safe
Cefotaxime	37	High	0.2	0.2*	—	—	—	Probably safe
Tetracyclines	Variable (35–93)	High	0.5–0.7	0.25–1.5*	Probably unchanged	Probably unchanged	Hepatotoxicity; pancreatitis; renal failure	Tooth discoloration and inhibition of bone growth
Tetracycline	65	High	0.6	0.25–1.5	—	—	As above	As above
Doxycycline	93	—	—	0.4	—	—	As above	As above
Minocycline	76	—	—	—	—	—	As above	As above
Chloramphenicol	50	High	0.7—1.0	0.6	Unchanged	↓ Hepatic conjugation (50% present as inactive metabolite)	Bone marrow depression; aplastic anemia	Bone marrow depression; possibly gray baby syndrome

TABLE 1. Pharmacokinetic and Toxicologic Characteristics of Selected Antimicrobial Agents During Pregnancy and Lactation (Continued)

Group, Agent	Approx. % Protein-Bound (Maternal)	Degree of Placental Transfer	Fetal/ Maternal Serum Level Ratio	Milk/ Maternal Plasma (M/P) Ratio	Pharmacokinetics		Potential Toxicity	
					Maternal	Fetal/ Neonatal	Maternal	Fetal/Neonatal
Metronidazole	20	High	High	1.0	Probably unchanged	Probably unchanged	Blood dyscrasia; neuropathy; intolerance to alcohol	No known teratogenicity in humans but avoidance in early pregnancy probably prudent
Erythromycin	70–75	Low	Low	0.5	↓ Serum level; ↓ absorption	Low penetration	Allergic reactions; cholestatic hepatitis (estolate > others)	Safe
Clindamycin	90	Moderate	0.4–0.5	0.1–3.0	Serum level unchanged; ↓ t½	Unchanged	Allergic reactions; diarrhea and pseudomembranous colitis	Safe
Sulfonamides	40–90	High	0.1–0.9	0.06–0.5	Serum level unchanged; ↓ t½	Unchanged	Allergic reactions; crystalluria	Kernicterus; hemolysis (G6PD deficiency)
Sulfisoxazole	85	High	—	0.06	Serum level unchanged	65%–70% protein-bound; ↑ VD	As above	As above
Sulfamethoxazole	70	High	0.7–1.0 (1.5–1.8 when used with trimethoprim)	—	Serum level unchanged	57% protein-bound; ↑ VD	As above	As above
Trimethoprim	44	High	0.7–0.8	1.25	Serum level unchanged; ↓ t½	Serum level unchanged; ↓ t½	Allergic reactions	Folate antagonism kernicterus; hemolysis (G6PD deficiency); potentially teratogenic
Nitrofurantoin	60	High	>1.0	Very low	↓ Serum level; ↑ excretion	↑ Excretion	Neuropathy; hemolysis (G6PD deficiency)	Hemolysis (G6PD deficiency)
Nalidixic acid	93	Low	—	0.08–0.13	Probably unchanged	↑ t½	Toxic psychosis and convulsions	As above

Aminoglycosides	0–6	Low to moderate	0.2–0.5	0.1–1.0*	↓ Serum level; ↑ VD: ↑ excretion	VD; excretion	Nephrotoxicity and ototoxicity	8th nerve toxicity (proved only for streptomycin); possible alteration of intestinal flora
Streptomycin	5	Moderate	—	0.5–1.0*	—	—	As above	As above
Gentamicin	0	Moderate	0.4	—*	↓ Serum level	—	As above	As above
Tobramycin	0	Moderate	0.5	0.1*	↓ Serum level; t½ unchanged	—	As above	As above
Amikacin	2–6	Moderate	0.2	low*	↓ Serum level	—	As above	As above
Vancomycin	55	—	—	—*	Unknown	Unknown	Ototoxicity and possible nephrotoxicity	Unknown
Antituberculous Drugs								
Isoniazid	0	Yes	High	1.0	Serum level unchanged	Unchanged	Hepatotoxicity	Neuropathy and convulsions
Ethambutol	40	Unknown	—	—	↑ Excretion	Unknown	Retrobulbar neuritis	Probably safe
Rifampin	85	High	0.3	0.1–0.4	Serum level unchanged	Probably unchanged	Hepatotoxicity; hypoprothrombinemia and bleeding	No known teratogenicity in humans; probably safe
Antifungal Drugs								
Amphotericin B	93	Yes	0.3–1.0	—*	Probably unchanged	Unknown	Hepatotoxicity; hypokalemia; anemia; idiosyncratic reactions	Reversible azotemia and hypokalemia; no known teratogenicity
Flucytosine	4	Unknown	—	—	Probably unchanged	Unknown	Hepatotoxicity; marrow aplasia	Potentially teratogenic
Miconazole	>90	Unknown	—	—*	Unknown	Unknown	Hyperlipidemia; hyponatremia and thrombocytosis	Safety not established
Ketoconazole	99	Unknown	—	—	Unknown	Unknown	Hepatitis	Safety not established; teratogenic in rats
Griseofulvin	—	Yes	0.5–1.0	—	↓ Serum level	—	Allergic reactions; hepatotoxicity	Teratogenic in mice; safety not established

TABLE 1. Pharmacokinetic and Toxicologic Characteristics of Selected Antimicrobial Agents During Pregnancy and Lactation (Continued)

Group, Agent	Approx. % Protein-Bound (Maternal)	Degree of Placental Transfer	Fetal/ Maternal Serum Level Ratio	Milk/ Maternal Plasma (M/P) Ratio	Pharmacokinetics Maternal	Pharmacokinetics Fetal/ Neonatal	Potential Toxicity Maternal	Potential Toxicity Fetal/Neonatal
Antiviral Drugs								
Amantadine	—	Unknown	—	low	Unknown	Unknown	Anxiety; hallucinations, and psychosis	Teratogenic in animals; rare report of cardiovascular lesion
Vidarabine	20–30	Unknown	—	—*	Unknown	Unknown	Neurotoxicity with tremor and hallucinations; thrombocytopenia and leukopenia	Teratogenic and carcinogenic in animal species
Acyclovir	9–22	Unknown	—	—	Unknown	↑ t½	Nephrotoxicity with dehydration and rapid infusion	No known teratogenicity but safety not established
Zidovudine	34–38	Unknown	—	—	Unknown	Unknown	Bone marrow depression, headache, nausea	Unknown

NOTE: Dashes indicate either no published data or no information known to authors.

↓ = Decreased; ↑ = increased; VD = volume of distribution; t½ = half-life; G6PD = glucose-6-phosphate dehydrogenase.

*These drugs are not significantly absorbed via the alimentary tract.

(Modified from Chow AW, Jewesson PJ. Pharmacokinetics and safety of antimicrobial agents during pregnancy. Rev Infect Dis 1985; 7:287–313.)

amoxicillin, will not achieve adequate concentrations in the infant to treat infection.

■ AMINOGLYCOSIDES

All aminoglycosides studied cross the placenta, achieving fetal serum levels of approximately 30 per cent to 50 per cent of maternal levels. Neither animal nor human data suggest that these drugs are teratogenic.[1,12]

Ototoxicity has been reported in the offspring of mothers receiving streptomycin (SM) or dihydrostreptomycin (DHSM) during pregnancy for the treatment of tuberculosis.[14] It has not been reported with other aminoglycosides. The association must be interpreted cautiously, since the majority of infants with congenital hearing deficits have not been exposed to SM or DHSM, and the majority of children exposed to these agents prenatally do not develop hearing deficits.[15] The weight of the evidence, however, suggests that the association is genuine, and since there are many alternative agents for the treatment of tuberculosis, SM and DHSM should be avoided, wherever possible.

Aminoglycosides are secreted in breast milk in concentrations approaching that in maternal plasma; however, they are not absorbed through the gastrointestinal tract and are considered safe during lactation.[11–13]

■ ERYTHROMYCIN

The base, stearate, and ethylsuccinate forms of erythromycin have been used during pregnancy for many years without evidence of greater toxicity than in nonpregnant patients. In a study of 161 women receiving erythromycin estolate for 3 to 6 weeks during the latter half of pregnancy, 16 (10 per cent) developed elevations of serum aspartate aminotransferase 3 or more standard deviations above the mean, compared with 3 of 163 women taking placebo.[16] This difference was statistically significant. There were no significant differences between symptoms reported by these two groups of women, and the enzyme elevations decreased shortly after cessation of therapy.

In pregnant patients, the estolate salt should be avoided, since the other forms of erythromycin appear to be safer, and there

is no evidence that any one form is more effective than others despite differences in oral absorption. Fetal toxicity has not been observed with any forms of erythromycin.

Erythromycin crosses the placenta; however, levels in fetal blood and tissues are low, probably never exceeding 10 per cent of the maternal blood level.[1,12]

Erythromycin is also excreted in breast milk, with measured milk/plasma (M/P) ratios of 0.5 to 3.0. Adverse effects have not been noted in breast-fed infants, and erythromycin is considered safe during lactation.[12,13]

■ CLINDAMYCIN

Clindamycin has been used during pregnancy for many years and does not appear to be harmful to the fetus. Clindamycin crosses the placenta readily, achieving fetal blood levels of approximately 20 per cent to 50 per cent of maternal levels.[1,12]

Clindamycin is excreted in breast milk in concentrations below maternal plasma levels. A single case report of bloody diarrhea in a nursing infant whose mother was receiving clindamycin and gentamicin is noted. *Clostridium difficile* was not implicated, and the cause of the diarrhea was not definitively established. Otherwise, experience has shown clindamycin to be safe during lactation.[12,13]

■ SULFONAMIDES

Sulfonamides have been used extensively in the treatment of urinary tract infections in pregnant women. These agents cross the placenta, achieving similar concentrations in fetal and maternal blood.[1,12] Although fetal toxicity has not been clearly demonstrated, a theoretical risk of hemolysis exists because of a relative deficiency of fetal glucose-6-phosphate dehydrogenase (G6PD) and glutathione. Additionally, sulfonamides compete for bilirubin-binding sites on plasma albumin. While excess unconjugated bilirubin may be cleared antenatally by the placenta, the presence of sulfonamide-induced hyperbilirubinemia in the neonate may predispose an infant to kernicterus. For this reason, sulfonamides, particularly long-acting sulfonamides, should be avoided near the end of pregnancy.

Sulfonamides are excreted into breast milk in low concentrations. Diarrhea and skin rash have been reported rarely in exposed nursing infants. Exposure to sulfonamides via breast milk should be avoided in premature infants, jaundiced infants, and those with G6PD deficiency. Breast-feeding is not contraindicated in healthy, full-term infants whose mothers are taking sulfonamides.

FOLIC ACID ANTAGONISTS

Trimethoprim and pyrimethamine both inhibit dihydrofolate reductase, an enzyme critical to the synthesis of folic acid. These agents are much more active against bacterial dihydrofolate reductase than is the human enzyme. Trimethoprim crosses the placenta readily and achieves therapeutic levels in both fetal blood and amniotic fluid. Although limited use of these drugs in human pregnancy does not provide any evidence of teratogenicity, high-dose trimethoprim is teratogenic in rats. Accordingly, these drugs should be avoided in pregnancy wherever possible.[1,12]

Both trimethoprim and pyrimethamine are excreted in breast milk in low concentrations, and there are no contraindications to their use during lactation.[12,13]

QUINOLONES

Nalidixic acid is the prototype agent of this class of drugs, which also includes oxolinic acid, cinoxacin, norfloxacin, and ciprofloxacin. Few data exist for the use of agents of this class during pregnancy, apart from nalidixic acid. No adverse effects on development were observed in 63 neonates whose mothers received nalidixic acid during pregnancy, including 6 who had been exposed during the first trimester.[17] Nevertheless, because adverse effects of the central nervous system have been associated with nalidixic acid in nonpregnant patients, particularly children, some investigators caution against its use during the first trimester of pregnancy, when the fetal brain is in its most crucial stages of development, although others do not. In addition, nalidixic acid and other quinolone antibiotics cause cystic lesions in the articular cartilage of developing

dogs. For these reasons, quinolone antibiotics are contraindicated during pregnancy.

Nalidixic acid is excreted in low concentrations in breast milk. A single case of hemolysis has been reported in a nursing infant with G6PD deficiency. Otherwise, adverse effects have not been reported. Data for other quinolones are not available.

It is preferable to avoid quinolones in lactating women, especially since there are usually safer alternatives. When quinolone therapy is unavoidable, we favor temporary formula feeding.

NITROFURANTOIN

Nitrofurantoin readily crosses the placenta, achieving fetal serum levels at least as great as maternal levels.[1,12] As in the maternal situation, drug levels outside the urinary tract are inadequate to treat infection. Nitrofurantoin has been used for many years in the treatment of urinary tract infection during pregnancy, and it appears to be quite safe, without any evidence of fetal toxicity. As with sulfonamides, a theoretical risk of hemolysis due to fetal G6PD deficiency exists; however, such toxicity has not been reported.

Trivial amounts of nitrofurantoin have been measured in breast milk, but adverse effects in breast-fed infants have not been reported.[12,13]

VANCOMYCIN

Vancomycin is a glycopolypeptide antibiotic that is used increasingly in the treatment of gram-positive infections. Little is known about its ability to cross the human placenta. Its high molecular weight of approximately 1450 daltons would present a substantial obstacle to placental transfer. On the other hand, in pregnant rabbits vancomycin has been shown to cross the placenta to enter fetal blood and amniotic fluid. Given the lack of human data, alternative agents should be selected when possible, but vancomycin should not be withheld in the case of serious infections caused by methicillin-resistant staphylococci.

Data regarding the excretion of vancomycin in breast milk are not available; however, vancomycin is not absorbed via the gastrointestinal tract. Therefore, we consider maternal vancomycin therapy compatible with breast-feeding.

■ CHLORAMPHENICOL

Chloramphenicol is currently rarely used in adults, but its use is indicated occasionally. Chloramphenicol has been shown to cross the placenta readily, achieving similar levels in fetal and maternal blood at term. [1,12] In addition to its well-known toxicity to the bone marrow, chloramphenicol can cause the gray baby syndrome when administered postnatally to neonates. This syndrome is related to excessive serum levels of chloramphenicol and would be very unlikely to occur in neonates who receive no further drug postnatally. Significant fetal adverse effects from maternal chloramphenicol have not been reported, and chloramphenicol is not contraindicated during pregnancy. [1,12]

Chloramphenicol is excreted into breast milk in approximately half the concentration found in maternal plasma. [11,12] Such quantities are inadequate to produce the gray baby syndrome, but theoretically could cause bone marrow depression, although this has not been reported. Minor adverse effects in infants exposed to chloramphenicol through breast-feeding have been reported, including refusal of the breast, falling asleep during feeding, intestinal gas, and vomiting. [12] There is a lack of consensus regarding the advisability of breast-feeding during maternal chloramphenicol use, and we favor avoiding breast-feeding during such exposure.

■ METRONIDAZOLE

Metronidazole crosses the placenta, achieving similar fetal and maternal blood levels. [1,12] Because metronidazole is mutagenic in bacteria and carcinogenic in some but not all animal species, some clinicians have been reluctant to use this drug in pregnant women, although it is not teratogenic in animals. Considerable clinical experience with metronidazole has not demonstrated any evidence of teratogenicity or carcinogenicity; [18] however, metronidazole should be avoided in the first trimester, if possible.

Metronidazole is excreted in breast milk in concentrations approximating those in maternal plasma; however, plasma concentrations in nursing infants are about 20 per cent of maternal levels. [12] Adverse effects in breast-fed infants have not been reported, except for a single case of diarrhea. The American Academy of Pediatrics recommends interrupting breast-feeding during maternal metronidazole therapy, [13] but we find no justification for this recommendation.

■ TETRACYCLINES

The tetracyclines cross the placenta readily. These drugs are contraindicated during pregnancy, since they frequently cause permanent discoloration of the developing teeth, much as they do when given to infants and young children. [19] Pancreatitis and fatty metamorphosis of the liver have been described in five pregnant women receiving tetracycline for the treatment of urinary tract infection. [20] All these women were azotemic, and since tetracycline is primarily excreted by the kidney, the toxicity may have been related to markedly elevated levels of drug. Whether or not there is increased maternal toxicity during pregnancy, tetracycline should be avoided for fetal reasons.

Tetracycline is excreted in breast milk, with reported M/P ratios of between 0.25 and 1.5; however, fetal serum levels are negligible or undetectable. It is presumed that the high concentration of calcium ions contained in the milk is sufficient to chelate the tetracycline and prevent its absorption. Adverse effects in infants exposed to tetracycline via breast milk have not been reported, and tetracycline is considered safe during lactation. [12,13]

■ ANTIMYCOBACTERIAL DRUGS

Isonicotinic acid hydrazine (INH), rifampin, and streptomycin all cross the placenta. [1,12,21] Streptomycin should be avoided during pregnancy because of its toxicity to the fetal ear. [14] INH has proved to be quite safe in pregnancy, [1,12,21,22] but it is recommended that pregnant women routinely receive pyridoxine while on this medication. Rifampin is teratogenic in rodents, but not rabbits. [21]

There are no convincing data that rifampin is teratogenic in humans, and indeed it is generally recommended for the treatment of tuberculosis during pregnancy.[21,22] Ethambutol is teratogenic in both rabbits and rats[21] but does not appear to be toxic in human fetal development.[21,22] INH, rifampin, and ethambutol are considered the safest antimycobacterial drugs for use in pregnancy.[21,22] The safety in pregnancy of pyrazinamide and third-line agents is unknown; therefore, these agents should be avoided.

Both INH and rifampin are secreted in breast milk, and adverse effects have not been reported in exposed infants.[12] Nevertheless, because of the prolonged duration of treatment, we favor avoiding breast-feeding during antimycobacterial therapy.

■ ANTIFUNGALS

Limited information is available regarding the use of systemic antifungal drugs during pregnancy. The experience with amphotericin B during pregnancy has been reviewed by Ismail and Lerner.[23] No evidence of teratogenicity was observed in 21 pregnancies. Twenty infants were normal and one died of coccidioidomycosis 19 days postpartum. Maternal toxicity was similar to that in nonpregnant individuals. Amphotericin B crosses the placenta, achieving fetal blood levels of about one third of maternal levels at term.

Flucytosine is teratogenic in rats. Although flucytosine has been used successfully in three pregnant women without adverse effects on fetal outcome, we believe that it is contraindicated during pregnancy.

Ketoconazole is teratogenic in rats and thus should be avoided during pregnancy, although data regarding human safety are lacking. Miconazole is not teratogenic in rats or rabbits, but since human data are unavailable, it should be avoided during pregnancy.

Griseofulvin is an oral agent used exclusively for dermatophyte infections, although it has been largely replaced by ketoconazole. Griseofulvin is both embryotoxic and teratogenic in rats and thus should be avoided during pregnancy.

Vaginal preparations of nystatin and various imidazoles have proved to be safe and effective in pregnancy. Slight systemic absorption of vaginally administered imidazoles has been observed, but the degree of placental transfer, if any, is unknown. Some clinicians choose to defer treatment of vaginal candidiasis during pregnancy until after the first trimester, if the symptoms are tolerable.

Data regarding excretion in breast milk and safety of breast-feeding during maternal antifungal therapy are not available. Given the fact that amphotericin B and miconazole are not absorbed orally, we consider these drugs compatible with breast-feeding. In addition, we would not interrupt breast-feeding for topical or vaginal antifungal therapy, but we would recommend against breast-feeding during maternal flucytosine or ketoconazole therapy.

■ ANTIVIRAL AGENTS

Few data exist regarding the safety of antiviral drugs during pregnancy. Since most of these agents are antimetabolites, they should be avoided whenever possible.

Amantadine, active against influenza A virus, is embryotoxic and teratogenic in animals. Accordingly, it should not be used in pregnancy. Vidarabine is also teratogenic in laboratory animals and should be avoided during pregnancy.

Acyclovir has been shown to cross the placenta in both rats and rabbits, and there is no evidence of teratogenicity in these two species. Its safety in human pregnancy is not established, although no adverse events have been observed in a small number of human pregnancies. It is recommended that acyclovir be used only in pregnancy for life-threatening situations, such as herpes simplex encephalitis.

Ribavirin is teratogenic in rabbits and rats, but not baboons. Accordingly, it should be avoided during pregnancy, except for the treatment of Lassa fever in which, despite the risk, the benefits of treatment may offset the known high mortality of untreated disease.

Zidovudine is contraindicated in pregnancy because of lack of data regarding safety.

Data regarding the safety of alpha-interferon during pregnancy are lacking, but as this is a natural product of human leukocytes, it is highly unlikely that interferon will present any hazard to the fetus.

Data regarding the safety of antiviral therapy during lactation are unavailable, and therefore, we recommend against breastfeeding during maternal antiviral therapy.

■ ANTIMALARIAL DRUGS

Chloroquine has been used extensively during pregnancy, without evidence of congenital malformations. Chloroquine crosses the placenta and occasionally has been reported to cause cochleovestibular damage in the fetus when given daily to treat rheumatic disease in the mother.[24] This has not been reported when given to treat or prevent malaria that can adversely affect the pregnancy. Its benefits, therefore, clearly outweigh its risks.[25]

Primaquine, used to eradicate hepatic hypnozoites of *Plasmodium vivax* and *P. ovale*, is not recommended during pregnancy, since it may precipitate hemolysis in individuals deficient in glucose-6-phosphate dehydrogenase and glutathione, such as the developing fetus. Maternal relapses may be prevented by weekly prophylactic chloroquine until the postpartum period, when primaquine can be given. Dapsone should be avoided for the same reasons.

Pyrimethamine and proguanil should be avoided, as they are folate antagonists. Sulfonamides should be avoided near term to reduce the likelihood of kernicterus. Tetracyclines are contraindicated, as discussed previously.

Quinine was formerly used in high dosage as an abortifacient. Hypoplasia of the optic nerve and congenital deafness were observed in the offspring of mothers treated unsuccessfully for this purpose; however, teratogenicity has not been observed when therapeutic dosages have been used. We recommend that quinine not be used prophylactically or to treat chloroquine-susceptible strains. Quinine, together with clindamycin, should still be used during pregnancy for proven chloroquine-resistant *P. falciparum* infection.

■ ANTIPROTOZOAL AGENTS

Considerably fewer data are available regarding placental transfer and safety of antiprotozoal drugs during pregnancy, compared with antibacterial drugs. The use of metronidazole (for amebiasis, giardiasis, and trichomoniasis), amphotericin B (for leishmaniasis), trimethoprim-sulfamethoxazole (for isosporiasis and pneumocystosis), pyrimethamine-sulfonamide (for toxoplasmosis), and antimalarial agents has been discussed.

The principal luminally active amebicides are diloxanide furoate, diiodohydroxyquin, and paromomycin. The safety of these agents during pregnancy is not well documented. Since diloxanide is well absorbed from the gastrointestinal tract whereas the other two are only trivially absorbed, diloxanide probably should be avoided, even though it is not teratogenic in laboratory animals. Asymptomatic amebic cyst passers should not be treated during pregnancy, but patients with invasive amebic disease should be treated with metronidazole.

Of the agents effective in giardiasis, metronidazole is safest for use in pregnancy. An increased fetal death rate has been demonstrated in rats after quinacrine exposure, but human data are lacking. Furazolidone is not teratogenic in laboratory animals but induces mammary neoplasia in rats and, in addition, is less effective than either metronidazole or quinacrine. Paromomycin, an aminoglycoside used orally as a luminal amebicide, also has been advocated for giardiasis during pregnancy. Paromomycin is likely to be safe; however, data regarding its efficacy in giardiasis are limited. As with intestinal amebiasis, patients with giardiasis who have few or no symptoms should not be treated until after delivery.

Pentamidine has been given to thousands of pregnant African women during chemoprophylactic campaigns against trypanosomiasis. In most instances, injections were limited to women in the latter half of pregnancy, and dose reduction was not uncommon. No increases in abortions, premature deliveries, or malformations were reported. However, in Africa, failure to recognize teratogenicity implies only that gross fetal damage has not occurred. Given the consequences of failure to treat trypanosomiasis in its early stages, and the observation that pentamidine is not an obvious teratogen, the benefits of pentamidine treatment outweigh its potential risks.

The safety of suramin, nifurtimox, melarsoprol, and stibogluconate during pregnancy is not well established; however, pregnant women with the trypanosomiases and invasive forms of leishmaniasis should be treated for maternal reasons. If the gestational age is suitably young, the option of terminating the pregnancy should be contemplated, not only because of possible fetal drug toxicity but also because congenital cases of Chagas' disease and kala-azar have been reported.

■ ANTHELMINTIC AGENTS

The great majority of helminth infections are unaccompanied by symptoms. When symptoms occur, they are frequently mild. Few worm infections will result in significant morbidity if treatment is delayed or even never administered. Furthermore, the safety of most anthelmintic agents during pregnancy is not established. Therefore, for most pregnant women infected with helminths, the prudent course of action is to defer treatment until after delivery. Expert consultation is recommended before using these agents during pregnancy.

■ Summary

In this chapter, we reviewed the physiologic changes of pregnancy that alter drug pharmacokinetic parameters from those of the nonpregnant state, and we reviewed the factors influencing transfer of drugs across the placenta and into breast milk.

We then examined the data available regarding the safety during pregnancy and lactation of specific antimicrobial agents. Insufficient data are available for too many of these agents. Accordingly, the clinician must be certain that antimicrobial therapy is truly indicated in a given patient, and then select the least toxic efficacious agent.

When newer agents that have not been evaluated for safety in pregnancy are deemed to be essential for maternal welfare, the treating physician should keep careful records regarding possible adverse effects, particularly on fetal outcome, or the lack thereof, and report the results to the appropriate drug regulatory agency, so that we will have better information in the future than we have now.

Most drugs are safe during lactation, but when there is uncertainty, temporary formula feeding during maternal drug therapy is recommended.

REFERENCES

1. Chow AW, Jewesson PJ. Pharmacokinetics and safety of antimicrobial agents during pregnancy. Rev Infect Dis 1985; 7:287–311.
2. Parry E, Shields R, Turnbell AC. Transit time in the small intestine in pregnancy. J Obstet Gynecol Br Commonw 1970; 77:900–901.
3. Mendenhall NW. Serum protein concentrations in pregnancy. I. Concentrations in maternal serum. Am J Obstet Gynecol 1970; 106:388–399.
4. Fever G. Action of pregnancy and various progesterones on hepatic microsomal activities. Drug Metab Rev 1979; 9:147–169.
5. Sims EAH, Krantz KE. Serial studies of renal function during pregnancy and the puerperium in normal women. J Clin Invest 1958; 37:1764–1771.
6. Moore KL. The Developing Human; Clinically Oriented Embryology. 4th ed. Philadelphia: WB Saunders, 1988.
7. Mirkin BL. Pharmacodynamics and drug disposition in pregnant women, in neonates, and in children. In Melmon KL, Morelli HF (eds). Clinical Pharmacology; Basic Principles in Therapeutics. 2nd ed. New York: Macmillan, 1978.
8. Juchau MR. Mechanisms of drug biotransformation reactions in the placenta. Fed Proc 1972; 31:48–51.
9. McCarthy T, Saunders P. The origin and circulation of the amniotic fluid. In Fairwether DVI, Eskes TKAB (eds). Amniotic Fluid—Research and Clinical Applications. 2nd revised ed. New York: Excerpta Medica, 1978.
10. Howard FM, Hill JM. Drugs in pregnancy. Obstet Gynecol Surv 1979; 34:643–653.
11. Wilson JT, Brown RD, Cherek DR, et al. Drug excretion in human breast milk: principles, pharmacokinetics and projected consequences. Clin Pharmacokin 1980; 5:1–66.
12. Briggs GG, Freeman RK, Yaffe SJ. Drugs in Pregnancy and Lactation. 2nd ed. Baltimore: Williams and Wilkins, 1986.
13. Committee on Drugs, American Academy of Pediatrics. The transfer of drugs and other chemicals into human breast milk. Pediatrics 1983; 72:375–383.
14. Robinson GC, Cambon KG. Hearing loss in infants of tuberculous mothers treated with streptomycin during pregnancy. N Engl J Med 1964; 271:949–951.
15. Warkany J. Antituberculous drugs. Teratology 1979; 20:133–138.
16. McCormack WM, George H, Donner A, Kodgis LF, Alpert S, Lowe EW, Kass EH. Hepatotoxicity of erythromycin estolate during pregnancy. Antimicrob Agents Chemother 1977; 12:630–635.
17. Murray EDS. Nalidixic acid in pregnancy. Br Med J 1981; 282:224.
18. Peterson WF, Stauch JE, Ryder CD. Metronidazole in pregnancy. Am J Obstet Gynecol 1966; 94:343–349.
19. Kutscher AH, Zegarelli EV, Tovell HMM, Hochberg B, Hauptman J. Discoloration of deciduous teeth induced by administration of tetracycline antepartum. Am J Obstet Gynecol 1966; 96:291–292.
20. Whalley PJ, Adams RH, Combes B. Tetracycline toxicity in pregnancy. JAMA 1964; 189:357–362.
21. Good JT Jr, Iseman MD, Davidson PT, Lakshminarayan S, Sahn SA. Tuberculosis in association with pregnancy. Am J Obstet Gynecol 1981; 140:492–498.

22. Snider DE Jr, Layde PM, Johnson MW, Lyle MA. Treatment of tuberculosis during pregnancy. Am Rev Respir Dis 1980; 122:65–79.
23. Ismail MA, Lerner SA. Disseminated blastomycosis in a pregnant woman. Review of amphotericin B usage during pregnancy. Am Rev Resp Dis 1982; 126:350–353.
24. Hart CW, Naunton RF. The ototoxicity of chloroquine phosphate. Arch Otolaryngol 1964; 80:407–412.
25. Centers for Disease Control. Health information for international travel 1988. Publication No. (CDC)88-8280):102–103. Washington, DC: US Public Health Service, Department of Health and Human Services, 1988.

Apnea and apparent life-threatening events in infancy

John E. Yount

For 1 in 500 infants aged 1 to 6 months, an episode of stopped breathing or unusual color will be observed.[1] These incidents become some of the most hard to accept and disquieting histories for the office practitioner or emergency room physician. The parent of an apparently healthy infant determinedly insists that the baby was found limp, motionless, and very pale, or even cyanotic, and was aroused only after vigorous effort. For several years these episodes were labeled "near-SIDS" or "aborted-SIDS"—relating the episode to the sudden infant death syndrome (SIDS), which is the most common cause of infant mortality after 2 weeks of age. Although there is some link between apnea and SIDS, there is enough uncertainty about the precise relationship that the current trend is to avoid names that overstress the threat of SIDS in the minds of parents. The terms *apnea of infancy* (AOI) and *apparent life-threatening event* (ALTE) have been coined and given support by a recent National Institutes of Health (NIH) panel of experts. ALTE presentations may have a treatable etiology or they may have no clear cause, in which case the infant is described as having AOI.[1]

■ Background

Probably there were many occurrences of infant apnea before the 1970s, but the condition was not reported in the medical literature except as a symptom secondary to other primary diseases. It now seems clear that prolonged apnea can be both a secondary symptom and a primary form of pathologic behavior particularly likely to occur in infants. As with convulsions, breath-holding, and a few other pediatric conditions, the occurrence of ALTE is apparently affected by neurologic predisposition, developmental age, underlying genetic factors, infection, and the random appearance of conditions in the environment that may influence the infant's behavior. Examples of the latter are room temperature changes, fever, and sleeping regularity. Apnea may be the first symptom of several treatable diseases (Table 1).[1-3] If the severity of ALTE symptoms is excessive for the degree of primary disease, observation with a monitor may be needed to confirm tolerance of the next similar disease exposure.

The risk of later sudden infant death syndrome has been shown to be higher in the group of infants who have had an ALTE. The risk may be as much as 30 to 50 times greater than the risk of 1.5 to 2.0 SIDS deaths per 1000 infants born in North America.[4] The association with unexplained death and recurrent ALTE has resulted in the use of infant monitors and medication at home.[1,5]

■ INFANTS AT HIGHEST RISK

The association of presenting symptoms and concurrent clinical or social conditions causes some infants an even greater risk of death and recurrent episodes. There is evidence of dramatically increased mortality (20 to 30 per cent) for infants with severe recurrent ALTE events and a later seizure disorder.[5] A comparable risk of death (20 to 25 per cent) is described for infants who have prolonged apnea documented on an overnight recording 37 weeks postconception and whose parents do not complete assessment of stress tolerance or contact their apnea program before discontinuing monitor use.[6] In one report describing nine such deaths among 40 infants, seven were thought to be "healthy," developing, preterm infants ready for discharge until a cardiorespiratory Holter recording showed unsuspected sleep apnea.[7] Preterm infants' parents seem to be less likely to be compliant in monitor use than parents whose infant has had an ALTE.[1,5,7] Infants surviving the neonatal period with chronic lung injury severe enough to require a prolonged interval of supplemental oxygen show evidence of both an increased risk for apnea during episodes of hypoxic stress[8] and an increased incidence (10 to 12 per cent) of death from SIDS.[9] Infants exposed to illicit drugs, especially cocaine, have been reported to have increased risk (15 to 17 per cent) of an early, unexpected death, but these data are unclear.[10]

Most apnea-prone infants will lose the tendency to have apneic events with growth and time, and a few will apparently adapt to becoming adults with sleep apnea of varying degrees of significance[11] (see article on Sleep Apnea). The purpose of this chapter is to outline a concise, practical management plan to deal safely with infants.

■ NORMAL VARIATIONS IN CARDIORESPIRATORY ACTIVITY

Normal Breathing Frequency and Heart Rate. For term infants, normal behavior in quiet sleep ranges from 20 to 60 breaths per minute and from 90 to 160 heart beats per minute on a 1-minute time base.[12,13] These frequencies normally would increase upon altered metabolic demand with acidosis, cold stress, or fever, and also upon decreased pulmonary efficiency from cardiac failure or respiratory illness. For the first few days after birth, the heart rate for term infants in quiet sleep is lower than at 2 to 6 weeks of age, when the lowest expected heart rate is slightly in excess of 110 beats per minute. The average resting heart rate for all term infants at 6 weeks of age ranges from 115 to 140 beats per minute and gradually declines over the next 6 months to 85 to 135 beats per minute.[13]

A small percentage of infants have sporadic ectopic beats (atrial, junctional, or ventricular) without apparent cause or harm.[13,18] One in several hundred infants presents with a congenital arrhythmia that requires management. The breathing frequency and heart rate of infants normally

increase 50 per cent to 100 per cent or more with altered activity and the sleep state.[12,13] Observation of the face and chest reveals little breathing movement for many infants. Maximal breathing motion at rest is usually at the abdomen due to the diaphragm pressing the contents of the abdominal cavity against a relaxed anterior muscle wall.[14]

Normal Apneic Pauses. Studies of normal infants recorded while sleeping either under laboratory conditions or in a normal environment show many short central apneas in the course of a full night's sleep. These pauses are commonly 4 to 12 seconds in duration and occur after deep sighs in quiet sleep or randomly in REM sleep. It would be extremely rare for a normal term infant older than 2 weeks to exhibit a breathing pause of 13 or more seconds.[12,13,15] Apneic pauses of 15 or more seconds have never been reported in healthy control infants over 2 weeks of age. A 15-second interval is used by many apnea programs as the division between normal and abnormal behavior.[16,26]

Periodic Breathing. At least a third of normal term infants may exhibit short intervals of three or more sequential apneic pauses within 20 seconds of each other in quiet sleep. This pattern of alternating pauses and breathing is called periodic breathing.[1] This periodic pattern occurs in 10 per cent or more of the quiet sleep of infants at postconceptional ages under 38 weeks and in up to 2 per cent of quiet sleep of normal term infants in the first 6 months of life.[15] This pattern is seen in sleeping older children or adults only when mild hypoxia (such as that due to high altitudes) or an alteration in body chemistry (as in ketoacidosis) is present.[17] At some undetermined time after 6 months of age, periodic breathing is not normally noted at sea level.

■ ABNORMAL BEHAVIOR

Abnormal Apnea

Three principal forms of abnormal events are recognized:

- (1) central apnea—no evidence of neural signals generating respiratory effort,
- (2) obstructive apnea—blockage of the airway and absence of airflow despite adequate effort because of incoordination in

pharyngeal or laryngeal supporting structures, and
- (3) mixed apnea—both absence of effort and airway occlusion are present during different stages or a single event.[1,16]

A fourth pattern of behavior, consisting of continuous forced exhalation and deep cyanosis, has been described recently in older pediatric patients and termed expiratory apnea.[18]

Among both term and preterm patients aged 42 or more weeks postconception, a few unusual infants can exhibit prolonged apnea, prolonged hypoventilation, or both intermittently. This tendency may not be present every night and usually will be exacerbated by intercurrent illness and sleep disruption. In the normal home, these episodes can and probably do occur repeatedly for this small group of infants, without any care provider seeing warning behavior. It has been suggested that ALTE "episodes" are simply the random detection of one apneic interval from among many recurrent events that have increased in frequency upon changes in the infant's health or environment.[16]

We know that some of these infants later die even if the condition is recognized and treated. Most often the deaths occur during a mild interval of illness or disrupted care when the infant has been removed from a monitor before the apnea program has given clearance for it. Very rarely, infants have died while undergoing presumably effective monitor surveillance.[1,5] Since apneic behavior may arise from a variety of conditions that all happen to have apnea or an ALTE as a common symptom, the prognosis may vary greatly, depending on the cause. Rarely, infants have presented with apnea and then months later manifested a clear neurologic disease or tumor.[1,18]

Abnormal Responses to Hypoxia and Hypercapnia

Some infants presenting with an ALTE history are observed to hypoventilate in sleep without apnea.

As they fall asleep, these infants with normal muscle strength develop elevated carbon dioxide and marginal oxygen levels without evidence of central or obstructed apnea, because of their failure to maintain an adequate depth and frequency of breathing despite normal muscle strength. This condition was felt to be extremely rare, but now that artificial ventilatory support facilities are widely available, it appears that a small number of infants who receive immediate ventilatory support at birth are not able to sustain normal CO_2 in sleep. Other infants with more marginal defects may present after several weeks of age.[19]

Most infants presenting with a history of ALTE behavior increase ventilation with slightly increased CO_2 and lowered O_2 in inspired air in a way that overlaps with the response of normal infants. The response to suddenly induced, profound hypoxia (11 per cent FIO_2) is arousal in a normal sleeping infant, but there is less evidence of arousal for most infants who have an ALTE history.[20] Many infants requiring supplemental oxygen for treatment of neonatal chronic lung injuries will develop apnea that lasts long enough to require stimulation after a profound hypoxic challenge.[8]

■ PATIENTS WHO SHOULD BE MONITORED

Plans for care of infants after an apneic episode changed in May, 1978, with an official statement by a special ad hoc committee of the American Academy of Pediatrics. The committee recommended home monitor use for all infants documented to have central apnea in excess of 20 seconds, or shorter apnea with associated bradycardia, cyanosis, pallor, or profound hypotonia. The NIH-sponsored Consensus Development Conference on Infantile Apnea and Home Monitoring in 1986 sorted through the complex issues of care, harm, and cost for the families expected to monitor infants at home. They also outlined the type of family education and social support system necessary to maintain effective monitoring in the home.[1]

Four groups of infants were listed as requiring routine monitor use at home on the basis of both medical need and cost-benefit:

- (1) infants found after a severe apparent life-threatening event, usually at home,
- (2) preterm infants with symptomatic behavior at the normal time for hospital discharge,
- (3) infants born into families in which two or more siblings had died of sudden infant death syndrome, and

- (4) infants with congenital or acquired diseases associated with an increased need for resuscitation.

Other groups with a relative potential need based on individual family and physician choice were:

- (1) infants in a home where one sibling had died of SIDS,
- (2) infants experiencing very mild ALTE behavior,
- (3) infants born to mothers who abused opiates or cocaine, and
- (4) infants with tracheostomies.

The consensus panel was particularly concerned about the potential for harm as well as benefit in using monitors, and stressed that families in these last four groups "should not be made to feel guilty" if they elected not to use an infant monitor. They also emphasized the harm that would be created by overuse of monitors, unsupervised over-the-counter sale of unproven monitor systems and general prescription of equipment for all preterm infants after discharge, and overanxious parents of term infants.[21]

■ Management

■ PROLONGED INFANT APNEA OR ALTE

In infants and very young children, apnea is a symptom known to be the product of several conditions (Table 1). Except when the infant involved in an ALTE is marginally resuscitatable and in shock, or requires support for obvious concurrent illness, it is often tempting to reject the need for further investigation because no abnormality is detected. Despite the benign appearance of most infants within minutes of the ALTE episode, there is now strong evidence that these infants are at significantly increased risk for both recurrent ALTE episodes and death from SIDS. After treatable conditions have been controlled or ruled out, routine monitor use is recommended for all patients with severe ALTE at risk for recurrence.[21]

With more complete diagnostic and treatment facilities now available in many communities, there is currently a need to deter-

mine carefully in each patient with ALTE admitted to hospital how many diagnostic studies should be done. Logical samples and studies for diagnosis of pertinent conditions in Table 1 should be obtained, depending on the history and physical examination. Sometimes detailed fluoroscopic studies of the effect of position and the neurophysiology of feeding are helpful. An electrocardiogram (ECG), electroencephalogram (EEG), and overnight sleep polygraph, including pulse O_2 saturation and end-tidal CO_2 or transcutaneous carbon dioxide ($TcCO_2$) level, are often performed following severe ALTE events.[1]

While the confirmation of prolonged apnea or hypoventilation syndrome is an important and valuable demonstration of the need for treatment, few infants with clearly abnormal histories have abnormal behavior. Depending on the methods used and the effect of some diagnostic techniques on the sleep state, abnormal activity in a few infants has been observed in several studies performed overnight from various centers, each assessing over 100 subjects within 24 to 48 hours of ALTE episodes.[1] Many of the documented instances of later deaths or severe recurrent ALTE episodes have occurred among those infants who had normal behavior as detectable by currently available clinical tests.[15] Deciding whether an infant needs to be watched at home with a monitor at present depends mostly on a careful, detailed analysis of the history of the presenting event.

Reviewing the History

It has usually been helpful to reconstruct the event fully, including the level of awareness of the person finding the infant, the reason for contact with the infant, and all the associated activity of the involved adults capable of accurately describing what they saw. If the event has just occurred and was severe, it is wisest to arrange hospitalization overnight to observe the infant, document the history, and educate the family.

If the infant is described to have had rather mild behavior, or when the event did not prompt immediate contact with medical care, then screening the infant's behavior at home with a multichannel recording, such as a tracing of pulse oxygen saturation, the pulse wave, breathing pattern at the abdomen, and ECG, is a much more cost-effec-

TABLE 1. Diseases Causing Central and Obstructive Apnea in Infants

	Preterm	*Term Neonate*	*Infant*
Anatomic and Developmental	Apnea of prematurity Respiratory distress syndrome Patent ductus arteriosus Transient hyperammonemia Gastric reflux	Pierre Robin syndrome Treacher Collins syndrome Goldenhar's syndrome Choanal atresia Nasopharyngeal dermoid Laryngeal atresia Gastric reflux	Apnea of infancy Arnold-Chiari syndrome Trisomy 21 Glossoptosis Expiratory apnea Gastric reflux

Neuromuscular	CNS hemorrhage, cysts, tumors
	Seizures of any type
		CNS hemorrhage, cysts, tumors
		Seizures of any type
		Dysautonomias
			CNS hemorrhage, cysts, tumors
			Seizures
			  Complex partial
			  Temporal
			  Alpha motor
			  ?Subcortical
			Dysautonomias
			Rett's syndrome
			Myopathy of beta-fibers

Infectious *Bacteremia-Septicemia*	Beta-streptococcus *Escherichia coli* *Klebsiella, Enterobacter* Coag-neg. staphylococcus	Beta-streptococcus *Escherichia coli* *Klebsiella* *Listeria*	*Bordetella pertussis* *Haemophilus influenzae* Beta-streptococcus *Meningococcus* *Escherichia coli*
Viremia-Septicemia	Respiratory syncytial virus Coxsackie virus Cytomegalovirus Herpes simplex	Respiratory syncytial virus Coxsackie virus Herpes simplex ECHO virus Cytomegalovirus	Respiratory syncytial virus Coxsackie virus Herpes simplex ECHO virus Cytomegalovirus
Parasitic	*Chlamydia*	*Chlamydia*	*Chlamydia*
Metabolic	Hypoglycemia Hyponatremia Hypocalcemia Hypomagnesemia B_6 deficiency	Hypoglycemia Hyponatremia Hypocalcemia Hypomagnesemia B_6 deficiency Adrenal hyperplasia	Hypoglycemia Hyponatremia Hypocalcemia Hypomagnesemia Adrenal hyperplasia
Genetic *Carbohydrate* *Amino Acid*	Lactic acidemias Nonketotic hyperglycinemia Tyrosinemia Methylmalonic acidemia	Lactic acidemias Nonketotic hyperglycinemia Tyrosinemia Methylmalonic acidemia	Lactic acidemias Branched chain defects Urea cycle defects (hyperammonemias)
Lipid			Acyl-CoA deficiencies
Iatrogenic	Anemia Hypermagnesemia Endotracheal tube kinking & blockage Nares blocked by NJ & NG tubes and tape and eye patches for phototherapy Head flexion Hyperthermia & hypothermia Hypoxia with bronchopulmonary dysplasia or chronic lung injury Benzyl alcohol poisoning	Anemia Hypermagnesemia Nares obstruction by eye patches for phototherapy Endotracheal tube kinking & blockage Hyperthermia & hypothermia Hypoxia with bronchopulmonary dysplasia or chronic lung injury	Foreign body aspiration Battered baby syndrome Hyperthermia & hypothermia Hypochloremic alkalosis Hyperphosphatemia Münchausen-by-proxy Hypoxia with bronchopulmonary dysplasia or chronic lung injury

tive method of attempting to be certain that there is no frequent occurrence of hypoxia. If the history is quite marginal and the recording at home shows over 12 hours of normal, quiet sleeping behavior with good oxygenation, there seems little reason for further concern or intervention.

For significant episodes lasting more than 20 seconds, with depression, slow arousal, pallor or cyanosis, and other suspicious behavior, the absence of recognized symptoms in hospital or later in the first several days at home does not alter the plan to watch with a monitor for several weeks. A single night's sleep in a strange, stimulating environment without showing unusual breathing does not mean that the infant will tolerate the next stress of infection or major disturbance in care. If abnormal patterns are recorded, the risk of SIDS may be increased[7] (also see Parental Compliance).

Reconstructing the Presenting Event

It is important to avoid providing "correct" answers to the questions and at the same time to elicit the full history of how severe the child's depression really was and how long it lasted. It is wisest not to accept any history at face value but to ask each person to describe what brought them to the baby, what the baby was last seen doing, the timing of feeding, and other data related to overall activity in the environment. It is always important to get individual histories from each person present during the ALTE. Be sure that there was adequate light and exposure of the infant to allow an accurate assessment before committing a specific duration or color change for the event on paper. Many infants will not exhibit color changes that are easily interpreted by parents in the available light of the home, but questions about appearance sometimes are helpful.

It is important to get a sense of how rapidly the baby first responded to contact, and any sounds or movements the baby made. Most healthy infants would not allow vigorous stimulation or resuscitation without prompt, vocal protest. A history of "blowing in the nose and mouth" may refer to simply blowing at the infant without lip contact. Ask for a demonstration without giving information.

The perception of time is not well developed for most observers. The time estimates

they initially provide will usually be far in excess of reality and should not be entered in the medical record until there has been an effort to have the observer "feel" measured time intervals for reference. Many parents are unaware of the fact that infants normally can have short breathing pauses in sleep. If it is not clear what they have seen, ask them to describe the length of the event and the resuscitation while checking a watch. Ask all persons providing an event history to sit quietly for 10 and 15 seconds to give them the "feel" of normal variations. It is sometimes helpful to have the person providing the history pantomime the movements and distances through which action occurred while the action is timed.

It is usually necessary to ask specific questions about the facial appearance (eyes open or shut), eye movements, muscle tone (limp, normal, or rigid), presence of emesis, evidence for shaking or recurrent movement, and other evidence for associated seizures, for most parents do not provide that information spontaneously. In each instance it is worthwhile inquiring about any previous spells the family may have seen in this child or in other family members. Some kindreds with multiple instances of ALTE and SIDS have been described as a result of metabolic defects.[2,4]

It is often revealing to ask whether any friends or other family have had infants who have experienced ALTE episodes or SIDS. Whereas a positive response may not be sufficient to discount a significant history, obviously there will be even greater need for careful education about normal apneic activity and the factors influencing SIDS risks. If the history does seem insignificant, the education may be the most appropriate intervention. A monitor may create as much anxiety as reassurance because of false alarms, and it is then a significant and purposeless expense, as well as a social albatross.

Awake ALTE Events

Some disruptions in breathing that cause parental concern are not associated with sleep. These usually divide into two distinct groups, based on severity. If the event is significant, usually it will be associated with more complex behavior, often with a component of seizure activity or productive of seizures. Monitors have a role for severe disruptions in breathing, awake or asleep, but additional diagnostic and treatment programs are often needed to sort out complex neurologic behavior. Insignificant awake events are usually the most benign behavior that prompts referral. This is possibly because overanxious parents tend to react to activity during periods of maximal contact, especially during care provision when the infant is awake much of the time. The prognosis for awake events is thought to be better than for sleep events.[1]

Apnea and Later SIDS Death

It is important from the outset to avoid labeling any living infant with terms referring to sudden infant death syndrome. Most infant apnea patients will not die. Many infants with an ALTE presentation in the era before monitors were introduced are alive now. The difficulty is in recognizing those who may be transiently dependent on monitoring until they mature. Fewer than 10 per cent of SIDS victims were observed to have an unusual breathing pattern.[1,4] It is unknown whether this means that most victims of SIDS do not have abnormal breathing control as a cause of death, or whether any transient warning spells are too subtle to be seen in routine care.

Münchausen-by-Proxy

A small number of parents have unusual psychopathologic needs that cause them to describe nonexistent episodes, or more rarely, to create life-threatening behavior by occluding their child's airway. These parents often will give the appearance of being extremely interested in pleasing the staff and initially may appear to be the epitome of concern. Key hints in recognizing these cases of Münchausen-by-proxy are the occurrence of repeated severe ALTE episodes in hospital when only the parent is present, and the refusal of the model parent ever to leave the child's side, sometimes not even for meals. This freakish and frightening parental behavior is present in fewer than 1 per cent of ALTE cases and has been associated with apparent later infanticide.[1,4,18]

■ SYMPTOMATIC PRETERM INFANTS AT DISCHARGE

Apnea of Prematurity. At least 30 to 50 per cent of preterm infants are found to have apnea that has no "cause" other than immaturity. Some preterm infants require weeks of ventilatory or medical support for apnea. Continuous physiologic recordings of infants confirm that abnormal transient apneic behavior often will escape the awareness of experienced medical personnel in an intensive care setting.[22] Nurses are sometimes told to note only events requiring stimulation, and they are often confronted with apnea or bradycardia alarms from apneic events that would be classified as ALTE in an older infant, but most of these are transient and self-resolving without apparent acute consequence. In addition, many current monitors produce only a very brief bradycardia alarm during mixed apnea or have imperfect alarm systems that delay the arrival of the nurse, or they even may fail to generate an alarm before the infant is breathing again.[22–26]

Most centers attempt to wean patients from methylxanthine treatment a week or more prior to discharge.[2,3] Following this, some short "bradycardias" (usually actually due to mixed apnea)[22] or central apnea alarms may be noted by the nursing staff. They also may see episodes of subtle cyanosis when the monitor is not connected, or the baby may require oxygen supplementation. Toward the end of hospitalization these may be the only symptoms despite hospital care costs of hundreds of dollars a day. On the basis of the 1978 AAP recommendation for monitor use with apnea and the realization that unrecognized apnea is a common occurrence in hospital,[16,22,26] some intermediate care nurseries have recorded activity from all infants approaching discharge. Others have tried to recognize the fraction that would be considered "symptomatic"[21] through a combination of nursing reports and recording. There is strong evidence that preterm infants have an increased risk of SIDS after discharge,[1] and evidence now links this to breathing patterns at discharge.[25] There is still need for a carefully structured prospective study to help decide the most appropriate method of discharging preterm infants.

Detection of Symptomatic Preterms at Discharge. Monitor use in many centers is now continued until the time of discharge, to detect the persistence and occasional onset of apnea late in the hospital course. There is uncertainty about the least harmful and most accurate means of defining a symptomatic preterm population. Information in the following paragraph is drawn largely from the empirically developed management plan at Oregon Health Sciences University, Portland, Oregon, in a state where infant mortality data have been matched to birth weight and hospital of birth for over 18 years. Two other approaches are also described from centers on the East Coast of America. The optimal management plan, including all social and risk factors, is uncertain at present.

Program at Oregon Health Sciences University (OHSU). In 1977 and early 1978, research to assess infants' response to inspired CO_2 began as a means of judging the maturity of the preterms ready for discharge. The result was recognition of infants with prolonged apnea and normal CO_2 response. Since the 1978 AAP committee report, sleep-related prolonged apnea of any form, or prolonged periodic breathing in uninterrupted intervals in excess of 5 minutes, especially with declining oxygen levels, has been regarded as symptomatic behavior warranting a further 5 to 7 days of observation in hospital. At the same time, the family has been given the option of taking the infant home with a monitor as an alternative. Prolonged periodic breathing causing marginal hypoxia without heart or breathing alarms has been treated with theophylline if the infant goes home with that behavior. No medication has been given to those being assessed for the rate at which they are maturing in hospital, unless extremely frequent episodes occurred without theophylline. Infants going home with medication also have been monitored. If the infant has reached 37 weeks postconception and is otherwise ready for discharge, then monitor use at home is advised if abnormal activity in sleep continues.

Method of Recording. Because of inaccuracies in signals produced by thoracic impedance monitors,[16,26] we have chosen recording systems employing abdominal respiratory effort, ECG, transcutaneous pO_2, or later oxygen saturation as diagnostic signals and avoided any sensors creating facial stimulation in our preterm assessment protocol unless special studies were being performed after the commitment to monitor had already been made. Studies were performed overnight toward the end of the week of observation after any methylxanthine therapy and usually lasted for at least 18 to 24 hours (see Medical Therapy of Apnea).

Frequency of Monitor Prescription. The number of preterm infants monitored at discharge is related to the postconceptional age. In a complete summary of all births from 1982 to 1985 at the University Hospital in Oregon, of 533 infants under 2 kg at birth and surviving to be discharged, studies were performed on 230 (43 per cent) who were considered potentially symptomatic 35 weeks postconception. Studies were performed at weekly intervals. If a monitor was indicated through testing, one was obtained and supported regardless of the family's resources.

SIDS Risk in Discharged Preterms. Based on the occurrence of apnea and/or prolonged periodic breathing in sleep at 35 to 37 weeks postconception, 130 (24 per cent) of all infants were monitored and 403 (76 per cent) were not. Nine SIDS deaths occurred among fewer than 40 families receiving monitors who did not maintain contact with the program before stopping monitor use.[7] The only SIDS death among over 90 families who apparently were using the monitors as requested occurred when one infant died 10 days after discharge while the parents slept through the alarm. To date there have been no deaths of infants in families in whom monitor use has been completed by assess-

TABLE 2. Protocol for Showing Stress Tolerance Before Stopping Monitor Use

Alarms are maintained at 15 sec for apnea and 80% of the heart rate in quiet sleep, or the most sensitive values producing no more than 2–3 brief alarms per day. There should be no increase in the previous rate of both heart or breathing alarms while the baby is sleeping during and after all three stresses:

- (1) Viral infection
- (2) At least one DPT-OPV immunization
- (3) Sleep disturbance, created by attempting to double usual awake activity during 1 day

If a questionable cluster of alarms occurs, then monitor use continues until the stress is repeated. A four-channel recording of abdominal breathing, ECG, thoracic impedance, and oxygen saturation is made at home for 24–48 hours of sleep until alarms occur. If alarms are false or no alarms occur, monitoring is discontinued. If real apnea occurs with oxygen desaturation, the monitor is continued until the same stress is tolerated (one sleep deprivation trial/month) without decompensation. Using this protocol, the average monitoring duration was less than 5 months; many infants never required studies; and no deaths occurred among several hundred high-risk infants with complete demonstration of stress tolerance. Inadequate compliance by parents in monitor use (14 infants) and by physicians using the protocol (3 infants) has been associated with SIDS.

ing stress tolerance (Table 2). Monitor brand has not altered compliance among the devices chosen to date.

The SIDS risk in the Northwest is the highest in the United States and among the highest in the world. From 1975 to 1985, the postdischarge risk statewide had risen with declining neonatal mortality to 16/1000 SIDS per discharged patient (1 in 60) for infants born weighing under 2 kg. The risk of SIDS postdischarge for our urban center was 25/1000 (1 in 40) in 1975 to 1977. It declined to 8 to 10/1000 for 3 years after the monitor program was started; there were four deaths among noncompliant families in 1983. Since 1978, deaths from SIDS have occurred predominantly among monitored patients not on equipment and in unstudied infants.

Although the occurrence of SIDS has declined among our discharged infants since this protocol was initiated in 1978, the occurrence of families who do not comply with monitor use has prevented the assertion that have monitoring significantly decreases the risk of death among the total population of preterm infants discharged (Fig. 1). In the first 3 years of the program, a threefold decline in SIDS death occurred when all family contact was by one person.[1,7,16] The monitoring program has grown in size and geographic referral area, which makes this level of personal contact difficult, and many families have limited resources for phone and transportation.[1,16] Parental contact and education are a very critical part of monitor use. Two other centers have

reported very good results when they were able to provide more complete family contact.[1]

Limitations of Recurrent Assessment in Hospital. The limited value of indefinite reassessment in hospital is shown by the reports of others and our own experience with four preterm infants abnormal at 37 weeks, who later each had normal recordings for 24 to 48 hours in a random unstressed interval for monitor adjustment, and then a few weeks later died of SIDS while off the monitor.

The Value of Confirming Stability Before 37 Weeks. The observation of early stability seems more useful. If a preterm infant of less than 37 weeks postconception has no evidence of transient apnea on an overnight recording, no monitor is considered necessary. Among several hundred assessed and unmonitored preterm infants over the past 11 years, one infant from the University Hospital in Oregon had a stable record under 37 weeks, which was followed by discharge without a monitor and later death from SIDS. That infant initially had bradycardias lasting more than 15 seconds, without any central or mixed apnea, and then developed a totally stable record within 7 days. We have seen some infants without apnea before 37 weeks who have been readmitted with ALTE and then monitored following severe infection. The low risk for stable young infants at discharge has been described in other populations.[1,25]

Education for Observation Without Monitor Use. Among preterm infants nearly

Figure 1. The pattern of SIDS incidence for infants under 2 kg born and discharged from Oregon Health Sciences University, 1975–1985. This figure illustrates the difficulty in showing benefit from monitor use. The reduction in SIDS if monitors worked among noncompliant families would be significant. The absence of SIDS (among numbers estimated through 1988) for infants whose families are compliant in monitor use and among those trained to observe during infection after discharge with intrafeeding apnea offers the possibility of testing these approaches prospectively using electronic compliance documentation.

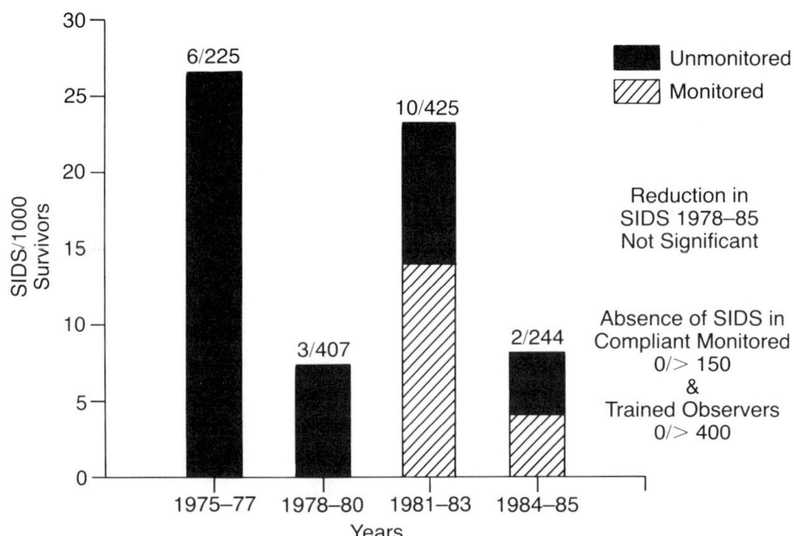

ready for hospital discharge, apnea can be classified by whether it occurs in sleep or during awake or care provision intervals, using combined recording transducers. At our center, infants with apnea occurring only during care provision have not had monitors routinely prescribed for use at home. Infants showing only apnea induced by feeding have been assigned an intermediate level of risk for postdischarge apneic events. Parents who could be contacted were taught to observe their infant's abdominal breathing patterns during 1-hour intervals of sleep at night when the infant contracted a respiratory illness (Table 3).

Of over 400 infants discharged by 37 weeks postconception whose parents were taught the protocol in Table 3, no SIDS deaths have occurred, and a dozen families are known to have recognized valid ALTE episodes confirmed by medical personnel or physiologic recording. Four SIDS deaths, three after the onset of a later mild infection and one postcongenital cytomegaloviral infection, have occurred among fewer than 100 infants with similar intrafeeding apnea behavior but whose families were not trained because of inability of the instructor to contact them.

TABLE 3. Home Observation of Preterm Infants with Intermediate Risk of Apnea After Discharge

Instructions for parents, after showing them their baby's recording done in the hospital:

1. Observe the baby's abdomen in feeding and withdraw the bottle if apnea occurs. Observe the baby in sleep only if a mild infection occurs. The recording done in the hospital (record shown) showed spells only when there was someone feeding the baby. Some babies like this start to have long breathing pauses or irregular breathing in sleep during infection.
2. During an infection with nasal congestion, watch through the 40- to 60-minute interval of sleep *before* three or four nighttime feedings, especially from 10:00 at night to 8:00 in the morning. Set an alarm if necessary.
3. Have enough light and use a watch with seconds to time breathing pauses.
4. The baby should wear a lightweight sleeper. Arrange the blankets to allow a view of the *abdomen*. The baby may wear a cap; the legs and chest can be covered.
5. Expect normal pauses of up to 15 seconds, and some pauses in a row, which is called periodic breathing. (Examples are shown and 15 seconds "felt" with the instructor.)
6. If any pause lasts more than 15 seconds, or if more than 3 minutes of periodic breathing without steady breathing is noted, contact the doctor or hospital promptly by phone.

■ ALTERNATIVE APPROACHES TO PRETERM DISCHARGE

In the same interval from 1982 to 1985 at Children's Hospital of Philadelphia, all preterm infants were recorded just before discharge regardless of reported activity. Thirty-one per cent of the studies in preterm infants before discharge were normal, with no attempt made to separate intrafeeding events from those in sleep. All abnormal infants were monitored, and those with periodic breathing of more than 10 per cent received theophylline as well. Among 589 preterm infants assessed by overnight recording of airflow, ECG, and chest movements, all 177 stable infants were unmonitored, and there were no deaths among either monitored or unmonitored infants. Two full-time nurses made frequent family contacts.[1]

Another approach in outpatient use of theophylline was done at Massachusetts General Hospital (MGH). From 1973 to 1986, the recordings of over 3000 preterm infants from many different hospitals were analyzed at MGH, which does not have a maternity unit. Those infants with the most unstable behavior were discharged on oral theophylline therapy without a monitor for 1 month, with weekly measurement of blood levels and adjusted theophylline dosage by local physicians. Infants were reassessed by recording with a monitor taken to the home 1 month after discharge just as drug treatment was abruptly stopped (see following section on Medical Therapy of Apnea). If that record was abnormal based on criteria for older infants,[5,15] then the monitor and/or medication was continued. A few deaths occurred when treatment was refused or medication reduced during the interval without simultaneous monitor use, but overall mortality has been as low as, or lower than, that for term infants. The report mentions that among all infants four deaths occurred when infants were off the monitor. Three were preterm infants. The investigators feel that parents of preterm infants may have lower compliance than other parents using monitors.[1]

■ MEDICAL THERAPY OF APNEA

Parenteral and oral methylxanthines and medications with greater side effects were widely used initially to reduce the severity of apnea and ventilatory dependency for preterm infants.[27] Oral methylxanthine compounds, either caffeine or theophylline, have been shown to reduce the frequency and severity of problems with breathing frequency control in mild cases of recurrent central, mixed, and obstructive apnea in term infants presenting with ALTE episodes.

A variety of methylxanthine treatments and levels of therapy have been suggested.[1,2,24,25] At discharge of preterm infants, we have used an oral loading dose of alcohol-free liquid theophylline, 4 to 6 mg/kg, followed by 2 to 3 mg/kg q 8 hours' maintenance. Therapeutic effects without significant side effects were gained rapidly. Those centers using caffeine recommend 1 oral dose of 10 mg/kg, followed by 2.5 mg/kg daily (based on weight of caffeine). For both drugs, the amount or timing is adjusted weekly, as natural growth shortens the half-life and increases body size. Some theophylline is normally metabolized to caffeine.[2]

Blood levels for both drugs, measured just prior to treatment, should be 10 to 18 mg/L for adequate effect and to allow a margin for growth. Ideal peak levels are no more than 20 to 25 mg/L to minimize side effects. Transient instability in breathing control when stopping therapy seems to be reduced by a tapered withdrawal (50 per cent reduction in 24 hours). Some infants are reported to have gastrointestinal or behavioral disturbances with theophylline, which are reported less frequently with caffeine therapy. Unmanaged overdosage causes tachycardia, seizures, fever, and occasionally death.[29] There is no commercial preparation of oral caffeine, but most pharmacies can prepare it. Blood level determinations need to be developed separately for caffeine. Some reports have mentioned using doxapram in preterm infants unresponsive to theophylline.[2]

Nontapered withdrawal of medical therapy can be followed by severe exacerbation of apnea or ALTE. The use of medication at home without monitoring the infant has been successful but carries the risk of the development of unrecognized ALTE behavior, as dosages become marginal with growth or with sudden withdrawal of treatment. A few sudden deaths, when the medication was not maintained and no monitor was present, have been reported.

■ PRESCRIBING A MONITOR

Communications About Monitoring

Parents are told the following:

- (1) All infants having experienced ALTE or born preterm are at increased risk for ALTE and SIDS.
- (2) There is a possible link between prolonged transient apneas, ALTE, and SIDS.
- (3) Their infant has a subtle problem with breathing control, like many others.
- (4) Most apnea-prone infants outgrow the problem.
- (5) Recordings for hours or days may not show the problem in older apnea-prone infants, and apnea still returns with stress.
- (6) The most likely outcome is a good one, but at our center 11 preterm infants with apnea at discharge and 7 term ALTE patients have died when off the monitor before being watched through all aspects of the stress tolerance protocol.
- (7) No infants in our experience have died after the stress protocol was followed, but some infants have died of SIDS after monitoring was stopped in other programs.

We make a firm recommendation that further tests in hospital offer less assurance and are more costly than documenting that the baby tolerates the stresses of infection and sleep disruption at home without decompensation. Parents are told and shown that the best equipment and care by in-hospital staff do not always clearly recognize all apnea and that some short alarms may be self-resolving events. The roles of the family and medical team starting to monitor their infant are delineated. Their job is to record all possible transient events. To keep the responsibility for any errors clearly on the doctors, we will tell them when to discontinue monitoring.

Monitor Choice

Monitors we use have included a portable ECG-only monitor, if bradycardia always occurred with apnea, and ECG and thoracic impedance monitors when this relationship was not certain.[16] In recent years, use of the existing heart rate–only devices has declined owing to the advantages of recognizing loose lead alarms more readily and more reliable detection of transient alarms. The chief advances have been the arrival of battery-powered heart and breathing monitors and improved reliability of home monitors to a level equal or superior to in-hospital units. The newest equipment has very flexible heart rate and sensitivity adjustments (changes in alarm level by 1 BPM) and is more stable in detecting the ECG during normal movements in sleep.

Apnea and Respiration Frequency Alarms

Studies from all centers that have ever reported recording infant behavior after 2 weeks of life reveal that central apnea longer than 15 seconds has never been documented in a randomly selected control infant.[26] It seems reasonable to use this value as the apnea delay interval on well-designed monitors, and many programs have done so successfully in observing thousands of infants. When respiration rate alarm options are present, a setting of 6 to 10 breaths per minute can be used with good equipment without excessive false alarms. This setting occasionally has been helpful in keeping track of seizures or airway obstruction episodes that produce slow, widely spaced gasping efforts. Careful attention to sensitivity adjustments and lead placement may be needed when using a respiration frequency alarm. Monitors without manual options appear more prone to false alarm.

A high likelihood of missed central apnea (varying from 0 to 98 per cent accuracy) occurs among devices currently on the market. This has been the source of clinical concern and some legal action when deaths have occurred. We have reduced that problem by using devices with the greatest flexibility for manual adjustment to individual infants and have used "automatic" settings only when the monitor reliability was greater than 95 per cent in tests developed at our center.[24,26] There is clear need for public labeling and grading of equipment reliability, and that process has slowly begun through voluntary agencies and the Food and Drug Administration.[16,24]

Heart Rate Alarms

A reflex decrease in heart rate is frequently present with both central and obstructed apneic events, making bradycardia the primary means of detecting most mixed and obstructed apnea with current equipment at home. The bradycardia alarm must be kept

above the heart rate plateau value sustained for each event. At the same time, normal heart rate decreases need to be avoided.[16] The Oregon Health Sciences University program has successfully monitored over 1100 infants at home using a low heart rate alarm setting at 80 per cent of the heart rate in quiet sleep. This is accomplished by choosing equipment that accurately detects the ECG signal even during movement, and adjusting the sensitivity level and/or changing lead positions in the presence of inappropriately frequent alarms.

Physicians at the Royal Alexandra Hospital in Calgary have recently reported the most definitive study to date that compares heart rate changes to apneas detected by hospital staff in an NICU setting.[22] They found heart rate to be the most useful factor in the detection of apneas and indicated that 25 per cent of apneas would not be detected unless the heart rate setting was in excess of 100 BPM. They used an alarm setting of 100 BPM or 70 per cent of the average previous day's rate, whichever was higher. Because it is difficult to determine the total average heart rate, especially in the home, we have suggested 80 per cent of the value in quiet sleep. The Calgary group found that 87 per cent of all apneas in the 1266 events studied had a 20 per cent or greater heart rate decrease. They felt that an alarm that recognized a 15 per cent decrease would be optimal in the NICU.

Most infants in our program initially are discharged with heart rate settings of 95 to 105 beats per minute, designed to be 5 to 10 BPM above the documented heart rate plateau reached during that infant's apneic events. A few older infants (5 to 10 per cent) with a normal resting heart rate in the range of 80 to 95 BPM or with repeatedly occurring ectopic heart beats may require settings as low as 65 to 75 BPM, and sometimes lower.

Some manufacturers recommend using lower heart rate alarm settings than these for all infants (80 BPM), and to change all infants' alarm levels arbitrarily to 60 BPM by 2 months postnatal age, rather than maintaining the alarm at a fraction of resting heart rate. Those less sensitive and presumably less safe settings were the product of trying to use older ECG detection circuitry. It is hoped they will no longer be needed as better heart rate detection circuitry becomes more widely available. It appears that infants who die of SIDS tend to have higher resting heart rates than controls, and apnea-prone infants may have less vagal reduction in heart rate.[15,18] Some infants with these patterns of behavior might have to suffer recurrent severe hypoxia before an alarm that is set that far from their usual heart rate would alert the parent.[16,18] An effort is being made to develop more effective standards in monitor design and use.[1,24,26]

High Heart Rate. The high alarm level is set above the rate reached with crying and agitation, usually 220 to 230 BPM. This setting serves to detect electrical interference that causes the appearance of false tachycardia and also detects a few infants with unsuspected tachyarrhythmias, usually paroxysmal atrial tachycardia.

Alternative Monitors

Some infants develop profound airway obstruction, persistent respiratory efforts, and significant cyanosis without a heart rate decline below 120 to 140 BPM. These episodes frequently are not associated with noisy breathing in very small infants. Most of these babies have required tracheostomy, and we have attempted to use end-tidal CO_2 monitors and pulse oxygen saturation monitors at home. The former have significant practical limitations after the infant is 3 to 4 months old.[22] Pulse oxygen saturation is better for providing a stable means of alarm for all behavior producing cyanosis.

Compliance in Monitor Use

Failure of parental compliance to document stress tolerance carries the greatest risk for an infant death after monitor use is prescribed. Some parental noncompliance results from excessive false alarms; in most cases, a 2- to 3-week interval without alarms has given noncompliant families in our program a false sense of security.[7]

There are no easy methods for ensuring appropriate monitor use. A balanced and accurate explanation of the benefits, risks, and problems experienced both nationally and in individual programs and maintenance of close contact with families seem to be the only means of ensuring maximal compliance. In most instances, both the need and the effective use of the monitor are based on faith in the capacity of the parent to give accurate information and respond appropriately. The goals for the medical team are always to remain in close, supportive communication with the family; to provide complete and, if necessary, repeated education of the parents; and to provide immediate, competent support in the event of technical problems.

Utility of Self-Documenting Monitors

In rare instances, failure of parental compliance in using monitors has occasioned temporary custody of the infant in medical foster care. This is justifiable only when the infant exhibits clear physiologic abnormalities and the parents have been unable to monitor effectively after understanding the need and agreeing to do so. The decision always has followed repeated and extraordinary efforts at education and social support in a setting of many features of neglect in care. With the availability of monitors that store in memory the exact time of use, setting changes, and the complete pattern of all alarms, it is quite difficult for negligent parents to disguise inadequate care. Some brands of monitor will store and transmit over the phone information to be interpreted by apnea program personnel.[26]

The systems do not represent a purely negative "Big Brother" supervision. Many parents who have been providing marginal care respond positively to the use of automatic alarm logging and recording systems, because of the capacity of these devices to show them the intervals of unusual behavior occurring within the intervals of questionable alarms. The most complete systems record other signals (abdominal breathing, oxygen saturation, and so on), which allow confirmation of the significance of short, self-resolving alarms. In many instances this allows anxious, overconscientious parents to stop the use of the monitor despite recurrent short false alarms.[16] Recordings consisting only of processed ECG and thoracic impedance signals from the monitor may simply produce the false signals generating an alarm.[16,26]

■ SURGICAL CORRECTION OF RECURRENT AIRWAY OBSTRUCTION

After an ALTE presentation, some infants gradually develop more severe symptoms of airway obstruction as lymphoid tissues proliferate in the pharynx. Many severe cases of recurrent obstructive apnea are not benefited by medication and produce unmanageably frequent alarms and severe arrest episodes requiring rehospitalization and surgical correction. The first effort is usually tonsillectomy and adenoidectomy, followed by mask continuous positive airway pressure (CPAP) if the patient is old enough to cooperate. If recurrent severe obstruction persists, then tracheostomy may be life saving.[1,11,27]

Effective treatment is followed by a growth spurt eliminating failure to thrive, reversal of cardiovascular changes, and resolution of behavioral defects from sleep disruption. Some associated sudden unexplained deaths in sleep have been described both in older children and in adults without treatment. This more severe pattern may occur with increased risk in some family groups.[27]

■ HYPOVENTILATION WITHOUT APNEA

Infants experiencing hypoventilation without apnea may present with unexplained cardiac failure, profound decompensation during respiratory infection, or ALTE episodes with cyanosis and continued breathing. Hypoventilation without apnea is demonstrated by increased carbon dioxide levels in sleep detected with continuous end-tidal CO_2 tests, transcutaneous CO_2 measurements, or sequential blood gases. There is evidence of an absent or inadequate increase in minute ventilation when a carbon dioxide challenge is given in the inspired air to the sleeping infant. Minute ventilation is usually increased normally to CO_2 challenges when the baby is awake. Many infants with this condition are not recognized immediately after birth. In some instances the diagnosis is not made until late in the first year of life.[19] Most described patients do not respond to medications and need artificial ventilation or phrenic nerve pacing in sleep.

cardia can prevent death from all forms of SIDS, they are often a consideration in a family with a new baby whose sibling has died. Very subtle but statistically significant differences in breathing patterns have been described for about 20 per cent of the brothers and sisters of infants who have died of SIDS, but this has not been confirmed in all other studies.[4] It appears that over 99 per cent of subsequent siblings, including most of these infants, are clinically asymptomatic and develop normally.[1,4]

There is an increased SIDS risk for subsequent siblings of approximately 1 in 150 sibling births, compared with the overall risk of 1 in 400 to 600 American births. If maternal age and position in family are considered, the risk is less unusual.[4] This may be due in part to the inclusion of a small number of families for whom the risk of SIDS is quite high. Some cohorts with multiple infant deaths within the span of two generations are described. Routine monitor use is recommended for subsequent infants in families in which two infants have died within the same sibling group.[21]

The decision to monitor a subsequent sibling after a family has lost a single infant to SIDS requires a full and careful exploration by the family of the social, emotional, and economic costs with a supportive individual who is capable of helping them reach their own best solution. No simple algorithms or flow charts cover the various needs of these parents. Social contacts, sleep, babysitting options, and family life all will be constrained by the monitor. For some, the relative reassurance provided will make life easier in balance, and the monitor may serve to recognize the very rare occurrence of real abnormality among many false alarms, if the family is well trained. The family choosing to monitor an infant after having lost a previous child should establish close contact with an experienced medical support person who anticipates and helps deal with the problems created by their choice, particularly during the interval when the monitor should be discontinued.

■ Issues and Risks

■ MONITOR USE FOR SUBSEQUENT SIBLINGS OF SIDS VICTIMS

Despite the absence of evidence that monitors for the recognition of apnea and brady-

REFERENCES

1. Apnea. *In* Infantile Apnea and Home Monitoring. Report of Consensus Development Conference, 1986. NIH publication No. 87–2905. Section II 2:1–25 and appendix B:23–51. Bethesda, MD: Department of Health and Human Services, 1987.

2. Marchal F, Bairam A, Vert P. Neonatal apnea and apneic syndromes. Clin Perinatol 1987; 14(3):509–529.

3. Martin RJ, Miller MJ, Carlo WA. Pathogenesis of apnea in preterm infants. J Pediatr 1986; 109(5):733–741.

4. Sudden infant death syndrome. *In* Infantile Apnea and Home Monitoring. Report of Consensus Development Conference, 1986. NIH publication No. 87–2905. Section 3:1–23. Bethesda, MD: Department of Health and Human Services, 1987.

5. Oren J, Kelly D, Shannon DC. Identification of a high-risk group for sudden infant death syndrome among infants who were resuscitated for sleep apnea. Pediatrics 1986; 77:495–499.

6. Yount JE, Lewman LE. Apnea and sudden infant death—monitor use may alter risk of death only if compliance is maintained (abstract). Clin Res 1987; 358(1):215A.

7. Yount JE. Optimal methods for apnea detection. J Perinatology. In press.

8. Garg M, Kurzner SI, Bautista D, Keens TG. Hypoxic arousal responses in infants with bronchopulmonary dysplasia. Pediatrics 1988; 82(1):59–63.

9. Shennon AT, Dunn MS, Ohlsson A, et al. Abnormal pulmonary outcomes in premature infants: prediction from O_2 requirement in the neonatal period. Pediatrics 1988; 82(4):527–532.

10. Bauchner H, Zuckerman B, McClain M, Frank D, Fried LE, Kayne H. Risk of sudden infant death syndrome among infants with in utero exposure to cocaine. J Pediatr 1988; 113:831–834.

11. Guilleminault C, Souquet M, Ariagno RL, Korobkin R, Simmons FB. Five cases of near-miss sudden infant death syndrome and development of obstructive sleep apnea syndrome. Pediatrics 1984; 73(1):71–78.

12. Carse EA, Wilkinson AR, Whyte PL, Henderson Smart DJ, Johnson P. Oxygen and carbon dioxide tensions, breathing and heart rate in normal infants during the first six months of life. J Dev Physiol 1981; 3(2):85–100.

13. Richards JM, Alexander JR, Shinebourne EA, et al. Sequential 22-hour profiles of breathing patterns and heart rate in 110 full-term infants during their first 6 months of life. Pediatrics 1984; 74(5):763–777.

14. Honma Y, Wilkes D, Bryan MH, Bryan AC. Rib cage and abdominal contributions to ventilatory response to CO_2 in infants. J Appl Physiol 1984; 56(5):1211–1216.

15. Oren J, Kelly DH, Shannon DC. Pneumogram recordings in infants resuscitated for apnea of infancy. Pediatrics 1989; 83(3):364–368.

16. Yount JE. Optimal detection sensitivity: a clinical perspective. *In* Medical Technology for the Neonate. AAMI Technology Assessment Report (TAR No. 9–84). Arlington, VA: Association for the Advancement of Medical Instrumentation, 1984.

17. Khoo MC, Kronauer RE, Strohl KP, Slutsky AS. Factors inducing periodic breathing in humans: a general model. J Appl Physiol 1982; 53(3):644–659.

18. Southall DP. Role of apnea in the sudden infant death syndrome. Pediatrics 1988; 80(1):73–84.

19. Guilleminault C, McQuitty J, Ariagno RL, Challamel MJ, Korobkin R, McClead RE Jr. Congenital central alveolar hypoventilation syndrome in six infants. Pediatrics 1982; 70(5):684–694.

20. van der Hal AL, Rodriguez AM, Sargent CW, Platzker ACG, Keens TG. Hypoxic and hypercapnic arousal responses and prediction of subsequent apnea in apnea of infancy. Pediatrics 1985; 75(5):848–854.

21. Consensus development statement on infantile apnea and home monitoring. *In* Infantile Apnea and Home Monitoring. Report of Consensus Development Conference, 1986. NIH publication No. 87–2905. Section I:1–12. Bethesda, MD: Department of Health and Human Services, 1987.

22. Muttit SC, Finer NN, Tierney AJ, Rossman J. Neonatal apnea: diagnosis by nurse versus computer. Pediatrics 1988; 82(5):713–720.

23. Yount JE. Apnea at discharge among low birthweight infants—evidence for accurate risk assessment for sudden infant death syndrome with doubled risk and greater neonatal survival (abstract). Clin Res 1986; 357(1):34A.

24. Yount JE. Technical problems in recognizing and monitoring infant apnea. Proceedings of the 11th Annual Conference of IEEE/Engineering in Medicine and Biology Society, Seattle, November, 1989; 11:325–326.

25. Yount JE, Richey SL, Phillips GK, Alexander JR, Stebbins VA, Southall DP. Apnea and prolonged periodic breathing in sleep precedes sudden infant death syndrome (SIDS)—a controlled blinded analysis of preterm infants at discharge (abstract). Pediatr Res 1988; 23(4):1551A.

26. Detecting apnea and establishing monitor settings. *In* Apnea Monitoring by Means of Thoracic Impedance Pneumography. AAMI Technical Information Report. AAMI TIR No. 4–02/89. Arlington, VA: Association for the Advancement of Medical Instrumentation, 1989:50–82.

27. Ross RD, Daniels SR, Loggie JMH, Meyer RA, Ballard ET. Sleep apnea—associated hypertension and reversible left ventricular hypertrophy. J Pediatr 1987; 111(2):253–255.

Ascites

Alex H. Bruckstein

Ascites is a serious complication in patients with chronic liver disease. It results when the rate of fluid entering the peritoneal cavity exceeds the capacity of the lymphatics and blood vessels to return it to the circulation. Several pathophysiologic factors appear to contribute to the development of ascites in patients with chronic liver disease.

Patients with massive ascites often have difficulty ingesting enough calories to maintain adequate nutrition because of early satiety. By elevating the diaphragm, massive ascites may impair respiratory function. Additionally, umbilical hernias can develop; these occasionally rupture. Finally, the presence of ascitic fluid within the peritoneum constantly exposes the patient to the risk of bacterial infection and peritonitis.

Background

DEFINITION

Ascites is defined as the accumulation of fluid within the peritoneal cavity. It may present as an isolated clinical finding or may present in a setting of generalized fluid retention with edema. Under normal conditions, the peritoneal cavity contains approximately 200 ml of fluid. As much as 1500 ml of fluid may accumulate before being detected on physical examination, especially in obese patients. Severe ascites, in addition to being a cosmetic problem, is uncomfortable and potentially hazardous. The mechanical effect of abdominal distention results in symptoms that adversely affect the quality of life.

Specifically, spontaneous peritonitis and pulmonary atelectasis with pneumonia are serious, potentially life-threatening complications of ascites. Patients will benefit from therapy of ascites because these symptoms and their consequences are minimized, despite the fact that the severity of the underlying liver disease and ultimate survival are not improved.

Alcoholic cirrhosis is the most common cause of ascites in North America and Europe, occurring in approximately 8 per cent to 15 per cent of the alcoholic population.[1] When ascites becomes refractory to therapy with diuretic agents, it is an ominous complication of cirrhosis, with a 50 per cent mortality within one year of its development.

MAKING THE DIAGNOSIS

The patient generally notes increasing abdominal girth and weight gain. Occasionally, the patient will note anorexia without weight loss, because the weight has shifted into the abdomen. Edema may be noted by the patient, although ascites can occur without recognizable edema. On physical examination, with the patient lying supine, percussion dullness of the flanks is noted. "Shifting dullness" is demonstrated when the same area of dullness becomes resonant as the patient rolls to the side. Generally, bowel floats on top of ascitic fluid, so the midabdomen will be resonant and the flanks will be dull. A fluid wave can be detected, although this is unreliable in obese patients.

No specific abnormalities in routine laboratory studies indicate ascites. Azotemia and hyponatremia may develop owing to chronic liver disease, especially in those treated with diuretics. The chest radiograph may reveal an elevated diaphragm and pleural effusion. X-ray of the abdomen will reveal a "ground-glass" diffuse abdominal haziness and loss of psoas margins, suggestive of ascites. Ultrasonography is useful in its ability to detect as little as 100 ml of fluid, to determine the presence of a mass, and to evaluate the size of the liver. Computed tomography provides similar information.

Diagnostic Paracentesis

Once ascites has been detected, a diagnostic paracentesis is indicated, unless there is a contraindication. In occasional patients, paracentesis may be risky if there are adhesions from previous surgery, in which case the bowel may be perforated. Ultrasound is useful in this setting to help guide management. In rare cases, a paracentesis may be omitted in the patient who has recurrent ascites of known cause in whom the likelihood of asymptomatic spontaneous bacterial peritonitis is not a consideration.

The diagnostic paracentesis should be performed with a small-bore needle within a plastic sheath, so that the steel needle can be removed and the plastic sheath retained in the peritoneal cavity. This permits the patient to move in various positions so that the fluid can be aspirated without risk of lacerating blood vessels or loops of bowel.[2] For a diagnostic paracentesis, removal of 50 to 100 ml is adequate. This fluid should be examined for its gross appearance and sent to the laboratory for determination of its protein and glucose content, lactic dehydrogenase (LDH) and amylase content, cell count and differential cell count, as well as Gram and acid-fast stains and culture. Cytology and cell-block examination are indicated as well.

The classification of ascitic fluid often serves as a useful guide in the initial evaluation of patients with ascites (Table 1). On the basis of protein concentration, ascitic fluid is separated into two broad categories: transudate, in which the protein content is less than 2.5 gm/dl, and exudate, in which the protein concentration is greater than 2.5 gm/dl. Chronic liver disease, congestive heart failure, and nephrosis are common causes of transudates. Disorders associated with inflammatory reactions, such as tuberculosis, tumors, and peritonitis, are among the frequent causes of exudates. Bloody ascitic fluid suggests neoplasm or trauma.

■ PATHOGENESIS

The accumulation of fluid within the peritoneal cavity of patients with chronic liver disease results from interaction of a number of factors. In alcoholic cirrhosis, fibrosis around the terminal hepatic venules is the initial lesion. Perhaps the most important factor in the development of ascites is an increase in sinusoidal pressure (intrahepatic hypertension) secondary to hepatic venous outflow obstruction. This is the basis for the "overflow" hypothesis.[3]

However, another equally important factor in the pathogenesis of ascites is the increased renal retention of sodium. This is the basis for the classic "underfill" theory of ascites.[4] With advanced cirrhosis, the urinary sodium excretion decreases, to such a degree that the most avid sodium retention state seen in renal pathophysiology occurs in patients with ascites. The renal abnormalities in salt-handling are mediated through several factors, including alteration in the renin-angiotensin-aldosterone system, decreased renal prostaglandin synthesis, and increased sympathetic nervous activity.[5]

TABLE 1. Classification of Ascites

Transudate	Exudate
Cardiac	***Tumors***
Congestive heart failure	Metastatic to liver
Cardiomyopathy	Metastatic to peritoneum
Constrictive pericarditis	Primary hepatoma
Tricuspid insufficiency	Lymphoma
Hepatic	***Inflammatory Disease of Peritoneum***
Alcohol-related liver disease	Tuberculous peritonitis
Chronic liver disease, any cause	Spontaneous bacterial peritonitis
Portal hypertension	Pancreatic ascites
Budd-Chiari syndrome	Bile peritonitis
Renal	
Nephrotic syndrome	
Other	
Hypoalbuminemia	
Meigs' syndrome	

Also important for the development of ascites is an imbalance between the formation and removal of hepatic and intestinal lymph. When lymphatic drainage does not compensate for increased lymphatic leakage, primarily as a result of elevated hepatic sinusoidal pressure, ascites develops.

Other factors that contribute to ascites formation include leakage of albumin into the abdominal cavity and impaired reabsorption of fluid across a thickened peritoneum. A decreased oncotic pressure from hypoalbuminemia, contrary to earlier concepts, does not seem to contribute significantly to ascites formation.

■ DIFFICULTIES ENCOUNTERED IN THERAPY

As mentioned, the most common cause of ascites is alcohol-related liver disease. The therapy of ascites involves self-control in the form of moderate-to-severe dietary sodium restriction, as well as abstinence from alcohol. Considering the fact that most chronic alcohol abusers have difficulty with self-control, a therapy that involves abstinence from alcohol as well as restriction of sodium intake will be difficult to adhere to. The aid of a dietitian will be useful in educating the patient regarding the sodium content of various foods and in evaluating the eating and cooking habits of the patient, especially one who works and dines out.

■ Management

■ DIETARY SODIUM RESTRICTION

The mere presence of ascites is not an indication for therapy, since mild-to-moderate ascites does no harm and does not warrant the potential complications of aggressive diuretic therapy. As a complication of liver failure, initial management of ascites should be an attempt to improve hepatic function. Therapy for impaired liver function depends on the nature of the dysfunction; thus, it may include abstinence from alcohol, provision of nutrients for hepatic regeneration, or therapy for certain forms of liver disease.

Therapy for ascites begins with dietary sodium restriction. However, considerable judgment must be used, since the more rigid the sodium restriction, the more items are eliminated from the patient's diet. Thus, given a patient with cirrhosis and ascites who is malnourished, effective nutritional therapy may be of greater benefit than severe restriction of sodium intake.[6] Additionally, severe sodium restriction in ambulatory patients makes the diet unpalatable and financially prohibitive. Thus, un-

---

TABLE 2. Management of Ascites

Determine the etiology of the ascites

Perform diagnostic paracentesis (see Table 1)

Treat underlying disease

If etiology is:
    Cardiac—cardiotonic regimen
    Tumor—oncology consult
    Infectious—antibiotics, drainage
    Hepatic—nutrition, drugs

Initial management

Bed rest
Dietary sodium restriction
    Mild/moderate ascites: 2 gm Na/day (outpatient)
    Severe ascites: 500 mg Na/day (hospitalized)
Assess response to above with daily weight
measurements
    Loss of 0.5 lb/day is fine
    If no weight loss:
        reassess diet
        "room search" for "snacks"
        evaluate other medications for Na content
        proceed to diuretic therapy

Diuretic therapy

Initial management
    Determine urine sodium and potassium
    concentration
    Spironolactone, 50 mg orally QID
    In 4 days, assess weight loss:
        0.5 lb/day loss is fine
    If weight loss inadequate, determine urine sodium:
        if urine sodium is less than urine potassium, spironolactone, 75 mg QID
    Every 4 days, repeat above steps
        may increase spironolactone by 25 mg QID, as long as urinary sodium is less than urinary potassium
Further management
    If weight loss is not adequate with the increased dose and urinary sodium drops below urinary potassium:
        cautiously add furosemide, 40 mg/day
        higher dose of furosemide needed if renal function is impaired

Aggressive therapy

If ascites is refractory to combination of spironolactone and furosemide, consider
    Large-volume paracentesis
    Peritoneovenous shunt

---

less the patient is compulsive, severe dietary restriction invites noncompliance with the therapy.

With these considerations in mind, the treatment of ascites generally begins with a sodium allowance of 2 gm per day (Table 2). It must be remembered that the amount of dietary sodium permitted is not necessarily the same as the amount actually ingested, because a portion of the diet might not be eaten. Sodium restriction alone initiates a safe, progressive diuresis, with loss of a half pound per day. A more rapid diuresis is acceptable only if the patient has peripheral edema and can be achieved only with drug therapy. Approximately 5 per cent to 15 per cent of cirrhotic patients with ascites can be managed with bed rest and moderate sodium restriction.[7]

■ FLUID RESTRICTION

Generally, the restriction of fluid intake is more likely to be punitive than helpful in cirrhotic patients; physiologic control of thirst is a reliable guide of fluid need. Additionally, fluid restriction is a potent stimulus for secretion of antidiuretic hormone and becomes counterproductive. Despite serum sodium concentrations as low as 126 mEq/L, cirrhotic patients remain asymptomatic. Fluid restriction is indicated only in the patient who is a compulsive water drinker (daily liquid intake above 2 liters), or in progressively worsening hyponatremia that is likely to become symptomatic.

■ DRUG THERAPY

Once a decision has been made that dietary sodium restriction has not been adequate, perhaps because the diet has been so restricted as to result in inadequate nutritional intake, then diuretics should be considered. A baseline measurement of serum and urine sodium concentration is obtained. Generally the urine sodium will be low (less than 10 mEq/L) and the urine potassium will be high. It is reasonable then to begin therapy with spironolactone (Aldactone) at an oral dose of 50 mg QID. This drug inhibits the aldosterone-mediated distal tubular reabsorption of sodium, so that an effective dosage can be titrated to urinary sodium excretion and overall diuretic response. Prac-

tically speaking, the drug works slowly, with maximal diuresis starting 3 to 4 days later. The diuretic is generally not toxic, but hyperkalemia must be looked for.

After the patient has been on this dose for a few days, if the diuretic response is not adequate for the clinical situation the decision to increase the dose of spironolactone is based upon a repeat urinary sodium determination. A spot urinary sodium and potassium determination is made; if the urinary sodium is still less than the urinary potassium, the dose of spironolactone may be increased gradually to as much as 400 mg daily. The patient is maintained on the new dose for a few days, and the clinical response is monitored. If the clinical response is not adequate, then a repeat urinary sodium and potassium determination is obtained. As long as the urinary sodium is below the urinary potassium, the effect of circulating aldosterone is still present, indicating that additional spironolactone may be added. Practically speaking, it is rare for this to occur above a dose of 400 mg of spironolactone per day, although occasionally double that amount may be given before the urinary sodium becomes higher than the urinary potassium. If the diuretic effect is still not adequate for the clinical situation when the urinary sodium becomes higher than the urinary potassium, an additional diuretic is indicated.

Before proceeding to additional diuretic therapy, the physician must consider certain principles. The maximal rate of peritoneal fluid reabsorption is limited to 700 to 900 ml/24 hr.[8] Peripheral edema is mobilized more rapidly than ascitic fluid. Thus, diuresis should not exceed 1 to 2 lb/day in the presence of edema and should only be about 0.5 pound per day in the absence of peripheral edema. Otherwise, attempts to mobilize more than 900 ml/day of ascitic fluid will be at the expense of the intravascular volume rather than the ascitic fluid, with loss of plasma volume and eventual hyponatremia, azotemia, and encephalopathy. Thus, the rate of diuresis, the serum electrolyte concentration, and the neurologic and renal function must be carefully monitored, with the dosage of diuretic adjusted according to response. Caution is especially important when dry weight is approached or when larger doses of diuretic are needed to obtain a response.

If the patient responds to spironolactone

with the loss of 300 ml of ascites fluid per day, this will result in a loss of 2 to 4 pounds per week. The therapy should be continued until the ascites is reduced sufficiently. It is better to let the patient retain some fluid than to continue diuretic therapy until the patient is "bone dry." Again, it must be realized that ascites is a symptom and a cosmetic problem; the purpose of diuretic therapy is to provide comfort—disappearance of ascites cannot improve the underlying liver disease. The physician should not attempt to dry the patient out, because the associated decrease of plasma volume will result in impaired renal perfusion and impaired hepatic blood flow, whereas improvement of hepatic function and reduction of hepatocellular necrosis require an improvement of hepatic blood flow.

■ OTHER DIURETIC THERAPY

Diuretics more potent than spironolactone are available. Thiazide diuretics interfere with sodium reabsorption primarily in the distal tubule. The loop diuretic furosemide (Lasix), which impairs sodium reabsorption in the loop of Henle, is generally the next drug that is tried. Furosemide is a drug that wastes potassium, so that its use in conjunction with spironolactone, which conserves potassium, is ideal. The drug should be administered intermittently and in the lowest effective dose so as to minimize the incidence of electrolyte abnormalities and azotemia. Generally, the higher the dose that will be required, the more severe the liver disease and the higher the potential complication rate from the drug. Furosemide may result in hypokalemic alkalosis, which may require potassium supplementation.

When spironolactone and furosemide are given in combination, the patient must be observed carefully for signs of excessive diuresis. These include a rising blood urea nitrogen determination, hyponatremia, and evidence of reduced plasma volume (orthostatic hypotension). Any one of these three signs implies that the ascitic fluid cannot replace the diuretic-induced decrease in plasma volume rapidly enough; at this point, diuretic therapy must be stopped. If deteriorating renal function (rising blood urea nitrogen) is recognized prior to major deterioration of renal cortical perfusion, expanding the circulating plasma volume may be suc-cessful in reversing the deterioration in renal function. If diuretic therapy results in an increase of blood urea nitrogen, the therapy must be reduced or eliminated and plasma volume expanded with 5 per cent albumin or fresh-frozen plasma at a rate of 250 to 750 mg/day, depending upon the central venous pressure (estimated by neck veins) and response of renal function.

For the great majority of patients, a combination of bed rest, dietary sodium restriction, and diuretic therapy titrated to the urinary sodium response and clinical response is adequate. Only the rare patient will be unresponsive to this therapy. It is important to evaluate the patient who does not respond to this therapy for overlooked sources of sodium intake, such as antacids containing sodium and intravenous antibiotics. Additionally, drugs that can interfere with renal sodium excretion should be discontinued; particularly important here are the nonsteroidal anti-inflammatory drugs. Beta-blockers that are useful for prophylaxis in patients with a history of variceal hemorrhage are culprits here, as well, and should be discontinued.

■ INVASIVE MEDICAL THERAPY

For the few patients in whom diuresis cannot be achieved with the foregoing measures, venous return, cardiac output, and renal blood flow may all be improved by paracentesis of tense ascites. There is some debate as to exactly how much is "too much" fluid to remove. Generally speaking, a paracentesis of 2 to 3 liters may be safely performed without the addition of plasma or albumin to expand the plasma volume. Removal of more fluid should be done only with the intravenous expansion of plasma volume with plasma or albumin.[9] In a recent study, several patients underwent a 5-liter paracentesis safely, without drop in plasma volume, despite the facts that there was no peripheral edema in these patients and albumin was not administered.[10]

■ SURGICAL THERAPY

An effective form of therapy for the patient who has "refractory" ascites is surgical implantation of an artificial conduit between the peritoneal fluid and the circulation. This is known as the LeVeen peritoneovenous shunt. The primary indication for the La-Veen shunt is progressive renal impairment with refractory ascites. Another indication is refractory ascites in a compliant patient and a questionable indication of refractory ascites in a noncompliant patient. Refractory ascites can be clinically defined as ascites in a patient who has had diuresis under rigidly controlled conditions in the hospital but who cannot live an acceptable life outside the hospital without reaccumulation of fluid in incapacitating amounts. Clearly, as mentioned, the simple presence of ascites that does not interfere with the patient's nutrition, activities of daily living, or respiration is acceptable and does not require intensive surgical therapy that can have potentially fatal complications.

Placement of a LeVeen shunt, or one of its modifications, results in mobilization of ascites, with increased clearance of both free water and sodium, but its use is limited by the increased frequency of postshunt coagulopathy, variceal bleeding, and shunt failure.[11] Uremic, pancreatic, and malignant ascites generally respond very well to LeVeen shunts when simpler measures are ineffective.

■ Issues and Risks

■ SIDE EFFECTS OF MANAGEMENT

As mentioned, ascites indicates severe liver disease and an associated poor prognosis. Treatment of the ascites per se does not improve survival, since progression of the underlying liver disease is unaffected. Additionally, therapy, whether conventional diuretic therapy or surgical shunting, has the risk of inducing clinically significant complications. Thus, vigorous attempts to remove ascites are not justified in patients with moderate, asymptomatic ascites. In these patients, salt restriction is generally adequate. Removal of ascitic fluid for cosmetic reasons alone is not indicated.

On the other hand, severe ascites is uncomfortable and can result in a variety of complications that necessitate therapy. These complications are generally related to the mechanical effects of the ascites, such as

(1) compression of the stomach, resulting in anorexia and inability to obtain adequate nutrition, (2) elevation of the diaphragm, resulting in the patient's having difficulty breathing when lying flat or in pulmonary atelectasis with recurrent pneumonia, and (3) increased intra-abdominal pressure, resulting in development of umbilical or inguinal hernias. The patient who has had general anesthesia will have difficulty in becoming extubated as a result of an elevated diaphragm. Rupture of an umbilical hernia is an uncommon but severe complication of ascites.[12] Bleeding esophageal varices are a complication of ascites insofar as they relate to increased plasma volume. Thus, there is justification for the therapy of severe ascites.

Medical management is successful in the majority of patients. Occasionally, bed rest and dietary sodium restriction suffice. However, for the majority of patients, diuretics are required to reduce ascites to clinically acceptable levels. Complications generally do not develop until vigorous therapy with diuretics is initiated. The complications include electrolyte disorders (hyperkalemia from spironolactone, hypokalemia from furosemide, hyponatremia from excessive diuresis), hypotension, prerenal azotemia, hepatorenal syndrome, and hepatic encephalopathy. The physician must remember that since diuretics act on the kidney, they directly eliminate salt and water only from the blood; when utilizing diuretics, the clinician assumes that the plasma volume contraction will result in ascitic fluid being absorbed from the abdomen to re-expand the diminished circulating blood volume. As mentioned, the maximal rate at which this can occur appears to be about 900 ml/24 hr. Thus, an optimal diuretic regimen cannot reduce ascites by more than 1 kg/day. More vigorous diuresis results in the hepatorenal syndrome and hepatic encephalopathy, either of which often becomes the mode of the patient's demise.

Spironolactone is a potassium-sparing diuretic. Therefore, the physician should be careful if prescribing a potassium-containing salt substitute for the patient taking spironolactone who is on a sodium-restricted diet.

Furosemide is a potent (loop) diuretic. When it is given, the risk of hypotension, hyponatremia, and impaired renal function is high. For the clinician, however, the strategy must remain that renal function takes priority over weight loss. Thus, given a patient who has progressive prerenal azotemia, it becomes more important to reverse this process and improve renal function than to mobilize ascitic fluid. In fact, the improvement of renal function is so significant that the clinician occasionally may increase the amount of ascitic fluid in the process of attempting to achieve improved renal function.

COMPLIANCE

As mentioned, patients with ascites are generally chronic alcohol abusers who have had difficulty with self-control during their entire life. Complying with a low sodium diet will be difficult. It is not uncommon for the attending physician to find potato chips and pretzels in the patient's hospital nightstand. The patient will claim that "the hospital food doesn't taste good" and that his or her family brought in a "snack."

Additionally, the highly motivated patient who strictly adheres to the dietary regimen in the hospital finds it very difficult outside the hospital. In this situation, the peritoneovenous shunt might be considered if the ascitic fluid reaccumulates.

NATURAL HISTORY

Ascites is a complication of portal hypertension that develops in patients whose disease is in an advanced stage. Clinically, ascites is easily correctable initially, but it has a tendency to recur; with each recurrence, its control becomes more difficult. One of the signs of an ominous prognosis is a rising blood urea nitrogen level, often related to therapy. The prognosis is even less favorable when it is accompanied with a rising serum creatinine concentration. The prognosis is ominous when signs of renal failure develop without diuretic therapy, or when discontinuing the diuretics does not result in improved renal function.

COST CONTAINMENT

In patients with ascites who are asymptomatic and clinically stable, the frequency of routine laboratory studies can be limited. On the other hand, in patients who are difficult to treat and who are on high-dose diuretic therapy, close observation of renal function is essential.

PREVENTION

The prevention of ascites requires prevention of the underlying etiology (see Table 1).

REFERENCES

1. Rocco VK, Ware AJ. Cirrhotic ascites: pathophysiology, diagnosis and treatment. Ann Intern Med 1986; 105:573–585.
2. Runyon BA. Paracentesis of ascitic fluid. A safe procedure. Arch Intern Med 1986; 146:2259–2261.
3. Lieberman FL, Denison EK, Reynolds TB. The relationship of plasma volume, portal hypertension, ascites, and renal sodium retention in cirrhosis: the overflow theory of ascites formation. Ann NY Acad Sci 1970; 170:202–212.
4. Epstein M. Deranged sodium homeostasis in cirrhosis. Gastroenterology 1979; 76:622–635.
5. Epstein M. The sodium retention of cirrhosis: a reappraisal. Hepatology 1986; 6:312–315.
6. Gauthier A, Levy VG, Quinton A, et al. Salt or no salt in the treatment of cirrhotic ascites: a randomized study. Gut 1986; 27:705–709.
7. Linas SL, Anderson RJ, Miller PD, Schrier RW. The rational use of diuretics in cirrhosis. In Epstein M (ed). The Kidney in Liver Disease. 2nd ed. New York: Elsevier Science Publishing Company, 1983:555–567.
8. Pocros PJ, Reynolds TB. Rapid diuresis in patients with ascites from chronic liver disease: the importance of peripheral edema. Gastroenterology 1986; 90:1827–1833.
9. Gines P, Arroyo U, Quintero E, et al. Comparison of paracentesis and diuretics in the treatment of cirrhotics with tense ascites: results of a randomized study. Gastroenterology 1987; 93:234–241.
10. Pinto PC, Amerian J, Reynolds TB. Large-volume paracentesis in nonedematous patients with tense ascites: its effect on intravascular volume. Hepatology 1988; 8:207–210.
11. LeVeen EG, LeVeen HH. Why cirrhotics should be treated by peritoneovenous shunt. Am J Gastroenterol 1988; 83:1086–1087.
12. Kirkpatrick S, Schubert T. Umbilical hernia rupture in cirrhotics with ascites. Dig Dis Sci 1988; 33:762–765.

Asthma, refractory

Judd Shellito

Asthma is a recurrent disease associated with wheezing and shortness of breath. A characteristic feature of asthma is widespread narrowing of lung airways with resultant obstruction to air flow, which can vary, both spontaneously and in response to treatment. Asthma is a common disease, affecting approximately 3 per cent of the population of the United States.[1] Recent epidemiologic data suggest that mortality from asthma may be increasing,[2] underscoring the importance of proper management of these often difficult patients. This chapter will focus on outpatient management of refractory asthma in the adult patient. The term *refractory* indicates the presence of persistent but not incapacitating symptoms in spite of a trial of inhaled beta-adrenergic agonist bronchodilators, oral theophylline, or both.

■ Background

In most cases, the asthmatic patient presents to the physician with complaints of episodic wheezing and sensations of chest tightness. Patients with asthma are usually categorized as having *extrinsic* or *intrinsic* asthma. Extrinsic asthma is characterized by a seasonal variation in severity and often coexists with seasonal allergic rhinitis. Such patients commonly experience asthma during childhood and have an atopic history. Intrinsic asthma is asthma occurring in the absence of a history of atopy. Many of these patients develop asthma for the first time as an adult and have perennial symptoms.

■ DIFFERENTIAL DIAGNOSIS

Proper management of the asthmatic patient begins with an accurate diagnosis. In this regard, the aphorism, "All that wheezes is not asthma," is appropriate. Common conditions that may mimic the clinical presentation of asthma are shown in Table 1. It is incumbent upon the clinician to exclude nonasthmatic disease, in order to avoid misdirected and possibly toxic therapy.

■ ATYPICAL PRESENTATIONS

Asthma may also present in an atypical fashion, as shown in Table 2. It is important to recognize the many forms of asthma, because the clinical presentation may have implications for therapy. For example, in exercise-induced asthma, patients wheeze shortly after exercise. Often they do not require continuous medication but respond to an inhaled bronchodilator (beta-adrenergic agonist or cromolyn sodium) just before the onset of exercise. Endurance sports, such as distance running, are best avoided, but swimming is particularly well tolerated. Some patients with asthma initially present not with wheezing but with complaints of cough or exertional dyspnea.

Occupational asthma is important to recognize, because the major goal of therapy in these patients is not to treat bronchospasm but to limit exposure to sensitizing antigen. Patients with occupational asthma develop symptoms in relation to their work, with improvement on weekends or holidays and recurrence of symptoms during the work week. Often coworkers also have experienced respiratory problems. The list of occupations that may result in asthma is extensive and has been recently reviewed.[3] The clinician should be suspicious of occupations that involve exposure to substances of animal origin (bird fanciers, animal handlers, farmers), of plant origin (grain handlers, wood workers, bakers), and of chemical origin (metal workers, chemical workers, fumigators). Diagnosis is difficult and involves documentation of work exposure and in

TABLE 1. Differential Diagnosis of Wheezing

Left ventricular failure ("cardiac asthma")
Chronic bronchitis/emphysema
Pulmonary embolism
Sarcoidosis
Central airway obstruction (tumor, extrinsic compression, retained foreign body)
Pulmonary aspiration
Cystic fibrosis
Bronchiolitis

many cases inhalation challenge with the suspect antigen. Patients with occupational asthma should change their occupation to eliminate exposure to the offending agent, because irreversible obstructive disease may result from continued low-level exposures.

Approximately 5 per cent of asthmatics will experience a worsening of symptoms after taking aspirin.[4] This reaction is idiosyncratic and occurs within minutes of ingesting the drug. Flushing, urticaria, and angioedema also may be observed. Many of the patients will have rhinitis with nasal polyps and sinusitis. When all three features are present—asthma, aspirin sensitivity, and nasal polyps—the syndrome has been termed *triad asthma*. The syndrome of triad asthma is important to recognize because asthma in these patients tends to be severe, and therapy should focus on avoidance of aspirin and education about the aspirin contained in many over-the-counter medications. Of particular importance is the likelihood that these patients also will develop adverse reactions to the widely prescribed nonsteroidal anti-inflammatory drugs.

Some patients may experience symptoms only at night (*nocturnal asthma*), often in association with sensations of heartburn. Reflux of gastric acid has been postulated to induce vagally mediated bronchoconstriction in susceptible asthmatics. Gastroesophageal

TABLE 2. Atypical Presentations of Asthma

Exercise-induced
Persistent cough
Exertional dyspnea
Occupational asthma
Triad asthma (asthma, nasal polyps, aspirin sensitivity)
Allergic bronchopulmonary aspergillosis
Sulfite sensitivity

reflux may be a more important trigger factor in asthma than is generally appreciated, with reflux being found in one half to two thirds of asthmatic patients.[5] Reflux of gastric contents and exacerbation of asthma also may be seen with esophageal diseases such as achalasia. Treatment of nocturnal asthma is directed toward decreasing reflux and neutralizing gastric acid. Commonly employed maneuvers include elevation of the head of the bed, weight loss, smoking cessation, and use of antacids and H_2 receptor blocking agents. It should be noted that theophylline lowers esophageal sphincter pressure and alternatives to theophylline should be employed in the treatment of patients with nocturnal asthma.

Allergic bronchopulmonary aspergillosis is a complicated form of asthma caused by sensitization of the patient to fungi of the genus *Aspergillus*. Most of these patients have severe asthma, and many note lumps or plugs in expectorated sputum. The chest radiograph may show migratory alveolar infiltrates as well as changes compatible with central bronchiectasis. The peripheral eosinophil count is almost always increased, and precipitating IgG antibodies may be demonstrable in the serum. Serum IgE levels are also markedly elevated beyond the atopic range. Allergic bronchopulmonary aspergillosis is important to recognize, because therapy with corticosteroids is always indicated. The response to therapy should be guided by serial measurement of serum IgE as well as by resolution of symptoms, shadows on chest radiograph, and improvement in pulmonary function.[6]

Food allergies are uncommon in adults, but some asthmatics do develop worsening asthma in response to sulfiting agents used in commercially prepared foods and beverages. Sulfiting agents are commonly used in salad bars to retard browning of the produce and are contained in wines and dried fruits. Adverse reactions to sulfites are rare, fortunately, but may be quite severe. Typically, a patient with pre-existing asthma develops wheezing with or without anaphylaxis within 30 minutes of ingesting processed foods, wine, or beer. Management of the sulfite-sensitive asthmatic patient involves provocative testing with controlled doses of sulfites, education regarding selective avoidance of certain foods/beverages, and self-administration of epinephrine.[7]

■ Management

■ DRUGS USED IN THE TREATMENT OF ASTHMA

Beta-Adrenergic Agonists. These drugs are the mainstay of asthma therapy at all stages of severity. Bronchodilation is mediated through stimulation of $beta_2$-adrenergic receptors in the airways, whereas tachycardia and palpitations may result from stimulation of cardiac $beta_1$-adrenergic receptors. Thus, the ideal agent for the treatment of asthma is a $beta_2$-selective agent, such as metaproterenol, terbutaline, albuterol, fenoterol, or bitolterol. There is little practical difference among these drugs, and prescribing habits should be based on cost and patient preference. There is currently little or no indication for the outpatient use of non-$beta_2$-selective agents such as isoproterenol, epinephrine, and isoetharine.

All the $beta_2$-adrenergic agonists are available for inhalation by metered-dose inhaler, and this is the preferred route of administration. Oral administration of beta-adrenergic agonists is associated with a higher risk of palpitations and tremor than inhaled administration and should be avoided in the treatment of asthma, with the exception of nocturnal asthma. Beneficial effects from the use of a metered-dose inhaler are critically dependent upon technique of administration, and all patients given an inhaler should be personally coached by the clinician in proper use. For elderly patients, patients with arthritis, or those with poor comprehension, a number of spacer devices are available for use with a metered-dose inhaler to enhance drug penetration to the airways.[8] Nebulization of beta-adrenergic agonists with an electrically powered air pump is no more effective in terms of drug delivery than a properly used metered-dose inhaler.

After inhaled administration, the $beta_2$-selective agonists have an onset of bronchodilation within 30 minutes, a peak effect at 2 to 4 hours, and a duration of action of up to 5 hours. Thus, a sustained effect requires inhaler use at least four times daily, but in practice beta-adrenergic agonists are prescribed for much more frequent use. Patients with asthma do not develop tolerance to the effects of inhaled beta-adrenergic agonists,[9] and all asthmatic patients should be encouraged to use their inhaler whenever they feel the need. Patients with mild and intermittent asthma may carry their inhaler with them for use on a prn basis, but most asthmatic patients require regular inhaler administration every 6 hours, with prn use at any time. The use of beta-adrenergic agonist inhaler immediately prior to exercise may be of value in the treatment of exercise-induced asthma, and inhaler use at bedtime may help some patients with nocturnal asthma.

Methylxanthines. This class of drugs includes aminophylline and anhydrous theophylline. The bronchodilating action of methylxanthines is directly proportional to the serum concentration, with the therapeutic range being accepted at 10 to 20 mg/L. This class of drugs is best employed as sustained-release tablets, which are available in many forms and may be administered every 12 hours. The average daily dose is 12 mg/kg for adults. Patients should be started at a lower daily dose and gradually work up to the therapeutic range to avoid nausea and abdominal discomfort. There is no need to employ an oral loading dose. Serum theophylline levels should be checked frequently, as there is wide interpatient variability in theophylline clearance. Unfortunately, as shown in Table 3, theophylline clearance is also influenced by a number of other drugs, by congestive heart failure, and by liver disease.[10] Side effects from methylxanthines include nervousness, nausea, vomiting, headache, and insomnia, as well as more serious toxic effects, including seizures and cardiac arrhythmias. Although commonly pre-

TABLE 3. Theophylline Clearance

Factors That May Increase Theophylline Blood Levels
  Advanced age
  Congestive heart failure
  Liver disease
  Drugs
    Cimetidine
    Troleandomycin
    Propranolol
    Erythromycin
    Allopurinol

Factors That May Decrease Theophylline Blood Levels
  Infants and children
  Smoking (tobacco, marijuana)
  Drugs
    Phenobarbital
    Phenytoin
    Isoproterenol

scribed, the methylxanthines are relatively weak bronchodilators in comparison to the beta-adrenergic agonists.[11] Because of this, and given the risk of toxic side effects, methylxanthines are recommended only as a second- or even third-line drug in the treatment of asthma.

Cromolyn Sodium. Cromolyn sodium is thought to interfere with the release of mediators from mast cells but probably has other mechanisms of action as well. It is not a bronchodilator but rather a prophylactic agent. When used properly, cromolyn will prevent immediate and late-phase bronchospasm after the inhalation of antigen. Cromolyn formerly was available only in a powder form, the inhalation of which often caused throat irritation. A metered-dose inhaler form of cromolyn is now available, and this is the preferred method of drug delivery. The usual adult dose is 2 puffs (800 μg cromolyn/puff) four times daily, although some practitioners use higher doses. It is important that both the clinician and the patient understand that cromolyn is a prophylactic agent and will not provide immediate relief of bronchospasm. Benefit from the drug requires regular use over a 2- to 4-week period, before a decrease in the severity or frequency of symptoms is appreciated. Cromolyn is remarkably free of toxic side effects. Because of its unique mechanism of action and lack of toxicity, cromolyn is recommended for use in all asthmatic patients who are not easily controlled with beta-agonist agents alone.

Corticosteroids. Corticosteroids are important agents in the treatment of asthma, but the potentially serious side effects associated with long-term corticosteroid therapy dictate that these agents be the last added to a treatment regimen and the first to be removed after optimization of nonsteroidal therapies. Corticosteroids have multiple and potent anti-inflammatory actions, which contribute to their effectiveness in the treatment of asthma. In addition, corticosteroids increase beta-adrenergic responsiveness of airway cells and lymphocytes. Intermediate-acting steroids, such as prednisone, prednisolone, and methylprednisolone, are recommended for use in asthmatic patients, because only these agents can be used in alternate-day therapy.

Corticosteroids can be delivered intravenously, orally, or by inhalation. Intravenous administration is reserved for hospitalized patients and will not be discussed here. Oral administration is usually employed as short-term or "burst" therapy in exacerbations of asthma, although many patients with severe disease will require long-term oral therapy. Inhaled corticosteroids are usually used continuously as prophylactic agents to prevent exacerbations, although they also may be employed in concert with oral steroids to reduce the oral dose of corticosteroid and the risk of side effects.

It is difficult to make dosage recommendations for corticosteroids in the treatment of asthma, because the initial dosage and duration of therapy depend upon the severity of asthma in an individual patient, a history of prior corticosteroid use, and the initial response to therapy. Rather than rely on fixed treatment schedules, the clinician should base reduction in corticosteroid dose on measured improvement in peak expiratory flow or spirometry (discussed later). For burst treatment of chronic or subacute asthma, patients rarely require more than a single morning dose of 40 mg of prednisone. The onset of improvement is generally within 6 to 8 hours after an oral dose, with maximal improvement reached in about a week. Assuming a good response to therapy, the daily dose of steroid can then be tapered slowly by 10 mg every 3 days. A shorter 1-week course of steroid therapy also has been reported.[12] For patients who have received long-term treatment with corticosteroids, a more prolonged reduction in dosage is necessary. These patients usually can be fairly rapidly tapered to 10 to 15 mg of prednisone daily, but subsequent dose reductions should be done in 1-mg steps at 1- to 2-week intervals. In patients who have required frequent courses of corticosteroids, consideration should be given to alternate day therapy to reduce deleterious side effects. Alternate day therapy should not be employed until symptoms have been well controlled on daily therapy. It consists of giving 2.5 times the minimum effective daily dose on alternate mornings.

Dosages of inhaled corticosteroids must be carefully considered because the available inhaled steroids vary in potency. Most clinicians do not start the use of inhaled steroids until symptom control has been achieved with oral corticosteroids, because inhaled steroids can precipitate cough and bronchospasm. The recommended dose for all available inhaled preparations is 2 puffs four times daily, but there is currently a trend to use higher doses (16 to 20 puffs of beclomethasone daily).[13] As with cromolyn, improvement in symptoms with the use of inhaled corticosteroids is not immediate but requires 2 to 4 weeks of regular use.

Side effects from corticosteroids are related to both the duration and dose of therapy. In adults, side effects are uncommon if the duration of therapy is kept to less than 2 weeks. This has made burst therapy a popular treatment regimen for asthma. Side effects are minimal for chronic therapy at daily prednisone doses of 5 mg or less, but with higher doses weight gain, cushingoid habitus, bruisability, fluid retention, and mental changes can be troublesome. With long-term therapy, osteopenia, aseptic necrosis of the hip, hyperglycemia, and cataract formation occur frequently. Adrenal suppression is a problem for patients being weaned from long-term high-dose therapy, and these patients should be aware of the need for "stress" doses of corticosteroids in the event of trauma or surgery. Inhaled corticosteroids have few systemic side effects, and adrenal suppression is uncommon even with high-dose therapy. Candidiasis of the mouth and throat is observed in some patients using inhaled corticosteroids and can be successfully treated without stopping the drug by using a spacer device with the inhaler and washing the mouth out after each use. Less cough has been reported after the inhalation of triamcinolone in comparison with beclomethasone.[14]

Anticholinergics. Anticholinergic therapy of asthma has received recent attention because of experimental evidence supporting a role for the parasympathetic system in the pathogenesis of bronchoconstriction and because of the introduction of a potent inhaled form of atropine, ipratropium bromide, which is free of systemic side effects. Studies in asthmatic patients generally have shown that ipratropium is a slightly less effective bronchodilator than the beta-agonists but has a more prolonged duration of action.[15] A trial of ipratropium should be considered in asthmatic patients who have not responded well to nonsteroidal therapy, particularly in the older age group. These agents are also of particular benefit in patients who have troublesome side effects from beta-adrenergic drugs or who have bronchospasm aggravated by beta-blocker

therapy. The usual starting dose is 2 puffs four times daily, and patients should be warned not to expect the rapid onset of action characteristic of the inhaled beta-adrenergic agonists.

Antibiotics. Expectoration of thick, eosinophil-laden sputum during an exacerbation of asthma can be mistaken for purulent bronchitis and prompt the administration of antibiotics. Unfortunately, antibiotics are rarely indicated in the treatment of asthma, because exacerbations are generally triggered by viral rather than bacterial infections.[16] Commonly implicated viruses in adults include rhinovirus and influenza A.

Mucus-Active Agents. A variety of preparations are available to facilitate the clearance of tenacious sputum in patients with asthma and chronic bronchitis. Expectorants such as guaifenesin and iodide act as gastric irritants and stimulate bronchial mucus secretion through a vagal reflex arc. Mucolytic agents, such as acetylcysteine, liquefy sputum by breaking down glycoprotein disulfide bridges. Unfortunately, there is little evidence that any of these agents do in fact alter either the volume or viscosity of sputum when administered to asthmatic patients. Aerosolized acetylcysteine can also precipitate cough and severe bronchospasm.

Steroid-Sparing Agents. This class of drugs includes troleandomycin, ketotifen, and methotrexate, all of which have been used in asthmatic patients to reduce the dose of corticosteroids necessary for symptom control. Troleandomycin is a macrolide antibiotic that appears to exert its effect by impairing clearance of methylprednisolone. Concurrent use with corticosteroids may reduce the dose of steroid necessary for asthma control, but it is unclear whether this will reduce toxic side effects. Ketotifen fumarate is an antihistamine-like drug that has reported efficacy as a prophylactic agent mainly in patients with extrinsic asthma. It is not available in the United States. A recent small study of asthmatic patients treated with the cytotoxic drug methotrexate showed that methotrexate therapy resulted in a small but statistically significant decrease in the amount of prednisone necessary for symptom control.[17] This study requires confirmation in larger groups of patients before methotrexate can be recommended for clinical use in the treatment of asthma.

Medications That Can Interfere with the Treatment of Asthma. A large number of beta-blocker drugs have been reported to precipitate bronchospasm in patients with asthma. Such reactions can occur at any time after the institution of therapy with these agents, and the resultant attack of asthma may be resistant to treatment with beta-adrenergic agonists. Asthmatic reactions also have been reported to beta-blocker eye drops used in the treatment of glaucoma.[18] Clinicians should avoid the use of beta-blocker medications in all asthmatic patients. A subgroup of asthmatic patients also may react adversely to oral aspirin or nonsteroidal anti-inflammatory drugs (see Background).

■ NONPHARMACOLOGIC TREATMENT OF ASTHMA

An important part of asthma treatment is recognition of those factors that precipitate symptoms in an individual patient. This may allow the patient to change job, hobby, or lifestyle to avoid exposures that aggravate asthma, and it may result in better overall control of symptoms. For example, exposure to cold air is a recognized trigger for bronchospasm and may be avoided by the use of a muffler or a paper mask. Patients also may be able to avoid exposure to pets or animals, if this worsens their asthma. The patient who experiences exercise-induced asthma may benefit from inhaler use immediately prior to exercise. Limiting exposure to dusts, fumes, smoke, and other respiratory irritants is good advice for any asthmatic patient, and the asthmatic patient who smokes should be encouraged to quit. Conservative measures that are important in the treatment of any chronic pulmonary disease include adequate hydration to facilitate clearance of secretions, avoidance of excess weight, adequate rest, and vaccination against influenzal and pneumococcal infection.

Immunotherapy or hyposensitization has proven value in the management of allergic disorders. The best evidence for such value is in patients with allergic rhinitis, but limited data suggest that immunotherapy may benefit some patients with extrinsic asthma.[19] This has been best demonstrated for patients with allergies to dust mites and pollens. There is no evidence that immunotherapy with bacterial vaccines, food extracts, or aspirin is of value in the treatment of asthma. Repetitive injection of appropriate allergens stimulates the production of an IgG "blocking" antibody and a fall in circulating IgE levels with long-term therapy. Evaluation of a patient for immunotherapy involves defining IgE-mediated sensitivity to relevant antigens by skin testing or other in vitro tests. This should be done by a qualified allergist. In many cases, a patient's environment can be modified to reduce exposure to a particular allergen. Dust control measures can be very helpful in those patients sensitized to dust mites. If environmental measures are unsuccessful, a regimen of immunotherapy is instituted based on the injection of escalating doses of antigen extracts once or twice weekly. Benefit is apparent after 6 months to a year of therapy. The length of therapy is poorly defined, and many patients are treated indefinitely. Evaluation for immunotherapy is recommended for all patients with extrinsic asthma who require corticosteroid therapy or are poorly controlled with medications alone.

Nasal and sinus disease is more common among asthmatics than is generally appreciated. Up to 30 per cent of asthmatic patients have nasal polyps, and occult sinusitis may be present in up to 40 per cent.[20] The presence of reflex pathways from the nose and sinuses that can trigger bronchospasm suggests that treatment of the asthmatic nose may help the asthmatic lung. Many patients do, in fact, report that their asthma is improved after surgical procedures to remove nasal polyps or improve sinus drainage. The clinician should consider the possibility of nasal and sinus disease in all asthmatic patients, and an otolaryngologic consultation is not unreasonable for patients with refractory asthma.

Because emotional stress can precipitate bronchospasm and because some patients have difficulty coping with a chronic disease, the notion persists that asthma is a psychologic disorder. Patients should be reassured that asthma is a disease of the lungs, not of the brain, and should be cautioned not to rely upon stress reduction or hypnotherapy to the exclusion of bronchodilators. Psychiatric therapy may be of value in some patients with personality disorders, extreme anxiety, or depression.

■ STRATEGIES OF ASTHMA THERAPY

General Principles of Asthma Therapy

The initial evaluation of the asthmatic patient should be directed toward establishing an accurate diagnosis and excluding conditions that may mimic asthma. A thorough history is important, particularly with respect to factors that precipitate symptoms and the distinction between extrinsic and intrinsic asthma. The clinician should be alert to atypical presentations of asthma, because these may require different therapies. Complete pulmonary function testing is recommended, with the initial evaluation to gauge the severity of obstruction and to serve as a basis of comparison with follow-up testing. A baseline chest radiograph is also helpful. The goal of treatment in asthma is to reduce the frequency of attacks and to improve lung function as much as possible without side effects from medications.

Asthma therapy should be initiated in a stepwise fashion, with serial assessment of both symptoms and pulmonary function tests. As a general rule, medications should not be discontinued if there is no response, but new drugs should be added to the existing regimen. Symptoms can be recorded by the patient in a symptom diary, and pulmonary function can be assessed either by peak flow measurement using a disposable device or by office spirometry. The importance of serial measurements of pulmonary function to guide therapy cannot be overemphasized; symptoms alone correlate poorly with expiratory air flow. Because the therapy of asthma relies heavily on inhaled medications, patients should be educated (and re-educated) regarding proper inhaler use, and a spacer device should be prescribed if necessary. All patients using inhaled corticosteroids should probably use a spacer device to decrease the risk of candidiasis.

Therapy According to Severity of Asthma

Patients with mild asthma that occurs only seasonally or in response to exercise may respond to an inhaled beta-adrenergic agonist used on a prn basis. However, most patients respond better to these agents when they are used on a regular basis. The initial dosage is 2 puffs every 6 hours, but the inhalers may be used much more frequently, and patients should be encouraged to use their inhaler whenever they feel it is necessary. If there is an inadequate response to inhaled beta-adrenergic agonists, an anti-inflammatory drug such as cromolyn or inhaled corticosteroids should be added to the regimen. Because of its lack of side effects, cromolyn is probably the first choice in therapy after beta-adrenergic agonist inhalers. A therapeutic response to cromolyn requires 2 to 4 weeks of treatment, and patients should be encouraged to continue treatment even if they perceive no immediate benefit. After a trial of cromolyn, inhaled corticosteroids should be added if needed. Burst therapy with oral corticosteroids is often necessary to treat exacerbations. If a patient requires frequent bursts or is on continuous low-dose oral corticosteroids, consideration should be given to alternate-day therapy. Systemic corticosteroid therapy will result ultimately in serious side effects, and aggressive management is indicated in these patients to allow systemic steroids to be discontinued altogether or to reduce the dose as much as possible. These patients should be evaluated for immunotherapy and for occult nasal and sinus disease. A trial of either inhaled ipratropium or high-dose inhaled corticosteroids also would be appropriate in these cases.

■ Issues and Risks

Asthma can be fatal. It has been estimated that 2000 deaths occur each year from asthma in the United States.[21] The majority of these deaths are preventable. Death in asthma is not caused by overuse of medications. In fact, most studies of asthma fatalities suggest that excessive use of bronchodilators is a reflection of worsening asthma and the need for more effective therapy.[22] A common theme in all studies of asthma mortality is poor appreciation by both patients and health care providers of the severity or progression of the asthmatic condition. All patients with asthma should be educated about the potential severity of asthma and know what to do if their condition worsens. Danger signs include the need for more frequent inhaler use and cough or breathlessness that occurs with minimal exertion or interferes with sleep. Clinicians need to approach the asthmatic patient reporting a change in symptoms with the same urgency as a patient complaining of chest pain. Frequent office or emergency room evaluations are recommended, and objective measurement of expiratory flow is essential. Hospitalization is absolutely indicated for the following: disturbances of consciousness, cyanosis, arterial oxygen tension of less than 60, any increase in arterial carbon dioxide tension, gross pulmonary overinflation on chest radiograph, and any degree of pneumothorax or pneumomediastinum.[23] Hospitalization should also be considered for asthmatic patients with fever and infiltrates on chest film. Particular caution is warranted for asthmatic patients who have required hospitalization or mechanical ventilation in the past or who have had a long period of poor control.

REFERENCES

1. Prevalence of Selected Chronic Respiratory Conditions—United States, 1970. Series 10, No. 84. Washington, DC: US Department of Health, Education and Welfare, 1973.
2. Burr M. Is asthma increasing? J Epidemiol Commun Health 1987; 41:185–189.
3. Chan-Yeung M, Lam S. State of the art: occupational asthma. Am Rev Respir Dis 1986; 133:686–703.
4. Samter M, Beers R Jr. Intolerance to aspirin: clinical studies and consideration of its pathogenesis. Ann Intern Med 1968; 68:975–983.
5. Ward P. Complications of gastroesophageal reflux. West J Med 1988; 149:58–65.
6. Ricketti A, Greenberger P, Mintzer R, Patterson R. Allergic bronchopulmonary aspergillosis. Chest 1984; 86:773–778.
7. Bush R, Taylor S, Busse W. A critical evaluation of clinical trials in reactions to sulfites. J Aller Clin Immunol 1986; 78:191–202.
8. Tobin M, Jenouri G, Danta I, Kim C, Watson H, Sackner M. Response to bronchodilator drug administration by a new reservoir aerosol delivery system and a review of other auxiliary delivery systems. Am Rev Respir Dis 1982; 126:670–675.
9. Harvey J, Tattersfield A. Airway response to salbutamol: effect of regular salbutamol inhalations in normal atopic and asthmatic subjects. Thorax 1982; 37:280–287.
10. Miller J, Baciewiz A, Bauman J, Self T. Factors modifying serum theophylline concentrations. Immunol Aller Prac 1983; 131:18–44.
11. Siegel D, Sheppard D, Gelb A, Weinberg P. Aminophylline increases the toxicity but not the efficacy of inhaled beta-adrenergic agonists in the treatment of acute exacerbations of asthma. Am Rev Respir Dis 1985; 132:283–286.
12. Fiel S, Swartz M, Glanz K, Francis M. Efficacy of short-tem corticosteroid therapy in outpatient treatment of acute bronchial asthma. Am J Med 1983; 75:259–262.
13. Smith M, Hodson M. High-dose beclomethasone inhaler in the treatment of asthma. Lancet 1983; 1:265–269.
14. Shim C. Cough and wheezing from beclomethasone dipropionate aerosol are absent after triamcinolone acetonide. Ann Intern Med 1987; 106:700–703.
15. Gross N, Skorodin M. The place of anticholinergic agents in the treatment of airways obstruction. Immunol Aller Prac 1986; 8:7–14.
16. Li J, O'Connell E. Viral infections and asthma. Ann Allergy 1987; 59:321–331.
17. Mullarkey M, Blumenstein B, Andrade P, Bailey G, Olason I, Wetzel C. Methotrexate in the treatment of corticosteroid-dependent asthma: a double blind crossover study. N Engl J Med 1988; 31:603–607.
18. Dunn T, Gerber M, Shen A, Fernandez E, Iseman M, Cherniack R. The effect of topical ophthalmic instillation of timolol and betaxolol on lung function in asthmatic subjects. Am Rev Respir Dis 1986; 133:264–268.
19. Lichtenstein L, Valentine M, Norman P. A reevaluation of immunotherapy for asthma. Am Rev Respir Dis 1984; 129:657–659.
20. Slavin R. Relationship of nasal disease and sinusitis to bronchial asthma. Ann Allergy 1982; 49:76–80.
21. Report of Task Force on Epidemiology of Respiratory Diseases. NIH Pub. No. 81-2019. Washington, DC: National Institutes of Heath, 1980.
22. Benatar S. Fatal asthma. N Engl J Med 1986; 314:423–429.
23. Rebuck A, Read J. Assessment and management of severe asthma. Am J Med 1971; 51:788–798.

Atrial fibrillation

Nicholas Z. Kerin ■ *Howard Frumin* ■ *Ira Seth Cohen*
Bruno Escaler ■ *Melvyn Rubenfire*

Atrial fibrillation (AF) is the most common of the supraventricular arrhythmias and is characterized by asynchronous atrial movement, to which the ventricles respond irregularly.

"The auricles pipe and the ventricles perforce must dance . . . a dance that sometimes leads to death."[1] Kannel and associates described a significant increase in the mortality rate of patients suffering from AF with or without cardiovascular disease.[2] The mortality rate in patients who developed AF was double that of control subjects, with an average time to death of 6 years after the appearance of this disorder. A healthy population has a 2 per cent chance of developing chronic AF in the first 20 years of life, with risk increasing dramatically with age. In the majority of instances, AF occurs in association with congestive heart failure, rheumatic heart disease, hypertension and diabetes mellitus. Only 31 per cent of the cohort developed AF without apparent clinical cardiovascular disease.[2]

■ Background

■ PRECIPITATING FACTORS AFFECTING THERAPEUTIC MANAGEMENT

Diagnosing the precipitating factors leading to AF is an important part of clinical evaluation, since abatement or correction of these factors may become an important step in management of the patient. The precipitating factors of AF, based on sporadic case reports, are listed in Table 1A.

Thyrotoxicosis. AF has been reported to occur in 10 to 28 per cent of patients with clinically overt thyrotoxicosis. The incidence of arrhythmia increases with advanced age, with an incidence of 20 per cent over age 50 years.[3] A significant proportion of patients (13 per cent) with idiopathic AF has biochemical abnormalities suggestive of thyrotoxicosis.

The incidence of embolic phenomena in patients with thyrotoxicosis and AF is high (40 per cent), with 53 per cent of the embolic episodes affecting the brain.[4] In hyperthyroidism, a hyperdynamic circulatory state occurs, resulting in an adrenergic stimulation of the heart. It is generally accepted that acute therapeutic intervention for the cardiac manifestations of hyperthyroidism should focus on the hyperadrenergic state. The definitive therapy for cardiac manifestation of hyperthyroidism is treatment with oral antithyroid drugs, radioactive iodine, or surgery.

Holiday Heart Syndrome. The alcohol-induced paroxysmal AF (holiday heart syndrome) has been reported to be as high as 35 per cent.[5] There are no complications as the result of paroxysmal AF in alcoholic patients, with the majority of patients converting spontaneously to sinus rhythm within 24 hours without intervention.

■ ETIOLOGIC FACTORS

The etiology of AF (Table 1B) is related to either atrial tissue damage or elevated atrial pressure. The incidence of the etiologic factors responsible for AF has changed during the last 50 years. In a 1930 report, Parkinson and Campbell noted hypertension as the etiology in 24 per cent of patients with paroxysmal AF, myocardial disease in 22.5 per cent, rheumatic valvular disease in 22 per cent, hyperthyroidism in 14 per cent, and idiopathic in 15 per cent.[6] In recent years, the number of patients with hypertension and coronary artery disease has increased to 64.9 per cent, while the percentage of patients who have valvular disease and hyperthyroidism has declined.[7]

TABLE 1. Factors Promoting Atrial Fibrillation

A. Precipitating Factors
   Thyrotoxicosis
   Alcohol, caffeine
   Metabolic imbalance
      Catecholamines
      Hypoglycemia
      Fever
      Electrolyte
      Blood gases
      Acid-base
   Neurogenic imbalance
      Emotion
      Exertion
      Vomiting
      Cerebrovascular events
   Miscellaneous
      Hypothermia
      Electrocution

B. Etiologic Factors
   Hypertensive heart disease
   Coronary artery disease
   Rheumatic valvular disease
   Cardiomyopathy (congestive, hypertrophic)
   Sick sinus syndrome
   Thyrotoxicosis
   Congenital heart disease
   Pericarditis
   Idiopathic (lone) atrial fibrillation
   Post heart surgery
   Pulmonary embolism

Hypertensive Heart Disease. AF associated with hypertensive cardiovascular disease is common[2] and is attributable to the presence of both atrial distention and sick sinus syndrome. With the development of left ventricular hypertrophy or congestive heart failure, there is an increased tendency for AF. Aberg reported that 25 per cent of patients who died of hypertensive heart disease had transient AF.[8] The therapeutic approach should be the control of hypertension to prevent the atrial dilatation.

Coronary Artery Disease. AF occurs in about 10 per cent of patients with myocardial infarction and is secondary either to atrial infarction or congestive heart failure via a dilated atrium. Atrial infarction has been reported to occur in 17 per cent of patients who died of myocardial infarction.[9] Supraventricular arrhythmia has been described in 74 per cent of cases of atrial infarction, with AF the most common type found.

The clinical diagnosis of AF is important and has practical significance, since mural thrombosis has been reported to develop in 80 to 84 per cent of cases and pulmonary embolism in 24 per cent of cases[9] concomitantly with the development of AF. AF secondary to atrial infarction is difficult to convert to sinus during the acute event, because of the involvement of the atrial tissue.

In the clinical setting of extensive myocardial infarction, AF is associated with the development of congestive heart failure. In general, AF related to acute congestive heart failure is transient and converts to sinus with the improvement of the left ventricular function.

AF also may develop as a result of post-myocardial infarction syndrome (Dressler's syndrome). In the few patients in whom the control of ventricular response becomes difficult with medication, the addition of steroids, indomethacin, or aspirin may be helpful.

Rheumatic Valvular Disease. One of the most common causes of AF is underlying rheumatic valvular disease.[1,6–8] AF is a common complication of mitral stenosis (37.5 per cent), but bears no direct relationship to the degree of stenosis or atrial enlargement, which suggests that the development of arrhythmia may be the result of rheumatic involvement in atrial and myocardial tissues.[1] Fraser and Turner found that clots occur in the left atrium at operation in 40 per cent of patients with AF, whereas clotting occurs in only 2 per cent of patients in sinus rhythm.[1] Congestive heart failure occurs more frequently in patients with AF than in those in sinus rhythm.[1] AF occurs very rarely (0.8 per cent) in patients with aortic valve disease, but carries a poor prognosis when present.

Cardiomyopathy. AF is a common arrhythmia, appearing in 20 per cent of patients with congestive cardiomyopathy (also see article on Congestive Heart Failure). The development of AF is accompanied by increasing congestive heart failure and evinces advancement in the course of the disease.[10] The morbidity associated with AF is either related to hemodynamic changes brought forth by arrhythmia or by the effects of systemic embolism.

The incidence of AF in patients with idiopathic hypertrophic subaortic stenosis points to a poor prognosis. The arrhythmia usually complicates the course of the disease in patients who have left ventricular dysfunction. The hemodynamic consequences occurring during the paroxysms of AF with rapid ventricular response may lead to hemodynamic embarrassment, manifested by hypotension or shock. Patients presenting with AF and left ventricular dysfunction may benefit from digitalis therapy. In the clinical setting of a normal or hyperkinetic left ventricular ejection fraction, digitalis may increase the outflow obstruction and therefore should be avoided.

Sick Sinus Syndrome. Patients who have sick sinus syndrome may present with recurrent episodes of AF. AF becomes the escape mechanism as the sinus node fails. The slow ventricular response occurring in 30 per cent of patients may be due to the co-existence of AV nodal disease.

Antiarrhythmic drugs such as quinidine, procainamide, and propranolol have not been effective in preventing episodes of AF in sick sinus syndrome and may worsen bradycardia. Engle and Schaal showed that digitalis does not have a significant effect on either sinus node recovery time or the sinus node rate in patients with sick sinus syndrome.[11] The presence of AV block might represent a relative contraindication for digitalis use.[11]

Idiopathic (Lone) Atrial Fibrillation. Idiopathic AF occurs without clinically preexisting heart disease. Cardiovascular disease will develop in more than 40 per cent of subjects who have lone AF. The occurrence of stroke increases fourfold in patients who have lone AF.[12]

Post Heart Surgery. Postoperative AF is common in patients following valve replacement and coronary artery bypass surgery, with a reported incidence of about 23 per cent.[1] Although these arrhythmias are transient and are not usually life threatening, they often require treatment of the rapid ventricular rate. Digoxin and propranolol have been administered to prevent the development of AF in the immediate postoperative period. The results have been conflicting, ranging from a dramatic reduction in the incidence of AF[13] to inconsistent results.

Pericardial Disease. Spodick reports a 5 per cent incidence of AF in patients who have acute pericarditis.[14] A higher prevalence of AF is encountered in patients who have uremic pericarditis.

Wolff-Parkinson-White (WPW) Syndrome. The incidence of AF is significantly higher in patients with WPW than in the general population, with a frequency ranging from 11 to 39 per cent.[15] The high frequency of AF in WPW, coupled with its risk of degenerating into ventricular fibrillation, mandates that patients with WPW be evaluated for the potential risk of sudden cardiac death.

The appropriate treatment of AF in patients with accessory bypass is direct current cardioversion. After cardioversion, procainamide should be administered intravenously to prolong the refractoriness of the bypass tract as well as to prevent the recurrence of AF. Drugs such as verapamil and propranolol, which produce a depressant effect on the AV node without any effect on the bypass tract, should not be used. After restoration of sinus rhythm, electrophysiologic studies should be performed to confirm the effectiveness of the chosen antiarrhythmic drug. Only amiodarone and encainide have been shown effective in preventing AF in WPW by lengthening the refractoriness of both the bypass tract and the atrioventricular node.

■ COMPLICATIONS

AF poses a substantial risk in patients with underlying organic heart disease. Either paroxysmal or chronic AF may precipitate heart failure or atrial thrombosis. The atrium, functioning like a booster pump with regard to ventricular filling, augments cardiac output by about 20 per cent. In patients who have no clinically recognizable heart disease, the arrhythmia has a slightly adverse hemodynamic effect. The salutary effect of sinus rhythm suggests that patients who have a diseased heart pump benefit significantly from the re-establishment of sinus rhythm.

The presence of AF, especially in association with ischemic heart disease or mitral valve disease, results in significant risk of developing atrial thrombosis, which in turn results in raising the risk for development of systemic emboli.

■ NATURAL COURSE

AF can be classified as transient or paroxysmal and chronic, persistent, or permanent. In more than 90 per cent of patients, the paroxysms of AF do not last more than 7 days.[16] Paroxysmal AF often precedes the establishment of a chronic form of arrhythmia. Long paroxysms lasting for more than 2 weeks are observed in few patients (7.4 per cent).[7] The development of a chronic AF is an unfavorable prognostic sign suggestive of significant underlying heart disease. Paroxysmal AF becomes permanent in one quarter of patients.[6] The tendency of arrhythmia to become chronic depends on the underlying cause. A permanent form of AF develops in all patients with rheumatic valvular disease within 2 years after the appearance of paroxysmal episodes.[6] A tendency to chronicity of this arrhythmia depends on the duration of the episodes of AF, the underlying pathology (rheumatic valvular disease, congestive cardiomyopathy, or congenital heart disease), lone AF, and left atrial size. The paroxysmal form of arrhythmia usually develops in treatable or transient causes, i.e., thyrotoxicosis, pericarditis, WPW, atrial infarction, acute myocardial infarction, pulmonary embolism, sick sinus syndrome, and postcoronary bypass surgery.

■ Management

■ RAPID ATRIAL FIBRILLATION

AF with rapid ventricular response may occur in a variety of etiologic settings, detailed in Table 1B. The therapeutic option selected depends on the patient's hemodynamic stability at the time of evaluation or the underlying heart disease. An unstable situation in a patient with AF and rapid ventricular response may be manifested by hypotension, left ventricular failure, or unstable angina. If an unstable pattern exists or is anticipated to develop because of the underlying disease, the patient is a candidate for options listed in Table 2A.

Electrical conversion should be attempted if the patient is unstable either clinically or hemodynamically. When AF appears as a consequence of atrial infarction, thyrotoxicosis, post heart surgery, digitalis toxicity, or uncorrected congenital heart disease, it is very unlikely that a sinus rhythm will be restored by cardioversion. In these cases, the hemodynamic stability should be restored by controlling the rapid ventricular response through intravenous administration of digitalis, verapamil, beta-blockers, or amiodarone (Table 2A). Electrical conver-

TABLE 2. Management of Rapid Atrial Fibrillation

A. Clinically and/or Hemodynamically Unstable
Cardioversion

Digoxin	IV	Loading dose 1–1.25 mg/24 hr, followed by maintenance of 0.25–0.50 mg/24 hr
Verapamil	IV	0.075–0.15 mg/kg body weight up to 10 mg over 2–3 min. If necessary, an IV infusion of 0.005 mg/kg/min. If LV dysfunction presents, add 10–20 mg 10% calcium gluconate
Beta-Blockers		
Esmolol	IV	1 min loading infusion of 500 μg/kg/min, followed by a 4-min maintenance of 50 μg/kg/min titrated to ventricular rate and blood pressure response
Propranolol	IV	4–8 mg over 10–15 min
Metoprolol	IV	10–15 mg over 10–15 min
*Amiodarone**	IV	12-hr loading of 2.3 mg/min, followed by a maintenance of 0.7 mg/min for the next 36 hr

B. Clinically and/or Hemodynamically Stable
Cardioversion

Digoxin	IV	See Table 2A
Verapamil	IV	See Table 2A
	PO	80–120 mg TID/24 hr
Beta-Blockers	IV	See Table 2A
Propranolol	PO	10–80 mg TID/24 hr
Metoprolol	PO	50–100 mg BID/24 hr
*Amiodarone**	IV	See Table 2A
	PO	Loading dose of 800 mg—1 gm/24 hr for 7 days, titrated to maintenance of 200–400 mg/day

*Investigational.

sion during an acute situation has been shown to be effective in restoring sinus rhythm in patients with the following underlying pathologies: WPW, rheumatic valvular disease, postmyocardial infarction, cardiomyopathy, sick sinus syndrome, and hypertensive heart disease.

If a contraindication to cardioversion exists (e.g., a recent meal), another therapeutic option is the administration of intravenous procainamide (Table 3). The procainamide is effective in converting AF present for 2 weeks or less (88 per cent), but quite ineffective (20 per cent) if the arrhythmia is of longer duration.[17] Intravenous verapamil is an excellent and well-tolerated drug for control of the ventricular response in rapid AF, with control occurring in 97 per cent of patients after a single bolus of 10 mg. Approximately 10 to 37 per cent of patients will convert to sinus mechanism with verapamil.[17] The rate of decrease is transient, lasting 30 minutes. A constant infusion of verapamil may be necessary to maintain control of the ventricular rate. Verapamil-related hemodynamic (hypotension) or rate (bradycardia) complications may be prevented or reversed by concomitant administration of calcium gluconate (Table 2A).

TABLE 3. Drug Regimens for Conversion of Atrial Fibrillation and Maintenance of Sinus Mechanism After Conversion

A. Regimens for Drug Conversion

Procainamide	IV	800–1000 mg over 30 min
	PO	300 mg q 3 hr for 6 doses
Quinidine sulfate	PO	200–300 mg q 3 to 6 hr for 6 to 8 doses
Disopyramide	PO	300 mg initially, followed by 200 mg q 6 hr for 4 to 6 doses
Flecainide*	IV	50 mg given over 10 min. If sinus rhythm is not restored, the bolus can be repeated, not exceeding 2 mg/kg. Four hours later, 100–200 mg twice/day
Amiodarone	PO	See Table 2B

B. Regimens for Drug Maintenance

Quinidine gluconate	PO	330 mg q 6 or 8 hr, maintaining blood levels >2 µg/ml
Quinidine sulfate (sustained release form)	PO	300 mg q 6 or 8 hr/day, maintaining blood levels >2 µg/ml
Procainamide (sustained release form)	PO	500–1000 mg q 6 hr/day, maintaining blood levels >4 µg/ml
Disopyramide	PO	100–200 mg q 6 to 8 hr/day
Flecainide acetate	PO	100–200 mg twice/day

*Investigational.

Intravenous beta-blockers (Table 2A) are effective in controlling the ventricular response in AF.[18] During administration, transient mild hypotension may develop. To avoid asystole, verapamil should not be administered close to the time of administration of beta-blockers.

Rapid digitalization is useful to slow the ventricular rate in rapid AF (Table 2A). This may not be the case in the presence of fever or hyperthyroidism. The role of digitalis in conversion is controversial. It has been maintained that digitalis promotes conversion to sinus rhythm by slowing the AV conduction and by hemodynamic improvement.

Cardioversion, digitalis, verapamil, or beta-blockers should be considered as first-line approaches in the control of fast ventricular fibrillation.

In resistant cases, intravenous amiodarone, an experimental drug, can produce swift control of the ventricular rate (Table 2A). Amiodarone is well tolerated hemodynamically and can be used safely in patients with impaired left ventricular function.

If any of these agents alone does not slow the ventricular rate sufficiently, a combination of two of these drugs (e.g., verapamil plus digoxin, esmolol plus digitalis) can be tried.

The therapeutic regimens are outlined in Table 2B for patients in a clinically and/or hemodynamically stable state.

■ ESTABLISHED ATRIAL FIBRILLATION

Once rate control is achieved, attempts should be made to restore sinus rhythm. Type IA antiarrhythmic drugs (e.g., procainamide, quinidine, disopyramide), type IC (e.g., flecainide), and type IV (e.g., amiodarone) have demonstrated efficacy in the conversion of AF to sinus rhythm.[19-21] Quinidine is the antiarrhythmic drug of choice in the conversion treatment of AF. The efficacy rate of conversion in chronic AF has been reported to be around 60 per cent.[20] In AF of recent vintage, quinidine and flecainide appear to be equally effective (86 per cent vs. 80 per cent conversion rates).[20] Amiodarone is also effective (86 per cent) in converting chronic AF to sinus rhythm. Usually the conversion to sinus rhythm occurs between the third and fifth days of treatment, when doses of 600 to 800 mg/day are employed for as long as required to complete conversion. If conversion does not occur within a month, the therapy is terminated.[21] Conversion to sinus rhythm also can be obtained with a low-dose amiodarone approach (Table 2*B*).

■ ELECTRICAL CARDIOVERSION

Electrical conversion is an effective (95 per cent) method of converting AF to sinus rhythm without significant complications.[22] The number of patients maintaining sinus rhythm gradually falls with the passage of time. At 1 and 2 years, 35 per cent and 20 per cent, respectively, of the patients studied reverted to AF. Prophylactic administration of quinidine did not improve these figures appreciably.[22] Chronic therapy with low-dose amiodarone has been shown to be more effective in maintaining sinus rhythm, with 72 per cent of patients maintaining sinus rhythm at 1 year.[23]

The failure to maintain sinus rhythm after cardioversion of chronic AF depends on the underlying heart disease, left atrial enlargement, the duration of the arrhythmia, advanced age of patients, and the previous use of antiarrhythmic agents. Echocardiographic studies have suggested that a left atrial diameter of greater than 4.5 cm is associated with a high recurrence rate of atrial fibrillation. A recent study[23] revealed a poor correlation between atrial size and the outcome of cardioversion. We advocate that cardioversion be considered at least once for a patient with AF, even in the presence of a large atrium.

Drugs employed for the maintenance of sinus rhythm in patients with paroxysmal AF or after cardioversion are listed in Table 3. Previous studies failed to show any advantages between placebo, quinidine, or disopyramide in maintaining sinus rhythm following electrical cardioversion in patients with valvular heart disease.[24] Low-dose amiodarone has been shown to be safe and effective in maintaining sinus rhythm in patients with AF refractory to type IA antiarrhythmic agents. During long-term treatment, sinus rhythm was sustained on an average of 16 months in 53 per cent of patients resistant to type IA agents.[25]

■ Issues and Risks

Chronic AF is associated with a high incidence of thromboembolic events. In the Framingham study, patients with AF without valvular heart disease had a 5.6 times higher incidence of stroke than individuals in sinus rhythm.[26] The risk of embolism is greater in the patients with AF and the following underlying heart diseases: ischemic heart disease, mitral valve disease, sick sinus syndrome, lone AF (?), and congestive or hypertrophic cardiomyopathy. Anticoagulant treatment should be considered in these patients.

In patients subjected to pharmacologic or electrical cardioversion of AF, there is an increased incidence of systemic emboli. Two to three weeks of anticoagulation therapy are suggested prior to conversion, which should be continued for at least one month after cardioversion.

The therapeutic approach to the patient with AF should be individualized according to the clinical setting, underlying disease, and the potential hemodynamic consequences of the arrhythmia on the patient's clinical stability.

REFERENCES

1. Fraser HRL, Turner RWD. Auricular fibrillation with special reference to rheumatic heart disease. Br Med J 1955; 28:1414–1418.
2. Kannel WB, Abbott RD, Savage DD, McNamara PM. Epidemiologic features of chronic atrial fibrillation: The Framingham Study. N Engl J Med 1982; 306:1018–1022.
3. Hoffman I, Lowrey RD. The electrocardiogram in thyrotoxicosis. Am J Cardiol 1960; 6:893–904.
4. Bar-Sela S, Ehrenfeld M, Eliakim M. Arterial embolism in thyrotoxicosis with atrial fibrillation. Arch Intern Med 1981; 141:1191–1192.
5. Lowenstein SR, Gabow PA, Cramer J, Oliva PB, Ratner K. The role of alcohol in new-onset atrial fibrillation. Arch Intern Med 1983; 143:1882–1885.
6. Parkinson J, Campbell M. Paroxysmal auricular fibrillation. A record of two hundred patients. Q J Med 1930; 23:67–100.
7. Takahashi N, Seki A, Imataka K, Fujii J. Clinical features of paroxysmal atrial fibrillation. An observation of 94 patients. Jap Heart J 1981; 22:143–149.
8. Aberg H. Atrial fibrillation. I. A study of atrial thrombosis and systemic embolism in necropsy material. Acta Med Scand 1969; 185:373–379.
9. Wartman WB, Hellerstein HK. The incidence of heart disease in 2,000 consecutive autopsies. Ann Intern Med 1948; 28:41–65.

10. Goodwin JF. Congestive cardiomyopathy. *In* Hurst JW (ed). The Heart. 4th ed. New York: McGraw-Hill, 1978:1567–1580.
11. Engle TR, Schaal SF. Digitalis in sick sinus syndrome. The effects of digitalis on sinoatrial automaticity and atrioventricular conduction. Circulation 1973; 48:1201–1207.
12. Brand FN, Abbott RD, Kannel WB, Wolf PA. Characteristics and prognosis of lone atrial fibrillation. Thirty year follow-up in the Framingham Study. JAMA 1985; 254:3449–3453.
13. Ivey MF, Ivey TD, Bailey WW, et al. Influence of propranolol on supraventricular tachycardia early after coronary artery revascularization: A randomized trial. J Thorac Cardiovasc Surg 1983; 85:214–218.
14. Spodick DH. Arrhythmias during acute pericarditis: prospective study of 100 consecutive cases. JAMA 1976; 235:39–41.
15. Garan H. Problems common to the evaluation and management of several different forms of cardiac disease. 5. Preexcitation syndromes. *In* Johnson R, Haber G, Austen WG (eds). The Practice of Cardiology. Boston: Little, Brown, 1980:132–154.
16. Brill IC. Auricular fibrillation. The present status with a review of the literature. Ann Intern Med 1937; 10:1487–1502.
17. Tommaso C, McDonough T, Parker M, Talano JV. Atrial fibrillation and flutter. Immediate control and conversion with intravenously administered verapamil. Arch Intern Med 1983; 143:877–881.
18. Gray RJ, Bateman TM, Czer LSC, Conklin CM, Matloff JM. Esmolol, a new ultrashort-acting beta-adrenergic blocking agent for rapid control of heart rate in postoperative supraventricular tachyarrhythmias. J Am Coll Cardiol 1985; 5(6):1451–1456.
19. Kayden HJ, Brodie BB, Steele JM. Procaine amide. Circulation 1957; 15:118–126.
20. Borget A, Goy JJ, Maendly R, Kaufman U, Grbid M, Sigwart U. Flecainide versus quinidine for conversion of atrial fibrillation to sinus rhythm. Am J Cardiol 1986; 58:496–498.
21. Santos AL, Alexio AM, Laudeivo J, Luis AS. Conversion of atrial fibrillation to sinus rhythm with amiodarone. Acta Med Port 1979; 1:15–23.
22. Donaldson P, Kavanagh-Gray D. Electrical cardioversion of atrial fibrillation. Can Med Assoc J 1969; 100:370–373.
23. Dittrich HC, Ericson JS, Schneiderman T, Blacky R, Savides T, Nicod PM. Echocardiographic and clinical predictors for outcome of elective cardioversion of atrial fibrillation. Am J Cardiol 1989; 63:193–197.
24. Lloyd EA, Gersh BJ, Forman R. The efficacy of quinidine and disopyramide in the maintenance of sinus rhythm after electroconversion from atrial fibrillation. South Afr Med J 1984; 65:367–369.
25. Blevins RD, Kerin NZ, Benederet D, Frumin H, Faitel K, Jarandilla R, Rubenfire M. Amiodarone in the management of refractory atrial fibrillation. Arch Intern Med 1987; 147:1401–1404.
26. Wolf PA, Dawber TR, Thomas HE, Kannel WB. Epidemiologic assessment of chronic atrial fibrillation and the risk of stroke: The Framingham Study. Neurology 1978; 28:973–977.

Attention-deficit hyperactivity disorder

William R. Yates ■ *Les L. Barrickman*

■ Background

Attention-deficit hyperactivity disorder (ADHD) is a common childhood psychiatric disorder, with prevalence rate estimates of 3 to 6 per cent in the general population.[1] This base frequency rate means a standard classroom can expect to have one or two children with ADHD; it is, therefore, one of the most common childhood psychiatric disorders seen in primary care. Young boys are much more likely (six to nine times) to be affected and usually present with more symptoms than do girls. The majority have symptoms beginning in the fourth to sixth year of life, which persist through childhood and early adolescence. Despite persistent childhood symptoms, outcome studies suggest a good prognosis for uncomplicated ADHD.[2] A poorer prognosis in ADHD is found for those with comorbid psychiatric disorders (especially conduct disorder), low IQ, and parents with severe mental disorder. Although environmental factors may influence severity, genetic factors appear primary in the development of an ADHD syndrome.

Previously, ADHD has had many synonyms, such as hyperkinetic syndrome, hyperactive child syndrome, and minimal brain dysfunction (MBD). The development of standardized psychiatric nomenclature, including the recent revision of The Diagnostic and Statistical Manual of Mental Disorders (DSM-III-R),[3] emphasizes the need for consistent diagnostic criteria for ADHD. It is one of three disorders (the other two are conduct disorder and oppositional defiant disorder) subclassified under the Disruptive Behavior Disorders category of child/adolescent psychiatric disorders in DSM-III-R. Disruptive behavior disorders as a group are characterized by socially disruptive behaviors that are frequently more distressing to those around the child than for the ADHD child.

■ DIAGNOSIS

Diagnostic Criteria

The DSM-III-R diagnosis of ADHD requires a child to display at least 8 of 14 possible symptoms for a minimum duration of 6 months. A symptom meets the criteria only when it is considerably more frequent than in most similar-aged children. Criteria listed in descending order of discriminating power include:

- (1) often fidgets with hands or feet or squirms in seat (in adolescents, symptoms may be limited to subjective feelings of restlessness),
- (2) has difficulty remaining seated when required,
- (3) is easily distracted by extraneous stimuli,
- (4) has difficulty awaiting turn in games or group situation,
- (5) often blurts out answers to questions before they have been completed,
- (6) has difficulty following through on instructions from others (not due to oppositional behavior or comprehension failure), e.g., fails to finish chores,
- (7) has difficulty sustaining attention in tasks or play activities,
- (8) often shifts from one uncompleted activity to another,
- (9) has difficulty playing quietly,
- (10) often talks excessively,
- (11) often interrupts or intrudes on others, e.g., butts into other children's games,
- (12) often does not seem to listen to what is being said to him or her,
- (13) often loses things necessary for tasks or activities at school or home (e.g., toys, books, assignments), and
- (14) often engages in physically dangerous activities without considering possible consequences (not for the purpose of

thrill-seeking), e.g., runs into street without looking.

In general, one can classify these cardinal features as involving developmentally inappropriate inattention, impulsivity, or hyperactivity. Onset, by definition, must be before the age of 7 years. Though the syndrome frequently is not identified until a child enters the school setting, almost half the children have onset of symptoms prior to 4 years of age. The final diagnostic criterion is one of exclusion, requiring the child to not meet criteria for a Pervasive Developmental Disorder such as autism. After the diagnosis is made, DSM-III-R also adds criteria for assessing severity: mild—few, if any, excess symptoms required for diagnosis and, at most, only minimal impairment in school and social functioning; moderate—symptoms or functional impairment between mild and severe; severe—many symptoms in excess of those required for diagnosis, with significant and pervasive impairment in functioning at home and school and with peers. Academic problems, mood lability, low frustration level, and temper are frequent associated features. Complications and impairment vary with severity and usually involve academic and social functioning.

Diagnostic Difficulties Affecting Management

Conduct disorder is a frequent coexisting (comorbid) psychiatric condition of children with ADHD.[4] Conduct disorder is characterized by aggressiveness, rule-breaking, juvenile delinquency, and early alcohol and drug abuse problems. Because ADHD and conduct disorder commonly coexist, attention to this diagnosis is important in the evaluation and treatment of ADHD. Conduct disorder appears to have a separate genetic mechanism and to not respond to medication management. Unlike ADHD, conduct disorder is often a harbinger of adult psychiatric problems, including alcohol and drug abuse, along with adult antisocial behavior.

■ Management

General Principles

Physicians frequently receive requests from parents or teachers to initiate or continue stimulant medication for children with ADHD. This request highlights the need for physicians to use a multidisciplinary approach for the assessment, treatment, and follow-up care of this disorder. The physician may need to use multiple sources of information to determine whether a trial of medication is indicated. Information from family members, teachers, and school psychologists, as well as special education specialists, may be helpful in determining the severity of the target problem. Rating scales such as the Connors scale also can be helpful in determining the baseline severity of the problem and monitoring any pharmacologic or psychotherapeutic intervention.[5] Physicians need to resist being only prescription writers in the care of ADHD syndrome patients. A coordinated assessment and treatment plan is the beginning of successful treatment of ADHD. Pharmacotherapy without attention to specific classroom and academic problems is unlikely to be helpful. Nevertheless, pharmacotherapy can be quite helpful, and an awareness of the pharmacotherapeutic options will allow physicians to add an important element to the total care of children with ADHD.

■ PHARMACOTHERAPY

Before beginning a medication trial, the physician should perform a comprehensive history and physical examination. Special attention should be paid to vital signs, height, and weight, as well as to the neurologic physical examination.

Education of family, teacher, and patient forms the basis for a good outcome for medication trials in ADHD. The goal of medication management is to improve the child's ability to attend to school tasks and improve classroom performance. Before starting a trial, parents and the child should be informed of the goal of medication use, as well as nonmedication alternatives. Parents and the child with ADHD should be told that medication is helpful for some but needs to be seen as only part of the treatment program. Any trial of medication is just that— an attempt to see whether beneficial results can be obtained with pharmacotherapy. The family should be aware of the time required to evaluate the efficacy of a medication trial, as well as possible problems. Medication trials do not mean a commitment to long-term medication management. If a trial of the first medication is unsuccessful, the medication is discontinued. A second medication trial or nonmedication intervention can then be considered. When a medication trial is successful, a plan for medication holidays also must be developed, with periodic reassessments of the efficacy of and need for medication.[6] Following the provision of a base of family and patient education, the specific medication approaches to management are often extremely helpful.

Stimulants

The drugs of choice for treatment of ADHD are the stimulants,[7] which include methylphenidate (Ritalin), dextroamphetamine (Dexedrine), and pemoline (Cylert) (Table 1). Methylphenidate is the most widely prescribed of the stimulants and is considered the prototype for the stimulant class. The superiority of stimulants over placebo has been consistently shown in numerous studies.[8] Although other classes of medications have been used with efficacy in ADHD, stimulants are the only class of agents with Food and Drug Administration approval for ADHD. Stimulants do require physicians to follow state and national scheduled drug class regulations. Physicians need to be aware that many states track physician prescription patterns, paying special attention to Class II agents.

Doses lower than the usual effective dose of stimulants should be given at first, with gradual increases based on side effects and response. Because methylphenidate and dextroamphetamine have relatively short half-lives, a twice-a-day dosing schedule is often necessary, with doses just before school and at noontime. This schedule helps avoid any stimulant-related problems with insomnia. Doses given at school will need to be supervised by appropriate personnel under individual school policies for medication administration at school.

Stimulants can be given every day and frequently are in severe ADHD, but also may be given only on school days. For severe cases, stimulants may be required during summer months and school vacations, for year-round treatment. Stimulants appear to have different behavioral effects in children with ADHD compared with normal adults. These children infrequently experience common adult stimulant effects, including increased energy, decreased fatigue, and euphoria. Initial positive responses to

stimulants do not usually decrease with time or tolerance to the drug. There does appear to be a dose-response relationship, with higher doses (within acceptable limits) being more efficacious.[9] Doses higher than the recommended 0.7 mg/kg/day are rarely additionally beneficial and usually result in more frequent and severe adverse effects. Failure to respond to one stimulant does not necessarily indicate treatment resistance to the entire stimulant class.

Most of the adverse effects from stimulants are directly due to their psychopharmacologic properties acting at both central and peripheral areas. These effects are often also dose related. A "behavioral rebound" effect can occur within a few (about 5) hours after medication administration and primarily consists of excitability and talkativeness.

The common adverse stimulant effects are noted in Table 1. Two concerns deserve attention and awareness. First, some reports of involuntary tics and Tourette's syndrome have been noted in children treated for ADHD with stimulants.[10] Although these reports lack the necessary controls to confirm a causal relationship, it is best to avoid stimulants in patients with tics and to monitor for this problem in children receiving stimulant medication. Second, delay of growth during stimulant medication also has been noted. However, long-term follow-up of stimulant-treated children reveals evidence of a growth rebound phenomenon without permanent growth retardation when stimulants are discontinued.[11]

Although stimulants are the basis of most treatment programs, additional agents have been used in ADHD with some success. For children not responding to stimulants or with contraindications to stimulant use, other agents can be considered. These alternate agents can be grouped into antidepressants and other medication categories.

Antidepressants

Both tricyclic antidepressants (TCAs) and monoamine oxidase inhibitors (MAOIs), have been utilized in the management of ADHD (see Table 1). With TCAs, imipramine is probably the most frequently used, although there is also some clinical experience with desipramine. The MAOIs primarily used have been clorgyline and tranylcypromine sulfate. Results of several studies have shown rather impressive response rates, ranging from 50 to 80 per cent, in both

110

TABLE 1. Pharmacologic Agents in Attention-Deficit Hyperactivity Disorder

Generic Name	Brand Name(s)	Scheduled Class	Dose by Weight	Typical Dose	FDA ADHD Indication	Lower Age Limit	Adverse Effects
Stimulants							
Methylphenidate	Ritalin	II	0.3–0.7 mg/kg/day	10 mg BID	yes	6	Nervousness, insomnia, growth retardation, increased blood pressure
Dextroamphetamine	Dexedrine	II	0.3–0.7 mg/kg/day	10 mg BID	yes	3	Same as for methylphenidate
Pemoline	Cylert	IV	0.9–1.5 mg/kg/day	56.25 mg daily	yes	6	Insomnia, anorexia, liver function abnormalities
Antidepressants							
Imipramine	Tofranil, SK-pramine	none	2.5 mg/kg/day maximum	50 mg hs	no	6 (for enuresis)	Dry mouth, constipation, sedation, cardiac conduction disorder, orthostasis
Desipramine	Norpramin	none	2.5 mg/kg/day maximum	50 mg hs	no	*	As imipramine, with possibly less anticholinergic effect
Tranylcypromine	Parnate	none	0.1–0.3 mg/kg/day	10 mg daily	no	*	Tyramine hypertensive crisis, dry mouth, orthostasis
Other Agents							
Clonidine	Catapres	none	0.002–0.004 mg/kg/day	0.05 BID	no	*	Dry mouth, sedation, hypotension

*Limited information regarding lower age limit in children.

medication groups.[12] Benefits have been noted in reduction of both overactivity and inattention, with less problem with sleep disturbance seen at times with stimulants use. The onset of beneficial effect appears much sooner in ADHD compared with the course of beneficial response in depression. The antidepressant dosage required for ADHD is usually less than corresponding antidepressant requirements. Treatment is initiated with a low dose, usually one fourth to one half the typical dose, followed by gradual increments until therapeutic response, maximum dose, or significant adverse effects are noted. TCAs have the advantage of once-a-day administration and are usually given at bedtime. MAOIs are usually given twice a day, with average dosage ranges between 8 and 15 mg/day.

Various potential adverse effects exist for both groups (see Table 1). Pre-existing heart disease or closed-angle glaucoma are contraindications to TCA use in children. Most adverse effects of TCAs, such as dry mouth, sedation, and constipation, are due to the anticholinergic properties. MAOIs require a special tyramine-free diet; high-tyramine foods, such as some cheeses and pickled food, can lead to hypertensive crisis in children on MAOIs. Younger children may have difficulty complying with a tyramine-free diet, especially in meals consumed outside of the home. TCAs and MAOIs are not scheduled drugs and do not carry the dependence and misuse concern of stimulants. Withdrawal of the antidepressant medications should be gradual. Switching between TCAs and MAOI classes requires up to a 2-week "wash-out" period.

There are some indications that a particular subgroup of children with ADHD who have comorbid anxiety or depressive disorders is more likely to respond to the antidepressant group. Stimulant nonresponders are also candidates for a trial of one of the antidepressant groups of medication.

Other Medication Agents

Various other classes of medications may have a limited utility in the treatment of ADHD. Clonidine has some support for efficacy and deserves consideration as an alternative agent. This may be especially true for children with pre-existing motor or vocal tics. Anecdotal experience with lithium carbonate, major antipsychotics such as chlor-

promazine (Thorazine), and benzodiazepines is available. Practically speaking, complete medication nonresponse to stimulants and antidepressants is unusual in ADHD, and third-line agents are rarely necessary in clinical practice.

Failure to Respond to a Medication Trial

Although most children with ADHD respond positively to medication trials, a few who do not form a difficult management subgroup. If a child appears not to be responding, two initial possibilities must be considered: noncompliance and misdiagnosis. For the child failing to respond, the accuracy of dosing and compliance should be questioned carefully. Additionally, if there is a concern about the child receiving the medication, a urine drug screen can be used to determine the presence of the stimulants methylphenidate and amphetamines in the child. Additionally, blood levels of imipramine and desipramine can be obtained to check for absorption and compliance when these antidepressants are prescribed.

Failure to respond also should raise the suspicion of a possibly more complicated diagnostic case. As mentioned, if a conduct disorder diagnosis is also present, aggressive behavior problems may complicate assessment of the treatment response. Atypical presentations may represent early subtle neurologic problems requiring neurologic referral. For the child with ADHD not responding to one or two medication trials, referral to a child psychiatrist or hospitalization may be necessary for implementation of a successful treatment plan.

Finally, a small group of children with ADHD, despite adequate attempts using different agents, fail to respond to medication. In these children, special educational and behavioral interventions may be necessary. Removal from the regular classroom to a smaller, specialized classroom may be helpful.

Psychotherapy

Behavioral and cognitive therapy techniques can be considered as adjuncts to medication management in the majority of cases or as primary therapies for families with a desire not to use medication. Unfortunately, extensive time-intense behavioral interventions have been found to be of limited long-term success in ADHD.[13,14] Cognitive and behavioral techniques are apparently more successful in the management of aggressive behaviors found in ADHD, complicated by conduct disorders. Because ADHD often results in experiences of academic and classroom failure, supportive counseling and encouragement for successful academic and home events may help increase the self-esteem of children with ADHD.

■ NONSTANDARD THERAPIES

Since at least the 1920s there have been hypotheses linking hyperactivity with diet. A variety of substances have been implicated, such as sweets/sugar, some meats/proteins, preservatives, additives, artificial colors/dyes, flavorings, and other compounds. The pathophysiology of the diet-behavior link has been postulated to be a result of allergic, toxic, or other adverse/intolerance reactions. In 1975, Benjamin Feingold published for ADHD patients a diet low in simple carbohydrates and low in preservatives, which received much attention in the popular press.[15] Although conceptually popular, the sugar/preservative-ADHD link has failed to be upheld in controlled scientific investigations. Likewise vitamin and mineral therapies are undocumented treatment approaches to ADHD. Parents should be encouraged to provide a balanced diet for their children, but to be cautioned that dietary measures are not the cause of ADHD, thus dietary manipulations are unlikely to provide sustained improvement.

■ Issues and Risks

Some criticism of the use of stimulants in children has focused on a possible increase in adult drug abuse through exposure to stimulants in childhood. This criticism has not been supported in follow-up studies of children with uncomplicated ADHD.[2] Physicians do need to be aware of the possibility of misuse of stimulants by family members of children presenting ADHD symptoms. Parents with drug abuse problems coaching their children in the signs of ADHD so as to

obtain prescriptions from physicians have been reported.[16] This problem should cause physicians to be suspicious of requests for stimulants from patients new or unfamiliar to the practice.

An additional controversial issue in ADHD is the proposal of a possible residual ADHD syndrome in adults.[17] Although there is some preliminary evidence of ADHD persisting into adulthood in selected cases, and possible beneficial adult response to stimulants, the majority of ADHD children have no significant residual problem. Because of possible stimulant abuse problems in adults, adults requesting stimulants for ADHD symptoms are probably best handled by referral to adult psychiatrists.

REFERENCES

1. Anderson JC, Williams S, McGee R, Silva PA. DSM-III disorders in preadolescent children. Arch Gen Psychiatr 1987; 44:69–76.
2. Mannuzza S, Gittelman Klein R, Bonagura N. Hyperactive boys almost grown up. II. Status of subjects without a mental disorder. Arch Gen Psychiatr 1988; 45:13–18.
3. American Psychiatric Association. Diagnostic and Statistical Manual of Mental Disorders, 3rd ed, revised. Washington, DC: American Psychiatric Association, 1987; 49–53.
4. Meller W, Yates WR. Hyperactivity and conduct disorder: changing criteria and course. Am Fam Physician 1988; 37:129–132.
5. Conners C. A teacher rating scale for use in drug studies with children. Am J Psychiatr 1969; 126:84–87.
6. Rutter M, Hersov L. Child and Adolescent Psychiatry; Modern Approaches. 2nd ed. Oxford: Blackwell Scientific Publications, 1985:424–437.
7. Meller W, Lyle K. Attention deficit disorder in childhood. Prim Care 1987; 14:745–759.
8. Connors CK, Werry JS. Pharmacotherapy; Psychopathological Disorders of Childhood. 2nd ed. New York: John Wiley, 1979:179.
9. Pelham WE, Bender ME, Caddell J, Booth S, Moorer SH. Methylphenidate and children with attention deficit disorder. Arch Gen Psychiatr 1985; 42:948–952.
10. Lowe TL, Cohen DJ, Detlor J, Shaywitz BA. Stimulant medications precipitate Tourette's syndrome. JAMA 1982; 247:1729–1731.
11. Gittelman Klein R, Mannuzza S. Hyperactive boys almost grown up. III. Methylphenidate effects on ultimate height. Arch Gen Psychiatr 1988; 45:1131–1134.
12. Zametkin A, Rapoport JL, Murphy DL, Linnoila M, Ismond D. Treatment of hyperactive children with monoamine oxidase inhibitors. Arch Gen Psychiatr 1985; 42:962–966.
13. Abikoff H, Gittelman R. Hyperactive children treated with stimulants. Is cognitive training a use-

ful adjunct? Arch Gen Psychiatr 1985; 42:948–952.

14. Abikoff H, Gittelman R. Does behavior therapy normalize the classroom behavior of hyperactive children? Arch Gen Psychiatr 1984; 41:449–454.

15. Feingold B. Why Your Child Is Hyperactive. New York: Random House, 1975.

16. Fulton AI, Yates WR. Family abuse of methylphenidate. Am Fam Physician 1988; 38:143–146.

17. Wender PH, Reimherr FW, Wood D, Ward M. A controlled study of methylphenidate in the treatment of attention deficit disorder, residual type, in adults. Am J Psychiatr 1985; 142:547–552.

Bacteremia and sepsis

Richard L. Harris

Bacteremia may be transient or continuous and symptomatic or clinically silent. Sepsis is defined as the physiologic alterations and clinical consequences of the presence of bacteria or their products in the circulation or tissues. Although symptomatic bacteremia by definition causes sepsis, not all septic patients will have documented bacteremia. Septic shock is defined as circulatory failure resulting in inadequate tissue perfusion due to an infectious process.

■ Background

The epidemiology of bacteremia varies from institution to institution, but the most common aerobic, gram-positive isolates are staphylococci, pneumococcus, and enterococcus; the most frequently isolated aerobic, gram-negative organisms are *Escherichia coli, Klebsiella* sp., *Pseudomonas aeruginosa, Proteus* sp., and *Enterobacter* sp.; *Bacteroides* sp. are the most frequent anaerobes.[1] Although gram-negative rods are the most common cause of septic shock, virtually any organism can produce this syndrome. The specific diagnosis of the etiologic agent cannot be confidently made based on clinical manifestations.

Nosocomial bacteremias account for approximately 50 per cent of the total community- and hospital-acquired bacteremias in some studies and tend to have a higher mortality.[2] The greatest risk factor for the development of nosocomial bacteremia is the placement of an intravenous catheter. The degree of risk varies with the specific device implanted, but in all devices, the risk increases the longer the device is kept in place.

■ MANIFESTATIONS OF SEPSIS

The clinical manifestations of bacteremia and sepsis are many and varied.[3] The myriad combinations of manifestations that patients present with emphasizes the important concept that the diagnosis may be obvious or subtle. The clinician must have a thorough knowledge of the manifestations of sepsis for two reasons. Firstly, this will allow prompt recognition of the presence of bacteremia and sepsis. Secondly, some of the manifestations of sepsis require specific intervention above and beyond the therapy of the underlying infection.[3] Table 1 lists many of the clinical manifestations of sepsis.

■ PATHOPHYSIOLOGY

It is important to understand basic concepts of the pathophysiology of bacteremia and sepsis to allow a more rational approach to therapy. The initial interaction of the host and bacteria that determines whether infection will occur includes bacterial adherence to host tissues and then bacterial avoidance of the host humoral and cell-mediated defenses. If this initial interaction is favorable to the bacteria, then the host may be damaged by the elaboration of exotoxins or by direct damage of the bacterial cell wall by endotoxin.[4]

The biochemical structures of lipopolysaccharides or peptidoglycans are termed endotoxins based on biologic activity. Endotoxin appears to effect its havoc by an intermediate mediator of sepsis released by monocytes and termed cachectin, or tumor necrosis factor.[5] Via numerous other mediators, cachectin produces the manifestations of sepsis by activation of the complement, coagulation cascade, fibrinolysin, and bradykinin systems.

Septic Shock. The initial hemodynamic manifestation of sepsis is the reduction of the systemic vascular resistance (Table 2). If the cardiac output is able to compensate, blood pressure and tissue perfusion will remain adequate. As the septic process progresses, the cardiac output will not be able to sustain adequate tissue perfusion. Late in

TABLE 1. Manifestations of Sepsis

Common	Less Common or Seen Only in Severe Sepsis
Fever, rigors, myalgias	Hypothermia
Tachycardia	Shock (see Table 2)
Tachypnea (respiratory alkalosis)	Lactic acidosis
Hypoxemia	Adult respiratory distress syndrome
Proteinuria	Azotemia, oliguria
Leukocytosis (left shift, toxic granules, Dohle bodies)	Leukopenia, leukemoid reaction
Eosinopenia	Thrombocytopenia
Hypoferremia	Disseminated intravascular coagulation
Irritability, lethargy	Anemia
Mild liver function abnormalities	Stupor, coma
Hyperglycemia in diabetics	Overt upper gastrointestinal tract bleeding
	Cutaneous lesions
	Funduscopic lesions
	Hypoglycemia

(Reproduced with permission from Harris RL, Musher DM, Bloom K, et al: Manifestations of sepsis. Arch Intern Med 1987; 147:1893–1906.

TABLE 2. Hemodynamics of Sepsis

	Preshock	Early Shock	Late Shock
Blood pressure	→↓	↓	↓↓*
Systemic vascular resistance	↓	↓↓	→ ↑
Cardiac output	↑↑	↑	↓
Volume responsive	+ +	+	−
Acid-base status†	RA	RA, MA	MA

*Often pressor dependent.
†RA indicates respiratory alkalosis; MA, metabolic acidosis.
(Reproduced with permission from Harris RL, Musher DM, Bloom K, et al. Manifestations of sepsis. Arch Intern Med 1987; 147:1893–1906.

septic shock there is profound, but potentially reversible, left ventricular dysfunction.[6]

■ Management

Antibiotics are usually the first thought in clinicians' minds for management of bacteremia and sepsis. Prompt initiation of appropriate antimicrobial therapy is the cornerstone of the management of serious bacterial infections; nevertheless, general medical or adjunctive therapeutic measures are often just as crucial for a successful outcome. Antibiotics alone are likely to be inadequate unless abscesses are drained, infected foci (such as intravenous catheters) are removed, and obstructions (genitourinary or gastrointestinal) are relieved. Certain manifestations of sepsis may require specific therapy (Table 3).

■ FEVER

An elevated temperature is likely to be part of the host response to bacterial infection. It

TABLE 3. Manifestations of Sepsis That May Benefit from or Require Specific Therapy*

Manifestations	Therapy
Fever, rigors, myalgias	Antipyretics, cooling blanket
Hypotension	Volume replacement, dopamine (naloxone)
Hypoxemia	Supplemental oxygen
Respiratory failure, ARDS	Mechanical ventilation (PEEP)
Lactic acidosis	Bicarbonate administration
Azotemia, oliguria	Fluid and electrolyte management, reduction of renally cleared drugs
Thrombocytopenia	Platelet and/or RBC transfusions if actively bleeding
DIC	Fresh-frozen plasma, platelet, and/or RBC transfusions if actively bleeding (heparin)
Altered mentation	Monitoring/restraint of patient to prevent self-harm
GI tract bleeding	Nasogastric lavage/suction, RBC transfusions as needed (antacids, H_2-receptor antagonists)
Hyperglycemia	Insulin administration
Hypoglycemia	Constant 10% dextrose infusion

*In parentheses are therapeutic maneuvers that are possibly effective. ARDS indicates adult respiratory distress syndrome; PEEP, positive end-expiratory pressure; RBC, red blood cell; DIC, disseminated intravascular coagulation; GI, gastrointestinal; and H_2, histamine$_2$.
(Reproduced with permission from Harris RL, Musher DM, Bloom K, et al. Manifestations of sepsis. Arch Intern Med 1987; 147:1893–1906.

is unclear whether lowering an elevated temperature by antipyretics (nonsteroidal anti-inflammatory agents or acetaminophen) or a cooling blanket is beneficial or harmful to the host; furthermore, it is unknown whether one method is superior to the other.[1,7] Lowering an elevated temperature usually makes the patient feel better, although a brisk diaphoresis may occur. The outcome of the majority of infections is probably not affected by lowering the temperature. It seems prudent to attempt to lower significant temperature elevations in patients with minimal physiologic reserves, such as severe coronary artery disease or markedly reduced left ventricular function.

■ PULMONARY MANIFESTATIONS

Hypoxemia and ventilatory failure will require supplemental oxygen and mechanical ventilation. Optimal management of sepsis-induced adult respiratory distress syndrome (ARDS) remains a major challenge and requires careful attention to volume status, ventilatory settings, and anticipation of potential complications. (Also see the first article in this book on The Adult Respiratory Distress Syndrome.) The mortality rate in patients with gram-negative bacteremia and ARDS is exceedingly high.[8] Positive end-expiratory pressure (PEEP) is often added to improve oxygenation, although it has not been proved to increase the rate of survival of patients with ARDS. PEEP can aggravate hypotension, reduce tissue oxygen delivery, and increase the risk of pneumothorax. Glucocorticoids have been shown to not benefit patients with ARDS[9] and are not recommended unless the patient requires steroids for other underlying illnesses.

■ SEPTIC SHOCK

As mentioned previously, reduction of systemic vascular resistance occurs early in the course of septic shock. At this stage, volume expansion is often beneficial. Septic patients are often relatively volume depleted due to increased insensible losses, the "polyuria of sepsis," decreased oral intake, increased vascular permeability, and increased venous capacitance.[3] A volume challenge is usually indicated to maximize cardiac output. As the septic process worsens, a vaso-

pressor will be required to maintain brain and heart perfusion (usually a systolic blood pressure of 90 to 100 mm Hg). Dopamine hydrochloride appears to be the drug of choice[10] and should be given by a constant intravenous infusion, preferably via a central intravenous catheter. The dopamine infusion rate should be titrated to the lowest dose that maintains an adequate filling pressure. Two prospective, double-blind, placebo-controlled trials demonstrated no benefit of glucocorticosteroid therapy in the management of septic shock[11,12] and therefore cannot be recommended unless steroids are needed for other underlying illnesses.

■ METABOLIC ACIDOSIS

Most patients with bacteremia and sepsis maintain a normal metabolic acid-base status until a late and very serious stage of septic shock occurs. The therapeutic approach to lactic acidosis in sepsis must include careful attention to volume status, oxygenation, and perfusion pressure. For profound acidosis (pH less than 7.10), supplemental bicarbonate infusion for partial normalization of pH may make treatment of hypotension easier.

■ ANTIMICROBIAL THERAPY

General Guidelines. The selection of an appropriate antibiotic regimen should be based on the likely infecting organisms and their antibiotic sensitivity patterns. An "educated guess" of this can be based on (1) recent cultural data on the patient, e.g., a urine culture from several days ago, (2) a properly interpreted Gram stain of clinical specimens, (3) knowledge of "expected" flora from a regional body site, e.g., staphylococcus on the skin, gram-negative rods and group D streptococci in the urinary tract, and (4) the specific hospital's antibiotic resistance pattern from previous microbiologic and epidemiologic studies.

As a general rule, bacteremia and sepsis are treated with at least two antibiotics unless the sensitivity pattern of the specific infecting organism is already known. Two drug regimens are based more on prescribing habits than on bona fide scientific data, but there are several theoretical reasons for multidrug regimens: (1) to broaden the spectrum of coverage, (2) to provide synergistic killing of the organisms (best documented in the therapy of enterococcal endocarditis and profoundly neutropenic patients), (3) to prevent the emergence of antibiotic resistance, and (4) to assure an adequate serum level of antibiotics at all times. The most common reason to use multiple antibiotics is to broaden the coverage.

Antimicrobial therapy should be initiated by the intravenous route to assure maximal serum and tissue levels. The oral and intramuscular routes are too unpredictable in the management of critically ill patients. Bactericidal therapy is of documented necessity in the therapy of meningitis, endocarditis, and sepsis in a profoundly granulocytopenic patient. Once the sensitivity pattern of the invading organism is available, the least toxic (and least expensive) regimen should be substituted.

The appropriate length of therapy for bacteremia and sepsis is based on surprisingly few data. Certainly the underlying age and conditions of the host are crucial in the "length of therapy equation." Furthermore, host response to therapy must be carefully assessed. A young, otherwise healthy patient who develops *E. coli* bacteremia from the urinary tract and responds rapidly to therapy will not require the prolonged intravenous therapy that a patient with *E. coli*

TABLE 4. Initial Antibiotic Selection Based on Likely Focus of Infection

Site of Infection	Organisms	Antibiotics
Urinary tract	GNR	Aminoglycosides, ceftazidime
	GDS	Ampicillin, vancomycin
Pneumonia*		
community-acquired	Pneumococcus, aspiration	Penicillin G
	H. influenzae	Ampicillin
	Legionella, atypical pneumonias	Erythromycin
nosocomial	GNR	Piperacillin, ceftazidime
	S. aureus	Nafcillin, vancomycin
	Legionella	Erythromycin
Endocarditis		
native valve		
non-IVDA	α-streptococci, *S. aureus*	Penicillin, nafcillin
IVDA	*S. aureus*	Nafcillin, vancomycin
	GNR	Ticarcillin or ceftazidime and aminoglycosides
Meningitis		
adult	Pneumococci, meningococci	Penicillin, chloramphenicol
postneurosurgery,	*S. aureus, S. epidermidis*	Vancomycin, nafcillin
immunosuppressed	GNR	Ceftazidime
Gastrointestinal and	GNR	Ceftazidime, aminoglycoside
genital tract	GDS	Ampicillin, vancomycin
	Anaerobes	Clindamycin, piperacillin, metronidazole, chloramphenicol
Wound infection	*S. aureus*	Nafcillin, vancomycin
	GNR	Ceftazidime, aminoglycoside
Intravascular line	*S. aureus, S. epidermidis*	Vancomycin
	GNR	Ceftazidime, aminoglycoside
Neutropenia	GNR	Ceftazidime or ticarcillin and aminoglycoside
	S. aureus, S. epidermidis	Vancomycin
Postsplenectomy	Pneumococcus, *H. influenzae*, meningococcus	Penicillin, ampicillin
Empiric	*S. aureus*, streptococcus	Vancomycin
	GNR	Ceftazidime, aminoglycoside
	Anaerobes	Clindamycin, metronidazole

*Gram stain of sputum may help direct initial therapy.
GNR, gram-negative rod; GDS, group D streptococcus; IVDA, intravenous drug abuse.

TABLE 5. Dosage of Selected Antibiotics in Adult Patients with Normal Renal Function

Antibiotic	Dose	Usual Dosing Interval
Penicillins		
Penicillin G	1–2 million units	4 hours
Ampicillin	1–2 grams	4–6 hours
Antipseudomonal Penicillins		
Ticarcillin	3 grams	4 hours
Piperacillin	3–4 grams	4–6 hours
Antistaphylococcal Penicillins		
Nafcillin	1–2 grams	4–6 hours
Methicillin	1–2 grams	4–6 hours
Penicillins with β-Lactamase Inhibitor		
Ampicillin/sulbactam (Unasyn)	1.5–3.0 grams	6 hours
Ticarcillin/clavulanic acid (Timentin)	3.1 grams	4 hours
First-Generation Cephalosporin		
Cefazolin (Ancef, Kefzol)	1 gram	8 hours
Second-Generation Cephalosporin		
Cefotetan (Cefotan)	1–2 grams	12 hours
Third-Generation Cephalosporins		
Ceftazidime (Fortaz, Tazidime, Tazicef)	1–2 grams	8–12 hours
Cefotaxime (Claforan)	1–2 grams	8 hours
Carbapenem		
Imipenem/cilastatin (Primaxin)	0.5–1.0 gram	6–8 hours
Aminoglycosides		
Gentamicin	1 mg per kg	8 hours
Tobramycin	1 mg per kg	8 hours
Amikacin	7.5 mg per kg	12 hours
Others		
Vancomycin (Vancocin, Vancoled)	15 mg per kg	12 hours
Clindamycin	300–600 mg	8 hours
Erythromycin	500–1000 mg	6 hours
Doxycycline (Vibramycin)	50–100 mg	12 hours
Metronidazole (Flagyl)	7.5 mg per kg	6 hours
Chloramphenicol	25 mg per kg	6 hours
Ciprofloxacin* (Cipro)	200–300 mg	12 hours

*Not yet available in the intravenous form.

bacteremia from an intra-abdominal abscess will require.

Specific Antimicrobial Recommendations. Table 4 contains various antibiotic choices based on the likely organisms at a given site of infection. Although the "antibiotic of choice" is a constantly changing reflection of scientific progress, the relationship of the various organisms and site of infection is relatively constant. There are certainly other reasonable choices of antibiotics available to the clinician. Table 5 provides guidelines for the dosage of selected antibiotics.

Empiric Therapy. If a careful clinical examination fails to demonstrate a likely site of infection, then broad-spectrum therapy directed at least at gram-positive and gram-negative aerobes is indicated. Vancomycin is a reasonable choice because of its universal activity against staphylococci and streptococci. A broad gram-negative spectrum beta-lactam (such as ceftazidime) or an aminoglycoside is a reasonable initial therapy for gram-negative rods. If an occult intra-abdominal source of sepsis is possible, anaerobic coverage should be added.

■ Issues and Risks

The best approach to the management of bacteremia and sepsis is prevention. This is often difficult to do in the community-acquired cases; there is more hope in lowering hospital-acquired cases. Prevention of nosocomial infections is a very complex, relatively new science that is undergoing considerable investigation. Certainly, minimizing invasive procedures and intravascular lines is of paramount importance.

When sepsis cannot be prevented, it is incumbent upon clinicians to detect its presence as early as possible in order to initiate prompt and appropriate therapy.[3] It can be argued that there are more deaths from sepsis because of late recognition of the diagnosis than from the inappropriate therapy of this serious syndrome.

It seems doubtful that new antibiotics will significantly lower the mortality rate of bacteremia and sepsis, since in the great majority of cases there are multiple antibiotics that are active in vitro against the invading organisms. New approaches to the management of sepsis include attempts to augment the host's immune response. Active and passive immunization against common bacterial agents is an attractive concept.[13] Passive immunization with monoclonal antibody to core lipopolysaccharide determinants is undergoing clinical investigation. In experimental animal studies, antibody to cachectin blocks virtually all of the host's response to endotoxin administration[14] and would have the advantage of being useful against many types of microorganisms.

REFERENCES

1. Weinstein MP, Reller LB, Murphy JR, Lichtenstein KA. The clinical significance of positive blood cultures: a comprehensive analysis of 500 episodes of bacteremia and fungemia in adults. 1. Laboratory and epidemiologic observations. Rev Infect Dis 1983; 5:35–53.
2. Hamory BH. Nosocomial bloodstream and intravascular device-related infections. *In* Wenzel RP (ed). Prevention and Control of Nosocomial Infection. Baltimore: Williams and Wilkins, 1987:283–319.
3. Harris RL, Musher DM, Bloom K, et al. Manifestations of sepsis. Arch Intern Med 1987; 147:1895–1906.
4. Hewlett EL. Toxins. *In* Mandell GL, Douglas RG Jr, Bennett JE (eds). Principles and Practice of Infectious Diseases. New York: John Wiley and Sons, 1985:1–6.
5. Beutler B, Cerami A. Cachectin: more than a tumor necrosis factor. N Engl J Med 1987; 316:379–385.
6. Parker MM, Shelhamer JE, Bacharach SL, et al. Profound but reversible myocardial depression in patients with septic shock. Ann Intern Med 1984; 100:483–490.
7. Klastersky J, Kass EH. Is suppression of fever or hypothermia useful in experimental and clinical infectious diseases? J Infect Dis 1970; 121:81–86.
8. Kaplan RL, Sahn SA, Petty TL. Incidence and outcome of the respiratory distress syndrome in gram-negative sepsis. Arch Intern Med 1979; 139:867–869.
9. Bernard GR, Luce JM, Sprung CL, et al. High-dose corticosteroids in patients with the adult respiratory distress syndrome. N Engl J Med 1987; 317:1565–1570.
10. Parker MM. Current management of septic shock. Infect Med 1989; 6:47–52.
11. Bone RC, Fisher CJ, Clemmer TP, et al. A controlled clinical trial of high-dose methylprednisolone in the treatment of severe sepsis and septic shock. N Engl J Med 1987; 317:653–658.
12. The Veterans Administration Systemic Sepsis Cooperative Study Group. Effect of high-dose glucocorticoid therapy on mortality in patients with clinical signs of systemic sepsis. N Engl J Med 1987; 317:659–665.
13. Ziegler EJ. Protective antibody to endotoxin core: the emperor's new clothes? J Infect Dis 1988; 158:286–289.
14. Beutler B, Milsark IW, Cerami AC. Passive immunization against cachectin/tumor necrosis factor protects mice from lethal effects of endotoxin. Science 1985; 229:869–871.

Borderline personality disorder

Michael K. Magill ■ *Ellen Berkowitz*

Patients with borderline personality disorder are seen in most medical practices that include care of adults. These patients' lives are a jumble of losses, painful disappointments, and deeply hurt feelings.[1] The patients are difficult to manage because of their demanding, angry, impulsive, unpredictable, and self-destructive behavior. They tend to disrupt physician attempts to provide care for their medical problems. They may not readily accept psychiatric referral despite ongoing psychologic turmoil and occasional psychotic episodes. They may have significant biologic illness that is more difficult to manage as a result of the personality disorder. The physician who chooses not to accept as patients people with this problem will still encounter them, as they tend to move from one doctor to another. Nonetheless, nonpsychiatric physicians who can recognize this disorder and use an organized strategy for its management can be very effective in helping some of them with their medical problems, as well as with the difficult task of living with this disorder.

■ Background

Borderline personality disorder is most often recognized after several encounters with a patient. The physician may begin care for the patient as for any other, not noticing any particularly unusual features of the patient's behavior. This is because borderline patients may function quite well in everyday life despite the presence of this major psychologic problem. They may hold regular jobs, including work as professionals such as physicians, nurses, attorneys, or other responsible positions. However, over time these patients begin to demonstrate emotional instability, demandingness, dependency, depression, rage, suicidal behavior, or chemical dependency. These manifestations should alert the physician to consider the diagnosis of borderline personality disorder.

Occasionally, the physician may recognize this disorder in the first moments after meeting a new patient, especially if the patient is in the midst of a crisis. The physician may note extremes of patient anger or affection for the physician early in the first encounter. The physician may experience anger or guilt. These patients are skilled at identifying others' emotional "soft spots" and can quickly elicit strong feelings, positive or negative, from the physician. Borderline patients in crisis can clinically "appear schizophrenic, manic, depressed, intoxicated, or delirious."[1]

This diagnosis may be suggested first by the behavior of hospital or office staff. For example, the staff may complain to the physician about the patient's excessive demands for attention, medication, or laboratory tests. A more indirect clue to the diagnosis may be staff disagreements about the patient. For example, the staff actually may develop conflict among themselves as a result of the patient's manipulative behavior, which may not be recognized as such by the staff.

Formal diagnosis of borderline personality disorder is based on the presence of at least five of the following characteristics: unstable relationships with other people in which the patient alternates between overidealizing and devaluing the other; impulsive, potentially self-damaging behavior, such as spending, sexual behavior, stealing, dangerous driving, or drug use; emotional instability, with rapid swings between extremes of depression and anxiety; excessive or inappropriate anger or rage; self-destructive or self-injurious behavior or threats, such as suicide attempts or self-mutilation; severe disruption of a sense of self-identity; long-standing empty or bored feelings; and desperate attempts to prevent abandonment, whether real or perceived.[2]

■ Management

Management of the borderline patient is difficult because of the strong feelings expressed by the patient and elicited in caregivers. It is especially difficult for those who work with them to tolerate the intensity of these patients' anger and neediness.[3] Physicians react especially strongly to challenges to their self-esteem or professional competence.[4] Because borderline patients are expert at identifying and exploiting the emotional "triggers" of those around them, they are adept at finding effective ways to challenge physicians' self-esteem. Caregivers often have the need to defend themselves and be in control.

Management of the borderline patient requires attention to biologic medical problems in conjunction with management of the personality disorder. The physician does not attempt to alter the patient's basic personality or to help the patient achieve insight or understanding of the psychiatric problem. Rather, the physician provides support for the patient's healthy adaptational skills, avoids challenging the patient's areas of weakness, and provides acute intervention, including short courses of psychotropic medications, when necessary for management of crises. Brief psychiatric hospitalization occasionally may be required.

■ SUPPORT

The physician must recognize that the disruptive behavior borderline patients exhibit serves a self-protective function. These patients have very poorly developed senses of who they are. This sense of self as separate from others normally develops over the first 2 or 3 years of life and is retained by psychologically healthy adults whether with others or alone.[5] Borderline patients, however, may have experienced a failure to develop this normal sense of self and thus require contact with others, so that they can have a point of reference. When alone, they cannot retain a sense of who "me" is. Lacking this most basic of emotional anchors, they panic, and frantically seek out human contact as a way to re-establish a sense of their own selfhood.

Unfortunately, once they contact another person, they cannot retain a sense of themselves as separate from that other. They quickly begin to lose the sense of self they seek, feel overwhelmed by the personality of the other, and push away to control their panic once again. Thus, it is fear both of distance from others and of closeness that launches these patients on an "emotional roller coaster" between closeness and distance from others. The physician sees this as wild swings between clinging dependency and hostile rejection of caregivers.

Alternatively, as another way to control panic, these patients may identify certain individuals in their environment as all "good" and others as all "bad." Sometimes they can covertly manipulate these others into conflict with each other. Other times, the assigned roles change rapidly or abruptly, leading to troublesome feelings of hostility from staff or physician.

Empathy. The first step in effective management of these patients is for physician and staff to recognize that the aforementioned process occurs. They must realize that such primitive, ineffective behavior is the best available to the patient for controlling fear. Such empathy is the basis for obtaining emotional distance from the feelings expressed by the patient, whether hostile or affectionate, and for more effective management. Caregivers can express their awareness of the patient's problems, recognition of the patient's pain, and an understanding of issues facing the patient. But they can also set up an environment in which the patient and family are active participants.[3] Empathy needs to be balanced by realistic limit-setting to try to avoid increasing the risk of magical expectations.[1]

Staff. Open communication among all persons in regular contact with the patient is essential to prevent the patient from splitting off the staff from each other. All involved should realize that they will be assigned "good" and "bad" roles by the patient, and that these must not be allowed to disrupt relationships among caretakers. It is important for staff to be aware of the feelings these patients elicit in them, but not to act on them. Staff often feel conflicting wishes to rescue the patients as well as to reject and withdraw from them, with feelings ranging from rage to depression.[3] To the extent that these patients engage in self-blame or in blaming others, staff often want to blame and punish the patient.[3] There is often internal conflict over the professional need to give and a personal wish to withhold.[6]

Whether in the office or on a hospital unit, it is important for physicians to provide support for the staff. This can be done in part through direct teaching of staff. In addition, physicians should model for the staff their integrity, respect, and care for them and their patients, as well as setting limits on staff and patients in a nonpunitive way. Physicians can show examples of how to manage their professional relationships without getting into blaming or punishing and without feeling excess guilt or idealization.[3]

Guidelines. Borderline patients are best managed on a regular schedule of brief physician encounters that do not require new symptoms to justify each visit. The physician who schedules the patient for a 10-minute office visit every 2 weeks may spend far less time with the patient than one who tells the patient to "make an appointment when you have a problem." Caretakers should provide consistent limits on patient behavior. For example, telephone calls may need to be limited to two per week, or a time limit may need to be set for individual calls. The physician should set, and stick to, a limit on duration of individual office visits. Physicians and staff should not allow excess closeness or excess hostility to be expressed toward any member of the health care team. Firm limits are needed for the patient to feel safe. Caregivers should respond to the patient who expresses excessive degrees of affection or rage with tolerance and simple restatement of limits, without allowing the patient to elicit either an overly affectionate or angry response from the caregiver. The caregiver may simply note the emotion, but not necessarily comment on it or discuss it extensively with the patient. Limit setting is neither negative nor punitive. Rather it is a complicated interaction of empathic awareness of the patient's needs and the staff and patient's expectations.[3]

Caregivers should seek consistency in communication with the patient. Two or three office staff members may be designated the sole contact persons for any phone call or office visit. When the physician or other key person will be unavailable for a significant period of time, as for a vacation, the patient should be told in advance of the planned absence, and the physician should designate someone to call the patient early in this interval.

It is often helpful to redirect the destructive behavior of specific subtypes of borderline patients into more effective doctor-patient relationships.[7] Some patients, "dependent clingers," demonstrate primarily a need for dependency. Nonpunitive limit setting is helpful for these patients, when offered in the context of a consistent and reliable doctor-patient relationship.

Other patients, entitled "demanders," show more overtly angry, confrontational behavior as they insist on excessive diagnostic evaluation, referrals or treatment. Health care providers should gently redirect the demanding behavior of these patients away from conflict with the people who are trying to help them and toward the shared goal of having them receive the high-quality care they deserve.

"Help-rejecters" are patients who do not get better when appropriately treated. In fact, their symptoms paradoxically may get worse. The physician should share openly the patient's expectation that he or she may never get completely well. This reassures patients that they will be permitted to maintain a needed relationship with the physician so that, again paradoxically, the symptoms actually may improve.

"Self-destructive deniers" are patients who continue self-injurious behavior, such as chemical abuse or suicide attempts, despite the physician's appropriate interventions. The physician should recognize that these patients' underlying illness is incurable, and that limited therapeutic goals are appropriate.

■ MEDICATION

Borderline patients may be quite demanding of prescription medications, especially potent narcotic analgesics and benzodiazepines. The physician should be wary of prescribing these agents for extended courses of more than a few days, as they are not likely to lead to significant symptom relief and are highly likely to lead to dependency in these patients.

Medications should not be used with the idea that one is treating the underlying personality disorder but should be chosen to address specific target symptom areas.[8] In general, this is best done in the patient who is in ongoing psychotherapy and with collaboration between the physician and therapist. In many cases, long-term use of medication is not useful. Medication can be most helpful when the patient's level of functioning has significantly decreased and when the safety of the patient or others must be protected (e.g., in the hospital).

Short courses of low-dose neuroleptics may be appropriate for times of higher stress or brief psychosis in these patients. In addition to helping control the psychotic symptoms these patients can have, the neuroleptics can reduce emotional lability and aggressive behavior. Thioridazine (Mellaril), up to 300 mg at bedtime, can be helpful, especially if there is a need for sedation, or comparable doses of trifluoperazine (Stelazine) or fluphenazine (Prolixin) can be used when less sedation is desired. Antidepressants may be appropriate if the patient has a coexisting major depression in addition to the personality disorder or at times for those with some emotional lability, but these also can lead to increased anger and irritability in some patients.[9] Lithium may be similarly appropriate, especially to help reduce assaultive or self-destructive behavior. However, borderline patients have a high potential for impulsive, self-destructive behavior, and these medications should be prescribed in tightly controlled amounts—for example, no more than 1 week's supply for a patient who is not well known to the physician or who is in a crisis. Other cautions include the risk of tardive dyskinesia with prolonged neuroleptic use and awareness of drug interactions in patients with other medical problems.

Some patients who present with borderline-like symptoms actually have other underlying psychiatric illness that might respond to medication. For example, patients with atypical depression are usually characterized by dramatic behavior, sensitivity to rejection, moodiness, demanding behavior, and suicidal threats. These patients often respond to monoamine oxidase inhibitors (MAOIs) (Parnate, Nardil), sometimes with the addition of a low-dose neuroleptic. Some patients may be suffering from a chronic overwhelming anxiety, and the cy-clic antidepressants, MAOIs, lithium, buspirone, and neuroleptics all might be useful.[9] If they are not, sometimes a benzodiazepine is the drug of choice. Some patients with chronic anxiety primarily have a panic disorder, with secondary anticipatory and phobic anxiety. These patients do best on cyclic antidepressants or MAOIs for the panic disorder. Behavioral therapy and occasional short courses of benzodiazepines are helpful for the secondary anxiety.[9]

■ THE EMERGENCY ROOM

The emergency room can be a particularly trying place to deal with borderline patients. They may present with somatic concerns, but often they are in chaos owing to a real or perceived loss or other interpersonal disruption. The emergency room is unrealistically seen often as a place where professionals can take care of their problems quickly and effectively. When this does not happen, the presenting emotional problems can escalate. The excitement of the emergency room environment itself can increase a patient's anxiety. In addition, the staff, because of a need to maintain adequate control and obtain as rapid a disposition as possible, may tend not to take the patient's concerns seriously enough. In the staff's need to control they may overreact by means of excessive physical restraints or medication, which may increase rather than decrease the patient's distress and the resulting turmoil in the emergency room.[1]

An active and direct style of interacting often can decrease the patient's anxiety and agitation. Caregivers should try to identify what assistance the patient may want. This may not be explicit in the presenting complaint.[1] The assessment should be done as quickly as possible to decrease the chance of regression, but it needs to include a good history, to evaluate the risk of self-destructive behavior, and a medical history, specifically including alcohol and drug use. A thorough mental status examination is needed to rule out other significant medical or psychiatric illness.[1]

The principles of management, discussed previously, also apply in the emergency room. Caregivers should help the patient maintain adaptive defenses, and help him or her realize that long-term problems cannot be resolved in the emergency room. The physician can focus on helping the patient gain some immediate emotional stability, without necessarily needing to resolve the presenting complaint, and encourage the patient to initiate or continue follow-up psychotherapy.[1]

In the emergency room and in the hospital ward, concern about the suicide potential of these patients can generate anxiety for caregivers. The first priority is to insure the safety of a patient until assessment can be made. This is best done by one-on-one observation with some backup personnel available. Depending on the situation, this may mean using family, staff, or security guards.[10] At times medication or physical restraints or both may be needed. For the patient who is clearly suicidal, voluntary or involuntary psychiatric hospitalization is needed. When a patient requires continued stay on a medical or surgical ward, arrangements must be made for restraint or constant observation. Specific treatment, depending on the presenting psychiatric symptoms, can then be initiated.

The majority of suicide attempts presenting to the emergency room are "gestures," meaning that death was not the patient's intent (though it can occur accidentally). The emergency staff's response to such a gesture may alter the patient's immediate risk of suicide. Some patients will respond to uncomfortable but necessary medical care (e.g., insertion of nasogastric tubes or intravenous lines) with a decreased risk; for others, the positive support of staff decreases the risk of suicide. These patients usually can be sent home with referral for follow-up. Sometimes a patient in this group will continue to voice suicidal threats. Careful assessment of other risk factors is essential. If the patient is medically stable and has favorable social support, if there is low lethality or low specificity of the suicide attempt used and the patient has a prior history of reduced suicidal behavior when provided increased support, then she or he may be a candidate for discharge home from the emergency room rather than admission to the hospital.[11] However, if patients cannot be evaluated fully for risk in the emergency room because of the nature of the attempt (i.e., drug overdose), they should be hospitalized until the drug effects have worn off and then assessed as they otherwise would have been in the emergency room.[11]

■ Issues and Risks

Borderline patients elicit the most intense emotional reactions from physicians of any problem commonly seen in a wide variety of medical practices. These patients can be confrontational, demanding, demeaning, insulting, and frustrating. They may attack openly physicians' credibility and competence. They may repeatedly "terminate" the doctor-patient relationship, only to try to return again and again to the same physician. Such behaviors cause emotional distress even to seasoned clinicians.[4]

Borderline patients challenge physicians' ability to recognize and use their own emotions as diagnostic clues to the nature of the patients' problems, yet not simply act on these emotions to the detriment of both patient and doctor. Physicians who try never to accept these patients into their practices will continue to see patients with the disorder, because they surface among patients of any functional or socioeconomic status, and they "bounce" from doctor to doctor within a community.

Physicians who decide to manage patients like this should set limits on the number of "active" borderline patients they can accept at any one time. Most physicians are likely to be able to care for only two to five such patients at a time in the typical medical practice. Physicians may need to transfer care of such patients to colleagues to prevent excess emotional burnout.

Physicians may be concerned about professional liability risks in caring for these demanding, angry patients. If so, the potential for litigation should be openly discussed with these patients, and limitations on threats of litigation should be included early in the doctor-patient contract.

A more common area of potential liability may be in the nature of physicians' responses to these patients' suicidal or other self-injurious behavior. Physicians should respond promptly and clearly to hints or open threats of self-injury and should not hestitate to insist that the patient accept prompt psychiatric referral or be committed involuntarily for psychiatric observation. Most often, such a prompt response will be reassuring to the patient, and the need to gain attention through such behavior will diminish. If ignored or minimized, the behavior may tend to escalate. If patients present with a suicide attempt or gesture, psychiatric consultation is recommended, although the patients often will resist evaluation, may no longer be actively suicidal, and may not require or benefit from psychiatric hospitalization once they are medically stable from the effects of their suicide attempt.

Physicians should be wary of misuse of the diagnosis of borderline personality disorder to label people whom they simply do not like, or who do not get better under their care.[12]

Use of the diagnosis should be tentative and subject to revision over time. Borderline patients can develop other psychiatric syndromes, such as major depression, which must be addressed in addition to the personality disorder. Development of major depression warrants use of medication, such as antidepressants, but with caution and in limited amounts owing to the potential for overdose by these patients.

In addition, as the individual becomes better known to the physician, the diagnosis for the patient may change over time. These patients may appear more clearly to have a different personality disorder, such as a histrionic or antisocial personality, for which a different management approach is appropriate. Some patients with clear borderline features actually may be suffering from posttraumatic stress disorder or atypical depression and respond to appropriate psychotherapy and medications.

The physician should develop skill in an explicit "trial and error" approach to management of these patients. The guidelines offered here are intended as starting points, which, if used, will increase the physician's success with these patients. Far more important than these guidelines, though, is the physician's skill in use of flexible styles of behavior with different patients. For example, with some borderline patients, and in some circumstances, the physician can help reduce the patient's distress most effectively by gently setting limits on behavior. With different patients, and at other times with the same patient, the doctor must respond promptly to the patient's dependency needs. A willingness to maintain a curious, thoughtful, and tolerant approach to interacting with these patients will help the doctor "fine tune" management to the individual patient and will increase the success and satisfaction possible from care of patients with borderline personality disorder.

REFERENCES

1. Beresin E, Gordon C. Emergency ward management of the borderline patient. Gen Hosp Psychiatr 1981; 3(3):237–243.
2. American Psychiatric Association. Diagnostic and Statistical Manual of Mental Disorders. 3rd ed, revised. Washington, DC: American Psychiatric Association, 1987:347.
3. Adler G. The borderline patient in the general hospital. Gen Hosp Psychiatr 1981; 3(4):297–300.
4. Smith RC, Zimny GH. Physicians' emotional reactions to patients. Psychosomatics 1988; 29:392–397.
5. Magill MK, Garrett RW. Borderline personality disorder. Am Fam Phys 1987; 35:187–195.
6. Groves JE. Psychotic and borderline patients. *In* Hackett TP, Cassem NH (eds). Handbook of General Hospital Psychiatry. St. Louis: CV Mosby, 1978:174–208.
7. Groves JE. Taking care of the hateful patient. N Engl J Med 1978; 298:883–887.
8. Sarwer-Foner GJ. An approach to the global treatment of the borderline patient. *In* Hartocollis P (ed). Borderline Personality Disorders. New York: International Universities Press, Inc, 1977:345–364.
9. Klein DF. Psychopharmacological treatment and delineation of borderline disorders. *In* Hartocollis P (ed). Borderline Personality Disorders. New York: International Universities Press, Inc, 1977:365–383.
10. Guggenheim FG. Suicide. *In* Hackett TP, Cassem NH (eds). Handbook of General Hospital Psychiatry. St. Louis: CV Mosby, 1978:250–263.
11. Taylor MA, Sierles FS, Abrams R. General Hospital Psychiatry. New York: The Free Press, 1985.
12. Reiser DE, Levenson H. Abuses of the borderline diagnosis: a clinical problem with teaching opportunities. Am J Psychiatr 1984; 141:1528–1532.

Breast cancer

Peng-Tiam Ang ■ *Aman U. Buzdar*

■ Background

Cancer of the breast is the leading cause of cancer-related death among American women; about one in ten American women will develop breast cancer. The American Cancer Society estimated 135,000 new cases would occur in the United States during 1988 and that 42,300 of those people would die from the disease.[1] With available diagnostic techniques and appropriate treatment, this figure can be significantly reduced. Factors associated with an increased risk of developing breast cancer include prolonged uninterrupted hormonal stimulation from early menarche, no children, pregnancy over age 30 years, late menopause, a personal or family history of breast cancer, exposure to radiation, and possibly a high-fat diet.

■ DETECTION

The prognosis of a patient with breast cancer depends on how early the disease is diagnosed. When the disease is small and localized to the breast, 90 per cent of patients survive more than 5 years; if the breast cancer is not invasive (in situ), survival approaches 100 per cent. Detection of early disease is crucial to cure. This can be achieved by monthly breast self-examination (BSE) and by mammography. Ultrasound of the breast may help differentiate a solid from a cystic breast lump but appears to have little value for screening.

In spite of advances in mammographic and other radiologic techniques, most breast cancers continue to be self-detected. Women who practice monthly BSE present with more favorable clinical and pathologic stages than women who do not.[2,3] However, physical examination has its limitations, as the tumor has to be of a certain size and of different consistency from adjacent tissue to be detected.

Mammographic examination supplements BSE in early detection. In the Breast Cancer Detection and Demonstration Project, mammography detected 95 per cent of the lesions that were under 1 cm, whereas physical examination could only detect 30 per cent of these lesions. Mammography may fail to detect any abnormality in a patient who presents with a palpable breast lump. False-negative mammography occurs in up to 35 per cent of premenopausal patients[4,5] Although less frequent, this also can occur among postmenopausal women. Patients with a palpable breast mass despite a negative mammogram should have an excision or needle biopsy for confirmation of diagnosis. In the presence of a lump in the breast, a physician should never reassure the patient because of a negative mammogram.

■ Management of Minimal Breast Cancer

Minimal breast cancer is defined as intraductal or minimally invasive lesions with a mass no more than 10 mm in diameter. In most patients with minimal breast cancer, the disease is detected by mammography. The detection of minimal breast cancer poses certain diagnostic and therapeutic problems. As most of these lesions are not palpable, fine-needle biopsy by palpation is often not possible. The use of mammographic, ultrasound-guided needle biopsies or stereotactic techniques has also been called into question because the resulting cytologic diagnosis is often unreliable. Repeated punctures destroy the pathologic lesions and lead to fat necrosis, creating further difficulty in making a histologic diagnosis.

It is recommended that minimal lesions be excised in toto for diagnostic purposes. This surgery is preceded by preoperative localization with mammography.[6,7] As these lesions are small, they are best studied by multiple sections of permanently fixed material, as there is no room for doubt in the diagnosis.

The primary goal of therapy in minimal breast cancer must be cure. Therapeutic options include partial mastectomy with radiotherapy, total mastectomy, and modified radical mastectomy. The choice is based mainly on whether the patient desires breast conservation.

■ Management of Invasive Carcinoma

Primary therapy in breast cancer essentially entails surgical removal of the tumor. Surgical techniques have evolved from radical and extensive surgery to less disfiguring operations, and surgical techniques that emphasize preservation of the breast can be used if the disease is diagnosed early. Each case should be discussed at multidisciplinary meetings by the surgeon, radiotherapist, and medical oncologist to coordinate and determine the proper sequence of treatment modalities for each patient.

The therapeutic options available to stages I and II patients (T1 or T2, N0 or N1) are radical mastectomy, modified radical mastectomy, total mastectomy, or partial mastectomy with postoperative radiotherapy. Modified radical mastectomy has largely replaced radical mastectomy as the standard operative procedure in the treatment of breast cancer. Prospective randomized trials have shown comparable results for these two procedures, with modified radical mastectomy having the advantage of improved limb function and better cosmetic results.[8,9]

In total mastectomy, previously called simple mastectomy, the whole breast inclusive of the axillary tail is removed. Patients with stage I disease can be treated with total mastectomy alone.[10] When isolated axillary metastases become apparent, axillary dissection can be performed. This approach does not appear to influence distant metastases or overall survival. In patients with stage II disease, total mastectomy with regional radiation is as efficacious as radical mastectomy in terms of disease-free and overall survival.

Partial mastectomy, also called local excision, lumpectomy, segmental mastectomy, and tylectomy, involves excision of the primary tumor without sacrificing the breast. The contraindications for its use include multicentric or poorly defined tumor, skin involvement, fixed nodal disease, previous irradiation of the chest, or a relatively large tumor in a small breast. In patients with stage I and small (4 cm or less) stage II tumors, partial mastectomy with radiotherapy has been shown to yield disease-free and overall survival and loco-regional control similar to that of modified radical mastectomy.

In patients with clinically node-positive stage II, the recommended treatment is a modified radical mastectomy. Although axillary dissection is not useful in prolonging survival, it is important for pathologic staging and prevention of regional recurrence. In patients with stage IIIa disease (tumors larger than 5 cm in diameter but without fixed axillary lymph nodes), preoperative chemotherapy can down-stage locally advanced tumor, and breast conservation may be feasible.

Patients with stage IIIb disease (skin ulceration, fixation to chest wall, edema or satellite lesions, and/or infraclavicular, supraclavicular, internal mammary or extensive axillary nodal involvement with arm edema) are usually technically inoperable at presentation. These patients should be given initial chemotherapy before local therapy. After surgery or irradiation, patients should receive additional chemotherapy. High response rates to chemotherapy and improved survival have been reported with this combined modality approach.

■ ADJUVANT THERAPY IN OPERABLE BREAST CANCER

Despite advances in early diagnosis and primary treatment modalities, about half the patients who present with disease apparently localized to the breast and axillary lymph nodes will develop and eventually die of metastatic disease. This failure reflects the inadequacy of local therapy. Breast cancer is a systemic disease by the time of initial diagnosis in a large number of patients. Hence, despite local therapy with surgery and radiation, the disease may not be cured.

Systemic adjuvant therapy can reduce the risk of recurrence as well as improve the survival of patients with stage II and stage III disease.[11,12] Patients with nodal involvement should be referred for additional therapy following surgery. Combination chemotherapy has been shown to be superior to single-agent treatment, and doxorubicin-containing regimens appear to be better than other regimens.[11,12]

Among patients with stage I disease (tumor less than 2 cm with no nodal disease), certain high-risk groups have been identified. These include patients with estrogen receptor–negative disease, lymphatic invasion, blood vessel invasion, a high nuclear grade, a high labeling index, and a high S phase on flow cytometry. These patients have a higher risk of recurrence, and adjuvant therapy should be considered.

In postmenopausal women with positive axillary nodes and positive estrogen receptors, treatment with tamoxifen has shown modest survival benefit. At the National Institutes of Health (NIH) Consensus Conference in 1985, Peto and associates presented pooled data of all tamoxifen randomized trials and showed that adjuvant tamoxifen was associated with reduced mortality in postmenopausal patients with lymph node involvement. The advantage of this hormonal therapy is its lack of side effects and simplicity of oral administration. The survival benefit does not appear to extend to premenopausal or negative receptor status patients. Other endocrine interventions, such as progestins or aminoglutethimide, also have been studied in a few clinical trials. However, the higher incidence of side effects and lack of adequate data limit their usefulness.

■ TREATMENT OF METASTATIC DISEASE

About 40 per cent of patients with breast cancer eventually develop metastatic disease. Their treatment planning requires that the extent and site of disease and receptor status be determined prior to embarking on specific therapy for the patients. Patients suspected of having an isolated recurrence should have that fact histologically confirmed, as local recurrences often cannot be distinguished clinically or radiologically from benign conditions or a second pri-

mary.[13] Depending on the site of involvement, local therapy may entail surgery, radiotherapy, or both. Surgery is useful in patients with local soft tissue recurrence. Cranial irradiation can relieve symptoms for patients with brain metastases.

After local therapy for isolated recurrence, it is recommended that patients receive combination chemotherapy. The use of such adjuvant chemotherapy has resulted in a significant fraction of patients remaining free of disease for extended periods.[14,15]

The systemic treatment of metastatic disease can be divided into hormonal therapy and chemotherapy. The choice for initial therapy depends on factors such as hormonal receptor status, site of recurrent disease, and tumor burden. In estrogen receptor–positive patients with nonlife-threatening disease, i.e., soft tissue disease or osseous disease or limited visceral involvement without organ dysfunction, it is appropriate to begin with hormonal agents. This also applies to patients in whom receptor status cannot be determined but whose disease has clinical characteristics suggestive of a hormonally responsive tumor—a long disease-free interval, nonvisceral metastases, previous response to hormonal agents— and postmenopausal patients.

However, in life-threatening disease, chemotherapy always should be given first because of the higher risk and more rapid response. After initial response, the patients with estrogen receptor–positive tumors can be treated with hormonal agents. In patients with estrogen receptor–negative disease, the modality of choice is always chemotherapy.

Endocrine Therapy

The responsiveness of some patients with metastatic breast cancer to endocrine manipulation has been recognized for nearly a century. About 25 to 30 per cent of unselected patients respond to endocrine therapy. Discovery of hormonal receptors has made selection of patients for hormonal treatment somewhat simpler. Hormonal receptors described in this disease include estrogen, progesterone, androgen, prolactin, corticosteroids, and aromatase receptors. Of these, estrogen and progesterone receptors have been extensively evaluated. Patients with both of these receptors on the tumor have a 50 to 60 per cent probability of response to endocrine therapy. Choices of endocrine therapy include antiestrogens, progestins, estrogens, androgens, adrenal-blocking agents, and luteinizing hormone–releasing hormone (LHRH) agonists. Each of the endocrine therapies has a similar probability of response in hormone receptor–positive tumor. The sequence of use, based on the side effects, is tamoxifen followed by megestrol acetate, aminoglutethimide, and androgens.

Tamoxifen, an antiestrogen, is the drug of choice for first-line endocrine therapy in premenopausal and postmenopausal women. Estrogen receptor–positive patients have about a 60 per cent response rate.[16] The median duration of response is 8 to 12 months (range, 4 months to more than 40 months). Administered at the usual dose of 20 mg daily, it is almost free of side effects. When therapy is first started, some patients with osseous metastases may complain of increasing bone pain. This transient flare in bone pain is not a reflection of progressive disease. Similarly, early hypercalcemia may occur in patients with extensive bone metastases, necessitating careful monitoring and treatment of serum calcium levels. Minor side effects include hot flushes, nausea, and, rarely, vomiting.

Megestrol acetate, a progestin, is an active hormonal agent in postmenopausal women with breast cancer. As patients who respond to one hormonal therapy tend to respond to another, megestrol acetate can be used as a second-line agent in patients who relapse on (or were resistant to) tamoxifen. The probability of response to progestins as secondary therapy is about 30 to 40 per cent, with median durations of response in the range of 6 to 9 months. The usual dose of megestrol acetate is 40 mg four times a day. The main side effects are edema and weight gain.

Traditionally, oophorectomy has been the first-line therapy in premenopausal patients with metastatic disease. Recent studies with tamoxifen and LHRH agonist as initial therapy instead of oophorectomy have shown comparable results. Patients who respond initially to tamoxifen but later regress may achieve another response with surgical oophorectomy. However, if patients fail to respond to tamoxifen or LHRH agonist, the chances of responding to oophorectomy are very slim.

Other hormonal modifications can be achieved with adrenalectomy, hypophysectomy, or such agents as aminoglutethimide. Estrogens and androgens can be used to induce response in some patients.

Chemotherapy

Chemotherapy is indicated in patients who have exhausted all endocrine options, in those with estrogen receptor–negative tumors, or life-threatening disease. Carcinoma of the breast is responsive to a wide variety of antineoplastic drugs; the more active are doxorubicin, cyclophosphamide, 5-fluorouracil, methotrexate, mitoxantrone, vincristine, and mitomycin. As single agents, the response rate ranges from 25 to 50 per cent. Doxorubicin is probably the most active single agent.[17] Combination chemotherapy, making use of nonoverlapping toxicities, has been shown consistently to be superior to single agents. The two most effective regimens available for general use are cyclophosphamide, methotrexate, 5-fluorouracil (CMF) and 5-fluorouracil, doxorubicin (Adriamycin), cyclophosphamide (FAC). Addition of vincristine to these combinations has not shown any advantage.[18] Doxorubicin-containing regimens appear to be superior to CMF.

The role of sequential administration of noncross-resistant combination chemotherapy is being studied. Initial data suggest no advantage in response rates. Dose intensity, a measure of the amount of drugs administered per unit time, has been shown in retrospective analyses to be an important factor in determining outcome.[19] Ongoing prospective trials are evaluating its significance.

■ Management of Special Problems

One common and potentially lethal problem encountered in patients on chemotherapy is fever and infection. Neutropenia usually occurs between the 10th and 14th days after chemotherapy and patients present around this time with fever. Neutropenic fevers should never be treated lightly. These patients require admission to a hospital and immediate therapy with broad-spectrum antibiotics. If treated appropriately, their mortality is extremely low. Currently, increasing numbers of patients are given chemotherapy on an outpatient basis. The chemotherapy is usually administered via an intravenous long line or a subclavian catheter. These indwelling intravenous catheters are potential sources of sepsis, and they must be replaced if the sepsis cannot be adequately controlled with the antibiotics.

Hypercalcemia may occur spontaneously in patients with bone metastases or during the course of hormonal therapy. As the early symptoms—nausea, vomiting, constipation, lethargy and headaches—are nonspecific, the diagnosis is often missed. It is important to check serum calcium levels in breast cancer patients. Hypercalcemia often can be corrected with intravenous hydration and diuresis. In resistant cases, steroids, plicamycin, diphosphonates, or calcitonin may be needed.

In following patients with a previous history of breast cancer, certain special considerations must be kept in mind. In patients who were treated with radiotherapy, fat necrosis of the breast may occur. On mammography, microcalcifications and mass lesions may be identified. This should not be mistaken for recurrent disease or a second primary. Resorption of the bones in the field of radiation may also occur. The lytic lesion closely mimics metastatic disease. Postradiation pleural and pulmonary changes also may cause confusion for the unsuspecting physician.

INFLAMMATORY BREAST CARCINOMA

Inflammatory carcinoma is an uncommon form of breast cancer and carries a bleak prognosis. Without treatment, the median survival is about 6.5 months. The hallmarks of inflammatory carcinoma are redness, heat, tenderness, and edema of the skin. As this closely mimics acute infection, the unwary physician may treat it with antibiotics for prolonged periods or even attempt to incise and drain the presumed abscess. Inflammatory carcinoma often runs a rapid course, progressing from mild erythema to gross tender swelling of the breast in a matter of weeks. Metastases to regional lymph nodes tend to occur early. Even distant metastases are not uncommon at the time of presentation.

The key to diagnosis is a high index of suspicion on the part of the physician. If the inflammatory skin changes do not resolve completely after a brief course of antibiotics, a mammogram should be performed. This should be followed by a biopsy that includes skin tissue in order to confirm the diagnosis. In inflammatory breast carcinoma, dermal lymphatic and capillary invasion by the tumor is characteristically found.

Earlier therapeutic strategies were aimed solely at loco-regional control. The singular use of radiotherapy or surgery met with miserable results. Patients invariably died of metastatic disease with or without local recurrence. Now these patients should be referred to major cancer institutions for care.

The current strategy is a multimodality approach using intensive multiagent chemotherapy given with loco-regional irradiation or surgery. The use of combination chemotherapy before surgery can often yield dramatic responses.[20,21] At M. D. Anderson Cancer Center, patients are treated with induction chemotherapy consisting of FAC, vincristine, and prednisone (FACVP). Depending on their response, patients have either surgery or radiation for local control of disease. This approach has proved effective in reducing local and systemic recurrences and improving overall survival.[22]

PAGET'S DISEASE

Paget's disease of the breast occurs in 1 to 4 per cent of patients with breast cancer. It usually presents as itching, burning pain, oozing, or bleeding of the nipple. As the condition mimics eczema, patients often get topical therapy for extended periods. The disease often responds temporarily to topical medications but invariably recurs.[23] Patients who fail to respond to brief symptomatic treatment or have recurrent problems should have a mammogram. A wedge biopsy of the nipple is a reliable method of confirming the diagnosis. Two thirds of patients will have a palpable lump in the breast. In patients with underlying tumor, the treatment of choice is modified radical mastectomy. Total mastectomy can be performed in those who have no underlying tumor. The experience with local excision with or without radiotherapy is limited.

REFERENCES

1. American Cancer Society Cancer Facts and Figures—1988. New York: American Cancer Society, 1988.
2. Foster RS, Lang SP, Costanza MC, Worden JK, Haines CR, Yates JW. Breast self-examination practices and breast-cancer stage. N Engl J Med 1978; 299:265–270.
3. Greenwald P, Nasca PC, Lawrence CE, et al. Estimated effect of breast self-examination and routine physician examinations on breast-cancer mortality. N Engl J Med 1978; 299:271–273.
4. McDivitt RW, Beahrs OH, Shapin S, et al. Report of working group to review the NCI/ACS breast cancer detection demonstration projects. J Natl Cancer Inst 1979; 62:641–659.
5. Kopans DB, Meyer JE, Sadowsky N. Breast imaging. N Engl J Med 1984; 310:960–967.
6. Frank HA, Hall FM, Steer ML. Preoperative localization of non-palpable breast lesions demonstrated by mammography. N Engl J Med 1976; 295:259–260.
7. Feig SA, Schwatz GF. Radiologic technique for biopsy of nonpalpable breast lesions. *In* Feig SA, McLelland R (eds). Breast Carcinoma: Current Diagnosis and Treatment. New York: Masson, 1983;265–290.
8. Turner L, Swindell R, Bell WGT, et al. Radical versus modified radical mastectomy for breast cancer. Ann R Coll Surg 1981; 63:239–243.
9. Maddox WA, Carpenter JT, Laws HL, et al. A randomised prospective trial of radical mastectomy versus modified radical mastectomy in 311 breast cancer patients. Ann Surg 1983; 198:207–212.
10. Fisher B, Redmond C, Fisher ER, et al. The contribution of recent NSABP clinical trials of primary breast cancer therapy to the understanding of tumor biology. Cancer 1980; 46:1009–1025.
11. Buzdar AU, Hortobagyi GN, Kau SW, et al. Breast cancer adjuvant therapy trials of M.D. Anderson Hospital: results of three studies. *In* Salmon SE (ed). Adjuvant Therapy of Cancer V. Orlando, FL: Grune & Stratton, Inc, 1987; 411–418.
12. Bonadonna G, Valagussa P, et al. Milan adjuvant trials for stage I–II breast cancer. *In* Salmon SE (ed). Adjuvant Therapy of Cancer V. Orlando, FL: Grune & Stratton, Inc, 1987; 211–222.
13. Harkins LA, Yap HY, Buzdar AU, et al. Benign versus malignant hepatic lesions: a diagnostic dilemma with breast cancer patients. Cancer 1983; 52:1308–1311.
14. Blumenschein GR, Pinnamaneni K, Buzdar AU, et al. Combined regional and systemic therapy in breast cancer patients; an isolated metastasis with or without prior chemotherapy. *In* Jones SE, Salmon SE (eds). Adjuvant Therapy of Cancer IV. Orlando, FL: Grune & Stratton, Inc, 1984; 311–318.
15. Beck TM, Hart NE, Woodard DA, et al. Local or regional recurrent carcinoma of the breast: results of therapy in 121 patients. J Clin Oncol 1983; 1:400.
16. Morgan LR, Schein PS, Woolley PV, et al. Therapeutic use of tamoxifen in advanced breast cancer: correlation with biochemical parameters. Cancer Treat Rep 1976; 60:1437–1443.
17. Ahmann DL, Bisel HF, Eagan RT, et al. Controlled evaluation of Adriamycin (NSC-123127) in patients with disseminated breast cancer. Cancer Chemother Rep 1974; 58:877–882.
18. Broder LE. Combination chemotherapy of carcinoma of the breast. Cancer Treat Rev 1974; 1:183–203.
19. Hryniuk W, Bush H. The importance of dose intensity in chemotherapy of metastatic breast cancer. J Clin Oncol 1984; 2:1281–1288.
20. Hortobagyi GN, Buzdar AU. Progress in inflammatory breast cancer: cause for cautious optimism. J Clin Oncol 1986; 4:1727–1728.
21. Rouesse J, Friedman S, Sarrazin D, et al. Primary chemotherapy in the treatment of inflammatory breast carcinoma: a study of 230 cases from the Institut Gustave-Roussy. J Clin Oncol 1986; 4:1765–1771.
22. Buzdar AU, Hortobagyi GN, Frye D, et al. Inflammatory carcinoma of the breast: preliminary results of the combined modality approach. Proceedings of International Congress on Chemotherapy, 1987, pp 438–440.
23. Rissanen PM, Holsti P. Paget's disease of the breast. The influence of the presence or absence of an underlying palpable tumor on the prognosis and on the choice of treatment. Oncology 1969; 23:209.

Cardiomyopathy

Nanette Kass Wenger

Cardiomyopathy denotes a primary disorder of heart muscle of unknown etiology. Of the three pathophysiologic categories of cardiomyopathy—dilated, hypertrophic, and restrictive—dilated cardiomyopathy is by far the most prevalent. All are characterized by a diverse spectrum of severity, and for all therapy is less than satisfactory.[1] The contemporary application of cellular and molecular biology methods and of immunologic techniques may improve our understanding of cardiomyopathy, may suggest therapeutic strategies, and potentially may enable prevention.

■ Dilated Cardiomyopathy

Dilated cardiomyopathy (DC) is characterized by cardiomegaly with prominent ventricular dilatation, impaired ventricular systolic function, and increased myocardial mass. Limitation of atrial emptying results in atrial dilatation. The prior designation of congestive cardiomyopathy is no longer used, as congestive symptomatology is not invariably present. Relative stasis of blood flow engenders ventricular apical thrombus formation, as well as thrombosis of the atrial appendages, with resultant pulmonary and systemic emboli. Although depression of left ventricular pump function is most frequent, right ventricular DC is increasingly recognized, at times with prominent ventricular arrhythmia.

■ BACKGROUND

Persisting immunologic responses to an antecedent viral infection are under intensive investigation as a cause of DC; this forms the basis for the controversial immunosuppressive therapy advocated by some to treat DC of recent onset. The genetic susceptibility of animal models both to viral myocarditis and to subsequent cardiomyopathy draws attention to the potential contribution of genetic factors in humans. Calcium overload or musculoskeletal spasm are among other postulated causes. Alcohol abuse, pregnancy, and a variety of drugs and toxins are also implicated. The contemporary identification of ischemic "hibernating myocardium" warrants exclusion of severe obstructive coronary disease as etiologic by noninvasive tests or by coronary arteriography, particularly among patients reporting exertional chest pain.

The advanced disease is characterized by severe biventricular failure, frequently complicated by pulmonary and systemic emboli and serious ventricular arrhythmias. Sudden death may occur. The exercise or activity capacity, however, correlates poorly with ventricular function.

The patient describes progressive dyspnea, fatigability, and peripheral edema; an elevated jugular venous pressure, often with a prominent regurgitant (V) wave, hepatomegaly with hepatojugular reflex, and at times ascites and pleural effusion are evident with advanced DC. Pulsus alternans may be detected. Sinus tachycardia is prominent, even at rest, as a compensatory mechanism to maintain the cardiac output. Lung rales are frequent. The cardiac apex impulse is diffuse and laterally displaced; a parasternal (right ventricular) impulse may be evident. Third and fourth heart sounds are often appreciated as a summation gallop when tachycardia supervenes. Both papillary muscle dysfunction and annular dilatation contribute to atrioventricular valvular regurgitation; the murmurs of mitral and tricuspid regurgitation decrease in intensity as cardiac compensation is improved by therapy.

The electrocardiographic abnormalities present in DC are nonspecific: atrial abnormalities, nonspecific repolarization changes, low QRS voltage, and Q waves

"

mimicking myocardial infarction. Supraventricular tachyarrhythmias and ventricular ectopic beats are frequent, with ventricular tachyarrhythmias often present. The role of ambulatory electrocardiogram (ECG) and electrophysiologic studies in guiding decisions for and choice of antiarrhythmic therapy remains controversial.[2] The chest radiograph shows cardiac enlargement, vascular redistribution reflecting pulmonary venous hypertension, and interstitial costophrenic (Kerley) lines; pleural effusion may be present. At echocardiographic examination, there is 4-chamber dilatation with globular, hypokinetic ventricles; atrioventricular valvular regurgitation is detectable by Doppler studies. Ventricular or atrial mural thrombi may be identified. Focal wall motion abnormalities at echocardiography and radionuclide ventriculography may be present with both ischemic heart disease and cardiomyopathy, as may perfusion defects on thallium exercise scanning. In patients with chest discomfort, coronary angiography should be considered.

Adverse prognostic features in patients with DC include the severity of the ventricular dysfunction, the presence of left bundle branch block on the ECG, and malignant ventricular arrhythmias. Left ventricular hypertrophy, adequate to preserve wall thickness, is described to favorably influence outcome. The clinical course is steadily downhill, with recurring episodes of heart failure becoming increasingly difficult to control; mean survival time, prior to recent therapies, was 3 years after the onset of symptoms, with sudden death characteristically due to ventricular arrhythmia or embolism.

■ MANAGEMENT

The therapy is that of congestive cardiac failure and includes sodium restriction, digitalis and other positive inotropic drugs, diuretics, and vasodilator drugs. A nutritious diet with vitamin supplementation is advised, and activity restriction is warranted for symptomatic patients. Alcohol should not be used. Pregnancy is inadvisable. Long-term anticoagulation appears to decrease systemic and pulmonary thromboembolic events.

Although several nondigitalis-positive inotropic agents (phosphodiesterase inhibitors) have improved symptoms and hemodynamic abnormalities in the short term, survival benefit has not occurred.

On the other hand, reduction of resistance to left ventricular ejection appears advantageous. Recent controlled clinical trials of vasodilator therapy, both with combinations of isosorbide dinitrate (10 to 20 mg four times daily) and hydralazine (50 to 300 mg/day) and with angiotensin-converting enzyme inhibitors, have resulted in symptomatic and functional improvement. Survival benefit from angiotensin-converting enzyme inhibitor use has been documented for congestive heart failure of varied etiologies; hence their use is recommended in the absence of specific contraindications.[3,4] Combined therapy to reduce preload and afterload may be beneficial.

Intravenous therapy with dopamine and dobutamine or dobutamine combined with vasodilator therapy may provide hemodynamic benefit in patients with advanced disease.

The role of selective beta-blocker therapy in patients with DC remains controversial, despite the described improvement in functional status and in survival reported with metoprolol.[5,6] Immunosuppressive therapy is not currently recommended (see below).

Patients unresponsive to medical management should be evaluated for cardiac transplantation. Five-year survival rates of up to 70 per cent are currently reported.[7]

■ ISSUES AND RISKS

Endomyocardial biopsy appears clinically indicated only when a specific etiology for the DC is suspected, amenable to biopsy-diagnosis. As noted, the role of immunosuppressive therapy using corticosteroid hormones, cyclosporine, or comparable drugs has not been established, relegating their administration to the setting of controlled clinical trials; endomyocardial biopsy is routinely undertaken under these circumstances.

Further, although arrhythmias are the presumptive mechanism underlying the frequent sudden cardiac death in patients with DC, the role of antiarrhythmic therapy is uncertain. These preparations uniformly depress ventricular function; the ability of invasive electrophysiologic studies to guide therapy is uncertain; and the efficacy of antiarrhythmic therapy in favorably altering prognosis has not been established. Implanted cardioverter/defibrillator therapy should be considered for patients with malignant symptomatic ventricular arrhythmias unresponsive to medical therapy. Beta-blocking drug therapy, advocated by some as favorable, also requires further study.

The data from animal models that verapamil enhances the cardiotoxicity of anthracycline antitumor drugs (and that the cardiotoxicity can be alleviated by amrinone and sulmazole, among others) suggest that modification of anthracycline toxicity in humans warrants attention. The prevention of left ventricular dysfunction from alcohol ingestion in experimental animals by the concomitant administration of verapamil lends further credence to the abnormal calcium bonding postulated as contributory to the cardiodepressant effects of alcohol.[8]

■ Hypertrophic Cardiomyopathy

Much has been learned about the pathophysiology and hemodynamic spectrum of hypertrophic cardiomyopathy (HC), from a variety of noninvasive and invasive studies, since this disorder was initially characterized in the late 1950s. Both obstructive and nonobstructive varieties are described, dominated by substantial myocardial hypertrophy and a lack of ventricular chamber dilatation. There is substantial diastolic dysfunction (impairment of myocardial relaxation) of the slitlike ventricular chamber.[9] Rarely, systolic dysfunction may supervene. A genetic contribution to HC has been reported, predominantly with the obstructive variety. The importance of abnormalities of coronary perfusion related to impaired coronary vasodilatator reserve awaits further study. Right ventricular hypertrophic cardiomyopathy has not been adequately investigated.

■ BACKGROUND[10]

In patients with the obstructive variety of hypertrophic cardiomyopathy (HOCM), the dynamic subaortic obstruction involves apposition in systole of the anterior mitral leaf-

let to the disproportionately thickened ventricular septum (asymmetric septal hypertrophy); an endocardial mural plaque may develop at the site of contact. The outflow gradient is dynamic and is enhanced following a ventricular premature beat, inotropic stimulation, decreased left ventricular cavity size, and reduced aortic diastolic pressure.[9] Initial systolic contraction is powerful and rapid, expelling most of the left ventricular volume, and resulting in a brisk initial carotid upstroke (tidal wave); a pressure gradient develops, delaying the ejection of the remaining systolic volume. The carotid pulse collapse is often interrupted by a tidal wave, giving the arterial pulse a bifid or bisferiens character. There is a prominent *a* wave in the jugular venous pulse. An apical form of HC, with a characteristic spade-like deformity of the left ventricular cavity, is also described.

Atrial dilatation results from decreased ventricular compliance with resistance to diastolic filling. The mitral valve leaflets are thickened, and most patients have some mitral regurgitation, apparently related to abnormal bending of the papillary muscles. Abnormalities of atrioventricular conduction are frequent. Associated mitral annular calcium, as well as conduction disturbances, are more common in elderly patients.

Dyspnea and chest pain, the most frequent presentations, are unrelated to the presence or severity of an outflow gradient; these symptoms are exacerbated by tachycardia that limits ventricular filling. Dyspnea reflects the raised pulmonary venous pressure resulting from ventricular diastolic dysfunction. Palpitations appear to be caused by atrial or ventricular arrhythmias. The chest pain may relate to abnormalities of the intramyocardial coronary arteries or to subendocardial hypoperfusion, reflecting impaired diastolic blood flow. Syncope may result from arrhythmias or from left ventricular underfilling, with a resultant increase in the outflow gradient. Malignant ventricular arrhythmias are considered to cause the sudden deaths.

The cardiac apex impulse in the obstructive variety is powerful but poorly sustained and often associated with a prominent presystolic impulse reflecting the powerful atrial contraction. An S_4, its auscultatory counterpart, is prominent. A spindle-shaped left sternal border systolic murmur, at times with an associated thrill, characterizes a systolic pressure gradient. Post extrasystolic potentiation of the murmur is typical, as is accentuation of the murmur on standing and with the Valsalva maneuver, all of which result in ventricular underfilling. Squatting and handgrip, which increase ventricular volume, decrease murmur intensity. An apical systolic murmur of mitral regurgitation may be present.

There are few abnormal physical findings in the absence of an outflow gradient, save for the powerful sustained apex impulse and a palpable parasternal impulse of left atrial dilatation.

The electrocardiogram (ECG) is that of left ventricular hypertrophy; also present are left atrial abnormality, frequent left anterior fascicular block, Q waves of massive septal hypertrophy that may mimic myocardial infarction, and occasional pre-excitation. The latter is also implicated in causing arrhythmias. A normal ECG is not compatible with significant HC. The cardiac silhouette may be normal on chest roentgenogram, but left atrial enlargement and at times interstitial pulmonary edema are evident with significant disease.

Echocardiography is diagnostic, with characteristic, albeit not specific, abnormalities, including ventricular hypertrophy (often with disproportionate septal thickness), vigorous free wall contraction with septal hypokinesis, enlarged papillary muscles, decreased ventricular systolic dimensions, anterior displacement of the anterior mitral leaflet toward the septum with systolic anterior motion of the mitral leaflet in patients with an outflow gradient, and mid-systolic aortic valve closure. Doppler flow studies can document diastolic dysfunction, assess the outflow gradient, and evaluate the severity of the mitral regurgitation. Comparable information is available from radionuclide ventriculography; myocardial perfusion abnormalities are common with thallium imaging and likely reflect myocardial fibrosis. Ambulatory ECG is indicated to evaluate the presence and severity of arrhythmias. Cardiac catheterization and endomyocardial biopsy are not indicated for clinical diagnosis.

The clinical course varies widely, from few symptoms to rapidly progressive diastolic dysfunction with pulmonary edema, arrhythmias, syncope, and sudden death. Young age of onset, family history of sudden death, syncope, and malignant ventricular arrhythmias are adverse prognostic features. The onset of atrial fibrillation is often heralded by pulmonary edema, owing to the rapid heart rate and loss of the atrial contribution to ventricular filling increasing left-sided diastolic pressures. Infective endocarditis, often on the mitral valve, may exacerbate the clinical course.

■ MANAGEMENT[11]

Beta-adrenergic blocking drugs and calcium blocking drugs, in maximal tolerated doses, can decrease symptoms, enhance exercise capacity, and improve hemodynamics and diastolic function in both obstructive and nonobstructive HC. The decrease in myocardial contractility and slowing of the heart rate improve diastolic compliance. Propranolol and verapamil, alone or in combination, are described as most effective. It is uncertain whether ventricular hypertrophy diminishes with these therapies. Careful surveillance for the development of conduction abnormalities and/or pulmonary congestion is indicated when therapy is initiated with beta-blocking or calcium blocking drugs.

Unfortunately, neither category of drug appears to suppress life-threatening ventricular arrhythmias and predictably lessen sudden death. Amiodarone has been described by some to do so, but its use entails substantial pulmonary, hepatic, and ocular toxicity. Pacemaker implantation may be necessitated if beta-blocking or calcium blocking drugs impair atrioventricular conduction; cardioverter/defibrillator implantation should be considered if antiarrhythmic therapy is ineffective. Atrial fibrillation should be considered a medical emergency and managed with electrical cardioversion, as severe hemodynamic decompensation usually occurs abruptly.

In severely symptomatic patients with substantial outflow gradients, unresponsive to medical management, septal incision or resection may be indicated. Surgical enlargement of the left ventricular outflow tract lessens or abolishes the outflow gradient. Earlier surgical series were characterized by operative and late postoperative mortalities of about 8 per cent each; more recent reports suggest a significantly lowered operative mortality and favorable 5- and 10-year survival with symptomatic improvement.

Prophylactic administration of antibiotics is recommended for dental and operative procedures, as patients with obstructive HC are prone to infective endocarditis of the mitral leaflet.

Inotropic drugs such as digitalis can intensify the outflow gradient in patients with the obstructive physiology and should be avoided; volume depletion, hypotension, and vasodilator drugs all increase the outflow gradient and produce a reflex tachycardia and are similarly to be guarded against.

Competitive sports should be avoided, particularly with obstructive HC.

■ ISSUES AND RISKS

The need for therapy is uncertain in asymptomatic patients with mild HC. Since the prognosis among elderly patients with HC is relatively favorable, the need for and intensity of their medical therapy require evaluation.[12]

Further, although sudden death in patients with HC appears due to ventricular arrhythmia, abnormalities detected at electrophysiologic testing are variable, and electrophysiologic characteristics imparting high risk have not been identified.[13]

■ Restrictive Cardiomyopathy

Restrictive cardiomyopathy is an increasingly recognized entity as Doppler echocardiographic studies improve the identification of ventricular diastolic dysfunction.[14] A poorly compliant ventricle, typically with normal dimensions and normal wall thickness, fills rapidly in early diastole, but has little subsequent filling. Systolic function can be either normal or depressed.

■ BACKGROUND

Restrictive physiology is encountered in Loeffler's cardiomyopathy and endomyocardial fibrosis (EMF), as well as in idiopathic restrictive cardiomyopathy (RC); EMF is predominantly a tropical disease, with Loeffler's cardiomyopathy more frequent in temperate zones; immunologically abnormal eo-

sinophils are implicated in the pathogenesis of both disorders.

Restrictive diastolic hemodynamic abnormalities are the initial presentation of RC, with atrial dilatation and ventricular systolic dysfunction encountered subsequently. Diffuse myocardial fibrosis is generally present, but occasionally ventricular hypertrophy accompanies mild myocardial fibrosis. Both atrioventricular valve dysfunction and conduction abnormalities may be seen. Thromboembolic complications are far less frequent with RC than with Loeffler's cardiomyopathy, endomyocardial fibrosis, or DC; nevertheless, the 5-year prognosis for survival with RC is poor.

Further, Doppler echocardiography may help distinguish constrictive from restrictive physiology. In contrast to the rapid completion of ventricular filling in early diastole that occurs with restrictive physiology, constriction is characterized by increased right ventricular filling with inspiration, accompanied by diminished left ventricular filling and left ventricular output. Doppler studies may better differentiate pericardial constriction and cardiac tamponade from RC than is possible by clinical and cardiac catheterization features.[15] Endomyocardial biopsy is also recommended to differentiate RC from constrictive pericarditis.[16] Magnetic resonance imaging is also described as helpful.[17]

Effort dyspnea is due to the pulmonary venous hypertension that results from left ventricular diastolic dysfunction. Peripheral edema results from right ventricular diastolic dysfunction.

On clinical examination, the steep x and y descents of the elevated jugular venous column are manifestations of the restriction to cardiac filling. The jugular venous pressure rises with inspiration. The carotid pulse volume is decreased. The precordium is quiet. An S_4 is characteristic. The systolic murmur of tricuspid regurgitation is often accompanied by a right-sided S_3. Tachycardia is characteristic, as stroke volume cannot increase to maintain the cardiac output. Ascites is frequent with advanced disease. Prominent right atrial P waves are evident on the ECG, often associated with right axis deviation of the QRS complex. Low QRS voltage may be evident on the ECG, with nonspecific repolarization abnormalities. Cardiac enlargement is due to both the right atrial dilatation and pericardial effusion; a normal heart size is typical in the early stages of disease.

■ MANAGEMENT

The management is that of heart failure, with anticoagulant drugs used to prevent thromboembolic complications. Diuretic drugs must be used cautiously to avert hypovolemia.

Endomyocardial resection with replacement of significantly regurgitant atrioventricular valves has had considerable recent short-term success;[18,19] the long-term prognosis, however, is not known.

■ ISSUES AND RISKS

The role of eosinophilia and mechanisms of damage attributable to eosinophils require delineation. Management of eosinophilia is controversial, both in regard to antimetabolic drugs (methotrexate, cyclophosphamide, and hydroxyurea) and immunosuppressive therapies.

The role of surgical therapy is uncertain, although short-term improvement related to enlargement of the ventricular cavity is described.

REFERENCES

1. Wenger NK, Abelmann WH, Roberts WC. Cardiomyopathy and specific heart muscle disease. *In* Hurst JW (ed). The Heart. 7th ed. New York: McGraw-Hill, in press.
2. Anderson KP, Freedman RA, Mason JW. Sudden death in idiopathic dilated cardiomyopathy. Ann Intern Med 1987; 107:104–106.
3. Cohn JN, Archibald DG, Ziesche S, Franciosa JA, Harston WE, Tristani FE, Dunkman WB, Jacobs W, Francis GS, Flohr KH, Goldman S, Cobb FR, Shah PM, Saunders R, Fletcher RD, Loeb HS, Hughes VC, Baker B. Effect of vasodilator therapy on mortality in chronic congestive heart failure. Results of a Veterans Administration Cooperative Study. N Engl J Med 1986; 314:1547–1555.
4. The CONSENSUS Trial Study Group. Effects of enalapril on mortality in severe congestive heart failure. Results of the Cooperative North Scandinavian Enalapril Survival Study (CONSENSUS). N Engl J Med 1987; 316:1429–1434.
5. Engelmeier RS, O'Connell JB, Walsh R, Rad N, Scanlon PJ, Gunnar RM. Improvement in symptoms and exercise tolerance by metoprolol in patients with dilated cardiomyopathy: a double-blind, randomized, placebo-controlled trial. Circulation 1985; 72:536–546.
6. Heilbrunn SM, Shah P, Bristow MR, Valantine HA, Ginsburg R, Fowler MB. Increased β-receptor density and improved hemodynamic response to catecholamine stimulation during long-term metoprolol therapy in heart failure from dilated cardiomyopathy. Circulation 1989; 79:483–490.
7. Kopecky SL, Gersh BJ. Dilated cardiomyopathy and myocarditis: natural history, etiology, clinical manifestations and management. Curr Prob Cardiol 1987; 12:569–647.
8. Garrett JS, Wikman-Coffelt J, Sievers R, Finkbeiner WE, Parmley WW. Verapamil prevents the development of alcoholic dysfunction in hamster myocardium. J Am Coll Cardiol 1987; 9:1326–1331.
9. Brigden W. Hypertrophic cardiomyopathy. Br Heart J 1987; 58:299–302.
10. Maron BJ, Bonow RO, Cannon RO III, Leon MB, Epstein SE. Hypertrophic cardiomyopathy. Interrelations of clinical manifestations, pathophysiology, and therapy. N Engl J Med 1987; 316:780–789, 844–852.
11. Wigle ED. Hypertrophic cardiomyopathy 1988. Mod Concepts Cardiovasc Dis 1988; 57:1–6.
12. Kenny J, McCarthy C, Blake S, McCann P, Counihan TB. Hypertrophic cardiomyopathy: ten years' experience. Ir J Med Sci 1987; 156:56–60.
13. Watson RM, Schwartz JL, Maron BJ, Tucker E, Rosing DR, Josephson ME. Inducible polymorphic ventricular tachycardia and ventricular fibrillation in a subgroup of patients with hypertrophic cardiomyopathy at high risk for sudden death. J Am Coll Cardiol 1987; 10:761–774.
14. Appleton CP, Hatle LK, Popp RL. Demonstration of restrictive ventricular physiology by Doppler echocardiography. J Am Coll Cardiol 1988; 11:757–768.
15. Appleton CP, Hatle LK, Popp RL. Cardiac tamponade and pericardial effusion: respiratory variation in transvalvular flow velocities studied by Doppler echocardiography. J Am Coll Cardiol 1988; 11:1020–1030.
16. Shoenfeld MH, Supple EW, Dec GW Jr, Fallon FT, Palacios EF. Restrictive cardiomyopathy versus constrictive pericarditis: role of endomyocardial biopsy in avoiding unnecessary thoracotomy. Circulation 1987; 75:1012–1017.
17. Sectem U, Higgins CB, Sommerhoff BA, Lipton MJ, Huycke EC. Magnetic resonance imaging of restrictive cardiomyopathy. Am J Cardiol 1987; 59:480–482.
18. Challenor VF, Conway N, Monro JL. The surgical treatment of restrictive cardiomyopathy in pseudoxanthoma elasticum. Br Heart J 1988; 58:266–269.
19. Cherian G, Krishnaswami S, Sukumar IP, John S, Jairaj PS, Bhaktaviziam A. Endomyocardial fibrosis: report on the hemodynamic data in 29 patients and review of the results of surgery. Am Heart J 1983; 105:659–666.

Cervical spine injury

L. B. Lehman

■ Background

Traumatic injuries of the cervical vertebral column and spinal cord are among the most devasting, shocking, and catastrophic of all injuries. These injuries frequently occur dramatically, unexpectedly, and suddenly. They may also result from an otherwise safe and pleasurable sport or recreational activity when such life-threatening injuries are not at all anticipated. They may result in transient or permanent neurologic impairment, which, in turn, may result in a profound and dramatic alteration of lifestyle, daily activities, and future goals and plans. The unpredictable, sporadic, and episodic nature of cervical vertebral column and spinal cord injuries and their subsequent potential impact on the individuals sustaining these injuries, their families, and society as a whole make a review of this subject an important one for all physicians. In addition, the commonly life-threatening secondary medical and surgical complications and management pitfalls will be discussed in an attempt to reduce the overall morbidity and mortality of those very unfortunate individuals who sustain cervical spine injuries.

Although precise statistics concerning the true national scope of cervical spine injuries are currently unavailable, estimates of a national annual incidence of 40 per million per year, with some 10,000 new cases of acute traumatic spinal cord injuries annually in the United States, seem reasonable.[1,2] Prevalence figures of 250,000 total cases in the United States also seem realistic.[2] Most victims of acute traumatic cervical spinal cord injury are young adolescents and adults between the ages of 10 and 30 years; men outnumber women in most studies four to one. Some 3000 additional patients each year succumb to their cervical spine injury before ever reaching medical attention.[2] Although a large number of causes of cervical vertebral and spinal injuries are commonly reported, motor vehicle accidents, falls, and sports injuries head the lists in most studies.[1-6]

Of the patients who survive to reach medical facilities, some 40 per cent have "complete" lesions or injuries, implying the total absence of motor, sensory, and reflex functioning below the suspected anatomic level of the injury. Some 60 per cent of patients have "incomplete" lesions or injuries, implying some preservation of motor, sensory, or reflex functioning below the suspected anatomic level of the injury. The latter group of patients may be expected to improve neurologically over time, to some degree; the former group usually do not. In most published series, a small but very important subgroup of patients who survive to reach medical attention subsequently deteriorate neurologically, frequently as a result of inappropriate, untimely, or suboptimal medical or surgical management.[7] However, the medical impact and medicolegal ramifications of this small subgroup are often quite staggering. It is also important to note that more than one half of patients admitted to a hospital with the diagnosis of a spinal cord injury also have an associated traumatic injury to the brain, chest, abdomen, pelvis, or extremities that should be evaluated and treated simultaneously.

Unlike many other medical and surgical conditions, the most troubling aspect of analyzing series of patients sustaining acute traumatic cervical spine injury is the relatively poor prognosis for complete recovery, or even significant improvement. This is because, in humans, regeneration of central nervous system tissue does not occur, and hence destroyed neurons and ascending and descending spinal cord tracts are not replaced. Therefore, measures designed to prevent the initial injury from occurring, reduce the severity of the injury, immediately support and strengthen damaged but potentially viable neural elements, and prevent the development of subsequent or secondary injuries and complications are of paramount importance.[1,2,7,8]

■ Diagnosis

The diagnosis of a cervical vertebral column and spinal cord injury must be seriously considered and investigated in any patient sustaining multiple trauma who is mentally impaired (e.g., intoxicated) or unconscious, in any awake patient who reports neck pain following an accident or injury, and in any patient who suffers an accident or injury in which the cervical spine is placed in potential jeopardy due to the described or presumptive mechanism of injury (e.g., motor vehicle accident, diving injury, fall from a significant height).[1,5,6,9] A patient with a prior history of a cervical injury who subsequently reinjures his or her neck should also be considered at potential risk, as should the elderly patient with a history of cervical degenerative osteoarthritis or stenosis.[1]

The evaluation of a patient with a suspected cervical spinal cord injury begins with a careful and thorough neurologic screening examination performed as soon after injury as possible. The patient is examined in the supine position with the neck immobilized.[8,10] The screening neurologic examination consists of several easily repeated components, including the mental status examination, examination of the cranial nerves, examination of motor, sensory, and reflex systems, and testing of coordination and balance. The neurologic examination, however, must be considered only a portion of the admission examination of the multiple trauma patient, which also includes the evaluation and assessment of all other organ systems. The neurologic examination is most important in anatomically defining and localizing an injury to specific cervical segments or levels involved, and physiologically characterizing the lesion as "complete" or "incomplete." Similarly, injuries of the brachial plexus, nerve roots, or peripheral nerves[11] can be differentiated from cervical spinal cord injuries.

Characteristically, an individual with a very high cervical injury (i.e., above C_4) will either die at the site of accident or injury or present to medical attention after sustaining a respiratory or cardiorespiratory arrest with quadriplegia. A patient with a C_5-level spinal cord injury will present with paralysis of deltoid muscle function and all more distal muscle groups. A patient with a C_6-level spinal cord injury will manifest paralysis of biceps and wrist flexion function and all more distal muscle groups. A patient with a C_7-level spinal cord injury will show paralysis of triceps and wrist extension function and all more distal muscle groups. One with a T_1-level spinal cord injury will show paralysis of finger movement and all more distal muscle group function.

The hallmark of a spinal cord injury is the presence of neurologic dysfunction below the anatomic area of injury, ranging from total and permanent absence of function (i.e., quadriplegia) to partial absence of function (i.e. quadriparesis) to minimal and transient compromise of function. Usually, these neurologic deficits are bilateral and may involve compromise of sphincter function of the bowels and bladder. However, other sometimes confusing clinical pictures may signal the presence of a spinal cord injury (i.e., Brown-Séquard hemisection syndrome, "central cord" syndrome, syndrome of the anterior spinal artery).[1] After a brief period of "spinal shock," characterized by *hypotonicity* and *flaccidity*, a more prolonged period of *hypertonicity* with *spasticity* may result, especially if the injury is partial in nature.

In distinction from a cervical spinal cord injury, the hallmark of a brachial plexus injury is that of a painful complete or partial monoparesis of an upper limb. An injury of the upper trunk of the brachial plexus (i.e., $C_{5,6}$) may produce paralysis of deltoid, biceps, and brachioradialis function and an absent biceps reflex; injury of the middle trunk of the brachial plexus (i.e., C_7) may produce paralysis of the triceps function and wrist extension with an absent triceps reflex; injury of the lower trunk of the brachial plexus (i.e., $C_8 T_1$) may cause paralysis or flexion of wrist and finger muscle groups. Traumatic injuries to specific isolated cervical nerve roots and peripheral nerves also have been well described.[11]

As important as neurologic and physical examinations is the lateral cervical radiograph, which should be obtained, whenever feasible, prior to moving the patient.[1,4–6] The radiograph should include all cervical vertebrae from occiput to the T_1 level. Gently pulling down the arms of the patient at the time of radiography usually permits full visualization of all cervical levels. If unsuccessful, the familiar "swimmer's view" film, taken with one arm of the patient elevated above the head (as if about to swim) may permit complete visualization of the cervical area. These films must be carefully reviewed prior to obtaining other radiographs of the spine that may require movement of the patient (e.g., "open-mouth" view, anteroposterior view). They should be inspected for signs of bony fractures or subluxations, soft tissue swelling of the prevertebral space, and malalignment. The patient with a suspected cervical spine injury and a normal neurologic examination and radiographic series may be reassured that the likelihood of a significant injury is low. The presence of persistent pain, however, may at times, warrant further neurodiagnostic studies, such as a computer-assisted tomographic scan (CAT), a magnetic resonance imaging scan (MRI), or a flexion and extension radiographic series. More subtle or occult bony lesions may be demonstrated by conventional tomography.

The patient with a neurologic defect suggestive of a spinal cord injury but without plain radiographic evidence of a fracture or subluxation may present a perplexing diagnostic dilemma and raise the question of

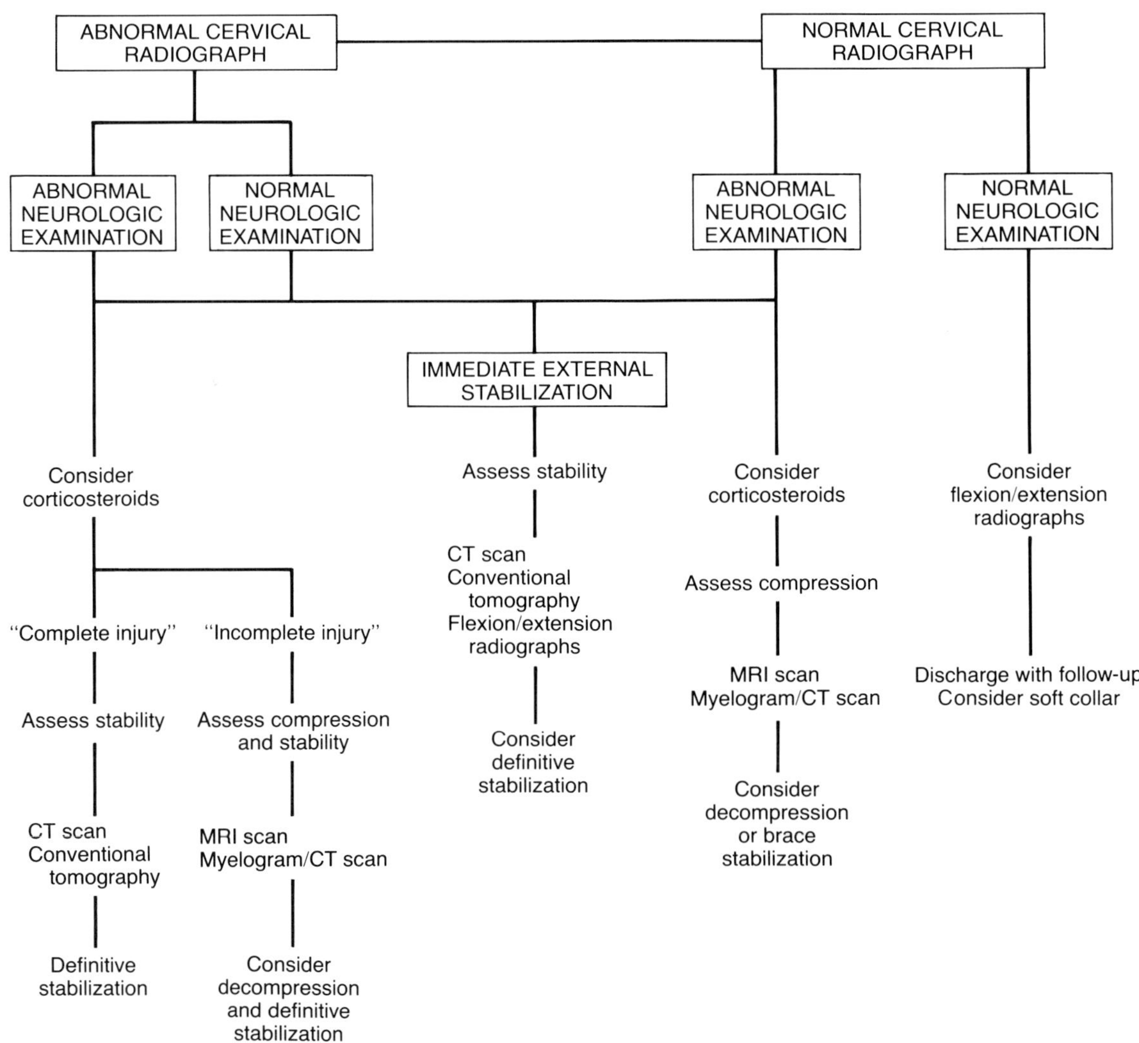

Figure 1. Management approach to the patient with a cervical spine injury, based upon radiographic findings and clinical examination.

whether he or she is showing a conversion reaction or is malingering. An MRI scan or myelogram with CAT scan[12] may be required to identify the presence of hematoma or extruded intervertebral disc. The patient with a documented cervical vertebral fracture with subluxation, either with or without a neurologic deficit, should undergo immediate cervical stabilization[13-18] prior to further neurodiagnostic tests, usually a CAT scan or a myelogram with CAT scan. Figure 1 is a flow diagram summary of the simultaneous diagnosis and management of the patient suspected of having a cervical spine injury.

■ Management

■ INITIAL MANAGEMENT

The management of the patient with a cervical vertebral column or spinal cord injury must be expert, timely, and comprehensive to avoid many of the complications of suboptimal management of these individuals.[3,7,8] The first step in management is the immediate and careful immobilization of the very fragile cervical spine. Physicians who are not formally trained in orthopedic surgery or neurologic surgery may perform this early, often prehospital, on-site care. For example, a young athlete who sustains a neck injury in gym class or at a football game may be so affected. A screening neurologic examination may demonstrate quadriparesis and cervical pain. Prior to evacuating and transporting the patient, the head and neck should be immobilized manually as a unit by the most senior and experienced clinician present at the scene. Whenever possible, the patient should be managed by those experienced in the care of patients with acute spinal injuries, such as physicians and physicians trained in advanced trauma care.[9] When available, a firm cervical support collar should be carefully applied while the injured patient's neck is maintained in a neutral position.

The patient should be moved from the site of injury, such as a firm gymnasium floor or dirt playing field, onto a firm transfer stretcher by several individuals, with the most senior and experienced clinician acting as the team captain and maintaining manual traction and the neutral positioning

of the head and neck.[8] "Logrolling," or rolling the patient as a unit akin to rolling a log, should be instituted to turn over an injured individual suspected of sustaining a cervical spine injury. Sandbags, books, or plastic water bags should be positioned on either side of the neck and held in place with a tape strip placed across the forehead to further immobilize the cervical spine.

In the rare event that the injured patient's neck is twisted to one side and he or she cannot straighten it, no manual efforts should be performed to place the neck in neutral position. Rather, the patient should be transported in the position of injury, because a rotatory subluxation may be present. Under no circumstance should the neck of an injured individual be forcefully manipulated at the scene of injury. The patient should be carefully and rapidly transported to the nearest facility having the capacity to care for spinal cord injury patients. At a minimum, such a facility should have immediately available orthopedic, neurosurgical, and general surgery consultants and equipment, and the capacity to perform emergency myelogram and CAT scan studies. An operating room with trained personnel, an intensive care unit with portable x-ray capability, and overall familiarity with and commitment to caring for patients in skeletal traction should be present.

When the patient arrives in the emergency area he or she should undergo a rapid general and neurologic assessment, as previously described, and a portable lateral radiograph of the cervical spine should be made and reviewed.[1,3,5,6,8] If a cervical fracture with subluxation is documented either with or without a neurologic deficit, cervical skeletal traction should be applied immediately. This is done both to further immobilize the neck and to gently reduce the area of subluxation in order to restore normal alignment. Traction equipment (e.g., "halo" rings, Gardner-Wells tongs, Crutchfield's tongs) is applied under local anesthesia as a bedside emergency room or intensive care unit procedure.[15-18] Radiographs are taken prior to and following the application of traction weight in order to assess radiographic alignment. Approximately 2 to 5 pounds of weight are applied for each cervical vertebral level involved (e.g., a $C_{5,6}$ subluxation may be reduced starting with 10 to 25 pounds of weight), and gradually increased until acceptable alignment is achieved. Periodic neurologic re-examinations are also important to insure that the adequate bony realignment is not accompanied by a paradoxic worsening of neurologic status, such as may occur with "over-reduction."

After the mechanical reduction is accomplished, application of a halo ring and vest[16,17] for a usual period of 3 months may be all that is required to effect an autologous natural fusion of the fractured bony elements. Very few orthopedic surgeons or neurosurgeons currently advocate prolonged bed rest with skeletal traction because of the significant number of associated medical problems. Occasionally, surgical wiring and fusion are indicated, particularly when severe ligamentous pathology exists in the absence of bony injury. Many of these considerations will be discussed under "Subsequent Management."

The management of the cervical spine injury patient with a neurologic deficit or deficits but a normal-appearing lateral radiograph depends largely upon the results of additional neurodiagnostic tests. If, for instance, a spinal epidural hematoma is discovered, a decompressive laminectomy with evacuation of the hematoma may be indicated. If a soft herniated disc is found, surgical discectomy with fusion should be considered. Rarely, if ever, should an exploratory operation on the cervical spine be performed prior to effecting adequate skeletal reduction and securing precise radiographic definition of the injury site.[7] The particular operative approach for decompression of the cervical spine is governed by the preoperative location of the offending bony compressive fragments (i.e., if anterior compressive fragments are present, the approach should be an anterior decompression and fusion; if posterior compressive elements are present, a posterior decompression, wiring, and fusion should be performed). Additional surgical considerations will be reviewed in the section on "Subsequent Management."

Unfortunately, all efforts to date to identify clinically useful pharmacologic adjunctive therapies to improve upon the neurologic outcome of the cervical spine injury patient have been unsuccessful, although many have held early promise in limited laboratory studies.[2,10,19,20] A large, multicenter, randomized, blind study to investigate the use of the corticosteroid methylprednis-olone, the most commonly administered pharmocologic agent in cervical spinal cord injury, showed no statistically significant benefit to its clinical application.[19] A number of potentially deleterious side effects have likewise been identified. While sound experimental bases underlie its use—namely, reducing edema of injured neural tissue, stabilizing membranes, and modulating the sodium-potassium membrane pump mechanism—a statistically significant clinical experience does not support its use. Steroids are still employed widely in spinal cord injury by clinicians who suspect that a small, but yet undefined, subgroup of patients might benefit from their use.

Naloxone has also been extensively investigated as an important potential adjunctive drug for acute spinal cord injury. The rationale for its experimental use is that the opiate receptor blocker may retard the destructive effects of endorphins released during spinal cord injury, which contribute to spinal cord ischemia. Ultimately, no statistically proved clinical benefit could be demonstrated by the use of naloxone.[20] Thyrotropin-releasing hormone has likewise been investigated and found to be clinically non-beneficial. Several other agents are currently under investigation, including the oxygenated perfluorocarbons, prostaglandin pathway intermediates and modulators, and dimethylsulfoxide.

■ SUBSEQUENT MANAGEMENT

The definitive surgical management of the patient with a cervical vertebral column and spinal cord injury must be specifically directed at a well-defined clinical and radiographic injury of known anatomic type and presumed physiologic mechanism.[2,14] Earlier attempts at performing indiscriminate and extensive cervical laminectomies, and, later, spinal cord "cooling" were notoriously unsuccessful. Contemporary cervical spinal surgery aims at neurologic improvement by decompression of a known compressive lesion, and at mechanical stability by fusing damaged skeletal elements.

Many investigators have previously addressed the specific surgical approaches and operations.[4,14] Others have extensively discussed the important supportive role of careful and expert anesthetic technique, including gentle intubation and positioning, in avoiding catastrophic intraoperative complications.

Patients sustaining and surviving injuries to the C_{1-2} complex, for the most part, are not treated surgically as they heal well with external support immobilization. Examples of such injuries are the Jefferson fracture (burst fracture of the arch of C_1), the "hangman's" fracture (bilateral pars interarticularis fracture of C_2), and the type I and type III odontoid fractures (fractures involving the tip of the dens and superior portion of the axis body, respectively). Because of the high rates of nonunion, patients with a type II odontoid fracture (fracture involving the dens above the axis body transversely) should be considered candidates for early posterior cervical wiring and fusion.

Patients sustaining injuries to the middle and lower cervical spine with significant bony fractures, and where adequate alignment is re-established and maintained by skeletal traction, also may be considered candidates for external support immobilization using the halo orthosis. When adequate reduction cannot be effected externally or a compressive bony lesion persists despite realignment, surgical decompression and simultaneous fusion should be considered. The surgical approach is dictated by the preoperative radiographic imaging studies. For example, a unilateral locked facet or posterior element fractures may be adequately reduced and stabilized via a posterior approach. A patient with a compression type of vertebral body fracture, with bone impacted into the spinal canal anteriorly, is best approached through an anterior cervical decompression and simultaneous fusion. Similarly, traumatic herniations or extrusions of cervical intervertebral discs are best handled by an anterior operative approach. Purely ligamentous injuries with cervical instability, often defined as vertebral body displacement, or nonalignment of more than 3.5 mm or angulation of more than 11 degrees is best treated by a posterior wiring and fusion, although advocates of anterior operative approaches also cite good results.

Very complex cervical injuries may require that a number of staged procedures be undertaken to accomplish both adequate decompression to restore the maximal return of neurologic functioning, and adequate fusion to restore a maximal amount of mechanical stability. These procedures may be performed at one or more operations. The

intraoperative recording of somatosensory evoked potentials allows the surgical team to monitor intrinsic spinal cord functioning even during the deepest stages of anesthesia. Serial intraoperative radiographs confirming the level of surgery, placement of hardware, and alignment of bony elements are also important in preventing intraoperative complications.

A number of externally worn cervical casts, braces, and orthoses are available to afford additional stability.[18,21] Clearly, the halo ring and vest afford the greatest degree of clinical stability, particularly for the upper cervical spine. Four-post braces, two-post braces, and molded plastic or plaster orthoses afford somewhat less stability in terms of rotational movement. Collar-type braces, such as the molded Philadelphia plastic collar and soft cervical foam collar, supply only a minimal amount of additional support but do remind the patient of the importance of limiting neck movement, particularly when they are worn conscientiously and correctly.

A well-structured and coordinated physical therapy and rehabilitation program[21] is also a central concern in the formulation of an overall cervical spine injury management program. The goals of such a multidisciplinary program are the early mobilization, reassimilation, and retraining of the injured patient. Physical therapists work largely to maintain lower extremity and upper extremity muscle tone, and with the assistance of supervising physiatrists and orthotists formulate braces and splints to prevent contractures. Occupational therapists work largely to help the neurologically impaired patient learn to adjust to a new deficit by employing special skills, techniques, and devices to perform the activities of daily living, such as feeding, personal hygiene, transfers from bed to chair, and the like. Skilled and compassionate physiatrists and therapists have assisted even the most profoundly impaired, ventilator-dependent quadriplegic patients in adopting as close to an independent lifestyle as possible.

The family physician or internist is also a key member of the spinal cord injury and rehabilitation team, and, along with the orthopedic surgeon, neurosurgeon, orthotist, physiatrist, therapists, and specially trained nurses and aides, must anticipate systemic problems before they occur and deal with them expeditiously when they do occur. Patients who sustain cervical spinal cord injuries are frequently in bed for prolonged periods of time and are therefore predisposed to develop pulmonary emboli, stasis ulcers, renal calculi, pneumonias, urinary tract infections, gastrointestinal tract ulcers or perforations, and a number of other problems. Such patients should be prophylactically placed on a bowel and bladder emptying regimen (e.g., antacids, stool softeners and enemas, intermittent urinary catheterization), kept well hydrated, turned and positioned carefully and frequently, and, in certain cases, anticoagulated. The use of many of the newer mattresses and beds also may be particularly helpful in selected cases.

Clearly, these individuals need to be examined frequently and meticulously in order to rapidly diagnose and treat common but often debilitating complications. A consultation and an on-going relationship with a psychiatrist, psychologist, or psychiatric social worker can do much in dealing with the profound reactive depression that frequently accompanies these devastating injuries. Similarly, "patient-to-patient" encounters with recovering or rehabilitated spinal injury patients and family support groups are also important components of the reassimilation process in the weeks and months following the injury.

■ Issues and Risks

Clearly, the greatest concern in the management of patients with a cervical vertebral column or spinal cord injury must be the prevention of these injuries and their secondary complications. This is truly an attempt at "preventive neurosurgery."

Many measures have been described to reduce the frequency and severity of these injuries.[22-24] The institution of a lower speed limit on highways, compulsory seat belt and shoulder harness laws in many states, and high-back seats with cervical rests in automobiles are examples of such efforts. A most impressive contribution to reducing cervical injuries in sports, most prominently football, has been made by the National Football Head and Neck Injury Registry, and in several other related sports as well. By identifying an array of particularly dangerous maneuvers and restricting or eliminating them,

the frequency and severity of cervical spine injuries in many of these sports have been dramatically reduced. The most notorious of these dangerous maneuvers is "spearing," or intentionally colliding with an opponent by using the helmeted flexed skull as a battering ram.[23,24] This places very strong forces on the vulnerable cervical spine and has resulted in literally hundreds of cases of cervical injury over the years. Individuals diving into shallow ponds or pools, usually while mentally impaired or intoxicated, is also a major source of severe cervical spine injuries, particularly during the warm summer months. Public awareness of these dangerous maneuvers and injury mechanisms is important but commonly absent.

Similarly, awareness and sensitivity about cervical vertebral column and spinal cord injury must be frequently raised among clinicians to reduce the risks of additional injury to the patient already sustaining a cervical injury. In one recent report,[18] some 3 to 25 per cent of spinal cord injuries occurred after the initial insult. The notion that patients sustaining a possible cervical spine injury must be evacuated and transported as rapidly and atraumatically as possible, with all possible precautions made to maintain complete and total immobilization of the head and neck unit should be emphasized.[2-6,9] Postinjury deterioration remains a major medical as well as medicolegal concern. This information, well known to the medical and paramedical community, also should be disseminated in schools and in the workplace. Individuals with particular vocational or avocational vulnerability for cervical injury should be so advised by their physicians and alerted to early signs and symptoms of injury.

Another important issue remains the early institution of measures to promote or enhance neurologic recovery after injury has occurred. Although most surgical and pharmacologic measures have thus far been less than successful clinically, newer experimental modalities may hold unexpected promise.[25] In vitro studies using nerve growth factor and other agents to stimulate the regeneration of damaged central nervous tissue, as well as surgical grafting experiments, are now being performed. Immunochemical and microvascular studies are also being done to study new ways to halt or reverse the sequelae of acute spinal cord injury at a molecular and biochemical level. New pharmacologic agents are also being developed for investigation.

The application of computer technology and robotics to the care of the spinal cord injury patient, while in very early stages, may hold a tremendous and revolutionary role in the future rehabilitation of injured patients.

■ Conclusions

Cervical spine injury remains a catastrophic and unforeseen sequela of many everyday activities, affecting largely young and previously healthy adults. Although some of these individuals do respond to immediate mechanical stabilization, early reduction and decompression of bony fractures and subluxations, and subsequent multidisciplinary team care, a large percentage of individuals remain neurologically devastated, physically handicapped, and psychologically and emotionally compromised.

The key to reducing the mortality and morbidity of cervical spinal cord injury is prevention. Increasing public awareness of the risks of quadriplegic injuries by outreach programs in the schools and workplaces should help dramatize the potential risks of casual diving, driving while intoxicated, high-risk gymnastics by those not trained and conditioned specifically for the maneuvers, and the like. Similarly, the increasing awareness of the medical community to the possibility of these injuries should reduce the incidence and frequency of secondary complications, both neurologic and systemic.

Cervical spine injuries remain a considerable challenge to clinicians on many levels. A comprehensive, team approach integrating many disciplines and viewpoints to custom design a management plan for each patient will optimize the chances for recovery of neurologic function, mechanical stability, and resumption of a productive and exciting life.

REFERENCES

1. Lehman LB. Injury of the cervical spine: some fundamentals of management. Postgrad Med 1987; 82:193–200.
2. Triggs KJ, Garfin SR, Marshall LF, et al. Spinal cord injury: advanced treatment concepts. Surg Rounds 1988; 11:39–41.
3. Sypert GW. Early management of spinal injuries. Am Fam Physician 1984; 29:113–122.
4. Fewer H. Management of acute spine and spinal cord injuries. Arch Surg 1976; 111:638–645.
5. Castillo RG, Bell J. Cervical spine injury: stabilization and management. Postgrad Med 1988; 83:131–132.
6. Saderstrom CA, Brumback RJ. Early care of the patient with cervical spine injury. Orthop Clin North Am 1986; 17:3–13.
7. Levine AM, Edwards CC. Complications in the treatment of acute spinal injury. Orthop Clin North Am 1986; 17:183–203.
8. Lehman LB. Preventing and anticipating neurologic injuries in sports. Am Fam Physician 1988; 38(4): 181–184.
9. Committee on Trauma, American College of Surgeons: Advanced Trauma Life Support Student Manual. Chicago: American College of Surgeons, 1984.
10. Luce JM. Medical management of spinal cord injury. Crit Care Med 1985; 13:126–131.
11. Lehman LB. Sports-related peripheral nerve injuries. Surg Rounds Orthop 1988; Sept:68–72.
12. Cooper PR, Cohen W. Evaluation of cervical spinal cord injuries with metrizamide myelography–CT scanning. J Neurosurg 1984; 61:281–289.
13. Crutchfield WG. Skeletal traction in the treatment of injuries to the cervical spine. JAMA 1954; 155:29–32.
14. White AA, Panjabi MM. The role of stabilization in the treatment of cervical spine injuries. Spine 1984; 9:512–522.
15. Gardner WJ. The principle of spring-loaded points for cervical traction. J Neurosurg 1973; 39:543–544.
16. Nickel VL, Perry J, Garrett A, et al. The halo: a spinal skeletal traction fixation device. J Bone Joint Surg 1968; 50:1400–1409.
17. Cooper PR, Maravilla KR, Sklar FH, et al. Halo immobilization of cervical spine fractures: indications and results. J Neurosurg 1979; 50:603–610.
18. Podolsky S, Baraff LJ, Simon RR. Efficacy of cervical spine immobilization methods. J Trauma 1983; 23:461–465.
19. Bracker MB, Collins WF, Freeman DF, et al. Efficacy of methylprednisolone in acute spinal cord injury. JAMA 1984; 251:45–52.
20. Flamm ES, Young W, Collins WF, et al. Phase I trial of naloxone treatment in acute spinal injury. J Neurosurg 1985; 63:390–397.
21. McCagg C. Postoperative management and acute rehabilitation of patients with spinal cord injuries. Orthop Clin North Am 1986; 17:171–182.
22. Lehman LB. Nervous system sports-related injuries. Am J Sportsmed 1987; 15:494–499.
23. Lehman LB. Reducing neurologic trauma in sports. New York State Med 1988; 88:15–17.
24. Torg JS, Vegso JJ, Sennett B, et al. The national football head and neck injury registry 1971–1984. JAMA 1985; 254:3439–3443.
25. Gunby P. From "regeneration" to prostheses: research on spinal cord injury. JAMA 1981; 245:1293–1297.

Cirrhosis of the liver in the alcoholic patient

Robert L. Mellman ■ *Robert Burakoff*

The alcoholic patient with cirrhosis of the liver can be difficult to manage because of the complications associated with cirrhosis and portal hypertension. At present, there is little hope of reversing the architectural derangements seen in the cirrhotic liver, although a few studies suggest that colchicine may be useful in halting or even reversing the relentless scarring of the liver. For now, however, we must encourage our patients to abstain from imbibing the spirits and promote good nutrition. In this chapter we focus on the pathophysiology and management of the five major complications of alcoholic cirrhosis: ascites, spontaneous bacterial peritonitis, variceal bleeding, hepatic encephalopathy, and the hepatorenal syndrome.

■ Ascites

■ BACKGROUND

The management of ascites presents a challenge to the physician because of the numerous problems caused by the increased intra-abdominal pressure, the risk of spontaneous bacterial peritonitis (SBP), and the risk of developing the hepatorenal syndrome (HRS), which occurs almost exclusively in patients with cirrhotic ascites.[1] The 5-year mortality rate is approximately 30 percent in patients with cirrhosis and ascites who stop drinking, and the percentage doubles in patients who continue to drink.[2] Although the treatment of ascites may not change the mortality rate, it will help change morbidity by relieving pain, dyspnea, and umbilical hernias; prevent atelectasis and pneumonia; reduce pleural effusions, portal hypertension, and variceal bleeding; increase cardiac output; and improve anorexia.

The pathophysiology of ascites has become quite complex in recent years. It is now recognized that a variety of factors contribute to the initiation and maintenance of ascites. At high intrasinusoidal pressures, hepatic lymph escapes via the surface lymphatics and accumulates within the peritoneal cavity once lymphatic drainage is overloaded.[3] Several hypotheses attempt to explain the maintenance of ascites. The underfill hypothesis, based on Starling's equation, requires portal hypertension and hypoalbuminemia to reduce the effective circulating plasma volume, which then results in the retention of sodium and water by the kidney.[4] In addition, there is a state of increased renin, aldosterone, antidiuretic hormone, and catecholamines in response to the decreased effective plasma volume. This response can be reversed by head out of water immersion as well as by reinfusion of ascitic fluid or saline into the venous system. Another theory, the overflow hypothesis, states that the defect is primarily renal and that the impaired sodium and water excretion is due to a baroreceptor reflex caused by increased intrahepatic sinusoidal pressure.[3,4] Lastly, the most recent hypothesis, peripheral arterial vasodilatation, proposes that arteriovenous fistulas and circulating hormones as yet unidentified cause decreased peripheral vascular resistance and decreased effective circulating plasma volume and result in sodium and water retention.[4] No one theory presently fully explains the pathogenesis of ascites.

The diagnosis of ascites is easily established by both physical examination and radiologic testing when more than 2 liters of fluid is present. When less than 2 liters is present, however, the physical examination and plain films of the abdomen do not have adequate sensitivity or specificity, and the best test to perform is abdominal ultrasound. Once it is established that ascites is present, a paracentesis should be performed.[5] Under sterile conditions, a 20-gauge 3- to 4-inch angiocatheter can be inserted under the umbilicus with the patient in a sitting position or in the right iliac fossa with the patient supine. If a difficult tap is anticipated, the paracentesis should be done with ultrasound or computed tomography guidance. Complications, which occur in less than 3 per cent of patients, include bowel perforation, hemorrhage, infection, or persistent leakage.[6] The fluid should be routinely evaluated for appearance, color, cell count and differential, total protein, lactic dehydrogenase (LDH), glucose, Gram stain, bacterial cultures, and cytology. If the ascitic fluid is turbid, triglyceride and cholesterol determinations should be ordered. If bacterial peritonitis is suspected, pH and lactate levels are needed, and if nonbacterial peritonitis is suspected, mycobacterial and fungal smear and culture should be obtained. In patients with ascites secondary to alcoholic liver disease, the ascites is a transudate (total protein less than 2.5 mg/dl or serum ascites–albumin difference more than 1.1 gm/dl) in 80 per cent of patients.

■ MANAGEMENT

The clinician must understand two important principles in order to safely manage cirrhotic ascites. First, the maximum amount of ascites that can be absorbed is 1000 ml/day if peripheral edema is present, and 500 ml/day if there is no edema.[5] If the patient with ascites and edema loses more than 1 kg/day or the patient with only ascites loses more than 0.5 kg/day, the loss will be at the expense of plasma volume depletion and possibly result in hypotension, prerenal azotemia, and the risk of hepatorenal syndrome.[3,5] Thus, a patient with 40 liters of ascitic fluid can lose 20 liters over 6 to 8 weeks, losing 1 to 2 pounds/day. Second, the goal is not to eliminate all the ascitic fluid; rather, it is to achieve a level of ascites consistent with patient comfort. Complications, therefore, can be minimized by avoiding overly aggressive diuresis, monitoring daily weights, and following blood urea nitrogen (BUN) and creatinine concentrations and serum and urine electrolytes, especially when using diuretics.

The treatment of ascites often begins with alcohol abstinence, bed rest, and sodium restriction. Bed rest allows mobilization of fluid, and sodium restriction (0.5 to 1 gm/day) is required to stop or reduce the accumulation of ascites. This therapy is most effective in about 10 to 20 per cent of patients whose urinary sodium excretion is greater than 10 mEq/day.[7] A problem, therefore, arises in the majority of patients who excrete less than 10 mEq/day and who cannot tolerate a diet of 10 to 20 mEq/day (250 to 500 mg of Na^+/day) in order to prevent positive sodium balance and fluid accumulation. For example, if a patient who has a urinary excretion of sodium of less than 10 mEq/day consumes a 2-gram sodium diet (80 mEq of Na^+), then he or she would retain about 400 to 500 ml of fluid. Therefore, most patients will require a diuretic to achieve a negative sodium balance and fluid loss. In the absence of significant hyponatremia (serum Na^+ less than 130), there is no need for fluid restriction, since many patients do not have impaired free water clearance, and because decreased fluid intake may lead to diminished renal blood flow and hepatorenal syndrome.[2,6,7]

Diuretics are the mainstay of therapy for the majority of patients with chronic cirrhotic ascites. Spironolactone (Aldactone) inhibits the synthesis and antagonizes the renal effects of aldosterone in the distal convoluted tubule and produces an effective diuresis in up to 75 per cent of patients.[1] The initial dose is 100 mg/day, which can be given in divided doses two to four times per day.[8] A maximum dose of 800 to 1000 mg/day has been reported to be safe and effective.[3] The urine Na^+ or urine Na^+-to-K^+ ratio can be used as a guide for selecting an initial dose. When the urine Na^+ is greater than 10 mEq or the urine Na^+-to-K^+ ratio is greater than 1, indicating a lesser degree of secondary hyperaldosteronism, a lower dose of spironolactone can be used.[3,6] It usually takes 2 to 4 days for diuresis to begin, and doses may be increased every 3 to 4 days if there is no response and the urine Na^+ is less than 10 mEq. Once a dose of 400 mg is reached with little or no response, then a loop diuretic should be added. This will increase flow to the distal convoluted tubule and enhance the effectiveness of spironolactone. One study has shown that spironolactone alone or in combination with furosemide (Lasix) was more effective and easier to use than furosemide alone.[9]

Approximately 50 per cent of patients

using furosemide alone will exhibit a satisfactory diuresis.[2] The loop diuretics are very effective natriuretics. Up to 25 per cent of the filtered sodium load may be excreted by impairing the transport of sodium and chloride in the loop of Henle. The starting dose is 20 to 40 mg/day, and the dose may be increased every 2 to 3 days, up to a maximum of 160 to 240 mg/day.[2,8] Complications are more frequent with the loop diuretics than with spironolactone, and in-hospital monitoring of daily weight, serum BUN and creatinine concentrations, and electrolytes is recommended when these drugs are initiated.

If combination diuretic therapy with spironolactone and a loop agent is ineffective, then spironolactone may be replaced by metolazone (Zaroxolyn) or hydrochlorothiazide (HCTZ). These two drugs by themselves result in a mild-to-moderate natriuresis, but when combined with the loop diuretics, produce a profound natriuresis. HCTZ may be initiated at 12.5 to 25 mg/day and metolazone at 2.5 to 5.0 mg/day. Careful monitoring of BUN and creatinine concentrations and electrolytes is mandatory. About 5 to 10 per cent of patients who have no response to diuretics or who respond only at the expense of worsening renal function have intractable ascites (Table 1). This small group of patients will require either repeated large-volume paracentesis or peritoneovenous shunting.

Large volume paracentesis, 4 to 6 liters, is ideal for patients who need rapid decompression of the abdomen: for example, with an incarcerated hernia, severe abdominal pain, or respiratory distress. When repeated abdominal paracentesis is used for refractory ascites, however, complications such as bleeding, infection, perforation, or hyponatremia are more likely to occur. The procedure is contraindicated in patients with infection, hemorrhage, hepatoma, hepatic encephalopathy, or hepatorenal syndrome. Removal of 4 to 6 liters of ascitic fluid over 30 to 90 minutes is safe in patients with peripheral edema, but if no edema is present, then intravenous infusion of 40 gm of albumin must be given to prevent plasma volume contraction and renal insufficiency. Since ascitic fluid accumulates rapidly, paracentesis may be required every 1 to 3 weeks. Sodium restriction, diuretics, or both may slow down the reaccumulation of fluid.

Peritoneovenous shunt can be of therapeutic value in about 5 per cent of cirrhotic patients with refractory ascites. There are numerous contraindications to the procedure, such as a serum bilirubin of greater than 8 mg/dl, congestive heart failure (CHF), pleural effusion, hepatic encephalopathy, peritonitis, a history of bleeding varices, coagulopathy, or disseminated intravascular coagulation (DIC). The shunt works by diverting ascitic fluid from the peritoneal cavity subcutaneously to the internal jugular vein via a pressure-activated one-way valve. Approximately 50 per cent of patients will have a reduction in the ascites for at least 1 year.[7] The problem with this form of therapy, however, is that it does not improve survival and the complication rate is quite high. Besides a high perioperative mortality (3 to 25 per cent), serious complications arise in greater than 10 per cent of patients, such as DIC, peritonitis, CHF, and variceal bleeding. Also, there is up to a 30 per cent chance of the shunt clotting.[3] Nevertheless, it may be the last option for some patients.

TABLE 1. Management of Cirrhotic Ascites

Initial management:
Bed rest and low sodium diet
Spironolactone, 100–400 mg/day
Furosemide, 40–200 mg/day added to spironolactone
Hydrochlorothiazide, 12.5–50 mg/day, or metolazone, 2.5–10 mg/day added to furosemide

Management of refractory ascites (unresponsive to diuretics or only at the expense of azotemia):
Correct problems
  Noncompliance with medication or diet
  Inadequate diuretic regimen
  Spontaneous bacterial peritonitis
  Hepatocellular carcinoma
  Hepatitis—viral, toxic, ischemic
  Budd-Chiari syndrome
  Hypokalemic alkalosis
Large-volume paracentesis (add albumin infusion if peripheral edema is not present)
Ultrafiltration and reinfusion
Peritoneovenous shunt

■ Spontaneous Bacterial Peritonitis

■ BACKGROUND

Spontaneous bacterial peritonitis (SBP) is an ominous complication that occurs in up to

10 per cent of patients with alcoholic cirrhosis and ascites. The mortality rate is between 60 and 90 per cent even when the diagnosis is not delayed. The diagnosis can be quite difficult to make because half of the patients present without any abdominal pain or tenderness. Therefore, clinical suspicion must be high in assessing cirrhotic patients with ascites and especially so in any patient showing a clinical deterioration such as hepatic encephalopathy, worsening of liver function, or hypotension.[1] The pathogenesis of primary SBP is thought to be due to gut flora migrating through edematous bowel and congested lymphatic and splanchnic vessels, bypassing a weakened hepatic reticuloendothelial system, and entering ascitic fluid low in antibody, complement, and opsonizing activity. Since nonenteric pathogens such as *Streptococcus pneumoniae* also cause SBP, hematogenous seeding may be important as well. The diagnosis is made by finding greater than 250 white blood cells per μl with at least 50 per cent polymorphonuclear leukocytes in the ascitic fluid. The Gram stain is positive in only about 25 per cent of cases, but cultures will be positive in up to 80 per cent of patients. Blood cultures are positive in about half the cases. Several features help distinguish primary from secondary bacterial peritonitis. SBP is caused by a single organism, most commonly *E. coli* or *Pneumococcus* in up to 80 per cent of cases, whereas bowel perforation and intra-abdominal abscesses usually have polymicrobial flora that frequently contain anaerobes.[6] In addition, secondary bacterial peritonitis tends to have a higher leukocyte count and protein concentration; if present, pneumoperitoneum suggests bowel perforation.

■ MANAGEMENT

Treatment with broad-spectrum intravenous antibiotics, such as ampicillin, along with an aminoglycoside or third-generation cephalosporin should be instituted immediately and then modified according to culture results. Adequate antibiotic concentrations are achieved in the peritoneal fluid parenterally, so that administration of intraperitoneal antibiotics as well as drainage of ascitic fluid is unnecessary.

■ Variceal Bleeding

■ BACKGROUND

Bleeding esophageal varices is the most serious complication of alcoholic cirrhosis. As many as 30 per cent of patients will not survive their initial bleeding episode, and only about one third of patients are alive at the end of 1 year.[2] Mortality for any given patient is closely linked to the degree of liver failure (Child's classification, Table 2) and the severity of bleeding, regardless of the specific treatment chosen. The Child's class A patient has a three to six times greater chance of surviving 2 years compared with a Child's class C patient.[10]

There are two critical factors in the development of bleeding esophageal varices. The first is portal hypertension, which tends to be higher in variceal bleeders. The second is the expanding size of the varices. According to Laplace's law, wall tension is directly proportional to pressure and radius; therefore, larger varices more commonly bleed. Since only 30 to 50 per cent of patients with varices will experience bleeding, other factors

TABLE 2. Modified Child's Classification

	Class A	Class B	Class C
Bilirubin	<2	2–3	>3
Prothrombin time	≤14	15–17	≥18
Albumin	≥3.5	2.8–3.4	<2.8
Ascites	negligible	mild	moderate-severe
Encephalopathy	negligible	mild	moderate-severe

(Adapted from DiMagno, EP, et al. Influence of hepatic reserve and cause of esophageal varices on survival and rebleeding before and after the introduction of sclerotherapy: a retrospective analysis. Mayo Clin Proc 1985, 60:149.)

must be involved as well. Early endoscopy is the procedure most often used to determine the etiology of upper gastrointestinal bleeding. In alcoholic cirrhotic patients, 40 to 50 per cent of bleeding will be from a source other than varices, such as a Mallory Weiss tear, peptic ulcer, gastric ulcer, or congestive gastropathy. Although emergency endoscopy has not been shown to improve survival, it will help direct appropriate therapy. At the time of endoscopy, only 20 per cent of patients who bled from their varices will be actively bleeding. Another 30 per cent will have stigmata of bleeding, such as cherry red spots, red whale markings, or hematocystic spots. Many patients, therefore, have no obvious source of hematemesis, and it is presumed that they are bleeding from their varices.[11]

■ MANAGEMENT

The management of variceal bleeding is divided into prophylaxis, emergency bleeding, and recurrent bleeding. It seems logical to try to prevent an initial episode of bleeding, which carries a substantial morbidity and mortality, and in two studies prophylactic sclerotherapy decreased the first episode of bleeding and increased survival.[11,12] However, a VA cooperative study has shown increased mortality in patients receiving prophylactic sclerotherapy versus controls.[13] As stated, only 30 to 50 per cent of patients with varices will bleed; therefore, the many complications of sclerotherapy may outweigh the benefits. Preliminary data show that propranolol may be effective for prophylaxis of variceal bleeding by reducing cardiac output and producing splanchnic vasoconstriction, but further studies will need to be performed before it can be recommended.[14,15] Prophylactic portosystemic shunts (PSS) have not been shown to improve survival and are definitely not recommended. Thus, at present there is no proven effective prophylactic treatment for variceal bleeding.

Bleeding varices can be treated in several ways. Intravenous vasopressin (antidiuretic hormone, ADH), given as a bolus of 10 to 15 μ in 100 ml of D5W over 15 minutes, followed by a continuous intravenous drip at 0.1 to 0.5 units/min, works via splanchnic vasoconstriction and esophageal muscular contraction. This has been shown to stop bleeding in 29 to 66 per cent of patients;

however, bleeding stops spontaneously in 33 to 66 per cent of patients, which questions the true value of ADH. Approximately one half of patients will rebleed with frequently ensuing complications, such as hypotension, hyponatremia, myocardial ischemia, and arrhythmias. Some of these complications may be reduced or prevented by simultaneously giving either IV nitroglycerin, 40 to 400 μg/min, or sublingual nitroglycerin, 0.6 mg every 30 minutes. ADH and nitroglycerin have been shown to work synergistically to lower portal pressure. Intravenous somatostatin, which also works via splanchnic vasoconstriction, has been found to be more effective than vasopressin and has a lower rate of complications. Its use is not yet approved for variceal bleeding.[16]

Balloon tamponade is as effective as the vasoactive drugs. Bleeding ceases in 50 to 70 per cent of patients, but rebleeding occurs in up to 50 per cent of patients. Balloon tamponade has several serious potential complications, such as aspiration pneumonia or esophageal perforation; these occur in up to 5 per cent of patients. Complications may be prevented by proper placement of the tube, verified by x-ray, and correct insufflation of the balloon, which should be tested prior to placing it into the patient. Several types of balloon tamponade devices are available; all require some expertise for proper use and placement. The Sengstaken-Blakemore tube (SBT) has an esophageal and stomach balloon with a port for stomach aspiration. The Minnesota tube is similar to the SBT but has an additional port for aspirating esophageal contents. A third type, the Linton Nachlas tube, has only a gastric balloon, with ports to aspirate from the stomach and the esophagus. This device is best suited for bleeding gastric varices. Both vasopressin and balloon tamponade provide temporary cessation of bleeding until definitive forms of treatment, such as sclerotherapy or portosystemic shunting (PSS), can be performed.

In four randomized trials,[17] sclerotherapy performed at the time of initial endoscopy was not shown to increase short-term survival (0 to 40 days), but there does appear to be a modest reduction in early rebleeding. The reason for this lack of effectiveness is thought to be due to the long time it takes for complete obliteration of varices. Whereas up to 80 to 90 per cent of patients will stop bleeding during the first sclerotherapy session, 25 to 30 per cent of patients will rebleed within the first 2 weeks. Sclerotherapy is contraindicated in patients who have fulminant bleeding, respiratory distress, or severe agitation.

Complications are divided into minor, moderate, and severe.[18] Minor complications include chest pain, fever, dysphagia, and pleural effusion. These problems are self-limited and usually subside in 48 to 72 hours. Esophageal stricture and ulceration are moderate complications that occur in up to 40 per cent and 50 per cent of patients, respectively. Ulcerations are mostly asymptomatic and are more likely to occur when a large amount of sclerosant is used. Most patients with strictures are symptomatic and can be treated safely and effectively with esophageal dilatation. Severe complications, fortunately, are rare and include esophageal perforation with mediastinitis, constrictive pericarditis, respiratory arrest, and spinal cord paralysis. Sclerotherapy is effective therapy for bleeding varices and, since it can be performed at the time of diagnosis, it is often the first step in controlling variceal bleeding. Three controlled studies show increased long-term survival (1 to 3 years) and a lower rate of rebleeding in the sclerotherapy-treated patients.[17] In all series, recurrence of varices occurs in approximately 60 per cent of patients. Therefore, sclerotherapy usually has to be repeated on a chronic basis. Cello and associates compared emergency sclerotherapy to portacaval shunt (PCS) in 52 Child's class C patients and found equal survival, but less rebleeding and a higher cost, in the PCS patients.[19] Both groups of patients had about a 60 per cent mortality rate in the first month, which relates to the severity of the underlying liver disease and not to the particular treatment.

Emergency portosystemic shunt (PSS) is the most effective way to stop variceal bleeding. Perioperative mortality (within 30 days), however, approaches 40 per cent, and postoperative encephalopathy develops in 20 to 30 per cent of patients. It is best, therefore, to avoid emergency PSS, especially in the Child's class C patient, at least until other methods have been tried. In the emergency setting, nonselective shunts, such as mesocaval and portocaval, should be performed. They are technically less difficult and take less time to perform; there are reports that if the patient survives the postoperative period, late mortality is quite low.[20] Elective PSS has been shown to reduce recurrent bleeding significantly and to improve long-term survival.[1] The best candidates for elective PSS are Child's class A and B patients who have hepatic vein pressure gradients over 12 mm Hg. All patients undergoing PSS should have a Doppler or venogram study to verify patency of the portal vein, superior mesenteric artery, and splenic vein prior to surgery. The distal splenorenal shunt (DSRS), a selective shunt, reduces portal hypertension while maintaining blood flow to the liver. There is a lower incidence of PSE, but the selectivity of the shunt wanes over time as collateral circulation develops. There is no difference in survival between the DSRS and PSS, and in some series rebleeding is more frequent in the DSRS patients.[1] Thus, proper patient selection and the operation that can be best performed by the surgeon are needed for an optimal result (Table 3).

TABLE 3. Treatment of Emergency Variceal Bleeding

	Cessation of Bleeding (%)	Rebleeding (%)	Complications
Vasopressin	29–66	50	25% morbidity, 3% mortality Myocardial ischemia, arrhythmias, hypertension, hyponatremia, ischemic bowel
Balloon Tamponade	40–80	46	15% morbidity, 3% mortality Aspiration, pneumonia, esophageal perforation
Sclerotherapy	80–90	20–30	50% morbidity, 1% mortality Esophageal perforation, respiratory arrest, pericarditis, paralysis, ulceration, stricture, pleural effusion, chest pain, fever, dysphagia
Portosystemic Shunts	>95	<1	40% perioperative mortality 20–30% postoperative encephalopathy

Propranolol at a dose of 40 to 400 mg/day, to decrease resting heart rate by 25 per cent, has been shown to reduce portal pressure in one half of patients. In one study by Lebrec and associates, 74 patients in Child's class A and class B were randomly assigned to propranolol or placebo after initial bleeding from varices had stopped.[14,15] They found a significant reduction in rebleeding and increased survival at 2-year follow-up in the propranolol group. Another study, comparing endoscopic sclerotherapy to propranolol showed no difference in the rate of rebleeding or death.[21] Only one study has looked at sclerotherapy and propranolol versus sclerotherapy alone; no significant difference in survival or rebleeding was found.[22] Larger randomized controlled trials are needed to confirm the usefulness of propranolol, but in certain patients in whom other forms of therapy are either contraindicated or refused, this offers some potential benefit. The drug should not be used in patients with asthma, severe congestive heart failure, or insulin-dependent diabetes.

■ RECOMMENDATIONS

Variceal bleeding is best treated at the time of initial endoscopy by sclerotherapy. This is especially true for Child's class C patients in whom portosystemic shunt surgery would carry a very high mortality rate. Adjunctive therapy may be required, such as vasopressin or balloon tamponade, to help stop the bleeding, but only until either sclerotherapy or surgery can be performed. For the patient with rebleeding, sclerotherapy may be reattempted, but if the bleeding should be uncontrollable, portosystemic shunting is usually the definitive treatment.

■ Hepatic Encephalopathy

■ BACKGROUND

Hepatic or portosystemic encephalopathy (PSE) is a syndrome characterized by alterations in the state of consciousness, neuromuscular function, intellectual function, personality, and behavior. The pathogenesis of the disorder is still unclear, but a number of toxins and metabolic derangements cause reversible cerebral dysfunction in the presence of portal hypertension and cirrhosis.

One toxin, ammonia, has been studied extensively and is found to be elevated in up to 90 per cent of patients. Although the serum level of ammonia does not strongly correlate with the degree of encephalopathy, reducing the level of it is associated with clinical improvement. Glutamine, which can be measured in the cerebrospinal fluid, and which is generated from serum ammonia, does correlate closely with the degree of encephalopathy. A second toxin, fatty acids, produced by gut flora, is increased in PSE, and at high doses will cause reversible coma in experimental animals. With treatment, there is a decline in the serum levels of free fatty acids. A third toxin, mercaptans, also produced in the gut via bacterial metabolism of methionine, accumulates in PSE, and elevated serum levels have been shown to correlate with the degree of PSE. The metabolites of mercaptans contribute to the sweetish odor of fetor hepaticus. It has been shown in animal studies that lesser quantities of these toxic substances are needed to produce PSE when they are given together than when each is given individually.[1]

In addition to toxins, there are several metabolic derangements. Branched-chain amino acids are catabolized in muscle, whereas the normal metabolism of aromatic amino acids in the liver is decreased. This results in an elevated aromatic amino acid–to–branched-chain amino acid ratio in the serum as well as in the brain. The increased aromatic amino acids may contribute to false neurotransmitter production (octopamine) and interfere with normal neurotransmitter function and concentration.[23] Gamma-aminobutyric acid (GABA), a potent inhibitory neurotransmitter, also has been shown to be elevated in the serum and brain of patients with PSE. The elucidation of its role in PSE is derived mainly from experimental animal studies that show a common neuronal receptor for GABA and benzodiazepines. The effects on visual evoked responses are similar for both molecules.[24]

The initial presentation of a patient with portosystemic encephalopathy can be quite variable. For example, a patient with mild encephalopathy (stage I) may present with a change in sleep pattern, decreased attention span, irritability, and tremor, whereas a patient with severe encephalopathy (stage III) may present with confusion or stupor, complete disorientation, bizarre behavior, asterixis, hyperreflexia, and fetor hepaticus. Patients with moderate disease have symptoms in between these extremes (stage II). Alcoholic patients who are comatose (stage IV) must be carefully evaluated to exclude all other causes of coma, such as subdural hematoma, alcohol withdrawal seizures, or drug overdose, before assuming a diagnosis of PSE.

Many precipitating factors contribute to the development of PSE. The more common ones are azotemia (caused by gastrointestinal bleeding, excessive dietary protein, overdiuresis, renal failure, and constipation), analgesics, sedatives, infection, metabolic alkalosis, hyponatremia, hypokalemia, and hypoglycemia.

The diagnosis of hepatic encephalopathy is based on clinical findings alluded to previously and laboratory testing. Although the arterial ammonia level is elevated in up to 90 per cent of patients, it is not pathognomonic for PSE, and levels do not correlate well with the degree of encephalopathy. An ammonia level obtained from a large vein is usually satisfactory and avoids arterial puncture. Electroencephalography may be useful in diagnosing PSE; however, as is the case with ammonia, it is sensitive but not specific. Findings include generalized slowing of cerebral electrical activity and theta waves with progression to delta waves as the comatose state is reached. Psychometric testing is helpful in supporting an early diagnosis of PSE and in following the response to treatment. The numbers connection test as well as standard mental status examinations should be performed daily.[1]

◾ MANAGEMENT

Management of PSE requires supportive care, removal of precipitating factors, diet, and drug therapy. Supportive care includes adquate intravenous hydration, correction of electrolyte and acid-base disorders, and evaluation for infection or trauma. Removal of precipitating factors is imperative. For example, a lethargic alcoholic patient who comes to the hospital with severe upper gastrointestinal bleeding may be hemodynamically unstable and acidotic and may have prerenal azotemia, in addition to the toxins

absorbed via bacterial breakdown of heme in the intestines. In addition to giving supportive care, the bleeding source must be found and controlled, and the patient should receive nasogastric lavage and cathartics to diminish absorption of nitrogenous products. Dietary protein must be limited initially to 40 gm/day or less, depending on the patient's stage of encephalopathy. Special formulations may be used that are rich in branched-chain amino acids and low in aromatic amino acids. Once the patient begins to improve, the protein should be gradually increased to about 60 to 100 gm/day, to allow reparative processes in the liver and reverse the catabolic state.

Lactulose, a nonabsorbable disaccharide, is given orally at a dose of 60 to 150 ml/day in divided doses or via enema made by mixing 300 ml of lactulose with 700 ml of water. The doses are adjusted to achieve two to three soft bowel movements per day. Lactulose is broken down by gut flora into lactic and acetic acid, reducing the luminal pH. This results in an osmotic diarrhea and the conversion of ammonia to ammonium, which does not get readily absorbed.[24,25] Lactulose also may change the bacterial flora to less ammonia-generating species. Side effects include nausea, vomiting, anorexia, cramps, bloating, and diarrhea. Lactulose is the treatment of choice for chronic as well as acutely encephalopathic patients. Patients who are unresponsive to protein restriction and lactulose also may be started on neomycin, a nonabsorbable aminoglycoside, which inhibits urease-producing bacteria. The antibiotic is given at a dose of 4 to 6 gm/day in divided doses or as a 1 per cent enema once or twice a day, if an ileus is present. Since 1 to 3 per cent of the drug gets absorbed, rental toxicity or ototoxicity is a risk. Neomycin may be beneficial when added to lactulose; however, eliminating the bacterial flora may increase the colonic pH, reducing the effectiveness of lactulose, which works best at a pH under 5.

◾ Hepatorenal Syndrome

◾ BACKGROUND

The hepatorenal syndrome (HRS) is a deterioration in renal function without any obvious histopathologic alterations in the kidney. It has been shown that kidneys from patients with HRS will function normally after transplantation into recipients without liver disease. HRS often occurs in alcoholic cirrhotic patients with or without jaundice but virtually always with ascites. It is characterized by oliguric renal failure without proteinuria and normal urinary concentrating abilities. The clinician must be attuned to the fact that HRS, which carries a mortality rate of up to 90 per cent, presents as prerenal failure that may have no precipitating cause. It often presents, however, in the setting of sepsis, hepatic encephalopathy, gastrointestinal bleeding, or overdiuresis. Several of these factors tend to worsen an already decreased effective plasma volume and further compromise renal function.

The pathogenesis of HRS has not been clearly elucidated, yet there is a definite relationship to renal hypoperfusion and renal cortical ischemia. Proposed mechanisms for sustaining renal hypoperfusion have been discussed in the section on the pathogenesis of ascites. Since not all patients with HRS have diminished intravascular volume or renal blood flow, there must be other mechanisms for maintaining renal cortical vasoconstriction and reduced glomerular filtration rate. Present hypotheses include alterations in intrarenal prostaglandin synthesis (decreased PGE_2—a vasodilator, and increased TxA_2—a vasoconstrictor), increased catecholamine and angiotensin activity, chronic endotoxemia, and false neurotransmitters, which may cause renal vasoconstriction in response to peripheral vasodilatation.[26,27]

The diagnosis of HRS is one of exclusion. It is imperative to seek out reversible causes of acute renal failure, which may be prerenal or postobstructive, and to remember that acute tubular necrosis (ATN), which also can occur in the setting of sepsis, gastrointestinal bleeding, overdiuresis, or nephrotoxic drugs, is a far more common diagnosis than HRS. HRS is marked by an output of less than 500 ml of urine per day, a normal urine sediment, a urine sodium of less than 10, and a fractional excretion of sodium of less than 1. In ATN, there are renal tubular epithelial cells and casts, with a urine sodium usually greater than 20 and a fractional excretion of sodium of greater than 1. The major difficulty comes in distinguishing prerenal azotemia from HRS which is often assumed to be prerenal azotemia when the patient responds to either fluid challenge or eliminating diuretics.

■ MANAGEMENT

There is currently no effective treatment for HRS. Supportive care includes identifying and eliminating any precipitating factors alluded to earlier, correcting electrolyte imbalances, treating infection, and avoiding or stopping nephrotoxic drugs or drugs that inhibit prostaglandin synthesis (NSAID, aspirin). Hypovolemia must be excluded by a fluid challenge, using either saline, salt-poor albumin, or fresh-frozen plasma, with central venous pressure monitoring to avoid precipitating variceal bleeding or congestive heart failure. Although a number of different drugs have been tried, including prostaglandins A and E, selective prostaglandin inhibitors, α_1-adrenergic inhibitors, low-dose dopamine, and calcium channel blockers, none have shown a consistent benefit.[28] Dialysis may be useful in patients with acute reversible forms of liver failure, but it will not improve survival in alcoholic cirrhotic patients with progressive liver disease. There are many case reports of reversal of HRS following peritoneovenous shunting. Although in theory it may be useful, a variety of serious complications may result from the shunt procedure, and presently there are no controlled studies to support its routine use. There are a few anecdotal reports in pediatric patients of reversal of HRS following orthotopic liver transplantation. Clearly, this is not an option for the alcoholic cirrhotic patient at this time.

REFERENCES

1. Conn HO, Atterbury CE. Major complications of cirrhosis. In Schiff L, Shiff E. Diseases of the Liver. 6th ed. Philadelphia: JB Lippincott, 1987:807–820.
2. Bender MD, Ockner RK. Ascites. In Sleisenger MH, Fordtran JS. Gastrointestinal Disease. 4th ed. Philadelphia: WB Saunders, 1989:428–447.
3. Rocco VK, Ware AJ. Cirrhotic ascites, pathophysiology, diagnosis and management. Ann Intern Med 1986; 105:573–585.
4. Schrier RW. Pathogenesis of sodium and water retention in high-output and low-output cardiac failure, nephrotic syndrome, cirrhosis, and pregnancy. N Engl J Med 1988; 319:1127–1131.
5. Kandel G, Diamant NE. A clinical view of recent advances in ascites. J Clin Gastroenterol 1986; 8:85–99.
6. Stassen MD, McCullough AJ. Management of ascites. Semin Liver Dis 1985; 5:291–306.

7. Boyer TD, Goldman ID. Treatment of Cirrhotic Ascites; Current Hepatology. Chicago: Year Book Medical Publishers, 1986:359–377.

8. Arroyo V, et al. Management of patients with cirrhosis and ascites. Semin Liver Dis 1986; 6:353–369.

9. Fogel MR. Sawhney K, Neal EA. Diuresis in the ascitic patient: a randomized controlled trial of three regimens. J Clin Gastroenterol 1981; (Suppl 1):73–80.

10. Bernuau J, Rueff B. Treatment of acute variceal bleeding. Gastroenterol Clin North Am 1985; 14:185–207.

11. Paquet KJ. Prophylactic endoscopic sclerosing treatment of esophageal varices; a prospective controlled randomized trial. Endoscopy 1982; 14:4–5.

12. Witzel L, et al. Prophylactic endoscopic sclerotherapy of esophageal varices; a prospective controlled study. Lancet 1985; 1:771–775.

13. Gregory P, et al. Prophylactic sclerotherapy for esophageal varices in alcoholic liver disease: results of a VA cooperative randomized trial. Gastroenterology 1987; 92 (Part 2):1414.

14. Lebrec D, et al. Randomized controlled study of propranolol for prevention of recurrent gastrointestinal bleeding in patients with cirrhosis: a final report. Hepatology 1984; 4:345–350.

15. Lebrec D. The medical prevention of variceal bleeding. Intens Care Med 1988; 97–99.

16. Gorden P. Somatostatin and somatostatin analogue (SMS 201–995) in the treatment of hormone-secreting tumors of the pituitary and gastrointestinal tract and non-neoplastic diseases of the gut; NIH Conference. Ann Intern Med 1989; 110:35–50.

17. Lieberman DA. Sclerotherapy for bleeding esophageal varices after randomized trials. West J Med 1986; 145:481–484.

18. Tabibian N. Sclerotherapy for esophageal varices. Am Fam Physician 1988; 37:147–152.

19. Cello JP, Grendel JH, Crass RA, et al. Endoscopic sclerotherapy versus portacaval shunt in patients with severe cirrhosis and variceal hemorrhage. N Engl J Med 1984; 311:1589–1593.

20. Orloff MD, Bell RH. Long-term survival after emergency portocaval shunting from bleeding varices in patients with alcoholic cirrhosis. Am J Surg 1986; 151:176.

21. Dollet JM, et al. Sclerotherapy versus propranolol after variceal hemorrhage in cirrhosis: a long-term controlled trial (abstract). Gastroenterology 1986; 90:1722.

22. Westaby D, et al. Selective and nonselective beta-receptor blockage in the reduction of portal pressure in patients with cirrhosis and portal hypertension. Gut 1984; 25:121.

23. Alexander WR, et al. The usefulness of branched chain amino acids in patients with acute or chronic hepatic encephalopathy. Am J Gastroenterology 1989; 84:91–96.

24. Fraser CL, Arieff AI. Hepatic encephalopathy. N Engl J Med 1985; 313:865–873.

25. MacMath TL, Pons PT. Hepatic encephalopathy. J Emerg Med 1985; 3:401–407.

26. Davidson E, Dunn MJ. Pathogenesis of the hepatorenal syndrome. Annu Rev Med 1987; 38:361–372.

27. Larsen HR, Henriksen JH. Pathogenesis of ascites formation and hepatorenal syndrome: humoral and hemodynamic factors. Semin Liver Dis 1986; 6:341–352.

28. Levy M. Pathophysiology of the hepatorenal syndrome and potential for therapy. Am J Cardiol 1987; 60:661–721.

Cluster headache

Robert B. Taylor

Cluster headache (also called Horton's headache or syndrome, histamine headache, migrainous neuralgia, and sphenopalatine ganglion neuralgia) is an uncommonly occurring type of headache that most often strikes men in the 20- to 45-year age group. The disease is called cluster headache because of episodes occurring in aggregates with prolonged pain-free intervals between clusters. Cluster headache is a difficult medical management problem because of the intense pain of the headache, the failure of most prophylactic regimens to prevent cephalgia, the lack of reliable abortive therapy, and the difficulty in evaluating the results of therapeutic interventions because of the episodic and relatively short nature of headache symptoms.

■ Background

The patient, who is often a tall man with ruddy complexion, describes a unilateral headache that is localized to the temporal or periorbital area and is markedly severe. The headache begins without warning, increases in intensity to reach a peak within 10 minutes, remains acute for approximately 60 to 90 minutes, and then abates over 10 to 15 minutes to leave no residual pain or neurologic deficit.[1]

In addition to the unilateral headache, the patient may exhibit engorged temporal vessels, unilateral nasal stuffiness, conjunctival injection or lacrimation, facial flushing, or a partial Horner's syndrome. The cluster, often appearing in the spring or fall of the year, lasts for several weeks or months. During this time, a headache occurs every day or two, often awaking the patient at night. When a cluster is present, the patient's headache may be triggered by various ingestants, notably alcohol and particularly red wine. At the end of a cluster of headaches, the recurrences cease, and the patient will be free of painful episodes for a long time, often years.

Eighty per cent of cluster headaches are episodic, and 20 per cent are chronic (no remission for at least 12 months). Chronic cluster headache patients have more frequent attacks and respond less well to prophylactic medication than do patients with the episodic type.

A rare variant, chronic paroxysmal hemicrania, is more common in women patients.[2] These individuals have headaches almost daily, usually lasting 10 to 30 minutes, and may report recurrences six or more times during the 24-hour period. Because therapeutic strategies differ, it is important to differentiate chronic paroxysmal hemicrania from migraine and cluster headache.

The cause of cluster headache, the reason for its episodic occurrence, and why it occurs chiefly in men are not well understood. Cluster headache is generally classified as a variant of migraine.[1] Its cyclic nature suggests a relationship to the circadian secretion of cortisol,[3] and baseline cortisol levels seem to be higher in cluster headache patients than in control subjects.[4] Another theory holds that cluster headache pain is related to activated parasympathetic and sensory nerve fibers in the sphenopalatine ganglion area and to the vasodilation of surrounding vessels in the pterygopalatine fossa.[5] Cluster headache onset after head trauma has been reported, suggesting that nerve injury may play a role.[6] A causal relationship with cigarette smoking has been postulated.[7]

The diverse etiologies postulated become important when considering the variety of therapeutic options available.

■ Management

The goals of therapy are pain relief and prevention of headaches during a cluster. No therapy is indicated between clusters.

■ EPISODIC THERAPY

Episodic therapy of cluster headache includes both vasoactive and analgesic medication; specific drugs, routes of administration, and common dosage recommendations are listed in Table 1.

The drugs most often used in attempted abortive therapy are the ergot alkaloids.[8] Although these drugs can be taken orally, sublingually, rectally, parenterally, or by inhalation, rapid absorption is important, and hence sublingual ergot tablets are generally the most useful preparations. For some patients, the physician may recommend an ergotamine aerosol inhaler or intramuscular self-administration of dihydroergotamine (D.H.E. 45) at the onset of headache. Ergotamine may be taken as a bedtime dose to prevent headaches beginning 1 to 2 hours after retiring. Overuse should be avoided, and the patient is generally limited to three sublingual ergot tablets in a 24-hour period, although the cluster nature of the headache is generally sufficient to prevent long-term overuse problems. Ergot preparations will be very useful for a few patients, but most cluster headache patients do not achieve satisfactory relief, and other therapeutic options must be tried.

Oxygen is a nonspecific cerebral vasoconstrictor that may abort cluster headaches.[9,10] Although sometimes cumbersome to have on hand when needed, oxygen is safe and relatively inexpensive. Approximately 75 per cent of patients will respond favorably to oxygen therapy.[2]

Sympathomimetic agents are useful for some patients. Midrin is a combination medication that combines a sympathomimetic drug with a sedative and a mild analgesic. An occasional patient will benefit from the use of an epinephrine aerosol preparation. As with all aborting medications, these products must be taken at the very first hint of headache pain.

Analgesic anti-inflammatory drugs may be used to relieve pain. Aspirin and other simple, non-narcotic analgesics can be prescribed safely. The use of narcotic analgesics is a problem in these patients, in whom the risk of habituation must be balanced against use of oral medications for a pain of 60 to 90 minutes' duration.

Other measures used to treat acute headaches include the local application of ice packs and the avoidance of bright light and loud noise. An uncommonly used treatment involves topical anesthesia of the sphenopalatine ganglion using 1 ml of a 4 per cent lidocaine solution or two to three drops of a 10 per cent cocaine solution.[11] The patient applies the solution while lying in a supine position with the head extended 30 degrees below the horizontal and turned toward the side of the headache.

TABLE 1. Episodic Therapy for Cluster Headache

Medication	*Dose*
Ergot Alkaloids	
Ergotamine tartrate, 2 mg, tablets (Ergomar, Ergostat)	One tablet sublingually at onset of attack, repeated at half-hourly intervals if needed, up to 3 tablets in 24 hr
Ergotamine tartrate, 0.36 mg per inhaled dose (Medihaler Ergotamine Aerosol)	One inhalation at onset of attack, repeated every 5 minutes, up to six inhalations in 24 hr
Dihydroergotamine, 1 mg/ml, ampules (D.H.E. 45)	Dose of 1 mg intramuscularly at onset of attack, repeated in 1 hour if needed
Oxygen	
Oxygen at 7 liters/min	Inhale using rebreathing bag, beginning at onset of attack
Sympathomimetic Agents	
Isometheptene, 65 mg, dichloralphenazone, 100 mg, and acetaminophen, 325 mg, capsules (Midrin)	One or two capsules orally at onset of attack
Epinephrine bitartrate, aerosol delivering 0.16 mg of epinephrine base per dose (Medihaler-Epi)*	One inhalation dose at onset of attack, may be repeated after 5 minutes
Analgesic Anti-Inflammatory Drugs	
Aspirin or acetaminophen	600 mg taken orally at the onset of pain
Ibuprofen (Nuprin, Motrin)*	400 to 800 mg taken orally at the onset of pain

*These drugs do not have FDA approval for use in vascular headaches.

TABLE 2. Ingestants to Be Avoided by Cluster Headache Patients

Alcohol, especially red wine
Aged cheese
Chocolate
Bacon, bologna, frankfurters, and other foods containing nitrites
Oriental and other foods containing MSG

■ PROPHYLACTIC THERAPY

Most patients will require prophylactic management. As an initial step, the patient should be advised to stop smoking and avoid all alcoholic beverages, as well as foods containing tyramine, phenylethylamine, nitrites, and monosodium L-glutamate (MSG). (See Table 2.)

Table 3 lists drugs used for prophylactic therapy of cluster headache.

Ergot derivatives, notably methysergide, represent a very appropriate first choice in the therapy of cluster headaches, especially in patients under age 30 years. Although methysergide use should not exceed 6 months, this prohibition is not a problem in the usual cluster headache patient who can discontinue the medication when the cluster disappears after 6 to 12 weeks, thus avoiding the fibrosis that can occur with long-term methysergide use. The drug is contraindicated in patients with arteriosclerotic vascular disease or coronary heart disease. Paresthesias, leg pain, and gastrointestinal symptoms are common side effects.

Lithium has been used to manage both episodic and chronic cluster headaches;[2,12,13] its greatest effectiveness has been reported in chronic headaches. It is especially useful in patients over age 45 years. About half of patients using the drug will report improvement.[2] The physician must monitor for toxic symptoms, such as vomiting, diarrhea, ataxia, tremor, or drowsiness, which may occur even at therapeutic serum levels. Rebound may occur when lithium is discontinued.[13]

Corticosteroids are often prescribed, especially for methysergide-refractory individuals. Corticosteroids frequently will stop a cluster of headaches, but may also "stop the clock";[14] that is, when the steroid medication is discontinued, the headaches recur and resume their previous course. The recommended course is generally about 3 weeks. Daroff and Whitney recommend use of corticosteroids for cluster headache patients in two circumstances: (1) to provide headache-free days when a special activity must be accomplished, and (2) to serve as a bridge until another prescribed medication, such as methysergide, becomes active.[14] The usual corticosteroid-related contraindications (e.g., gastrointestinal bleeding, current infection) and concerns (e.g., fluid retention, elevated blood glucose, suppressed immunity) must be observed.

Indomethacin (Indocin) is the drug of choice in chronic paroxysmal hemicrania and may also be useful in episodic cluster headache.[12] Nonsteroidal anti-inflammatory

TABLE 3. Prophylactic Therapy for Cluster Headache

Medication	*Dose*
Ergot Derivatives	
Methysergide (Sansert), 2-mg tablets	One tablet taken three to four times daily PO
Lithium*	
Lithium carbonate (Lithane), 300-mg tablets	900 mg daily PO; monitor blood levels to maintain range of 0.6–1.2 mEq/L
Corticosteroids*	
Prednisone	5 mg four to six times daily PO
Nonsteroidal Anti-Inflammatory Drugs*	
Indomethacin (Indocin)	25–50 mg taken three times daily PO
Beta-Adrenergic Blockers	
Propranolol (Inderal)	30–320 mg daily in divided doses PO
Calcium channel blockers*	
Diltiazem (Cardizem)	30–60 mg four times daily PO
Verapamil (Calan, Isoptin)	80–120 mg three times daily PO
Nifedipine (Procardia)	10–20 mg three times daily PO

*These drugs do not have FDA approval for use in the treatment of vascular headache.

drugs can cause abdominal distress, gastro-intestinal bleeding, and renal damage.

Beta-blockers such as propranolol, nal-dolol, or metoprolol may be prescribed, but generally they are less effective in cluster headache prophylaxis than in preventing classic migraine headaches.[14] Their use may be limited by patients' complaints of lassi-tude, depression, or insomnia.

There are increasing reports of the effi-cacy of calcium entry blockers in treating cluster headache. These drugs provide a highly selective calcium entry blockade of cephalic smooth muscle receptors. Meyer and colleagues report greatest success with nimodipine, with less therapeutic efficacy reported for verapamil and nifedipine.[15]

A number of other modalities may be helpful. Biofeedback, particularly the tem-perature-sensitive method, may be useful in some patients. Antihistamine/antiseroto-nin drugs such as cyproheptadine (Periactin) have proved useful in migraine prophylaxis and may be worth a trial in cluster head-ache; the usual adult dose is a 4-mg tablet taken three or four times daily. Other indi-viduals might gain relief from a trial on a tri-cyclic antidepressant such as amitriptyline (Elavil), 30 to 75 mg taken daily in a single bedtime dose; tricyclic antidepressants ap-pear to have a beneficial effect in vascular headaches that is independent of their anti-depressant action. Kuritzky and colleagues have advocated the use of sodium valproate to affect the circadian rhythms by increasing the central nervous system action of the in-hibitory transmitter gamma-aminobutyric acid (GABA).[16] One study reported benefi-cial results with cyproterone, a synthetic steroid with antiandrogenic action.[17] For pa-tients in whom drug therapy is unsuccessful or untolerated, the use of transcutaneous electrical nerve stimulation (TENS) may be helpful.

Some patients with chronic cluster head-ache have been treated surgically.[18-20] A ra-diofrequency procedure involving the tri-geminal nerve is most commonly used, and more than 50 per cent of patients report sat-isfactory-to-excellent results.[18] Retrogasser-ian glycerol injection has been used to treat chronic cluster headaches.[21] Watson and colleagues have concluded that no single procedure gives consistent long-lasting re-lief; patients should have a full trial of med-ical therapy before being considered for surgery; a radiofrequency or avulsion procedure is a reasonable first choice; and both the V root sections and petrosal neu-rectomy appear to be useful as second-stage procedures.[19] Apparently, achievement of a long-term pain-free state requires total an-algesia of the first and second divisions of the trigeminal nerve and dense or complete corneal numbness, although achievement of these goals does not guarantee a headache-free state.[18]

■ Issues and Risks

Because abortive therapy and prophylactic therapy often prove unsuccessful and oral medicines are too slow and not potent enough to provide effective analgesia, the management of patients with cluster head-aches is frustrating. The patient experienc-ing recurrent pain may demand increasingly potent analgesics or begin to visit hospital emergency rooms during headache epi-sodes. The result may be analgesic abuse and drug-seeking behavior. The best pro-phylaxis against analgesic habituation is an early contract between patient and physi-cian stating that one provider will direct all medication changes, and that emergency room visits will be avoided except in ex-treme emergencies.

Emotional support of the patient is an im-portant part of management. The physician must be willing to listen attentively to the patient's description of agonizing pain, which often seems belied by the healthy-ap-pearing young adult giving the history. It is important to discuss stressors in the pa-tient's life. Because these persons are often high achievers, the physician may give per-mission for them to lower their productivity goals. The physician must be willing to see the patient when needed, which may call for weekly visits during cluster episodes. During these times, the physician must be willing to try various medication combina-tions, offer continuing support, and reassure the patient that a wide variety of options are available and that, eventually, episodic clus-ter headache will run its course.

References

1. Taylor RB. Headache, acute. *In* Taylor RB (ed). Difficult Diagnosis. Philadelphia: WB Saunders, 1985:208–217.

2. Kudrow L. Cluster headache: diagnosis, management, and treatment. *In* Dalessio DJ (ed). Wolff's Headache and Other Head Pain. 5th ed. New York: Oxford University Press, 1987:122–130.
3. Waldenlend E, Gustafsson SA, Ekbom K, Wetterberg L. Circadian secretion of cortisol and melatonin in cluster headache during active cluster periods and remission. J Neurol Neurosurg Psychiatry 1987; 50:207–213.
4. Frediani F, Lamperti E, Leone M, Boiardi A, Grazzi L, Bussone G. Cluster headache patients' responses to dexamethasone suppression test. Headache 1988; 28:130–132.
5. Hardebo JE, Elner A. Nerves and vessels in the pterygopalatine fossa and symptoms of cluster headache. Headache 1987; 27:528–532.
6. Reik L. Cluster headache after head injury. Headache 1987; 27:509–510.
7. Sadjadpour K. Cluster headache. *In* Bergen Migraine Symposium, Suppl 1. Norway: Bergen, 1975.
8. Olenick JS, Taylor RB. Emergency evaluation and treatment of headache. Primary Care 1986; 13(1):97–107.
9. Eversole LR, Stone CE. Vasogenic facial pain (cluster headache). Int J Oral Maxillofac Surg 1987; 16:25–35.
10. Fogan L. Treatment of cluster headache. A double blind comparison of oxygen vs. air inhalation. Arch Neurol 1985; 42:362–363.
11. Kittrelle JP, Grouse DS, Seybold ME. Cluster headache: local anesthetic and abortive agents. Arch Neurol 1985; 42:496–498.
12. Geaney DP. Indomethacin-responsive episodic cluster headache. J Neurol Neurosurg Psychiatry 1983; 46:860–861.
13. Ekbom K. Lithium for cluster headache: review of the literature and preliminary results of long-term treatment. Headache 1981; 21:132–139.
14. Daroff RB, Whitney CM. Treatment of vascular headaches. Headache 1986; 26:470–472.
15. Meyer JS, Nance M, Walker M, Zetusky WJ, Dowell RE. Migraine and cluster headache treatment with calcium antagonists supports a vascular pathogenesis. Headache 1985; 25:358–367.
16. Kuritzky A, Hering R. The treatment of cluster headache with sodium valproate. Headache 1987; 27:301.
17. Sicuteri F. Antiandrogenic medication of cluster headache. Int J Clin Pharmacol Res 1988; 8:21–24.
18. Onofrio B, Campbell K. Surgical treatment of chronic cluster headache. Mayo Clin Proc 1986; 61:537–544.
19. Watson CP, Morley TP, Richardson JC, Schutz H, Tasker RR. The surgical treatment of chronic cluster headache. Headache 1983; 23:289–295.
20. Watson CPN, Evans RJ. Chronic cluster headache: a review of 60 patients. Headache 1987; 27:158–165.
21. Ekbom K, Lindgren L, Nilsson BYU, Hardebo JE, Waldenlend E. Retro-gasserian glycerol injection in the treatment of chronic cluster headache. Cephalgia 1987; 7:1–7.

Congestive heart failure

Peter J. Boosalis ■ *Thomas H. Johnson* ■ *Gary S. Francis*

Congestive heart failure, although relatively easy to diagnose, defies simple definition. It is not a disease but a constellation of physical signs and symptoms that reflects the heart's inability to provide a cardiac output commensurate with the metabolic requirements of the body. The incidence of this often refractory syndrome is very high and increasing. Fortunately, a number of proven therapeutic regimens have emerged during the past decade.

■ Background

The number of hospital discharges for congestive heart failure nearly tripled between 1970 and 1982, from 570,000 to 1,557,000, based upon estimates from the National Center for Health Care Statistics.[1] Furthermore, it is estimated that 2.3 million Americans suffer from congestive heart failure, with about 400,000 new cases being diagnosed annually.[2] The incidence of congestive heart failure increases dramatically with age, approximately doubling for each successive 10-year age span between the ages of 45 and 74.[3] A plausible explanation for the increase in the prevalence of congestive heart failure is that more persons are surviving myocardial infarction and living longer with coronary insufficiency and hypertension. Unfortunately, congestive heart failure, which is frequently the final clinical expression of these problems, has a poor prognosis, with only 50 per cent of patients surviving 5 years after the onset of symptoms, depite modern therapy.[4] The enormous increase in cases and the high morbidity and mortality of heart failure may be contributing substantially to the escalating cost of cardiovascular disease in the United States[5] (Figure 1).

Although the prognosis for congestive heart failure is grim, recent studies indicate that it can be improved by therapy.[6-8] Before specific treatment can be selected, however, clinicians must determine the etiology of the patient's heart failure. A history, physical examination, chest radiograph, electrocardiogram, and echocardiogram are frequently essential to this determination. Cardiac catheterization is sometimes necessary. The selection of therapy also depends on each patient's degree of disability. Exercise testing and a careful history can help establish a patient's level of disability.

Congestive heart failure has many causes (Table 1). The primary or precipitating causes of heart failure often can be successfully treated before chronic congestive heart failure develops, thus improving the prognosis for patients treated. For instance, acute congestive heart failure from valvular disease may be corrected by surgery or valvuloplasty before the heart muscle is damaged. Heart failure associated with hypertension may be prevented with drug therapy. Often heart failure manifests only when precipitating factors are added to pre-existing primary lesions, thereby placing an additional load on a myocardium that has reduced functional reserve. For example, tachyarrhythmias may precipitate congestive heart failure in patients with underlying yet fully compensated heart disease. If underlying causes cannot be found or if those existing cannot be resolved, an attempt must be made to control the congestive heart failure state.

Clinical symptoms of congestive heart failure may be due to diastolic as well as systolic dysfunction. In systolic, or "classic" heart failure, an impaired inotropic state leads to weakened systolic contraction, cardiac dilatation, a reduced ejection fraction, and the clinical symptoms that define congestive heart failure, such as fatigue and breathlessness. In diastolic heart failure, an impaired relaxation of the ventricle leads to an elevation of ventricular end-diastolic pressure, resulting in breathlessness. Patients with diastolic heart failure may have normal systolic function, as determined by

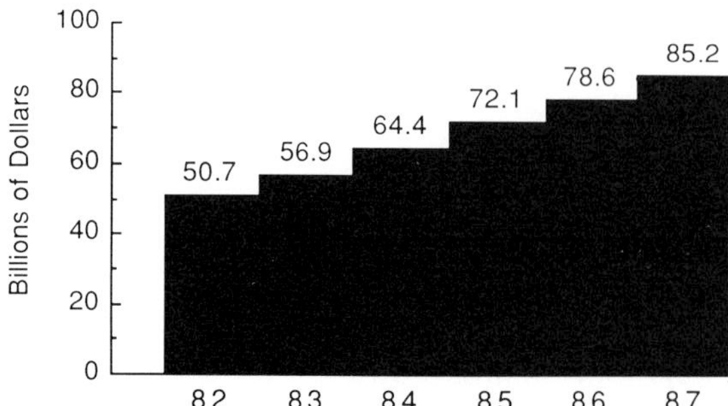

Figure 1. The cost of drugs, hospital care, outpatient care, and lost employee output, attributable to cardiovascular disease in the United States, escalated from 50.7 billion dollars in 1982 to 85.2 billion dollars in 1987.

echocardiography or radionuclide scanning techniques. Although it is generally agreed that diastolic dysfunction is a common cause of congestive heart failure, no such consensus exists as to its treatment. Therefore, discussion will focus on classic congestive heart failure for which drug regimens that prolong and improve life have been established.

■ THE PATHOGENESIS OF "CLASSIC" CONGESTIVE HEART FAILURE—A WORKING HYPOTHESIS

Classic congestive heart failure can occur as a consequence of virtually any form of heart disease and evolves from a reduction in myocardial performance. Pumping functions may be maintained initially by compensatory mechanisms that enhance myocardial performance. However, these mechanisms increase end-diastolic volume (preload) and resistance to ventricular emptying (afterload). An increasing preload leads ultimately to pulmonary and circulatory congestion, whereas a rising afterload eventually results in heightened cardiac wall tension and reduced pump performance. The endocrine and autonomic nervous systems are programmed to respond to a decrease in effective circulating volume. These systems cannot distinguish among shock, exercise, or heart failure. Increased levels of norepinephrine, renin, angiotensin II, aldosterone, and arginine vasopressin cumulatively stimulate excessive vasoconstriction while promoting sodium and water retention. The resulting additional increases in afterload and preload impair myocardial performance and thus further stimulate the secondary compensatory mechanisms that sustain the vortical course of congestive heart failure (Figure 2).

Drug regimens may stem the impelling force of these mechanisms. Optimal results depend upon the appropriate use of these drug regimens. Therapeutic strategies are based upon an understanding of the interaction between the pathophysiology of classic congestive heart failure and the pharmacology of the drugs proved effective in its treatment.

TABLE 1. Etiology of Congestive Heart Failure

Common Primary Causes of Congestive Heart Failure
Coronary artery disease with destruction of contractile muscle tissue
Systemic hypertension
Idiopathic dilated cardiomyopathy
Valvular heart disease
Diabetes mellitus
Chronic alcoholism

Common Precipitating Causes of Congestive Heart Failure
Pulmonary embolism
Dietary, environmental, and emotional changes
Myocardial infarction
Arrhythmias
Thyrotoxicosis and pregnancy (rare)
Anemia (rare)
Infection
Systemic hypertension

■ Management

■ CHRONIC CONGESTIVE HEART FAILURE—THERAPY

Although there is no specific formula for the treatment of chronic congestive heart failure, evidence supports an approach anchored on the simultaneous use of diuretics, vasodilators, and, for selected patients, digitalis (Table 2). Other oral inotropic agents and beta-adrenergic blocking drugs are considered experimental therapies.

Diuretics

Patients with congestive heart failure who exhibit signs and symptoms of fluid overload (e.g., edema, jugular venous distention, pul-

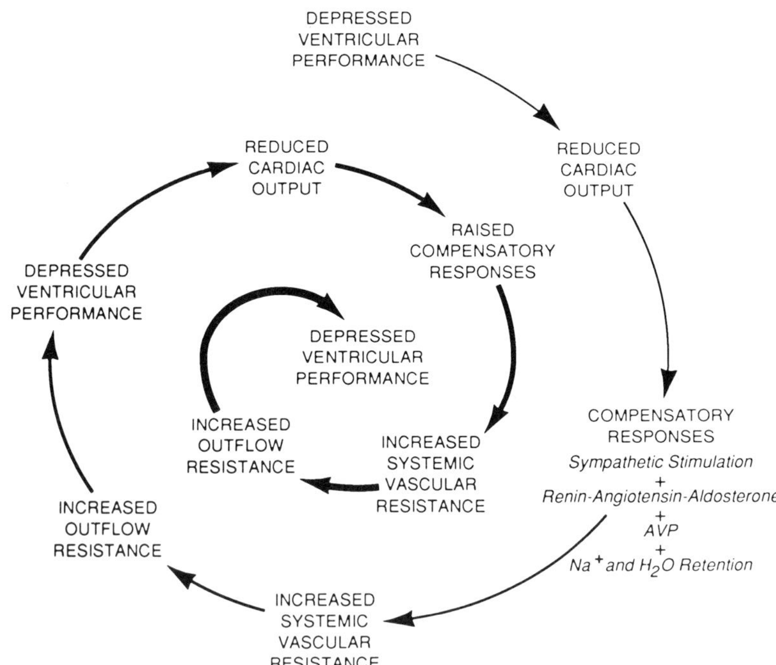

Figure 2. Congestive heart failure. A significant cardiac lesion will result eventually in decreased forward flow. Reduced forward flow leads to the activation of neuroendocrine mechanisms that are intended to be compensatory. However, in the long-term these mechanisms are maladaptive; they result in increased impedance to left ventricular ejection, as well as in sodium and water retention. These mechanisms thereby further impair myocardial performance and sustain the vortex-like course of congestive heart failure.

monary vascular congestion) should be placed on a low-sodium diet and treated with a diuretic.

Thiazide diuretics may reduce preload sufficiently in patients with *mild* congestive heart failure. Hydrochlorothiazide (Esidrix, HydroDIURIL, Oretic) is effective at an oral dose of 25 to 100 mg per day; however, the range of effective oral dose varies greatly depending on the thiazide. The thiazide diuretics act on the distal convoluted tubule of the kidney to cause a maximal increase in sodium excretion of approximately 8 per cent of the filtered load. They also increase potassium excretion. Because thiazide diuretics act directly on the renal vasculature

TABLE 2. Treatment of Chronic Congestive Heart Failure

Generic Name	Trade Name	Starting Dose	Usual Maintenance Dose Range	Limiting Factors	Comments
Digoxin	Lanoxin		0.125–0.375 mg/day	toxicity	Still debate about its usefulness
Furosemide	Lasix	40 mg/day	40–100 mg/day	hypokalemia	
Metolazone	Zaroxolyn	2.5 mg/day		dehydration, hypokalemia	Should be used as an intermittent supplement
Hydralazine	Apresoline	25–75 mg QID	300–400 mg per day	lupoid syndrome, hypotension, nausea and vomiting, edema	Dose is highly variable
Isosorbide dinitrate	Isordil, Sorbitrate	10–20 mg TID	10–60 mg TID	headache, hypotension	Headaches usually respond to Tylenol
Captopril	Capoten	6.25 mg TID	6.25–50 mg TID	hypotension, cough, rash, hyperkalemia	Renal function and K+ should be monitored
Enalapril	Vasotec	2.5 mg BID	2.5–10 mg BID	hypotension, cough, rash, hyperkalemia	Renal function and K+ should be monitored

to reduce gomerular filtration, they should not be used to treat patients with moderate-to-severe renal insufficiency (glomerular filtration rate below 30 ml/min). Therefore, thiazide diuretics have no role in the treatment of patients with advanced heart failure.

Potassium-sparing diuretics, such as spironolactone (Aldactone), triamterene (Dyrenium), and amiloride hydrochloride (Midamor), which act on the distal tubule, can potentiate the somewhat limited action of the thiazide diuretics while generally decreasing the potassium loss. This approach may be made easier by the use of fixed-dose combination tablets consisting of hydrochlorothiazide and either spironolactone (Aldactazide), triamterene (Dyazide, Maxzide), or amiloride (Moduretic).

Metolazone (Zaroxolyn), a quinethazone derivative, has a site of action and diuretic efficacy similar to those of the thiazides but, at the normal dose of 2.5 to 5 mg per day does not reduce renal blood flow or the glomerular filtration rate. Therefore, metolazone is effective even in patients with severe heart failure and markedly reduced renal glomerular filtration. Metolazone has a long duration of action (24 to 48 hours) and also may be a useful adjunct to a loop diuretic for reducing refractory edema in patients with more severe heart failure. Volume depletion may be avoided by the intermittent, rather than fixed and constant, use of supplemental metolazone. Therefore, it is appropriate for patients to add a predetermined dose of metolazone when they gain weight or feel edematous, and to discontinue the dose when they stabilize at their control weight.

Loop diuretics, which are capable of increasing the fractional sodium excretion to more than 20 per cent of the filtered load, are usually required for the treatment of more advanced heart failure. Furosemide (Lasix) and ethacrynic acid (Edecrin) enhance the excretion of sodium and water by inhibiting chloride transport in the thick ascending limb of the loop of Henle. These powerful diuretics may increase renal blood flow and, if so, shunt blood from the medulla to the cortex of the kidney. Loop diuretics tend to promote hypokalemia and, as with the thiazides, supplemental potassium (20 to 40 mEq per day) is often a necessary adjunct to diuretic therapy. Furosemide is prescribed more often than is ethacrynic acid. The prescribed dose of loop diuretic should

be incrementally increased until the signs and symptoms of vascular overload are eliminated. Determining the minimum effective dosage in this manner will reduce the effects of overtreatment (hypokalemia and volume depletion). A combination of diuretics may be needed for the treatment of heart failure patients whose vascular congestion is particularly refractory. For example, the addition of intermittent doses of a supplemental diuretic (metolazone) to a fixed dosage of loop diuretic may eliminate resistant sodium and water retention.

Patients with truly refractory edema and hypokalemia should have a "spot urine" measured for K^+/Na^+. If the ratio is greater than 1, secondary hyperaldosteronism is likely present. Amiloride, added to a loop diuretic at a dose of 5 or more milligrams per day, usually will counteract the influence of the hyperaldosteronism and frequently will help initiate a needed diuresis.

Vasodilators

The Vasodilator Heart Failure Trial (V-HeFT) was the first study to show that the natural course of heart failure can be altered by a specific vasodilator regimen. This trial demonstrated that a combination of isosorbide dinitrate (Isordil, Sorbitrate) plus hydralazine (Apresoline) substantially improved survival for class II and class III heart failure patients.[6] Furthermore, this combination modestly improved exercise tolerance.[7] More recently, the Cooperative North Scandinavian Enalapril Survival Study (Consensus) demonstrated that survival is improved for class IV patients treated with enalapril (Vasotec).[8] These studies provide the basis for the use of vasodilators with diuretics as the primary treatment for congestive heart failure.

Nitrates, particularly long-acting nitrates like isosorbide dinitrate, have an established role in the treatment of congestive heart failure. Their dominant effect is venodilation; oral nitrates lower right and left filling pressures at rest and during exercise.[9,10] Although nitrates are effective in lowering filling pressure and lack serious side effects, they should not be used as a vasodilator monotherapy for chronic congestive heart failure. There is no evidence that long-acting nitrates by themselves improve survival or exercise tolerance. Furthermore, continuous or frequent dosing may result in resistance to their action. Tolerance to the action of nitrates may be reduced by TID dosing. It is appropriate to combine isosorbide dinitrate (10 to 60 mg TID) with a direct arteriolar dilator (hydralazine) for the treatment of patients with symptomatic heart failure.

Hydralazine, by directly relaxing arteriolar smooth muscle, decreases peripheral vascular resistance and afterload. It markedly improves cardiac output and regional distribution of flow without changing left ventricular filling pressure. Hydralazine is associated with many adverse effects and, when used as monotherapy, does not demonstrate long-term efficacy.[11] The usual dose is 300 to 400 mg per day in divided doses. It is customary to initiate therapy with 75 to 100 mg QID. Although systemic vascular resistance falls, cardiac output usually rises to maintain blood pressure. Systolic blood pressures of 80 to 90 mmHg are not uncommon in severe heart failure and should not dissuade practitioners from using vasodilators.

A combination of hydralazine and isosorbide dinitrate reduces vasoconstriction in systemic arteries and veins. Impedance to left ventricular ejection is reduced, thereby enhancing left ventricular performance while reducing venous congestion. The prescribed doses of hydralazine and isosorbide dinitrate should be incrementally increased until sufficient clinical improvement occurs without side effects. As much as 2 grams of hydralazine per day has been used with success. With rare exception, a fluorescent antinuclear antibody (FANA) test will be positive for patients taking hydralazine in doses exceeding 300 mg per day. However, the drug is normally not discontinued unless clinical side effects develop (e.g., lupoid syndrome).

The angiotensin-converting enzyme (ACE) inhibitors are considered by many the preferred therapy for heart failure. They act to interfere with the secondary compensatory mechanisms that significantly contribute to the pathophysiology of heart failure. The renin-angiotensin-aldosterone and sympathetic nervous systems are activated in response to impaired cardiac function. Renin acts on renin substrate (angiotensinogen) to produce angiotensin I. The angiotensin-coverting enzyme acts on angiotensin I to produce angiotensin II. High levels of angiotensin II directly increase vasoconstriction and plasma aldosterone. Aldosterone

enhances kaliuresis, as well as sodium and water retention. Hypokalemia may result from increased plasma aldosterone. Angiotensin II also facilitates the release of norepinephrine from sympathetic nerve terminals and thus indirectly promotes additional vasoconstriction. Hypokalemia and increased sympathetic nervous system activity may set the stage for the ventricular arrhythmias that often accompany congestive heart failure. ACE inhibitors successfully counteract these detrimental metabolic consequences of heart failure.

Captopril (Capoten) and enalapril (Vasotec) are the only ACE inhibitors currently approved for the treatment of congestive heart failure in the United States. Either drug can be used in combination with or as an alternative to the combination of hydralazine and isosorbide dinitrate. Captopril and enalapril are similar in their basic mechanism of action but vary in their pharmacokinetics and pharmacodynamics. They have similar side effect profiles and efficacy. Captopril is started at a dose of 6.25 mg TID; the dose is gradually increased to 25 to 50 mg TID. Enalapril is started at a dose of 2.5 to 5 mg BID. The dose is gradually increased to a maximum of 10 mg BID. Because enalapril is a pro-drug and must be de-esterified by the liver to its active form, enalaprilat, it has a more gradual onset of action (3 to 4 hours) and a longer duration of action than that of captopril.

Captopril and enalapril are vasodilators, but they do not markedly improve cardiac output or ejection fraction. However, they produce a sustained reduction in left ventricular filling pressure[12–14] and improve exercise tolerance.[15,16] Captopril alleviates the symptom of breathlessness experienced with congestive heart failure.[15] Because captopril and enalapril indirectly inhibit sodium and water retention, they reduce the need for diuretic therapy and increase serum potassium levels. ACE inhibitors may also reduce the occurrence of complex ventricular arrhythmias.

Physicians should monitor their patients carefully while establishing the optimal dosage of ACE inhibitor. Patients who are hyponatremic, hyperkalemic, or hypotensive should be maintained on a lower dosage of ACE inhibitor. When possible, the concomitant use of potassium-sparing diuretics should be avoided, to prevent hyperkalemia. ACE inhibitors are usually well tolerated, but symptomatic hypotension and deterioration in renal function may occur. Hypotension may be avoided by the reduction or discontinuation of diuretics. However, ACE inhibitors probably should not be used to treat patients whose systolic blood pressure is less than 80 mm Hg. Patients with severe congestive heart failure may depend on angiotensin II to maintain intraglomerular pressure.[17] Therefore, severely ill patients with low blood pressure, hyponatremia, and renal insufficiency may exhibit abrupt deterioration in renal function when given ACE inhibitors. ACE inhibitors should be initiated in these marginal patients while they are under observation in the hospital. However, most patients can be successfully initiated on ACE inhibitors without being hospitalized.

In choosing vasodilator therapy, the physician is guided by the existence and nature of renal and vascular disease, as well as additional heart dysfunction, which complicate a patient's congestive heart failure. For example, because isosorbide dinitrate is an antianginal and a venodilating agent, patients with congestive heart failure complicated by angina may benefit more from isosorbide dinitrate than from captopril, enalapril, or hydralazine. Isosorbide dinitrate and hydralazine may be better tolerated than enalapril or captopril by patients with moderate-to-severe renal insufficiency. Enalapril, captopril, and the isosorbide dinitrate–hydralazine combination also can control hypertension. A study comparing hydralazine–isosorbide dinitrate with enalapril in the treatment of patients with heart failure is underway (V-HeFT II).

Diuretic and Vasodilator Regimen

Instituting furosemide with captopril, enalapril, or the combination of isosorbide dinitrate and hydralazine may dramatically relieve the patient's symptoms. However, breathlessness, fatigue, and edema eventually may return. When this occurs, transient increases in furosemide or the addition intermittently of a second type of diuretic (metolazone) may relieve the re-emergent symptoms. If additional diuretic does not adequately relieve symptoms, the vasodilator program not previously instituted should be added to the therapeutic regimen. Because frequent visits are usually required for the adjustment of medication, a close physician-

patient rapport develops. This rapport allows the physician to nurture efforts by the patient to monitor and respond to indications of symptomatic deterioration. For instance, based upon increases in weight or peripheral edema, patients can intermittently self-administer additional diuretic while coincidently increasing their potassium supplementation as they experience a diuresis.

Inotropic Agents

Digitalis (digoxin) is the only oral inotropic agent approved for the treatment of chronic congestive heart failure. Although digoxin is widely used, whether it improves survival in patients with heart failure is not known. In fact, many patients on digitalis probably do not derive enough benefit to offset the associated risk of toxicity. However, patients with more severe heart failure, as evidenced by greater left ventricular dilatation, a more reduced ejection fraction, and a third heart sound, may benefit from the inotropic action of digitalis.[18] It is likely, therefore, that most patients with heart failure will benefit from digitalis. The usual dose of digoxin is 0.25 mg per day. The dose should be reduced for patients with renal insufficiency. It is appropriate to prescribe digitalis, diuretics, and vasodilators (ACE inhibitors or hydralazine–isosorbide dinitrate) for nearly all patients with heart failure.

Beta-Adrenergic Blockers

Although short-term trials do not consistently demonstrate clinical improvement, preliminary studies suggest that as many as 70 per cent of patients with chronic heart failure may benefit from long-term therapy with beta-blocking drugs.[19,20] Sympathetic nervous activity can be detrimental to the failing heart. Norepinephrine may damage the myocardium directly. The benefits of chronic beta-adrenergic blockade are under investigation, and this form of therapy must be considered investigational at this time.

■ ACUTE CONGESTIVE HEART FAILURE (PULMONARY EDEMA)—THERAPY

Acute congestive heart failure is a medical emergency, whether it results from a large myocardial infarction or the decompensation of previously stable chronic congestive heart failure. There is no fundamental distinction between acute and chronic failure despite the difference in clinical presentation. In acute failure, the sudden reduction in cardiac output causes pulmonary edema. Systemic hypotension may also occur. The physical examination will reveal a cyanotic, diaphoretic patient whose breathing is rapid and laborious. The patient will refuse to lie flat and often will be unable to give a history because of respiratory distress. The differential diagnosis should include acute asthma and the exacerbation of chronic obstructive lung disease. Acute heart failure can be distinguished by the evaluation of a chest radiograph, an electrocardiogram, an echocardiogram, and arterial blood gases. Treatment must vary depending upon the mechanisms operative at the time of the patient's presentation (Table 3).

When acute heart failure and accompanying pulmonary and systemic congestion result from a recent lesion, such as an acute myocardial infarction or valve rupture, and blood pressure is adequate (e.g., systolic pressure greater than 90 mm Hg), treatment with low-flow oxygen, intravenous morphine, intravenous furosemide (Lasix), and intravenous nitroprusside (Nipride) should begin immediately. Sublingual nitroglycerin (Nitrostat) is also very useful in treating acute pulmonary edema in its earliest stages.

Low-flow oxygen (50 to 60 per cent), administered with a Venturi mask, should provide the patient with adequate oxygenation. If arterial blood gases indicate inadequate oxygenation, the patient may have to be intubated and mechanically ventilated.

Morphine, in intravenous doses of 2 to 5 mg, should be given every 15 minutes. The total dose should not exceed 15 mg. This drug reduces anxiety and adrenergic stimuli to the arteriolar and venous beds. Morphine also may cause respiratory depression. The respiratory depression may be reversed by naloxone (0.4 mg) given every 2 to 5 minutes for as long as necessary.

Furosemide (40 to 100 mg) should be given intravenously over 2 to 3 minutes to rapidly establish diuresis, reduce circulating volume, and relieve pulmonary edema. If the blood urea nitrogen is elevated, more than 100 mg of furosemide may be required. Oral furosemide is poorly absorbed in acute heart failure. Intravenous furosemide normally results in diuresis within 1 hour in patients who have normal renal function.

The extraordinary effectiveness of nitroprusside in the treatment of acute congestive heart failure and pulmonary edema is probably due to its quick onset, short half-life, and lack of direct effect on the myocardium and sympathetic nervous system. Nitroprusside is a potent smooth muscle dilating agent that has a balanced effect on afterload and preload. Therefore, it lowers

TABLE 3. Treatment of Acute Pulmonary Edema

Generic Name	Trade Name	Route of Administration	Average Dose	Limiting Factors	Comments
Furosemide	Lasix	IV	40–100 mg		Correct hypokalemia
Oxygen		Venturi mask	50–60%	CO_2 narcosis	Monitor blood gases
Morphine SO_4		IV	2–5 mg every 10–15 min	respiratory depression	May reverse respiratory depression with naloxone 0.4 mg every 2–5 min
Nitroprusside	Nipride	IV	15–300 μg/min	hypotension	May be combined with dopamine if BP stable
Nitroglycerin	Nitrostat	SL	1/150 gr	hypotension	May repeat as often as necessary if BP stable
Dopamine	Intropin	IV	3–20 μg/kg/min	tachycardia, arrhythmias	Use for hypotension, combine with nitroprusside if BP stable
Dobutamine	Dobutrex	IV	3–20 μ/kg/min	tachycardia, arrhythmias	Not useful for hypotension
Heparin		SQ	5000 U every 8 hr	bleeding, thrombocytopenia	

impedance to ejection and reduces end-diastolic volume and pressure. Ideally, nitroprusside will improve cardiac output substantially without causing a marked fall in blood pressure.

Nitroprusside should be started at a dose of 10 to 15 μg per minute. The dose should be increased until breathlessness is controlled. Most patients respond to doses of less than 150 μg per minute and rarely is a dose greater than 300 μg per minute required. The infusion should be maintained for 24 to 48 hours. Blood pressure, arterial blood gases, urine output, electrolytes, and renal function must be closely monitored. The dose must be reduced or stopped if the systolic blood pressure falls below 90 mm Hg.

If hypotension develops or is present from the onset, dopamine (3 to 20 μg/kg/min) (rather than dobutamine) should be used to restore perfusion pressure.[21] Once systolic pressure is restored, nitroprusside should be added as previously described. Dopamine is a potent peripheral vasoconstrictor and inotrope. Dobutamine, although an inotropic agent, lacks vasoconstrictor activity and therefore is relatively ineffective in raising blood pressure.

The acute decompensation of congestive heart failure is a common cause of symptomatic pulmonary edema. However, other causes of respiratory distress must be considered before the initiation of therapy. Loop diuretics, nitroprusside, supplemental oxygen, and morphine should be initiated. Because systolic blood pressure normally remains between 100 and 120 mm Hg after the acute decompensation of chronic heart failure, high doses of dopamine normally are not required. However, if systolic blood pressure falls below 90 mm Hg, dopamine should be administered as previously outlined. If blood pressure is normal, the addition of dobutamine and low-dose dopamine to the regimen may result in sustained improvement in the patient's condition. Low-dose dopamine (less than 3 μg/kg/min), by dilating arteries of the kidney, may improve sodium and water excretion in patients refractory to loop diuretics. Dobutamine can be added to nitroprusside to augment cardiac output. It is initially administered at an infusion rate of 2 to 5 μg/kg/min, which is increased every 30 minutes to a maximum rate of 20 μg/kg/min. The normal effective dose is 5 to 10 μg/kg/min. The use of do-

butamine may be limited by tachycardia, arrhythmias, headache, nausea, and tremor.

Patients with unstable heart failure should be hospitalized in the intensive care unit. Hemodynamic monitoring and consultation with a cardiologist are helpful. Such patients should be treated with dobutamine and nitroprusside for 48 to 72 hours and then switched to oral vasodilators. Many such patients demonstrate remarkable improvement.

■ Issues and Risks

Patients with mild congestive heart failure may be managed without hospitalization on a low-sodium diet (two gm or less); furosemide, 20 to 40 mg per day; supplemental potassium chloride (20 to 40 mEq/day); and vasodilators (ACE inhibitors or hydralazine–isosorbide dinitrate). Digitalis is effective in treating mild heart failure but is perhaps of most benefit to patients with advanced cardiomegaly. Calcium channel blockers should be avoided in patients with overt heart failure as they are myocardial depressants and stimulate the release of renin. In general, asymptomatic ventricular arrhythmias in patients with heart failure should not be treated, although this is a controversial topic that is in need of more study. The successful treatment of difficult cases can best be accomplished in a hospital where therapy can be tailored to the specific needs of each patient.

It is not known whether vasodilator therapy benefits patients without symptoms but with left ventricular dysfunction. This issue should be resolved at the conclusion of a large trial comparing enalapril to placebo in the treatment of asymptomatic patients with left ventricular dysfunction (Studies of Left Ventricular Dysfunction [SOLVD]). There is evidence that remodeling of the left ventricle after myocardial infarction leads to unfavorable changes in left ventricular cavity configuration and eventually to ventricular dilation.[22] Vasodilator therapy may reduce afterload and changes in cavity configuration, thereby preventing congestive heart failure. This concept is being studied in a large clinical trial (Survival and Ventricular Enlargement [SAVE]).

The selection of patients for cardiac transplantation is fraught with controversy and the complexities of organ procurement and lifetime immunosuppression. However, patients less than 65 years of age and refractory to intensive medical therapy should be considered for transplantation.

REFERENCES

1. Furberg CD, Yusuf S, Thom T. Potential for altering the natural history of congestive heart failure: need for large clinical trials. Am J Cardiol 1985; 55:45A–47A.
2. Francis GS. Heart failure management: the impact of drug therapy on survival. Am Heart J 1988; 115:699–702.
3. Smith WM. Epidemiology of congestive heart failure. Am J Cardiol 1985; 55:3A–8A.
4. McKee PA, Castelli WP, McNamara PM, Kannel WB. The natural history of congestive heart failure: the Framingham study. N Engl J Med 1971; 285:1441–1446.
5. Data on file with American Heart Association. Dallas, Texas.
6. Cohn JN, Archibald DG, Ziesche S, et al. Effect of vasodilator therapy on mortality in chronic congestive heart failure: results of a Veterans Administration Cooperative Study. N Engl J Med 1986; 314:1547–1552.
7. Cohn JN, Archibald DG, Johnson G. Effects of vasodilator therapy on peak exercise oxygen consumption in heart failure; V-HeFT (abstract). Circulation 1987; 75 (Suppl II):IV-443.
8. CONSENSUS Trial Study Group. Effects of enalapril on mortality in severe congestive heart failure: results of the Cooperative North Scandinavian Enalapril Survival Study (CONSENSUS). N Engl J Med 1987; 316:1429–1435.
9. Franciosa JA, Goldsmith SR, Cohn JN. Contrasting immediate and long-term effects of isosorbide dinitrate on exercise capacity in congestive heart failure. Am J Med 1980; 69:559–566.
10. Leier CV, Huss P, Magorien RD, Unverferth DV. Improved exercise capacity and differing arterial and venous tolerance during chronic isosorbide dinitrate therapy for congestive heart failure. Circulation 1983; 67:817–822.
11. Franciosa JA, Weber KT, Levine TB, et al. Hydralazine in the long-term treatment of chronic heart failure: lack of a difference from placebo. Am Heart J 1982; 104:587–594.
12. Kramer BL, Massie BM, Topic N. Controlled trial of captopril in congestive heart failure: a rest and exercise hemodynamic study. Circulation 1983; 67:807–816.
13. Sharpe DN, Murphy J, Coxon R, Hannan SF. Enalapril in patients with chronic heart failure: a placebo controlled, randomized, double-blind study. Circulation 1984; 70:271–278.
14. Packer M, Medina N, Yushak M, Meller J. Hemodynamic patterns of response during long-term captopril therapy for severe chronic therapy. Circulation 1983; 68:803–812.
15. Captopril Multicenter Research Group. A placebo-controlled trial of captopril in refractory congestive heart failure. J Am Coll Cardiol 1983; 2:755–763.
16. Franciosa JA, Wilen MM, Jordan RA. Effects of enalapril, a new angiotensin-converting enzyme inhibitor, in a controlled trial in heart failure. J Am Coll Cardiol 1985; 5:101–107.
17. Packer M, Lee WH, Kessler PD. Preservation of glomerular filtration rate in human heart failure by activation of the renin-angiotensin system. Circulation 1986; 74:766–774.
18. Lee DCS, Johnson RA, Bingham JB, et al. Heart failure in outpatients: a randomized trial of digoxin versus placebo. N Engl J Med 1982; 306:699–705.
19. Engelmeier RS, O'Connell JB, Walsh R, Rad N, Scanlon PJ, Gunnar RM. Improvement in symptoms and exercise tolerance by metoprolol in patients with dilated cardiomyopathy: a double-blind, randomized, placebo-controlled trial. Circulation 1985; 72:536–546.
20. Swedberg K, Waagstein F, Hjalmarson A, Wallentin I. Prolongation of survival in congestive cardiomyopathy by beta receptor blockade. Lancet 1979; 1:1374–1376.
21. Francis GS, Sharma B, Hodges M. Comparative hemodynamic effects of dopamine and dobutamine in patients with acute cardiogenic circulatory collapse. Am Heart J 1982; 103:995–1000.
22. Pfeffer MA, Lamas GA, Vaughan DE, Parisi AF, Braunwald E. Effect of captopril on progressive ventricular dilatation after anterior myocardial infarction. N Engl J Med 1988; 319:80–86.

Coronary artery disease in the surgical patient

Harold G. Olson ■ *Oddvar A. Myhre*

Despite recent major advances in diagnosis and therapy, coronary artery disease continues to be the major cause of death in the United States. The disease begins in childhood and usually becomes clinically manifest in middle and late life, a time when the patient is likely to undergo a surgical procedure. Coronary artery disease in the surgical patient is a difficult medical problem, because it increases the risk of the surgical procedure and complicates the management of the perioperative period. With present-day techniques of perioperative monitoring, the risk of operation can be greatly decreased even in patients who have had recent myocardial infarction, provided these patients are recognized as being at greater risk.

mechanism of perioperative myocardial infarction is multifactorial, requiring the presence of coronary artery disease plus the rapidly changing internal environment during and following surgery. It is possible that manipulation of perioperative factors may be critical in promoting a favorable outcome in the coronary artery disease patient undergoing surgery. These factors include preoperative, intraoperative, and postoperative ischemia and hypotension; the effect of anesthesia on the circulation; pulmonary complications; fluid and electrolyte shifts; and the effects of the perioperative period on catecholamines, platelets, and other thrombotic factors.

■ Background

The presence of coronary artery disease increases the risk of perioperative myocardial infarction. Moreover, it is estimated that the coronary patient with a prior myocardial infarction has a ten- to fiftyfold increased risk of another myocardial infarction following a surgical procedure and anesthesia. The mortality rate of a perioperative infarction is high, ranging from 30 to 60 per cent.[1,2] A large study from the Mayo Clinic, involving over 30,000 patients older than 30 years of age who underwent general anesthesia and surgery, showed that the incidence of perioperative myocardial infarction was 6.6 per cent in patients with a history of prior myocardial infarction, compared with a perioperative infarction rate of 0.13 per cent in patients without prior infarction.[2]

It is of interest that 70 per cent of perioperative myocardial infarctions occur during the first week after the surgical procedure, with the peak incidence on the third postoperative day. This indicates that the

■ Management

■ PREOPERATIVE RISK ASSESSMENT

The primary physician is frequently consulted regarding the risk of surgery for a patient with known coronary artery disease. The physician must assess the risk-benefit ratio of the surgical procedure. The surgical risk for the coronary artery disease patient can be defined by the nature of the surgical procedure performed, the clinical stability of the patient's disease, the status of ventricular function, the extent of coronary atherosclerosis, the sophistication of the anesthesiologist, and postoperative nursing care.

■ NATURE OF THE SURGICAL PROCEDURE

It is noteworthy that emergency surgery in the coronary artery disease patient results in a much higher mortality rate than if the same surgery is performed on an elective basis. Studies indicate that there is a two- to fourfold increased risk of death for emergency versus elective surgery in the coronary artery disease patient.[4] Accordingly, elective surgery should be planned to avoid the increased risk that is apparent if the same surgery has to be performed on an emergency basis. It is obvious that if the patient needs an emergency surgical procedure, such as abdominal surgery for a ruptured viscus, the patient must be referred for surgery and the increased risk accepted.

In general, intracavitary surgery, involving the abdomen or thorax, and especially surgery on the great vessels are associated with increased risk for the patient with coronary artery disease.[4,5] On the other hand, ophthalmic operations, noncardiac operations after successful coronary artery bypass grafting, and other minor operations with local anesthesia in patients with coronary artery disease are considered low-risk procedures.[6,7]

■ CLINICAL STABILITY: CLINICAL FACTORS TO ASSESS RISK

Goldman and associates studied 1001 patients, aged 40 years and over, who underwent elective surgery.[4] They noted that patients over 70 years of age, patients with recent myocardial infarcts (myocardial infarction within the previous 6 months), patients with evidence of clinical heart failure (neck vein distention or S_3 gallop), and patients with more than five premature contractions on electrocardiogram (ECG) were associated with an increase in cardiac mortality and morbidity. These investigators generated a point scale that can be used to predict cardiac morbidity (Tables 1 and 2).[4] These data have been confirmed by other workers.[8] Accordingly, Goldman Class IV patients should have surgery deferred; if this is not possible, aggressive management should be practiced during the perioperative period. Reports in 1972 and 1977 indicated that the risk of perioperative myocardial infarction or death had been as high as 30 per cent if surgery was performed within 3 months of a myocardial infarct. The risk decreased to approximately 15 per cent if the operation was performed between 3 and 6 months after infarct. Risk further decreased to 5 per cent when the surgery was performed 6 or more months after myocardial infarction.[2,4]

More recent studies indicate that death or reinfarction can be reduced to approxi-

TABLE 1. Computation of the Cardiac Risk Index

Criteria	Points
History:	
(a) Age > 70 yr	5
(b) MI in previous 6 mo	10
Physical examination:	
(a) S_3 gallop or JVD	11
(b) Important VAS	3
Electrocardiogram:	
(a) Rhythm other than on last preoperative ECG	7
(b) >5 PVCs/min documented at any time before operation	7
General status:	
$Po_2 < 60$ or $Pco_2 > 50$ mm Hg; K < 3.0 or $HCO_3 < 20$ mEq/ liter; BUN > 50 or Cr > 3.0 mg/dl; abnormal SGOT; signs of chronic liver disease; or patient bedridden from noncardiac causes	3
Operation:	
(a) Intraperitoneal, intrathoracic, or aortic operation	3
(b) Emergency operation	4
TOTAL POSSIBLE	53

BUN, blood urea nitrogen; Cr, creatinine; ECG, electrocardiogram; HCO_3, bicarbonate; JVD, jugular vein distention; K, potassium; MI, myocardial infarction; PACs, premature atrial contractions; Po_2, partial pressure of carbon dioxide; PVCs, premature ventricular contractions; SGOT, serum glutamic oxaloacetic transaminase; VAS, valvular aortic stenosis.

(From Goldman L, Caldera DL, Nussbaum SR, et al. Multifactorial index of cardiac risk in noncardiac surgical procedures. Reprinted with permission from The New England Journal of Medicine 1977; 297:845–850.)

TABLE 2. Cardiac Risk Index

Class	Point Total	No or Only Minor Complication (N = 943)	Life-Threatening Complication* (N = 39)	Cardiac Deaths (N = 19)
I (N = 537)	0–5	532 (99)†	4 (0.7)	1 (0.2)
II (N = 316)	6–12	295 (93)	16 (5)	5 (2)
III (N = 130)	13–25	112 (86)	15 (11)	3 (2)
IV (N = 18)	≥26	4 (22)	4 (22)	10 (56)

*Documented intraoperative or postoperative myocardial infarction, pulmonary edema, or ventricular tachycardia with progression to cardiac death.
†Figures in parentheses denote per cent.

(From Goldman L, Caldera DL, Nussbaum SR, et al. Multifactorial index of cardiac risk in noncardiac surgical procedures. Reprinted with permission from The New England Journal of Medicine 1977; 297:845–850.)

mately 6 per cent if surgery is performed within 3 months after infarction when invasive hemodynamic monitoring is utilized during the perioperative period.[3,9] Notwithstanding these interesting data, some workers recommend that elective surgery should be delayed whenever possible for at least 6 months after a myocardial infarction. The risk of perioperative myocardial infarction in a coronary disease patient without a history of myocardial infarction is less than 5 per cent.[1,2]

■ NONINVASIVE STUDIES TO ASSESS RISK

Electrocardiogram (ECG)

Although there is no consensus on the indications for obtaining an ECG on adult patients prior to surgery, a baseline ECG may be useful in the identification of a recent unrecognized myocardial infarction. If a recent infarction is recognized, elective surgery should be delayed until further studies, such as treadmill stress testing, can be performed to identify high-risk ischemia.

In addition, the ECG may reveal unsuspected arrhythmias, such as frequent premature ventricular contractions, which have been correlated with an increased surgical risk.[4] A recent study has shown that the presence of an abnormal preoperative ECG identified 88 per cent of patients who went on to develop a perioperative myocardial infarction.[10] Accordingly, an ECG should be obtained in all patients with known or suspected coronary artery disease prior to surgery.

Exercise Stress Testing

To assess the clinical stability, functional status, and extent of myocardial ischemia, exercise stress testing should be considered in some coronary artery disease patients prior to elective surgery. In a prospective study involving 200 patients older than 40 years of age, Carliner and associates showed that 27 per cent of patients with an ischemic response to preoperative exercise study had one or more cardiac end-points during the perioperative period (death, myocardial infarction, or severe myocardial ischemia), compared with 14 per cent of patients with a nonischemic response.[11] In this study, a multivariant analysis revealed that preoperative exercise study did not provide significant independent prognostic information, and that the baseline ECG was the only significant independent predictor of a cardiac end-point.

Nevertheless, patients found to have high-risk myocardial ischemia on exercise stress testing, manifested by either marked ST segment depression equal to or greater than 2 mV, prolonged time of recovery from ST segment depression, limited exercise capacity less than 5 METS, or exertional hypotension, should be considered candidates for coronary angiography prior to elective surgery.[12] If severe coronary artery disease is demonstrated at angiography, such as left main disease or three-vessel coronary artery disease with left ventricular dysfunction, it may be prudent to recommend a revascularization procedure prior to surgery.[13,14]

A report from the Coronary Artery Surgery Study (CASS) Registry indicated that the operative mortality was 2.4 per cent in patients with significant coronary artery disease who had noncardiac surgery without prior coronary artery bypass graft surgery, compared with 0.9 per cent in patients with similar coronary artery disease who had coronary artery bypass surgery prior to elective noncardiac surgery.[7] However, if one considers that the operative mortality for coronary artery bypass surgery is approximately 2 per cent, the apparent advantage that the bypass patients have in this study may be somewhat negated.

It is obvious that large, randomized, controlled trials are needed to determine whether prophylactic bypass surgery should be performed in patients with high-risk coronary artery disease prior to elective surgery. Although coronary angioplasty has been shown to be a safe and effective procedure in the management of single vessel coronary artery disease, there are no large studies that assess whether this modality will decrease perioperative ischemic events in the coronary artery disease patient undergoing surgery.

Finally, exercise treadmill studies should provide the anesthesiologist with information, such as the heart rate and blood pressure at which the patient became ischemic. The anesthesiologist can use these parameters to facilitate hemodynamic monitoring during the perioperative period.

Dipyridamole Thallium Scanning

Patients who are candidates for major vascular surgery and cannot perform exercise treadmill studies should be considered for intravenous dipyridamole thallium imaging. Eagle and associates evaluated 111 patients undergoing vascular surgery by dipyridamole thallium imaging.[15] Perioperative ischemic events occurred significantly more frequently in the patients who showed reversible thallium defects, compared with patients who showed no thallium redistribution. Moreover, dipyridamole thallium scanning added significantly to the risk stratification of the high-risk subgroup of patients who were already identified by clinical markers. Accordingly, patients with evidence of reversible ischemia by dipyridamole thallium should be considered for coronary angiography prior to elective major surgery.

Other Radionuclide Exercise Stress Studies

Although exercise thallium scintigraphy and exercise radionuclide angiography have been useful in the diagnosis and management of patients with coronary artery disease, studies indicate that they add nothing in routine risk assessment of the patient prior to surgery.[16] Accordingly, these studies should be reserved only for cases when standard exercise stress testing cannot be interpreted because of the presence on the ECG of such conditions as bundle branch block, resting ST-T wave changes, and hypertrophy patterns.

■ INVASIVE STUDIES TO ASSESS RISK

Coronary artery disease patients with unstable coronary artery disease (i.e., unstable angina) and high-risk ischemia, as determined by exercise stress testing, and those patients undergoing major vascular procedures, such as abdominal aneurysm repair, should be considered for coronary angiography prior to elective surgery. If severe coronary artery disease is found at angiography, such as left main artery disease, a revascularization procedure should be performed prior to surgery.

■ CARDIAC MEDICATIONS

Antianginal Therapy. Coronary artery disease patients should continue their antianginal drugs throughout the perioperative period. In most cases patients can take medications with a small sip of water on the day of the operation. In the postoperative period, antianginal drugs may be given via the nasogastric tube, topically, or in some cases intravenously. Doses should be adjusted accordingly to the status of the patient. Table 3 lists the common antianginal drugs and their doses.[17]

Antiarrhythmic Therapy. There is no evidence that prophylactic antiarrhythmic therapy alters the perioperative risk. Accordingly, it is not recommended to start antiarrhythmic therapy prior to surgery for the suppression of premature atrial or ventricular contractions. Indeed, it is possible that such therapy may cause worsening of the ar-

TABLE 3. Drug Therapy for Angina Pectoris

	Preparation	*Dose*	*Dosing Frequency*
Organic Nitrates			
Nitroglycerin	Parenteral	5–100 μg/min*	—
	Sublingual	0.15–0.6 mg	5–30 min
	Buccal	1–5 mg	4–6 hr
	Oral	1.3–9.0 mg	4–8 hr
	Topical	2% over 5–20 cm^2	4–5 hr
	Aerosol	0.4–0.8 mg	5–30 min
Isosorbide dinitrate	Sublingual	2–5 mg	2 hr
	Chewable	5–10 mg	30–240 min
	Oral	5–60 mg	4–6 hr
Beta-Adrenergic Blockers			
Propranolol	Parenteral	0.1 mg/kg over 20 min (loading dose)	—
	Oral	10–80 mg	4 times daily
Metoprolol	Parenteral	15 mg IV over 15 min (loading dose)	—
	Oral	25–100 mg	twice daily
Atenolol	Oral	25–100 mg	twice daily
Nadolol	Oral	40–240 mg	once daily
Pindolol	Oral	5–10 mg	four times daily
Esmolol	Parenteral	500 mg/kg over 1 min (loading dose)	50–200 mg/kg per min (maintenance)
Calcium Entry Blockers			
Verapamil	Parenteral	5–10 mg over 2–5 min	—
	Oral	80–120 mg	3 or 4 times daily
Nifedipine	Sublingual	10–30 mg	3 or 4 times daily
	Oral	10–30 mg	3 or 4 times daily
Diltiazem	Oral	30–90 mg	3 or 4 times daily

*Start with 5 μg/min, increase every 2 minutes by 10 μg/min until hemodynamic response (either systolic blood pressure drop of 10 mm Hg or increase in heart rate of 10 beats/min).
(Extracted from Drug Information 1988. Bethesda, MD: American Society of Hospital Pharmacists, 1988:764–959.)

rhythmias, the so-called proarrhythmia effect. Patients taking antiarrhythmic therapy for arrhythmias, especially those associated with cardiac arrest, should be maintained on drug therapy during the perioperative period.

Preoperative prophylactic digitalization should be considered, especially in older patients with a history of supraventricular arrhythmias.[18]

Antihypertensive Therapy. To mitigate the hectic blood pressure swings that occur in approximately one quarter of hypertensive patients who undergo surgery, blood pressure should be controlled prior to surgery.[19] Antihypertensive medication should be given up to and including the day of surgery. Patients on chronic diuretic therapy should be examined for postural hypotension and hypokalemia. These patients may require increased fluids during surgery because of blood volume contraction. Postoperative hypertension is usually caused by pain, hypoxia, anxiety, cessation of positive pressure ventilation, fluid and sodium over-load, and failure to resume preoperative antihypertensive medications.[20] Supplemental oxygen, diuretics, morphine, sodium nitroprusside, and intravenous nitroglycerin are useful in the treatment of postoperative hypertension.

Congestive Heart Failure Medications. As indicated by the Goldman cardiac risk index, congestive heart failure is a powerful predictor of adverse outcome following surgery.[4] Therefore, surgery should be deferred in patients with decompensated congestive heart failure. Patients should be optimally managed with diuretics, digitalis, and vasodilators prior to surgery in all cases. Patients with decompensated congestive heart failure and patients over 65 years of age with compensated congestive heart failure should be considered candidates for invasive monitoring during the perioperative period.

Antiplatelet Therapy. Many coronary artery disease patients are taking aspirin to prevent reinfarction or to maintain the patency of saphenous vein grafts. Aspirin

TABLE 4. Anticoagulant Management of Patients at High Risk for Thrombotic Events

Discontinue warfarin at least 5 days prior to surgery.

On the first day of warfarin withdrawal, begin intravenous heparin and maintain the activated partial thromboplastin time between 1.5 and 2.0 times control.

Discontinue heparin 6 hours prior to surgery.

Twenty-four to forty-eight hours after surgery, restart heparin and maintain activated partial thromboplastin time 1.5 to 2.0 times control.

Restart oral warfarin 2 days after surgery.

Discontinue heparin when prothrombin time is at therapeutic level.

alters platelet function and facilitates postoperative bleeding. It should be discontinued at least 1 week prior to elective surgery. If this is not possible, platelet transfusions may be used to stop excessive bleeding in the perioperative period.

Anticoagulants. Many coronary artery disease patients are receiving chronic oral anticoagulants such as warfarin to prevent thrombotic events. Warfarin should be discontinued at least 5 days prior to surgery to reduce the risk of bleeding. In some of these patients, disruption in chronic anticoagulation therapy is deemed deleterious. Table 4 shows the perioperative management of anticoagulants in those patients thought to be at high risk for thrombotic events.

■ ANESTHESIA

General anesthetics such as halothane cause myocardial depression and autonomic reflex suppression. They place the patient at risk for intraoperative hypotension, which may lead to perioperative myocardial infarction. Spinal and epidural anesthesias cause sympathetic denervation, thereby resulting in vasodilation. These anesthesias have no direct cardiac depressant effects and may be useful in the patient with profound ventricular dysfunction.[21] However, studies indicate that there is no difference in the incidence and severity of intraoperative hypotension comparing general versus spinal anesthesia.[22]

A recent randomized, controlled study indicates that epidural anesthesia plus analgesia significantly reduced postoperative morbidity in high-risk surgical patients. Further studies are needed to determine whether this anesthetic approach will be beneficial in the high-risk coronary artery disease patient.[23] In the final analysis, the decision about the anesthetic agent and the rate of delivery must be left to the anesthesiologist after consulting with the surgeon and the primary physician.

■ INVASIVE MONITORING DURING THE PERIOPERATIVE PERIOD

In 1983, Rao and associates reported that invasive monitoring, with prompt treatment of any hemodynamic perturbations during the perioperative period, resulted in a reduced perioperative infarction rate in patients operated on within 6 months of an acute myocardial infarction.[3] In that study, patients who received invasive hemodynamic monitoring had a perioperative infarction rate of 1.9 per cent, compared with a perioperative infarction rate of 7.7 per cent in patients who did not receive hemodynamic monitoring.

Moreover, when the myocardial infarction was 0 to 3 months old, perioperative infarction occurred in 5.7 per cent of patients who received hemodynamic monitoring, compared with 36 per cent of patients who did not have hemodynamic monitoring during the perioperative period. In the 4- to 6-month period following infarction, perioperative myocardial infarction occurred in 2.3 per cent of patients who received hemodynamic monitoring, compared with 26 per cent of patients who did not have hemodynamic monitoring during this same perioperative period.[3] Based on these findings, it is recommended that all high-risk surgical patients have Swan-Ganz catheters and arterial lines inserted preoperatively to monitor circulatory hemodynamics during the perioperative period.

Rao showed that patients who became hypotensive, hypertensive, and tachycardic were more likely to suffer a perioperative myocardial infarction. Accordingly, it is recommended that hemodynamic variables, such as pulmonary artery pressure, arterial pressure, and heart rate, should not deviate more than 20 per cent from preinduction values.[3] Rapid-acting intravenous agents like nitroglycerin, beta-blockers, digitalis, and catecholamines can be used to regulate these hemodynamic variables. Table 5 lists criteria for invasive monitoring in patients undergoing surgery.

TABLE 5. Criteria for Invasive Hemodynamic Monitoring During the Perioperative Period

Goldman cardiac risk index IV
Emergency surgery
Myocardial infarction within past 3 months
Unstable angina pectoris
Decompensated congestive heart failure
Major surgery in a patient more than 70 years of age

It must be emphasized that hemodynamic monitoring should be extended for 48 to 72 hours in the postoperative period. Studies indicate that the perioperative myocardial infarcts occur during the first 3 days after surgery.[3] Additionally, the incidence of postoperative heart failure occurs in a bimodal distribution, with peak incidence on the day of operation and on day 3 following surgery when fluid is released from third space sources.[23]

REFERENCES

1. Topkins MJ, Artusio JF. Myocardial infarction and surgery. Anesth Analg 1964; 43:716–720.
2. Tarhan S, Moffitt JH, Taylor WF, Gioliana ER. Myocardial infarction after general anesthesia. JAMA 1972; 220:1451–1454.
3. Rao TLK, Jacobs KH, El-Etr AA. Reinfarction following anesthesia in patients with myocardial infarction. Anesthesiology 1983; 59:499–505.
4. Goldman L, Caldera DL, Nussbaum SR, et al. Multifactorial index of cardiac risk in noncardiac surgical procedures. N Engl J Med 1977; 297:845–850.
5. Jeffrey CC, Kunsman J, Cullen DJ, Brewster DC: A prospective evaluation of cardiac risk index. Anesthesiology 1983; 58:462–464.
6. Backer CL, Tinker JH, Robertson DM, Vliestra RE. Myocardial reinfarction following local anesthesia for ophthalmic surgery. Anesth Analg 1980; 59:257–262.
7. Foster ED, Davis KB, Carpenter JA, Abele S, Fray D, and principal investigators of CASS and their associates. Risk of noncardiac operations in patients with defined coronary disease: the Coronary Artery Surgery Study (CASS) Registry Experience. Ann Thorac Surg 1986; 41:42–50.
8. Zeldin RA. Assessing cardiac risk in patients who undergo noncardiac surgical procedures. Can J Surg 1984; 27:402–408.
9. Wells PH, Kaplan JA. Optimal management of patients with ischemic heart disease for noncardiac surgery by complementary anesthesiologist and cardiologist interaction. Am Heart J 1981; 102:1029–1037.
10. Charlson ME, MacKenzie CR, Ales K, Gold JP, Fairclough G, Shires GT. Surveillance for postoperative myocardial infarction after noncardiac operations. Surg Gynecol Obstet 1988; 167:407–414.
11. Carliner NH, Fisher ML, Plotnick GD, et al. Routine preoperative exercise testing in patients undergoing major noncardiac surgery. Am J Cardiol 1985; 56:51–57.
12. Ellestad MH. Stress Testing Principles and Practice. 3rd ed. Philadelphia: FA Davis, 1986:316–337.
13. Takaro T, Pifarre R, Fish R. Left main coronary artery disease. Prog Cardiovasc Dis 1985; 28:229–232.
14. Killip T, Passamani E, Davis K, and the CASS Principal Investigators and their associates. Coronary Artery Surgery Study (CASS): a randomized trial of coronary bypass surgery: eight-year follow-up and survival in patients with reduced ejection fraction. Circulation 1985; 72:102–105.
15. Eagle KA, Singer DE, Brewster DC, Darling RC, Mulley AG, Boucher CA. Dipyridamole thallium scanning in patients undergoing vascular surgery, optimizing preoperative evaluation of cardiac risk. JAMA 1987; 257:2185–2189.
16. Morise AP, McDowell DE, Savrin RA, et al. The prediction of cardiac risk in patients undergoing vascular surgery. Am J Med Sci 1987; 293:150–158.
17. Drug Information 1988. Bethesda, MD: American Society of Hospital Pharmacists, 1988:764–959.
18. Selzer A, Walter RM. Adequacy of preoperative digitalis therapy in controlling ventricular rate in postoperative atrial fibrillation. Circulation 1966; 34:119–121.
19. Prys-Roberts C, Meloche R, Foex P. Studies of anesthesia in relation to hypertension: cardiovascular responses of treated and untreated patients. Br J Anesthesiol 1971; 43:122–126.
20. Goldman L. Anesthesia and surgery in the hypertensive patient. *In* Amery A (ed). Hypertensive Cardiovascular Disease: Pathophysiology and Treatment. The Hague: Martinus Nijhoff Publishers, 1982:916.
21. Hug CC Jr. Anesthetic agents and the patient with cardiovascular disease. *In* Ream AK, Fogdall RP (eds). Acute Cardiovascular Management: Anesthesia and Intensive Care. Philadelphia: JB Lippincott, 1982.
22. Deron SJ, Kotler MN. Non-cardiac surgery in the cardiac patient. Am Heart J 1988; 15:831–838.
23. Yeager MP, Glass DD, Neff RK, Johnson TB. Epidural anesthesia and analgesia in high-risk surgical patients. Anesthesiology 1987; 66:729–736.

Cystic fibrosis

Robert B. Fick, Jr. ■ *M. L. Reichardt-Fick*

Cystic fibrosis (CF) is a genetic disease with systemic manifestations. Hardly any organ is spared, and there is extreme variability in the expression of this genetic disorder. All fields of medicine may be touched by this disease, and a truly interdisciplinary approach is necessary for the optimal management of these complex patients.[1] Management, then, transcends traditional specialty lines and is further complicated by the fact that many therapeutic options have not been rigorously studied. Their efficacy remains unproved.

It is possible for the astute physician to discover CF patients presenting primarily with chronic sinusitis, asthma, pancreatic insufficiency, spruelike symptoms, azoospermia, or cirrhosis and portal hypertension (Table 1). A high index of suspicion must be applied. The differential diagnostic exercise is lengthy and often confusing, causing some patients to be misdiagnosed for years.

Although there is great variability in the course of this disease, with deterioration occurring at different rates, it is a uniformly disabling disease. Pulmonary disease appears in all patients with CF, frequently dominates the clinical picture, and is progressive. There is no relationship between disease in the extrapulmonary sites and the extent or severity of pulmonary disease. In the end, cor pulmonale and respiratory failure uniformly contribute to the premature demise.[2]

■ Background

Cystic fibrosis is now a grown-up pediatric disease, with one third of patients who are registered in the 127 United States CF Centers surviving to the third decade of life;[3] the median survival age of CF patients is now 26 years.[4] While up to 15 per cent of CF patients may be diagnosed in adulthood, owing to a misdiagnosis as a child or a very mild disease early in life, the majority of adults with CF were diagnosed within the first 2 years of life. Indeed, it is often stated that increased survival of CF patients into adulthood is attributed to two developments: (1) diagnosis at an earlier age, making possible expectant therapy, and (2) management of these complex patients in specialized CF centers where pediatricians, internists, nurse clinicians, respiratory and physical therapists, and social workers combine skills for optimal care.

Molecular biologists using recombinant DNA techniques have identified the CF gene on the long arm of chromosome 7.[5] The protein product is, at this time, referred to as the cystic fibrosis transmembrane regulator protein. Although the chromosomal localization of the CF gene is the first step in using recombinant DNA technology to identify the primary biochemical disorder in this disease, prenatal diagnosis and heterozygote screening are still not generally available. Glimpses, though, of what the future holds are available in reports of first trimester prenatal diagnosis by means of linked DNA markers in conjunction with microvillar intestinal enzyme analysis in those with well-defined family risks.[6]

Despite the promise that molecular biology holds for an earlier diagnosis and for the ultimate therapy of CF, standard care for this disease remains based on prompt initiation of effective treatment of the infective airways lesion that contributes much of the morbidity and virtually all the excess mortality of this disease. Hallmarks of CF include chronic bronchopulmonary infection, chronic sinusitis, pancreatic insufficiency, high levels of sodium and chloride in sweat, and a family history of CF, but not all patients possess all these, and no consistent abnormalities emerge from routine hematologic and biochemical tests. Involvement of the respiratory tract dominates the clinical picture as the patient grows older, and gas-

TABLE 1. Systemic Involvement in Cystic Fibrosis

Opacification of paranasal sinuses 100%*
Chronic lung disease 85–90%
  Cor pulmonale and respiratory failure 9/10†
  Recurrent *Pseudomonas* respiratory infections 8/10
  Bronchiectasis 8/10
  Blood-streaked sputum 5/10
  Intermittent wheezing 3/10
  Pneumothorax 2/10
Gastrointestinal disease 70–84%
  Pancreatic insufficiency 9/10
    Steatosis 3/10
    Diabetes mellitus 1/10
  Partial small bowel obstructions 5/10
  Focal biliary cirrhosis 2/10
  Cholelithiasis 1/10
Aspermia 95%
Hypertrophic pulmonary osteoarthropathy 20–30%
Heat stroke 10%

*Per cent of young adults at the time of diagnosis with this organ involved.
†Pulmonary and gastrointestinal complications from most frequent to least common, expressed as relative risk of developing these complications in those with chronic lung or GI disease.

trointestinal and pancreatic symptoms become less prominent.

■ MICROBIOLOGY

Historically, the CF airway is infected with *Staphylococcus aureus* and *Haemophilus influenzae* during the first few years of life. The mucoid variant of *Pseudomonas aeruginosa* appears infrequently during the first year of life, with only 2 of 84 infants affected in one series.[7] With increasing age of the CF patient, mucoid *P. aeruginosa* becomes the predominant pathogen, being present in up to 85 per cent of cultures obtained from patients with advanced disease. The mucoid variant of *P. aeruginosa* is associated with an extensive exopolysaccharide glycocalyx. It is thought that mucoidy plays a role in adhesion of the pseudomonas organism to the tracheal epithelium, a process which is potentially important to early colonization of the CF airway. Furthermore, the polyanionic glycocalyx may offer protection by preventing incorporation of antibiotics into the bacterial cell.[8]

Although *P. aeruginosa* is the most common bacterial isolate obtained from the airway of adult patients with CF, recently new multiresistant organisms have emerged.

One non-aeruginosa pseudomonas strain, *P. cepacia*, has been associated with increased morbidity and premature death in some centers. During acute flare-ups of pulmonary symptoms, 5 to 15 per cent of bacterial strains isolated from sputa may be non–aeruginosa pseudomonas. Effective recovery of this pseudomonas species requires use of selective media of polymyxinbacitracin-lactose agar or *P. cepacia* isolation agar. Notably, *P. cepacia* is associated with greater impairment of pulmonary function compared with *P. aeruginosa*.[9] The clinical importance of *P. cepacia* is greatly magnified by its resistance to commonly used antipseudomonas antibiotics, including ticarcillin (Ticar), ceftazidime (Fortaz, Tazicef, Tazidime), piperacillin (Pipracil), and the aminoglycosides.[9]

In addition to bacterial pathogens, respiratory viruses can promote clinical deterioration of the CF patient. These etiologic agents remain an important consideration when deciding therapeutic options. In a prospective trial evaluating CF patients and their healthy normal siblings, Wang and colleagues evaluated serologic changes diagnostic of adenoviruses; parainfluenza, types 1, 2, and 3; respiratory syncytial virus; and influenza viruses A and B.[10] A significant correlation existed between the incidence of viral infection and decrements in clinical scores and pulmonary function in the CF group when observed over a 2-year period of time.

■ PRESENTATION OF CF LUNG DISEASE

CF pulmonary disease may present acutely with staphylococcal pneumonia or insidiously with persistent cough following an upper respiratory viral infection. Respiratory infection in CF follows a smoldering course punctuated by acute exacerbations (in part caused by viral agents), superimposed upon a baseline of chronic productive cough and bacterial colonization most commonly caused by mucoid *P. aeruginosa*. Greater than 90 per cent of CF deaths occur during one of these pulmonary infections.

The clinical signs and symptoms of pulmonary infection in the CF patient are notoriously variable. Curiously, temperature elevations are uncommon, routine blood counts are generally not helpful, and positive blood cultures are practically unknown. In general, an acute exacerbation is associated with an increasingly productive cough, occasional wheezing, and decreased appetite with subsequent weight loss. Of less value are other classic indices of infection, such as an elevated leukocyte count, fever, and an increased erythrocyte sedimentation rate.

The chest radiograph in established CF lung disease (Figure 1) shows hyperinflation with peribronchial infiltration and generalized bronchiectasis with cystic changes.[11] Typical findings of bronchial pneumonia are infrequent. Pulmonary function tests in the CF patients show airway obstruction with decreased peak expiratory flow rate (PEFR), low vital capacity (VC), and a diminished ratio of forced expiratory flow rate in 1 second to forced vital capacity (FEV_1/FVC ratio). The ratio of residual volume to total lung capacity (RV/TLC) is typically increased, suggesting air trapping. Although many patients complain of wheezing, reversible airflow obstruction or increased

TABLE 2. Differential Diagnosis of Airways Obstruction in Young Patients

With Copious Chronic Sputum Production
Cystic fibrosis
Immotile cilia syndrome (Kartagener's)
Gastroesophageal aspiration
Bronchiectasis following pneumonia*
Bronchiectasis in association with host defense abnormalities†
Congenital tracheobronchomegaly

With Fibrotic Chest Radiographic Picture
Lymphangioleiomyomatosis
Eosinophilic granuloma (histiocytosis-X)
Hypersensitivity pneumonitis
Allergic bronchopulmonary aspergillosis
Idiopathic sarcoidosis

*Caused by *M. tuberculosis*, viral agents, fungi, or, rarely, following necrotizing bacterial pneumonia.
†E.g., hypogammaglobulinemia, IgG subclass deficiency, familial complement deficiencies.

bronchomotor tone is present in only 20 to 30 per cent of those tested. A practical differential diagnosis to consider when young patients present as described above is given in Table 2.

■ CF LUNG PATHOLOGY

CF lungs are morphologically normal at birth, and the onset of pulmonary pathology may occur at any time after birth, with varying severity of the resulting respiratory signs and symptoms. Nevertheless, only 2 per cent of adults with CF lack evidence of pulmonary disease by history, chest radiographic examination, or pulmonary function tests. Although the exact role of bacteria in the initial pathogenesis of the pulmonary lesion has never been defined, it is the bacterial infection that most commonly leads to irreversible damage. Particularly prominent are bronchiolitis, peribronchiolar inflammation, and bronchiectasis. However, careful light and electron microscopic studies have failed to identify a single lesion specific for CF. Epidermoid metaplasia, large dilated bronchial glands, copious surface mucus, and alveolar destruction are seen in a wide variety of chronic obstructive lung diseases and are not unique findings in CF lungs. Recent morphometric work performed on CF lungs obtained at autopsy indicates that the lung disease and remodeling are irregularly dis-

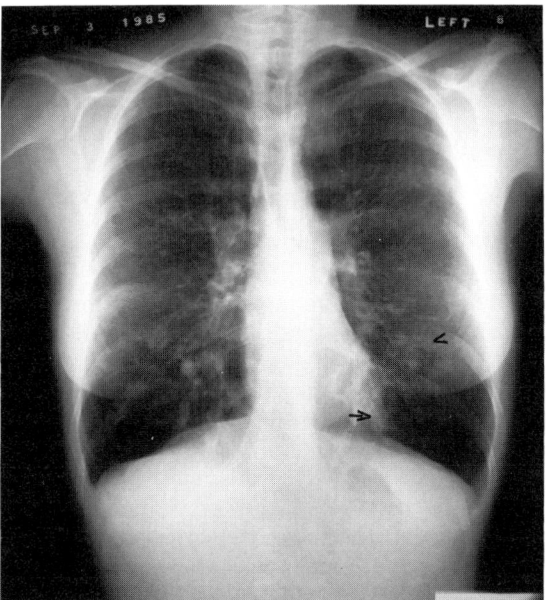

Figure 1. PA chest radiograph of an adult with marked CF lung disease. Predominant radiographic findings of bronchiectasis are cystic "ring" shadows (arrowhead); "tramtracks" of mucosal edema and dilatation (arrow); mucous plugging and atelectasis; and cicatrization and distortion of pulmonary architecture.

tributed and that upper lobe segments are disproportionately involved.[12]

■ PULMONARY COMPLICATIONS

Five to ten per cent of cystic fibrosis patients are troubled by clinically evident pneumothoraces; 25 per cent are multiple, and 58 per cent of these pneumothoraces subside spontaneously, not requiring tube drainage. Hypertrophic pulmonary osteoarthropathy (ossifying periostitis) occurs as a complication in older children with severe CF lung disease and causes long bone pain, arthralgias, and occasional joint effusions. Hemoptysis usually amounts to blood streaking of sputum but may be massive (greater than 300 ml per episode). There is disagreement in the literature as to the prognosis portended by hemoptysis.

■ Management

Because the clinical course of CF is so variable, large numbers of patients must be followed over long periods of time in order to evaluate the effects of chronic treatment interventions. Prospective follow-up with appropriate controls is the best way to demonstrate whether or not a particular treatment or management is beneficial. Yet many of the widely applied treatment protocols for CF have not, unfortunately, been rigorously evaluated. There is little room for dogma. Despite the paucity of therapies proved by prospective, case-controlled studies, the general approach in CF clinics is to stress *nutritional* management and *exercise*, which directly affect respiratory physiology; apply standard *vaccine* therapies to avoid respiratory illness; and use prompt (expectant), aggressive management of *acute pulmonary infections*. Each of these therapies will be discussed in the sections that follow.

■ NUTRITIONAL MANAGEMENT

At routine semiannual visits, weight and height are recorded, and caloric intake can be approximated through a 3-day diet recall. An estimate of the degree of malabsorption can be obtained by the consistency and number of stools per day. It is important to inquire about abdominal pain. This may be related to malabsorption or possibly may be an indication of intermittent intestinal obstruction (meconium ileus equivalent). A list of current treatments should include pancreatic enzyme supplements, fat-soluble vitamin supplements, and other nutritional caloric supplements. Yearly laboratory assessment should include hemoglobin/hematocrit, as anemia may result from vitamin E deficiency; albumin and serum cholesterol determinations may give additional indications of the nutritional status.

Replacement of deficient pancreatic enzymes is required in the majority of patients even if steatorrhea is not a symptom, because pancreatic enzymes will correct the lithogenic bile, tend to prevent gallstones, and lessen chances of meconium ileus equivalent. Patients taking pH-sensitive microspheres, such as pancrelipase (Creon, Pancrease), experience significantly less dyspeptic symptoms, decreased stool frequency, better appetite, and greater increments in weight gain than do those treated with older, powdered pancreatic enzyme preparations. It is known that frequently duodenal postprandial pH in CF patients is too acidic to permit rapid dissolution of current enteric-coated dosage forms of these enzymes, so bicarbonate may be used (5.2 gm/ m^2 body surface/meal) to enhance the enzymatic activities. Cimetidine (Tagamet), 200 to 400 mg half an hour before meals, may be substituted. Fat-soluble vitamins must also be replaced, and during hot weather some increase in salt intake should be encouraged.

Meconium ileus equivalent is managed conservatively by adjustments to diet and supplemental pancreatic enzymes. More persistent, disruptive symptoms of small bowel obstruction may be treated with N-acetylcysteine (Mucomyst), 5 to 20 ml of 10 per cent solution three times daily. Meglumine diatrizoate (Gastrografin) by enema may be effective in relieving severe obstruction and simultaneously will permit radiographic definition of the site of the obstruction.

Patients who have less pancreatic dysfunction and less malabsorption have longer survival.[13] However, it is not clear that nutritional rehabilitation will either reverse or prevent ongoing pulmonary deterioration.

Studies documenting improved nutritional status by means of central venous hyperalimentation[14] or by enteral feedings[15] suggest that improved growth contributes to fewer pulmonary exacerbations and perhaps contributes to better pulmonary function tests.

Continuous nocturnal feedings via a nasogastric tube or by gastrostomy tube can provide the extra calories needed to promote growth.[15] Most children learn to tolerate the NG tube easily and feel good about their improved body habitus. Many adults prefer gastrostomy feeding tubes, which can be inserted by the percutaneous endoscopic technique. It remains to be determined whether aggressive nutritional support in the short term can lead to long-lasting nutritional and pulmonary improvement, or whether lifelong support is necessary.[14] Perhaps improved nutrition lessens the rate of decline in pulmonary function.

CHEST PERCUSSION AND POSTURAL DRAINAGE

In an effort to facilitate mucociliary clearance and to prevent mucous plugging, postural drainage and chest percussion (chest physiotherapy, CPT) have been advocated on a daily basis. Even though the benefits of this therapy have been documented,[16] routine CPT is inconvenient and time consuming. It is not known whether CPT will have a prophylactic effect in infants with little evidence of lung involvement at the time of diagnosis. For adult patients, who may not have family members available to assist with percussion, it may be difficult to reach all lung areas, therefore exercise may be substituted (see next section).

Aerosolized beta-agonists (isoproterenol [Isuprel, Proternol] or metaproterenol [Alupent]) prior to CPT may increase the effectiveness of this therapy by increasing ciliary beat frequency and causing bronchodilatation.[17] Mucolytics are occasionally recommended but without clear evidence of benefit; many patients subjectively feel their sputum is more readily expectorated after N-acetylcysteine, however. In the face of doubtful effectiveness and potential detriment, mucolytics should be used only for the selected patients who feel the subjective need for them.

EXERCISE

Exercise-conditioning programs improve exercise tolerance in adolescents and adults with CF (ages 10 to 30 years).[18] An exercise program consisting of three 1-hour sessions per week continued for 3 months produced significantly increased exercise tolerance, lower heart rates for submaximal work loads, and increased respiratory muscle endurance. An added benefit of exercise is that deep breathing facilitates effective clearance of thick respiratory secretions, thereby substituting for more mundane postural drainage. The exercise sessions consist of stretching exercises and jog-walks lasting 30 minutes that are designed to raise heart rates to 70 to 80 per cent of peak (mean HR_{max} 175 bpm). There were no adverse effects of this program. However, constant supervision was provided, and very hypoxic CF patients with cor pulmonale were excluded.

It is known that falls in oxygen saturations of 5 per cent or greater may occur in those CF patients with an FEV_1 of less than 50 per cent of FVC, or a diffusing capacity for carbon monoxide of less than 80 per cent of predicted. These patients should have supervised exercise testing with ear oximetry before undertaking solo exercise programs.

ANTIMICROBIAL THERAPY

In large measure, the improvement in CF survival reflects timely use of newer, more potent antimicrobials. Noting the central role pseudomonas plays in the pathogenesis of the CF lung disease, many of these new antibiotic protocols are directed at this pathogen (Table 3).

Clinicians are best advised to prescribe antimicrobial chemotherapeutic agents at high doses, because the serum–airway partition coefficient for many classes of antibiotics has reproducibly been shown to approximate 5:1. That is, the level in airways will be only 20 to 30 per cent of a simultaneously obtained serum concentration.[19] The newly released quinolones and the much older agent chloramphenicol appear to be exceptions to this formula.

Finally, the value of quantitative sputum cultures in many clinical settings has been argued, but they may be of value in the CF

TABLE 3. Antimicrobial Agents in the Treatment of CF Airway Bacterial Infections

Class	Specific Agents	Usual Dose	Remarks
Penicillins	Dicloxacillin (Dycill, Dynapen, Pathocil)	250 mg q 6 hr PO	Cleared more rapidly by CF patients
	Ticarcillin	50 mg/kg q 4–6 hr IV	Adjust dosage for renal insufficiency. May induce hypokalemia
Fluoroquinolones	Ciprofloxacin (Cipro)	500–750 mg q 8–12 hr PO	Not recommended in children or pregnant women, as animal studies show quinolone accumulation in joints; dose adjustment in renal insufficiency
Aminoglycosides	Tobramycin (Tobrex, Nebcin)	80 mg/m^2 q 6 hr IV	Aim for peak levels 5–12 mg/L; trough level < 2 mg/L.
Ureidopenicillins	Piperacillin (Pipracil)	3–4 gm q 4–6 hr IV	In vitro activity against *P. aeruginosa* most increased
	Azlocillin (Azlin)	3–4 gm q 4–6 hr IV	Resistance may be rapidly acquired
	Mezlocillin (Mezlin)	3–4 gm q 4–6 hr IV	
Third-generation cephalosporins	Ceftazidime (Fortaz, Tazicef, Tazidime)	2 gm q 8 hr IV	Dose adjustment needed in renal insufficiency
	Cefsulodin (Cefomonil)	60 mg/kg q 8 hr IV	Investigational in USA; CF patients have altered renal clearance of this agent
Carbapenems	Imipenem/ Cilastatin (Primaxin)	250–500 mg q 6 hr IV	Dose adjustment in renal insufficiency
Monobactams	Aztreonam (Azactam)	2 gm q 6 hr IV	Resistance in gram-positive and anaerobic organisms
Others	Trimethoprim-sulfamethoxazole (Bactrim, Cotrim, Co-Trimoxazole, Septra)	80–160 mg trim 400–800 mg sulfa q 12 hr PO	Useful for staphylococcus or *H. influenzae*
	Chloramphenicol (Chloromycetin)	750 mg q 6 hr PO	Rare hematologic complications

patient. Several clinical studies have demonstrated that the bacterial species identified in the culture of an expectorated sputum specimen are representative of the bacteriology obtained from resected lung segments, protected catheter brushes, and percutaneous needle aspirates of the lungs of CF patients. Quantifying the bacterial burden is useful in following response to therapy and confirming the clinical impressions of worsening or improvement in patients with bronchiectasis.[20] The presence of pseudomonas in the sputum has been related to the severity of lung disease, as shown by clinical deterioration and death, and by pulmonary function tests and chest radiographs. Having said this, it is important to emphasize that the greatly distorted airways of these patients continuously harbor bacteria and will infrequently yield a sterile sputum culture despite aggressive antibiotic treatment, although there may be a decrease in the density of organisms in the sputum.[20]

Oral Agents

The fluoroquinolones (ciprofloxacin [Cipro]) are bactericidal antibiotics that may be efficacious in the treatment of bronchopulmonary exacerbations of cystic fibrosis. These agents offer broad-spectrum coverage with significant activity against commonly associated CF pathogens, including *Pseudomonas aeruginosa* as well as *Staphylococcus aureus* and *Haemophilus influenzae*. Ciprofloxacin's oral bioavailability and longer serum half-life allow for twice daily dosing, an advantage for outpatient therapy of the adult CF patient. The high volume of distribution of this class of antibiotics offers good penetration into bronchial secretions. The concomitant use of the fluoroquinolones can result in increased concentrations of theophylline and coumadin by affecting hepatic clearance of these commonly used medications.

Clinical studies generally have shown oral ciprofloxacin to be comparable to conventional intravenous antimicrobial therapy in bronchopulmonary exacerbations of cystic fibrosis. Although clinical response was apparent, ciprofloxacin rarely eradicated the pseudomonas organism, or, if it did, this was a transient finding. When used chronically on a daily basis rather than intermittently or sporadically, a disturbingly high rate of resistance is acquired. As with many new chemotherapeutic agents, high expectations generally have not been realized.

Older oral agents include trimethoprim/sulfamethoxasole and the penicillinase-resistant penicillins. Although virtually all *P. aeruginosa* strains are resistant to trimethoprim (Proloprim, Trimpex), this drug is commonly administered to CF patients when *S. aureus* or *H. influenzae* predominate in sputum. Similarly, dicloxacillin (Dycill, Dynapen, Pathocil) is administered orally for the suppression of *S. aureus* colonization in the sputum of patients early in the course of CF lung disease.

Parenteral Agents (see Table 3)

Imipenem, like ciprofloxacin, is an extremely potent pseudomonicidal antibiotic but with chronic use may fail through acquisition of resistance. Ceftazidime is a third-generation cephalosporin that has the best activity against *P. aeruginosa* of all the available cephalosporins, and ticarcillin has been combined with clavulanic acid to enhance activity against β-lactamase–producing bacteria, e.g., *H. influenzae* or *S. aureus*, frequently found in CF airways concurrently or antedating pseudomonas infections.

Azlocillin, mezlocillin, and piperacillin exhibit an extended spectrum against *P. aeruginosa*. These drugs are derived from the ampicillin molecule with side chain adaptations but are not absorbed after oral administration and must be administered parenterally. Potential advantages of these agents over carbenicillin and ticarcillin include a lower sodium load, decreased drug-associated platelet dysfunction, and minimal need for dosage adjustment in renal failure. In combination with an aminoglycoside in vitro, these drugs show a synergistic inhibitory effect. The clinical significance of these benefits to cystic fibrosis patients requires further investigation.

Aztreonam represents the initial entry of the monobactam class of antibiotics, which has specific activity against gram-negative aerobic organisms, including *P. aeruginosa*. Gram-positive organisms, including the staphylococci and streptococci, as well as anaerobes, appear to be resistant to aztreonam. As with the aminoglycosides, aztreonam requires intravenous delivery, but unlike aminoglycosides, it is not associated with nephrotoxicity or ototoxicity. In a clinical study by Scully and colleagues, 12 cystic fibrosis patients with 26 exacerbations of their disease thought to be caused by *P. aeruginosa* were treated with intravenous aztreonam.[21] The apparent rate of clinical improvement of 85 per cent suggested potential clinical efficacy in the treatment of the *P. aeruginosa* infection associated with cystic fibrosis exacerbations. Because of the lack of comparative drug trials, the question of whether aztreonam offers a significant advance over conventional therapy (for example, the aminoglycosides) remains unanswered.

Frequently, the aminoglycosides are administered parenterally in an attempt to decrease the pseudomonas burden. It is important to note that altered gentamicin disposition, peculiar to CF,[22] precludes application of the standard guidelines widely used in adults. A higher dose, administered more frequently, is usually required, and peak and trough blood levels must be monitored.

Dosing Regimens

The most effective protocol for administration of these potent antimicrobial agents in the CF patient has not been defined. Should these agents be administered parenterally or by nebulizer? If the parenteral route is selected, should the antibiotics be given only to hospitalized patients, or can these antibiotics be safely administered in the outpatient home setting? Should antimicrobials be prescribed chronically or for the first week of each month?

With improvements in the availability of home-health care, parenteral antibiotic therapy can be achieved easily at home, with success equal to that of in-hospital treatment in selected patients.[23] This can be achieved with either peripheral intravenous access or indwelling central venous access. It should be noted that antibiotic therapy alone, without appropriate attention to concomitant chest physiotherapy and nutrition, will have less than optimal results. Donati and associates, in a controlled, prospective trial, compared home and hospital antibiotic therapy.[23] The patients (41 in each group) were matched for age, sex, pulmonary function, and arterial blood gases. Intravenous antibiotics, usually a semisynthetic penicillin and an aminoglycoside, were employed with intravenous catheters ("heparin locks") maintained by registered nurses. The home care compared favorably with hospital care, and was significantly less costly, and allowed the individual patient a greater opportunity to participate in work or school activities. Before implementation of outpatient parenteral antibiotics, the physician must consider (1) the patient's degree of illness and ability for self-care; (2) the potential for ancillary support, including chest physical therapy and nutritional supplementation; (3) the availability of individuals to care for the intravenous catheters; and (4) availability of close medical follow-up, because day-by-day physician contact is generally terminated when the patient returns home.

Nebulizers have been used to deliver aminoglycosides, broad-spectrum penicillins (Table 4), and cephalosporins. A particular advantage is that this therapy may be used at home. Several relatively small clinical trials have demonstrated the safety, absence of untoward effects, and low rate of development of bacterial resistance. This presents an alternative to the rather short list of oral pseudomonicidal agents used in daily outpatient maintenance therapy.

Recently, investigators have analyzed an inexpensive, commercially available aerosolizer (Centimist, Intec Corp) and, using an immunoenzymatic assay for gentamicin, calculated that 7.7 per cent of the original amount of antibiotic placed in the chamber was deposited in airway secretions.[24] The peak sputum levels (mean, 377 μg/ml) greatly exceeded MIC and MBC levels for clinical isolates of *P. aeruginosa*, and yet serum levels were not detected. Therefore, high concentrations of pseudomonicidal antibiotics may be safely and selectively delivered to the CF airways, thus avoiding nephrotoxicity.

It is interesting to note the generally favorable results of these protocols employing nebulized antimicrobials in CF patients, despite the fact that *P. aeruginosa* rarely has been eradicated from the airway secretions. This should not be surprising, because we seldom sterilize the sputum with any treatment, including parenteral pseudomonicidal antibiotics delivered in-hospital. Sterilization of secretions in these patients with distorted airways is seldom possible and suggests that an appropriate goal of therapy in CF patients may be simply reduction of the bacterial burden rather than eradication of pseudomonas.

Because of the ongoing bacterial load in airway secretions, many have advocated either chronic and continuous or regular and cyclic administration of oral antibiotics. These approaches are supported by a double-blind cross-over study using cephalexin (Keflex) that demonstrated improved growth, fewer pulmonary exacerbations, and fewer nonpseudomonas organisms in the sputum in the treated group. However, more mucoid pseudomonas species were isolated in the treatment group, suggesting that there may be adverse long-term sequelae of chronic therapy.[25] In fact, the change in predominant flora from staphylococcus to pseudomonas in CF patients was postulated to be due to oral antibiotics selecting for the pseudomonas. Currently, a

TABLE 4. Nebulized Antibiotic Protocols for Recalcitrant Pseudomonas Infection in CF Airways

Gentamicin (Apogen, Garamycin, V-Gencin)	20–40 mg in 2 ml of 0.125% phenylephrine and propylene glycol delivered BID–TID
Tobramycin (Nebcin)	40–80 mg in 2 ml of normal saline delivered BID–TID
Ticarcillin (Ticar) and Tobramycin (Nebcin)	80 mg of tobramycin plus 1 gm of ticarcillin delivered BID*

*Aminoglycoside has been reported to be inactivated by broad-spectrum penicillins. Best advised to administer separately.

multicenter trial of chronic oral antibiotic therapy is underway to help answer the question of whether this is beneficial.

■ CORTICOSTEROIDS

A randomized, double-blind placebo-controlled study of alternate day prednisone [Deltasone] 2 mg/kg to a maximum of 60 mg daily in CF children (ages 1 to 12 years) concluded after a 4-year follow-up that the prednisone-treated group had significant advantages for height, weight, vital capacity, FEV_1, peak flow, and number of hospitalizations required.[26] It remains unclear whether the same chronic corticosteroid treatment protocol would prove beneficial in adolescent and adult CF patients with a great deal more structural lung disease. It is known that acute daily doses of prednisone (20 to 30 mg/day for 3 weeks) do not significantly increase pulmonary function in those with more advanced disease and, further, may expose these patients to an increased risk of developing a pneumothorax.

■ IMMUNIZATION

Despite new generations of antibiotics, truly effective therapy has not yet been achieved, and immunotherapy has been considered. Parenteral administration of polyvalent pseudomonas vaccines to children before acquisiton of pseudomonas and to CF adults colonized with pseudomonas failed to delay the onset of pseudomonas infections in the children and did not clear the adult airways of this bacterium. Similarly, local respiratory immunization by intranasal administration of the pseudomonas lipopolysaccharide vaccine to a small number of adult CF patients troubled by chronic pseudomonas infections of the airways did not result in clinical improvement or eradication of the pathogen. Although many different pseudomonas vaccines are in preparation, it seems unlikely that any will be widely used in the treatment of CF patients in the near future.

Exacerbations of CF respiratory disease may be triggered by viral infections; measles and influenza are especially devastating, so immunization against these viruses is crucial. Other childhood immunizations should also be given on schedule. Pneumococcal vaccine is not necessary for patients with cystic fibrosis.

■ Issues and Risks

CF is the most common lethal genetic disease in the United States, and the socioeconomic impact is enormous: the mean annual expenditure for health care throughout the life of a CF patient is estimated to be $25,000. As reviewed, treatment of this chronic systemic and disabling disease is complex. Optimal management requires a joint coordinated effort by the patient and family members. Social-psychologic costs are significant as well: guilt, fear, anxiety, and stress disrupt the CF family. However, most of the funded research has focused on elucidation of pathophysiologic mechanisms, diagnosis, treatment, and management of the physiologic disease. Studies of psychologic adaptation and development of valid coping mechanisms are incomplete.

Physicians caring for CF patients must recognize four sources of stress, each with the potential to cause emotional disturbance: altered physical appearance causing a distorted body image and sexual denial; strained interpersonal relationships leading to social isolation; heightened conflicts with parents; and fears about death.[27] To achieve optimal management of the CF patient, each must be addressed by a sensitive health care provider.

The nature of the relationship between CF patients and their physicians deserves study.[28] Extension of the caretaking role may deter the patient from maturing and developing independence. Conversely, remaining aloof and distant precludes optimal management of social-psychologic factors. The proper posture, leading to an improvement in independent functioning and compliance, will be difficult to define.

Several studies have identified the factors that increase compliance: educating patients regarding their medical regimen; reducing the cost, complexity, duration, and amount of behavioral change required by the management protocol; improving the patient-provider relationship; monitoring compliance; and utilizing patients' social support networks.[29] Coping mechanisms may be employed to influence compliance with the treatment program.

Family assessment in CF centers should include identification of coping strategies and other variables that promote adaptation to illness. The routine availability of psychologic support is often cited by patients as an important facet of total care[1] and investigators have identified adaptive coping behaviors used by families.[30] These reports are increasing our understanding of the relationship between variables of successful family adaptation and life pattern adjustments dictated by the disease of cystic fibrosis.

REFERENCES

1. Davis PB, di Sant' Agnese PA. Diagnosis and treatment of cystic fibrosis. An update. Chest 1984; 85:802–809.
2. Fick RB. Pseudomonas in cystic fibrosis: sylph or sycophant? Clin Chest Med 1981; 2:91–102.
3. Arehart-Treichel J. Lengthened survival raises problems in cystic fibrosis. JAMA 1984; 252:2526–2527.
4. Cystic Fibrosis Foundation. Report of data registry, 1986.
5. Kerem B, Rommens JM, Buchanan JA, et al. Identification of the cystic fibrosis gene: genetic analysis. Science 1989; 245:1073–1080.
6. Spence JE, Buffone GJ, Rosenbloom CL, et al. Prenatal diagnosis of cystic fibrosis using linked DNA markers and microvillar intestinal enzyme analyses. Hum Genet 1987; 76:5–10.
7. Huang NN, Doggett RG. *Pseudomonas Aeruginosa: Clinical Manifestations of Infection and Current Therapy*. New York: Academic Press, 1979.
8. Costerton JW. *Pseudomonas aeruginosa: In* Sabath LD (ed). *Pseudomonas aeruginosa—The Organism, Diseases It Causes, and Their Treatment*. Bern, Switzerland: Hans Huber Publishers, 1980:15–25.
9. Isles A, MacClusky I, Corey M, et al. *Pseudomonas cepacia* infection in cystic fibrosis: an emerging problem. J Pediatr 1984; 104:206–210.
10. Wang EEL, Prober CG, Manson B, et al. Association of respiratory viral infection with pulmonary deterioration in patients with cystic fibrosis. N Engl J Med 1984; 311:1653–1658.
11. Murphy S. Cystic fibrosis in adults: diagnosis and management. Clin Chest Med 1987; 8:695–710.
12. Tomashefski JF, Bruce M, Goldberg HI, Dearborn DG. Regional distribution of macroscopic lung disease in cystic fibrosis. Am Rev Respir Dis 1986; 133:535–540.
13. Gaskin K, Gurwitz D, Durie P, Corey M, Levison H. Improved respiratory prognosis in patients with cystic fibrosis with normal fat absorption. J Pediatr 1982; 100:857–862.
14. Mansell AL, Andersen JC, Muttart CR, et al. Short-term pulmonary effects of total parenteral nutrition in children with cystic fibrosis. J Pediatr 1984; 104:700–705.
15. Shepherd RQ, Holt TL, Thomas BJ, et al. Nutritional rehabilitation in cystic fibrosis: controlled studies of effects on nutritional growth retardation, body protein turnover, and course of pulmonary disease. J Pediatr 1986; 109:788–794.
16. Reisman JJ, Rivington-Law B, Corey M, et al. Role of conventional physiotherapy in cystic fibrosis. J Pediatr 1988; 113:632–636.
17. Sutton RP, Gensel HG, Innes N, et al. Use of nebulized saline and terbutaline as adjuncts to chest physiotherapy. Thorax 1988; 43:57–60.
18. Orenstein DM, Franklin BA, Doershuk CF, et al. Exercise conditioning and cardiopulmonary fitness in cystic fibrosis. Chest 1981; 80:392–398.
19. Fick RB, Stillwell PC. Controversies in the management of cystic fibrosis lung disease. Chest 1989; 95:158–164.
20. Smith AL, Redding G, Doershuk C. Sputum changes associated with therapy for endobronchial exacerbation in cystic fibrosis. J Pediatr 1988; 112:547–554.
21. Scully BE, Ores CN, Prince AS. Treatment of lower respiratory tract infections due to *Pseudomonas aeruginosa* in patients with cystic fibrosis. Rev Infect Dis 1985; 7(S4):669–674.
22. Kearns GL, Holman BC, Wilson JT. Dosing implications of altered gentamicin disposition in patients with cystic fibrosis. J Pediatr 1982; 100:312–318.
23. Donati MA, Guenetti G, Auerbach H. Prospective controlled study of home and hospital therapy of cystic fibrosis pulmonary disease. J Pediatr 1987; 111:28–33.
24. Ilowite JS, Garvoy JD, Smaldone GC. Quantitative disposition of aerosolized gentamicin in cystic fibrosis. Am Rev Respir Dis 1987; 136:1445–1449.
25. Loening-Bauke VA, Mischler E, Myers MG. A placebo-controlled trial of cephalexin therapy in the ambulatory management of patients with cystic fibrosis. J Pediatr 1979; 95:630–637.
26. Auerbach HS, Williams M, Kirkpatrick JA. Alternate-day prednisone reduces morbidity and improves pulmonary function in cystic fibrosis. Lancet 1985; 2:686–688.
27. Boyle IR, di Sant' Agnese PA, Sack S, Millican F, Kulczyoki LL. Emotional adjustment of adolescents and young adults with cystic fibrosis. J Pediatr 1976; 88:318–326.
28. Eigen H, Clark NM, Wolfe JM. Clinical-behavioral aspects of cystic fibrosis: directions for future research. Am Rev Respir Dis 1987; 136:1509–1513.
29. Becker MH, Maiman LA. Strategies for enhancing patient compliance. J Community Health 1980; 6:113–135.
30. Gibson C. How parents cope with a child with cystic fibrosis. Nurs Papers/Perspec Nurs 1986; 18:31–45.

Depression in the elderly patient

H. Michael Zal

Depression is the most common psychiatric illness in the geriatric population. Epidemiologic estimates are confusing, with incidence estimates ranging from 10 to 50 per cent. Expert opinion varies. Some agree that "the incidence of depressive disorders rises with age."[1] The Epidemiologic Catchment Area Project, conducted by the National Institute of Mental Health (1980), showed that depression was less common in elderly people than in younger persons. However, the clinician cannot help but be aware of both the significant incidence of mood changes in those over age 65 years and the ability of these emotional changes to cause distress and suffering. Depression in elderly people presents a diagnostic challenge and often proves difficult to manage.

■ Background

Growing older may not always conform to the Robert Browning line, "Grow old along with me! The best is yet to be. . . ." However, it need not be a time of frustration, pain, and helplessness. Most people fall within the middle range. Many physicians assume that feeling sad is a natural reaction to be expected in elderly people and dismiss depression as being age-appropriate. Some have difficulty recognizing clinical depression and differentiating it from the temporary response to the many changes and losses found in the normal aging process.

■ DIAGNOSIS

Depression is often loosely defined. It "is a term applied to everything from transitory unhappiness to incapacitating suicidal despair."[2] In clinical depression, the dysphoric mood lasts for at least 2 weeks and is accompanied by many symptoms: decreased energy; changes in appetite and weight; difficulty in sleep pattern; feelings of guilt, loneliness, hopelessness, helplessness, and worthlessness; somatic complaints; difficulty in concentration and making decisions; crying easily; loss of sexual interest or pleasure; feeling everything is an effort; and recurrent thoughts of death or suicide.

A full range of mood disorders can affect the aged. The DSM-III-R includes uncomplicated bereavement, adjustment disorder with depressed mood, depressive disorders (dysthymia; major depression) and bipolar disorders.[3] The classification of mood disorders has undergone major changes in the last 10 years. Traditionally, we spoke of a neurotic-psychotic distinction and an endogenous-reactive dichotomy. Mood disorders are now divided into bipolar disorders and depressive disorders. Qualifiers include with psychotic features, melancholic type, and seasonal pattern.

Major affective disorder with psychotic features includes the older diagnosis of psychotic depressive reaction. Here the clinical characteristics described previously are seen but in a more intense and severe form. In addition, there is impairment in reality testing. Delusions (false beliefs) are present, usually involving a somatic preoccupation. There are intractable insomnia, suicidal ruminations, and much guilt. Marked changes in bodily functions are seen, including severe anorexia, weight loss, constipation, and psychomotor retardation. The patient's ability to function is impaired.

Another type of mood disorder is manic depressive illness, or bipolar disorder. These disorders in elderly people are usually recurrences of previously existing illnesses but can represent late-onset disorders in some. The episodes are not related to a precipitating life experience but are considered to be endogenous, with definite genetic and familial factors. The disorder of mood (rather than thought) dominates the mental life of the patient and is responsible for whatever loss of contact or impairment of reality testing he or she has with the environment. Delusions are in keeping with the manifest affect—either depressed or manic. There is impairment in the ability to function. Patients with bipolar disorder, depressed, usually will show psychomotor retardation and many of the aforementioned clinical characteristics of general depression.

PRESENTATION

Masked Depression. Another reason for underdiagnosis of depression in elderly people is the symptom variation that they often show. Masked depression is a common presentation in the geriatric patient. Here multiple, vague, nonspecific somatic complaints in several body systems eclipse the dysphoric mood. "Depressive equivalents" include headache, chronic pain, gastrointestinal upsets (constipation, nausea), and decreased energy or drive. Other barometers of depression in elderly people include sleep disturbances or an internal feeling of nervousness or restlessness. Apathy with subtle ideation of failure, pessimism, loneliness, and hopelessness can be silent indications of underlying depression.

Pseudodementia. Geriatric patients with major depression may present subjective complaints of deteriorating memory, difficulty in concentration, or difficulty in thinking. They may appear demented. If this cognitive impairment is reversible when the true depression is treated, the diagnosis is depression-induced organic mental disorder, or "pseudodementia." Jarvik has noted that as many as one third of patients diagnosed as demented may suffer from depression.[4] "It is important to mention that a combination of depression with dementia in varying quantities is a very frequent occurrence."[5]

PSYCHOSOCIAL STRESSORS

"Loss is a predominate theme in characterizing the emotional experience of older people."[1] Forgetfulness and impairment in cognitive ability produce psychologic losses. Physical and physiologic losses follow changes in health, strength, and appearance. Economic losses are caused by reduced income, property loss, and employment reduction or retirement. A predominate theme in geriatric communication involves the stress of living on a "fixed income." Social losses may occur through possible changes in prestige, status, and respect. Changes in sexual ability also may serve as a loss. The death of family members and friends creates additional interpersonal losses.[6] Depression is a natural reaction to loss and change. However, it is wrong to assume that being depressed is just a normal consequence of aging. The physician must be sensitive to the continuum between existential sadness and clinical depression.

MEDICAL CAUSES OF DEPRESSION (Table 1)

Physical illness and polypharmacy often share a relationship with depression in elderly people. Giannini and associates have listed 91 possible medical disorders that can present as depression.[7] Various endocrine and metabolic disorders, certain neoplasms, and some central nervous system disorders may be accompanied by, be confused with, or precipitate depression. Depression also may follow a stroke.

The first line of defense in treatment of late-life depression is a thorough diagnostic medical workup, including physical examination, laboratory tests, and electrocardiogram (ECG), to rule out these conditions, many of which can be corrected. Goff and Jenike, in discussing treatment-resistant depression, suggest that "if [depressed] patients fail to improve despite optimal treatment, reconsider an undiagnosed medical etiology."[8]

A review of current medications should also be part of the initial evaluation if depression is suspected. Drug-induced depressions are often seen in the geriatric population. These medications include antihypertensive agents, hormones, antiparkinson drugs, and anticancer drugs (Table 2). Patients should be asked about drug and alcohol use, because substance abuse is often a hidden disorder among elderly people and may be associated with depression.

TABLE 1. Medical Diseases Associated with Depression

Endocrine/Metabolic Disorders
Hypothyroidism/hyperthyroidism
Diabetes/hypoglycemia
Hyperparathyroidism/hypoparathyroidism
Addison's disease
Cushing's disease
Porphyria
Conn's disease
Menopause
Acromegaly
Uremia/urinary tract infection
Gout

Malignant Disease
Pancreatic carcinoma
Brain tumor
Oat cell carcinoma
Lymphoma

Central Nervous System
Parkinson's disease
Multiple sclerosis
Dementia
Stroke
Head trauma
Temporal lobe seizures
Myasthenia gravis
Huntington's disease
Normal pressure hydrocephalus

Nutritional Deficiencies
Thiamine
Vitamin B_{12}
Folate
Pyridoxine
Iron
Protein
Vitamin C

Infections
Influenza
Hepatitis
Viral pneumonia
Tuberculosis
Viral encephalitis

Collagen-Vascular Disease
Rheumatoid arthritis
Systemic lupus erythematosus
Giant cell arteritis
Polyarteritis nodosa

Gastrointestinal Disease
Cirrhosis
Inflammatory bowel disease
Celiac disease/Whipple's disease

Miscellaneous
Hypoxia
Sleep apnea
Congestive heart failure/myocardial infarction
Alcoholism
Sensory deprivation (visual/hearing loss)
Heavy metal intoxications

■ Management

Treatment options for depression in the elderly include education, individual and group psychotherapy, chemotherapy, and electroconvulsive therapy (ECT).

■ EDUCATION

An important function of the clinician is to help educate the depressed patient about the nature of the illness, its time-limited character, and its potential responsiveness to therapy. When pharmacotherapy is appropriate, education about its mechanism and possible side effects will enhance compliance. It is the job of the physician to disseminate information, correct misconceptions, give perspective, and help patients correct obstructive ways of communicating their basic needs. Education also should include the patient's family members and

TABLE 2. Drugs Associated with Depression

Antihypertensive Drugs
Reserpine
Methyldopa
Propranolol hydrochloride
Guanethidine
Hydralazine
Clonidine

Cardiac Drugs
Digitalis
Propranolol
Lidocaine

Hormones
Estrogen
Progesterone

Antineoplastic Drugs
Vincristine sulfate
Vinblastine sulfate

Antiparkinson Drugs
Levodopa
Amantadine hydrochloride

Psychotropic Drugs
Benzodiazepines
Chlorpromazine, other aliphatic phenothiazines

Miscellaneous
Corticosteroids
Cimetidine
Timolol maleate
Cycloserine
Alcohol/disulfiram
Sedatives
Stimulants

friends in order to encourage their support and dispel counterproductive assumptions and misconceptions.

PSYCHOTHERAPY

Individual Psychotherapy. Psychotherapeutic intervention with dysphoric elderly patients can run the gamut from the psychoanalytic to behavioral to supportive, depending on patients' emotional and cognitive resources. However, more important than specific choice of therapeutic discipline are various common goals and attitudes. The therapeutic relationship is the cornerstone of any treatment plan. The doctor-patient relationship is a powerful therapeutic force. An atmosphere of acceptance, empathy, and neutrality is essential to help patients relax and express painful feelings. Take the patient seriously and try to understand the meaning of a particular event for each individual. What may be stressful to one person may not be an issue to another.

The supportive, nonjudgmental milieu of individual therapy can give the depressed patient an opportunity to talk and release anger. It encourages relationships and decreases isolation. It reduces the stress of separation and fulfills some of the older person's emotional needs. It can decrease feelings of guilt. It can help place things in perspective, suggest alternatives, and provide a degree of reality testing by acting not so much as the echo of conscience as the quiet voice of reason.

The depressed geriatric patient may feel helpless, hopeless, and overwhelmed. An optimistic therapeutic attitude will help reduce these feelings. The therapist, acting as a surrogate parent or protective helping person, must take charge of the situation. Having established rapport in this way, the therapist can work to re-establish self-confidence and self-esteem in the patient and encourage her or him to develop new interests. This goal-directed behavior, in turn, will help restore a sense of identity and direction.[6]

Environmental manipulation to alter conditions to bring about relief is often appropriate. This can include helping the patient increase the capacity to make and retain new friendships and reintegrate into a social network. This goal can be achieved by introducing the patient to others, providing necessary transportation, and making the person aware of neighborhood resources. Motivate the patient by encouragement and continued interest to increase activity within the limits of remaining resources. Try to evoke a desire to be maximally productive and creative. Support systems play an important role in helping the patient follow through on professional advice. A total support system includes family members, friends, and any interested parties in the community. Attention and love can help increase security and improve behavior.

Group Psychotherapy. Jarvik and associates recommend group psychotherapy as effective treatment for the loneliness and isolation experienced by many depressed elderly patients.[9] Here they can share their experiences and problems and learn that they are not alone or different. Group psychotherapy can foster self-expression and ventilation, as well as better interpersonal relationships and communication. This approach is particularly helpful in institutions, nursing homes, and health-related facilities.

Transference-Countertransference. A special difficulty in treating late-life depression is the issue of transference. Sometimes the age of the therapist is a factor. He or she may be too young to gain the respect of the older patient, who unconsciously sees the therapist as the good or frustrating child or grandchild. However, for the most part, the elderly person will accept the therapist and be grateful for the attention. The therapist's attitude toward age is even more significant. Countertransference issues can block good therapy. To work with elderly people, one's own feelings about parents and grandparents must be resolved. If one acts as though old people should be obeyed and feared, it may be difficult to work with them therapeutically. One also will have difficulty if threatened by old age or if one overidentifies with the lonely, fearful, depressed elderly patient.[6]

CHEMOTHERAPY

Pharmacokinetics

Keep in mind various age-related physiologic changes to avoid the risk of side effects and toxic reactions. Hepatic, renal, cardiac, and lung changes may contribute to altered metabolism and elimination of tricyclic antidepressants. Decreased liver enzyme activity can result in a longer half-life of medication. Diminished renal blood flow, glomerular filtration rate, and tubular secretion can delay the excretion of lithium and metabolites of cyclic antidepressants and increase plasma concentrations. There is also a decrease in plasma proteins with age, causing a decrease in total antidepressant binding and an increase in the availability of unbound medication.

Diminished cardiac output may delay circulation time and affect the tissue distribution of drugs. Lee reminds us that old people are smaller than they look.[10] Their body mass is deceptive, because the wasting of muscle tissue is often masked by the substitution of fat. Drug dosage of lipid-soluble antidepressants, therefore, should be related to lean body mass. There also may be altered sensitivity of the target organ. Neuronal changes in the aging brain cause drug receptor sites to be more sensitive to antidepressants.

Tricyclic Antidepressants. These medications potentiate the action of catecholamines by blocking the re-uptake of norepinephrine or serotonin. Common side effects include sedation and the anticholinergic effects of dry mouth, constipation, tremor, and blurred vision. Tricyclic antidepressants also may cause orthostatic hypotension, cognitive impairment, weight gain, nausea, urinary retention, and tachycardia. "The drugs may induce central anticholinergic toxicity leading to a dose-related atropine-like psychosis."[11]

They are contraindicated in the acute recovery phase following a myocardial infarction or in patients with atrial or ventricular arrhythmias. Avoid these compounds if there is a history of acute (narrow) angle glaucoma, significant prostatic hypertrophy, or cardiac conduction defects. They differ very little in therapeutic effectiveness but do vary in relation to their potential for anticholinergic and sedative side effects and cardiovascular toxicity. A baseline ECG, pulse count, and sitting and standing blood pressure measurements should be obtained before initiating treatment.

The tricyclic tertiary amines (amitriptyline, imipramine, trimipramine [Surmontil], and doxepin [Adapin, Sinequan]) have a high degree of sedation and may be helpful in the agitated and depressed patient who is having difficulty in sleep pattern. Less sedating drugs such as the tricyclic secondary amines (despiramine [Norpramin, Pertofrane], protriptyline [Vivactil], and nortriptyline [Aventyl, Pamelor]) may be useful with the more withdrawn depressive with psychomotor retardation. Amitriptyline and imipramine are more likely to cause orthostatic hypotension than the secondary amines. Amitriptyline has the most potent anticholinergic effects, and desipramine, the least. The tricyclic dibenzoxazepine amoxapine [Asendin] is moderate in reference to both sedation and anticholinergic effects, but it can cause extrapyramidal symptoms. It may be useful in psychotic depression. "On the basis of differential side effects . . . desipramine and nortriptyline are the preferred cyclic antidepressants for older patients."[12]

The tetracyclic agent maprotiline [Ludiomil] has a high sedative effect and low anticholinergic properties. It usually does not cause orthostatic hypotension and has a low incidence of cardiovascular side effects. However, seizures have been reported with its use.[13] The triazolopyridine derivative trazodone [Desyrel] has minimal anticholinergic side effects. Although it has a relatively benign cardiac side effect profile,[14] it should be used with caution in patients with preexisting cardiac disease because of the possibility of cardiac toxicity. It is very sedating and can produce hypotension. Fluoxetine hydrochloride [Prozac], a stimulating antidepressant, has no measurable anticholinergic side effects.

Monoamine Oxidase Inhibitors (MAOIs). MAOIs, such as phenelzine sulfate [Nardil], are used at times for depressed patients who fail to respond or have medical contraindications to tricyclic antidepressants. They have also been used with atypical symptoms, such as hypochondriasis, phobia, anxiety, and irritability. Although they do not produce anticholinergic or cardiac side effects, orthostatic hypotension is common. MAOIs can be a problem, however, because they can trigger a hypertensive crisis or cerebrovascular accident if a tyramine-free diet is not maintained or if medications containing phenylethylamine are used. Elderly people may be more susceptible to these complications because of the presence of atherosclerotic vascular disease and decreased circulatory compliance.

Many foods and drugs that exhibit indirect sympathomimesis need to be avoided.

Dietary restrictions include red wine, fava (broad) beans, and all spoiled, decayed, overripe, old, aged, or fermented foods, especially proteins. Drug prohibitions include ephedrine, phenylephrine, and phenylpropanolamine (which may be found in cold or sinus medications), as well as some nasal sprays, suppositories, stimulants, and diet pills.[15] Reliable, compliant patients need to be chosen. If the patient adheres to the diet, side effects are limited to postural hypotension, insomnia, and weight gain.

Lithium Carbonate. Lithium is the treatment of choice for manic-depressive illness. It is also helpful in some forms of recurrent unipolar depression. It is rare for bipolar disorder to begin after age 65 years. However, since it can continue into later life, the bipolar population beyond this age can be substantial. Special precautions are needed when using lithium in elderly people. It is contraindicated in the medically impaired older patient. Lithium is almost exclusively excreted by the kidneys. The glomerular filtration rate decreases with advancing age. Renal disease can impair lithium excretion and may increase the risk of lithium-induced nephrotoxicity. Dementing illness may sensitize a patient to lithium-induced neurotoxicity and also decrease ability to comply with dosing schedules. Cardiovascular disease may make patients vulnerable to fluid and electrolyte alterations and may increase the risk of cardiotoxicity.[16]

Pretreatment workup should include a baseline ECG, thyroid profile, serum electrolytes, and BUN and creatinine concentrations.

Therapeutic serum levels for lithium are 0.6 to 1.2 mEq/L. In elderly people, "plasma-lithium levels of 0.6 to 0.7 mEq/L are often satisfactory for maintenance treatment and even for the treatment of some acute episodes. These levels are usually achieved with doses of 600 to 900 mg per day, although higher doses may be required for the more severe manic attacks."[11] Signs of lithium toxicity, indicating that the medication should be stopped, include persistent diarrhea, vomiting or severe nausea, coarse trembling of hands or legs, frequent muscle twitching, blurred vision, confusion, marked dizziness, slurred speech, difficulty in walking, and swelling of the feet or lower legs.

Lithium may be useful as an adjuvant to improve response to tricyclic antidepressants or MAO inhibitors.[17]

Combination Drug Therapy. A major affective disorder with psychotic features may require the combined use of antidepressant-antipsychotic drug therapy to control symptoms of agitation and delusions. Problems can arise if both drugs have anticholinergic effects. Perphenazine (Trilafon) and haloperidol (Haldol), which have low anticholinergic activity, may be helpful here.

Psychostimulants. The stimulants methylphenidate (Ritalin) and dextroamphetamine may be helpful with the apathetic, withdrawn, depressed elderly patient. They are used in the medically ill or postoperative older adult. "Therapeutic effects are usually achieved with daily doses of 20 to 40 mg of methylphenidate or 10 to 20 mg of dextroamphetamine, given orally in two divided doses, preferably 30 minutes before meals."[18] Methylphenidate may be used initially for 7 to 10 days to augment the action of the tricyclic antidepressants. These drugs should be given before 4 P.M. to avoid insomnia. Other problems include brief duration of action, rebound depression, development of tolerance, and side effects such as anorexia, hyperactivity, hypertension, and premature ventricular contractions.

Triazolobenzodiazepine. Alprazolam (Xanax) may be a viable choice in treating depression in elderly people, particularly in those who cannot tolerate other agents. It has been shown to have significantly fewer anticholinergic side effects than tricyclic antidepressants like imipramine.[19] Being free of cardiovascular side effects, it may be helpful with dysphoric patients with cardiac conduction disease.[8]

L-Triiodothyronine (T3). T3 can be an effective adjuvant potentiating tricyclic antidepressants in treatment-resistant patients. Goodwin and colleagues went so far as to suggest that a trial of a tricyclic should not be considered a failure until T3 potentiation has been tried.[20]

■ ELECTROCONVULSIVE THERAPY (ECT)

ECT is a treatment option in severe and psychotic depression, especially if the elderly patient is intolerant or resistant to antidepressant or other pharmacologic therapy. It may be the treatment of choice in the self-destructive, depressed older patient who is a suicidal risk or who refuses to eat. It is well tolerated in this age group. The procedure has become more humane. The use of anticholinergic premedication, short-acting barbiturates for anesthesia, muscle relaxants, low-energy stimulus wave forms, and unilateral stimulus electrode placements all have helped reduce the risks and side effects of ECT without diminishing its therapeutic efficacy.[21] Excellent results are often seen after six to eight treatments.

Contraindications to ECT include a recent myocardial infarction and a space-occupying lesion within the skull. The presence of an aortic aneurysm, recent fractures, or bone disease is not a strict contraindication if the patient is premedicated. ECT can be used in hypertension and orthostatic hypotension. Cardiac conduction disorders or other abnormal electrocardiographic changes are not contraindications, provided there is good cardiac reserve.

Memory loss following treatment continues to be an area of controversy. This is particularly relevant in the older patient with cognitive impairment. Unilateral ECT given through the nondominant hemisphere, usually the right, has been shown to cause less confusion and amnesia. Memory loss may still be a concern in older people with dementia. "However, in the elderly patient suffering from a life-threatening or disabling psychotic depressive disorder, such a risk must be balanced against the often clear, and sometimes dramatic, benefits of ECT."[22] "Its use among older persons without signs of irreversible dementing illness, however, should not produce long-term untoward effects."[23]

■ Issues and Risks

■ SUICIDE

Suicide is the most serious consequence of depression. It is a real possibility in elderly people. "Those older than age 65 account for 25 per cent of all suicides, although comprising only 12 per cent of the population. The suicide rate peaks for men between the ages of 80 and 90 and for women between 50 and 65."[24] "Predictors of suicide risk include age, male sex, widowed or divorced status, isolation, alcohol or drug abuse, and the presence of debilitating diseases."[25]

Evaluation of a depressed patient should always involve direct questioning about suicidal thoughts and previous threats or attempts. If you suspect that someone is thinking of committing suicide, be direct. Talking about suicide will not cause a person to commit suicide. Talking helps relieve a person's emotional pain. Show concern and urge the person to get help. Your caring and interest will help break down the sense of isolation and alter the cycle of depression and anger. Lastly, do something. It is better to be wrong than sorry. A patient's threatening suicide is a warning that should never be ignored.

To understand clearly and manage depression in elderly people, one must take a holistic approach. Biologic and physiologic correlates as well as psychologic and social factors must be considered in etiology and treatment. A multidisciplinary team approach needs to include medical and psychiatric representatives, social and community workers, and a support system made up of family and friends and other interested people. Consider the whole person and his or her individual needs and problems. "Older people . . . want the same thing they have always wanted, the same things that younger people want: affection, intimacy, love, tenderness, comforting and nurturing, sex, and above all relief from pain."[12] They are usually much appreciative of your help and attention. Be somewhat aggressive in your approach. Remember, depression in elderly people is treatable.

REFERENCES

1. Butler RN. Geriatric psychiatry. *In* Kaplan HI, Sadock BJ (eds). Comprehensive Textbook of Psychiatry. 4th ed. Baltimore: Williams & Wilkins, 1985:1953–1959.
2. Thomas P. Primary care: depressed elderly's best hope. Med World News, July 13, 1987:39–54.
3. Diagnostic and Statistical Manual of Mental Disorders. 3rd ed, revised. Washington, DC: American Psychiatric Association, 1987.
4. Jarvik LF. Depression: a review of drug therapy for elderly patients. Consultant 1982; 22:141–146.
5. Thienhaus OJ. Depression in the elderly: phenomenology and pharmacotherapy. Geriatr Med Today 1989; 8:34–45.
6. Zal M. Geriatric psychiatry: growing older in the 80's. Osteopath Ann 1983; 11:50–56.

7. Giannini AJ, Black HR, Goettsche RL. Psychiatric, Psychogenic, and Somatopsychic Disorders Handbook. New York: Medical Examination Publishing Company, 1978.

8. Goff DC, Jenike MA. Treatment-resistant depression in the elderly. J Am Geriatr Soc 1986; 34:63–69.

9. Jarvik LF, Mintz J, Stever J, et al. Treating geriatric depression. A 26 week interim analysis. J Am Geriatr Soc 1982; 30:713.

10. Lee PC. Drug therapy: avoiding the pitfalls. Geriatrics 1972:27–28.

11. DiGiacomo J, Prien R. Pharmacologic treatment of depression in the elderly. In Crook T, Cohen GD (eds). Physicians' Guide to the Diagnosis and Treatment of Depression in the Elderly. Madison, CT: Mark Powley Associates, Inc., 1983:39–51.

12. Berezin MA, Liptzin B, Salzman C. The elderly person. In Nicholi AM Jr (ed). The New Harvard Guide to Psychiatry. Cambridge, MA: The Belknap Press of Harvard University Press, 1988:665–679.

13. Dominiquez RA. Evaluating the effectiveness of the new antidepressants. Hosp Community Psychiatr 1983; 34:405–407.

14. Himmelhoch JM. Cardiovascular effects of trazodone in humans. J Clin Psychopharmacol 1981; 1:765.

15. Zisook S. A clinical overview of monoamine oxidase inhibitors. Psychosomatics 1985; 26:240–251.

16. Jenike MA. Depression in the Elderly: Diagnosis, Treatment and Management. Clinical Perspectives on Aging. Number 7 in a series, produced under an educational grant from Wyeth-Ayerst Laboratories, 1988:10–12.

17. Jefferson JW, Avd FJ. Combining lithium and antidepressants. J Clin Psychopharmacol 1983; 3:303.

18. Kaufman MW, Murray GB, Chassem NH. Use of psychostimulants in medically ill, depressed patients. Psychosomatics 1982; 23:817–819.

19. Weissman MM, Prusoff BA, Sholomskas AJ, Berry C. The pharmacologic treatment of the depressed elderly: a pilot study of alprazolam (Xanax), imipramine (Tofranil) or placebo. In Burrows GD, Norman TR, Maguire KP (eds). Biological Psychiatry: Recent Studies. London: John Libbey, 1984:167–174.

20. Goodwin FK, Prange AJ, Post RM, et al. Potentiation of antidepressant effects of L-triiodothyronine in tricyclic nonresponders. Am J Psychiatr 1982; 139:34–38.

21. Jenike MA. Electroconvulsive therapy: what are the facts? Geriatrics 1984; 38:33–38.

22. Fink M. Guidelines for electroconvulsive therapy in the elderly. In Crook T, Cohen GD (eds). Physician's Guide to the Diagnosis and Treatment of Depression in the Elderly. Madison, CT: Mark Powley Associates, Inc., 1983:55–59.

23. American Psychiatric Association Task Force on ECT. No. 14. Washington, DC: American Psychiatric Association, 1979.

24. Resnick H, Cantor J. Gerifacts. Geriatrics 1967; 22:68.

25. Avant R. Diagnosis and management of depression in the office setting. Fam Pract Recert 1983; 5(Suppl 1):41–48.

Diabetes mellitus in pregnancy

Donald R. Coustan

■ Introduction

Pre-existing diabetes mellitus complicates approximately three of every thousand pregnancies in the United States.[1] Prior to the discovery of insulin in 1921, diabetic pregnancies were accompanied by a maternal mortality rate of 30 per cent and a perinatal mortality rate of 65 per cent.[2] Maternal mortality rates plummeted once insulin became available; it is no longer necessary to warn young women with diabetes that if they get pregnant they will be "taking their life in their hands," with the exception of diabetic women who have previously suffered a myocardial infarction. Progress in the last quarter century has centered on the prevention of perinatal mortality and morbidity in such pregnancies. The result is that perinatal mortality rates are now reported to be well under 5 per cent in virtually all centers specializing in the management of pregnancy in such women.

Management of overt diabetes in pregnancy is best accomplished by a multidisciplinary team approach, in which various health care providers work together to help the woman with diabetes and her fetus achieve an optimal outcome. Such teams vary in composition but often consist of an obstetrician with expertise in maternal-fetal medicine, an internist with expertise in diabetes, a pediatrician with expertise in neonatology, nurse clinicians, diabetes nurse educators, social workers, nutritionists; ready access to specialists in nephrology, ophthalmology, neurology, cardiology, and so on, also is usually available. There are no hard-and-fast rules about who must be on the team and who should take primary responsibility, as various models have been successful.

A team approach provides optimal care, yet in some regions the relative paucity of women with diabetes who become pregnant prevents the formation of such a team, and long travel distances make it difficult for diabetic women to reach the nearest perinatal center. Physicians caring for patients in such areas must deal with the problems at hand. If the patient prefers to remain in her own locale for treatment, after careful counseling about the existence of such teams for high-risk care, the primary physician may undertake the management of the pregnancy, perhaps with telephone consultation from the nearest perinatal center. The details of management of diabetic pregnancy are beyond the scope of this chapter, and the reader is referred to a recent treatment of the subject.[3]

With the lowering of maternal and perinatal mortality rates, the most troubling problem remaining in diabetic pregnancy is the significantly increased incidence of congenital malformations in the offspring. Prevention of these malformations is possible for every practitioner who provides health care to women with diabetes; therefore that prevention shall be the focus of this article. No better opportunity is presently available for the prevention of disabling and sometimes fatal birth defects.

■ Background

Congenital malformations have long been known to occur with increased frequency in the offspring of diabetic mothers, with various series reporting incidences of 7 to 10 per cent, compared with 2 to 3 per cent in the general population. All types of anomalies are found, with the most common being cardiovascular, skeletal, and central nervous system problems and the most specific (but rare) being the caudal regression syndrome[4]

TABLE 1. Birth Defect Risk Among Infants of Diabetic Mothers and Gestational Age of Occurrence

Type of Birth Defect	Relative Risk*	Weeks Postovulation
Central nervous system	2	4
Cardiac	4	5–6
Caudal regression syndrome	252	3

*Compared with nondiabetic population.
(Adapted from Mills JL, Baker L, Goldman AS. Malformations in infants of diabetic mothers occur before the seventh gestational week: implications for treatment. Diabetes 1975; 11:23–29.)

(Table 1). Since, by tradition, prenatal care does not usually commence until after the second missed menstrual period (i.e., approximately 6 weeks postconception), the possible teratogenic influences responsible for the increased number of malformations among offspring of diabetic mothers have been very difficult to characterize, because of lack of opportunity to make observations about the metabolic milieu during human organogenesis. A number of recent developments have allowed a much greater understanding of potential causes of congenital malformations in diabetic pregnancy.

Although a genetic predisposition toward birth defects has been postulated, studies of the offspring of diabetic fathers (and nondiabetic mothers) show no increased frequency of malformations, which suggests that the intrauterine environment is in some way responsible.[5,6] Although there have been frequent speculations that insulin taken by the mother may be responsible for the observed birth defects, this appears highly unlikely. Animal data show that the direct application of insulin to the developing embryo is associated with malformations. However, exogenous insulin administered to the mother does not appear to cross the placenta to any appreciable extent.[7] It is also unlikely that fetal endogenous hyperinsulinemia is causally related, since insulin does not appear to be present in the fetal pancreas until approximately 9 weeks' menstrual age,[8] and the beta-cell mass in the pancreata of fetuses of diabetic mothers is not different from that of normal control fetuses until 16 to 20 weeks' gestation.[9]

Most recent attention has focused on the maternal metabolic milieu bathing the developing conceptus, with hyperglycemia, hypoglycemia, and hyperketonemia as leading contenders for causation of human birth defects. Studies using whole embryo tissue culture of the developing rodent fetus have demonstrated each of the aforementioned metabolic aberrations to be associated with developmental and structural disruptions,[10] and in vivo insulin replacement in the streptozotocin diabetic rat mother has been shown to prevent the development of congenital anomalies.[11,12] What has not been shown to date is exactly how "normal" the metabolic milieu must be, and whether there is any increase in anomalies when environmental hypoglycemia occurs.

The development of assays for glycosylated hemoglobin enabled clinical researchers to obtain a retrospective view of glucose control during the previous months. Because, as mentioned, pregnant women with diabetes are not usually available for observation during the period of organogenesis, the existence of such assays made it possible to correlate metabolic events during the first 2 months of gestation with the development of congenital malformations in human offspring. In the first report of this relationship, a British group noted an association between high glycosylated hemoglobin levels in early pregnancy and congenital malformations in the offspring of diabetic mothers.[13] Three of the five diabetic women with hemoglobin A_1 levels above 12 per cent in the first trimester later gave birth to babies with lethal congenital malformations. In a later, larger retrospective review, the group at the Joslin Clinic reported a strong association between elevated hemoglobin A_{1c} levels in the first trimester and major congenital malformations,[14] as shown in Table 2. Similar studies from other parts of the world followed, and

TABLE 2. Association of Birth Defects and Hemoglobin A_{1c} Levels

First Trimester HbA$_{1c}$ (%)	N	Number with Anomalies	Per Cent*
<8.6	58	2	3.4
≥8.6	58	13	22.4

*p<0.01.
(Data from Miller E, Hare JW, Cloherty JP, et al. Elevated maternal hemoglobin A_{1c} in early pregnancy and major congenital anomalies in infants of diabetic mothers. N Engl J Med 1981; 304:1331–1334.)

it soon became apparent that improvement of metabolic control around the time of conception might offer the chance to reduce the likelihood of congenital malformations.

In the late 1970s, the group at Karlsberg in the German Democratic Republic began a program to enroll women with diabetes prior to, or during the early weeks of, pregnancy in order to normalize metabolic control. Their experience, published in the mid-1980s, showed that early intensification of diabetic control was associated with a major malformation rate of 1.1 per cent in 185 diabetic pregnancies, compared with a rate of 6.6 per cent in the pregnancies of 473 diabetic women who enrolled for care after the eighth week of gestation.[15] Similar results have subsequently been reported from Israel,[16] and similar studies are currently under way in various parts of the world.

Recently, the results of the Diabetes in Early Pregnancy (DIEP) study were reported.[17] In this multicentered observational study, women with overt diabetes and normal control subjects were enrolled prior to or during very early pregnancy, and data were collected on glucose and glycosylated hemoglobin levels throughout the first trimester. A second control group of diabetic women who were enrolled after the 21st postconceptional day (5 weeks' gestational age) was also included. All subjects with diabetes were given equipment and instructions for self blood glucose monitoring four or more times per day; weekly measurements of glycosylated hemoglobin and various metabolites were made. Management of the diabetes and the pregnancy was undertaken by the patient's own health care team, and no specific goals for metabolic control were promulgated. This was to be a strictly observational study. The 389 individuals in the normal control group manifested a major malformation rate of 2.1 per cent, compared with 4.9 per cent for the 347 early-entry diabetic women and 9.0 per cent for the 279 late-entry diabetic women.

Because there was no apparent relationship between maternal glucose levels or glycosylated hemoglobin levels during organogenesis and congenital anomalies, the title of the article raised concern that early glycemic control might not be as important as previously believed. However, it is important to point out that the group of subjects investigated had neither excellent nor exceedingly poor metabolic control, since 90 per cent had a mean glucose value in the first trimester of between 140 and 235 mg/dl. Had a larger group of patients with excellent metabolic control (mean values below 120 mg/dl) and with very poor control been studied, a clearer relationship might have emerged. Most important, this study demonstrated that early enrollment, preferably preconception, with frequent metabolic monitoring was associated with a roughly 50 per cent reduction in the likelihood of congenital abnormalities. Similarly reassuring was the finding of no association between maternal hypoglycemia during organogenesis and congenital abnormalities.

A second report from the DIEP Study showed similar spontaneous abortion rates among early-entry diabetic subjects and controls.[18] However, there was a marked increase in the spontaneous abortion rate when glycosylated hemoglobin levels exceeded 7 to 9 standard deviations above the mean for normal pregnant women, suggesting that there might be a continuum of poor control, with mild degrees leading to congenital malformations and more severe degrees associated with spontaneous abortion. The reports of the DIEP Study can best be viewed as supporting the concept of prepregnancy counseling and metabolic control while leaving open the questions of how normal control must be in order to reduce risks and whether glucose is the only important variable to be considered.

▪ Management

Every health care provider seeing female patients with diabetes should be aware of the background just discussed. Primary caregivers have a unique opportunity to prevent congenital malformations but can take advantage of this only if they counsel their patients *before* conception takes place. This means that every woman with diabetes who is old enough to menstruate must be counseled about diabetic pregnancy and informed of the importance of conception being planned, not accidental. Appropriate contraceptive advice should be offered. Informational materials are available,[19] and should be recommended to patients prior to pregnancy.

■ COUNSELING

Ideally, counseling about diabetic pregnancy should begin at the time of puberty for adolescent girls with diabetes. Many adolescents become pregnant, apparently without plan, often out of ignorance about reproductive function. This is doubly tragic if the patient has diabetes, because the fetus in such pregnancies is much more likely to suffer from a congenital anomaly, since maternal periconceptional metabolic control is unlikely to be optimal. Our patients need to know about the increased risk of birth defects and about ways of increasing the likelihood of having a healthy baby, because organogenesis occurs so early in pregnancy that improving control after conception is too late to prevent anomalies. When a woman with diabetes conceives without benefit of prepregnancy counseling, we have lost an unparalleled opportunity to prevent human suffering.

■ METABOLIC CONTROL

If a particular individual with type I diabetes desires to conceive, the health care provider should begin to work with her to achieve good metabolic control. Although controversy exists as to the most appropriate goals for metabolic control during the periconceptional period, it is clear that "near-normalization" is better than poor metabolic control. In our center, we consider an appropriate goal to be the achievement of circulating glucose values generally below 150 mg/dl during the prepregnancy period. If a particular patient is not "brittle," and glucose values similar to those strived for during pregnancy (50 to 120 mg/dl) can be easily achieved prior to conception, so much the better. If a particular health care provider is uncomfortable with such a responsibility or does not have the necessary time to devote to it, the patient may be referred to a center specializing in high-risk pregnancy care at this point.

To assess metabolic control prior to pregnancy, it is necessary for every individual with type I diabetes to learn self glucose monitoring.[20] A number of different meters are available, and it is also possible to use visual inspection of glucose strips without the aid of a reflectance meter. A number of different schedules are available for self glucose monitoring. In our center we ask patients to check their glucose level prior to breakfast each morning and approximately 2 hours after each meal. Other proposed schedules include fasting and 1-hour postprandial values and premeal values throughout the day. All have their proponents and all seem to be successful when used consistently. Close telephone contact with the physician or diabetes nurse clinician helps the patient learn how to improve her metabolic control. One extremely helpful recent advance in maintaining good metabolic control is the availability of meters with a memory chip, which allows verification of all self glucose monitoring values.[21]

Most individuals with type I diabetes will require multiple-dose insulin regimens to achieve near-normalization. The regimen we use as a starting point is the mixed, split-dose approach, in which a combination of intermediate-acting and short-acting insulins is administered approximately 30 minutes before breakfast and before dinner.[22] The total morning dose is twice the total evening dose. The ratio of intermediate to short-acting insulins is 2:1 in the morning and 1:1 in the evening. Adjustments in the individual components are then made in response to glucose levels at the appropriate time of day. For example, if the 2-hour postbreakfast glucose level is above the goal, the morning dose of short-acting insulin is increased the next day. If the 2-hour postlunch level is high, the morning intermediate-acting insulin is adjusted. If the fasting glucose is outside the planned range, the predinner intermediate-acting insulin is adjusted. Many diabetic individuals will require the splitting of their evening insulin into predinner short-acting doses and bedtime intermediate-acting doses, in order for enough insulin to be present in the circulation by the time of awakening the next morning to avoid fasting hyperglycemia.

The aforementioned insulin regimen is only one of many that have been proposed. Others, including short-acting insulin before each meal, with intermediate-acting insulin in the morning and/or at bedtime, and the use of continuous subcutaneous insulin infusion pumps,[23] have been equally successful. What is generally not successful is the use of a single injection of intermediate-acting insulin each morning. Such a regimen may appear to be successful if circulating glucose levels are measured only in the afternoon, when absorption of intermediate-acting insulin is at its peak, but glucose levels at other times of the day are bound to be high if measured.

Once the patient has demonstrated glucose values in or near the desired range, glycosylated hemoglobin measurement should be performed to confirm that prepregnancy control is adequate. Values below the upper limit of normal for nondiabetic individuals are most desirable, and when such levels are achieved the patient can be advised to try to conceive.

■ CONTRACEPTION

Individuals with diabetes who do not desire pregnancy should be offered options for contraception if they are sexually active. Even if a diabetic female is not currently sexually active, the choices should be outlined and instructions given to return for contraceptive advice when commencement of sexual activity is contemplated. Obviously, abstention from sexual intercourse is the only absolutely effective contraception. However, in modern society many individuals are not willing to practice celibacy, and the health care provider has an obligation to inform patients about their choices.

Oral contraceptives are highly effective, but carry the risk of vascular complications, which many diabetologists believe can compound the vascular problems that may occur with long-standing type I diabetes. In addition, combined oral contraceptives apparently can interfere with diabetic control, although much less so now that lower-dose pills are available. While not absolutely contraindicated in diabetic individuals, oral contraceptives should be prescribed only when close monitoring of glucose levels and blood pressure is planned.

The diaphragm, if used correctly and faithfully, is approximately 95 per cent successful in preventing pregnancy. Although some couples find that diaphragm use is intrusive, it is an ideal method for many diabetic individuals, since it carries no particular medical risks. Condoms and foam are similarly free of medical risks but appear to be somewhat less effective than diaphragms. The intrauterine contraceptive device (IUCD), available again in the United States, has the advantage of being relatively "maintenance-free," that is, it is effective without any effort on the part of the couple. There does appear to be a higher rate of pelvic infection with IUCD use compared with other types of contraception, but this risk may be considered acceptable by some couples. Some data, based upon very small numbers, suggest an increased failure rate for IUCDs in diabetic women,[24] whereas others have reported more favorable results.[25] Variations on the rhythm method are also commonly utilized, but are considerably less effective. The choice of method is up to the particular couple involved, but every provider who cares for women with diabetes has an obligation to explore this topic with them.

Currently, the high rate of congenital malformations is the most disturbing problem confronting diabetic pregnancy. It is within the capability of primary health care providers to reduce this risk considerably and does not require anything more than the communication of information and the utilization of currently available techniques for improving metabolic control. This is truly the challenge of the 90s.

REFERENCES

1. US Department of Health and Human Services, Public Health Service, Centers for Disease Control, Center for Prevention Services, Division of Diabetes Control. Public Health Guidelines for Enhancing Diabetes Control through Maternal and Child Health Programs. Atlanta: 1986.
2. Williams JW. The clinical significance of glycosuria in pregnant women. Am J Med Sci 1909; 137:1–4.
3. Reece EA, Coustan DR (eds). Diabetes Mellitus in Pregnancy: Principles and Practice. New York: Churchill Livingstone, 1988.
4. Mills JL, Baker L, Goldman AS. Malformations in infants of diabetic mothers occur before the seventh gestational week: implications for treatment. Diabetes 1979; 28:292–293.
5. Chung CS, Myrianthopoulos NC: Factors affecting risks of congenital malformations. II. Effect of maternal diabetes on congenital malformations. Birth Defects 1975; 11:23–29.
6. Comess LJ, Bennett PH, Burch TA, Miller ML. Congenital anomalies and diabetes in the Pima Indians of Arizona. Diabetes 1969; 18:471–478.
7. Adam P, Teramo K, Raiha N, Gitlin D, Schwartz R. Human fetal insulin metabolism early in gestation. Diabetes 1969; 18:409–415.
8. Stefan Y, Grasso S, Perrelet A, Orci L. A quantitative immunofluorescent study of the endocrine cell populations in the developing human pancreas. Diabetes 1983; 32:293–301.
9. Reiher H, Fuhrmann K, Noack S, et al. Age-dependent insulin secretion of the endocrine pancreas in vitro from fetuses of diabetic and nondiabetic patients. Diabetes Care 1983; 6:446–451.

10. Freinkel N. Diabetic embryopathy and fuel-mediated organ teratogenesis: lessons from animal models. Horm Metab Res 1988; 20:463–475.
11. Baker L, Egler JM, Klein SH, Goldman AS. Meticulous control of diabetes during organogenesis prevents congenital lumbosacral defects in rats. Diabetes 1981; 30:955–959.
12. Eriksson UJ, Dahlstrom E, Hellerstrom C. Diabetes in pregnancy: skeletal malformations in the offspring of diabetic rats after intermittent withdrawal of insulin in early gestation. Diabetes 1983; 32:1141–1145.
13. Leslie RDG, Pyke DA, John PN, White JM. Hemoglobin A_1 in diabetic pregnancy. Lancet 1978; 2:958–959.
14. Miller E, Hare JW, Cloherty JP, et al. Elevated maternal hemoglobin A_{1c} in early pregnancy and major congenital anomalies in infants of diabetic mothers. N Engl J Med 1981; 304:1331–1334.
15. Fuhrmann K, Reiher H, Semmler K, Glockner E. The effect of intensified conventional insulin therapy before and during pregnancy on the malformation rate in offspring of diabetic mothers. Exp Clin Endocrinol 1984; 83:173–177.
16. Goldman JA, Dicker D, Feldberg D, Yeshaya A, Samuel N, Karp M. Pregnancy outcome in patients with insulin-dependent diabetes mellitus with preconceptional diabetic control: a comparative study. Am J Obstet Gynecol 1986; 155:293–297.
17. Mills JL, Knopp RH, Simpson JL, et al. Lack of relation of increased malformation rates in infants of diabetic mothers to glycemic control during organogenesis. N Engl J Med 1988; 318:671–676.
18. Mills JL, Simpson JL, Driscoll SG, et al. Incidence of spontaneous abortion among normal women and insulin-dependent diabetic women whose pregnancies were identified within 21 days of conception. N Engl J Med 1988; 319:1617–1623.
19. American Diabetes Association. Diabetes and Pregnancy: What to Expect. Washington: American Diabetes Association, Inc., 1989.
20. Consensus Development Panel, American Diabetes Association, Centers for Disease Control, Food and Drug Administration, National Institute of Diabetes and Digestive and Kidney Diseases. Consensus statement on self-monitoring of blood glucose. Diabetes Care 1987; 10:95–99.
21. Langer O, Mazze RS. Diabetes in pregnancy: evaluating self-monitoring performance and glycemic control with memory-based reflectance meters. Am J Obstet Gynecol 1986; 155:635–637.
22. Lewis SP, Murray WK, Wallin JD, et al. Improved glucose control in nonhospitalized pregnant diabetic patients. Obstet Gynecol 1976; 48:260–267.
23. Coustan DR, Reece EA, Sherwin RS, et al. A randomized clinical trial of the insulin pump vs. intensive conventional therapy in pregnant diabetics. JAMA 1986; 255:631–636.
24. Gosden C, Ross A, Steel J, Springbett A. Intrauterine contraceptive devices in diabetic women. Lancet 1982; 1:530–535.
25. Skouby SO, Molsted-Pedersen L. Intrauterine contraceptive devices for diabetics. Lancet 1982; 1:968–970.

Diabetes mellitus in the surgical patient

David S. Schade

■ Background

Surgical treatment of the diabetic patient is common, not only because diabetic patients are living longer but also because diabetes predisposes to conditions requiring surgical intervention. It has been estimated that 50 per cent of all diabetic patients will undergo major surgery during their lifetime.[1] Unfortunately, the diabetic patient is at greater risk during surgery not only because of the propensity for metabolic decompensation but also because underlying complications of diabetes, such as atherosclerosis, may enhance postoperative morbidity and mortality.

Many perioperative regimens for treating diabetic patients have been published.[2-14] Most of these studies separate diabetes into three categories: (1) the type II diabetic patient, well controlled on diet alone; (2) the type II diabetic patient requiring sulfonylurea or insulin therapy; and (3) the type I diabetic patient. Most authorities do not give insulin to the first category of patients if the surgery is minor and no concurrent stress is present.[3,7] There is no consensus on how to treat the second category, and the third category always is treated with intravenous or subcutaneous short- or long-acting insulin. The primary reason for this lack of consensus on therapy is the lack of controlled investigative studies involving sufficiently large numbers of patients to demonstrate an improved outcome. Furthermore, it is not even clear what end-points for improvement should be measured: for example, length of hospital stay, cost of hospitalization, surgical complication rate, duration of

This work was supported by National Institutes of Health Grants 5-MO1, RR-997-05, 5-RO1 AM-31973-02, IP50-11327-08, and Research Allocation 8007 and is adapted from David S. Schade, Surgery and Diabetes, Med Clin North Am, 1988; 72:1531–1543, copyright W. B. Saunders Company.

intensive care, to cite just a few possibilities. All agree that blood glucose concentration must be measured (directly or indirectly) in order to regulate the insulin dose and to avoid hypo- and hyperglycemia.

The tendency for diabetic patients to develop hyperglycemia during acute illness, necessitating surgery, may be caused by several mechanisms, including increased glucose production, decreased tissue glucose utilization, and decreased renal clearance of glucose [Figure 1]. Overproduction of glucose is probably the most important pathogenic mechanism. The detrimental effects of hyperglycemia are secondary to the osmotic activity of glucose, which causes water shifts between body compartments and induces an osmotic diuresis. The water shifts occur because water moves freely throughout the body tissues, whereas glucose transport across cellular membranes depends on multiple factors, particularly insulin. Significant osmotic diuresis occurs whenever the plasma glucose concentration exceeds the patient's renal glucose threshold (approximately 180 to 250 mg/dl). An osmotic diuresis induces a loss of water, resulting in dehydration. Multiple ions are excreted with the water (sodium, potassium, chloride, magnesium, and phosphate), which may have detrimental effects on vascular volume and cellular function.

The term *ketone bodies* commonly refers to three different but related molecules: acetone, acetoacetic acid, and beta-hydroxybutyric acid.[15] Acetoacetic acid and beta-hydroxybutyric acid are not toxic per se but induce harmful effects by their dissociation (ionization) at physiologic pH (that is, 7.4) into hydrogen ions and the anions acetoacetate and beta-hydroxybutyrate. If allowed to accumulate, the hydrogen ions lower the blood pH, resulting in systemic acidosis that eventually induces cardiovascular collapse (Figure 1).

Several factors in the perioperative period

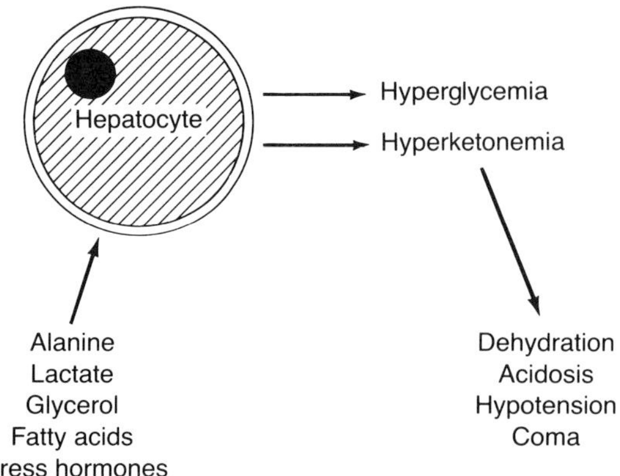

Figure 1. Consequences of insulin deficiency in the diabetic patient. The stress of surgery inevitably enhances hepatic glucose and ketone production, which will require additional insulin to suppress. An intravenous infusion of insulin is the simplest method of preventing metabolic decompensation.

predispose the diabetic patient to metabolic decompensation, including (1) absolute or relative insulin deficiency, (2) stress hormone excess, (3) fasting, and (4) dehydration.[16] During periods of stress, nondiabetic individuals increase basal insulin secretion to counteract the insulin resistance produced by the effects of stress hormones. In the diabetic patient, insulin resistance also occurs, which must be counteracted by appropriate adjustment of the insulin dose. Because all individuals respond differently to the stress of surgery, it is not feasible to prescribe a specific change in dosage. For this reason, the diabetic patient's glucose must be monitored frequently, preferably by capillary blood glucose measuring techniques. Furthermore, because intermediate- or long-acting insulin (lente, neutral protamine Hagedorn, or ultralente) cannot be adjusted rapidly for acute changes in insulin sensitivity, their use during the perioperative period is discouraged.

Major stress induces the secretion of stress hormones (glucagon, epinephrine, norepinephrine, cortisol, and growth hormone) that counteract the effects of circulating insulin. The mechanism(s) whereby the secretion of these hormones increases undoubtedly is complex, involving not only changes in circulating substrates but also central nervous system mediation. Fever, which is not uncommon during the postoperative period, has been studied in detail, and secretion of the stress hormones precedes the rise in blood glucose and ketone body concentra-

tion.[17] Even in nondiabetic humans, the synergistic effects of the stress hormones may induce hyperglycemia.[18] Because these hormones may change rapidly in concentration, frequent changes in insulin dosage may be needed to maintain the diabetic patient in metabolic balance.

To prevent aspiration, patients usually are fasted for at least 8 hours prior to surgery. Because certain tissues cannot utilize fatty acids for energy (for example, central nervous system, red blood cells, and adrenal medulla), a decrease in enteral glucose results in stimulation of endogenous production of glucose by glycogenolysis or gluconeogenesis or both and mobilization of fatty acids from adipose tissue to enhance hepatic ketone body production and provide tissues with an alternative energy source. A relative deficiency of insulin decreases the peripheral utilization of ketone bodies, further increasing their plasma concentration. Thus, fasting sets the stage for the development of ketoacidosis.

Dehydration almost invariably occurs during stress-induced hyperglycemia. The sites of fluid loss are multiple, although the kidney is the most important, and attempts must be made to reduce the loss as much as possible. Fluid losses cause cellular dehydration, which may alter cerebral function. Massive loss of sodium results in intravascular contraction, with consequent decreased cardiac output and diminished glomerular filtration (prerenal azotemia). Although this kidney dysfunction eventually results in oliguria and thus restricts the loss of water, the net consequence is a further increase in glycemia because large quantities of glucose no longer can be excreted by the kidney. In fact, in the well-hydrated patient with intact renal function it is almost impossible to induce severe, prolonged hyperglycemia (blood glucose greater than 350 mg/dl), even with severe insulin deficiency, because the kidney acts as a major site of glucose disposal. Dehydration also is accompanied by stress hormone secretion, which in turn exacerbates the metabolic disturbance.[19]

■ Management

Although much has been written on the perioperative care of the diabetic patient, no consensus exists. The reasons for this are multiple. First, recent advances in glucose monitoring technology and fluid infusion pumps have outdated previous therapeutic approaches. Second, diabetic patients undergo many types of surgery, and one perioperative approach may not be appropriate for different types of operations. Third, diabetic patients are a heterogeneous group, and different subgroups may need different perioperative care. Fourth, the resources available for perioperative diabetic care may vary greatly from the large urban hospital to the small rural hospital. And, fifth, the financial resources of the patient may dictate a minimum duration of hospitalization. This chapter offers a reasonable compromise that is suitable for the majority of diabetic patients.

Should insulin be administered subcutaneously, intravenously, or perhaps not at all in some type II diabetic patients? There is no single answer to this question, but three points must be considered. First, all diabetic patients are characterized by at least relative insulin deficiency, even when not undergoing surgery. Second, anesthesia and surgery are a stress that increases the insulin requirements in all patients. Third, there is no proven method to predict a priori whether an individual diabetic patient will require insulin during surgery. For this reason, a safe approach is to plan to give insulin to all patients (except the diet-controlled type II patient) based on a sliding scale such as that shown in Table 1. The route of insulin administration (subcutaneously or intravenously) in the type II diabetic patient probably is a matter of preference. The intravenous approach is easier and more predictable, although some investigators have used subcutaneous insulin successfully. In the type I diabetic patient, intravenous insulin clearly is the route of choice. Of more importance than the route of insulin delivery is the necessity to monitor blood glucose frequently, to enable appropriate adjustment of the insulin dose.

The blood glucose concentration ideally should remain within a specified narrow range throughout surgery, because hypoglycemia can be hazardous and hyperglycemia may inhibit normal leukocyte function and wound healing. Unfortunately, this goal rarely is achieved for several reasons. First, most operating rooms do not have the equipment (such as a closed-loop insulin infusion system) or the personnel to operate feedback intravenous blood glucose–regulating equip-

TABLE 1. Appropriate Intravenous Insulin Infusion Rate to Maintain Metabolic Homeostasis

Patient A:	Patient B:
Thin	Obese
Minimum illness, minimum surgery	Severe illness, major surgery
Usual insulin requirement < 50 U/day	Usual insulin requirement > 50 U/day
Infusion fluid: 1 L sodium chloride (0.45 mol/L) plus 20 mEq/L potassium chloride plus 500 U heparin* plus 50 U rapid-acting insulin.	Infusion fluid: 1 L sodium chloride (0.45 mol/L) plus 20 mEq/L potassium chloride plus 500 U heparin* plus 100 U rapid-acting insulin.

Blood Glucose Concentration (mg/dl)	Infusion Rate (ml/hr)	Pt. A Insulin (U/hr)	Pt. B Insulin (U/hr)
0–50	5	0.25	0.50
50–100	10	0.50	1.00
100–150	15	0.75	1.50
150–200	20	1.00	2.00
200–250	25	1.25	2.50
250–300	30	1.50	3.00
300–350	35	1.75	3.50
350–400	40	2.00	4.00
> 400	50	3.00	6.00

Insulin always should be delivered by a reliable self-regulating fluid pump; for example, an IVAC or IMED.

Blood glucose should be measured by finger prick and BG Chemstrips (Boehringer Mannheim, Indianapolis, IN) or Dextrostix (Miles Laboratories, Elkhart, IN)) every 1 to 2 hours to readjust the insulin infusion rate.

We do not add protein or blood to the fluid to prevent adsorption of insulin to the bottle or tubing because we have found this unnecessary. We do, however, discard approximately 20 ml of the insulin solution prior to infusing it into the patient to block the insulin adsorption sites on the plastic tubing.

*Does not anticoagulate the patient but does maintain the intravenous line patent.

ment. Second, preparation of the diabetic patient may be less than optimal, either because of an emergency condition (trauma, acute abdomen, and so on) or because the patient does not have the resources to afford a hospital day prior to surgery. Third, capillary blood glucose monitoring has been adopted only recently for general use by medical specialties other than internal medicine.

The widespread availability during the past several years of capillary blood glucose monitoring has greatly simplified the perioperative management of the diabetic patient. Not only can blood glucose values be obtained within minutes at the patient's bedside, but also the cost of the measurement (compared with the clinical laboratory) has been reduced significantly. Although not essential, the use of a glucose meter to read the glucose oxidase strips is recommended for two reasons: (1) the meter removes bias by medical personnel and corrects any visual deficiencies (such as color blindness) that may be present; and (2) the newer meters automatically record the time and date of the glucose reading so there is no doubt about the patient's preoperative glucose status. These machines can be downloaded to a personal computer, which provides a permanent record of the patient's perioperative glucose control.

Because capillary blood glucose monitoring is available so readily, there is no reason not to monitor the patient's blood glucose concentration frequently before, during, and after surgery. The frequency depends on the stability of the patient and the current blood glucose level. However, a reasonable maintenance rate would be a minimum of once per hour for several hours prior to and several hours after surgery. If the patient is a brittle diabetic patient, this may have to be increased to every 30 minutes.

The lack of morbidity and mortality data demonstrating the superiority of one therapeutic approach versus another in preparing a patient for surgery favors the most simple and least demanding approach. A single approach can be utilized for all diabetic patients undergoing surgery, eliminating the need for different approaches for type I versus type II diabetes, single versus complex surgeries, emergencies versus elective surgeries, and so forth (see Table 1).

Several general principles simplify the care of the patient undergoing surgery (Table 2). First, all diabetic patients should

TABLE 2. Treating the Diabetic Patient During Acute Surgery

Admit the patient to the hospital 24 to 48 hours prior to surgery to ensure metabolic stabilization.

Prolonged glucose concentrations above 250 mg/dl must be prevented by administration of short-acting (regular) insulin (preferably intravenously).

Urinary ketone bodies in the ill diabetic patient indicate that additional insulin is needed, and carbohydrate may have to be ingested to permit insulin to be safely administered.

In the ill diabetic patient, the following parameters must be monitored: (1) weight, (2) mental function, (3) respiratory rate, (4) pulse, (5) temperature, (6) glucose, (7) urine ketone bodies, (8) insulin dose, (9) oral intake, (10) electrolytes, (11) renal and hepatic function, and (12) electrocardiogram.

All diabetic patients should be in good metabolic balance prior to surgery.

At least 12 hours should elapse between food intake and surgery in the diabetic patient.

The best index of fluid status in the surgical diabetic patient is the patient's stable preoperative weight.

Capillary blood glucose monitoring should be routine in the preoperative, operative, and postoperative periods.

be in good metabolic balance prior to surgery. Good metabolic balance means normal vital signs and electrolytes (sodium, potassium, chloride, and carbon dioxide) and a blood glucose concentration of between 100 and 200 mg/dl. A chemistry profile always should be obtained to assess renal and hepatic function, because abnormalities in either of these two systems will alter fluid therapy in the perioperative period. A preoperative electrocardiogram is essential in all adult diabetic patients, because of the increased prevalence of atherosclerosis in diabetes. Patients should be stabilized preoperatively because significant metabolic deterioration takes longer when starting at normality. Although this approach has been emphasized by Alberti and Thomas,[3] patients undergoing surgery are usually hyperglycemic immediately before and during surgery. The easiest approach to achieving normal metabolism is to admit the patient to the hospital the day before surgery and to discontinue all intermediate- and long-acting insulins and oral antidiabetic agents (chlorpropamide should be discontinued at least 36 hours before surgery because of its very long half-life). After admission, the patient is placed on a sliding scale, using intravenous insulin as outlined in Table 1 with appropriate adjustments individualized to the patient. The disadvantage of this approach (that the patient is admitted 1 day before surgery) is offset by the improved safety and ease of diabetic control that result.

A second general principle relative to surgery in the diabetic patient is the timing of food ingestion. The standard procedure for most patients undergoing surgery usually is no food or drink after midnight; however, this may not be appropriate for the diabetic patient. At least 12 hours should elapse between food intake and surgery in the diabetic patient. The reason for this approach is that the diabetic patient may have undiagnosed gastroparesis that may prolong retention of food in the stomach, increasing the danger of aspiration pneumonia during anesthesia induction. Obviously, if the diabetic patient is continued on long-acting insulin or oral hypoglycemic agents prior to surgery, a 12-hour fast may induce hypoglycemia. Thus discontinuation of these agents and initiation of intravenous insulin, utilizing a sliding scale (with intravenous glucose as needed for hypoglycemia), is the approach of choice (see Table 1). Another advantage of using intravenous insulin is to permit continued metabolic control of the diabetic patient, even if the surgery is delayed. This is a rather frequent event, because the start of surgery can be altered by several unanticipated factors. When an intravenous insulin infusion is used to maintain homeostasis, no major changes in diabetic management are needed during an unanticipated delay.

It is emphasized that the approach outlined in Table 1 necessitates frequent blood glucose monitoring (every 1 to 2 hours) to adjust the insulin infusion rate. Furthermore, in those patients with relatively low blood glucose levels (less than 100 mg/dl) it may be necessary to add glucose to the intravenous fluid regimen (10 gm/hr). Blood glucose is measured at least every hour throughout the operation and postsurgery, until the patient has left the recovery room. If this is done, severe hyperglycemia or hypoglycemia never should be encountered.

■ MANAGEMENT DURING ROUTINE SURGERY

As discussed, many "successful" regimens can be used to treat the diabetic patient undergoing surgery. These range from giving one half the dose of subcutaneous insulin on the day of surgery to the continuous intravenous infusion of insulin, glucose, and potassium. The latter regimen makes physiologic sense and has been used successfully by Husband and colleagues.[8] The theory upon which this approach is based is that by supplying glucose, the need for protein catabolism to meet gluconeogenic needs in the diabetic patient is reduced, and a less negative nitrogen balance results. In our experience, infusion of this solution (from one bottle) does not permit variation in the glucose-to-insulin infusion rate, and we therefore infuse glucose and insulin separately, using different infusion pumps. We recommend that blood glucose concentration be monitored every hour during surgery (by use of glucose reagent strips). A recent review encourages the anesthesiologist to monitor blood glucose by the fingerstick method rather than by sending the blood to the clinical laboratory and encountering a long delay.[20] Thus, no changes need to be made in the preoperative regimen until the patient returns from the recovery room, when the caloric needs must be considered. Depending on the nature of the surgery, this may range from a clear liquid diet to total parenteral nutrition. A fixed intravenous dose of insulin is not recommended during surgery, because the development of hypoglycemia or hyperglycemia is possible.

The most difficult aspect of perioperative diabetic care undoubtedly is correct fluid management, because compromised renal function and cardiovascular insufficiency (manifested by angina or congestive heart failure) are common in diabetic patients. The best index of fluid status in the surgical diabetic patient is the patient's stable, preoperative weight. Thus, daily weight measurements are a necessity in all diabetic patients undergoing surgery, even if a bed scale must be used. Other indices of hydration—for example, dry skin and dry mucous membranes—and records of fluid intake and output are not nearly as reliable as the patient's weight.

The fluid regimen must be individualized to the patient. For minor surgery in which the patient is ingesting fluid orally within hours afterward, 5 per cent glucose in 0.45 M sodium chloride (D5/0.5NS) is acceptable at 100 ml/hr postoperatively. In contrast, for the diabetic patient who undergoes abdominal surgery and will not be ingesting fluid for several days, a more variable regimen is needed. In this patient, serum electrolytes must be measured at least daily and more often if potassium abnormalities are present. In general, 2 to 3 liters of fluid (that is, approximately 100 ml/hr) should be infused to replace insensible losses and to provide a urine output of at least 40 ml/hr. Obviously, additional fluid also may be needed if nasogastric suction or wound drainage is significant. Furthermore, sufficient glucose must be given to prevent ketosis (approximately 150 gm/day). This amount of carbohydrate can be provided by having all intravenous fluids contain 5 per cent glucose. Thus, a patient who receives 3 liters of fluid per day also will receive 150 gm of glucose. It should be remembered that "free" water is lost in the urine, so that hypotonic fluids (that is, relative to sodium) are indicated. An acceptable (and easy) fluid regimen in the diabetic patient is to alternate 1 liter of 5 per cent dextrose in water (D5W) with 1 liter of D5/0.5N saline, remembering to add 10 to 20 mEq of potassium chloride to each liter of fluid infused. This regimen will maintain a diabetic patient in balance for several days if intravenous insulin also is infused according to Table 1.

■ MANAGEMENT DURING EMERGENCY SURGERY

Infrequently, the diabetic patient may require emergency surgery.[9] If he or she is in metabolic balance upon admission (for example, after an automobile accident), the same rules apply as if the patient were admitted for surgery electively; that is, all subcutaneous insulin is discontinued, and an intravenous insulin infusion is begun. It must be remembered, however, that the patient probably has already injected the insulin dose for that day, and hypoglycemia may occur. Thus, not only should an insulin infusion be begun, but also intravenous glucose may be required if the blood glucose concentration is less than 100 mg/dl. An acute method to administer glucose to the hypoglycemic patient is to rapidly give 10 ml of 50 per cent glucose intravenously and to repeat as necessary. This solution is available commercially and is available routinely in all emergency rooms. Blood glucose concentration will increase transiently approximately 50 mg/dl after this dosage.

Emergency surgery may need to be performed in the unstable diabetic patient admitted in diabetic ketoacidosis with an abdominal catastrophe, for example, a ruptured appendix. In this condition, aggressive fluid and insulin administration must be begun immediately, utilizing standardized therapy for diabetic ketoacidosis. An indepth discussion of the pathogenesis and treatment of this condition is beyond the scope of this chapter. The reader is referred to several recent monographs on the subject.[17,21] However, it may be advisable that the patient's physician accompany the patient to the operating room and make the therapeutic decisions during surgery regarding the patient's metabolic state. Because of the complexity of the patient's condition, a team approach is required, and the patient's physician must assume responsibility for the patient's metabolic condition. Consultation with an endocrinologist or diabetologist should be obtained.

■ POSTOPERATIVE THERAPY

The treatment of the patient in the postoperative period depends on the surgery involved. In the majority of patients, a progressive diet from liquids to solids is feasible within 48 hours. Until the patient is taking solid foods, the insulin infusion should be continued, utilizing a sliding scale and adjusting the dose every 2 to 4 hours (see Table 1). Once the patient can ingest solid foods, the usual dose of subcutaneous insulin is begun, and the intravenous insulin infusion is terminated 30 minutes after the first short-acting insulin injection is given. This delay in termination of the intravenous insulin prevents a period of acute insulin deficiency, because 30 minutes may be required before subcutaneous insulin is absorbed and exerts significant hypoglycemic activity.

During the postoperative period, insulin resistance caused by surgical stress still is present, and adjustments in the subcutaneous dose will be needed, as determined by the patient's blood glucose concentration, food intake, and the presence of surgical complications such as fever and infection. If infection is present, maintenance of the intravenous insulin infusion is the easiest method to normalize the metabolic state. If major abdominal surgery is performed and several weeks of no oral ingestion of food are anticipated, total parenteral nutrition must be begun according to standard guidelines. Again, an infusion of intravenous insulin is the best approach to ensure reasonable metabolic control.

■ Issues and Risks

This article has focused on the perioperative management of the adult diabetic patient. Alternative strategies may be required when planning perioperative therapy for other categories of diabetic patients. For example, the geriatric patient may have other serious medical problems that necessitate parenteral pharmaceutical agents.[6] The diabetic patient undergoing open heart surgery may require 2 to 4 U of intravenous insulin per hour.[22] The child undergoing surgery will need to have fluids and insulin therapy calculated on a weight or body surface area formula. The pregnant diabetic patient will experience a sudden decrease in insulin requirements upon delivery, when the placenta no longer is active metabolically.[3]

These problems emphasize why many authorities favor providing insulin by continuous intravenous infusion, which allows rapid changes in dosage to meet changing metabolic needs. In the type II diabetic patient, however, well-controlled on diet only and undergoing minor surgery, insulin is not required because the stress is minimal. A glucose-containing solution should not be infused into these patients, nor should lactate (a precursor of gluconeogenesis).[23] It is imperative, however, that appropriate preoperative evaluation be performed, because most of these patients are elderly and have some degree of atherosclerosis.

Appropriate perioperative management of the diabetic patient is not difficult but does require planning and oversight by the patient's physician. The key to success is not the choice of a specific regimen but the frequent monitoring of the patient's metabolic status and appropriate responses to the metabolic state. Physicians should adopt a standard management plan for diabetic patients and become thoroughly familiar with its use. They also must be certain that the other physicians who participate in the patient's care understand this approach. With frequent glucose monitoring of the patient,

there is no reason that metabolic decompensation should be encountered in the diabetic patient undergoing surgery.

REFERENCES

1. Root HF. Preoperative care of the diabetic patient. Postgrad Med 1966;40:439–444.
2. Schade DS. Surgery and diabetes. Med Clin North Am 1988; 72:1531–1543.
3. Alberti KGMM, Thomas DJB. The management of diabetes during surgery. Br J Anaesth 1979; 51:693–706.
4. Barnett AH, Robinson MH, Harrison JH, et al. Minipump: method of diabetic control during minor surgery under general anesthesia. Br Med J 1980; 128:78–79.
5. Bovington MM, Spies ME, Troy PJ. Management of the patient with diabetes mellitus during surgery or illness. Nurs Clin North Am 1983; 18:661–671.
6. Crosby DL. Management of the elderly surgical patient. Br J Hosp Med 1987; 38:135–138.
7. Galloway JA, Shuman CR. Diabetes and surgery. Am J Med 1963; 34:177–191.
8. Husband JD, Thai AC, Alberti KG. Management of diabetes during surgery with glucose-insulin-potassium infusion. Diabetic Med 1986; 3:69–74.
9. Johnston DG, Alberti KGMM. Diabetic emergencies: practical aspects of the management of diabetic ketoacidosis and diabetes during surgery. Clin Endocrinol Metab 1980; 9:437–456.
10. Lum CT, Sutherland DE, Goetz FC, et al. Management of the diabetic patient before, during, and after surgery, with special emphasis on uremic patients and kidney transplant recipients. Minn Med 1985; 68:693–696.
11. Marble A, Steinke J. Physiology and pharmacology in diabetes mellitus: guiding the diabetic patient through the surgical period. Anesthesiology 1963; 24:442–447.
12. Meyers EF, Alberts D, Gordon MO. Perioperative control of blood glucose in diabetic patients: a two-step protocol. Diabetes Care 1986; 9:40–45.
13. Schade DS. Acute medical illness and surgery in the diabetic patient. In Olefsky JM, Sherwin RS (eds). Contemporary Issues in Endocrinology and Metabolism. Vol 1: Diabetes Mellitus: Management and Complications. New York: Churchill Livingstone, 1985:331–352.
14. Thompson J, Husband DJ, Thai AC, et al. Metabolic changes in the noninsulin-dependent diabetic undergoing minor surgery: effect of glucose-insulin-potassium infusion. Br J Surg 1986; 73:301–304.
15. Schade DS, Eaton RP. Differential diagnosis and therapy of hyperketonemic states. JAMA 1979; 241:2064–2065.
16. Schade DS, Eaton RP. Prevention of diabetic ketoacidosis. JAMA 1979; 242:2455–2458.
17. Schade DS, Eaton RP. The temporal relationship between endogenously secreted stress hormones and metabolic decompensation in diabetic man. J Clin Endocrinol Metab 1980; 50:131–136.
18. Shamoon H, Hendler R, Sherwin RS. Synergistic interactions among anti-insulin hormones in the pathogenesis of stress hyperglycemia in humans. J Clin Endocrinol Metab 1981; 52:1235–1241.

19. Waldhausl W, Kleinberg G, Korn A, et al. Severe hyperglycemia: effects of rehydration on endocrine derangements and blood glucose concentration. Diabetes 1979; 28:577–584.
20. Roelofse JA, Erasmus FR. Anaesthesia and the diabetic patient. S Afr Med J 1985; 68:872–875.
21. Schade DS, Eaton RP, Alberti KGMM, Johnston, DG. Diabetic Coma: Ketoacidotic and Hyperosmolar. Albuquerque: University of New Mexico Press, 1981.
22. Gill GV, Sherif IM, Alberti KGMM. Management of diabetes during open heart surgery. Br J Surg 1981; 68:171–172.
23. Thomas DJB, Alberti KGMM. Hyperglycaemic effects of Hartman's solution during surgery in patients with maturity-onset diabetes. Br J Anesth 1978; 50:185–188.

Diabetes mellitus, type I

Kay F. McFarland

■ Background

Type I diabetes mellitus, characterized by insulin deficiency and dependence on injected insulin to prevent ketosis and sustain life, is due to autoimmune destruction of the pancreatic beta cells in genetically susceptible individuals.[1] Although the disorder may begin at any age, the onset is usually before age 30 years. The diagnosis generally is not difficult, because patients present with polyuria, polydipsia, weight loss, a serum or plasma glucose of over 200 mg/dl, and ketonuria. Other more nonspecific symptoms include blurred vision, fatigue, malaise, headache, and vaginitis. Frequently, the only abnormal physical finding is hepatomegaly.

The major objectives of therapy are prevention of ketosis and elimination of symptomatic hyperglycemia.[2] To accomplish these goals, patients should learn enough of the pathophysiology of diabetes to be able to recognize, differentiate, and appropriately manage the symptoms of hyperglycemia and hypoglycemia. They need to understand the basic principles of a healthy diet, the rational use of insulin, the effects of exercise and intercurrent illness on glucose levels, the procedures for monitoring blood sugar, the rationale for checking urine ketone levels, and appropriate foot care in order to assume primary responsibility for their disease.

Uncertainty still exists regarding how treatment affects the development of vascular complications,[3,4] and there is evidence to show that intensive treatment increases the risk of hypoglycemia. Therefore, the effort and commitment expended to maintain as near-normal glucose levels as possible depends largely on the patient's and physician's beliefs regarding these issues. In order to minimize the impact of diabetes on the patient and his or her family, the treatment plan must be adapted to the needs and lifestyle of each individual.

■ Management

■ INSULIN

Insulin is the mainstay of treatment of type I diabetes. Most patients may be started on insulin without hospitalization except when another condition such as ketoacidosis or a surgical emergency necessitates in-hospital care. Particularly early in treatment, concise written instructions by the physician and ready accessibility of the physician by phone do much to allay the anxiety and misunderstanding that may occur regarding the insulin dose, as well as the other aspects of management.

Lente or NPH insulin, which has an intermediate range of action, may be used initially, with 0.4 to 0.6 unit/kg body weight given before breakfast and 0.2 to 0.3 unit/kg before supper. The exact amounts of the A.M. and P.M. doses, as well as the ratio of short-acting (Regular, Semilente), intermediate-acting (NPH, Lente), or long-acting (Ultralente) insulin, then are adjusted, based on glucose levels obtained by home glucose monitoring (Table 1). The usual total dose will not exceed 1 unit/kg, except during adolescence and pregnancy when doses of between 1 and 1.5 units/kg are common. Some patients experience a "honeymoon phase" soon after the diagnosis, during which exogenous insulin need drops dramatically. During this phase, which may last a month to a year or more, the insulin dose may be decreased, or rarely, even discontinued.

In regulating the type and timing of insulin administered, the major objective is to prevent hyperglycemia from occurring, rather than to treat an already elevated glucose level. Usually NPH or Lente plus a short-acting insulin is given before breakfast and before supper. When fasting glucose levels are persistently elevated or nighttime reactions occur, the afternoon NPH or Lente insulin may be given at bedtime rather than

TABLE 1. Insulin Therapy

Insulin Action	Onset (hr)	Peak (hr)	Usual Duration (hr)
Regular	0.5–1	2–3	3–6
NPH or Lente	2–4	4–12	10–18
Ultra Lente	6–10	—	18–30
Animal insulin: 0–6 hr later onset, peak, and/or duration			

Beginning Therapy—0.5–0.7 unit/kg/day

Time	Dose Proportion	Ratio Intermediate:Short-Acting Insulin
Before breakfast	2/3 dose	2:1 NPH or Lente:Regular
Before supper	1/3 dose	1:1 NPH or Lente:Regular

Modifying Dose—Average maintenance dose 0.6–0.8 unit/kg/day*

Time	Dose to Be Changed	Ways to Change Dose
Before breakfast	P.M. NPH or Lente	↓ insulin 10% for glucose < 60 mg/dl, or ↑ insulin 10% for
Before lunch	A.M. Regular	glucose > 200 mg/dl × 3 days. Consider covering
Before supper	A.M. NPH or Lente	with 1–2 units Regular before meals when glucose is
Before bedtime	P.M. Regular	> 200 mg/dl

*Higher maintenance dose during pregnancy and adolescence

Other Considerations

P.C. glucose ↑	↑ time interval between insulin injection and meal
Nighttime reactions	Give P.M. Lente or NPH at bedtime rather than before supper
Wide variation—glucose day-to-day	Check timing/consistency of meals and exercise Inquire about recent lifestyle changes (shift work, emotional stress, alcohol, drugs, technique of monitoring)
Acetone moderate to strong—plus ↑ glucose	Give 4–8 units Regular insulin q 4 hr until blood sugar is <250 mg/dl and acetone negative. Call MD if two extra doses needed

before supper. To increase the flexibility in meal timing, some patients prefer to take regular insulin three times a day, combining the morning and before supper insulin with NPH. Alternatively, Ultra Lente may be used once or twice daily with a short-acting insulin before meals.

Changes in the intermediate-acting insulin dose usually are made no more than twice weekly. The goal is to keep the fasting glucose level between 60 and 140 mg/dl and other levels below 200 mg/dl at least 80 per cent of the time. Higher levels must be accepted, however, when hypoglycemic reactions are common. Regular insulin may be added before meals to counteract the intermittent effects of stress, infection, and dietary changes. An example of a coverage scale that may be used is 1 to 2 units of regular insulin for every 50 mg/dl increase in the blood sugar over 150 mg/dl, with that dose being doubled if moderate-to-strong acetone is present in the urine. It is easier to increase the diet or add snacks than to reduce the amount of insulin taken prior to strenuous exercise.

The same amount or even more basal insulin than ordinary usually is required during times of illness. If patients are not eating much, the intermediate-acting insulin dose is not decreased, but the short-acting insulin taken before meals may need to be reduced. Whenever patients are ill, they should check their urine for acetone. Extra Regular insulin is given every 4 hours as long as acetonuria plus hyperglycemia persists.

An insufficient amount of insulin is usually the cause of persistently elevated glucose levels, but occasionally paradoxic glucose elevation may follow hypoglycemia caused by excessive insulin administration. Clinical clues that the insulin dose may be too high include hypoglycemia followed within a few hours by marked hyperglycemia; weight gain in a patient receiving insulin; development of extreme brittleness unrelated to meals or activities; significant glycosuria or ketonuria or both in the early morning with a history of nocturnal sweating and headache; unexplained increase in insulin requirements; and an insulin dose exceeding 1.2 units/kg/day. Therefore, rather than continually increasing insulin doses in patients with widely fluctuating glucose levels, the proportion of short-acting, intermediate-acting, and long-acting insulin may need to be altered and the total dose decreased. Frequent glucose measurements are critical in determining whether hyperglycemia results from previous hypoglycemic reactions or from insulin deficiency, which is treated by exactly the opposite recommendation: increasing the insulin dose.

When glucose levels are consistently elevated or reactions occur, the patient will need to be seen or at least be in contact with his or her physician weekly or even more frequently. Intervals between visits may be extended to once or twice per year when levels are stable. Patients should be encouraged to call whenever hyperglycemia with ketonuria persists for greater than 4 hours or repeated vomiting or a severe insulin reaction occurs.

Hypoglycemia is a major complication of treatment with insulin. It is often caused by the omission or delay of meals, insulin overdose, or unusually heavy exercise occurring that day or even sometimes 1 or 2 days prior to the reaction. Changing the site of insulin administration from the leg to the arm, administering insulin after a hot shower, or massaging the injection site may increase the rate of insulin absorption and lead to hypoglycemic reactions. Frequent hypoglycemic episodes that continue after the insulin dose has been decreased substantially suggest the possibility of renal insufficiency, hypothyroidism, adrenal insufficiency, or early pregnancy.

Mild reactions detected at glucose levels of around 60 mg/dl[5] may only be a nuisance, but more severe ones are hazardous both to the health and morale of the patient. Because of the unpredictability of insulin reactions, insulin-dependent patients should be instructed to have immediate access to sugar in some form and to wear a bracelet or a necklace identifying them as having diabetes. During hypoglycemic reactions, a commercially available glucose solution may be squeezed into the patient's mouth, or a patient may be urged to drink a sweetened beverage. When there is danger of aspiration, 25 grams of 50 per cent intravenous glucose or 0.5 to 1.0 mg of intramuscular glucagon should be given.

Fortunately, systemic reactions to insulin are quite rare. They are characterized by generalized urticaria and dyspnea and should be treated like any severe allergic reaction, with epinephrine and steroids. In patients who are ketoacidosis prone, insulin therapy is essential, and desensitization is indicated. Special kits provided on consultation with the pharmaceutical company may be used to assist with desensitization.

Reactions such as redness and itching that occur at the site of insulin injection are relatively rare now that human insulin is widely used. If local reactions are of concern and the patient is not taking human insulin, a change to this form should be tried. If Lente insulin is used, then the patient may be switched to NPH insulin or vice versa. Another option is to switch the patient to insulin manufactured by another company, as the diluent is slightly different and may be less irritating.

Lipoatrophy, the loss of subcutaneous tissue at the injection site, is treated by switching patients to human insulin if a beef or pork insulin had been used. The lesions usually fill out within 2 or 3 months when human insulin is repeatedly injected into the atrophy sites. Insulin hypertrophy is the thickening of subcutaneous tissue at the insulin injection site. To treat this condition, the area of hypertrophy is avoided and other injection sites used.

A rare and infrequently recognized complication of insulin treatment is fluid retention, or "insulin edema." This may occur in patients who have been hyperglycemic for some time and follows restoration of glucose to near-normal levels. Most cases clear spontaneously in a few days without specific therapy.

In spite of experimental use of alternative methods of insulin delivery, subcutaneous intermittent insulin injections, using disposable syringes and needles, continue to be the most widely accepted method of treatment. Administering insulin by jet injection has gained popularity; from available data, this appears to offer a mechanically reliable alternative to the use of syringes, though precision and patient acceptability need to be further assessed.[6] The insulin pump provides another method for delivering insulin subcutaneously. Although effective, and with few complications, the pump is poorly accepted by most patients as it is expensive, requires a great commitment to use, and psychologically requires considerable adjustment. Pancreatic transplantation, particularly in patients undergoing renal transplantation, has been studied at selected centers but again is not widely applicable.[7]

Intranasal and other forms of insulin administration are investigational and not practical at this time.[8]

■ DIET

The dietary emphasis for insulin-dependent diabetic patients is on good nutrition and regular timing of meals and snacks.[9] The recommended dietary content is the same as for the nondiabetic individual, with 50 per cent or more of calories from carbohydrate and less than 30 per cent from fat. It is advisable to eliminate fried foods, reduce the intake of red meat and eggs to twice weekly or less, substitute skim milk for whole milk, and limit the amount of cheese and butter eaten, to reduce dietary cholesterol. It is wise to substitute foods with more nutritional value and lower calories for those high in sugar content, such as candy, cake, pie, soft drinks, ice cream, sherbet, beer, and wine. When the patient is of normal weight, the appetite is a more reliable indicator of caloric requirements than any technique of calculation.

Actually, in patients with widely fluctuating glucose levels, the timing of meals may be more important than the content. As much as possible, patients with insulin-dependent diabetes should eat their meals within a half hour of the same time each day. Often a mid-afternoon snack of fruit and a bedtime snack high in protein may be added to prevent hypoglycemic reactions. Special diet foods are expensive and generally are not needed, although unsweetened or artificially sweetened canned fruits, carbonated beverages, chewing gum, and desserts may replace those that contain sugar. Recommendations regarding the limitation of alcohol intake to 2 ounces per day are the same for patients with and without diabetes.

■ MONITORING CONTROL

Numerous home devices are available for measuring blood glucose levels. With proper technique, the meters are quite accurate and provide the most efficient and reliable means of monitoring glucose on a regular basis. Many insulin-dependent patients find it reassuring to measure their glucose daily and several times per day during times of stress, illness, and pregnancy and when their daily routine has changed. Reasons for errors in monitoring include inadequate blood on the strip, poor technique in removing blood, inaccurate timing, old strips, or improper functioning of the meter, as, for example, from a low battery charge.

The reason for monitoring is to provide a basis for recommendations regarding the insulin dose. Some patients modify the short-acting insulin given before each meal, depending on their glucose level. The amount of extra insulin taken depends on the patient's sensitivity to insulin but usually is in the range of 5 to 10 per cent of the total daily dose. Urine glucose testing is easy and inexpensive but should not be used to regulate the amount of insulin given. Urine ketones need to be measured when the patient is ill or glucose levels are over 300 mg/dl,[10] as acetonuria does alert one to the necessity of increasing the insulin dose, the caloric intake, or both.

Glycosylated hemoglobin measurements and other forms of glycated hemoglobin, such as HbA_{1c}, serve as a useful index of glucose levels over a 4- to 8-week period. Values that are within 1 or 2 percentage points of the upper range of normal often may be obtained with intensive therapy, but here again individual patient goals must be considered. Some physicians and patients find it reassuring to check glycated hemoglobin levels every 6 to 12 months to assess control, whereas others become discouraged when values are above the target level. Thus, to some patients glycated hemoglobin may be a positive motivating factor and to others a form of judgment or sign of failure. Although fewer studies are available to assess its value, fructosamine, a glycated protein measurement, also is used as an index of glucose levels present over a 2-week period.[11]

Effective monitoring requires that the patient maintain records, which include the insulin dose administered, glucose levels, weight, changes in diet and exercise, and other factors that may influence glucose levels. For example, the time of insulin administration, medications taken, and unusual exercise help decipher the glucose variability. The pattern of glucose changes is of much more importance than a single high or low reading. Also, the physician will want to note in the office records the weight, blood pressure, insulin dose, medications taken, number of glucose levels that are high or low during a specific time period, frequency of hypoglycemic reactions, glucose, and glycated hemoglobin measurements. Also, notations should be made in the chart periodically of the funduscopic examination, peripheral pulses, and vibratory sensation in the lower extremity.

Reviewing the records with the patient and keeping a duplicate of home glucose readings for the office chart provides assurance to the patient that the physician takes commitment seriously. When records are incomplete, the physician should not disapprove but should encourage the patient, empathizing with the difficulty in paying daily attention to the unceasing demands of diabetes. It takes a great deal of motivation for a patient to continue checking glucose levels indefinitely on a daily basis; possibly the most motivating factor is having a supportive physician with whom he or she can consult regarding problems that arise periodically.

Stress may lead to inconsistency in food intake, heavier use of alcohol, a change in activity, and hormonal changes, all of which may affect glucose levels. Therefore, dealing with everyday stresses is as important a factor in the management as is attention to insulin, diet, and exercise. Causes of nonadherence include lack of knowledge, fear of hypoglycemia, and difficult occupational or social circumstances. Most patients will follow the recommended program when the effort to them does not exceed the potential benefit.

■ KETOACIDOSIS

Patients with diabetic ketoacidosis usually present with nausea, vomiting, polyuria, tachypnea, and occasionally alterations in consciousness. Severe abdominal pain may be present, particularly in children and young adults. On physical examination, the most striking abnormalities are profound dehydration with dryness of the mucous membranes, poor skin turgor, rapid respirations with a fruity odor of the breath, hypotension, and a rapid heart rate.

Early diagnosis and close monitoring of the patient are the critical factors in influencing the successful outcome of diabetic ketoacidosis. The diagnosis is established by finding a plasma glucose level of over 300 mg/dl, a strongly positive reaction for ketones in the urine, and acidosis with a pH of 7.3 or less or bicarbonate below 18 mEq/L. Initial laboratory studies should include a plasma or serum glucose determination, bicarbonate and potassium measurements, BUN, and urinalysis. For the first few hours, glucose levels are followed every 1 to 2 hours and bicarbonate and potassium levels every 3 to 4 hours. When the bicarbonate rises to 18 mEq/dl and the patient is eating, bicarbonate and potassium levels may be monitored every 6 to 12 hours until normal.

Treatment with insulin should begin immediately upon diagnosis, with 10 units of Regular insulin (or 0.15 unit/kg) given by IV push followed by a continuous infusion of 10 units of Regular insulin every hour (or 0.1 unit/kg/hr). If glucose levels do not fall at least 75 mg/dl per hour, the rate of insulin administration should be increased. Intermediate-acting insulin is begun when the patient is alert and eating, and the bicarbonate level is equal to or greater than 18 mEq/dl. Extra Regular insulin may be needed every 4 hours for several hours in order to maintain the glucose levels within the normal range (Table 2).

Initially, normal saline is used to expand the intravascular volume, with the first liter being infused within 2 hours. The rate is decreased then to about 300 ml/hr. When the serum glucose level falls to 250 mg/dl, the fluids are changed to 5 per cent dextrose in water or 0.45 per cent sodium chloride. Bicarbonate is rarely needed as there is little evidence of benefit when the pH is above 6.9; the ketoacidosis will correct simply with adequate fluids and insulin.[12]

Potassium is given as soon as it is verified that the serum potassium is not elevated. Usually, potassium is infused slowly at a rate no greater than 20 mEq/hr, although serum potassium levels below 3 mEq/L may necessitate an infusion rate as high as 0.5 mEq/kg/hr. Potassium chloride rather than potassium phosphate is given unless the serum phosphorus level is less than 1 mg/dl.

■ NEUROPATHY

The most common form of diabetic neuropathy is characterized by symmetric, slowly progressive sensory loss affecting the distal portion of the lower extremity, or, paradox-

TABLE 2. Diabetic Ketoacidosis

Dx: BS ≥ 300 mg/dl; urine acetone strong; pH ≤ 7.3; HCO₃ ≤ 18 mEq/L

Insulin
1. Initially 10 units Regular insulin IV bolus, or 0.15 unit/kg
2. Follow with Regular insulin infusion, 10 units/hr or 0.1 unit/kg/hr; increase dose if glucose falls
   < 75 mg/dl/hr
3. Decrease insulin infusion rate to 1–5 units/hr when glucose is < 250 mg/dl
4. Start NPH or Lente plus Regular insulin when patient eating, glucose < 250 mg/dl, and HCO₃ ≥ 18 mEq/L

Fluids and Electrolytes
1. 0.9% NaCl—500 ml/hr × 1 liter; then 300 ml/hr until hydrated
2. KCl—adjust rate by serum K level. Start when hyperkalemia excluded. K₃HPO₄ may be used when phosphorus
   is 1 mg/dl or less
3. D5W or D5/0.45 NaCl—200–300 ml/hr after glucose < 250 mg/dl; discontinue IV fluids when patient is eating
   and HCO₃ is > 18 mEq/L
4. Bicarbonate rarely if ever needed (consider if pH < 6.9)

Laboratory Studies
1. Serum or plasma glucose initially every 1–2 hours, then every 3–4 hours when glucose is < 250 mg/dl
2. Bicarbonate, potassium, BUN initially q 3–4 hr until HCO₃ > 18 mEq, then q 6–12 hr until normal
3. Blood gases optional
4. Urinalysis initially
5. ECG if age > 40 years or chest pain present
6. X-ray films as clinically indicated
7. Cultures as clinically indicated, especially when fever present

ically, by hyperesthesia and pain with nocturnal intensification. Ulcers may develop on the feet from repeated minor trauma but may go unrecognized and untreated because they usually are not painful. Almost all ulcers caused by neuropathy are over pressure points and surrounded by callus. The diagnosis of symmetric peripheral neuropathy may be verified by noting the absence of ankle reflexes and decreased vibratory sensation in the ankles and toes.

The treatment is not satisfactory. There is some evidence that normalization of serum glucose is associated with increased nerve conduction velocity; however, the symptoms actually may get worse during initial normalization of the glucose level. A number of drugs have been used in an attempt to relieve the pain and dysesthesias, but their efficacy is difficult to evaluate. Amitriptyline may be effective in promoting sleep and reducing symptoms; carbamazepine and imipramine also have been found helpful in some patients. Phenytoin, aldose reductase inhibitors, vitamins, gangliosides, and dietary myoinositol supplementation are not clinically used, for data regarding their effectiveness and toxicity are inconclusive.[13] Narcotics, also, should be avoided.

Probably the most important aspect of treatment is education of the patient in proper foot care. Patients need to examine their feet carefully for evidence of trauma, since the reduction in sensation may result in small lesions being overlooked. Shoes should be worn at all times; open-toed shoes and sandals should be avoided. The temperature of bath water should be checked with the hand before placing the feet into it. Heating pads are contraindicated, and the patient should leave cutting calluses to the physician or podiatrist.

Treatment of autonomic neuropathy is empiric and supportive. The best treatment for bladder neuropathy is to encourage frequent urination with suprapubic pressure. Bethanechol, 10 to 20 mg three times a day may be tried, but repeated catheterizations may be needed if no other method is effective. Treatment of orthostatic hypotension is difficult, although increased dietary sodium, elastic stockings, and elevation of the head of the bed have been advocated. Other suggested drugs include indomethacin 25 to 50 mg three times a day, diphenhydramine, cimetidine, metoclopramide, and pindolol.

There are a number of other autonomic neuropathies. Gastric retention may be relieved with 10 to 20 mg of metoclopramide hydrochloride given before meals and at bedtime. Diabetic diarrhea may be related to altered gastrointestinal motility and occasionally will respond to a 10- to 14-day course of a broad-spectrum antibiotic such as tetracycline. Clonidine, 0.1 to 0.4 mg twice daily also may be tried.[14] Treatment of impotence due to autonomic dysfunction is usually disappointing, but repeated penile injections of papaverine or the use of a surgically placed penile implant may produce satisfactory results. A mechanical device, Erec-Aid, also is marketed. Brompheniramine, 8 mg twice daily; imipramine, 25 mg three times a day; or phenylephrine, 60 mg intravenously, may reverse retrograde ejaculation.

NEPHROPATHY

The first sign of diabetic renal disease is proteinuria, followed by a decrease in creatinine clearance within 5 years. Treatment is similar to the management of other forms of chronic renal disease. Hypertension should be treated early and vigorously and urinary tract infections managed aggressively. Therapeutic principles for the treatment of hypertension include limiting the use of diuretics and beta-blockers and favoring the use of alpha-blockers, calcium channel blockers, and angiotensin-converting enzyme inhibitors, with monotherapy whenever possible.[15] Research continues on the use of a low-protein diet to prevent progression or development of diabetic nephropathy, but results are still inconclusive. Radiographic contrast material should be avoided in diabetic patients with renal insufficiency.[16] End-stage disease is treated with dialysis and renal transplantation.

RETINOPATHY

Retinopathy occurs in about 50 per cent of patients by 10 years after diagnosis. Therefore, careful retinal evaluation using the direct ophthalmoscope should be done at least annually. High-risk characteristics, which include new vessels covering 25 per cent of the optic disc, new vessels on the disc, or new vessels equal to 50 per cent of the disc area in other retinal areas, with preretinal or vitreous hemorrhage, necessitate urgent treatment with photocoagulation. Also, immediate referral is strongly advised when proliferative retinopathy of any degree is present or when preproliferative changes are noted, with dilated irregular veins, cotton wool spots, multiple dot and blot hemorrhages, and intraretinal microvascular abnormalities.

Panretinal photocoagulation with the argon laser is the standard therapy, with focal photocoagulation recommended for macular edema. Vitrectomy is used to remove vitreous humor filled with blood, cut fibrous traction bands, peel contractile fibrous membranes, and repair some types of retinal detachments. Treatment by these modalities is highly effective in preserving or salvaging vision. Pancreatic transplantation and subsequent normoglycemia neither reverse nor prevent the progression of diabetic retinopathy.[17]

EMOTIONAL FACTORS

Insulin-dependent diabetes, like all serious chronic illnesses, invariably produces significant emotional stress. No single therapeutic plan can meet the psychologic needs of all diabetic patients, as they are from a wide range of age groups and social classes, and have unique personalities and coping styles. When the physician acts in a consultative rather than a directive manner, it not only makes the treatment plan more realistic to the patient's circumstances but it also encourages the patient to seek information about problems instead of concealing failure; it actually improves adherence. Education is important, but perhaps even more important is acceptance by physicians that their role is to work with the patient to decrease elevated glucose levels by balancing food intake, exercise, and insulin, rather than by dictating treatment schedules. In this manner the physician acts as an ally with the patient in his or her struggle to prevent delayed complications, which is certainly the greatest fear of both the patient and physician. This reminds us that it is of the greatest importance to treat the individual and not the disease.[18]

REFERENCES

1. Eisenbarth GS. Type I diabetes mellitus. N Engl J Med 1986; 314:1360–1368.
2. American Diabetes Association. Physician's Guide to Insulin-Dependent (Type I) Diabetes: Diagnosis and Treatment. Alexandria, VA: American Diabetes Association, 1988.
3. The DCCT Research Group. Are continuing studies of metabolic control and microvascular complications in insulin-dependent diabetes mellitus justified? N Engl J Med 1988; 318:246–250.

4. Nathan DM. Modern management of insulin-dependent diabetes mellitus. Med Clin North Am 1988; 72:1365–1378.
5. Boyle PJ, Schwartz NS, Shah SD, Clutter WE, Cryer PE. Plasma glucose concentrations at the onset of hypoglycemic symptoms in patients with poorly controlled diabetes and in nondiabetics. N Engl J Med 1988; 318:1487–1492.
6. American Diabetes Association. Position statement on jet injectors. Diabetes Care 1988; 11:600–601.
7. Corry RJ. Vascularized pancreas transplantation. Diabetes 1989; 38:321–322.
8. Sussman KE. Diabetes—The road ahead. Am J Med 1988; 85:166–171.
9. American Diabetes Association. Position statement: Nutritional recommendations and principles for individuals with diabetes mellitus: 1986. Diabetes Care 1987; 10:126–132.
10. Singer DE, Coley CM, Samet JH, Nathan DM. Tests of glycemia in diabetes mellitus: their use in establishing a diagnosis and in treatment. Ann Intern Med 1989; 110:125–137.
11. Smart LM, Howie AF, Young RJ, Walker SW, Clarke BF, Smith AF. Comparison of fructosamine with glycosylated hemoglobin and plasma proteins as measures of glycemic control. Diabetes Care 1988; 11:433–436.
12. Morris LR, Murphy MB, Kitabchi AE. Bicarbonate therapy in severe diabetic ketoacidosis. Ann Intern Med 1986; 105:836–840.
13. Harati Y. Diabetic peripheral neuropathies. Ann Intern Med 1987; 107:546–559.
14. Fedorak RN, Field M, Chang EB. Treatment of diabetic diarrhea with clonidine. Ann Intern Med 1985; 102:197–199.
15. Kaplan NM, Rosenstock J, Raskin P. A differing view of treatment of hypertension in patients with diabetes mellitus. Arch Intern Med 1987; 147:1160–1162.
16. Parfrey PS, Griffiths SM, Barrett BJ, Paul MD, Genge M, Withers J, Farid N, McManamon PJ. Contrast material–induced renal failure in patients with diabetes mellitus, renal insufficiency, or both. N Engl J Med 1989; 320:143–149.
17. Ramsay RC, Goetz FC, Sutherland DER, Mauer SM, Robison LL, Cantrill HL, Knobloch WH, Najarian JS. Progression of diabetic retinopathy after pancreas transplantation for insulin-dependent diabetes mellitus. N Engl J Med 1988; 318:208–214.
18. McFarland K, Schell B, McCullough T. Helping diabetic patients avoid guilt when 'out of control.' Postgrad Med 1989; 5:243–248.

Dialysis patient, medical management of

D. Kaji ■ *A. Malik*

■ Background

Uremia encompasses a host of clinical manifestations as a result of end-stage renal failure. The syndrome is due to accumulation of uremic toxins, deficiency of factors produced by normal kidneys, and disturbances of homeostatic mechanisms that control water and electrolyte balance. Although almost all organ systems are affected, the degree of organ involvement varies from patient to patient.

■ CARDIOVASCULAR ABNORMALITIES

Congestive heart failure (CHF) is a major cause of morbidity and mortality in the dialysis patient. Fluid retention remains the most common cause of CHF. Less commonly, low-pressure pulmonary edema caused by increased permeability of the alveolar capillaries ("uremic lung") may be seen in the inadequately dialyzed patient.[1]

The incidence of accelerated atherosclerosis in dialysis patients is much greater than in the general population. Hypertension, glucose and lipid abnormalities, metastatic vascular calcification, and high cardiac output all may be responsible.[1]

Pericarditis in the dialysis patient is either "uremic" or due to viral infection or systemic diseases. The term *uremic pericarditis* refers to pericarditis of unknown etiology in association with uremia, which is seen in the inadequately dialyzed patient and is associated with hemorrhagic effusion.[2]

Hypertension is the most common complication in the dialysis patient. Sodium retention and volume expansion are the most important contributing factors. The absolute levels of plasma renin activity (PRA) are variable, but the renin values are believed to be inappropriately elevated for the degree of sodium and volume retention.[1]

■ NEUROLOGIC ABNORMALITIES

Many neurologic signs and systems, such as asterixis, coma, or altered consciousness, are believed to reflect inadequate dialysis and to signal the need for increasing dialysis therapy. Similarly, the presence of peripheral neuropathy in a nondiabetic dialysis patient should suggest the possibility of inadequate dialysis. In contrast, dialysis dementia, a progressive neurologic disorder characterized by dyspraxia, myoclonus, dementia, seizures, and characteristic electroencephalographic (EEG) changes, does not respond to increased dialysis.[3] Aluminum toxicity has been implicated in some cases.[4] The incidence of intracranial hemorrhage is high, especially in patients with polycystic kidney disease. Muscle weakness is common and may be related to vitamin D deficiency. Increased deposition of β_2-microglobulin in the transverse carpal ligament leads to a new form of amyloidosis and carpal tunnel syndrome.[5]

■ GASTROINTESTINAL COMPLICATIONS

The conversion of urea to ammonia by oral bacteria results in "uremic fetor," an unpleasant odor to the breath. Aluminum hydroxide, given routinely to dialysis patients to bind oral phosphate, predisposes the patient to severe constipation, which at times may result in fecal impaction and even cecal perforation. The incidence of diverticulosis, peptic ulcer disease, and viral hepatitis is increased in the dialysis patient. Episodes of gastrointestinal bleeding are frequent because of increased incidence of peptic ulcer disease, arteriovenous malformation, and heparin administration during dialysis. An occasional dialysis patient presents with idiopathic ascites.[6]

■ HEMATOLOGIC PROBLEMS

Anemia, defective hemostasis, and leukocyte dysfunction are commonly observed in the dialysis patient.[7] Anemia is usually normocytic and normochromic and is secondary to decreased erythropoietin synthesis by the diseased kidney. Increased blood loss and shortened erythrocyte life span also contribute to anemia in some patients. The dialysis patient shows a hemorrhagic diathesis with abnormal platelet aggregation and increased bleeding time. Enhanced susceptibility to infection is a major problem in the dialysis patient. Leukocyte dysfunction, a defect in response to acute inflammation, and a defect in delayed hypersensitivity response are commonly observed. The vascular access created for dialysis serves as a portal of entry for bacteria. In response to acute bacterial infections, fever and leukocytosis are less common in the dialysis patient. Because of the increased susceptibility to infections and the difficulty in diagnosing infections, uremic patients should be treated as soon as the clinician suspects infection.

■ RENAL OSTEODYSTROPHY

This term encompasses a variety of skeletal abnormalities, including changes due to osteitis fibrosa from hyperparathyroidism, osteomalacia, osteoporosis, and osteosclerosis.[4] The role of increased bone deposit of aluminum has recently received greater recognition.[4] The retention of phosphorus in dialysis patients inhibits the conversion of vitamin D into 1,25-dihydroxycholecalciferol, depresses serum calcium, and leads to metastatic calcification. Both hypocalcemia and low levels of 1,25-dihydroxycholecalciferol lead to hyperparathyroidism.[4]

■ ENDOCRINE AND METABOLIC DISTURBANCES

In nondiabetic uremic patients, the catabolism of insulin is reduced, leading to prolonged insulin action. A postreceptor defect results in insulin resistance and an abnormal glucose tolerance. Seventy per cent of men on dialysis are impotent, and women on dialysis frequently report a decrease in the frequency of orgasm during intercourse.[8] Both psychologic and endocrine dysfunctions contribute to this problem. Menstrual cycles are anovulatory, and only a few cases of successful pregnancies have been reported. Sexual maturation and growth are often impaired in adolescent children on dialysis. Of the various lipid abnormalities in the dialysis patient, a modest increase in total triglyceride with an inconsistent rise in cholesterol (type IV hyperlipidemia) is the commonest.[8]

The psychologic impact of end-stage renal disease and life-sustaining dialysis therapy is enormous. Patients on dialysis are often depressed and anxious. They are afraid of cumulative illnesses, reduced socioeconomic status, sexual dysfunction, and dependence on dialysis therapy.[9]

■ Management

The management of the dialysis patient is divided into four sections: (1) general principles, (2) treatment of uremic complications, (3) selected aspects of dialysis and dialysis-related complications, and (4) vaccinations.

■ GENERAL PRINCIPLES

Diet. Most dialysis patients are severely oliguric or anuric and therefore require strict restriction of sodium (1 to 2 gm/day), potassium (2 to 2.5 gm/day), and fluids (800 to 1500 ml/day).[10] Although unable to excrete toxic metabolites that contribute to uremia, some dialysis patients continue to excrete near-normal quantities of urine. A more liberal diet is permitted and recommended for these patients. A mild protein restriction (0.5 to 1 gm/kg body weight per day) is recommended for hemodialysis patients, but patients on peritoneal dialysis may be permitted a near-normal (1 to 1.2 gm/kg/day) intake. Adequate caloric intake must be maintained to prevent malnutrition.

Ancillary Treatment. Supplemental water-soluble vitamins (B and C) and folic acid are required for all patients because of dialysis-related loss of these nutrients.[10] Many patients will require oral or intravenous iron and periodic transfusion of blood.

Treatment of Pruritus. Severe, persistent pruritus is a vexing problem for the dialysis patient. Antihistamines such as chlorpheniramine maleate or diphenylhydramine are most commonly employed, but control of hyperphosphatemia, high doses (4 to 6 gm/day) of activated charcoal, ultraviolet phototherapy, and removal of offending allergens (ethylene oxide, beef or pork insulin, and so on) all may be useful.[11]

Use of Drugs. Because of impaired renal excretion or altered metabolism, many drugs may have toxic effects in the dialysis patient if given in doses that are optimal for the patient with normal renal function. For a detailed discussion of drugs in renal failure, the reader is referred to more comprehensive nomograms and tables for modifying drug dose.[12] Medications to be avoided outright include sulfonylureas (severe hypoglycemia), phenformin (lactic acidosis), and nitrofurantoin (peripheral neuropathy). Medications requiring decreased dosage, along with monitoring of drug levels when possible, include digoxin, cimetidine, insulin, barbiturates, cytotoxic agents, clofibrates, and antibiotics, especially aminoglycosides and vancomycin. We wish to emphasize that infections occur frequently and have a devastating morbidity and mortality in dialysis patients. When the physician is confronted with the possibility of an infection that will respond best to aminoglycosides or vancomycin, the right approach is not to avoid these antibiotics but to treat the patient vigorously with appropriately reduced doses or frequency of the desired antibiotics and to monitor drug levels frequently.

Special care is needed to treat insomnia in dialysis patients. Drugs such as phenobarbital or meprobamate may lead to prolonged obtundation, but chloral hydrate and flurazepam are relatively safe.

■ UREMIC COMPLICATIONS

Cardiovascular Complications

The general principles of treatment of congestive heart failure in the dialysis patient are the same as those in the nondialysis patient. Fluid removal is usually achieved by ultrafiltration on dialysis rather than by diuretics, since diuretics are generally ineffective in the oligoanuric dialysis patient. Despite appropriate reduction in dose and frequency of digoxin administration, digoxin toxicity remains a significant hazard. Frequent monitoring of serum digoxin levels is strongly recommended.

The diagnosis of pericarditis requires a re-evaluation of the adequacy of dialysis and a vigorous search for systemic causes, such as tuberculosis. Uremic pericarditis is best treated with daily dialysis and fluid removal. There is no good evidence that indomethacin is effective. Intrapericardiac injection of steroids has been employed at some centers, with variable results. Pericardiectomy is needed when pericarditis fails to respond to dialysis or is associated with cardiac tamponade.[2]

Most hypertensive patients have sodium and fluid retention and respond to vigorous ultrafiltration on dialysis. When antihypertensive drugs are needed, they are best given 4 to 6 hours prior to dialysis or after dialysis to prevent hypotensive episodes on dialysis. Some drugs, such as atenolol and pindolol, accumulate in dialysis patients and should be used with caution. Hyperkalemia may be seen with the use of beta-blockers, especially in dialysis patients who indulge in vigorous exercise.[13] Selective $beta_1$-blockers may be considered for these patients.

Neurologic Complications

There is no specific therapy for peripheral neuropathy. Increasing the duration or frequency of dialysis helps only occasionally, but renal transplantation may result in striking improvement. In contrast, uremic encephalopathy usually responds to increased dialysis.[3] Dialysis dementia is generally associated with poor prognosis and is unresponsive to intensive dialysis.[3] In the patient with dialysis dementia and documented aluminum toxicity, vigorous chelation with deferoxamine may help (see Renal Osteodystrophy below). Carpal tunnel syndrome is most effectively treated with surgical decompression of the nerve. Patients with intracranial hemorrhage are prone to sudden clinical deterioration when heparin is administered routinely during hemodialysis. Therefore, these patients are best hemodialyzed with minimal or no heparin or switched to peritoneal dialysis.

Gastrointestinal Complications

Uremic fetor and decreased taste sensation may be ameliorated by mouthwash with half-strength hydrogen peroxide, which kills oral bacteria converting urea to ammonia, or by small amounts of lemon juice, which neutralizes ammonia.

Hematologic Diseases

Moderate-to-severe anemia (hematocrit, 20 to 30 per cent) remains a major problem in dialysis patients. Patients should be investigated for iron, B_{12}, and folic acid deficiency, hemolysis, and metal (lead and aluminum) intoxication. The major cause of anemia is erythropoietin (EPO) deficiency. Increased dialysis and anabolic steroids may stimulate the bone marrow and improve anemia on occasion, but the definitive treatment with recombinant human EPO awaits Federal Drug Adminstration approval. In clinical trials, EPO administration has resulted in adverse side effects such as hypertension, increased tendency to clot, and even seizures.[14] Packed red cell transfusions are of transient benefit only and may suppress the bone marrow, lead to iron overload, and cause transmission of hepatitis B and acquired immunodeficiency syndrome. Therefore, transfusions are indicated only for anemic dialysis patients with cerebrovascular disease, angina, or CHF. It is worth emphasizing that even severe anemia is well tolerated by most dialysis patients.

The hemorrhagic diathesis generally responds to increased dialysis. The administration of vasopressin (desamino-8-D-arginine vasopressin, DDAVP) may result in normalization of bleeding time in the dialysis patient who requires emergency surgery.[15]

Renal Osteodystrophy

The mainstay of therapy of renal osteodystrophy is the control of elevated serum phosphorus combined with strategies to normalize serum calcium and parathormone (PTH) levels.[4] Although aluminum-containing phosphate binders (aluminum hydroxide gels) have been widely used, they have been shown to contribute to aluminum toxicity. Nonaluminum phosphate binders, such as calcium carbonate, are now gaining popularity.[4] Suppression of parathyroid gland may be achieved by raising serum calcium to the high-normal range by oral calcium carbonate, or by oral administration of 1,25-dihydroxycholecalciferol, 25 to 50 μg/day. The administration of thrice weekly 1,25-dihydroxycholecalciferol intravenously has been shown to suppress hyperparathyroidism, possibly by direct binding of the vitamin D analog to receptors on the parathyroid gland. Bone disease secondary to aluminum toxicity is treated with deferoxamine, 85 mg/kg per week, given IV over the last two hours of dialysis in divided doses.[4]

Metabolic, Endocrine, and Psychologic Complications

Asymptomatic hyperuricemia in the moderate range (7 to 13 mg/dl) is best left alone. Frequent attacks of gout may be prevented with prophylactic colchicine. Because of increased toxicity, allopurinol, if used, should be administered in reduced amounts (100 mg/day).

It is difficult to ameliorate sexual dysfunction in the dialysis patient. The treatment of impotence with oral zinc (50 mg of elemental zinc/day) has met with only mixed success,[8] and the benefit of zinc is controversial at present. In one small study, bromoergocriptine led to improved libido and erections. Antihypertensive agents that interfere with potency should be avoided. Increasing dialysis is rarely useful, but renal transplantation, if successful, may restore libido, improve spermatogenesis and fertility in men, and lead to impregnation in women.[8]

Metabolic acidosis should be treated with supplemental oral bicarbonate when predialysis serum bicarbonate is below 15 mEq per liter, to replenish the base reserve, to prevent skeletal demineralization, and to enhance cardiovascular function. Hyperkalemia (predialysis K^+ above 5.5 mEq/L) is generally due to dietary indiscretion. Dietary compliance is not feasible. Decreasing dialysate K^+ to 0 to 1 mEq/L and/or administration of Kayexalate, 15 to 30 gm/day, at least for a short interval, may be of help in preventing life-threatening hyperkalemia.

Psychologic problems are best fought by encouraging participation in exercise, and in group activities such as those of the NAPHT (National Association of Patients on Hemodialysis and Transplantation), encouraging self-reliance by offering home hemodialysis or continuous ambulatory peritoneal dialysis (CAPD), and family support. Individual and group psychotherapy is also useful.[9]

■ SELECTED ASPECTS OF DIALYSIS

Dialysis involves the removal of small and middle-sized molecular substances (clearance) and removal of water (ultrafiltration) from the blood across a semipermeable membrane. In peritoneal dialysis, this procedure takes place across the peritoneal membrane, and the dialysate instilled in the peritoneum is removed periodically. In hemodialysis, blood is circulated through an extracorporeal circuit and is dialyzed by an artificial semipermeable membrane.

Choice of Modality

Because of frequent episodes of peritonitis, continuous ambulatory peritoneal dialysis (CAPD) has not replaced hemodialysis as the primary mode of treatment for patients with end-stage renal disease (ESRD). CAPD may be preferred for patients who develop frequent hypotension or arrhythmias on hemodialysis, who refuse blood transfusions (Jehovah's Witnesses), or in whom it is impossible to construct a vascular access. For patients on hemodialysis, home hemodialysis offers several advantages, such as the flexibility of schedule, lesser risk of hepatitis, and a sense of self-reliance. However, performing home hemodialysis can be stressful for the patient and the spouse.

Dialysis Prescriptions

A precise definition of adequate dialysis is still not universally agreed upon. However, it is clear that relatively low predialysis BUN (less than 100 mg/dl) and serum creatinine (less than 10 mg/dl) concentrations may be associated with inadequate dialysis, especially if dietary protein intake (and therefore the rate of urea generation) is low. For patients with no residual renal function, dialyzed three times a week, the dialyzer clearance (K in ml/min) and time on single dialysis (t, in minutes) should be adjusted according to the body weight so that Kt/v is 1 to 1.2, where v = volume of urea distribution in ml. The value v in ml can be roughly estimated by the equation v = 0.6 × body weight in kg × 1000.[16]

Treatment of Dialysis-Related Complications

Several investigators have reviewed dialysis-related complications in detail.[17,18] Most of these complications are handled by the medical and nursing staff in the dialysis unit. Only a few comments are in order here.

The primary physician should ensure that the arm with the vascular access is not used for venipunctures, IV fluids, or blood pressure measurements, all of which may lead to thrombosis or infection.

Cramps are frequent, both on dialysis and in the interdialytic period. On dialysis, intravenous hypertonic glucose or saline ameliorates cramps effectively. Oral quinine sulfate, 325 mg just before dialysis, reduced the incidence of cramps in one double-blind controlled study.[19]

Hypotension during dialysis is common and is caused by removal of large quantities of fluid relative to the intravascular volume. Therefore, hypotension in a patient who has just returned from the dialysis unit to the ward should be treated with volume expansion. Drugs such as norepinephrine (Levophed) are almost never indicated.[14,18]

Headache, nausea, and vomiting also occur commonly and may be related to sudden osmolar shifts (dysequilibrium syndrome). Increasing dialysate Na concentration to 140 mEq/liter and reducing blood flow during the first 30 minutes of dialysis may be of help.

The treatment of seizures is no different from that in a patient not on dialysis. Special attention should be given to exclude hypotension, intracranial bleeding, and electrolyte or acid base imbalance.

First-use syndrome refers to a constellation of symptoms on dialysis with new (not reused) dialyzers. Dyspnea, a burning sensation, itching, sneezing, and abdominal cramps may all be seen, singly or in combination. Using preprocessed or reused dialyzers or dialyzers sterilized without ethylene oxide (by gamma rays) may be helpful. Antihistamine, steroids, and epinephrine have been tried and may be beneficial.

Dialysis with cellulose membranes can result in complement activation, hypoxemia, and neutropenia. Therefore, blood for diagnostic blood counts should be drawn predialysis or 4 to 6 hours after dialysis.

■ VACCINATIONS

Vaccinations currently recommended for dialysis patients are influenza A and B every year, diphtheria and tetanus booster every 10 years, pneumococcus once followed by revaccination depending on antibody response, and hepatitis B (in double doses) in the deltoid muscle at 0, 1, 5, and 6 months. Except for hepatitis B, the doses of vaccines are similar to those used in the general population.

■ Issues and Risks

Despite effective measures to exclude hepatitis B virus from the blood supply, the incidence of infection is 0.4 per cent for patients and 0.5 per cent for staff members in the dialysis unit, higher than in the general population.[20] Hepatitis B carriers traditionally have been confined to special areas of the dialysis unit. We recommend protective eyewear, gowns, and gloves for staff members in charge of patients who are positive for hepatitis B surface antigen (HB_sAg). Eating, drinking, and smoking are forbidden in the dialysis unit. All contaminated material should be autoclaved and all blood spills on surfaces washed with 1 per cent sodium hypochlorite. Handwashing after all patient contacts is mandatory. Patient and staff members should be screened for HB_sAg and anti-HB_s every 3 months.

In contrast to hepatitis B, non-A,non-B hepatitis is rare in dialysis staff members, even though most dialysis patients with hepatitis have non-A,non-B hepatitis.[20] Reducing blood transfusions is the only way to prevent its spread.

Patients who were on hemodialysis and received transfusions before 1986 are at increased risk for human immunodeficiency virus (HIV) infection.[20] The Centers for Disease Control (CDC) recommends that routine screening for HIV infection should not be performed in dialysis patients without clinical evidence of acquired immunodeficiency syndrome (AIDS), but many centers routinely screen all dialysis patients. The

CDC also does not recommend a special dialysis machine for HIV-positive patients, does not forbid dialyzer reuse in these patients, and suggests only that body fluid precautions routinely observed on dialysis be followed. Because of uncertainty about HIV, many nephrologists believe that the CDC recommendations are too liberal. Most units take at least the same precautions with HIV-positive patients that they take with patients who are HB_sAg-positive.

■ OUTCOME AND SURVIVAL

After segregating risk factors, the survival for dialysis patients is 90 and 84 per cent at 4 and 5 years for 20 to 60 year old patients.[18] The death rate for this group is 2.7 deaths per 1000 patient months. For patients 46 to 60 years old, the death rate is 4.1 deaths per 1000 patient months.[18] The death rate is higher for blacks and for diabetic patients. The degree of rehabilitation achieved by these patients is controversial. Some workers have claimed that a majority of dialysis patients are disabled, whereas others have found that most patients were able to work part-time.[18] Medicare regulations require proof of disability before providing benefits, and this may have provided a disincentive to patients for accepting part-time or full work.

REFERENCES

1. Kim KE, Swartz C. Cardiovascular complications of end-stage renal failure. *In* Schrier RW, Gottschalk CW (eds). Diseases of the Kidney. Boston: Little, Brown, 1988:3093–3126.
2. Suki WN. Pericarditis. Kidney Int 1988; 33(Suppl 24):S10–S12.
3. Fraser CL, Arieff AI. Nervous system complications in uremia. Ann Intern Med 1988; 109:143–153.
4. Sherrard DJ, Ott S, Maloney N, et al. Renal osteo-dystrophy: classification, cause and treatment. *In* Frame B, Potts JT (eds). Clinical Disorders of Bone and Mineral Metabolism. Amsterdam: Excerpta Medica, 1983:254–276.
5. Kleinman KS, Coburn JW. Amyloid syndromes associated with hemodialysis. Kidney Int 1989; 35:567–575.
6. Johnson WJ. The digestive tract. *In* Daugirdas JT, Ing TS (eds). Handbook of Dialysis. Boston: Little, Brown, 1988:486–494.
7. Anagnostou A, Fried W, Kurtzman N. Hematological consquences of renal failure. *In* Brenner W, Rector FC (eds). Diseases of the Kidney. Boston: Little, Brown, 1981.
8. Lim VS. Endocrine disturbances. *In* Daugirdas JT, Ing TS (eds). Handbook of Dialysis. Boston: Little, Brown, 1988:373–381.
9. Levy NB. Chronic renal dialysis and transplantation. *In* Stondemire A, Fogel BS (eds). Principles of Medical Psychiatry. New York: Grune and Stratton, 1987:583–593.
10. Mitch WE. Nutritional therapy and the progression of chronic renal insufficiency. Annu Rev Med 1984; 35:249–256.
11. Gilchrest BA, Stern RS, Steinman TI, Brown RS, Arndt KA. Clinical features of pruritus among patients undergoing maintenance dialysis. Arch Dermatol 1982; 118:154–156.
12. Bennett W, Blythe WB. Use of drugs in patients with renal failure. *In* Schrier RW, Gottschalk CW (eds). Diseases of the Kidney. Boston: Little, Brown, 1988:3437–3506.
13. Rastegar A, DeFronzo RA. Disorders of potassium metabolism associated with renal disease. *In* Schrier RW, Gottschalk CW (eds). Diseases of the Kidney. Boston: Little, Brown, 1988:2921–2945.
14. Eshbach JW. The anemia of chronic renal failure: pathophysiology and the effects of recombinant erythropoietin. Kidney Int 1989; 35:134–148.
15. Shapiro M, Kelleher SP. Intranasal deamino-8-D-arginine vasopressin shortens the bleeding time in uremia. Am J Nephrol 1984; 4:260–263.
16. Gotch FA, Sargent JA. A mechanistic analysis of the National Cooperative Dialysis Study (NCDS). Kidney Int 1985; 28:526–534.
17. Bregman H, Daugirdas JT, Ing TS. Complications during hemodialysis. *In* Daugirdas JT, Ing TS, (eds). Handbook of Dialysis. Boston: Little, Brown, 1988: 121–145.
18. Friedman EA. Outcome and complications of chronic hemodialysis. *In* Schrier RW, Gottschalk CW (eds). Diseases of the Kidney. Boston: Little, Brown, 1988:3323–3343.
19. Kaji DM, Ackad A, Nottage WC. Prevention of muscle cramps on hemodialysis. Lancet 1976; 2:66–69.
20. Lentino JR, Leehey DJ. Infections. *In* Daugirdas JT, Ing TS, (eds). Handbook of Dialysis. Boston: Little, Brown, 1988:353–372.

Diarrhea, infectious

Christopher D. Truss

Management of diarrhea may be specific or not, depending on several factors. Isolated cases are usually impossible to diagnose when first seen, and therapeutic trials and symptomatic therapy are often used. The evaluation of diarrhea should be approached with restraint because it is often difficult to complete on an outpatient basis, and a clear diagnosis may be forthcoming only for infectious causes. Prospective series of acute, nonepidemic adult diarrhea from around the world report remarkably similar results. In most sporadic diarrheas, an infectious etiology is found in only 20 to 50 per cent of cases.[1] There are two key questions to ask when considering infectious diarrhea: is the diarrhea acute or chronic, and is it dysentery? If the diarrhea has lasted less than a week or two, it will probably resolve without specific treatment, and symptomatic therapy can be emphasized unless the patient is extremely ill. Chronic diarrhea will require specific treatment to cure the infection, and a diagnostic evaluation is necessary.

■ Background

Infectious diarrheas are caused by viruses, bacteria, or parasites. Viruses cause acute diarrhea only. Bacteria, whether invasive or toxigenic, usually cause only acute diarrheas. The parasites are more commonly diagnosed during chronic diarrheas. In approaching acute diarrhea, it is important to look for features of dysentery, which are pus or blood in the diarrheal stool. Dysentery is caused by microbial invasion of the mucosa; the more distal its site in the gastrointestinal tract, the more likely the patient will see bloody or purulent diarrhea. Chronic infectious diarrhea is usually not a dysentery and is more often caused by parasites than bacteria.

■ VIRAL GASTROENTERITIS

The viruses are not routinely cultured, and specific diagnosis is rarely made outside research institutions. Two viruses, Norwalk virus and rotavirus, are responsible for most gastroenteritis. Norwalk is the predominant agent causing diarrhea in infants and young children. Gastroenteritis caused by these viruses is an acute, self-limited illness with diarrhea or vomiting and cannot be distinguished clinically. Management is symptomatic, to control vomiting and diarrhea and correct dehydration.

■ BACILLARY DYSENTERY

Only a few bacteria can be cultured or diagnosed by current clinical laboratory techniques, and many of the bacterial agents listed in treatises are not relevant to most practicing physicians because they are not seen in the United States or because they cannot be cultured and the diarrhea is self-limited. Bacillary dysentery in the United States is usually caused by *Campylobacter jejuni*, *Salmonella* species, and *Shigella* species. *Yersinia* will cause disease but much less frequently than the first three.[2] These same organisms are responsible for most acute bacterial diarrhea in all developed countries. In comparable studies of adults with acute diarrhea from Switzerland (119 patients), San Francisco (113 patients), and New Zealand (60 patients), the number of proven cases of infectious diarrhea has ranged from 38 to 50 per cent,[2–4] and the remainder are culture negative. The largest portion of these diagnosed infections are the bacillary dysenteries caused by *Campylobacter jejuni* (12 to 25 per cent), *Shigella* sp. (up to 16 per cent), and *Salmonella* sp. (2 to 12 per cent). In the two studies that did not exclude cases with recent antibiotic exposure, *Clostridium difficile*–induced pseudomembranous colitis was the next most common cause of bacterial diarrhea after the three bacillary dysenteries, accounting for about 5 per cent of acute diarrheas. There were one or two cases of *Giardia lamblia* infection in each series but no cases of amebic dysentery in San Francisco or Switzerland and only one in New Zealand. Two cases of *Yersinia* were diagnosed in the San Francisco study but none in the other two, and only two *Vibrio* infections were seen, both in New Zealand. Thus a quick review of three areas of the "developed" world suggests that our diagnostic efforts need to focus on only a handful of "treatable" infectious causes of acute diarrhea. Many of the undiagnosed cases in these series are probably viral, but these are self-limited and cannot be diagnosed by readily available techniques. The other point is that there is a host of rare and undiagnosable organisms that the clinician need not be concerned with, e.g., the enterotoxigenic *E. coli* and *Vibrio cholerae* organisms, which are not acquired in the United States.[2]

The usual course of bacillary dysentery lasts less than 1 week and is associated with fever and blood or pus in the stool. If these signs are present, the yield on stool culture will approach 80 per cent;[2,6] however, by the time the culture is positive, most cases will have resolved. The clinical characteristics of these dysenteries are similar and cannot be used to distinguish one from another.[5]

Clostridium difficile is a bacterium that colonizes the colon but is kept suppressed by the normal flora, unless the latter is destroyed by broad-spectrum antibiotics. A toxin produced by proliferating *C. difficile* can induce mild diarrhea or an inflammatory pseudomembranous colitis (PMC). Recent prospective data show that up to 75 per cent of patients admitted to hospitals may become colonized by *C. difficile*, and about a third of those subsequently exposed to antibiotics will develop diarrhea.[7] *C. difficile* probably accounts for half of antibiotic-related diarrhea, the rest being due to nonspecific alteration of colonic flora or overgrowth of *Candida albicans*.

■ FOOD POISONING

Bacteria can also cause food poisoning. The three most common organisms are *Salmonella* sp., *Staphylococcus aureus*, and *Clostridium perfringens*.[8] In practice, a specific diagnosis is rarely made because the symptoms are short lived and the remaining food not ingested is usually not available for culture when the patient becomes symptomatic. The diagnosis is suspected by history, and management is similar to that for viral gastroenteritis. *Salmonella* sp. always lead the list of agents but may be overrepresented because they can be cultured from the stool. The usual course of disease lasts only 24 to 48 hours and may be a dysentery. There are suggestive patterns for each organism, such as a short incubation of 7 hours and profuse vomiting for *Staphylococcus* and *Bacillus cereus*. The former is usually associated with meats and the latter, which is rare in the United States, with rice. *Salmonella* poisoning has been acquired from so many sources (milk, poultry, pork, marijuana, pet turtles) that a history is rarely of any use. *C. perfringens* is associated with meat or fish; it causes a diarrhea without fever that runs its course in 24 hours. The *Vibrio* species include the agent of epidemic cholera, *Vibrio cholerae*, but it is not seen in the United States. Other *Vibrio* species include *V. parahaemolyticus* and *V. non-01 cholerae*, which are found in Gulf Coast waters and which will cause an occasional gastroenteritis. These cases are rare (three in 10 years in one large medical center), and unless a specific history of shellfish ingestion is obtained, these organisms probably can be ignored;[9] however, they can be detected on routine stool examinations, or specialized techniques can be used. Treatment of all bacterial food poisoning is symptomatic.

■ PARASITIC DIARRHEAS

Parasites cause a disproportionate amount of chronic infectious diarrhea, compared with the bacteria and viruses. In most areas of the United States, there are only two or three offending parasites, and the more exotic organisms may not be recognized by inexperienced technicians. Local laboratories in smaller hospitals often will have experience with only a few, such as *G. lamblia*, *E. histolytica*, or *Strongyloides stercoralis*.[10] The key to diagnosis is to suspect parasites and to be aware of those that local laboratories commonly detect. We do not have reliable tests to exclude parasitic infestations, so therapeutic trials of reliable and safe antimicrobials are part of the diagnostic evaluation of chronic diarrhea.

The most common parasites that cause diarrhea are the protozoans *Giardia lamblia* and *Entamoeba histolytica*. Intestinal helminths, except for *Strongyloides stercoralis*, do not cause as much diarrhea as the protozoans. Of these three parasitic infestations, amebiasis is not common and is usually limited to the Southwest or is found in patients with a history of travel to endemic areas. By contrast, giardiasis is ubiquitous in this country, and, contrary to textbook lore, the patient rarely gives a history of travel or of drinking contaminated water.[11]

Giardia lamblia is currently the most common parasite causing gastroenteritis in the United States. This appears to be true for all areas of the country, whether rural or urban.[10,11] This parasite is not related to socioeconomic conditions or racial groups and probably has little to do with sanitation, except for infants in daycare centers. It dominates other parasites statistically and will account for 50 to 97 per cent of all parasites isolated in most areas of the United States. *G. lamblia* infection probably is self-limited in many cases that go unrecognized. It can cause chronic diarrhea, and *Giardia* is the main organism that should be considered when chronic diarrhea is evaluated. In one prospective series of chronic diarrhea, *G. lamblia* was thought to be the cause in 24 per cent of cases.[12] Giardiasis symptoms appear to evolve as the infection becomes chronic, with diarrhea becoming slightly less prominent and abdominal pain, flatulence, bloating, and nausea or anorexia becoming more bothersome. Chronic infestation can cause significant weight loss, which is not clearly due to malabsorption in all cases but may be secondary to profound anorexia.

Strongyloides stercoralis occurs in most areas of the United States. As a helminth, it will usually induce eosinophilia. Diarrhea is a common presenting symptom, but in many cases there will be upper intestinal symptoms of epigastric pain, anorexia, nausea, and bloating.[13] The worms burrow into the intestinal wall and are a cause of visceral larvae migrans, with cough, wheezing, or rash. The rash may be urticaria. An overwhelming dissemination can occur in immunosuppressed patients on steroids. Diagnosis can be made on stool examination or intestinal biopsy. The stool may contain Charcot-Leyden crystals, which are degenerated eosinophils.

Entamoeba histolytica causes amebic dysentery. This is a colitis with blood and pus and occasional ulceration of the colonic epithelium. However, most cases of *E. histolytica* are nondysenteric and produce only watery diarrhea. Both types are usually self limited, but they can be chronic or life threatening. It is unusual to have eosinophilia, but in colitis cases the patient will have fever and leukocytosis. Endemic areas tend to be the Southwest United States, Mexico, and Latin America.

Blastocystis hominis recently has been classified as a pathogen causing a giardiasis-like syndrome. It may also occur in asymptomatic people. This organism has not been well studied but may be fairly common.

Cryptosporidium should be mentioned only because it is found in AIDS patients. In normal people it produces a self-limited infection with diarrhea. It is difficult to diagnose, and there is no effective treatment for it. In patients with AIDS, the diarrhea may be chronic and debilitating.

■ TRAVELERS' DIARRHEA

Travelers' diarrhea is a separate entity that encompasses all the aforementioned causes as well as agents not endemic to the United States. Most cases are bacterial and are self limited. Enterotoxigenic *E. coli* may be responsible for half of all cases and will cause a watery diarrhea that usually lasts 4 days.[14] *Salmonella* and *Shigella* tend to produce a dysentery, but this is probably much less common than once was suspected. Because antibiotic prophylaxis can reduce the rate of diarrhea by 90 per cent in prospective studies, it is probably fair to assume that most travelers' diarrhea is due to bacterial pathogens. Amebic dysentery is rare. There may also be a postinfectious diarrhea that can cause chronic diarrhea.[15] This may be due to persistent infection with *Giardia*, *Salmonella*, *Shigella*, or *E. histolytica* or may be secondary to lactase deficiency following an infection or tropical sprue. Giannella refers to a "postdysenteric irritable bowel syndrome" that he feels develops in some patients after a bout with travelers' diarrhea.[15]

Travelers' diarrhea usually occurs in a visitor from a "developed" country going to a less developed country. The more primitive the sewage disposal system, the more likely there is to be fecal contamination of food and water. The attack rate of travelers' diarrhea is 25 to 50 per cent, depending on the traveler's origin and the country he or she visits.

■ Management

Ninety per cent of acute diarrhea resolves spontaneously. Chronic diarrhea by definition has not resolved, and the physician will be obligated to attempt to make a diagnosis. Chronic idiopathic diarrheas have a natural history of eventual resolution over a period of months rather than weeks.[1] The limited number of treatable and diagnosable causes for diarrhea must also be kept in mind. Among bacterias, only the *Salmonella* sp., *Shigella* sp., *Campylobacter jejuni*, and *Yersinia* sp. can be cultured by routine laboratory techniques, and the parasites identifiable by stool examination are limited by technician experience. Most laboratories should be able to recognize *Giardia lamblia* and *E. histolytica. Strongyloides* is fairly easy to identify in fresh stool because it is highly motile and very large (visible on low power).

■ SYMPTOMATIC THERAPY

Almost all acute diarrhea should be treated symptomatically. Indeed, most patients never consult physicians but tolerate the symptoms until they resolve. A physician should avoid the temptation to do extensive evaluations because of the low yield of diagnostic evaluation.

Therapy should be directed at maintaining proper hydration and electrolyte balance—these are usually a problem only in infants or in those with intractable vomiting as part of their gastroenteritis. Pediatricians have a variety of diets, some with interesting names, such as the "brat diet" (bananas, rice, applesauce, and toast), that assure the child will be well hydrated and provided with glucose and electrolytes. The basis of diet therapy for diarrhea is to reduce agents that stimulate motility, avoid complex and poorly absorbed carbohydrates, and provide adequate water and electrolytes. Caffeine-containing products such as coffee and colas

should be avoided. Poorly absorbed carbohydrates include lactose products (milk, cheese, ice cream) and fructose sweeteners (many soft drink beverages). Milk products like yogurt should also be avoided since the lactose degradation is variable. Certain fruits, such as grapes and prunes, have poorly absorbed sugars such as sorbitol and xylitol in them. Many people regard fruit juice as a staple of diarrhea therapy and I think simply making them aware that it might exacerbate the problem is better than absolute prohibition. Simple sugar, glucose, is easily absorbed and facilitates absorption of electrolytes and can be obtained in a variety of products, including honey. Heavy meals with a large fat content may exacerbate diarrhea by stimulating motility reflexes, so multiple small meals should be encouraged.

Vomiting or inability to eat and drink due to dehydration and obtundation are indications for intervention with drugs or intravenous fluids. For adults, antiemetics by suppository are usually adequate. For young children I would not allow unsupervised use of suppositories longer than one day. If the diarrhea and vomiting are not reduced or signs of dehydration develop, close observation in hospital may be indicated. Elderly or malnourished individuals may also develop more severe problems because of inability to use oral therapy to maintain fluid and electrolyte balance during gastroenteritis.

The use of antiperistaltic drugs is controversial if the patient has a dysentery, but if the patient does not have fever or bloody, purulent diarrhea then loperamide (Imodium) is recommended to decrease the frequency of stools. Loperamide is now available over the counter and should be taken on a regular schedule of every 8 to 12 hours as needed.

■ ACUTE SEVERE DYSENTERY

Patients with fever, bloody diarrhea, and early signs of dehydration require further evaluation. Most of them will have a bacillary dysentery caused by *C. jejuni, Salmonella* sp., or *Shigella* sp. if they have not had prior antibiotics. The finding of leukocytes in the stool will confirm the impression of dysentery and should lead to an initial stool culture. If a patient has taken antibiotics, a stool specimen should be sent for detection of *C. difficile* toxin. If the patient is suspected of having pseudomembranous colitis, a proctoscopic examination can be diagnostic, and initial therapy can be started with metronidazole, 250 mg three times a day. If bacillary dysentery is suspected and the patient is severely ill, a broad-spectrum agent such as ciprofloxacin, 500 mg twice a day, trimethoprim-sulfamethoxazole (TMP-SMX), twice a day, or ampicillin, 500 mg four times a day, can be started. In most cases, by the time the stool culture is reported the symptoms will be resolving and antibiotics can be discontinued. On the other hand, if the patient is still ill more specific therapy can be used. For *C. jejuni*, use erythromycin, and for enteric fever from salmonellosis or shigellosis, culture sensitivity should probably guide therapy if the patient is not responding to TMP-SMX or ampicillin. *Yersinia* sp. are usually sensitive to TMP-SMX.

Pseudomembranous colitis must be treated because it is potentially fatal. The first step in treating PMC is to discontinue the offending antibiotic if the patient is still receiving it. Metronidazole or vancomycin, the latter in a dose of 125 mg three times a day, is given for 10 days to kill *C. difficile.* Vancomycin is very expensive, it tastes bad, and it cannot be given intravenously for pseudomembranous colitis because it does not produce any measurable fecal levels. Metronidazole is effective orally or intravenously.[16] The initial use of vancomycin for this disorder was based on the erroneous assumption that it was caused by *Staphylococcus aureus.* PMC has a relapse rate of about 15 per cent with both antimicrobials, so patient follow-up is important. Cholestyramine, 4 gm four times a day, has long been a useful drug that works by binding the toxin and allowing the natural regrowth of the colonic flora to suppress the *C. difficile.* I think this drug is most useful in patients with mild disease or relapse. Relapses often can be multiple and may require a prolonged tapering dose of suppressive drugs.[17]

Antibiotic-related diarrhea that is not due to *C. difficile* will usually resolve within 1 week of discontinuation of antibiotic use. If the diarrhea has not resolved, I have found useful nystatin, 500,000 units orally four times a day combined with *lactobacillus* powder twice a day. Symptoms can be suppressed safely with loperamide.

Occasionally a patient with proctitis will present with diarrhea due to gonorrhea, herpes simplex, or rarely cytomegalovirus (CMV). Infectious proctitis should be suspected in patients with bloody diarrhea, tenesmus, or a history of rectal intercourse. A rectal swab for gonococcal culture should be obtained. Herpes and CMV are self-limited and do not require specific therapy, although acyclovir, 200 mg every 4 hours, has been used to shorten the duration of herpetic proctitis.

■ CHRONIC NONDYSENTERIC DIARRHEA

In patients whose diarrhea has persisted longer than 4 to 6 weeks, further evaluation is necessary. Dysentery persisting this long usually will fall into the category of idiopathic inflammatory bowel disease. Crohn's disease, or ulcerative colitis (see Inflammatory Bowel Disease). It is rare to diagnose an infectious cause of chronic dysentery. If the diarrhea is not a dysentery, the most common infectious etiologies will be parasitic disorders or a postinfectious diarrhea. For this reason, the evaluation will center on ova and parasite (O&P) examination rather than culture, although culture is usually obtained but has low yield. A history of travel should be sought and a complete blood count done to look for eosinophilia. Traditionally, three stool specimens are obtained for O&P. These should be done on separate days and *prior to* any barium studies. In addition, any physician can obtain intestinal samples with the use of the "string test" (Enterotest). An encapsulated string is swallowed with water and then retrieved 4 hours later. Bile-stained fluid is then squeezed into a test tube and examined by the laboratory or in the office. I usually have patients wake about 4 A.M., swallow the string, then return to bed and come to the laboratory about 8 A.M. NPO.

If no diagnosis is made with these steps, I usually consider a therapeutic trial of antimicrobials. If the patient has no eosinophilia and no suspicious travel history, I treat for giardiasis. This therapy is guided by a knowledge of the frequency and types of parasites indigenous to my location in Alabama; however, a physician can obtain similar information by asking the parasitology laboratory which organisms are found most commonly. For giardiasis, there are three treatments: metronidazole, 250 mg three times a day, or quinacrine hydrochloride, 100 mg three times a day for adults, both for 7 days, and for children who cannot take pills, furazolidone, 1.25 mg/kg four times a day for 7 days. *Blastocystis hominis* is also treated with this dose of metronidazole. If the patient has eosinophilia and suspected strongyloidiasis, I proceed to duodenal sampling with biopsy and wet prep examination of the fluid. If these tests are negative and I still suspect *Strongyloides,* then a trial of thiabendazole, 25 mg/kg twice a day for 2 days, is administered. Thiabendazole is relatively safe, but two cases of Stevens-Johnson syndrome have been reported. If the patient vomits the medication, then an additional dose is given. Amebiasis is so rare in most areas of the United States that a therapeutic trial should not be used without reasonable proof of infection. This might include positive serology or stool examination in addition to a history of travel to endemic areas. Treatment for amebiasis is usually metronidazole, but in a large dose of 750 mg three times a day or 50 mg/kg/ day in three divided doses. Lower doses have been used for mild cases, and a variety of alternative antimicrobials are available.

Certain esoteric infectious diarrheas, such as Whipple's disease or tropical sprue, require small bowel biopsy and are rare enough that evaluation can be reserved for patients referred to a gastroenterologist. Bacterial overgrowth cannot easily or reliably be diagnosed and is also best left for specialist evaluations.

■ Issues and Risks

Antibiotics for Bacillary Dysentery

Antibiotics for bacterial diarrheas are routinely used only for *C. difficile*–induced pseudomembranous colitis. Reports of prolongation or induction of the carrier state have caused concern about treating salmonellosis with antibiotics.[18] Nevertheless, treatment is recommended when the patient is severely ill with "enteric fever" and possible bacteremia.

Antiperistaltic Drugs

A tradition has developed not to treat dysentery with antimotility drugs for fear of exacerbating the infection. This has been reported, in controlled trials of shigellosis, to prolong fever and prevent clearance of the organism.[19] However, most patients with dysentery are never seen by physicians and are undoubtedly self-medicated with opiate-like drugs such as paregoric and loperamide without evidence of any problem. I reserve use of these agents in dysentery for cases in which the frequency of loose stools is intolerable and diet therapy is not effective.

Travelers' Diarrhea Prophylaxis

Antibiotic prophylaxis is undoubtedly effective in preventing diarrhea, but the side effects probably outweigh the advantages.[14] The two drugs shown to be effective are TMP-SMX double-strength and doxycycline, 100 mg; however, since prolonged use of these can be associated with antibiotic-related diarrhea, it probably is best to avoid them. A reasonable approach is to allow the patient to take a 3-day supply of one of these antibiotics on the trip and to take one tablet twice daily at the first sign of diarrhea. This will shorten the course from 4 days to 1 day.[14] A supply of loperamide can also be taken on the trip and used to suppress diarrheal symptoms.

Referral

Cases of chronic diarrhea in which initial diagnostic evaluations have failed should be referred to a gastroenterologist. Because the disease is chronic, symptom suppression is no longer adequate. On the other hand, acute or subacute cases in which the symptoms are mild or easily suppressed may reasonably be observed. Most will resolve, and extensive evaluations have low yield and are expensive.[1] Patients with weight loss, vomiting, or nocturnal diarrhea probably should be referred.

REFERENCES

1. Blaser MJ. Infectious diarrheas: acute, chronic, and iatrogenic. Ann Intern Med 1986; 105:785–787.
2. Siegel D. Predictive value of stool examination in

acute diarrhea. Arch Pathol Lab Med 1987; 111:715–718.

3. Loosli J, Gyr H, Stalder GA, Stalder W, et al. Etiology of acute infectious diarrhea in a highly industrialized area of Switzerland. Gastroenterology 1985; 88:75–79.

4. Chancellor AM, Ellis-Pegler RB. A clinical and aetiological study of adult patients hospitalised for acute diarrheal disease. NZ Med J 1982; 95:154–156.

5. Blaser MJ, Wells JG, Feldman RA, Pollard RA, Allen JR. *Campylobacter* enteritis in the United States: a multicenter study. Ann Intern Med 1983; 98:360–365.

6. Koplan JP, Fineberg HV, et al. Value of stool cultures. Lancet 1980; 1:413–416.

7. McFarland LV, Mulligan ME, Kwok RYY, Stam WE. Nosocomial acquisition of *Clostridium difficile* infection. N Engl J Med 1989; 320:204–210.

8. Snydman DR. Bacterial food poisoning. In Gorbach SL (ed). Infectious Diarrhea. Boston: Blackwell Scientific Publications, 1986:201–218.

9. Bonner JR, Coker AS, Berryman CR, Pollock HM. Spectrum of *Vibrio* infection in a Gulf Coast community. Ann Intern Med 1983; 99:464–469.

10. Pearson R, Coleman S, Truss C. Giardiasis in Alabama. Ala J Med Sci 1988; 25:137–141.

11. Carr MF, Ma J, Green PHR. *Giardia lamblia* in patients undergoing endoscopy: lack of evidence for a role in nonulcer dyspepsia. Gastroenterology 1988; 95:972–974.

12. Bolin TD, Davis AE, Duncombe VM. A prospective study of persistent diarrhoea. Aust NZ J Med 1982; 12:22–26.

13. Milder JE, Walzer PD, Kilgore G, Rutherford I, Klein M. Clinical features of *Strongyloides stercoralis* infection in an endemic area of the United States. Gastroenterology 1981; 80:1481–1488.

14. NIH Consensus Conference. Travelers' diarrhea. JAMA 1985; 253:2700–2704.

15. Giannella RA. Chronic diarrhea in travelers: diagnostic and therapeutic considerations. Rev Infect Dis 1986; 8:S223–S226.

16. Teasley DG, Olson MM, Gerhard RL, Ferraro MJB, Rosenberg ML. Prospective randomized trial of metronidazole versus vancomycin for *Clostridium difficile*–associated diarrhea and colitis. Lancet 1983; 2:1043–1046.

17. Tedesco FJ. Treatment of recurrent antibiotic-associated pseudomembranous colitis. Am J Gastroenterol 1982; 88:220–221.

18. Rosenthal SJ. Exacerbation of salmonella enteritis due to ampicillin. N Engl J Med 1969; 280:147–148.

19. DuPont HL, Hornick RB. Adverse effect of Lomotil therapy in shigellosis. JAMA 1973; 226:1525–1528.

Endocarditis, infective

Michael E. Assey ■ *E. Edward Proctor*

■ Background

Prior to the availability of antibiotics, infective endocarditis was a highly fatal disease, with most patients dying from uncontrolled sepsis. Today, despite widely available and effective antimicrobial therapy, mortality and morbidity remain high, and infective endocarditis is responsible for many hospital admissions.[1] Earlier, this was a disease of relatively young people, who had underlying rheumatic or luetic heart disease. In the modern era, the affected population is older, with a distinctly different risk profile. The continued prevalence of infective endocarditis results from drug abusers who use drugs intravenously, the creation of a new population at risk (those who have undergone corrective surgery for congenital or acquired cardiac disease), and the increased use of medical invasive procedures.

■ Management

■ CLINICAL PRESENTATION

As classically described, infective endocarditis presents as a febrile illness with prominent constitutional symptoms, anemia, a new or varying heart murmur, splenomegaly, and signs of peripheral embolization. In the modern era, however, this classic presentation is seen in as few as 10 per cent of cases.[2,3] The physician must be aware of the potential for varying clinical presentations and multisystem involvement. Cardiac manifestations may predominate, as when infective endocarditis produces severe valvular insufficiency and pulmonary edema. Embolic complications may present as hematuria, abdominal pain, peripheral pulse deficits, or neuropsychiatric symptoms ranging from headache to completed stroke.

Acute and *subacute bacterial endocarditis* were terms primarily used in the preantibiotic era. Patients who died less than 8 weeks from the onset of the illness were classified as acute and usually were infected with virulent organisms, such as *Staphylococcus aureus* and *Neisseria gonorrhoeae*. These organisms could infect and quickly destroy even normal cardiac valves, producing dramatic cardiovascular decompensation. Subacute bacterial endocarditis applied to patients who survived longer and presented in a chronic manner, with fever, anemia, and constitutional symptoms. The infecting organisms included viridans streptococci and other less virulent bacteria. Infection usually occurred on valves that were already structurally altered from congenital or rheumatic heart disease.

Although marginally useful in a descriptive sense, the terms acute and subacute endocarditis have largely been abandoned. Survival is uniformly expected, although not always realized, and the clinical presentation can overlap. The effective treatment of endocarditis caused by virulent organisms can convert an acute illness to a subacute presentation. The inappropriate treatment of low-virulence organisms can result in serious cardiac complications more typical of acute bacterial endocarditis.

■ DIAGNOSIS

Prompt and proper identification of the infecting organism is the cornerstone of diagnosis and effective management. The bacteremia of infective endocarditis is qualitatively continuous as organisms are constantly seeded into the blood stream from vegetations on valves or other intravascular sites. In most cases, three sets of blood cultures, properly obtained by using alternate venipuncture sites with sterile preparation of the skin, allow an identification of the infecting organism. Larger numbers of blood cultures (six or more) may be needed if there has been prior antibiotic use or if more culture material is needed to identify slow-growing or nutritionally fastidious organisms.

The incidence of culture-negative endocarditis ranges between 3 and 15 per cent and is largely related to prior antibiotic use. In such cases, other diagnostic tests may be useful.[4] Nonspecific markers include an elevated sedimentation rate and C-reactive proteins, along with cryoglobulinemia. The rheumatoid factor is an IgM antibody directed against the fragment crystalline part of an IgG antibody. It is present in up to half of the patients who have had symptoms of infective endocarditis for longer than 6 weeks. Circulating immune complexes against the infecting organism can be identified as well. Unfortunately, the titers of these immune complexes are related to the duration of the disease, making them less useful in acute illnesses of shorter duration. The presence of teichoic acid antibodies suggests that a staphylococcal bacteremia is the result of a deep-seated infection. It does not, however, allow differentiation of infective endocarditis from other types of serious *Staphylococcus aureus* infections, such as osteomyelitis.

Echocardiography may be the only means of confirming the diagnosis of endocarditis when blood cultures are persistently negative. Vegetations as small as 2 mm can be identified and characterized by two dimensional echocardiography.[5,6] Smaller vegetations are not visualized; consequently, echocardiography cannot be used to rule out endocarditis. The technique cannot reliably differentiate new from old lesions and may be hampered in identifying endocarditis on prosthetic valves or other echogenic intracardiac structures. Figure 1 shows a typical vegetation present on a native aortic valve.

In addition to identifying the site of intracardiac infection, echocardiography can elucidate important complications, including ring abscess formation, anatomic disruption, and clinically unanticipated involvement of other intracardiac structures.[7,8] Doppler echocardiography, particularly color flow Doppler imaging, provides a semiquantitative assessment of the degree of valvular insufficiency resulting from the infective endocarditis. Doppler imaging also may identify abnormal fistulous tracts resulting from deep-seated cardiac infections.

While M-mode echocardiography is less sensitive than the two-dimensional technique in identifying valvular vegetations, it

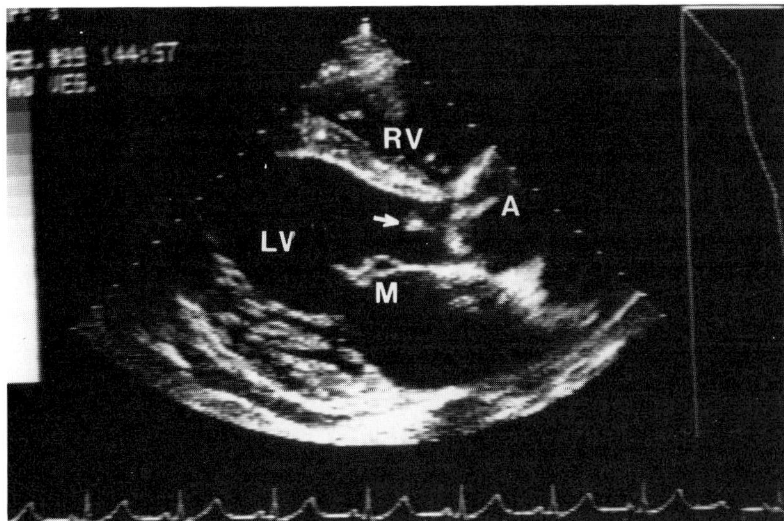

Figure 1. Two-dimensional echocardiogram in the parasternal long axis view. Arrow points to an echogenic vegetation on the aortic valve (A). During diastole, the vegetation prolapses down into the left ventricular outflow tract. (LV, left ventricle; RV, right ventricle; M, mitral valve.)

can play an important role in the management of infective endocarditis, when the aortic valve is involved. When acute aortic insufficiency results from aortic valve endocarditis, there is a dramatic increase in left ventricular pressure. This may result in closure of the mitral valve prior to the onset of ventricular systole, an event that can be accurately identified by M-mode echocardiography.[9] This finding, even in the absence of obvious clinical deterioration, constitutes a strong indication for emergency surgery, as these patients are at great risk of sudden cardiovascular deterioration and death. As demonstrated in Figure 2, sodium nitroprusside, given to reduce the amount of aortic

insufficiency, can attenuate or reverse the premature closure of the mitral valve. In this way, M-mode echocardiography provides important noninvasive hemodynamic information that in the past could be acquired only by invasive techniques.

The 12-lead electrocardiogram is also helpful in the assessment of patients with endocarditis.[10] The development of a prolonged PR interval, particularly in the absence of cardiac glycoside therapy, new bundle branch block, or ventricular ectopy, suggests the possibility of an annular or myocardial abscess. Such a finding generally indicates a need for surgery, as discussed later.

Figure 2. M-mode echocardiogram in a patient with acute aortic insufficiency secondary to staphylococcal endocarditis. The mitral valve (MV) closes prior to the onset of ventricular systole (before the QRS of the electrocardiogram). Nitroprusside therapy stabilized the hemodynamic abnormality and moved the mitral valve closure time back toward normal. (ECG, electrocardiogram; IVS, interventricular septum; PW, posterior left ventricular wall.) (From Assey ME, Usher BW. Echocardiography in diagnosing and managing aortic valve endocarditis. Reprinted with permission from the Southern Medical Journal 1981; 74:563.)

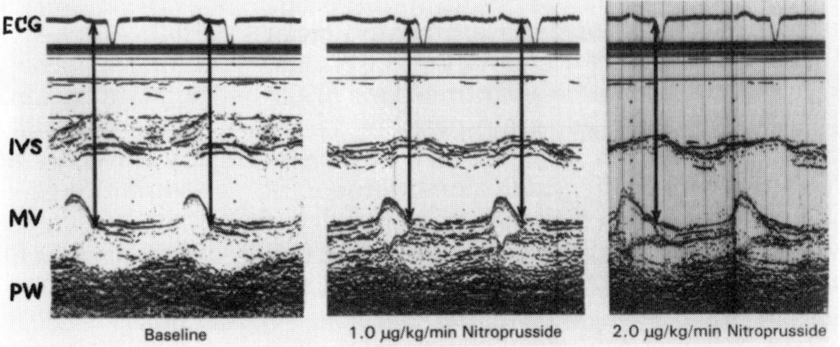

■ CARDIAC CATHETERIZATION

The benefits and risks of cardiac catheterization performed during active infective endocarditis remain controversial. Early reports focused on the need to insure that the operating surgeon had as much information as possible prior to intervening in these seriously ill patients. However, many patients with infective endocarditis tolerate cardiac catheterization poorly, particularly those with severe aortic or mitral insufficiency and decompensated congestive heart failure. This fact, coupled with the coming of age of noninvasive tools (particularly echocardiography and Doppler echocardiography) has obviated the need for acute catheterization in most patients.

Today, most patients undergo cardiac catheterization later to establish the presence and degree of residual valvular lesions. When cardiac catheterization is required during active infective endocarditis, consultation between the interventional cardiologist and cardiac surgeon is essential. Limited procedures—such as restricting the catheterization to a determination of right heart pressures and oxygen saturations, along with coronary angiography—allow one to obtain vital information while reducing the risks inherent in the catheterization of such patients.

■ ANTIMICROBIAL THERAPY

For antimicrobial therapy to be effective, the drug must be given in an appropriate dose over a period of time long enough that it will be able to kill the infecting organism and clear it from the blood stream. Identification of the infecting organism by the bacteriology laboratory and measurement of serum bactericidal levels have greatly enhanced our ability to treat this disease.

Infective endocarditis can be caused by diverse species of bacteria, fungi, and other microorganisms. The majority of microbiologically confirmed cases of infective endocarditis are due to gram-positive cocci, including viridans streptococci, staphylococci, enterococci, and nonenterococcal Group D streptococci, such as *Streptococcus bovis.* Recent recommendations for treatment have been made based on clinical and experimental data.[11]

The term *viridans streptococci* refers to a variety of streptococcal species. In the preantibiotic era, these streptococci were responsible for the majority of all cases of endocarditis, but recent studies have suggested that staphylococci are now more common. Penicillin is the drug of choice for viridans streptococci. The dose depends on the susceptibility of the particular strain, as some strains of viridans streptococci exhibit penicillin tolerance in the laboratory. Some cases of highly penicillin-sensitive viridans streptococci can be treated with a combination of penicillin and streptomycin for 2 weeks with a very high bacteriologic cure rate. The 2-week regimen should be confined to susceptible organisms in patients with uncomplicated endocarditis who are at low risk for aminoglycoside toxicity. It is not appropriate for prosthetic valve endocarditis or when intracardiac or extracardiac abscess formation is suspected. Vancomycin is generally recommended for penicillin-allergic patients. For viridans streptococci relatively resistent to penicillin, a 4-week course is recommended, in combination with streptomycin or gentamicin for the first 2 weeks.

Infective endocarditis due to *Staphylococcus epidermidis* frequently occurs on prosthetic valves and is discussed later. *Staphylococcus aureus* infection is characterized by a high incidence of cardiac and extracardiac abscess formation and is particularly prevalent in intravenous drug abusers. Most staphylococci are highly resistant to penicillin and require treatment with penicillinase-resistant penicillins. Nafcillin for 6 weeks, combined with gentamicin for the first 2 weeks, causes a rapid clearing of the bacteremia, although there is an increased risk of renal toxicity. Rifampin is sometimes used in combination with penicillinase-resistant penicillins and aminoglycosides. Vancomycin, again, is recommended for the penicillin-allergic patient.

The enterococci are Group D streptococci that normally inhabit the gastrointestinal tract. They are more resistant to penicillin than the other streptococci and relatively resistant to aminoglycosides. The combination of penicillin (alternatively ampicillin or vancomycin) and certain aminoglycosides (streptomycin or gentamicin) exerts a synergistic bactericidal effect.[12] Therapy should be continued for a minimum of 4 weeks.

Streptococcus bovis and *Streptococcus mutans* are Group D streptococci distinct from the enterococci. Both are killed effectively by penicillin, and treatment regimens are similar for viridans streptococci endocarditis. A particularly important aspect of *Streptococcus bovis* endocarditis is its association with conditions of the gastrointestinal tract, including carcinoma and inflammatory bowel disease. Patients with *S. bovis* endocarditis should undergo a thorough search for these underlying diseases.

■ LESS COMMON CAUSES OF ENDOCARDITIS

In the preantibiotic era, pneumococcal endocarditis was relatively frequent. Today it is seen occasionally in immunosuppressed patients, often in combination with pneumonitis and meningitis. *Haemophilus parainfluenzae* can form large valvular vegetations that may embolize and occlude a large peripheral vessel. Large-vessel embolization is also seen with fungal endocarditis. Gonococcal endocarditis is classically associated with sternoclavicular joint tenderness and a twice-daily temperature spike. Endocarditis caused by fungi and yeast occurs in immunosuppressed patients, including those on chronic steroid therapy, and in patients with indwelling intravenous catheters, in whom *Candida* infection is particularly prominent.

■ INDICATIONS FOR SURGERY DURING INFECTIVE ENDOCARDITIS

Surgery sometimes must be performed in a patient with active infective endocarditis in an effort to limit morbidity and mortality.[13] Table 1 lists the most common indications for surgical intervention. The major indication is congestive heart failure, particularly when it does not respond to simple maneuvers such as the addition of diuretics. Surgery also may be needed when the causative organism is extremely virulent or resistant, in which case antimicrobial therapy would not be expected to control the infection successfully. This is most likely to occur with fungal endocarditis, culture-negative endocarditis, or infections caused by certain strains of *Staphylococcus aureus*. This latter organism may cause extravalvular infection (myocardial or annular abscess, heart block, purulent pericarditis) and coronary embolism. Some investigators have suggested that native valve endocarditis due to *S. aureus* be

TABLE 1. Indications for Surgery During Active Infective Endocarditis

Congestive heart failure not responding to simple therapy

Recurrent systemic embolization
   may operate after a single embolic episode, particularly if large vegetation persists on mitral or aortic valve by echocardiography

Failure to clear bacteremia despite appropriate antimicrobial therapy

Infection secondary to medically resistant organisms
   fungal endocarditis
   ? *Staphylococcus aureus*

Extravalvular extension
   myocardial or annular abscess
   purulent pericarditis
   extracardiac abscess

Loss of anatomic integrity of native aortic or mitral valve while on antimicrobial therapy

Prosthetic valve endocarditis, particularly if there is anatomic disruption of the valve

operated regardless of the hemodynamic status.[14] An important exception is when *S. aureus* infects the tricuspid valve, as is often seen with intravenous drug abusers. Medical therapy is generally effective in this setting, and surgery is not usually indicated.

The risk of cardiac abscess formation must be emphasized. In a small study at our institution, 19 patients with native valve endocarditis were operated early (15 because of poorly controlled congestive heart failure, 2 with systemic emboli, and 2 with abscess and mild congestive heart failure). At surgery, eight patients were found to have a cardiac abscess, and only two survived hospitalization. Of the group of 35 operated patients, six patients died, of whom four had cardiac abscess formation.[15]

Other strong indicators for surgery in active endocarditis include recurrent systemic emboli or even a single embolic event when echocardiography demonstrates a large residual vegetation on a left-sided cardiac valve. Failure of medical treatment despite appropriate antimicrobial therapy and anatomic disruption of the valve constitute strong indications for surgery regardless of the duration of antibiotic therapy. The incidence of prosthetic valve endocarditis following surgery for native valve endocarditis is only around 5 per cent. This supports an aggressive surgical approach when native valve endocarditis is associated with these important cardiac and extracardiac complications.

Issues and Risks

INCREASING INCIDENCE OF RIGHT-SIDED ENDOCARDITIS

Infective endocarditis involving the tricuspid valve and, less frequently, the pulmonic valve is usually a complication of intravenous drug abuse. As this behavior has become more prevalent, the relative frequency of right-sided infective endocarditis has increased. The most frequently encountered infecting organism is *Staphylococcus aureus*, but outbreaks of enterococcal and *Pseudomonas* infection and fungal endocarditis have occurred in addicts sharing drug paraphernalia in various communities. For many years, it was thought that the source of the bacteremia was the infected equipment or contaminants within the drug itself. However, sophisticated bacteriologic studies using phage analyses have concluded that the drug user is usually the source of the infecting organism.

In most circumstances, the infected valve is structurally normal. Perhaps repeated exposure to foreign contaminants in the injected drug damages the endothelial lining of the valve leaflets and promotes bacterial colonization. Fever and a new cardiac murmur (tricuspid insufficiency or pulmonic insufficiency) are the usual presentations, but there are other typical characteristics. Drug abusers with endocarditis are generally younger in age, have many more respiratory symptoms and pulmonary infiltrates on chest radiograph, have a shorter duration of symptoms prior to hospitalization, and are less likely to present with congestive heart failure.[16] The prominence of pulmonary symptoms and chest film abnormalities is due to septic embolization from the right-sided cardiac valve vegetations. We have seen cases in which acute dyspnea, bronchospasm, and hemoptysis were temporally associated with a dramatic reduction in the size of the vegetation as demonstrated by echocardiography.

PROSTHETIC VALVE ENDOCARDITIS

This serious complication of valve replacement is also increasing as a result of the increased number of patients undergoing valve replacement. The overall incidence is between 2 and 4 per cent.[17] Earlier reports demonstrated a much higher risk of this complication, and it is assumed that the reduction in incidence has been due to the use of prophylactic antibiotics at the time of cardiac surgery. The value of these prophylactic regimens, however, has not been proved in prospective, controlled studies. Prosthetic valve endocarditis is divided into those events that present within 60 days of valve insertion and those that occur after that period of time. This temporal classification seems appropriate since the clinical presentations and microbiologic patterns are different.[18] Although the mitral valve is most commonly affected in cases of native valve endocarditis, prosthetic valve endocarditis usually occurs on the aortic valve.

Staphylococci are the most frequent causative organisms when prosthetic valve endocarditis occurs within 60 days of surgery. The most common single isolate is *Staphylococcus epidermidis*. Other organisms responsible for early prosthetic valve endocarditis (e.g., diphtheroids) grow very slowly and require prolonged incubation times before identification is possible. Fungal organisms may cause prosthetic valve endocarditis, with *Candida* species being the most frequent, followed by *Aspergillus*.[19] Late prosthetic valve endocarditis has a greater preponderance of streptococcal organisms, particularly non-Group D streptococcus. The variable microbiology reflects the specific hospital flora, as prosthetic valve endocarditis occurring within 60 days of surgery generally is due to contamination.

Prosthetic valve endocarditis is very difficult to manage with antibiotics alone, and surgery is usually necessary. The presence of even mild heart failure is an ominous prognostic sign. The loss of structural integrity, identified by the presence of paravalvular leaks at the time of echo/Doppler studies or rocking of the prosthesis on fluoroscopy, is a strong indication for early operative intervention.

Early death from prosthetic valve endocarditis exceeds that of native valve endocarditis, and the overall long-term prognosis is generally less favorable. Prosthetic valve endocarditis is often complicated by deep tissue involvement, with a high incidence of myocardial or annular abscess. Additionally, the infecting organisms are less antibiotic responsive.

■ PREVENTION

In one large study, almost three fourths of patients with endocarditis had evidence of pre-existing structural cardiac abnormalities.[20] This suggests that most of the population at risk for infective endocarditis can be defined by careful history and physical examination. Cardiac structural abnormalities that are particularly prone to endocarditis include implanted prosthetic devices and congenital or acquired heart disease (Table 2). Bacteria are usually deposited in areas of high blood flow velocity with decreased lateral pressure.[21] Vegetations develop most frequently on insufficient rather than stenotic valves, and in the case of insufficient valves they lodge on the low-pressure side of the regurgitant jet. Accordingly, ventricular septal defects and mitral insufficiency (in which case an abnormal communication exists between a high-pressure chamber and a low-pressure chamber) are at high risk for infective endocarditis. In contrast, an atrial septal defect in which the size of the communication is large and exists between two low-pressure chambers carries a low risk for endocarditis.

Equally important to the rationale for infective endocarditis prophylaxis is the ability to identify procedures that are prone to result in sustained bacteremia and infection of a structurally abnormal intravascular structure. Table 3 lists some of the more frequent procedures that are associated with important bacteremias. A final justification for prophylaxis is the observation that the incidence and duration of postprocedure

TABLE 2. Cardiac Conditions Requiring Endocarditis Prophylaxis

Rheumatic heart disease with stenotic or regurgitant murmurs

Congenital heart disease
  uncomplicated atrial septal defects do not require prophylaxis, except for 6 months following surgical closure

Prosthetic heart valves—mechanical or biologic

Surgically constructed systemic-pulmonic shunts

Idiopathic hypertrophic subaortic stenosis

Mitral valve prolapse with mitral regurgitation

Prior history of infective endocarditis

(Modified from Shulman ST, Amren DP, Bisno AL, et al. Prevention of bacterial endocarditis. Circulation 1984; 70:1123A–1127A.)

TABLE 3. Procedures That Frequently Produce Bacteremia and Require Endocarditis Prophylaxis in Susceptible Patients

Dental procedures likely to induce bleeding

Surgical procedures, including tonsillectomy, adenoidectomy, incision and drainage of infected tissue, and biopsy of the respiratory mucosa

Rigid bronchoscopy

Urethral catheterization, cystoscopy, and any prostate or urinary tract surgery

Gallbladder or colon surgery

Esophageal dilation or sclerotherapy of varices

Upper gastrointestinal tract endoscopy with biopsy

Colonoscopy

Proctosigmoid direct biopsy

(Modified from Shulman ST, Amren DP, Bisno AL, et al. Prevention of bacterial endocarditis. Circulation 1984; 70:1123A–1127A.)

bacteremia can be reduced by appropriate antimicrobial therapy.[22]

The specific prophylactic antimicrobial regimen depends on the intended procedure and therefore the expected type of bacteremia.[23–25] In patients with native valve abnormalities, dental procedures that cause gingival bleeding should be pretreated with penicillin. We recommend 2 gm of oral penicillin 1 hour before the anticipated bacteremia, followed by 1 gm 6 hours later. Patients unable to take oral penicillin can be given aqueous penicillin G (2 million units intramuscularly or intravenously) 60 minutes before the procedure, followed by a parenteral dose of 1 million units 6 hours after the procedure. Penicillin-allergic patients may be given oral erythromycin or parenteral vancomycin.

Patients with prosthetic valves deserve added protection, and the antibiotic regimen is increased, even for dental procedures and respiratory tract surgery. Such coverage includes parenteral ampicillin (1.0 to 2.0 gm) plus gentamicin, 1.5 mg/kg, 30 minutes before and 8 hours after the procedure. These dosages are for adult patients. The dosing intervals are the same in children, but the pediatric dose is based on weight, although the peak dose should not exceed the maximum recommended adult dose.

Proper prophylaxis for genitourinary and gastrointestinal tract procedures is different, reflecting the varying bacteriologic flora of those mucosal surfaces. The standard regimen recommends 2 gm of parenteral ampicillin plus gentamicin, 1.5 mg/kg, 30 to 60 minutes prior to the procedure. A single follow-up dose, 8 hours after the procedure, is recommended. Penicillin-allergic patients should substitute vancomycin for ampicillin. Patients undergoing repeated genitourinary or gastrointestinal procedures who are felt to be at low risk for endocarditis can be treated with 3 gm of oral amoxicillin 1 hour prior to the procedure, followed by 1.5 gm 6 hours later.

A frequently asked question concerns the need for endocarditis prophylaxis in patients with mitral valve prolapse, which may affect up to 10 per cent of the population at large. Although these patients are clearly at risk for infective endocarditis, the magnitude of the risk appears low and must be balanced against the potential risk of prophylactic antimicrobial therapy. The risk is reportedly higher in patients with mitral valve prolapse with an associated mitral insufficiency murmur.[26] It has been suggested that restricting prophylaxis to mitral valve prolapse patients with a systolic murmur would provide coverage for almost 90 per cent of prolapse patients.[27] Since the risk of a serious adverse reaction to parenteral penicillin exceeds the risk of oral penicillin, only oral prophylaxis is recommended.

REFERENCES

1. Garvey GJ, Neu HC. Infective endocarditis—An evolving disease. A review of endocarditis at The Columbia-Presbyterian Medical Center, 1968–1973. Medicine 1978; 57:105–127.
2. Weinstein L, Rubin RH. Infective endocarditis—1973. Prog Cardiovasc Dis 1973; 16:239–274.
3. Weinstein L, Schlesinger JJ. Pathoanatomic, pathophysiologic and clinical correlations in endocarditis. N Engl J Med 1974; 291:832–837.
4. Miller MH, Casey JI. Infective endocarditis: new diagnostic techniques. Am Heart J 1978; 96:123–128.
5. Dillon JC, Feigenbaum H, Konecke LL, Davis RH, Chang, S. Echocardiographic manifestations of valvular vegetations. Am Heart J 1973; 86:698–704.
6. Gilbert BW, Haney RS, Crawford F, McClellan J, Gallis HA, Johnson ML, Kisslo JA. Two-dimensional echocardiographic assessment of vegetative endocarditis. Circulation 1977; 55:346–353.
7. Mintz GS, Kotler MN, Segal BL, Parry WR. Survival of patients with aortic valve endocarditis. The prognostic implications of the echocardiogram. Arch Intern Med 1979; 139:862–866.
8. Sareli P. Klein HO, Schamroth CL, et al. Contribution of echocardiography and immediate surgery to the management of severe aortic regurgitation from active infective endocarditis. Am J Cardiol 1986; 57:413–418.
9. Botvinick EH, Schiller NB, Wickramasekaran R, Klausner SC, Gertz E. Echocardiographic demonstration of early mitral valve closure in severe aortic insufficiency. Its clinical implications. Circulation 1975; 51:836–847.
10. Hutter AM Jr, Moellering RC. Assessment of the patient with suspected endocarditis. JAMA 1976; 235:1603–1606.
11. Bisno AL, Dismukes WE, Durack DT, Kaplan EL, Karchmer AW, Kaye D, Rahimtoola SH, Sande MA, Sanford JP, Watanakunakorn C, Wilson WR. Antimicrobial treatment of infective endocarditis due to viridans streptococci, enterococci, and staphylococci. JAMA 1989; 261:1471–1477.
12. Sande MA, Scheld WM. Combination antibiotic therapy of bacterial endocarditis. Ann Intern Med 1980; 92:390–395.
13. Dinubile MJ. Surgery in active endocarditis. Ann Intern Med 1982; 96:650–659.
14. Richardson JV, Karp RB, Kirklin JW, Dismukes WE. Treatment of infective endocarditis: a 10-year comparative analysis. Circulation 1978; 58:589–597.
15. Assey ME, Usher BW, Crawford FA. Surgical considerations in the diagnosis and management of infective endocarditis. Infect Surg 1983; 6:418–430.
16. Chambers HF, Korzeniowski OM, Sande MA. *Staphylococcus aureus* endocarditis: clinical manifestations in addicts and non addicts. Medicine 1983; 62:170–177.
17. Baumgartner WA, Miller DC, Reitz BA, et al. Surgical treatment of prosthetic valve endocarditis. Ann Thorac Surg 1983; 35:87–104.
18. Dismukes WE, Karchmer AW, Buckley MJ, Austen WG, Swartz MN. Prosthetic valve endocarditis: an analysis of 38 cases. Circulation 1973; 48:365–377.
19. Cowgill LD, Addonizio VP, Hopeman AR, Harken AH. Prosthetic valve endocarditis. Curr Probl Cardiol 1986; 11:617–664.
20. Pelletier LL Jr, Petersdorf RG. Infective endocarditis: a review of 125 cases from the University of Washington hospitals 1963–72. Medicine 1987; 56:287–313.
21. Rodbard S. Blood velocity and endocarditis. Circulation 1963; 27:18–28.
22. Baltch AL, Schaffer C, Hammer MC, et al. Bacteremia following dental cleaning in patients with and without penicillin prophylaxis. Am Heart J 1982; 104:1335–1339.
23. Shulman ST, Amren DP, Bisno AL, et al. Prevention of bacterial endocarditis. A statement for health professionals by the Committee on Rheumatic Fever and Infective Endocarditis of the Council on Cardiovascular Disease in the Young. Circulation 1984; 70:1123A–1127A.
24. Kaye D. Prophylaxis for infective endocarditis: an update. Ann Intern Med 1986; 104:419–423.
25. Clemens JD, Horwitz RI, Jaffe CC, Feinstein AR, Stanton BF. A controlled evaluation of the risk of bacterial endocarditis in persons with mitral-valve prolapse. N Engl J Med 1982; 307:776–781.
26. Bisno AL. Antimicrobial prophylaxis for infective endocarditis. Hosp Pract 1989; 24:209–226.
27. MacMahon SW, Hickey AJ, Wilcken DEL, Wittes JT, Feneley MP, Hickie JB. Risk of infective endocarditis in mitral valve prolapse with and without precordial systolic murmurs. Am J Cardiol 1986; 58:105–108.

Endocrine manifestations of cancer

Thomas E. Lad ■ *Subhash C. Kukreja*

Tumors commonly produce various hormones that are not normally produced by the tissue of origin. The term *ectopic hormone production* has been used to denote this phenomenon. However, it has been demonstrated recently that many normal tissues contain small quantities of hormones, such as human chorionic gonadotropin (hCG) and adrenocorticotropic hormone (ACTH), and therefore the production of these hormones by cancer tissue may not be truly ectopic.[1] Notwithstanding this observation, the concept of ectopic hormone production is still clinically useful. The tumors in this situation produce hormone in sufficient quantities so that it either can be detected in the serum or results in the clinical syndrome of excessive hormone production. Besides the classic endocrinopathies, several other manifestations of cancer, such as fever, digital clubbing, neuropathy, cerebellar atrophy, and myopathy, also may be caused by production of humoral substances by the tumors.[2] Table 1 presents a partial list of hormones produced by tumors and the clinical manifestations. Several of these do not result in any clinical syndromes. Common clinical endocrine syndromes associated with cancer are hypercalcemia, ectopic ACTH syndrome, and syndrome of inappropriate antidiuretic hormone secretion (SIADH). These will be discussed in detail. Other less common syndromes will be briefly discussed.

■ Background

■ HYPERCALCEMIA

Hypercalcemia is the most common of the endocrine manifestations of cancer. Lung cancer is the most common cancer in the Western world, and about 15 per cent of lung cancer patients develop hypercalcemia during the course of their illness. Hypercalcemia is also seen in breast cancer, the most common cancer in women. Consequently, a primary care physician is likely to encounter this problem with some frequency.

The clinical presentation of hypercalcemia is one of confusion, lethargy, polyuria, dehydration, and constipation. Since most of these symptoms are somewhat nonspecific and occur in malnourished and debilitated cancer patients, one's index of suspicion for hypercalcemia depends upon the primary site and histology of the tumor.

Hypercalcemia occurs in patients with cancers of the lung (usually squamous, but not small cell in which it virtually never occurs), ENT region, esophagus, cervix, ureter and bladder, kidney, prostate (unusual), and breast, and in multiple myeloma and T-cell

TABLE 1. Hormones Produced by Neoplasms and Their Manifestations

Hormones	Clinical Features
Antidiuretic hormone	SIADH
Adrenocorticotropic hormone	Ectopic ACTH syndrome
Calcitonin	None
Chorionic gonadotropin	Gynecomastia, precocious puberty, hyperthyroidism
Growth hormone	? Clubbing
Growth hormone–releasing hormone	Acromegaly
Transforming growth factors	? Hypercalcemia
Insulin-like growth factors	Hypoglycemia
β-Lipotropin, proopiomelanocortin	Hyperpigmentation
Hypophosphatemia-producing factor	Hypophosphatemia, osteomalacia
Parathyroid hormone–related protein	Hypercalcemia
Osteoblast-inducing factor	Hypocalcemia
Prolactin	Galactorrhea

237

lymphoma. In other cancers, hypercalcemia is quite rare.

The diagnosis of hypercalcemia is easily made by measuring the serum calcium level. Normal homeostatic mechanisms maintain serum calcium levels within a narrow range, and any elevation is significant. In general, cancer-associated hypercalcemia produces higher levels of serum calcium than does primary hyperparathyroidism. Since calcium is protein-bound, hypoalbuminemia will increase ionized calcium levels for a given total calcium value. Ionized calcium is the biologically active moiety, and various formulas have been espoused to correct for hypoalbuminemia in an attempt to reflect ionized calcium levels more accurately. However, these formulas do not correlate very well with measured ionized calcium levels.[3] Ionized calcium is more costly to assay than is total calcium, and the latter will suffice for routine clinical use.

The mechanism for the development of hypercalcemia varies with the type of cancer, but the common denominator for all the mechanisms is bone resorption.[4] This can occur locally at the site of bone metastasis, as in breast cancer when bone resorption by tumor cells has been reported, or throughout the skeletal system, which is mediated by circulating hormone-like substances. Prostaglandin E_2 has been implicated in this regard but is quite rare as a cause of hypercalcemia. Cytokines, including interleukin-1, cachectin, and lymphotoxin, collectively referred to as *osteoclast-activating factor*, are operative in hematologic neoplasms. Most recently, the newly characterized peptide called *parathyroid hormone–related peptide* has been demonstrated to be the likely cause of most cases of humorally mediated hypercalcemia observed in solid tumors of all kinds.[4]

■ ECTOPIC ACTH SYNDROME

Biologically active ACTH is derived from a large-molecular-weight protein of 26,000 MW, which is called proopiomelanocortin.[5] β-Lipotropin, enkephalins, and endorphins are also derived from this larger precursor molecule.[5] β-Lipotropin and ACTH both contain sequences for melanocyte-stimulating activity. The cancers that are commonly associated with ectopic ACTH syndrome are of the lung (especially small cell), pancreas,

and thymus. Benign tumors such as bronchial carcinoid and pheochromocytoma are also associated with this syndrome. In one study, plasma ACTH levels were elevated in 53 of 74 (72 per cent) of patients with lung cancer.[6] However, in a majority of patients, this molecule exists in the precursor form and is biologically inactive. The clinical syndrome is seen in about 3 per cent of patients with small cell carcinoma of the lung.

Ectopic ACTH production associated with benign tumors, such as bronchial carcinoid, can result in classic Cushing's syndrome with central obesity, moon facies, and striae. However, in malignant tumors, the manifestations of ectopic ACTH production are superimposed on the underlying features of cancer, and the clinical features of the Cushing's syndrome are modified. Common presenting features are severe muscle weakness, hypokalemia, edema, hypertension, impaired glucose tolerance, and hyperpigmentation. A patient with cancer who has these clinical features should be tested for this syndrome. The most accurate means to establish the diagnosis is to perform the classic dexamethasone suppression test. Patients with ectopic ACTH syndrome do not suppress serum cortisol, urine 17-hydroxysteroids, or urinary free cortisol with either the low (2 mg/day for 2 days) or the high dose (8 mg/day for 2 days) of dexamethasone. This test takes several days to perform, and in case of a strong clinical suspicion may be simplified as follows: After obtaining a baseline A.M. serum cortisol value, the patient is given 8 mg of dexamethasone at night. Serum cortisol determinations are repeated the next morning. A less than 50 per cent suppression from the base value indicates that the patient has either an adrenal tumor or an ectopic ACTH syndrome.[7] A plasma ACTH level measurement then would differentiate between these two entities; the levels are suppressed in adrenal tumors and are high (usually greater than 100 pg/ml) in ectopic ACTH syndrome.[8]

■ SYNDROME OF INAPPROPRIATE ADH SECRETION

Diagnosis of the syndrome of inappropriate antidiuretic hormone (SIADH) is made by (1) hyponatremia, (2) low serum osmolality, (3) inappropriately high urine osmolality (usually the urine osmolality is higher than the plasma osmolality; however, the diagnosis can still be made if the urine is less than maximally dilute, i.e., its osmolality is greater than 150 mOsm/kg), (4) a urine sodium excretion rate greater than 20 mEq/L, (5) normal renal function, (6) normal adrenal and thyroid functions, and (7) absence of intravascular volume depletion.[9] Intravascular volume is moderately expanded, with low BUN and low serum uric acid levels. In a patient with cancer, SIADH may result from either excessive production of ADH by the tumor or the presence of pneumonia or brain lesions, or it may be an effect of antitumor (cyclophosphamide, vincristine) or analgesic therapy (morphine). The symptoms of hyponatremia are predominately related to the central nervous system: patients show lethargy, progressing to mental confusion, seizures, and coma. Patients are often hyporeflexic and may have focal neurologic deficits. The symptoms are correlated with the rate of fall in serum sodium concentration and the degree of hyponatremia. Subclinical hyponatremia may be present, which becomes overt after the patient receives excessive fluids either in intravenous or oral form. This is a special problem in patients receiving cyclophosphamide, in whom large amounts of fluids may need to be given to prevent cystitis. Small cell lung cancer is the most common tumor associated with SIADH. Other types of lung cancer; prostate, esophageal, adrenocortical, and pancreatic carcinoma; and Hodgkin's disease are also associated with the syndrome.

■ HYPOGLYCEMIA

Hypoglycemia seen in patients with cancer is most commonly spurious and is due to the blood being collected improperly. In a patient with normal hematocrit, blood cells utilize glucose at a rate of approximately 6 to 7 mg/dl/hr at room temperature. Therefore, if there is any doubt about the manner in which the blood has been collected, a repeat measurement should be obtained in which the sample is either refrigerated or collected in specialized tubes that contain an inhibitor of glycolytic enzymes. The tumors associated with hypoglycemia are often large mesenchymal tumors, such as mesothelioma, fibrosarcoma, or rhadomyosarcoma. The other tumors associated with

this syndrome are adrenocortical and hepatocellular carcinomas. The factor responsible for hypoglycemia in these tumors is immunologically different from insulin but is related in its biologic activity to insulin. This factor has been termed nonsuppressible insulin-like activity (NSILA). More recently, it has been shown that this factor may be an insulin-like growth factor II (IGF II).[10]

■ ECTOPIC HCG PRODUCTION AND HYPERTHYROIDISM

Large quantities of human chorionic gonadotropin (hCG) are produced by hydatidiform mole and choriocarcinoma. HCG binds weakly to the TSH receptor and results in its stimulation. Therefore, when large quantities of this hormone are present, hyperthyroidism with goiter and increased ^{131}I uptake may result.[11] Other tumors, which produce smaller amounts of hCG, are germ cell tumors of the testis and ovary, large cell carcinomas and adenocarcinomas of the lung, hepatomas, adenocarcinoma of the stomach and pancreas, and islet cell tumors. Precocious puberty in children, gynecomastia in men, and oligomenorrhea in premenopausal women may result from excessive hCG production. However, in a majority of patients, there are no clinical manifestations related to hCG production.

■ OTHER ENDOCRINE SYNDROMES ASSOCIATED WITH CANCER

Elevation in serum calcitonin (CT) has been reported in 20 to 60 per cent of patients with various cancers, especially carcinoma of the lung. Elevated serum CT levels may be due to the production of CT by the tumor or to alterations in physiologic control of CT secretion. There are no symptoms related to elevated serum CT levels. In general, measurement of serum CT levels has not been found to be a useful marker for follow-up of cancer patients.

Ectopic production of growth hormone (GH) has been suggested as a cause of clubbing seen in patients with lung cancer, but in follow-up studies, no clear-cut associations were found. Recently, production of classic acromegaly has been reported with ectopic production of growth hormone–releasing hormone (which in turn stimulated the pituitary to release excessive GH) by bronchial carcinoid. Removal of the primary tumor resulted in regression of the acromegalic symptoms.

Elevated serum prolactin levels have been reported in a few patients with cancer and may be associated with galactorrhea.

Hypocalcemia based on total calcium measurement is commonly seen in cancer patients. In most of these patients, the ionized calcium measurement is normal and hypocalcemia is spurious due to low serum albumin levels. True hypocalcemia may be seen either because of hyperphosphatemia during cell lysis in chemotherapy (especially in hematologic malignancies) or during cisplatin therapy (hypomagnesemia and increased urine calcium loss). A few patients with extensive osteoblastic metastases due to prostate, breast, or bronchial carcinoma with severe hypocalcemia have been reported. In these patients, hypocalcemia may be related to extensive accretion of calcium into the skeleton owing to the release of factors that activate osteoblasts.

A few patients with renal phosphate wasting and osteomalacia have been reported in association with benign mesenchymal, usually cutaneous or bone, tumors. Its association has also been reported with prostate cancer. The nature of the factors responsible for the phosphaturia is not known. These patients usually need large amounts of oral inorganic phosphorus (1 to 3 gm/day) to control the hypophosphatemia.

■ Management

■ HYPERCALCEMIA

Since the common denominator mechanism for cancer-associated hypercalcemia is bone resorption, the drugs used to control this problem are bone resorption inhibitors. However, before these are discussed, some general statements about the treatment of hypercalcemia need to be made. First, the most obvious way to control cancer-associated hypercalcemia would be to eradicate the cancer. Unfortunately this is usually not possible because hypercalcemia characteristically occurs in patients with metastatic disease, and these cancers are usually not curable at that stage, the exception being some of the lymphomas. Nonetheless, if the cancer is one that responds favorably to systemic therapy, the hypercalcemia can be controlled by chemotherapy or hormonal manipulation. Breast cancer and myeloma are good examples of such a situation. Second, it is sometimes stated that hypercalcemia should not be treated in patients with advanced cancer. This is certainly an issue of judgment on a case-by-case basis. The symptoms of hypercalcemia—confusion, polyuria, and constipation—make care of hypercalcemic patients difficult, particularly at home, and control of these symptoms can be very helpful to the caregiver. However, it is also true that treatment would be inappropriate at the time of imminent death. The primary care physician must weigh all these factors when deciding whether and how vigorously to treat.

Dehydration is a prominent feature of hypercalcemia. Significant hypercalcemia causes hypercalciuria, which results in a water diuresis. Dehydration ensues, followed by increasing proximal tubular stimulus for calcium reabsorption, worsening hypercalcemia, more diuresis, and so on. If water loss is replenished, the renal calcium reabsorption stimulus is lessened, and a significant reduction in serum calcium level can be achieved by hydration alone. Consequently, the initial therapeutic intervention should be intravenous normal saline. Although huge volumes of saline (over 20 liters per day) and several gram doses of furosemide (Lasix) have been reported to result in a significant lowering of serum calcium,[12] one can achieve a reasonable initial reduction with 3 or 4 liters of saline over a 24-hour period.[13] Furosemide will inhibit distal tubular calcium resorption but is probably not necessary, since the relative contribution of this to the overall picture is small. Once replacement of the water loss is achieved, there is often a significant improvement in the condition of the patient. At this point, bone resorption–inhibitor therapy can begin.

Until the advent of diphosphonates, mithramycin was generally considered the most effective treatment for cancer-associated hypercalcemia. This was demonstrated in a prospective randomized trial comparing the effectiveness of mithramycin, prednisone, oral phosphate, and indomethacin.[14] Calcitonin plus steroids is also an effective regimen, but benefit is very transient. Prompt (within 24 hours) reduction of the serum calcium level can be achieved with either mithramycin or calcitonin plus steroids, but the latter regimen loses its efficacy within a day or two despite continued administration.[15] Mithramycin's effect is also short-lived, its mean duration of benefit being around 5 days, after which it must be repeated. Mithramycin is given at a dose of 25 μg/kg IV bolus daily for 3 days, or until the serum calcium level begins to fall. The toxicities of mithramycin include azotemia, thrombocytopenia, and elevations of serum transaminase levels. These effects are more common with prolonged daily administration and are usually not a problem when the dosage is as specified. In addition, the toxicity of uncontrolled hypercalcemia is worse than potential toxicity from mithramycin therapy.

Diphosphonates are pyrophosphate analogs that are incorporated into the hydroxyapatite structure of bone and can inhibit resorption of bone by a number of agents, including parathyroid hormone, lymphokines, and prostaglandins. A number of experimental diphosphonates have shown clinical activity, and clinical trials of diphosphonates are current. Disodium-1-hydroxethylidene-1,1-diphosphonate (etidronate disodium, or Didronel) is the only diphosphonate commercially available in the United States at this time. It has been used in its oral form for Paget's disease, but the oral route is not effective in controlling hypercalcemia of malignancy.[14] The intravenous route is effective, however at a dose of 7.5 mg/kg/day given for at least 3 days. About three quarters of patients achieve normocalcemia within 5 days of treatment.[16] The duration of effect is probably in the range of a few weeks, but accurate data regarding this issue are difficult to obtain for a variety of reasons.

Acute toxicity from etidronate is minimal and consists of mild diarrhea in some patients. Long-term toxicity, osteomalacia, is not an issue at the dose recommended, especially for patients with limited survival probability. It is likely that newer disphosphonates that are easier to give, more effective, or both will be introduced in the near future. Dichloromethylene diphosphonate is already in use in Europe, and other compounds are in preclinical stages of development.

The transitional metal compounds gallium nitrate and cis-diamminedichloroplatinum (cisplatin, Platinol) have also been reported to control malignant hypercalcemia as well as inhibit bone resorption. These compounds are potentially more toxic than etidronate or even mithramycin, and although they can safely be administered by those who are experienced with the use of cytotoxic chemotherapy, their use is best left to oncologists.

Management of hypercalcemia is difficult. The survival of patients with hypercalcemia due to cancer is limited, one or two months on the average, and none of the treatments available today are of sufficient activity and long-term effectiveness to prevent hypercalcemia from continuing to be a major problem for a patient for the duration of his or her life. Since hydration status is so important, the adequacy of fluid intake for hypercalcemic patients cannot be overstressed. However, oral intake is usually poor in these patients because of anorexia and immobility caused by cancer, and these patients tend to require frequent hospitalizations for intravenous fluids and repeated treatment of hypercalcemia. Eventually the physician must decide when treatment becomes inappropriate. Often this decision is not difficult, since the hypercalcemia becomes refractory to attempts at control.

■ ECTOPIC ACTH SYNDROME

Removal of the primary tumor will result in normalization of cortisol secretion and an amelioration of the clinical signs and symptoms. However, in the case of malignant tumors, this is often not possible. Small cell lung carcinomas respond well to chemotherapy. The response of the endocrine abnormalities will parallel that of the primary tumor. However, it is often necessary to block the synthesis of adrenal steroids. The drugs most often used for this purpose are metapyrone, aminoglutethimide, or ketoconazole. Metapyrone is an 11-hydroxylase inhibitor, an enzyme needed for the final step in the synthesis of cortisol. The drug can be used therapeutically and is administered orally in 4 to 6 divided doses of 250 mg each. The most common side effect is the gastrointestinal intolerance. At higher doses, hypertension and hypokalemic alkalosis may be seen. When used alone, metapyrone is not a very effective agent. Aminoglutethimide (Cytadren) is an inhibitor of enzymes needed for the conversion of cholesterol to pregnenolone and is an effective therapeutic agent. It is given initially at a dose of 250 mg orally twice daily and then gradually increased to a total dose of up to 2 gm per day. Common side effects include skin rash (usually transient), gastrointestinal intolerance, and neurologic side effects such as lethargy, sedation, and blurred vision. The toxicity can be minimized by combining metapyrone (1 mg/day) and aminoglutethimide at a lower dose (500 to 750 mg/day).[17] Glucocorticoid synthesis may be completely blocked and can be easily followed by measurement of serum cortisol or 24-hr urine free cortisol. Symptoms of adrenal insufficiency—nausea and vomiting—may be similar to the symptoms caused by toxicity of the drugs. In case of doubt, the patient should be given a maintenance dose of cortisone acetate (25 mg in the morning and 12.5 mg in the afternoon) or hydrocortisone (20 mg in the morning and 10 mg in the afternoon).

Ketaconazole (Nizoral), an antifungal agent, blocks the cytochrome P-450–dependent enzymes in the steroidogenesis. The dose needed for this effect is higher than that required for its antifungal effects; to achieve an adequate suppression, the drug must be administered twice daily. The usual starting dose is 200 mg q 12 hr. The dose can then be increased up to 600 mg q 12 hr. The most common side effects include nausea, vomiting, abdominal pain, and pruritus. Hepatocellular dysfunction has been reported in a significant number of patients, and liver function tests should be monitored before and during therapy. Of the various antiadrenal drugs, ketoconazole appears to be the best tolerated. Plasma or urine cortisol should be monitored to determine the effectiveness of the therapy and to adjust the dose of the drug.[18]

■ SYNDROME OF INAPPROPRIATE ADH SECRETION

Asymptomatic patients with mild hyponatremia (serum Na > 130mEq/L) often can be left untreated, with precautions being taken so as not to give large amounts of fluids. Fluid restriction (less than 1000 ml) is the primary mode of therapy in SIADH and results in normalization of the serum sodium levels in a period of 3 to 7 days. In

emergency situations and in a severely symptomatic patient, the serum sodium may need to be corrected in a rapid manner. This can be achieved by administration of either normal or hypertonic saline along with furosemide. The serum Na should be brought up to a level of 125 mEq/L. Furosemide administration will result in a diuresis of hypotonic urine. Replacing this loss with normal saline (154 mEq/L) or 3 per cent saline (513 mEq/L) will result in a relatively rapid correction of serum Na.[19] A convenient formula to calculate the amount of sodium required is:

$$[125 \text{ mEq/L} - \text{measured serum Na}]$$
$$\times 0.6 \text{ body weight} = \text{required mEq of Na}$$

The patient should be carefully observed for development of pulmonary edema. A few patients with SIADH have been shown to develop central pontine myelinolysis and other central nervous system defects during rapid correction of hyponatremia. Effort should be made to avoid increasing the serum Na to normal or hypernatremic range in the first 48 hours in order to prevent this complication.[20] Lithium carbonate and demeclocycline (Declomycin) block the effect of vasopressin on the renal tubules and can correct the hyponatremia of SIADH. In lithium, the toxic-to-therapeutic dose ratio is low, and therefore this drug is not commonly used. If fluid restriction therapy has failed or is difficult to achieve, chronic therapy with demeclocycline should be considered.[21] The usual starting dose is 300 mg twice daily, which may be increased to 600 mg twice daily. Serum creatinine should be monitored, as impairment in renal function may occur with long-term use, especially at higher doses.

■ HYPOGLYCEMIA

The treatment of hypoglycemia can be difficult. Often patients will require large amounts of continuous intravenous glucose administration (5 or 10 per cent dextrose with appropriate electrolytes) to maintain their serum glucose level in the normal range. Chemotherapy or surgical debulking of the primary tumor may be necessary to reverse the hypoglycemia. Glucagon and glucocorticoids may be helpful in maintaining euglycemia on a long-term basis.

■ ECTOPIC HCG PRODUCTION AND HYPERTHYROIDISM

Removal of the gestational tumor will result in amelioration of hyperthyroidism. Prior to surgery, if necessary, the patient may be treated with β-adrenergic blockade or antithyroid therapy with propylthiouracil or both. Precocious puberty and gynecomastia will respond to therapy directed at the primary tumor. No therapy for the elevated hCG is required in asymptomatic patients. Measurement of βhCG, however, is a useful marker to gauge the response of tumors (especially germ cell) to therapy.

■ Issues and Risks

In general, endocrine manifestations of cancer, as well as other paraneoplastic syndromes, are found in patients in whom the diagnosis of cancer has already been made and is obvious. The paraneoplastic syndrome may be the presenting complaint, but one does not usually have to look very far for an explanation. However, occasionally the associated malignancy is occult. In such cases, knowledge of the associations between the various types of syndromes with the corresponding types of cancer will guide the physician in deciding which diagnostic tests to perform.

Therapy is best directed toward the primary tumor if it is one that is responsive to treatment. Often this is not the case, and knowledge of the appropriate endocrinologic mechanisms and interrelationships will help one to arrive at a rational attempt at palliation of the syndrome in question.

REFERENCES

1. Odell WD, Saito E. Protein hormone-like materials from normal and cancer cells—"ectopic hormone production." *In* 13th International Cancer Congress. New York: Alan R. Liss, 1983:247–258.
2. Odell WD. Humoral manifestations of cancer. *In* Wilson JD, Foster DW (eds). Williams' Textbook of Endocrinology. 7th ed. Philadelphia: WB Saunders, 1985:1327–1343.
3. Shemerdiak WD, Kukreja SC, York PAJ, et al. Evaluation of routine ionized calcium in cancer patients. Clin Chem 1981; 27:1621–1622.
4. Broadus AE, Manein M, Ikeda K, et al. Humoral hypercalcemia of cancer. Identification of a novel parathyroid hormone-like peptide. N Engl J Med 1988; 319:556–563.
5. Wolfsen AR, Odell WD. Pro ACTH: use for early detection of lung cancer. Am J Med 1979; 66:765–772.
6. Kato Y, Ferguson TB, Bennett DE, et al. Oat cell carcinoma of the lung. A review of 138 cases. Cancer 1969; 23:517–524.
7. Tyrell JB, Findling JW, Aron DC, Fitzgerald PA, Forsham PH. An overnight high-dose dexamethasone suppression test for the rapid differential diagnosis of Cushing's syndrome. Ann Intern Med 104:180, 1986.
8. Besser GM, Edwards CRW. Cushing's syndrome. Clin Endocrinol Metab 1977; 45:1108.
9. Bartter FC, Schwartz WB. The syndrome of inappropriate secretion of antidiuretic hormone. Am J Med 1967; 42:790–806.
10. Axelrod L, Ron D. Insulin-like growth factor II and the riddle of tumor-induced hypoglycemia. N Engl J Med 1988; 319:1477–1479.
11. Nisula BC, Ketelsegers JM. Thyroid-stimulating activity and chorionic gonadotropin. J Clin Invest 1974; 54:494–499.
12. Suki WN, Yium JJ, Von Minden M, et al. Acute treatment of hypercalcemia with furosemide. N Engl J Med 1970; 283:836–840.
13. Hosking DJ, Cowley A, Bucknall CA. Rehydration in the treatment of severe hypercalcemia. Q J Med 1981; 200:473–481.
14. Mundy GR, Wilkinson R, Heath DA. Comparative study of available medical therapy for hypercalcemia of malignancy. Am J Med 1983; 74:421–432.
15. Ralston SH, Dryburgh FJ, Cowan RA, et al. Comparison of aminohydroxypropylidene diphosphonate, mithramycin, and corticosteroids/calcitonin in the treatment of cancer-associated hypercalcemia. Lancet 1985; 2:907–910.
16. Ryzen E, Martodam RR, Troxel LM, et al. Intravenous etidronate in the management of malignant hypercalcemia. Arch Intern Med 1985; 145:449–452.
17. Bondy PK. Diseases of the adrenal cortex. *In* Wilson JD, Foster DW (eds). Williams' Textbook of Endocrinology. 7th ed. Philadelphia: WB Saunders, 1985:868.
18. Shepherd FA, Hoffert B, Evans WK, Emery G, Trachtenberg J. Ketoconazole. Use in the treatment of ectopic ACTH production and Cushing's syndrome in small cell lung cancer. Arch Intern Med 1985; 145:863–864.
19. Hantman D, Rossier B, Zohlman R, et al. Rapid correction of hyponatremia in the syndrome of inappropriate secretion of antidiuretic hormone. Ann Intern Med 1973; 78:870–875.
20. Ayus JC, Krothapalli RK, Arieff AI. Treatment of symptomatic hyponatremia and its relation to brain damage. N Engl J Med 1987; 317:1190–1195.
21. DeTroyer A, Demanet JC. Correction of antidiuresis by demeclocycline. N Engl J Med 1975; 293:915–918.

Endometriosis

Ronald C. Strickler

■ Background

Endometriosis is occurrence of the normal lining of the uterus in an ectopic location. The pathogenesis has been theorized to be reflux menstruation or other direct transport of endometrial tissue;[1] hematogenous or lymphatic metastasis;[2] or coelomic metaplasia.[3] Sampson's theory of retrograde menstrual flow explains most cases of endometriosis mechanically. Evidence that these patients also have an immune deficiency[4,5] or a genetic predisposition[6] suggests why reflux menstruation is observable in all women whereas endometriosis is found in only 20 per cent of laparotomies. Adenomyosis, sometimes called internal endometriosis because endometrial glands and stroma have grown deeply into myometrium, is a separate condition and is not discussed here.

Although the commonest sites for endometriosis are in the pelvis (cul de sac, uterosacral ligaments, ovaries), and the commonest symptoms are gynecologic (dysmenorrhea, dyspareunia, infertility), the disease can have many presentations: diarrhea, painful defecation, melena, rectal bleeding, and bowel obstruction from colonic endometriosis; dysuria, hematuria, ureteral obstruction from urinary implants; discolored masses that may bleed onto the surface of skin, umbilicus, vagina; sciatica, sensory/motor changes mimicking vertebral disc disease from paraspinal lesions; or hemoptysis, catamenial pneumothorax/hemothorax from lung metastases. The usual signs and symptoms are summarized in Table 1.

The prevalence of endometriosis is unknown: 7 to 15 per cent of women is a reasonable estimate. It should be suspected in menstruating women of any age; there is no racial immunity; women with a family history of endometriosis are seven to ten times more likely to develop this disease; the slim, tense achiever who postpones childbearing for a professional career is a caricature.

The fact that the level of the antigen CA-125 is elevated in the peripheral blood of women with endometriosis stirred hope for a noninvasive diagnostic test.[7] Unfortunately, CA-125 elevations are found in many conditions and the test has a low sensitivity (that is, a positive result is not diagnostic for endometriosis). However, since the specificity is very high (i.e., a negative test rules out endometriosis), the antigen is a useful marker for recurrence of disease in women treated for endometriosis.

The improved resolution of modern ultrasound scanners and innovations like the vaginal transducer have increased the value of pelvic sonography for the diagnosis of ovarian diseases.[8] An ovarian endometrioma (Figure 1) is suspected when a cystic or mixed cystic/solid lesion has a shaggy, irregular interior border, a thick, rindlike capsule, low-level fine echoes, especially in the dependent or peripheral portions of the mass, occasional septation, and a fluid level. These patterns also can be found with cystadenoma, teratoma, corpus luteum hematoma, tubo-ovarian abscess, and ectopic ges-

TABLE 1. Endometriosis

Symptoms (Per Cent of Patients)		Signs (Per Cent of Patients)	
Asymptomatic	>33	Normal examination	>50
Infertility	66	Retroverted uterus	40
Dysmenorrhea	66	Uterosacral nodules	33
Deep dyspareunia	33	Adnexal mass	15
Menstrual irregularity	15		

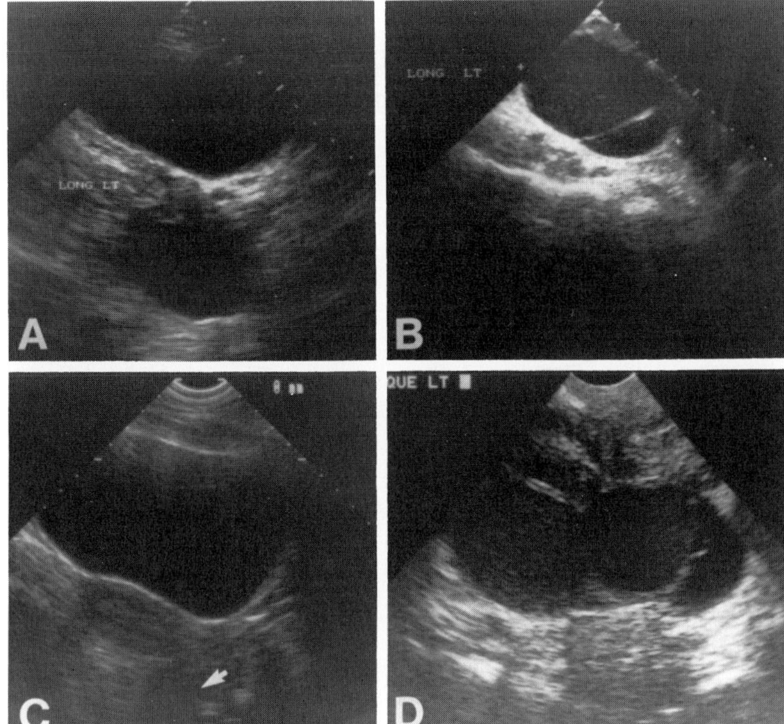

Figure 1. Sonographic identification of endometriosis. *A,* Transabdominal longitudinal scan of a left ovarian endometrioma. Other than an irregular, indiscrete outline, the sonolucent cyst has no distinguishing features. *B,* Transvaginal sonogram of the left ovarian endometrioma in *A.* Septation and a homogeneous echo pattern resembling a snowfall are seen. *C,* Midline longitudinal scan in a second patient shows a poorly defined, nonspecific cystic mass (arrow) displacing the uterus against the bladder wall. *D,* Transvaginal image of the cyst in *C.* The triple-loculated endometrioma shows a range of internal echo densities and an irregular, thickened wall. (Courtesy of Carolyn Martin, MD, Washington University Obstetrics and Gynecology Ultrasonography Division.)

tation. Conversely, endometrioma can appear as a simple cyst or a solid tumor. Transabdominal scans are less detailed and hence less diagnostic in comparison with transvaginal images. Ultrasonography is unable to identify peritoneal endometriosis implants.

Endometriosis can be suspected from the history, clinical examination, and noninvasive studies, but a diagnosis can be made only when typical lesions are seen. Rarely, the disease breaks through skin. Endoscopy, most commonly laparoscopy, reveals (1) *fleshy implants:* poorly demarcated, reddish, velvety superficial plaques of tissue; (2) *tobacco stains:* yellow/brown tissue discoloration of hemosiderin; (3) *powder burn/burnt match head lesions:* gray/blue/black circumscribed marks; (4) *blue-domed cysts:* discrete blisters of menstruum beneath the tissue surface; (5) *chocolate cysts:* walled-off collections of brown-black menstrual debris, usually in the ovary; (6) *stellate/sunbeam/spider scars:* a central pucker-point with radiating fibrosis; and (7) *depigmented lesions:* clear vesicles and white plaques. Biopsy is often disappointing: the pathologist requires endometrial glands as well as stroma for diagnosis. Frequently only one component of

the histology, perhaps combined with scar and hemosiderin, is present and thus reported "consistent with, but not diagnostic of, endometriosis." Pelvic adhesions and patent fallopian tubes with normal fimbria in a woman who has never had abdominal surgery or worn an intrauterine device suggests endometriosis rather than pelvic inflammatory disease.

There is poor correlation between the amount of pelvic endometriosis and the severity of patient symptoms. Resolution of a few implants can relieve incapacitating pain while a frozen pelvis can be asymptomatic and permit pregnancy. Accurate staging depends on (1) meticulous observation at a laparoscopy, which includes general/regional anesthesia, placement of a uterine manipulator, and double-puncture technique so that every millimeter of abdominal-pelvic tissue is exposed; (2) a detailed operative note; and (3) a pictorial record such as a diagram (Figure 2), still photographs, or videotape. Staging of endometriosis (Figure 3) is important: treatments are best compared when disease is measured with the same yardstick. Increasing severity of disease does correlate with decreasing effectiveness of medical therapy and increasing need for

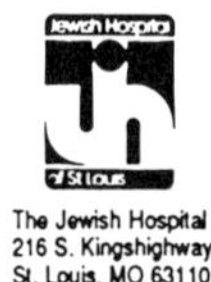

Jewish Hospital at Washington University Medical Center
Obstetrics and Gynecology

The Jewish Hospital
216 S. Kingshighway
St. Louis, MO 63110

REPORT OF LAPAROSCOPIC EXAMINATION

Patient: Indication:

Age: G.   P.   Ab.

LNMP:

Menses: Date: Surgeon:

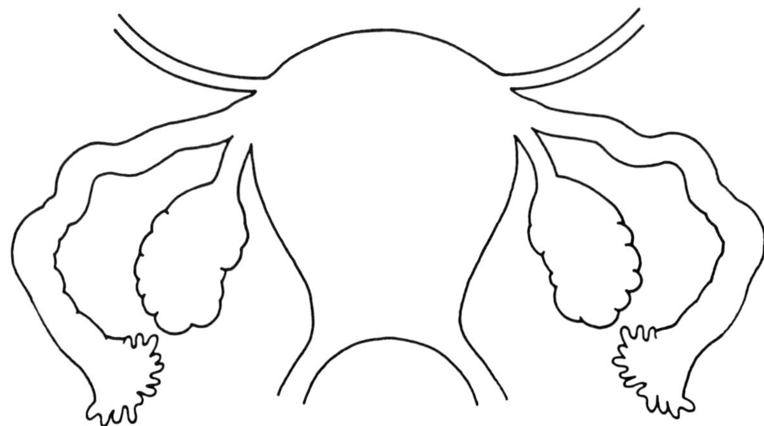

Diagnosis and Comments:

Plan:

Recorded by:

Figure 2. Sample of a pictorial record of a laparoscopic examination. (Courtesy of Jewish Hospital at Washington University Medical Center.)

		< 1 cm	1-3 cm	>3 cm
PERITONEUM	**ENDOMETRIOSIS**			
	Superficial	1	2	4
	Deep	2	4	6
OVARY	R Superficial	1	2	4
	Deep	4	16	20
	L Superficial	1	2	4
	Deep	4	16	20

	POSTERIOR CUL DE SAC OBLITERATION	Partial	Complete
		4	40

	ADHESIONS	< 1/3 Enclosure	1/3 - 2/3 Enclosure	> 2/3 Enclosure
OVARY	R Filmy	1	2	4
	Dense	4	8	16
	L Filmy	1	2	4
	Dense	4	8	16
TUBE	R Filmy	1	2	4
	Dense	4	8	16
	L Filmy	1	2	4
	Dense	4	8	16

Figure 3. The American Fertility Society Revised Classification of Endometriosis.

Stage I   (Minimal)   - 1-5
Stage II   (Mild)   - 6-15
Stage III (Moderate)   - 16-40
Stage IV   (Severe)   - >40

246

surgery. Before and after treatment assessments become objective measurements more than subjective impressions.

■ Management

Endometriosis treatment is requested to (1) relieve symptoms, especially pelvic pain; (2) protect or enhance fertility, because scar can mechanically disrupt tube-ovary relations, or because active disease seems to secrete factors that impair egg release, sperm function, embryogenesis, and tubal functions; and (3) differentiate severe endometriosis with anatomic distortion from pelvic malignancy.

■ NO THERAPY

Endometriosis is the incidental finding during laparoscopic tubal sterilization of a 35 year old mother. A 45 year old woman whose dysmenorrhea is adequately relieved by nonsteroidal anti-inflammatory drug has uterosacral ligament nodularity believed to be endometriosis. A career-oriented woman investigated for pelvic mass has asymptomatic endometriosis. These are clinical settings in which endometriosis may be managed by observation and/or symptom therapy. Since reflux menstruation is universal, it is likely that many women develop endometriosis that will be resolved by normal host defense mechanisms. Menopause deprives endometriosis of its obligatory hormone support and for most women cures active disease. Women who have no symptoms and who do not desire pregnancy may carry their disease to menopause without ever requiring therapy.

In infertile, otherwise asymptomatic women, minimal endometriosis management is controversial. Treatment in this setting is predicated on the clinical impression that there is an association between endometriosis and infertility[9] and on reports that fertility has been enhanced by danazol ($\approx$40 per cent pregnancy rate) and laparoscopic vaporization ($\approx$60 per cent pregnancy rate). However, since the original report of Garcia and Davis that 62 per cent of 17 untreated women conceived within 6 months of laparoscopic diagnosis of mild endometriosis,[10] other studies have observed a 55 per cent

pregnancy rate without treatment in approximately 350 patients. Thus, the investigative evidence argues that most couples conceive despite small amounts of disease. However, the ease with which minimal or mild endometriosis can be vaporized at diagnostic surgery, using a laparoscope-directed laser source, has been a pragmatic argument for therapy.

■ BIRTH CONTROL PILLS

The amelioration of disease during pregnancy stimulated birth control pill regimens named *pseudopregnancy,* because the formulations delivered continuous, increasing doses of estrogen and progestin to sustain amenorrhea.[11] Symptomatic improvement was expected in at least 60 per cent of patients, but there was objective resolution of disease in barely one half of the symptom responders, a high recurrence rate, and a poor pregnancy rate in infertile patients. In addition, there were frequent side effects, appetite stimulation, weight gain, breast tenderness, abdominal discomfort, and constant worries about major drug reactions such as thromboembolism. Pseudopregnancy has been replaced by newer therapies.

Cyclic therapy, as used for contraception, has long been promoted to hold endometriosis in check and to prevent disease recurrence after pregnancy or medical/surgical treatments. Since birth control tablets create an atrophic endometrium with a decreased volume of flow, there is a good theoretic basis for belief, but no evidence scientifically substantiates this prophylaxis.

■ PROGESTIN ONLY

As the serious side effects of oral contraceptives are estrogen-related, and as progestins induce endometrial atrophy, medroxyprogesterone acetate (MPA), megesterol acetate, norethindrone acetate, and dydrogesterone became popular. Symptomatic improvement occurs in about 67 per cent of patients and objective improvement in about 50 per cent. Moghissi's early work suggesting a 90 per cent pregnancy rate after MPA, 10 mg three times daily for 3 months, stimulated enthusiasm for progestins. Moghissi and colleagues recently reported a 71 per cent cumulative pregnancy rate in the 30 months after finishing MPA, compared with 55 per cent in a control group.[12] Side effects include breakthrough bleeding, bloating, appetite stimulation, and mood lability. The cost of therapy is about $120 per month.

■ METHYLTESTOSTERONE

The endometrial atrophy induced by androgen has long been known and was used to suppress endometriosis medically before oral contraceptives had been developed. Methyltestosterone, 5 mg daily, relieves symptoms as effectively as progestin compounds but does not block menstruation. Acne, hirsutism, and mild virilization trouble approximately 10 per cent of women. Objective regression of disease and conception rates are similar to those of birth control pills.

■ DANAZOL

This isoxazole derivative of 17α-ethinyltestosterone was originally believed to inhibit gonadotropin stimulation of the ovary and thus to cause a "pseudomenopause." Subsequent studies suggest a complex action, including stimulation through androgen and progesterone receptors to induce endometrial atrophy, as well as blocking enzymes in the steroid hormone cascade. Danazol became the benchmark therapy in the late 1970s because 70 per cent of women studied experienced subjective and objective improvement lasting 3 years and the corrected pregnancy rate was 72 per cent.[13]

Therapy is initiated within 3 days of the onset of menstrual flow. Patients are weaned onto the full dose, 200 mg four times daily, to limit gastrointestinal side effects. Danazol has a short half-life, and although many women have no breakthrough bleeding using the package insert–recommended twice daily dosage, a four-tablet daily regimen is necessary in others. Equally, 400-mg and 600-mg daily doses improve some patients, but 800 mg daily gives consistent amenorrhea and disease control. A minimum trial of therapy is 2 months if one judges only symptom improvement and 4 months if one wishes significant symptom relief or objective disease regression. It requires 6 months to resolve most peritoneal disease and 9 to 12 months to shrink ovarian

disease in the minority of patients who respond. Therapy is of limited value in women with ovarian endometriomas and does not resolve adhesions. Disease resolution can be followed clinically if there are palpable lesions and by ultrasonography if there are endometriomas. In most women, a "second look" laparoscopy is required to prove disease resolution.

Side effects occur in three fourths of women: appetite stimulation, weight gain, muscle cramps, headache, loss of energy, gastrointestinal disturbances, decrease in breast fullness, vaginal bleeding, decreased libido, vaginal dryness, acne, and seborrhea. In a minority of women these prompt patients to abandon this treatment. In a very few patients, androgenic side effects, such as hirsutism and voice change, force discontinuance of the drug. Liver enzyme changes can be demonstrated in women on this medication, but there is no clinical correlate to this observation and the changes reverse when danazol is stopped. Danazol is teratogenic, and although most women are amenorrheic on drug, barrier contraception during therapy and afterward until the first normal menstrual period is obligatory. The cost of therapy is approximately $200 per month.

■ GONADOTROPIN-RELEASING HORMONE ANALOGS

Long-acting analogs of the hypothalamic decapeptide gonadotropin–releasing hormone (GnRH) block the hypothalamic-pituitary-ovarian axis, interrupt both gonadotropin and steroid hormone production, and thereby create a "pseudomenopause" state, also described as "medical oophorectomy." GnRH agonists (GnRHa) down-regulate the pituitary LH/FSH secreting cells, a poorly understood process in which the cell surface receptor system is internalized and uncoupled from the second messenger system. Antagonists of GnRH occupy the receptor and exclude the endogenous hormone signal.

In 1989, GnRH antagonists are being clinically evaluated, but side effects are dampening enthusiasm for the current products. One GnRHa, leuprolide acetate, is available, although its approved indication is palliation of prostatic carcinoma. Other analogs, nafarelin and buserelin, should be marketed soon. GnRHa is now competing with danazol to become the treatment standard. They also give 90 per cent symptom relief, 60 per cent objective disease resolution, and promote fertility in 50 per cent of patients.[14]

During the first 2 weeks of GnRHa therapy, the agonist action stimulates gonadotropin output and may temporarily exaggerate symptoms. Thereafter, the hormone deprivation begins, signaled often by menopause-like symptoms such as hot flushes, vaginal dryness, decreased breast fullness, and nonspecific emotional changes. The severe hypoestrogenic state may contribute to osteoporosis; therefore, therapy should be complemented by 1500 mg of calcium daily and regular exercise. The daily subcutaneous injection sites are rotated as in a diabetic person, as bruising and pruritus at these sites can be annoying. The cost of therapy is approximately $300 per month. Depot injections lasting 2 to 4 weeks and nasal spray formulations are being evaluated.[15,16]

■ LAPAROSCOPIC SURGERY

Early attempts to correct endometriosis using the laparoscope relied on scissors and electrocoagulation. The extensive tissue injury caused by electrocoagulation severely limited use around the fallopian tubes and overtop sidewall blood vessels and ureter.

Carbon dioxide (CO_2) laser therapy allows precise varporization of tissue with injury limited to 500 microns from impact and sealing of vessels up to a few millimeters in diameter. The laparoscope is placed through an umbilical incision, and secondary punctures are placed into the lower abdomen. The laser beam may be directed through the operating channel of the laparoscope or through the secondary ports. Since the CO_2 laser energy is rapidly attenuated by water and is diffused by glass, backstops of irrigation or quartz rod protect adjacent tissues. Adhesions can be lysed, peritoneal implants vaporized, ovarian endometriomas opened and drained, and the lining laser-coagulated. Partial transsection of the uterosacral ligaments reduces sensation from the uterus and cul de sac analogous to a presacral neurectomy. Operating time is comparable to, or even somewhat longer than, laparotomy, but the postoperative recovery is usually complete within a week.

Three other lasers that can be delivered through a flexible fiberoptic cable and can pass through fluids are also in use. The Nd:YAG (neodymium:yttrium-aluminum-garnet) laser strongly coagulates tissues, but energy scatter increases the extent of tissue necrosis. The argon laser's energy is absorbed by hemoglobin and is therefore useful to coagulate active implants of endometriosis selectively. The KTP 532 (potassium-titanium-phosphate) laser has a wavelength of 0.532 micron and properties similar to those of the argon laser.

Excellent relief from symptoms, a 10 per cent recurrence rate of disease each year, and a 50 per cent pregnancy rate all compare favorably to conservative surgery,[17] but without the prolonged recovery time. Equally, laser surgery is as effective as drug without months of hormone suppression and drug side effects.[18] Since laparoscopy is necessary for accurate diagnosis and staging of endometriosis, and the addition of laser treatment often adds little morbidity to the surgery or the recovery, it is rapidly becoming the preferred therapy. Unfortunately, this same ease of therapy makes it difficult to enroll patients in control groups or in other therapy regimens to prove scientifically the benefits ot this new tool.

■ CONSERVATIVE SURGERY

To preserve or enhance fertility and relieve the pain or bleeding of endometriosis in women whose disease is unsuited to laparoscopic surgery, laparotomy is performed to resect disease and preserve as much normal tissue as possible.[19,20] As a working rule, the first attempt at such surgery gives the best hope for effective treatment; second operations most often are disappointing. To reduce the volume of disease that must be resected and to reduce vascularity within the pelvis, often medical suppressive therapy is administered for 3 to 4 months preoperation. Principles of conservative surgery include magnification for the best definition of tissue planes; heparinized irrigation to moisten and cool tissues while inhibiting formation of clots that act as fibrin bridges for adhesion formation; avoidance of sponges, which cause surface abrasions; meticulous hemostasis with microcautery or laser; gentle handling of tissues; fine, nonreactive suture materials; raw surfaces covered by reperitonealization or laser eschar; and chemical adjuncts to reduce adhesions, such as macromolecular dextran, dextrose solution, nonsteroidal anti-inflammatory drugs, steroids, and antibiotics. Many surgeons routinely perform a presacral neurectomy to assure relief of dysmenorrhea, to insure against pain if there is disease recurrence, and, although controversial, to enhance fertility. After 5 years, approximately 50 per cent of women have achieved pregnancy and at least 33 per cent have recurrence of their disease.[21]

■ HYSTERECTOMY AND OOPHORECTOMY

Based on the long-known fact that menopause corrected endometriosis, castration is the only cure of endometriosis. Radiation-induced ovarian destruction is rarely warranted because of radiation injury to adjacent tissues. Although as much diseased tissue as possible is removed at the surgery, it is acceptable to leave difficult-to-dissect areas and allow the surgical menopause to "starve away" remnant disease.

■ ALTERNATE CONCEPTION TECHNOLOGIES

When endometriosis-directed therapy fails to promote conception, techniques to bypass the presumed effects of endometriosis are available.

Superovulation, using clomiphene or menopausal gonadotropins combined with intrauterine insemination of husband's sperm, addresses two premises: (1) multiple eggs, like multiple lottery tickets, increase the chances of winning; and (2) endometriosis "toxins" may interfere with sperm capacitation/transport or early embryogenesis.

Gamete intrafallopian transfer (GIFT) involves stimulating multiple follicle development with drugs and placing harvested eggs and washed sperms into the fallopian tubes. If endometriosis has subtly disturbed the ovum pickup mechanism or induces luteinized unruptured follicles, GIFT can overcome such effects.

In vitro fertilization and embryo transfer (IVF/ET) completely bypass the peritoneal/tubal environments. The drug-stimulated crop of eggs is harvested at laparoscopy or ultrasound-directed capture, fertilization and early conceptus growth occur in a laboratory environment, and the 4- to 8-cell embryos are transferred across the cervix and into the uterus.

A living baby results from 15 to 20 per cent of GIFT and up to 25 per cent of superovulation/insemination treatment cycles. These outcomes are similar for couples with unexplained infertility and endometriosis. Couples with blocked fallopian tubes and endometriosis take home a baby in 10 to 15 per cent of IVF/ET treatment cycles.[22] Damewood and Rock observed that 28 per cent of patients who did not achieve an IVF/ET pregnancy conceived on their own within one year.[23] This cycles us back to our beginning thought: about one third of patients with endometriosis are fertile.

■ Issues and Risks

■ ASYMPTOMATIC ENDOMETRIOSIS, FUTURE FERTILITY IMPORTANT

The goals of treatment are to hold current disease in check, promote disease regression if possible, and forestall the appearance of new disease. Perhaps some women will do this on their own, but short of repetitive laparoscopy to evaluate possible progression, there is no practical way to select this group. Hence, therapy is recommended for all. Birth control pills are the least expensive, best-tolerated therapy. It is unproved that aggressive treatment at the time of diagnosis is better than attempts to forestall progression, even if aggressive treatment is required later.

■ SYMPTOMATIC ENDOMETRIOSIS, FUTURE FERTILITY IMPORTANT

Laparoscopic surgery followed by birth control pill cycles to forestall disease recurrence is often possible at the time of initial diagnosis. Symptomatic therapy using birth control pills may be effective, but often aggressive medical therapy to bring the process under control, followed by birth control pill cycles, is necessary. Extended use of medroxyprogesterone, 30 mg daily, or danocrine, at the lowest dose that blocks menses, is an alternative approach.

■ INFERTILITY

Endometriosis blocks pregnancy in 66 per cent of affected women and increases the likelihood for early miscarriage to 25 per cent.[24] In women during the decade of their 30s who have never been pregnant, laparoscopy demonstrates endometriosis in 16 to 33 per cent of otherwise unexplained infertility.

Laparoscopic surgery at the time of diagnosis to erase disease and minimize the delay in continuing attempts at pregnancy is widely practiced. It is unclear whether women with minimal-to-moderate endometriosis that has not caused adhesions that mechanically disadvantage the tube-ovary relationship need treatment (see No Therapy).

Laparoscopic surgery combined with 3 to 4 cycles of medical suppression therapy is promoted by some because microscopic endometriosis—disease present but not yet of a size that can be recognized—has been left untreated. The incidence of this problem is unknown.

Other surgeons recommend preoperative medical therapy. They argue that this treats microscopic disease and reduces the size and vascularity of all lesions, thereby making surgery easier. Furthermore, most conceptions occur during the first year following surgery, and months during which adhesions may be forming are not squandered on medical therapy.

When laparoscopic surgery is not possible, medical therapy for 6 to 9 months and medical therapy/conservative surgery are options. In women under 30 years of age, medical therapy alone uses up months but keeps the surgical option for use lest medicine alone is insufficient. Women aged 30 to 35 years are in transition between medical and surgical recommendations. In women over 35 years of age, combined medical therapy/ conservative surgery saves valuable months in which to attempt pregnancy.

The success of both medical and surgical therapies to correct endometriosis-associated infertility, even with severe disease which has caused significant pelvic scarring, exceeds the success currently achieved with alternate conception technologies. It is not logical to bypass time-tested endometriosis therapies and immediately embrace new technology. Rather, GIFT and IVF/ET are reserved for couples in whom specific therapies have failed to achieve pregnancy.

■ SYMPTOMATIC, FERTILITY UNIMPORTANT

Assuming symptomatic therapies have failed, extended medical therapies are unacceptable, and menopause is not imminent, hysterectomy with bilateral oophorectomy is curative. Hysterectomy removes the endometrium that has seeded the disease, and ovariectomy deprives any residual disease of the hormonal nourishment that could continue it and its symptoms.

■ ESTROGEN REPLACEMENT THERAPY

If estrogens fuel endometriosis progression, then estrogen replacement therapy (ERT) should be contraindicated for women who have undergone castration surgery as therapy or who are recently menopausal. For women troubled with vasomotor symptoms and unwilling to risk endometriosis reactivation, medroxyprogesterone, 20 mg daily, and clonidine, 0.2 mg daily, are effective treatments. Osteoporosis risk can be reduced with 1500 mg/day of calcium combined with exercise; osteoporosis can be prevented with calcitonin.

However, empiric observation does not support theory. Very few patients reactivate their disease taking ERT such as 0.625 mg of conjugated estrogens, the minimum required to prevent osteoporosis. Thus, a useful approach to the menopausal syndrome in women with endometriosis is to withhold estrogens in favor of other treatments for 6 to 12 months, assume that this interval of severe hypoestrogenism has starved any residual disease, and then begin ERT.

■ RUPTURED ENDOMETRIOMA

Classic teaching has been laparotomy to wash the abdomen and often adnexectomy to remove the cause of the peritoneal cavity soilage. Endometrioma fluid is very irritating to abdominal cavity surfaces and does incite inflammation that causes adhesions. However, the abdomen can be extensively lavaged using Ringer's lactate solution directed by the laparoscope. Also, the laparoscope-directed laser beam can be used to unroof small endometriomas and coagulate the cyst lining.[25] Dextran and other flotation fluid left in the abdomen and nonsteroidal anti-inflammatory drug therapy (e.g., ibuprofen, 600 mg four times daily for 3 days) reduce the likelihood for significant adhesion formation.

■ Summary

Endometriosis often explains pelvic pain and infertility. The diagnosis and management are captured in a few "pearls":

1. Never exclude endometriosis as explanation for infertility or pain because a woman is otherwise asymptomatic, clinical examination is normal, or the amount of disease is small.
2. Never treat for endometriosis without visualizing the disease, to make a firm diagnosis.
3. Laparoscopy-directed laser vaporization of endometriosis treats the disease at the time of diagnosis with low morbidity and good efficacy.
4. Medical suppression is the backbone of therapy to relieve symptoms, preserve fertility, complement surgery to enhance fertility, and manage disease recurrence.
5. Although we must be surgically aggressive with advancing patient age and with advancing stages of disease that causes adhesions, it is the first surgeon who likely will determine the patient's pregnancy potential.

REFERENCES

1. Sampson JA. Development of the implantation theory for origin of peritoneal endometriosis. Am J Obstet Gynecol 1940; 40:549–557.
2. Javert CT. Pathogenesis of endometriosis based on endometrial homeoplasia direct extension, exfoliation and implantation, lymphatic and hematogenous metastasis. Cancer 1949; 2:399–410.
3. Meyer R. Eine Unbekannte Art von Adenomyom des Uterus mit einer kritischen Besprechung der Urnierenhypothese von Recklinghausen's. Ztschr Geburtsh Gynak 1903; 49:464–507.
4. Dmowski WP. Immunologic aspects of endometriosis. Contr Gynec Obstet 1987; 16:48–55.
5. Halme J, Becker S, Haskill S. Altered maturation and function of peritoneal macrophages: possible role in pathogenesis of endometriosis. Am J Obstet Gynecol 1987; 156:783–789.
6. Simpson JL, Elias S, Malinak LR, Buttram VC. Hereditable aspects of endometriosis: genetic studies. Am J Obstet Gynecol 1980; 137:327–331.
7. Barbieri RL, Niloff JM, Bast RC, Scaetzi E, Kistner RW, Knapp RC. Elevated serum concentrations of CA-125 in patients with advanced endometriosis. Fertil Steril 1986; 45:630–634.
8. Boog G, Penot P, Momber A. Ultrasound as a diagnostic aid in endometriosis. Contr Gynec Obstet 1987; 16:119–124.
9. Strathy JH, Molgaard CA, Coulam CB, Melton LJ. Endometriosis and infertility: a laparoscopic study of endometriosis among fertile and infertile women. Fertil Steril 1982; 38:667–672.
10. Garcia CR, David SS. Pelvic endometriosis: infertility and pelvic pain. Am J Obstet Gynecol 1977; 129:740–744.
11. Barbieri RL, Kistner RW. Hormonal therapy of endometriosis. In Raynaud J-P, Ojasoo T, Martini L (eds). Medical Management of Endometriosis. New York: Raven Press, 1984:27–40.
12. Hull ME, Moghissi KS, Hull ME, Magyar DM, Hayes MF. Comparison of different treatment modalities of endometriosis in infertile women. Fertil Steril 1987; 47:40–44.
13. Dmowski WP, Cohen MR. Antigonadotropin (danazol) in the treatment of endometriosis. Evaluation of posttreatment fertility and three-year follow-up data. Am J Obstet Gynecol 1978; 130:41–48.
14. Steingold KA, Cedars M, Lu JKH, Randle D, Judd HL, Meldrum DR. Treatment of endometriosis with a long-acting gonadotropin-releasing hormone agonist. Obstet Gynecol 1987; 69:403–411.
15. Lemay A. Monthly implant of luteinizing hormone-releasing hormone agonist: a practical therapeutic approach for sex-steroid dependent gynecologic diseases. Fertil Steril 1987; 48:10–13.
16. Henzl MR, Corson SL, Moghissi K, Buttram VC, Berqvist C, Jacobson J, for the Nafarelin Study Group: Administration of nasal nafarelin as compared with oral danazol for endometriosis. A multicenter double-blind comparative clinical trial. N Engl J Med 1988; 318:485–489.
17. Gast MJ, Tobler R, Strickler RC, Odem R, Pineda J. Laser vaporization of endometriosis in an infertile population: the role of complicating infertility factors. Fertil Steril 1988: 49:32–36.
18. Adamson GD, Lu J, Subak LL. Laparoscopic CO_2 laser vaporization of endometriosis compared with traditional treatments. Fertil Steril 1988; 50:704–710.
19. Buttram VC Jr. Surgical treatment of endometriosis in the infertile female: a modified approach. Fertil Steril 1979; 32:635–640.
20. Dargent D. General rules for surgery in the treatment of endometriosis. Contr Gynec Obstet 1987; 16:271–279.
21. Rock JA, Guzick DS, Sengos C, Schweditsch M, Sapp

KC, Jones HW Jr. The conservative surgical treatment of endometriosis: evaluation of pregnancy success with respect to the extent of disease as categorized using contemporary classification systems. Fertil Steril 1981; 35:131–137.

22. Frydman R, Belaisch-Allart JC. Results of in vitro fertilization for endometriosis. Contr Gynec Obstet 1987; 16:328–331.

23. Damewood MD, Rock JA. Treatment-independent pregnancy with operative laparoscopy for endometriosis in an in vitro fertilization program. Fertil Steril 1988; 50:463–465.

24. Wheeler JM, Johnston BM, Malinak LR. The relationship of endometriosis to spontaneous abortion. Fertil Steril 1983; 39:656:660.

25. Reich H, McGlynn F. Treatment of ovarian endometriomas using laparoscopic surgical techniques. J Reprod Med 1986; 31:577–584.

Esophageal motility disorders

Joseph W. Griffin ■ *Rex L. Gomez*

■ Background

Esophageal motility disorders (EMD) are a group of either primary or secondary dysmotility conditions affecting the smooth and striated muscles of the esophagus. The clinical hallmarks of these disorders are dysphagia, chest pain, and gastroesophageal reflux. Dysphagia is present with both liquids and solids and may be slowly progressive. Food impactions may occur, but, unlike an obstruction resulting from a structural lesion, they can be relieved with repeated swallowing or Valsalva maneuvers. The sensation of food sticking may be located anywhere from the suprasternal notch to the gastroesophageal junction. There is no diagnostic pattern of dysphagia for a specific motility disorder.

Chest pain is an alarming symptom that causes the patient to seek help, frequently in the emergency room. This pain is usually substernal, varying from dull and aching to acute, severe pressure or even to a bursting sensation. The pain may radiate into the neck or left arm, as does cardiac pain, because of the common vagal innervation of the esophagus and pericardium.

Before embarking on a workup for an esophageal etiology of chest pain, a cardiac source for the pain must be excluded. In adults who present with substernal chest pain, approximately 30 per cent will not have significant coronary artery disease (CAD).[1] Even when significant CAD is found, approximately 20 per cent of these patients will have concomitant esophageal disorders.[2] A further confusing aspect of these patients' pain is that in almost two thirds of those with esophageal disease, the pain is exacerbated by exercise.[3] Whereas many patients may develop their pain while eating or can identify certain "triggering" factors, as in dysphagia, there is no diagnostic pain pattern for a specific esophageal disorder.

The third predominant symptom is gastroesophageal reflux; it occurs predominantly in secondary esophageal motility disorders. Patients note a substernal burning with regurgitation, water brash, and hoarseness. Symptoms are usually worse in the recumbent position, when bending, when lifting heavy objects, and after a large meal. There is usually poor clearance of the refluxed acid from the esophagus, which contributes to acid-peptic damage to the mucosa, resulting in ulceration and stricture. In patients with scleroderma, 60 per cent have erosive esophagitis caused by involvement of the distal esophageal muscle and the lower esophageal sphincter.[4]

Table 1 lists the most common motility disorders, and the manometric and radiographic features of each.

TABLE 1. Radiologic and Manometric Findings for Primary Esophageal Motility Disorders

	Radiologic Findings	Manometric Findings
Achalasia	Chest radiograph: Widened mediastinum Absence of a gastric air bubble An air fluid level within a dilated esophagus Barium esophagogram: Beaklike tapering at the esophagogastric junction Esophageal dilation supporting column of barium Aperistalsis of body	Aperistalsis of esophageal body* Incomplete LES relaxation Elevated LES pressure (> 45 mm Hg)
Diffuse Esophageal Spasm	Barium esophagogram: Tertiary contractions Segmentation in the distal esophagus (corkscrew esophagus)	Simultaneous contractions (> 10% wet swallows)* Intermittent normal peristalsis Repetitive contractions (> 3 peaks) Spontaneous contractions ↑ duration of contraction (> 6 sec)
Nutcracker Esophagus	Normal or nonspecific	Normal peristaltic contraction with ↑ distal amplitude (> 180 mm)* ↑ duration (> 6 sec)
Hypertensive Lower Esophageal Sphincter (LES)	Nonspecific but may support barium column	Elevated LES pressure (> 45 mm Hg)* Normal LES relaxation* Normal peristalsis
Nonspecific Esophageal Motility Disorder	Normal, nonspecific findings	↑ nontransmitted contractions (> 6 sec) Prolonged duration of contractions (> 6 sec) Triple peaked contractions Spontaneous contractions Decreased amplitude of esophageal peristalsis (> 30 mm Hg)

*Required manometric criteria to confirm diagnosis.

■ Management

The goal of therapy in patients with esophageal motility disorders is the alleviation of their symptoms of chest pain, dysphagia, and gastroesophageal reflux. Equally important is reassurance of these patients that sudden death or catastrophe is very unlikely when the esophagus is the cause of their symptoms. Treatment of esophageal motility disorders can be divided into four areas: reassurance, pharmacology, forceful dilation, and surgical intervention (Table 2).

■ REASSURANCE

The first line of therapy is to reassure the patient that the symptoms are not secondary to malignancy or significant cardiac disease. Reassurance must be based on a thorough history, careful physical examination, and appropriate diagnostic studies. After complete evaluation, patients who understand and who are reassured that the esophagus is the cause of their symptoms do not show a significant difference in pain pattern, but do significantly decrease their disability and the continued need for physician evaluation of their pain.[5] In a study of the patients with nutcracker esophagus, a 77 per cent decrease in physician and emergency room visits resulted after patients were shown that the esophagus was responsible for the pain and given reassurance that their pain was noncardiac.[6]

■ PHARMACOLOGIC THERAPY

Psychotropic Agents

Useful pharmacotherapy for motility disorders may include antidepressants and antianxiolytics. As high as 84 per cent of patients with EMD may be found to have an

TABLE 2. Treatment Modalities of Primary Esophageal Motility Disorders

Treatment	Medication Dosage
Psychotropics	
Trazodone	50–150 mg PO daily
Diazepam	5–15 mg PO daily
Nitrates	
Nitroglycerin	0.4 mg SL, ac and hs
Isosorbide	10–40 mg PO 30 min ac
Calcium channel blockers	
Nifedipine	10–30 mg SL or PO TID or QID, ac and hs
Diltiazem	60–90 mg PO QID, ac and hs
Other smooth muscle relaxants	
Hydralazine	25–50 mg PO QID
Anticholinergics	
Dicyclomine	20–40 mg PO QID
Bougie dilation	50–54 Fr prn
Pneumatic dilation	3–3.5 cm prn
Esophagomyotomy	
Reassurance	

underlying psychiatric diagnosis.[7] This agrees with an observation of patients with the colonic motility disorder of irritable bowel syndrome, leading some authorities to term these problems the *irritable esophagus*.[8] Trazodone (Desyrel), 100 to 150 mg, which has a minimal manometric effect on esophageal motility, has been found to effect a significant reduction in patients' chest pain.[9] Diazepam (Valium), 10 to 15 mg daily, or other benzodiazepines may be tried as adjuvant therapy.

Smooth Muscle Relaxants

The goal with smooth muscle relaxants is to obtain smooth muscle relaxation with a resultant decrease in amplitude and duration of distal esophageal contractions and, additionally, relaxation of the lower esophageal sphincter tone.

Nitrates. Nitroglycerin (NTG) is a potent smooth muscle relaxant. Its effects are not restricted to the vascular smooth muscle. In healthy male volunteers, there is a significant decrease in the lower esophageal sphincter pressure in as early as 3 minutes after sublingal nitroglycerin administration.[10] NTG has been shown to decrease the

amplitude and number of repetitive contractions in patients with diffuse esophageal spasm.[11] In patients with mild symptoms, 0.4 mg of sublingual NTG is effective in aborting acute chest pain. Isosorbide (Isordil), 10 to 40 mg PO QID, offers significant long-term clinical relief in some patients with diffuse esophageal spasm.[12]

In achalasia, isosorbide, 5 mg sublingually, has been found to be effective in significantly decreasing the LES pressure. Clinically, 13 of 15 patients had symptomatic relief of dysphagia and 8 of these had adequate esophageal emptying of a radioactive meal after isosorbide administration.[13] However, many times the patient is unable to tolerate the adverse side effects of headaches, orthostatic hypotension, and tachyphylaxis, and nitrate therapy is not recommended for long-term management of achalasia.

Calcium Channel Blockers. Recent work has demonstrated the efficacy of nifedipine (Procardia) and diltiazem (Cardizem) in treatment of esophageal motility disorders. Nifedipine has been shown to decrease the LES pressure as well as producing a dose-dependent decrease in the amplitude of esophageal contractions. In this same study, nifedipine, 10 to 30 mg PO TID yielded a dose-dependent decrease in the duration and amplitude of contractions in patients with nutcracker esophagus, but this did not always correlate with resolution of the chest pain.[14]

In patients with diffuse esophageal spasm, nifedipine, 10 mg sublingually 15 to 30 minutes before meals, is effective in preventing the dysphagia and choking sensation often accompanying meals.[15] Diltiazem, 30 to 90 mg PO QID, may result in both clinical and manometric improvement in patients with esophageal spasm, nutcracker esophagus, and hypertensive LES.[16]

Nifedipine has been shown to be effective in decreasing the lower esophageal spasm pressure by as much as 47 per cent in patients with achalasia.[17] Clinical improvement has been documented, with about two thirds of patients having good-to-excellent results in esophageal emptying with nifedipine, 10 to 20 mg sublingually before meals. Results of long-term use with any of these pharmacologic modalities are not available.

Other Smooth Muscle Relaxants. Anticholinergics (propantheline bromide [Pro-Banthine], 50 mg PO) have been found to decrease the LES pressure as well as the contraction amplitude in the body of the esophagus. It is also shown that when given in combination with nifedipine there was an additive effect on both LES and esophageal body pressures.[18] Anticholinergics should be considered as an adjuvant therapy in chest pain patients who do not fully respond to either a calcium channel blocker or nitrates alone.

Hydralazine (Apresoline), another smooth muscle relaxant used primarily as an antihypertensive, in dosages of 75 to 200 mg PO per day, has been shown to significantly blunt the response of bethanechol (Urecholine) to produce prolonged esophageal contractions and chest pain. Hydralazine was found to be more effective than isosorbide in preventing chest pain and on long-term follow-up had more favorable symptomatic response in patients with esophageal motility disorders.[19]

■ FORCEFUL DILATION

In achalasia, no therapy is available to restore peristalsis of the esophagus. Therefore, to improve esophageal emptying, lowering of LES pressure by forceful stretching or pneumatic dilation of the LES is the nonsurgical therapy of choice. This is accomplished by passing a 3- to 3.5-cm diameter pneumatic balloon under fluoroscopic guidance across the LES. The balloon is inflated to 12 to 15 pounds per square inch and held for 1 to 3 minutes. Pneumatic dilation is usually associated with significant chest pain, but prolonged chest pain should alert the physician to the possibility of perforation, the most common complication of the procedure. Good-to-excellent immediate results can be obtained in 48 to 76 per cent of patients with a single dilation. Good-to-excellent late results are seen in 65 to 70 per cent.[20] Repeat pneumatic dilation has less than a 50 per cent rate of good-to-excellent results. The patients who appear to have the best results are over 45 years of age, have had symptoms less than 20 years, and have only a moderately dilated esophagus (< 5 to 8 cm). Complications with this procedure are esophageal perforation (1 to 5 per cent), acute hemorrhage (1 per cent), and long-term reflux esophagitis (1 per cent).

Other types of esophageal motor disorders that respond well to pneumatic dilation are vigorous achalasia, which is probably in a spectrum between diffuse spasm and acha-

lasia, and hypertensive LES. Following pneumatic dilation, up to 84 per cent of these patients have good-to-excellent results.[20] Diffuse spasm, on the other hand, does not seem to respond as well, with only 45 per cent having results being classified as excellent to good, but pneumatic dilation may be offered to those patients not responding to pharmacologic therapy.

Other Dilation Therapy

Mercury-weighted esophageal bougies have been used in various esophageal motility disorders. In a comparison of a 54 French and a 24 French dilator in patients with nutcracker esophagus, there was a slight but not significant improvement in the relief of chest pain with the larger dilator.[21] In fact, both groups improved equally over baseline, again pointing to the benefits of reassurance and physician-patient interaction in these patients. For those patients who do not respond to medical therapy, dilation with a 50 French bougie may be beneficial. Both bougie dilation and pneumatic dilation in symptomatic patients with hyertensive LES may be effective.[22]

■ SURGICAL MYOTOMY

Patients with achalasia who are unable technically to be dilated or who do not respond to pneumatic dilation should be offered surgical myotomy. An anterior cleavage of the musculature to the mucosa is made from a few millimeters below the LES to 5 to 8 cm above it. Excellent-to-good results are usually achieved in 75 to 85 per cent of these patients. The complications, however, are more frequent than those seen in pneumatic dilations. Perforation is the most common and serious early complication of surgery, with an approximate 2 per cent incidence of fistula formation or free perforation. Long-term, gastroesophageal reflux is the major significant complication (18 per cent), leading to the suggestion that an antireflux procedure should be done, especially in any patient with an associated hiatal hernia.[20] Surgical myotomy also may be offered as a last resort to patients with diffuse esophageal spasm who have truly intractable symptoms and who have failed in all other therapies. The myotomy is extended from the LES to above the level of manometric involvement, usually to the aortic arch. Good-to-excellent results can be seen in one half to two thirds of these patients.[23]

Secondary Esophageal Motility Disorders

Disorders of the esophagus affecting the striated and/or smooth muscles which are a result of systemic disease are classified as secondary motility disorders. Dysphagia and gastroesophageal reflux are the predominant symptoms. Progressive systemic sclerosis, or scleroderma, is the most common disorder affecting the esophagus and involves the distal two thirds of the esophagus (smooth muscle) and the LES. The complication of severe, prolonged gastroesophageal reflux is peptic esophagitis, which is seen in 60 per cent of patients with scleroderma.[4] Peptic strictures frequently occur and complicate management. As there is no specific treatment for progressive systemic sclerosis, therapy is directed at treating the severe reflux and its complications. An antireflux regimen consisting of elevation of the head of the bed, nothing by mouth 3 hours before lying down, eating several small meals daily, and strict avoidance of smoking, caffeine, chocolate, and mints is the first line of therapy. H_2-blockers in high doses are often required and are best given twice daily.[24] The newest, most potent antisecretory agent is omeprazole, a H^+,K^+ ATPase inhibitor that promises to be very useful in refractory esophagitis.[25] Omeprazole was recently approved for use in the United States. Medical therapy must be maintained indefinitely.[25] Sucralfate (Carafate) slurries, 1 gm 1 hour before meals and at bedtime, also may promote healing of peptic esophagitis. Adjuvant therapy with prokinetic agents to increase LES tone and to stimulate esophageal and gastric peristalsis may be attempted with a cholinergic such as bethanechol or a dopaminergic antagonist such as metoclopramide. Cisapride, a new prokinetic agent, also has been shown to improve esophageal and gastric emptying, improving reflux symptoms.[26] Details of medication doses are given in Table 3.

Those who develop peptic stricture will require dilation with mercury bougies or di-

TABLE 3. Treatment of Gastroesophageal Reflux in Scleroderma

Antireflux measures	
Eat small meals; elevate the head of the bed; NPO 3 hr before sleep; avoid caffeine, chocolate, smoking, alcohol	
H_2-Blockers*	
Cimetidine	300 mg PO QID
	400 mg PO BID
Ranitidine	150 mg PO BID
Famotidine	20 mg PO BID
Nizatidine	150 mg PO BID
Carafate	1 gm slurries, 1 hr ac and hs
Antacids	30 ml 1 hr pc, hs, and prn
Omeprazole	20–40 mg PO daily
Prokinetics	
Metoclopramide	10 mg PO, ac and hs
Bethanechol	10–25 mg PO, ac and hs
Cisapride	10 mg PO QID
Dilation of strictures	
Antireflux surgery	

*Larger doses (1.5–2 × usual amounts) frequently required.

lations over guidewires or endoscopically placed balloons. In refractory patients or in those with pulmonary complications of their reflux, an antireflux procedure should be considered with a "loose" fundic wrap.

OTHER SECONDARY MOTILITY DISORDERS

A large number of other systemic diseases can affect esophageal motor function. Neurologic and neuromuscular disease such as myasthenia gravis, amyotrophic lateral sclerosis, dermatomyositis, and bulbar palsies frequently produce problems in the striated muscle of the hypopharynx and upper third of the esophagus. Aspiration is a common complication, and therapy is directed toward the underlying neurologic disorder.

Diabetes mellitus, alcoholism, and advancing age (presbyesophagus) may produce impressive radiographic abnormalities of motility, but fortunately clinical dysfunction is uncommon. These conditions generally do not require treatment.

Issues and Risks

Esophageal motility disorders produce significant symptoms and morbidity. They represent a diverse clinical group of diseases of unknown etiology. Therapy is directed at alleviation of symptoms and prevention of complications. Because the disorders are of minimal-to-no risk of mortality, safety of therapy is of paramount importance.

Many patients are able to cope with the fear of their chest pain once they have been appropriately evaluated. This usually requires referral to a swallowing or esophageal study center at a major medical center. Subsequently, patients may require minimal or intermittent medication. Those patients requiring therapy must be fully informed that the therapeutic end-points are usually not complete relief of all symptoms but improvements in general well-being and daily functional level. Medications utilized are often nonspecific in their actions and have a variety of side effects, ranging from mild annoyance to significant and incapacitating adverse events. Therefore, the lowest doses of drugs are recommended initially, and incremental increases are employed carefully.

For those conditions requiring the more invasive and riskier treatments, the experience and expertise of the treating physician are paramount. Usually the patient is referred to a medical or surgical specialist. Again, full understanding by the patient of the risks of any procedure is mandatory and contrasted with the likelihood of progression and long-term complications of the untreated disorder. Obviously, vigorous treatment of reflux esophagitis in patients with scleroderma is indicated. Also, efforts to improve emptying of the esophagus in achalasia should be attempted, because of the long-term consequences of pulmonary aspiration.

In other motility disorders, therapy is predicated more on relief of symptoms as opposed to preventing long-term complications, and careful weighing of benefits versus risks of any therapy must be considered.

REFERENCES

1. Richter JE, Bradley LA, Castell DO. Esophageal chest pain: current controversies in pathogenesis, diagnosis, and therapy. Ann Intern Med 1989; 110:66–78.
2. Cattau EL, Castell DO. Symptoms of esophageal dysfunction. Adv Intern Med 1982; 27:151–181.
3. Henderson RD, Wigle ED, Sample K, Marryatt G. Atypical chest pain of cardiac and esophageal origin. Chest 1978; 73:24–27.
4. Zamost BJ, Hirschberg J, Ippoliti AF, Furst DE, Clements PJ, Weinstein WM. Esophagitis in scleroderma: prevalence and risk factors. Gastroenterology 1987; 92:421–428.
5. Ward BW, Wu WC, Richter JE, Hackshaw BT, Castell DO. Long-term follow-up of symptomatic status of patients with non-cardiac chest pain. Am J Gastroenterol 1987; 82:215–218.
6. Richter JE, Dalton CB, Bradley LA, Castell DO. Oral nifedipine in the treatment of noncardiac chest pain in patients with the nutcracker esophagus. Gastroenterology 1987; 93:21–28.
7. Clouse RE, Lustman PJ. Psychiatric illness and contraction abnormalities of the esophagus. N Engl J Med 1983; 309:1337–1342.
8. Young SJ, Alpers DH, Norland CC, Woodruff RA Jr. Psychiatric illness and the irritable bowel syndrome: practical implications for the primary physician. Gastroenterology 1976; 70:162–166.
9. Clouse RE, Lustman PJ, Eckert TC, Ferney DM, Griffith LS. Low-dose trazodone for symptomatic patients with esophageal contraction abnormalities. A double-blind, placebo-controlled trial. Gastroenterology 1987; 92:1027–1036.
10. Kikendall JW, Mellow MH. Effect of sublingual nitroglycerin and long-acting nitrate preparations on esophageal motility. Gastroenterology 1980; 79:703–706.
11. Orlando RC, Bozymski EM. Clinical and manometric effects of nitroglycerin in diffuse esophageal spasm. N Engl J Med 1973; 289:23–25.
12. Swamy N. Esophageal spasm: clinical and manometric response to nitroglycerin and long-acting nitrates. Gastroenterology 1977; 72:23–27.
13. Gelfond M, Rozen P, Gilat T. Isosorbide dinitrate and nifedipine treatment of achalasia: a clinical, manometric and radionuclide evaluation. Gastroenterology 1982; 83:963–969.
14. Richter JE, Dalton CB, Buice RG, Castell DO. Nifedipine: a potent inhibitor of contractions in the body of the human esophagus. Studies in healthy volunteers and patients with the nutcracker esophagus. Gastroenterology 1985; 89:549–554.
15. Nasrallah SM. Nifedipine in the treatment of diffuse oesophageal spasm. Lancet 1982; 2:1285.
16. Silverstein BD, Kramer CM, Pope CE II. Treatment of esophageal motor disorders with a calcium-blocker, diltiazem (abstract). Gastroenterology 1982; 82:1181.
17. Bortolotti M, Labo G. Clinical and manometric effects of nifedipine in patients with esophageal achalasia. Gastroenterology 1981; 80:39–44.
18. Hongo M, Traube M, McCallum RW. Comparison of effects of nifedipine, propantheline bromide, and the combination on esophageal motor function in normal volunteers. Dig Dis Sci 1984; 29:300–304.
19. Mellow MH. Effect of isosorbide and hydralazine in painful primary esophageal motility disorders. Gastroenterology 1982; 83:364–370.
20. Vantrappen G, Hellemans J. Treatment of achalasia and related motor disorders. Gastroenterology 1980; 79:144–154.
21. Winters C, Artnak EJ, Benjamin SB. Esophageal bougienage in symptomatic patients with the nutcracker esophagus. JAMA 1984; 252:363–366.
22. Traube M, Lagarde S, McCallum RW. Isolated hypertensive lower esophageal sphincter: treatment of a resistant case by pneumatic dilatation. J Clin Gastroenterol 1984; 6:139–142.

23. Ellis FH, Olser AM, Schlegel JF. Surgical treatment of esophageal hypermotility disturbances. JAMA 1964; 188:862–866.
24. Handel L, Aggestrup S, Stenfoft P. Long-term ranitidine in progressive systemic sclerosis (scleroderma) with gastroesophageal reflux. Scand J Gastroenterol 1986; 21:799–805.
25. Hetzel DJ, Dent J, Reed WD, et al. Healing and relapse of severe peptic esophagitis after treatment with omeprazole. Gastroenterology 1988; 95:903–912.
26. Horowtiz M, Maddern GJ, Maddox A, Wishart J, Chatterton BE, Shearman DJC. Effects of cisapride on gastric and esophageal emptying in progressive systemic sclerosis. Gastroenterology 1987; 93:311–315.

Fibromyalgia syndrome

Thomas J. Romano

▪ Background

The patient with pain, fatigue, and loss of motivation, in association with sleeping problems, headaches, and other complaints, may have a chronic soft tissue rheumatism known as fibromyalgia syndrome (FS). FS is one of the most common, yet ironically one of the most overlooked, musculoskeletal problems facing physicians today. This entity, also known as *fibrositis, myofibrositis, tension rheumatism, muscular rheumatism,* and a host of other terms has been the subject of intense interest and much debate in recent years. It causes misery and concern for literally millions of patients. Delay in diagnosis (and, thus, proper treatment) can prolong the patient's suffering, causing frustration and confusion for the FS patient and treating physician alike. Hence, its inclusion in this text is not only appropriate but quite necessary, as FS can truly be a difficult medical management problem.

FS is the subject of much debate and disagreement among rheumatologists and the cause of a great deal of misery and concern for patients.[1–4] It has been called the "epitome of the soft tissue rheumatic pain disorders,"[5] and, though the term *fibrositis* was introduced to the medical literature by Gowers in 1904,[6] it remains a relatively little known and poorly understood disorder. Each of us has experienced, at one time in our lives, a form of soft tissue rheumatism. It may have been an attack of "tennis elbow" (lateral epicondylitis) or subacromial bursitis after engaging in a home improvement project. Other terms, such as tendinitis, muscle spasm, and low back sprain represent common, but often self-limited problems.

Musculoskeletal pain that does not remit in a few weeks becomes cause for concern, however. When a patient presents with a nagging subacute or chronic musculoskeletal problem, many different entities need to be considered in the differential diagnosis, including better known conditions such as inflammatory arthritis and degenerative joint disease. However, if joint warmth, swelling, and deformity are absent and pain is the most prominent problem, FS also should be considered.

▪ Management

▪ DIAGNOSIS

The diagnosis of primary FS is reserved for those patients who possess all the following attributes: (1) periarticular or soft tissue aching that may be associated with paresthesias, numbness, or burning sensations in numerous anatomic areas, which has persisted for 3 or more months, (2) the presence of tender points or trigger points that can be reliably and reproducibly demonstrated in a given patient at different points in time, and

(3) normal laboratory tests. Additional features that may be noted in individual patients are not necessary for the diagnosis. Patients with chronic diseases, such as rheumatoid arthritis or tuberculosis, can acquire FS, which is then termed secondary FS.[7] Because many of the symptoms of the underlying malady and FS are very similar, confusion can arise as to how best to manage the patient.

FS is about ten times more common in women than in men (hence the frequent use of the feminine pronoun for patients), and the age at diagnosis is usually between 35 and 60 years.

A recent review article[8] has attempted to standardize the diagnosis of FS, since in the past FS was used as a "wastebasket term" for rheumatologic entities that did not fit criteria for such better-defined diseases as rheumatoid arthritis, osteoarthritis, and so on. Table 1, adapted from reference 8, stresses the importance of chronicity of the condition, multiple reproducible tender points, and the absence of other systemic conditions that could cause musculoskeletal pain and stiffness. Diagnosis can be made with reasonable confidence if all of three obligatory criteria and three of five minor criteria are fulfilled.

The presence of a sleep disorder is considered by many rheumatologists a sine qua non for the diagnosis of primary FS,[9,10] although debate continues on this issue. The complaints of subjective swelling or numbness, chronic headaches, and/or irritable bowel syndrome can figure prominently in the clinical presentation of many FS sufferers.

TABLE 1. Criteria for Diagnosis of Primary Fibromyalgia Syndrome

Obligatory Criteria
    Chronic, diffuse aching or stiffness affecting three
      or more areas for more than 3 months
    Tender points at multiple characteristic locations
    Absence of other conditions to explain musculo-
      skeletal symptoms

Minor Criteria
    Chronic headache
    Disturbed sleep
    Pain in neck, shoulders, or upper back
    Generalized fatigue or malaise
    Subjective swelling, numbness, or morning stiffness

(Adapted from Goldenberg DL: Fibromyalgia syndrome. An emerging but controversial condition. JAMA 1987; 257:2782–2787.)

To evaluate a patient properly for the presence of FS (or, for that matter, any medical problem), a careful history must be taken. The history, however, takes on added importance when FS is in the differential diagnosis, since laboratory testing of the FS patient does not help confirm the diagnosis, but rather is useful in excluding other conditions. The physician who suspects FS should inquire about quality as well as amount of sleep, fatigue, arthralgias, myalgias, neuropathic symptoms such as numbness and tingling, the presence of stress (emotional, environmental, physical), gastrointestinal symptoms, presence and quality of headache, and any other chronic complaints. Often, clues from a carefully taken history can alert the physician to the presence of FS, abrogating the need for costly, time-consuming, and possibly even dangerous invasive testing.

A common thread running through the histories of the majority of FS patients is the presence of a sleep disorder. Typically, there are complaints of difficulty in falling asleep, intermittent sleep, and/or early morning awakening. When the FS patient arises in the morning, she often is fatigued and feels like she has not slept at all. This nonrestorative sleep pattern is typical of a defect in stage 4 non-REM delta wave sleep.

Figure 1 demonstrates the different electroencephalographic patterns found in sleep. The top tracing shows delta waves normally found in stage 4 sleep. The middle tracing is that of a fibromyalgia patient. This demonstrates some delta waves, but these are interrupted by the presence of alpha waves seen in arousal. The bottom tracing is seen in the undisturbed sleep of FS patients and also in normal volunteers whose sleep is interrupted by an external stimulus (bell, electric shock). The similarity of the sleep patterns of these two disparate groups led some investigators to believe that the FS patients had an internal arousal mechanism that prevented uninterrupted restorative sleep.[11,12]

When examining the patient suspected of having FS, a careful "point count" should be made. This entails manual palpation of several areas of the body (Fig. 2) for unusual tenderness or sensitivity to pressure. All these areas are tender in normal persons but are much more so in patients with FS. The syndrome is strongly suspected if at least six points are tender.

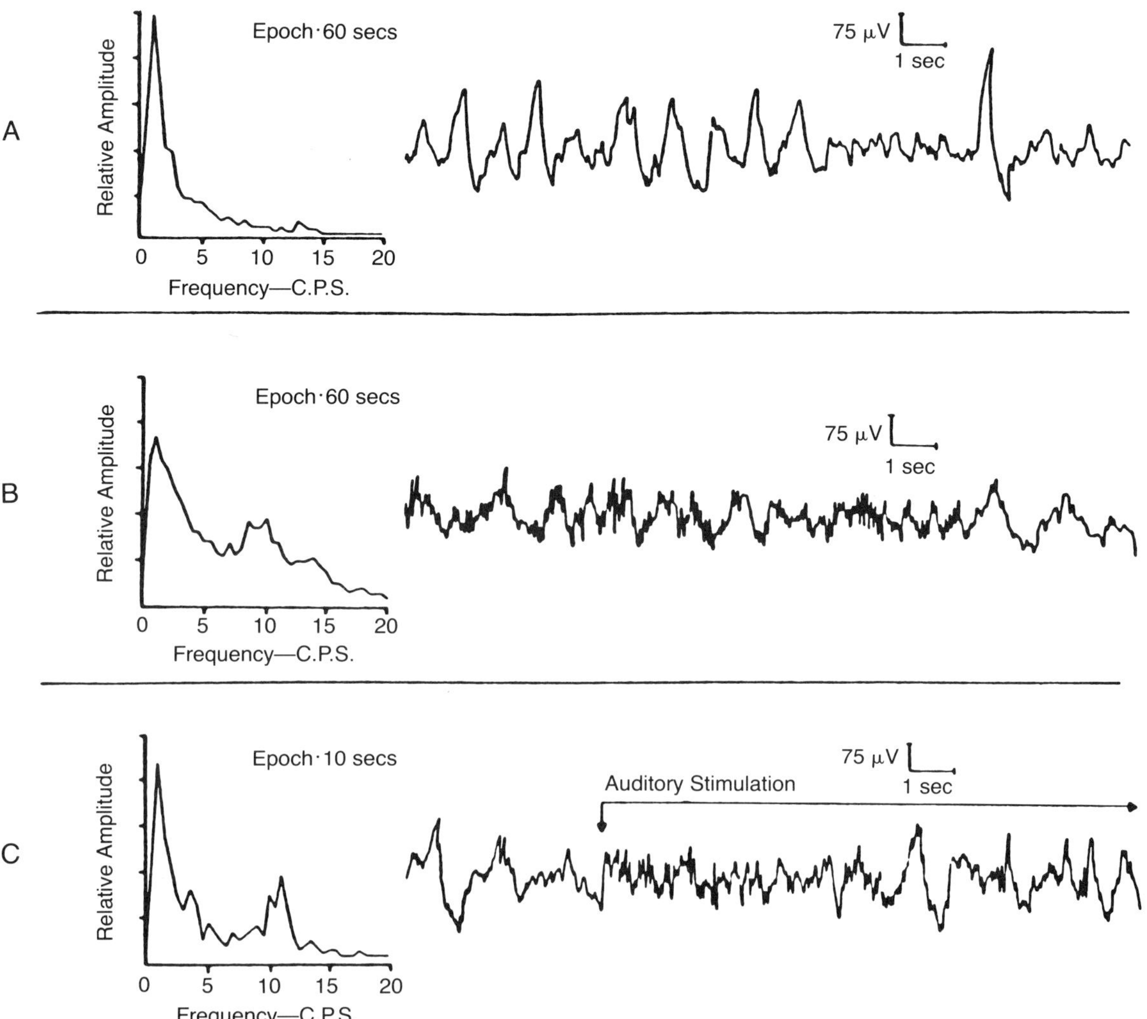

Figure 1. *A*, Frequency spectra and raw EEG from NREM (stage 4) sleep in a healthy 25-year-old subject. The spectrum shows that most amplitude is concentrated at 1 cps (delta). *B*, NREM sleep in a 42 year old "fibrositis" patient. The spectrum shows amplitude at both 1 cps (delta) and 8 to 10 cps (alpha). *C*, NREM sleep of a healthy 21 year old subject during stage 4 sleep deprivation. In the EEG, there is a clear association between external arousal (auditory stimulation) and alpha onset. Again, the frequency spectrum (obtained by 10-second analysis from stimulus onset) shows amplitude concentrated in the delta and alpha bands. (Reprinted by permission from Schumacher HR Jr (ed): Primer on the Rheumatic Diseases. 9th ed. New York: Elsevier Science Publishing Company, Inc., 1989, p 229.)

A dolorimeter, an instrument for measuring the precise amount of pressure applied over an anatomic site, can be used to quantify sensitivity to tender points. The instrument is not needed to evaluate the patient or to make the diagnosis but is useful to increase the degree of objectivity in the examination. FS needs to be clearly differentiated from psychogenic rheumatism and malingering. In such cases, patients may report tenderness over almost every area palpated or pressed on by the examiner or may exhibit one pattern of tenderness on the first examination and a far different one on subsequent examination.[7] In contrast, patients with FS have tenderness over specific anatomic sites, and results of examinations tend always to be similar. In fact, many patients with the syndrome help the physician by locating the exact area of musculoskeletal tenderness. Pressure over control points such as fingers, tarsals, or forehead does not cause pain in patients with FS but may elicit complaints of discomfort or cause withdrawal in the malingerer or patient with psychogenic rheumatism. Of course, in the process of ex-

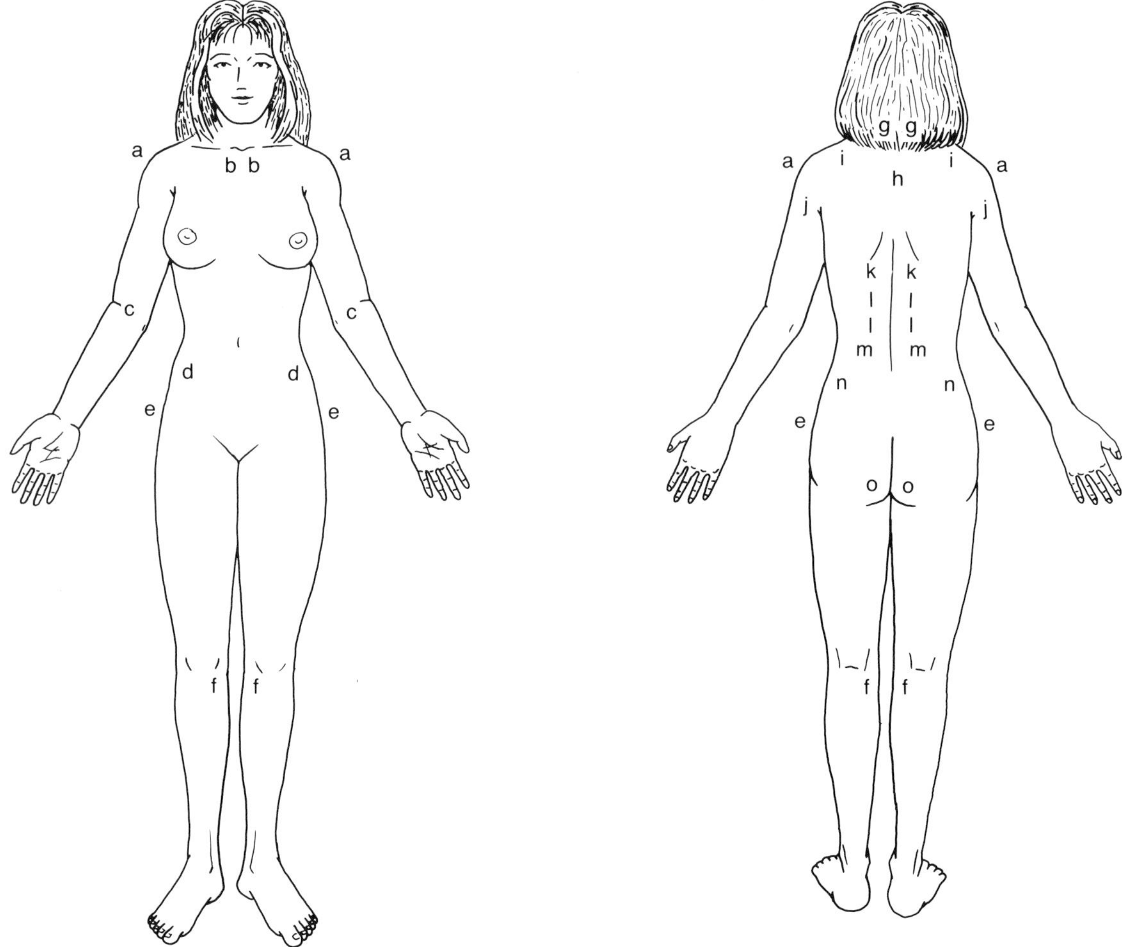

Figure 2. Myofascial trigger points for fibromyalgia syndrome. If six points are unusually tender, the diagnosis is likely.

Key

a Supraspinatus tendon
b Costochondral junction (especially at second rib)
c Lateral epicondyle of humerus
d Iliac crest
e Greater trochanteric bursa of femur
f Medial fat pad of knee
g Splenius muscle of head
h Nuchal ligament

i Trapezius muscle
j Infraspinatus tendon
k Rhomboid muscle
l Erector muscle of lumbar spine
m Multifidus muscle
n Middle gluteus muscle
o Piriformis muscle

amination, the physician notes any other pertinent physical findings that could contribute to the diagnosis.

Because the symptoms of primary FS are similar to those of other maladies, a careful search for other causes (Table 2) is needed in all cases. When warranted by additional history and physical findings in patients who complain of diffuse aching and stiffness, the following studies should be done: erythrocyte sedimentation rate (ESR) (Westergren), rheumatoid factor with titer, antinuclear antibody (ANA) and complete blood count (CBC). Patients who complain of numbness, tingling, and burning need neurologic evaluation; electromyography and nerve conduction studies are done when indicated.

Additional laboratory procedures, such as urinalysis, serum liver and muscle enzyme determinations, hormone studies, radiography, and radionuclide scanning, should be performed if other signs and symptoms point to a disorder in a particular anatomic area or organ system. If the rheumatoid factor is of high titer and the patient has symmetric

**TABLE 2. Conditions Other Than
Fibromyalgia Syndrome in Differential
Diagnosis of Patients with Chronic Aches
and Pains**

Metabolic Problems
Bone disease (e.g., osteomalacia)
Hypothyroidism

Inflammatory Conditions
Early rheumatoid arthritis
Polymyalgia rheumatica
Systemic lupus erythematosus
Polyarteritis nodosa
Seronegative spondyloarthropathies

Infections
Viral prodromes
Subacute bacterial endocarditis
Sequelae of viral infections or vaccinations
Brucellosis and other unusual infections
Acute leukemias

Anatomic Problems
Hypermobility syndromes
Idiopathic edema
Muscle overuse syndrome
Paget's disease

Neurologic Conditions
Early multiple sclerosis
Early Parkinson's disease

small-joint polyarticular arthritis, FS is considered secondary to rheumatoid arthritis. However, if results of all the standard laboratory tests are negative, as is often the case, then, and only then, can a diagnosis of primary FS be made.

The symptoms of malaise, fatigue, myalgia, and arthralgia accompany many connective tissue diseases. Patients with early rheumatoid arthritis may have positive tests for rheumatoid factor despite evanescent physical findings of synovitis or other evidence of articular inflammation. The response of the patient with rheumatoid arthritis to large doses of salicylates is greater than that of the patient with FS, although the latter may obtain some relief.

Patients with FS often complain of muscle aching, and the diagnosis of polymyositis or dermatomyositis may be considered. However, these entities can be excluded if muscle enzyme level determinations and electromyography are normal, and objective evidence of proximal muscle weakness is lacking. Polymyalgia rheumatica is characterized by shoulder and pelvic girdle aching and must be considered in elderly patients with these complaints. The ESR is elevated with polymyalgia rheumatica but normal in elderly patients with primary FS. Patients

with polymyalgia rheumatica respond dramatically to relatively low doses of corticosteroids, whereas patients with FS do not improve.

Other entities, such as hypothyroidism, multiple sclerosis, and early Parkinson's disease, can be confused with FS, but these and other similar problems are accompanied by findings on physical examination or laboratory analysis that point to their existence.

At present, interest is intense in developing an objective test that is both sensitive and specific for FS. Promising reports on objectively measurable abnormalities were presented at the 1988 meeting of the American Rheumatism Association. One study showed that patients with FS exhibit abnormal lymphocyte activity that can be normalized with therapy.[13] A second study showed that patients with primary FS have abnormalities in current perception thresholds as measured by neurometer testing.[14] The significance of these findings is unclear at this point, and more research is needed before definite conclusions can be made.

However, abnormalities noted by sophisticated immunologic or neurologic testing of FS patients should lend more credence to the view that FS is a musculoskeletal problem that can be influenced by psychologic factors and not the converse.

■ TREATMENT

The clinician who is aware of how FS presents can often make the diagnosis or suspect it at the patient's initial office visit. Workup can then be done promptly and a treatment plan initiated relatively quickly. Not only does this save the patient needless worry and expense, but it also renews the patient's faith in traditional medical approaches. If treatment is to be effective, this faith is essential, as is rapport between patient and physician.

First and foremost, these patients need reassurance that their pain is real and that their problem is a cause for concern but not for alarm or worry. I tell my patients that FS does not kill or cripple but can cause pain that will be intense at times. They are advised that good treatment strategies are available (Table 3).

I stress that patients themselves can participate in their care. This is crucial because the patient must be an active partner in

TABLE 3. Treatment of Fibromyalgia

Explain and reassure

Counsel spouse/family

Correct sleep disorder

A	B
Amitriptyline	Temazepam
Nortriptyline HCl	Chloral hydrate
Cyclobenzaprine	Triazolam
Doxepin	Flurazepam
Trazodone	

Muscle relaxants
Orphenadrine
Cyclobenzaprine
Chlorzoxazone, acetaminophen

Antianxiety agents
Alprazolam
Lorazepam
Prazepam
etc.

NSAIDs
Salicylates
  Aspirin
  Nonacetylated salicylates
  Salsalate
  Choline magnesium trisalicylate
  Magnesium salicylate
Nonsalicylates
  Ibuprofen
  Piroxicam
  Naproxen
  Phenoprofen
  Sundilac
  Indomethacin
  etc.

treatment and not merely a passive recipient of medical care. Support from family members, especially a spouse if the patient is married, is essential. If the spouse is carefully educated about the ailment and its treatment, he or she can often be included in the therapeutic effort.

No single "miracle drug" cures FS, and the approach to treatment varies from patient to patient. One must remember that FS is not a form of arthritis, although patients with arthritis may also have FS. Consequently, the rationale behind the use of nonsteroidal anti-inflammatory drugs (NSAIDs) for FS is different than that for arthritis. In FS, the NSAIDs are used for their analgesic rather than their anti-inflammatory properties because, as noted before, true inflammation is not present. Because many FS patients also have irritable bowel syndrome[15] or other gastrointestinal disorders, I prefer to prescribe low doses (400 to 600 mg) of ibuprofen (Motrin, Rufen) orally three times a day with meals or 500 to 750 mg of a nona-

cetylated salicylate (Trilisate, Disalcid) orally three or four times a day.

In addition, the use of tricyclic antidepressants at bedtime helps prevent early morning awakening, partially inhibits REM sleep (thus allowing a deeper sleep), and has an indirect muscle relaxant effect. Most commonly used are amitriptyline (Amitril, Elavil, Endep) and nortriptyline (Aventyl, Pamelor), the active metabolite of amitriptyline. Both are effective, but I start with amitriptyline because it is less expensive and is known to be effective.

Amitriptyline is given at bedtime in an initial dose of 10 to 50 mg. If tachycardia, visual blurring, or other anticholinergic side effects become a problem, I switch to 10 to 25 mg of nortriptyline, which has been reported to have a better side effect profile. The doses may be increased slowly as needed and as tolerated to a total maximum bedtime dose of 150 to 200 mg of amitriptyline or 75 to 100 mg of nortriptyline nightly. Blood levels of these medications are monitored to avoid toxicity.

Other medications for bedtime use include doxepin (Adapin, Sinequan), trazodone (Desyrel), and imipramine (Janimine, SK-Pramine, Tofranil). I recommend starting at very low doses and making increments cautiously. Recent studies have advocated the use of cyclobenzaprine (Flexeril), a muscle relaxant that is structurally related to tricyclic medication. Recommended doses are 10 to 20 mg as a one-time dose after supper or at bedtime. In addition to its sleep-promoting action, cyclobenzaprine also modulates efferent activity to muscle spindles, thus reducing muscle tension in a direct way.

Many patients who take these drugs have morning grogginess and sluggishness. I reassure them that these annoying but harmless side effects generally pass in less than a week. It is important that patients be told that although these medications are commonly used for depression, they are being prescribed for FS and not for depression. Patients with significant depression need to be referred for psychiatric help.

Muscle relaxants, such as 100 mg of orphenadrine citrate (Neocyten, Norflex) twice a day or 500 mg of chlorzoxazone (Paraflex) three or four times a day, may help selected patients.

Traditional pharmacotherapy may be unsuccessful in patients with FS if they cannot tolerate NSAIDs or tricyclic agents because of side effects or because they fear becoming dependent on medication. For these patients, 100 mg of pyridoxine (vitamin B_6) daily, may be preferable. Pyridoxine is thought to potentiate peripheral nerve receptor responses to endorphin.

Many patients with FS find it "hard to relax" and describe themselves as "worriers." They may be under stress either at work or at home and often push themselves to finish tasks even when they are in pain. These patients need to change their lifestyle and set aside time for relaxation and recreation. They must see to it that they "wind down" for an hour before bedtime.

If patients with FS cannot learn to relax on their own, psychologic consultation may be necessary. I stress to patients that I am not sending them to see a psychologist because they are mentally unstable, but rather because I think that the psychologist is best suited to help with stress management and teach them relaxation techniques, such as biofeedback.[16]

Physical therapy modalities such as massage, acupressure, ultrasound, hotpacks, and "spray-and-stretch" treatments are useful for some patients with FS but should be combined with pharmacotherapy for best results.[17,18] Systemic corticosteroids and narcotics are to be avoided; they do not work, and the risk of undesirable side effects or dependence is too great.

Despite treatment, many patients continue to have active FS, with tenderness of specific muscles or muscle insertions and muscle tautness and stiffness. These patients are good candidates for injection of a local anesthetic, with or without a glucocorticoid preparation, into tender or trigger points.[17] I usually inject the affected areas with 2 ml of 1 per cent lidocaine (Xylocaine) or 1 per cent procaine (Novocain), with or without 2 to 5 mg of triamcinolone hexacetonide (Aristospan). This usually gives prompt, albeit temporary, relief and should be followed by local application of heat and avoidance of such aggravating factors as overuse of muscles and insufficient sleep. In some patients, the beneficial effects of these injections last for weeks or months, which far exceed the half-life of the injected medications. Interruption of a pain-spasm-pain cycle is thought to be a mechanism of action of these injections.

Moderate exercise is to be encouraged in FS patients. In the beginning, mild forms of exercise such as walking and cycling should be encouraged. As the FS patient improves, more vigorous forms of exercise should be introduced. In addition to its conditioning effects, a graduated buildup to intensive physical exertion may tend to promote further endogenous endorphin production. Swimming is the best overall exercise for patients with generalized pain and FS. The words of Maimonides seem to be as relevant today as they were in the twelfth century: "If one leads a sedentary life and does not take exercise, neglects the calls of nature, or is constipated—even if he eats wholesome food and takes care of himself in accordance with medical rules—he will, throughout his life, be subject to aches and pains and his strength will fail him."[19]

■ Issues and Risks

The fibromyalgia syndrome (FS) affects millions of persons in the United States. While some investigators believe that FS is not a discrete musculoskeletal problem, an increasing number of rheumatologists are reporting that it is one of the most common diagnoses being made in their practice, and recent studies demonstrate neurologic and immunologic abnormalities in FS patients.

Until recently, few careful, scientifically controlled studies dealt with FS, and, until more is learned, we should all greet our patients' complaints with an open mind.

A simple evaluation in the office often leads to a speedy diagnosis, and conservative outpatient treatment is frequently successful. Time must be taken to perform a directed physical examination; "laying on of hands" is essential for an accurate determination of myofascial tender or trigger points. In an age with tremendous advances in diagnostic testing, it is essential that these tests be used as an adjunct to, but not a substitute for, a careful physical examination done after a detailed medical history is obtained.

The physician needs to explain the nature and cause of FS and to reassure the patient that the disorder is benign and treatable. Alerting our colleagues in other specialties to the nature of FS will expedite management of these patients.

REFERENCES

1. Wood PH. Rheumatic complaints. Br Med Bull 1977; 27:82–88.
2. Nuki G, Brooks R, Buchanan WW. Economics of arthritis. Bull Rheum Dis 1972/73; 23:726–733.
3. Allander E. Prevalence, incidence, and remission rates of some common rheumatic diseases or syndromes. Scand J Rheumatol 1974; 3:145–153.
4. Mazanec DJ. First year of a rheumatologist in private practice (letter). Arthritis Rheum 1982; 25:718–719.
5. Sheon RP, Moskowitz RW, Goldberg VM. Fibrositis syndrome. *In* Soft Tissue Rheumatic Pain. Recognition, Management, Prevention. Philadelphia: Lea & Febiger, 1982:241–252.
6. Gowers WR. Lumbago: its lessons and analogues. Br Med J 1904; 1:117–121.
7. Beetham WP Jr. Diagnosis and management of fibrositis syndrome and psychogenic rheumatism. Med Clin North Am 1979; 63:433–439.
8. Goldenberg DL. Fibromyalgia syndrome. An emerging but controversial condition. JAMA 1987; 257:2782–2787.
9. Yunus M, Masi AT, Calabro JJ, Miller KA, Feigenbaum SL. Primary fibromyalgia (fibrositis). Clinical study of 50 patients with matched normal controls. Semin Arthritis Rheum 1981; 11:151–172.
10. Campbell SM, Clark S, Tindall EA, Forehand ME, Bennett RM. Clinical characteristics of fibrositis. I. A "blinded" controlled study of symptoms and tender points. Arthritis Rheum 1983; 26:817–824.
11. Moldofsky H, Scarisbrick P, England R, Smythe H. Musculoskeletal symptoms and non-REM sleep disturbance in patients with "fibrositis syndrome" and healthy subjects. Psychosom Med 1975; 37:341–351.
12. Moldofsky H, Scarisbrick P. Induction of neurasthenic musculoskeletal pain syndrome by selective sleep stage deprivation. Psychosom Med 1976; 38:35–44.
13. Russell IJ, Vipraio GA, Michalek J, Fletcher E. Abnormal T cell subpopulations in fibrositis syndrome (abstract C113). Arthritis Rheum 1988; 31:S99.
14. Romano TJ. Abnormal cutaneous perception in primary, secondary and post traumatic fibromyalgia patients (abstract C112). Arthritis Rheum 1988; 31:S99.
15. Romano TJ. Coexistence of irritable bowel syndrome and fibromyalgia. West Virginia Med J 1988; 84:16–18.
16. Peck CL, Kraft GH. Electromyographic biofeedback for pain related to muscle tension. Arch Surg 1977; 112:889–895.
17. Travell J. Myofascial trigger points: clinical view. *In* Bonica JJ, Albefessard D (eds). Advances in Pain Research and Therapy. Vol I. New York: Raven Press, 1976:919–926.
18. Travell J. Ethyl chloride spray for painful muscle spasm. Arch Phys Med Rehabil 1952; 33:291–298.
19. Maimonides M. *In* Hyamson M (ed). Mishnah Torah (1177), The Book of Knowledge. Boys Town, Jerusalem: Israel Publishers, 1962.

Head injury

Aizik L. Wolf ■ *Michael Salcman*

Trauma is the leading cause of prolonged disability, and the leading cause of death, in all population groups under 40 years of age.[1] Acute head injury plays a major role in trauma. In fatal motor vehicle accidents, injury to the brain is present in 75 per cent of the victims at autopsy.[2] This does not even begin to reflect the disability incurred by many of the survivors, who in general are young adults. It has been estimated that up to 65 per cent of fatalities occur at the scene of an accident[3] or en route to a medical facility, allowing only one third of potentially lethal head injuries to be evaluated and treated by a physician. The medical management of head injury is challenging because of a variety of factors related to age, pre-existing disease, associated multiple trauma, delay in treatment, severity of injury, neurologic function, and type of lesion.[4]

Medical management of head injury is aimed at preventing further damage from secondary pathology, such as hemorrhage, edema, infection, or seizures. In essence, one attempts to maintain an optimal environment to promote recovery of the brain. Much of the difficulty in treating head-injured patients is due to our inability to distinguish between reversible and irreversible damage in the immediate postinjury period. We are not yet able to treat the primary brain injury, only prevent the progression of neural damage.

▪ Background

It has been estimated that approximately 500,000 individuals each year suffer from a head injury: skull fractures, intra- and extracerebral hematomas, and primary injury to the brain parenchyma, such as contusions and lacerations that result in direct damage to neural and supporting tissues. Widespread damage to the brain, often not radiographically visible, is referred to as diffuse axonal injury and is secondary to acceleration-deceleration and rotational forces, resulting in shearing of nerve fibers and reactive axonal swelling.[5] Currently there is no treatment for this primary injury, although experimental therapy now being tested holds some promise.[6]

Management of head injury is aimed at the secondary injury. Secondary injury results from an inability to meet the brain's metabolic and perfusion demands, resulting in further insults to an already compromised brain. These insults are often a result of hypoxia, hypotension (ischemia), hypercapnia, elevated intracranial pressure, infection, and other metabolic abnormalities (hypoglycemia, hyponatremia), caused by alterations in brain metabolism, intracranial hemodynamics (inadequate cerebral perfusion pressure, secondary to low cerebral compliance and high intracranial pressure), and brain water compartmentation during the hours following the injury. A satisfactory outcome for the head-injured patient requires recognition and successful treatment of these derangements.[3] Treatment is aimed at the common pathway of neuronal injury,[3] the impaired oxygen delivery, and decreased metabolic substrate. It is vital to avoid changes in the pressure-volume relationship to prevent resultant intracranial hypertension and subsequent brain herniation.

The hallmark of traumatic head injury is an altered level of consciousness; in the acute stage this is an indicator of severity. The challenge has been to quantify the level of consciousness in a manner that would correlate with the severity of injury and the patient's ultimate outcome. Use of the Glasgow Coma Scale (GCS) (Table 1) as a numerical method of defining the level of con-

TABLE 1. Glasgow Coma Scale

Parameter	Score
EYE OPENING	
Spontaneously	4
To verbal command	3
To pain	2
No response	1
BEST MOTOR RESPONSE	
To verbal command:	
Obeys	6
To painful stimulus:	
Localizes pain	5
Flexion—withdrawal	4
Flexion—abnormal	3
Extension	2
No response	1
BEST VERBAL RESPONSE	
Oriented and converses	5
Disoriented and converses	4
Inappropriate words	3
Incomprehensible sounds	2
No response	1
GCS Total	3–15

sciousness allows one to quantify mild and severe degrees of altered consciousness.[7] The scale consists of three components: eye opening, motor response, and verbal response. Many studies have reported a correlation between the GCS and neurologic outcome and survival. The GCS is easy to administer and repeat. The score is the sum of elements in the three components and varies from 3 to 15; 3 corresponds to unresponsive coma. The standard definition of coma—inability to open the eyes, make any recognizable sound, or follow commands—corresponds to a score of 8.

The most sensitive of the three components, the motor response, is the factor used to separate different levels of coma when the score is 3 to 7. This portion of the examination distinguishes the ability to integrate information and process motor tasks correctly by being able to follow verbal commands (motor score 6) from local cerebral communication, as ultimately demonstrated by the ability to localize a painful pinch (motor score 5).[7] The ability to follow commands indicates that large areas of the cortex are functioning correctly. The rubrospinal pathway subserves flexion responses but innervates only the upper extremities in humans, thus a flexor response reflects a physiologic level of injury or disconnection between the cortex and the red nuclei, resulting in a motor score of 3. A motor score of 2, or decerebration (extension of all 4 limbs), reflects a level of injury between the red nuclei and vestibular nuclei, as this pathway subserves extension in all four extremities. Such a response is thought to occur when there is damage to the midbrain–upper pontine area. Absence of motor response, or flaccid extremities, indicates that the functional level of injury is below the vestibular nuclei, at the pontomedullary junction in the brain stem.

Patients with a moderate head injury (defined as a GCS of 9 to 12 at the time of admission) usually do not suffer obvious neurologic deficits; however, more than two thirds of these patients are rendered moderately or severely disabled 3 months

NEUROLOGICAL ASSESSMENT–MARYLAND COMA SCALE

EYE OPENING
SPONTANEOUSLY	3
TO SOUND	2
TO PAIN	1
NONE	0
UNTESTABLE	U

ORIENTATION
TIME, PLACE, PERSON	3
2 OF THE 3	2
1 OF THE 3	1
NONE	0
UNTESTABLE	U

PUPIL, CORNEAL & CALORIC REFLEXES AND GRIMACE
NORMAL	2
DECREASED OR ABNORMAL	1
ABSENT	0
UNTESTABLE	U

STIMULUS
VOICE	3
SHAKE OR SHOUT	2
PAIN	1
CENTRAL PAIN	0

VERBAL RESPONSE
ORIENTED	4
CONFUSED	3
INAPPROPRIATE	2
INCOMPREHENSIBLE	1
NONE	0
UNTESTABLE	U

LEG MOTOR RESPONSE
NORMAL	2
ABNORMAL OR EXTENSOR	1
NONE	0
UNTESTABLE	U

ARM MOTOR RESPONSE
DEXTROUS AND STRONG	5
PARETIC	4
LOCALIZES	3
ABNORMAL FLEXION	2
EXTENSION	1
NONE	0
UNTESTABLE	U

DATE	
TIME	
SEDATION MEDS	
PARALYTIC AGENTS	
SEIZURES	
BP	
HR	
RESP	
TEMP	
EYE OPENING	
ORIENTATION	
PUPILS (R/L)	
CORNEALS (R/L)	
FACIAL GRIMACE (R/L)	
CALORICS (R/L)	
STIMULUS	
VERBAL RESPONSE	
ARM MOTOR (R/L)	
LEG MOTOR (R/L)	

Figure 1. Flow chart of the Maryland Coma Scale. This flow chart allows one to record and score all the variables of the Glasgow Coma Scale with the addition of the important brainstem reflexes, right-left asymmetry and other clinical variables that may affect the evaluation of the neurologic examination. (Reproduced with permission from Salcman M, Schepp RS, Ducker TB. Calculated recovery rates in severe head trauma. Neurosurgery 1981; 8:301–308.)

postinjury, probably secondary to cognitive impairment. With these patients, initial therapeutic efforts should concentrate on cognitive rehabilitation.[8]

The Maryland Coma Scale (MCS) (Fig. 1) is used at our institute to compensate for some of the deficiencies in the GCS, including absence of brain stem reflex testing, inadequate accountability of variables (i.e., intubated patient unable to verbalize), and not differentiating between the two sides in motor responsiveness. One of the advantages of the MCS is that it does not penalize patients when data cannot be assessed secondary to other associated injuries. Since it tests brain stem function from the midbrain to the medullary-cervical junction, it is more accurate in the prediction of recovery rates from severe head injury than is the GCS.[9]

Many studies have concluded that the severity of the initial injury is the major determinant for prognosis. Despite this, since the early 1970s, increased knowledge of the nature of brain injury and its contributing factors has resulted in improved brain injury therapy, a lower mortality rate, and fewer patients left in the vegetative state.[10]

The role of emergency medical services in the prehospital phase of brain injury is self-evident. Studies reveal that anywhere from 20 to 70 per cent of motor vehicle accident victims could be saved with adequate treatment before arriving at a hospital. Prehospital care providers should focus on effective resuscitation and treatment of the patient, so that further damage to an already injured and compromised brain is minimized.

■ Management

The first rule in intensive management of head trauma is to prevent hypoxia and ischemia. It is estimated that up to 50 per cent of patients in coma from a brain injury are suffering from either one or both of these secondary insults when first seen in an emergency room. The most common cause of impaired ventilation in the comatose, brain-injured patient is upper respiratory tract obstruction. Maintaining the airway is paramount; skillful intubation should avoid damage to the larynx, aspiration, or high airway pressures that would further aggravate intracranial pressure. A high inspired oxygen concentration is imperative. Spontaneous hyperventilation is not a substitute for this, as severe ventilation-perfusion mismatch is a frequent complication. If difficulty arises in ventilating and/or intubating the patient with severe facial and neck injuries, then early tracheostomy or cricothyroidotomy is indicated.

The second step in the management of the brain-injured patient is control of hypotension. It is important to understand that brain injury per se *does not cause hypotension*. When shock is present, it is essential to investigate the cause elsewhere in the body. Patients with brain injury may have significant blood loss from scalp lacerations or from an open depressed skull fracture that must be controlled by digital compression of the source of hemorrhage, followed by definitive surgical repair. By treating hypotension, we can avoid one of the factors contributing to brain ischemia. Management of brain injury focuses on providing an adequate environment for neurons to survive by assuring adequate blood flow to the brain. It is imperative to remember that though intracranial hematomas in adults do not reach a volume sufficient to cause hypovolemic shock, such loss of blood in an infant may produce profound hypotension.[11]

Cerebral perfusion is a vital factor in the resuscitation of the brain-injured patient. Elevated intracranial pressure secondary to brain swelling and its concomitant dysfunctional cerebral autoregulation must always be considered. Cerebral perfusion pressure (CPP) is approximated by the difference between mean systemic arterial pressure and mean intracranial pressure. Since we attempt to keep CPP between 65 and 90 torr, hypotension in these patients must be treated in order to maintain an adequate blood pressure and avoid an increase in intracranial pressure that further reduces the CPP.

■ INTENSIVE CARE UNIT MANAGEMENT OF INTRACRANIAL PRESSURE

The most frequent cause of death in head-injured patients is uncontrollable intracranial pressure (ICP). Secondary insults must be controlled first to avoid uncontrollable ICP. Earlier and more aggressive treatment of modest elevations of ICP (>15 mm Hg) will also reduce the incidence of uncontrolled ICP.[12,13]

It is our policy to monitor ICP in all patients who have a GCS of 8 or less, and in any patient who cannot be followed by neurologic examinations, such as those requiring paralysis for respiratory difficulties. An ICP greater than 40 mm Hg in a patient with a severe head injury appears directly responsible for brain ischemia and severe, if not fatal, neurologic dysfunction.[13] Thus, there is a consensus that patients in coma, postoperative patients after intracranial surgery, those with abnormal CT scans on admission, and those with continuous pressures of over 20 mm Hg need ICP monitoring. All patients have immediate CT scanning after cardiopulmonary stabilization and subsequently are transferred to the intensive care unit if no surgical lesion is found. Treatment for ICP then follows.

After the prevention of hypoxia and hypercapnia, proper patient positioning is imperative. We elevate the head to approximately 30 degrees, avoiding rotation or flexion, to maximize cerebral venous drainage. A Philadelphia collar is useful for this purpose. Hyperventilation should be instituted to attain a $PaCO_2$ of 25 to 30 mm Hg in the acute setting. Extremes of hyperventilation may be deleterious, as a $PaCO_2$ of less than 25 mm Hg may produce severe cerebral vasoconstriction and worsen focal ischemia. Despite globally impaired cerebral autoregulation, most severely head-injured patients maintain some degree of cerebral vasoreactivity to $PaCO_2$.

Meticulous attention to fluid management maintains blood pressure without worsening cerebral edema. The goal is to produce euvolemia without hypo-osmolality. Solutions containing dextrose should be avoided, as invariably there is a hyperglycemic response to injury that may increase cerebral lactic acidosis and potentially worsen outcome.

ICP Control

Mechanical hyperventilation is a powerful means of acutely lowering ICP, by causing cerebral vasoconstriction and thereby decreasing cerebral blood volume. Hypocapnia is also thought to correct brain acidosis.[14] Significant decreases in intracranial pressure may be seen despite a risk of promoting vasogenic edema formation in vasoparalyzed and injured tissue. We maintain the patient on hyperventilation until the intracranial pressure stabilizes at normal values. We do not use it as prophylactic management to avoid the potential risks of ischemia secondary to cerebral vasoconstriction and "inverse steal," resulting in focal edema and secondary brain injury.[15] We prefer to maintain $PaCO_2$ levels in the range of 32 to 35 torr acutely and then wean the patient from hyperventilation gradually, as tolerated.

After hyperventilation, the initial management of ICP is with mannitol, in doses of 0.25 to 1 mg/kg, achieving a peak effect in 12 to 17 minutes. Smaller doses have the same ICP-reducing effect as larger ones but are less sustained. Several concerns about the use of mannitol are rarely seen, such as acute increases in cerebral blood volume and a rebound phenomenon of mannitol ingress via damaged endothelium leading to a paradoxic increase in brain swelling. In fact, increases in cerebrospinal fluid pressure that are seen in normal patients upon rapid mannitol infusion are not observed in those with elevated pressure. Mannitol may reduce cerebrospinal fluid (CSF) formation and increases cerebrovascular constriction as a reflex response to the decrease it produces in blood viscosity; these effects are probably of minor importance relative to the osmotic mechanism. The goal of mannitol therapy is to produce and maintain a hyperosmolar state in the range of 310 to 315 mOsm/liter. Electrolyte abnormalities such as hypernatremia and hypokalemic alkalosis must be sought and treated aggressively.

The use of furosemide (Lasix) also has been advocated to treat elevated ICP. Its effectiveness when used alone seems to be less than that of mannitol, and there is considerable risk of dehydration. In spite of this, some have maintained that furosemide given in a bolus of 1 mg/kg is superior to mannitol because it produces less alteration of electrolytes and yields an immediate decrease in ICP.[16] In combination with mannitol, it seems to hasten the onset of ICP reduction and to sustain the effects of a low dose of mannitol. The combination of albumin and furosemide is useful for chronic maintenance of the euvolemic, hyperosmolar state after an initial mannitol bolus.

The use of cerebrospinal fluid (CSF) drainage for head injury is routine in our institution. Because of its quick therapeutic effectiveness, it is one of the modalities most often used to treat ICP problems. If repeat CT scans of patients with elevated ICP demonstrate increasing ventricular size, a ventricular catheter is inserted and the patient's ventricles are decompressed and drained to a pressure of 10 mm Hg. By changing catheter sites every 5 days, we have kept our complication rate (including meningitis and ventriculitis) at approximately 2 per cent. We do not use antibiotic prophylaxis. It is clear, however, that CSF volumes do not account for the majority of ICP elevations after severe head injury and that other means besides CSF drainage are necessary for controlling ICP elevation.[11,17]

Barbiturates have been reported to be effective in reducing ICP following severe head injury in some patients, as well as in improving outcome.[18-20] This has been hypothesized to be secondary to membrane stabilization,[21] changes in cerebrovascular resistance, reduction of cerebral metabolic requirements, and protection from generalized and focal cerebral ischemia.[22] Although a randomized, prospective study on the prophylactic use of barbiturates failed to show a therapeutic effect,[23] barbiturates may be indicated as a last resort in controlling ICP in a select group of patients. For short episodes of ICP greater than 20 mm Hg, thiopental in doses of 2 to 4 mg/kg is usually effective. Longer-term management is usually performed with pentobarbital. An effective protocol involves loading the patient with 5 to 10 mg/kg/hr for 4 hours, and then giving a maintenance dose of 1.6 mg/kg/hr to achieve plasma levels of 2.5 to 3.5 mg per cent. The goal of this therapy is to decrease ICP to less than 20 mm Hg while maintaining a cerebral perfusion pressure of greater than 60 mm Hg.

Barbiturate therapy has several problems, including cardiovascular instability, profound hypotension, pulmonary complications, and hypothermia. The decision to use this modality requires an intracranial pressure monitor, the ability to monitor serum barbiturate levels, a commitment to support the patient a minimum of 5 to 7 days, and cardiac monitoring capabilities, preferably with a Swan-Ganz catheter.

Decisions related to the patient's neurologic status, especially in regard to the presence or absence of brain function, cannot be made accurately until the barbiturate levels fall to normal. The latter usually requires up to 96 hours after barbiturates have been discontinued. Barbiturates are discontinued when the ICP is less than 20 mm Hg for 72 hours or there is evidence of progressive neurologic deterioration. Multiple CT scans are performed to help monitor intracerebral events.[19]

Moderate hypothermia (32 to 33°C) is used in cases in which other methods have been or become ineffective. A decrease in core temperature to 32°C decreases ICP by reducing the cerebral metabolism approximately 35 per cent and therefore decreasing blood flow and volume. The incidence of cardiac arrhythmia increases at temperatures below 32°C, and temperatures below 30°C are to be avoided.[11] Problems have not been encountered with hypothermic therapy with or without barbiturates. Rewarming, however, is the most dangerous time because of the possibility of further cardiac problems, and cardiac depression may be observed.

When all medical management fails, surgical decompression, though rarely performed, may be indicated. Large bifrontal craniectomies can be performed to allow the frontal lobes to expand upward and forward in an attempt to lower intracranial pressure and prevent herniation. Bitemporal craniectomies also have been used to assist in controlling ICP. Temporal and frontal lobectomy also may be indicated as a last-ditch attempt in the management of intracranial hypertension. The role of surgical decompression as a means to control elevated ICP when no focal mass lesion is present has been less than satisfactory,[24,25] and we do not recommend large surgical decompressions for a severely swollen hemisphere.

■ SURGICAL MANAGEMENT

The timely identification and removal of intracranial mass lesions and acute respiratory support of the coma patient have offered the greatest improvement in outcome. The tools of prognostication, including ICP data, CT images, GCS, age, and brain stem findings, make decisions regarding surgical removal of lesions identified on CT scanning complex and difficult. It is still not possible to predict results for the majority of patients, and even at the extremes of presentation, there may be surprisingly good and poor outcomes. Early surgical intervention (within 4 hours of injury) has been reported to significantly decrease mortality from acute subdural hematoma, compared with later intervention.[26] Though intracranial hematomas account for a small percentage (<10 per cent) of severe head injuries, they are found in more than 50 per cent of patients treated for coma. Immediate diagnosis of these mass lesions with CT scanning and surgical decompression as soon as possible may prevent ischemia secondary to brain swelling with transtentorial herniation, and thus contribute to optimal results. Nevertheless, there appears to be general agreement that patients with intracranial mass lesions have a poorer outcome than those with diffuse injuries.[10,27]

Epidural hematomas occur in approximately 1 per cent of all head-injured patients, in 8 per cent of those unable to follow commands or verbalize, and in anywhere from 5 to 15 per cent of those with fatal injuries.[28] Early surgical intervention can reduce the mortality rate of this lesion to only 8 per cent, with the potential for good neurologic outcome. It is important to realize that though 90 per cent of epidural hematomas are associated with a skull fracture, CT is the diagnostic test of choice. Underestimating the seriousness of delayed intracranial events caused by what is initially felt to be a minor head injury is a common error in the management of epidural hematomas.[29]

Subdural hematomas also make up about 1 per cent of all head injuries and occur in up to 63 per cent of *severe* head injuries. Subdural hematomas are classified as simple or complicated, depending on whether there are associated lacerations or bursting of brain substance.[29] The overall mortality rate of acute subdural hematomas ranges from 45 to 90 per cent.[30,31] This high mortality rate may reflect secondary cortical and brain stem damage more than the hematoma's direct mass effect.[27,29] Compared with epidural hematomas and diffuse axonal injury, the worst head injury is clearly a subdural hematoma, with increased mortality rates in both the GCS 3 to 5 and GCS 6 to 8 categories. It not only causes a greater percentage of deaths but also the worst quality of survival.[28]

Surgical management of a subdural hematoma depends on the size of the clot, the degree of shift of midline structures (greater than 5 mm), and the hematoma's absolute volume. Since the hematoma may result from bleeding from lacerated brain, torn bridging veins, or torn cortical vessels, a large decompressive craniotomy should be used to evacuate the clot. Adequate decompression may require frontal and temporal lobe debridement, and these areas should be included in the exposure. It is also mandatory to have access to the midline to repair torn bridging veins.[32] In neurosurgical trauma, a craniotomy flap should not be restrictive, so that the exposure allows the injured brain to be handled and retracted as gently as possible. Surgical decompression of intracerebral hematomas should not be performed through small flaps or burr holes, as both are an inadequate means of detecting and evacuating lesions[32,33] and may invite postoperative complications. In all surgical decompressions, the immediate goals are a reversal of brain shift and a lowering of ICP.[33]

Intracerebral hematomas can be isolated or combined with other lesions. As with cerebral contusions, which are most often located on the surface, intracerebral hematomas are most often located in the frontal and temporal regions. Any combination of lesions that have shifts of greater than 2 cm, increasing ICP, or deteriorating neurologic function should have early surgery.

■ SKULL FRACTURES

Basilar skull fractures occur in up to 24 per cent of head injuries[29] and may be associated with a persistent CSF fistula. Such a CSF leak may predispose the patient to meningitis. In the presence of a CSF leak, the patient should be observed for up to 7 days and monitored for signs of meningitis. If the leak does not stop with bed rest, the first form of treatment is diversion of CSF flow by lumbar drainage if the CT scan is negative. If the leak persists beyond 72 hours, then a formal exploratory craniotomy should be performed to repair the fistula. Prophylactic antibiotics should not be used, as they have not been shown to prevent meningitis and may select resistant organisms.[34]

Depressed skull fractures are considered surgical lesions if the inner table fragments are depressed by at least the thickness of the skull, if there is an associated scalp laceration, or if CT scanning reveals a dural tear. The main objective of surgical treatment is the prevention of infectious complications, as inadequate debridement is the most common cause of infection.[35] Skin debridement and closure should be accomplished as soon as possible, and surgical exploration always should include closure of dural tears and removal of devitalized tissue. Closed depressed skull fractures in patients who are neurologically intact should be elevated only for cosmetic reasons.[29,35] Treatment of depressed fractures may decrease the incidence of post-traumatic seizures.

Medical Sequelae of Head Injury

Post-traumatic seizures may be seen in all age groups but especially in children. Approximately 1 per cent of all patients will have a seizure at the time of injury. This is felt to result from direct injury to the brain. Immediate (within minutes) and early (within 1 week) seizures are especially apt to be seen in childhood (from 2.5 to 7 per cent). Early seizures are characterized by a relatively favorable long-term prognosis, with less than one third of patients developing epilepsy.[36] By the end of the first year, 70 per cent of delayed seizures have occurred. A correlation of high significance has been made between the frequency and persistence of seizures; the greater the frequency, the greater the probability of persistence. Prompt attention to seizures is thus warranted, though data are suggestive that prophylaxis is not successful in preventing onset.[37]

Our pharmacologically paralyzed patients receive anticonvulsant medication to decrease the incidence of unrecognized seizures; otherwise, we do not administer prophylactic treatment. Our preferred treatment of post-traumatic seizures is a loading dose of intravenous phenytoin (17 mg/kg) given at a rate not to exceed 50 mg/kg, followed by 300 to 400 mg/day in divided doses.[29] Every attempt is made to maintain therapeutic levels in the range of 10 to 20 mg/ml. If no further seizure activity occurs following an early seizure, therapy can be discontinued after 6 months, unless an electroencephalogram shows localized spikes or spikes and waves.[38]

Fulminant pulmonary edema may develop after head injury and is characterized by marked pulmonary vascular congestion, intra-alveolar hemorrhage, and protein-rich edema fluid. It most often occurs in the absence of underlying cardiopulmonary disease. It is thought that a massive sympathetic discharge caused by increased ICP affects the pulmonary vascular bed directly. Intensive management of respiratory dysfunction in the head-injured patient includes oxygen to correct hypoxemia, positive end-expiratory pressures (PEEP) to decrease the need for high oxygen concentration and to decrease pulmonary shunting, chest percussion, and postural drainage.

The hematologic system is also potentially deranged after head injury. The high thromboplastic activity of brain tissue and the increased fibrinolysis seen after trauma[39] are thought to account for the 8 per cent rate of disseminated intravascular coagulation observed in head injury. These coagulation derangements place patients at risk for recurrent intracranial hemorrhage[40] and increased hypoxemia and acute respiratory failure. We usually treat coagulopathies with fresh-frozen plasma and cryoprecipitate and platelet transfusions, as dictated by clotting studies.

Head-injury patients face a myriad of other medical complications, including fluid and electrolyte abnormalities (secondary to alteration of antidiuretic hormone secretion or diabetes insipidus), gastrointestinal complications (ulcerations, nutritional deficiencies), as well as skin, myocardial and genitourinary tract difficulties. It is essential to deal effectively with these potential complications quickly and aggressively if patients with head injury are to be given the best possible chance for recovery.

Issues and Risks

Far more work needs to be done for the head-injured patient. More intensive forms of rehabilitation should be investigated at the same time that possibly harmful intervention is examined. As Lawrence Marshall has stated, the concept that we can't do any harm is not necessarily correct. At the same time that diagnostic capabilities such as magnetic resonance imaging are allowing us to classify primary and secondary forms of injury along with clear anatomic localization, we need to go further in treating the primary form of the injury. Rather than concentrating just on monitoring the patient and treating secondary events, we need to focus on intervening at early stages of primary injury, such as axonal shearing. That is why clinical trials using drugs that are aimed at intervening during the dynamic process of the injury are important and should be encouraged. Ultimately, specific pharmacologic agents will serve to salvage or spare brain neurons from the traumatic injury, as well as enhance cognitive and functional recovery.

■ THERAPEUTIC ADVANCES

The central hypothesis underlying all theoretic treatment plans for severe head injury is that the central nervous system can suffer *reversible injury* and that appropriate treatment aimed at specific pathophysiologic processes can reverse it. Severe head injury has been shown to produce generalized and focal brain tissue and CSF acidosis, which can irreversibly damage otherwise potentially viable brain cells. Lactate levels and the CSF pH correlate with the severity of the injury.[41] Acidosis within the injured brain has been proposed to lead to altered cell membrane structure and function, breakdown of the blood-brain barrier, brain edema, and widespread injury to brain tissue.

Acidosis and acute brain swelling have been reversed or altered in a dog model of head injury treated with tris(hydroxymethyl) aminomethane (THAM). THAM is thought to buffer lactate by causing a hypocapnic alkalosis as well as by intracellular effects. Published reports have shown that the drug is effective in controlling ICP and improving the EEG power spectrum and survival in head injury models.[42] THAM also may overcome the potential and theoretic problem of using hyperventilation to create a respiratory alkalosis, without the theoretic danger of cerebral vasoconstriction that could lead to hypoxia and ischemia.[41].

A randomized, controlled trial aimed at reversing brain tissue acidosis with THAM has been ongoing at the Medical College of Virginia and at the University of Maryland's Institute for Emergency Medical Services Systems. Positive findings of the study are (1) that prophylactic hyperventilation results in poor outcome for patients at 3 and 6 months but not at 1 year, and (2) that THAM used with prophylactic hyperventilation re-

sults in the same outcome as for patients using standard management. In other words, the drug protects the patient from the deleterious effects of hyperventilation in the acute postinjury period. Further clinical studies are evaluating THAM for its efficacy in ICP control. If THAM can be shown to be effective, it may be an important addition to the care of severely head-injured patients.

Pathologic investigations of head injuries have revealed classic vascular abnormalities,[43] and research has shown that accelerated arachidonate metabolism is partly responsible for the production of some of these abnormalities. Experimental models have shown that treatment with appropriate oxygen radical scavengers can eliminate the radicals generated by the prostaglandin-stimulated hydroperoxidase reaction.[44] Since vascular factors are thought to provide the major contribution to ICP problems in the head-injured patient,[17] this finding clearly has significant clinical relevance. A clinical trial using superoxide dismutase (SOD) (Enzer Company) in a stable form as PEG-SOD (monomethoxy polyethylene glycol) is presently undergoing evaluation at the Medical College of Virginia and at the University of Maryland. This long-acting, available, safe, and easy to administer drug may yield profitable therapeutic results.

REFERENCES

1. Gissane GW. The nature and causation of road injuries. Lancet 1963; 2:659–698.
2. Accidental Death and Disability. The Neglected Disease of Modern Society. Report of the National Academy of Sciences. Washington, DC: National Research Council, 1966.
3. Neave V, Weiss MH. Neurological evaluation of a patient with head trauma: coma scales. *In* Wilkins RH, Rengachary RH (eds). Neurosurgery. New York: McGraw-Hill, 1985:1570–1578.
4. Ward JD, Gadisseux P, Wood CO, Young HF. Intensive care of the head-injured patient. *In* Landolt AM (ed). Progress in Neurological Surgery. Basel: S. Karger, 1987:15–52.
5. Adams JH, Graham DI, Murray LS, Scott G. Diffuse axonal injury due to nonmissile head injury in humans: an analysis of 45 cases. Ann Neurol 1982; 12:557–563.
6. Stein DG, Sabel BA (eds). Pharmacological Approaches to the Treatment of Brain and Spinal Cord Injury. New York: Plenum Press, 1988.
7. Teasdale G, Jennett B. Assessment of coma and impaired consciousness. A practical scale. Lancet 1974; 2:81–84.
8. Marshall LF, Marshall SB. Current clinical head injury research in the United States: Part II. *In* Becker DP, Povlishock JT (eds). Central Nervous System

Trauma Status Report. Bethesda, MD: National Institutes of Health, 1985:45–51.

9. Salcman M, Schepp RS, Ducker TB. Calculated recovery rates in severe head trauma. Neurosurgery 1981; 8:301–308.

10. Miller JD, Butterworth JF, Gudeman SK, Faulkner JE, et al. Further experience in the management of severe head injury. J Neurosurg 1981; 54:289–99.

11. Robinson WL, Wolf AL. Pediatric neurosurgical emergencies. *In* Salcman M (ed). Neurologic Emergencies. 2nd ed. New York: Raven Press, in press.

12. Miller JD, Sweet RC, Narayan R, Becker DP. Early insults to the injured brain. JAMA 1978; 24:439–442.

13. Cooper PR, Bellegarrigeu R, Ducker TB. Control of intracranial pressure in severe head injury. *In* Ishlie VS, Nagai H, Brock M (eds). Intracranial Pressure. New York: Springer Verlag, 1983:567–571.

14. Gordon E, Rossanda M. The importance of the cerebrospinal fluid acid-base status in the treatment of unconscious patients with brain lesions. Acta Anaesth Scand 1968; 12:51–75.

15. Darby JM, Yonas H, Marion DW, Latchaw RE. Local "inverse steal" induced by hyperventilation in head injury. Neurosurgery 1988; 23:84–88.

16. Cottrell JE, Robustelli A, Post K, Turndorf H. Furosemide- and mannitol-induced changes in intracranial pressure and serum osmolality and electrolytes. Anesthesiology 1977; 47:28–30.

17. Marmarou A, Maset AL, Ward JD, Choi S, Brooks D, Lutz H, et al. Contribution of CSF and vascular factors to elevation of ICP in severely head-injured patients. J Neurosurg 1987; 66:883–890.

18. Marshall LF, Bruce DA, Bruno L, et al. Role of intracranial pressure monitoring and barbiturate therapy in malignant intracranial hypertension. J Neurosurg 1977; 47:481–485.

19. Marshall LF, Smith RW, Shapiro HM. The outcome with aggressive treatment in severe head injuries. II. Acute and chronic barbiturate administration in the management of head injury. J Neurosurg 1979; 50:26–30.

20. Rockoff MA, Marshall LF, Shapiro HM. High-dose barbiturate therapy in humans. A clinical review of 60 patients. Ann Neurol 1979; 6:194–199.

21. Smith AL, Margne JJ. Anesthetics and cerebral edema. Anesthesiology 1976; 45:64–72.

22. Himwich WA, Hornburger E, Maresca R, et al. Brain metabolism in man unanesthetized and in "pentothal" narcosis. Am J Psychiat 1947; 103:689–696.

23. Ward JD, Becker DP, Miller JD, et al. Failure of prophylactic barbiturate coma in the treatment of severe head injury. J Neurosurg 1985; 62:383–388.

24. Clark K, Nash TM, Hutchinson GC. Failure of circumferential craniectomy in acute traumatic cerebral swelling. J Neurosurg 1968; 29:367–371.

25. Cooper PR, Rovit RL, Ransohoff J. Hemicraniectomy in the treatment of acute subdural hematoma: a reappraisal. Surg Neurol 1976; 5:25–28.

26. Seelig JM, Becker DP, Miller JD, Greenberg RP, Ward JD, Choi SC. Traumatic acute subdural hematoma. N Engl J Med 1981; 304:1511–1518.

27. Becker DP, Miller JD, Ward JD, et al. The outcome from severe head injury with early diagnosis and intensive management. J Neurosurg 1977; 47:491–502.

28. Gennarelli TA, Spielman GM, Langfitt TW, Gildenberg PL, et al. Influence of the type of intracranial lesion on outcome from severe head injury. A multicenter study using a new classification system. J Neurosurg 1982; 56:26–32.

29. Geisler FG, Salcman M. Management of the head injury patient. Hosp Med 1988; 24:104–128.

30. Fell DA, Fitzgerald S, Moiel RH, et al. Acute subdural hematomas. Review of 144 cases. J Neurosurg 1975; 42:37–42.

31. Jamieson KG, Yelland JDN. Surgically treated traumatic subdural hematomas. J Neurosurg 1972; 37:137–149.

32. Gudemin SK, Ward JD, Becker DP. Operative treatment in head injury. Clin Neurosurg 1982; 29:326–345.

33. Hoff J, Grollmus J, Barnes B, Margolis MT. Clinical, arteriographic and cisternographic observations after removal of acute subdural hematoma. J Neurosurg 1975; 43:27–31.

34. Ignelzi RJ, Vander Ark GD. Analysis of treatment of basilar skull fractures with and without antibiotics. J Neurosurg 1975; 43:721–726.

35. Miller JD, Jennett B. Complications of depressed skull fracture. Lancet 1968; 2:991.

36. Jennett B, Teather D, Bennie S. Epilepsy after head injury. Residual risk after varying fit-free intervals since injury. Lancet 1973; 2:652–653.

37. Caveness WF, Meirowsky AM, Rish BL, Mohr JP, Kistler JP, Dillon JD, Weiss GH. The nature of posttraumatic epilepsy. J Neurosurg 1979; 50:545–553.

38. Courjon J. A longitudinal electro-clinical study of 80 cases of post-traumatic epilepsy observed from the time of the original trauma. Epilepsia 1970; 11:29–36.

39. Kaufman HH, Moake JL, Olson JD, Miner ME, duCruet RP, Pruessner JL, Gildenberg PL. Delayed and recurrent intracranial hematomas related to disseminated intravascular clotting and fibrinolysis in head injury. Neurosurgery 1980; 7:445–449.

40. Touho H, Hirakawa K, Hino A, Karasawa J, Ohno Y. Relationship between abnormalities of coagulation and fibrinolysis and postoperative intracranial hemorrhage in head injury. Neurosurgery 1987; 19:523–531.

41. Becker DP. Brain acidosis in head injury: a clinical trial. *In* Becker DP, Povlishock JT (eds). Central Nervous System Trauma Status Report. Bethesda, MD: National Institutes of Health, 1985:229–242

42. Rosner MJ, Becker DP. Experimental brain injury: successful therapy with the weak base, thromethamine. J Neurosurg 1984; 60:961–971.

43. Rosenblum WI, Povlishock JT, Wei EP, Kontos HA, Nelson GH. Ultrastructural studies of pial vascular endothelium following damage resulting in loss of endothelium-dependent relaxation. Stroke 1987; 18:927–930.

44. Wei EP, Kontos HA, Dietrich WD, Povlishock JT, Ellis EF. Inhibition by free radical scavengers and by cyclo-oxygenase inhibitors of pial arteriolar abnormalities from concussive brain injury in cats. Circ Res 1981; 48:95–103.

Hepatitis, chronic active

Robert T. Manning

The treatment of chronic liver injury is determined in large measure by definition of the underlying cause of the persistent cytotoxicity. Some origins are common, e.g., hepatitis B, but do not respond well to intervention, whereas some, for example autoimmune hepatitis (lupoid hepatitis), frequently respond to immunosuppression. For a few diseases such as Wilson's disease and hemochromatosis, early intervention may be lifesaving.

■ Background

Chronic active hepatitis (CAH) is defined as continuing biochemical evidence of liver cell injury without improvement for more than 6 months. Clinical symptoms may be absent or, if present, are most often nondescript fatigue, malaise, or mild anorexia. The differentiation of CAH from chronic persistent hepatitis (CPH) requires liver biopsy.

■ COMMON ETIOLOGIES

Hepatitis B, spread by infected blood or blood products and by intimate mucous membrane contact, is the major detectable cause of CAH. From 3 to 15 per cent of acute infections progress to the chronic state throughout the world. Part of the variation in frequency may relate to the high incidence of delta virus superinfection (discussed later) in certain geographic locales.

The presence of hepatitis B surface antigen (HB_sAg) in the serum is the marker of acute or chronic infection. In 75 to 85 per cent of patients with acute infection, the antigen disappears from the serum in 4 to 12 weeks and eventually anti-surface (anti-HBS) antibody appears. Surface antigen persists in the remaining 15 to 25 per cent and ultimately disappears over ensuing months to years in 50 to 75 per cent of these individuals. Persistence of HB_sAg beyond 3 to 4 months suggests that the patient is at increased risk for evolution of the chronic active state. Men are at 6 to 10 times the risk for development of chronic HB_sAg antigenemia and CAH as are women.

Hepatitis E antigen (HB_eAg), present only if the patient is HB_sAg-positive, is a marker of viral replication and infectivity. Its associated antibody (anti-HBE) reflects immunologic response and decreased infectivity risk. HB_eAg appears to represent a modification of the hepatitis B core antigen (HB_cAg). Antibody to HB_cAg, anti-HBC, appears early after acute infection as an IgM fraction and persists for months to years as an IgG antibody.

The *delta agent*, a most peculiar small RNA viroid, infects only individuals who are HB_sAg serum–positive.[1] It may occur as a simultaneous infection with hepatitis B, in which case the concomitant infection is associated with a striking increase in the frequency of acute fulminant hepatitis, or as a superinfection in an HB_sAg-positive patient, producing an exacerbation of "hepatitis" symptoms, sharp increase in transaminase levels, and conversion to a more active or aggressive injury to the liver. The prevalence of delta infection is greatest in geographic areas in Italy and the Arabian areas and among intravenous drug users and hemophilics in other parts of the world.

The presence of delta antigen or antidelta antibody is necessary for diagnosis. In the near future, an IgM-antidelta serum measurement may be available, as well as detection by nucleotide technology.

Following the introduction of HB_sAg testing of all donated blood in the United States, it was hoped that post-transfusion hepatitis would be eliminated. However, post-transfusion hepatitis continued to occur, but now without evident serologic markers for either hepatitis A or hepatitis B, *non-A, non-B hepatitis* (NANB),[2] currently called hepatitis C.

The frequency of CAH-NANB following acute infection is between 15 and 20 per cent, with equal sex distribution.

Autoimmune CAH (CAH-AI) is more common in women than in men and is not related to any known viral infection.[3] The term *lupoid hepatitis* arose from the observation that this form of chronic liver injury is associated with markers shared with systemic lupus erythematosus, such as the LE cell phenomenon and positive antinuclear antibody. The onset is insidious and may begin around the time of menarche or menopause, which suggests an influence of hormonal changes.

Alcoholic hepatitis may follow a clinical course quite similar to that of other forms of CAH.[4] Usually a history of chronic, excessive alcohol consumption is evident. Clues in the asymptomatic patient without characteristic physical findings include a macrocytic hyperchromic anemia, markedly elevated gamma-glutamyl transpeptidase (GGTP), a level of aspartic aminotransferase (AST) greater than that of alanine aminotransferase (ALT), and the presence of alcohol in the blood even when the patient denies alcohol consumption.

■ DRUG REACTIONS

Isonicotinic acid hydrazide (INH) and acetaminophen may produce acute and chronic injury. Any halogenated hydrocarbon may be associated with cytotoxic effects. These agents are commonly metabolized by the mixed enzyme oxidizing system, with associated free radical production and membrane injury.

Drug toxicity may reflect a direct injurious effect as with many halogenated hydrocarbons, e.g., carbon tetrachloride, or may be an idiosyncratic reaction in a given patient. Idiosyncratic reactions are not dose-related and occur with varying incidence in the population. Phenytoin and sulfonamides, in my experience, are more than occasional offenders.

The drugs to think of when you encounter a patient with acute or chronic liver cell injury are

Phenytoin
Nitrofurantoin
Alpha-methyl DOPA
Oxyphenacetin
Isonicotinic acid hydrazide

Halothane
Sulfonamides
Any halogenated hydrocarbon
Chlorpromazine
C_{17}-alkylated steroids.

The last two agents most commonly produce a cholestatic lesion, e.g., increased alkaline phosphatase and lesser transaminase elevations, and, uncommonly, lead to CAH.

■ LESS COMMON CAUSES

Primary biliary cirrhosis (PBC) is a disorder of unknown etiology associated with clinical and anatomic findings of CAH and typified by injury to the small, intrahepatic bile ducts.[5] It occurs with greater frequency in women than men, with onset in the 4th to 5th decade of life, and is characterized by the presence of antimitochondrial antibody (AMA) in the serum and, frequently, striking elevations of alkaline phosphatase. Clinically, patients with PBC commonly present because of generalized pruritus or jaundice or because an elevated alkaline phosphatase is discovered on a screening examination.

Wilson's disease, an inherited disorder of copper metabolism, may produce the CAH syndrome.[6,7] It is usually diagnosed early in life, up to the second decade, and should be suspected in any youngster with obvious hepatocellular injury who has no markers for other causes. Affected individuals also may show a hemolytic disorder caused by cytotoxic accumulation of copper in erythrocytes.

Alpha-1 antitrypsin deficiency, an inherited disorder of intracellular enzyme synthesis, produces CAH in children and chronic pulmonary disease in adults.[8]

Hemochromatosis, an inherited disorder of iron metabolism, is usually diagnosed in men in the 4th to 5th decade of life and in women in the 5th to 6th decade.[9] It produces the CAH syndrome and is associated with excessive iron accumulation, as detected by transferrin saturation or serum ferritin determinations. Transferrin saturation of more than 64 per cent, i.e., serum iron divided by total iron-binding capacity, is an effective laboratory screening test. Recently, it has been estimated that the gene frequency in men is 0.067.[10]

Occasionally, persistent enzyme elevations will be found in obese women without evidence of alcoholism, viral injury, medication etiology, or evidence of an immune disorder. Such patients with *steatohepatitis* are invariably hyperglycemic and, in addition, have elevated serum insulin levels disproportionate to the simultaneous level of glucose.[11] Biopsy specimens show microvesicular fatty infiltration with variable evidence of liver cell injury. The liver and clinical findings usually respond over time to weight reduction and do not require direct management of the hyperglycemia.

Primary sclerosing cholangitis (PSC), an uncommon disorder, appears more frequently in men than in women and is usually associated with inflammatory bowel disease.[12] Clinically, pruritus, jaundice, abdominal pain, transaminase elevation, and a moderate-to-marked increase in alkaline phosphatase are present. An apparent immunologically mediated injury involves the extrahepatic and larger intrahepatic bile ducts.

■ ANATOMIC CRITERIA

Piecemeal Necrosis and Bridging. The key pathologic elements defining CAH of any etiology are piecemeal necrosis (disruption of the limiting plate of cells surrounding the portal areas), severe mononuclear cell infiltration of the portal area, with lymph follicle formation, central portal bridging necrosis, and entrapment of single liver cells or groups of cells within zones of necrosis. There also may be a pronounced plasma cell infiltration in the portal and intralobular areas.[13]

Chronic persistent hepatitis lacks piecemeal necrosis, and the lobular architecture is well preserved. The portal areas show increased numbers of mononuclear cells and are well demarcated. Lobular infiltration is slight.

Nodular Regeneration and the Cirrhotic Process. The hallmark of the evolution of chronic hepatic injury caused by cirrhosis is the appearance of nodular regeneration, completing the triad of the cirrhotic process: injury, fibrosis, and nodular regeneration.

Markers of Hepatitis B. The presence of "ground glass" hepatocytes characterizes CAH-B. The Shikata stain may be used to identify such cells laden with surface antigen particles. The HB_sAg carrier state without elevation in transaminase values is associated histologically with lack of inflam-

mation or only mild inflammatory cell infiltration.

NANB Hepatitis. No clear differentiating features for CAH-NANB/hepatitis C from other causes are described in the literature. In general, the anatomic injury is not as dramatic as with hepatitis B; more bile duct injury is evident, and a degree of microvesicular fatty change may be present.

■ MARKERS OF UNCOMMON CAUSES

The typical changes of CAH may be evident with drug injury or less common etiologies, since all share a common pathogenetic mechanism of injury. Staining for iron, copper (Shikata stain), and for diastase-resistant PAS inclusion may define hemochromatosis, Wilson's disease, and alpha-1 antitrypsin deficiency, respectively. Primary biliary cirrhosis in early to mid stages is associated with intralobular duct injury and granuloma formation in the portal areas.

■ CLINICAL LABORATORY FINDINGS

The biochemical hallmark of liver cell injury is elevation of serum transaminase activity. In general, acute viral hepatitis increases the alanine transaminase (ALT) more than the aspartic transaminase (AST). In contrast, the reverse relationship is more common with alcoholic liver injury, i.e., AST > ALT. Reflecting the often obscure etiology of increased transaminase determination, the ICDA-9M manual has a specific code for "transaminasemia"—790.4.[14]

The primary marker of duct injury or proliferation is the serum alkaline phosphatase (SAP). Characteristically, any injury to the liver will be associated with a modest (< two times upper normal) increase in SAP activity. Bile duct obstruction, sclerosing cholangitis, primary biliary cirrhosis, and "cholestatic" drugs are associated with greater increases in SAP, e.g., more than three times normal.

Gamma-glutamyl transpeptidase (GGTP), another membrane enzyme, usually will parallel the alkaline phosphatase. Chronic alcoholism with associated alcoholic hepatitis typically produces much higher levels of GGTP—500 to over 1000 units.

Impairment of the multifunctional synthetic activities of the liver is not a hallmark of CAH. Usually these functions, such as albumin synthesis, remain within the physiologic range unless compounded by the evolution of cirrhosis, nutritional inadequacies, or other compounding variables in the patient's clinical state.

Hematologic parameters are usually within the expected range. Leukopenia may be present early in the course of viral hepatitis or with some drug interactions. The red cell mass is preserved unless compounded by hemolysis, as with alpha-methyl DOPA toxicity, Wilson's disease, or, occasionally, viral hepatitis due to hepatitis B, Epstein-Barr virus, or cytomegalovirus infection. Platelets remain normal in numbers.

Alcoholism frequently leads to abnormalities of absorption and metabolism of folic acid with a macrocytic, hyperchromic anemia. The combination of a mean corpuscular volume of over 100 and an elevation of GGTP of more than ten times normal always should be taken as an indicator of alcoholism until proved otherwise.

■ IMMUNOLOGIC MEASUREMENTS

CAH-B is associated with persistent viral replication in the liver cell. The continued presence of surface antigen or IgM anti-HB_c is frequent. The presence of HB_eAg indicates continuing viral replication, and, as noted, is a marker of high infectivity.

Immunologic markers associated with the varying forms of CAH include antinuclear antibody (ANA), antismooth muscle antibody (ASM) and antimitochondrial antibody (AMA). T-cell and B-cell abnormalities also may be detectable.

Increased titers of antinuclear antibody and antismooth muscle antibody are typical of CAH-AI (lupoid hepatitis) but may be present in low titer in all forms of CAH. Antimitochondrial antibody is characteristic of primary biliary cirrhosis. The diagnosis of primary biliary cirrhosis is always questionable in the absence of a positive antimitochondrial antibody titer done in a good reference laboratory.

■ IMAGING TECHNIQUES

Sonography of the upper abdomen, with particular attention to the gallbladder, biliary tract, and head of the pancreas, is an invaluable initial screening examination to assist in differential diagnosis. The presence or absence of gallstones, the dimensions of the common bile duct, and the presence or absence of pancreatic enlargement are necessary observations so that anatomic abnormalities will not be missed. Metastatic disease also may be detected with high-quality imaging of the liver.

Isotope studies are seldom of differential diagnostic value in CAH. If sonography is technically difficult or of poor quality, isotope studies with tracer-labeled materials may help in judging the patency of the biliary system and whether or not the gallbladder is diseased. If the excretory functions of the liver are impaired by CAH, the isotope excretion may be so defective that adequate imaging cannot be obtained.

CAT and MRI scans are occasionally indicated when mass lesions are suspected as with malignancy, hemangiomas, cysts, and so on, or for a noninvasive evaluation of common duct size.

Transhepatic cholangiography (THC) and endoscopic retrograde cholangiopancreatography (ERCP) are useful if an anatomic abnormality is suspected but not yet confirmed by other techniques. In suspected primary sclerosing cholangitis or primary biliary cirrhosis it is mandatory that the extrahepatic biliary system be anatomically studied, in the former to prove the process and in the latter to eliminate the possibility that the injury is related to an extrahepatic obstruction.

■ Treatment[15-19]

■ GENERAL PRINCIPLES

No specific dietary intervention provides clear benefit. The indolent anorexia and nausea that CAH patients may experience compound the functional derangement in the liver. I am more concerned *that* patients eat than about *what* they eat. Positive nitrogen balance is very difficult to maintain in most patients.

There is little evidence that activities of daily living alter outcome at all. I suggest to patients that they should avoid strenuous exertion, a recommendation they accept readily since many have a general sense of malaise and easy fatigue. They should not be "put to bed," however, just because they have CAH.

There is no clear evidence that patients with CAH have an increased susceptibility to medications or other injurious factors. It is prudent, I believe, that they abstain from all alcohol, and I recommend that they take no medication without my concurrence. Functional impairment of the liver may influence the individual's response to medications, e.g., prolongation of half-life in drugs that are metabolized in large measure by the liver.

■ PHARMACOLOGIC AGENTS

Corticosteroids

Autoimmune Hepatitis.[20–22] Corticosteroid administration is most beneficial in persons with CAH-AI in whom no etiology has been found and in whom immunologic markers, such as a positive ANA, suggest an autoimmune process. I begin with 40 mg of prednisone daily for 1 week and then decrease the daily dose by 5 mg at weekly intervals until the patient is taking 20 mg per day. During the dose reduction schedule, measure the transaminase levels at weekly intervals to follow the clinical response. Usually there is a prompt decline in levels toward 50 to 100 units. Dose reduction schedules may need to be held at a given level for more than 1 week, depending upon the rate of fall in transaminase values.

Once the dose is reduced to 20 mg per day and the transaminase values are stable for 3 to 4 weeks, try a dosing schedule of 40 mg every other day. If the transaminase levels remain reasonable, then decrease the every-other-day dose by 5 mg at weekly intervals, aiming for a target dose of 7.5 to 10 mg every other day. It is hoped that the every-other-day dose minimizes long-term side effects of corticosteroid use.

Once a given dose level has been reached, maintain that level, with periodic measurement of transaminase levels, for at least 6 months. Between 6 and 12 months, depending on response and side effects, discontinuance of corticosteroid use may be tried, again carefully following the clinical and biochemical markers for reactivation of the process. A minority of patients will not show a rebound and can be without corticosteroids for long periods of time. The majority will show varying reactivation of the hepatitis process and will need reinstitution of corticosteroid administration. Some believe that the second time around is associated with a lessened response to therapy (see later discussion of azathioprine).

Hepatitis B CAH.[23–25] Corticosteroid use in CAH-B remains controversial. There is no clear evidence that the natural history of the disease is altered by corticosteroid use. Transaminase values usually decrease during corticosteroid administration, but never to normal in my experience. Patients who are ill because of the hepatitis usually feel better, have improved appetite, and diminished jaundice, but no lasting benefit follows. Cessation of corticosteroid use is commonly followed by a sharp increase in transaminase values and reappearance of clinical symptoms.

The cellular injury with hepatitis B infection is thought not to be due to the virus but to a T-cell cytotoxic antibody-driven response. Corticosteroids may suppress this reaction but do not eliminate the virus from the liver and may enhance viral replication in the liver.

NANB Chronic Active Hepatitis. No convincing evidence has been presented that CAH-NANB responds to cortocosteroid administration.

Antimetabolites

Azathioprine may be used in conjunction with prednisone to allow smaller doses of corticosteroids while achieving a good clinical response with less steroidal side effects.[26] There is no evidence that its use alone has any benefit. A dose of no more than 50 mg per day is appropriate in combination with the aforementioned dose schedule for prednisone. Azathioprine may be hepatotoxic in some individuals and may cause pancreatitis, so careful clinical and biochemical follow-up is essential.

Methotrexate, an antimetabolite used in cancer chemotherapy and for chronic refractory psoriasis, has been tried in a small number of patients with primary sclerosing cholangitis (PSC) and primary biliary cirrhosis (PBC).[15] These initial case studies show encouraging results, occasionally dramatic, in improved laboratory values, symptomatic benefit and histologic improvement. Controlled trials are underway in both sclerosing cholangitis and primary biliary cirrhosis.

The use of methotrexate to treat liver disease is confounded by evidence that it may lead to diffuse hepatic fibrosis following long-term use. When used in patients for psoriasis, the recommendations are for 50 mg per week with a total accumulated dose over time of less than 2000 mg. The promising case reports, particularly in patients with primary biliary cirrhosis, suggest that despite its potential hepatotoxicity methotrexate may be a significant advance in therapy for PBC and PSC.

Antiviral Agents and Immunomodulators

Alpha-interferon use is based on its antiviral and immunomodulatory effects.[27-31] Used alone, it produces a clinical and biochemical response during the therapy period, but rebound occurs following cessation of the injections, with no clear long-term benefits. Side effects during treatment are uniform, with malaise and flulike symptoms.

Corticosteroid administration, then withdrawal followed by alpha-interferon, may prove to be effective in CAH-B.[32] Controlled trials of such a sequential regimen demonstrate disappearance of HB$_e$Ag and rarely of HB$_s$Ag, with biochemical improvement.

Alpha-interferon has been reported to decrease transaminase levels in a few patients with CAH-NANB during the period of administration. Further trials are being undertaken.

The use of *adenine arabinoside monophosphate (AAM)* in patients with CAH-B is predicated on its antiviral effects as well as potential suppression of T-cell cytotoxicity.[33-35] Use of AAM alone produces a variable response. Its combination with a pre-treatment course of corticosteroids in controlled trials revealed a promising response in some patients, with disappearance of DNA polymerase (DNAp) and HB$_e$Ag from the serum. Used alone or in combination with interferon in a controlled trial, no benefit was demonstrated.

Controlled trials of *cyclosporin* are presently underway to evaluate the effectiveness of this agent in PSC, PBC, and CAH-B.[36,37] Single case reports in patients with CAH-B show diminution of symptoms and decrease in transaminase levels. Preliminary results in PSC suggest no benefit and, in PBC, possible improvement in biochemical abnormalities. Its use is severely limited because of the frequent occurrence of renal dysfunction and hypertension.

Thymic hormone extracts (Thymostimulun) have been administered to CAH-B as well as CAH-AI patients.[38,39] No benefit was observed in a controlled trial in CAH-AI patients, whereas clinical and biochemical response was observed in a similar trial in CAH-B individuals. Long-term benefits are unknown.

Levamisole, an immunomodulator of T-cell activity, has been used in uncontrolled trials in CAH-B.[40] Seroconversion and regression of biopsy changes have been demonstrated in some patients.

Suramin has been shown to inhibit duck hepatitis B DNA polymerase (DNAp) in vitro.[41] A pilot, uncontrolled trial in three patients with CAH-B was without benefit and was accompanied by significant side effects.

Colchicine, long used in the management of acute gout, has been found to increase long-term survival in patients with primary biliary cirrhosis treated over a number of years.[18,42] Survival in the treated patients in one study was 47 per cent at 4 years in the colchicine group and 21 per cent in the placebo group. Although the mortality rate was favorably reduced, there is no clear evidence that the biochemical or clinical aspects are benefited.

Membrane Protectors/Stabilizers

Cyanidandol-3 **(Catergen)** may have a stabilizing effect on lysosomal membranes and provide some protection against hepatotoxins.[43,44] It is interesting that it appears to produce clinical benefit in patients with alcoholic injury. No benefit was demonstrated in a small group of patients with CAH-B.

Arginine thiazolidinecarboxylate (ACTA) also may affect cell membranes.[45] A brief controlled trial of CAH-B and CAH-NB suggests biochemical resolution during the trial period.

Miscellaneous Agents

Extracts of Phyllanthus amarus, an agent that apparently inhibits viral replication, have been reported to have potential value in CAH-B.[46]

Cell wall extracts of Propionibacterium granulosum (KP-45) injected intravenously in CAH-B patients in an uncontrolled trial were reported to produce good clinical and biochemical results in 3 of 12 patients studied.[47]

Tioprin (2-mercaptopropionyl glycine) has some protective benefits against chemical hepatotoxicity.[48] A randomized trial in CAH-B and CAH-NB patients revealed improvements in biochemical measurements without effect on HB_sAg titers.

Chloroquine was studied in 7 patients with CAH-B (anti-HB_e negative) for 6 to 16 months.[49] Biochemical improvement was noted. It is interesting that three of the patients who showed a decrease in transaminase activity inadvertently stopped the medication, with a rebound rise in transaminase levels that returned toward normal with reinstitution of therapy.

Copper accumulation in the liver of patients with primary biliary cirrhosis (PBC) is uniform. *Penicillamine,* a chelating agent that increases urinary copper excretion, has been tried in large trials of PBC without any evidence of benefit.

■ Summary

Treatment of chronic active hepatitis requires a clear definition of the etiologic-pathogenetic factors in any given patient, since this clinical, biochemical, and pathologic entity has diverse causes.

Promising trials of corticosteroids followed by alpha-interferon in patients with hepatitis B chronic active hepatitis may lead to methods for seroconversion, if not eradication, of the virus in the liver. Individuals with autoimmune etiology usually respond well to immunomodulation with corticosteroids in combination with other agents such as azathioprine. Drug-related chronic liver injury commonly responds to elimination of the offending agent. Colchicine may prove to benefit patients with primary sclerosing cholangitis or primary biliary cirrhosis. Rare but life-threatening diseases, such as Wilson's disease and hemochromatosis require early intervention in order to protect the patient. DIAGNOSIS IS THE KEY TO THERAPY.

REFERENCES

1. Rizetto M, Geriv JL, Purcell RH (eds). The hepatitis delta virus and its infection. *In* Progress in Clinical and Biological Research. Vol 234. New York: Alan R. Liss, 1987.
2. Gitnick G. Non-A, non-B hepatitis: etiology and clinical course. Annu Rev Med 1984; 35:265–278.
3. Manns MP, Nakamura RM. Autoimmune liver diseases. Clin Lab Med 1988; 8:281–301.
4. Mihas AA, Doos WG, Spenney JG. Alcoholic hepatitis—a clinical and pathological study of 142 cases. J Chron Dis 1978; 31:461–472.
5. Taal BG, Schalm SW, ten Kate FWJ, Hermans J, Geertzen RGM, Feltkamp BEW. Clinical diagnosis of primary biliary cirrhosis: a classification based on major and minor criteria. Hepatogastroenterology 1983; 30:178–182.
6. Scott J, Gollan JL, Samourian S, Sherlock S. Wilson's disease, presenting as chronic active hepatitis. Gastroenterology 1978; 74:645–651.
7. Walshe JM. Diagnosis and treatment of presymptomatic Wilson's disease. Lancet 1988; 2:435–437.
8. Sharp HL. Alpha-1-antitrypsin: an ignored protein in understanding liver disease. Semin Liver Dis 1982; 2(4):314–328.
9. Crosby WH. Hemochromatosis: current concepts and management. Hosp Pract 1987; 17:173–192.
10. Edwards CQ, Gritten LM, Goldgar D, et al. Prevalence of hemochromatosis among 11,065 presumably healthy blood donors. N Engl J Med 1988; 318:1355–1362.
11. Adler M, Schaffner F. Fatty liver hepatitis and cirrhosis in obese patients. Clin J Med 1979; 67:811.
12. Wiesner RH, LaRusso NF. Clinicopathologic features of the syndrome of primary sclerosing cholangitis. Gastroenterology 1980; 79:200–206.
13. Bianchi L. Liver biopsy interpretation in hepatitis. II. Histopathology and classification of acute and chronic hepatitis: differential diagnosis. Pathol Res Pract 1983; 178;180–213.
14. Hay JE, Czaja AJ, Rakela J, Ludwig J. The nature of unexplained chronic aminotransferase elevations of a mild to moderate degree in asymptomatic patients. Hepatology 1989; 9(2):193–197.
15. Payne JA. Chronic hepatitis: pathogenesis and treatment. Dis-a-Month 1988; 36:3.
16. Cooksley WGE, Bradbear JW, Halliday JW, et al. Chronic hepatitis: aetiology and current management. Drugs 1984; 27:579–584.
17. Czaja AJ. Diagnosis and treatment of chronic hepatitis. Compr Ther 1984; 10:58–63.
18. Kaplan MM. Chronic liver diseases: current therapeutic options. Hosp Pract 1989; 15:83–102.
19. Koff RS, Seef LB. Therapy for chronic active hepatitis. Adv Intern Med 1984; 2:109–145.
20. Maggiore G, Bernard O, Hadchouel M, et al. Treatment of autoimmune chronic active hepatitis in childhood. J Pediat 1984; 6:839–844.
21. Czaja AJ, Beaver SJ, Shiels MT. Sustained remission after corticosteroid therapy of severe hepatitis B surface antigen–negative chronic active hepatitis. Gastroenterology 1987; 92:215–219.
22. Chase WF, Winn RE, Mayes GR. Oral pulse prednisone therapy in the treatment of Hb_sAg-negative chronic active hepatitis. Gastroenterology 1982; 83:1292–1296.
23. MacKay IR. Treatment of chronic active hepatitis and other liver diseases with corticosteroid agents. Med J Austr 1987; 146:370–374.
24. Tanno H, Fay OH, Rojman JA, Palazzi J, Bessone F. HBeAg/anti-HBe seroconversion during and after protracted immunosuppressive treatment in type B chronic hepatitis. Hepatology 1988; 8(3):487–492.

25. Tong MJ, Liu S, Co RL. Persistence of serum hepatitis B virus deoxyribonucleic acid in hepatitis B surface antigen–positive patients with chronic persistent hepatitis treated with prednisone. Gastroenterology 1987; 92:862–866.

26. The Copenhagen Study Group for Liver Disease. Azathioprine versus prednisone in chronic active hepatitis and non-alcoholic cirrhosis. Scand J Gastroenterol 1982; 17:817–824.

27. Anderson MG, Harrison TJ, Alexander G, Zuckerman AJ, Murray-Lyon IM. Randomised controlled trial of lymphoblastoid interferon for chronic active hepatitis B. Gut 1987; 28:619–622.

28. Carreño V, Porres JC, Mora I, Gutiez J, Quiroga JA, Cajal R, et al. A controlled study of treatment with recombinant alpha interferon in chronic hepatitis B virus infection: induction and maintenance schedules. Antiviral Res 1987; 8:125–137.

29. Matsumura N, Yoshikawa T, Kondo M, Imanishi J, Kishida T. Effect of low dosage of interferon on natural killer activity in patients with HB_sAg-positive chronic active hepatitis. Digestion 1984; 30:195–199.

30. Matsumura N, Yoshikawa T, Kondo M, Kawakami H, Kishida T. Therapeutic effect of a low dosage of human leukocyte interferon on chronic hepatitis B virus infection. Digestion 1983; 26:206–212.

31. Carreño V, Porres JC, Mora I, Bartolomé J, Bas C, Gutiez J, et al. Prolonged (6 months) treatment of chronic hepatitis B virus infection with recombinant leukocyte A interferon. Liver 1987; 7:325–332.

32. Perrillo RP, Regenstein FG, Peters MG. Prednisone withdrawal followed by recombinant alpha interferon in the treatment of chronic type B hepatitis: a randomized, controlled trial. Ann Intern Med 1988; 109:95–100.

33. Weller IVD, Lok ASF, Mindel A, Karayiannis P, Galpin S, Monjardino J, et al. Randomised controlled trial of adenine arabinoside 5′-monophosphate (ARA-AMP) in chronic hepatitis B virus infection. Gut 1985; 26:745–751.

34. Garcia G, Smith CI, Weissberg JI, Eisenberg M, Bissett J, Nair PV, et al. Adenine arabinoside monophosphate (vidarabine phosphate) in combination with human leukocyte interferon in the treatment of chronic hepatitis B. Ann Intern Med 1987; 107:278–285.

35. Perrillo RP, Regenstein FG, Bodicky CJ, Campbell CR, Sanders GE, Sunwoo YC. Comparative efficacy of adenine arabinoside 5′-monophosphate and prednisone withdrawal followed by adenine arabinoside 5′-monophosphate in the treatment of chronic active hepatitis type B. Gastroenterology 1985; 88:780–786.

36. Mistilis SP, Vickers CR, Darroch MH, McCarthy SW. Cyclosporin, a new treatment for autoimmune chronic active hepatitis. Med J Austr 1985; 143:463–465.

37. Hyams JS, Ballow M, Leichtner AM. Cyclosporine treatment of autoimmune chronic active hepatitis. Gastroenterology 1987; 93:890–893.

38. Hegarty JE, Nouri-Aria KT, Eddleston ALWF, Williams R. Controlled trial of a thymic hormone extract (thymostimulin) in "autoimmune" chronic active hepatitis. Gut 1984; 25:279–283.

39. Romeo F, Arcoria D, Palmisano L, Polosa P. Effectiveness of thymostimulin treatment in hepatitis B surface antigen–positive chronic active liver disease. Drug Res 1985; 35(8):1317–1322.

40. Fattovich G, Cadrobbi P, Crivellaro C, Pornaro E, Alberti A, Realdi G. Virological changes in chronic hepatitis type B treated with levamisole. Digestion 1982; 25:131–137.

41. Loke RHT, Anderson MG, Coleman JC, Tsiquaye KN, Zuckerman AJ, Murray-Lyon IM. Suramin treatment for chronic active hepatitis B—toxic and ineffective. J Med Virol 1987; 21:97–99.

42. Kershenobich D, Vargas F, Garcia-Tsao G, Tamayo RP, Gent M, Rojkind M. Colchicine in the treatment of cirrhosis of the liver. N Engl J Med 1988; 318:1709–1713.

43. Fehér J, Toncsev H, Stréter L, Cornides Á, Kiss Á. Effect of cyanidanol-3 on lysosomal enzyme activity of serum and granulocytes in chronic liver disease and active hepatitis. Int J Tiss Reac 1984; VI(1):75–80.

44. Halmy L, Dávid K, Nagy I, Stotz G, Kelemen JT. Clinical, enzymological and histological changes in chronic diffuse liver diseases following (+)-cyanidanol-3 (catergen) treatment. Acta Physiol Hung 1984; 64:461–470.

45. Miracco A, Iodice G, Peluso C, Quarentelli A, Selce P, Tedesco A, et al. Arginine thiazolidinecarboxylate in the treatment of chronic active hepatitis: double-blind comparison with placebo. J Int Med Res 1984; 12:35–39.

46. Thyagarajan SP, Subramanian S, Thirunalasundari T, Venkateswaran PS, Blumberg BS. Effect of *Phyllanthus amarus* on chronic carriers of hepatitis B virus. Lancet 1988; 1(Oct):764–766.

47. Gil J, Ziemka J, Brzosko WJ, Dabrowski M, Dabrowska-Bernstein B, Szmigielski S, et al. Immunotherapy of chronic active viral hepatitis B with *Propionibacterium granulosum*. Hepatogastroenterology 1984; 31:109–118.

48. Ichida F, Shibasaki K, Takino T, Suzuki H, Fujisawa K, Inoue K, et al. Therapeutic effects of tiopronin on chronic hepatitis: a double-blind clinical study. J Int Med Res 1982; 10:325–332.

49. Kouroumalis EA, Koskinas J. Treatment of chronic active hepatitis B (CAH-B) with chloroquine: a preliminary report. Ann Acad Med 1986; 15(2):150–152.

Herpes simplex virus infections

David M. Arbesfeld ■ *George Kihiczak* ■ *Robert A. Schwartz*

Herpes simplex virus infection (also called cold sores, fever blisters, herpes facialis, herpes labialis, herpes genitalis, and herpes progenitalis) is one of the most commonly occurring viral infections of humans. The causative organism is herpes hominis, which consists of two closely related viruses called herpes simplex virus type 1 (HSV-1) and herpes simplex virus type 2 (HSV-2). Both types have a double-stranded linear DNA genome of molecular weight 160×10^6 surrounded by a protein coat and lipid envelope.[1,2] The two genomes share approximately 50 per cent of the nucleotide sequence. The overall size of the virus is approximately 180 nm. The viral genome, by encoding for several specific glycoproteins that are present on the viral surface and on the surface of virus-infected cells, enables the immune system to induce an antibody response against virus-infected cells. The two viral types are indistinguishable on clinical grounds; differentiation of the types requires laboratory study. However, in general, HSV-1 produces infections above the waist (brain, eye, nose, mouth, face), whereas HSV-2 produces infections below the waist (cervix, vulva, buttocks, penis, anus, sacrum). See Table 1.

■ Background

A characteristic of infections caused by HSV is that they initially occur in mucocutaneous locations and then remain dormant in ganglional nerve cells.[1] When the virus reactivates and migrates peripherally via axons to skin and mucous membranes, active disease or recurrence is produced. Infections can be classified as (1) a primary episode when it is the first HSV infection occurring in a seronegative patient, (2) a nonprimary first episode when the first apparent episode of HSV occurs when the patient is seropositive, and (3) recurrent HSV infection, when reactivation of latent HSV occurs. Primary infections are contracted in most cases by close personal contact. Twenty to fifty per cent of patients with primary HSV infection are asymptomatic, with the symptoms of the remaining patients ranging from mild-to-severe symptoms with high fever, toxicity, and pronounced local discomfort. Classically, one sees grouped vesicles in erythematous patches, which from several days to 4 weeks erode and ulcerate, form crusts, desiccate, and heal, usually without scarring (Table 2). When one sees persistent erosions or ulcerations failing to heal, one should think of acquired immunodeficiency syndrome (AIDS) or other immunosuppressive diseases, such as Hodgkin's disease.

■ PRIMARY HERPETIC GINGIVOSTOMATITIS

Primary herpetic gingivostomatitis is the most common type of clinically apparent primary herpetic infection, with half a million new cases per year in the United States.[2] It is estimated that 70 million to 100 million recurrences occur per year. The peak of the disease occurs between the ages of 1 and 5 years. The patient presents with fever, sore throat, painful vesicles, and ulcerative erosions on the tongue, palate, gingiva, buccal mucosa, and lips. The gums and lips may be swollen, and tender regional lymphadenopathy is usually present. The patient may have a foul odor to the breath, and drooling may be present. The patient and family members should be informed that viral shedding will occur for 15 to 16

TABLE 1. Types of Herpetic Infections

Primary herpetic gingivostomatitis
Pharyngeal, tonsillar, and upper respiratory
  infection
Vulvovaginitis, cervicitis, balanitis, urethritis, proctitis
Keratoconjunctivitis
Herpetic whitlow—primary cutaneous inoculation
  herpes
Eczema herpeticum
Meningoencephalitis
Disseminated herpes of the newborn
Recurrent disease of all the preceding

TABLE 2. Diagnosis of HSV Infection

Mucocutaneous location
Grouped vesicles
Erythematous base
Prodromal burning or itching (in recurrent disease)
Reactivation along cutaneous nerves (in recurrent
  disease)

days. One can suspect the diagnosis when one sees the rapid extension of the local grouped vesicles to cover the entire buccal mucosa. Confirmation of the diagnosis can be obtained by laboratory techniques, which will be discussed later.

■ PRIMARY HERPETIC VULVOVAGINITIS

Patients with herpetic vulvovaginitis and balanitis make up 4 per cent of visits to sexually transmitted disease clinics.[2] Approximately half a million new cases occur per year in the United States. Clinically, one sees widely spread, bilateral vesicles that rapidly extend from mucosal surfaces to adjacent skin. Ten to fifteen per cent of patients with primary genital HSV infection have exudative or ulcerative pharyngitis. Symptoms include vaginal discharge, backache, and dyspareunia. Urethritis may occur, producing urinary retention. In men with urethritis, one should think of HSV urethritis when one sees dysuria out of proportion to the urethral discharge. Perianal infections and proctitis are seen more commonly in homosexual men. Anogenital infections in children should raise suspicion of child abuse. Genital HSV infections are more common in adults than in children, which is a reflection of the sexual transmission of the disease.

Primary cutaneous inoculation herpes, affecting any small area of skin on the body, presents as 1- to 2-mm vesicles on an erythematous base, progressing to pustules and crusts, with healing within a few days to 4 weeks. When occurring on the skin of the fingertips and around the nails, such an infection is known as herpetic whitlow, which presents as a very painful vesicopustular inflammation simulating a pyogenic infection. Herpes gladiatorum is a widespread primary inoculation herpes affecting wrestlers, in which the virus is rubbed into the skin by physical contact during wrestling. Scattered grouped vesicles are usually seen on the right side of the face and hand, although they may appear on any part of the body. Epidemics have been reported among members of wrestling teams.

■ RECURRENT HSV

The recurrent nature of the disease is what is most troublesome to the patient. Any site of acquired primary HSV infection can be the site of recurrent disease. In recurrent HSV infection, unlike in primary HSV infection, there is an initial symptom of burning or itching at the site where erythema and vesicles will occur. Recurrences usually occur at sites of previous infections. Vesicles often progress to crusts, with healing occurring over several days to three weeks, usually without scarring. Recurrent infection is seen most commonly on the lips and face, the anogenital region (HSV-2 in 98 per cent of cases), and the sacrum and buttocks, in decreasing order of frequency. It is not uncommon for a patient to have multiple areas of recurrent HSV infection simultaneously. Lymphadenopathy with lymphangitis can be seen rarely in recurrent disease.

The number and frequency of recurrences are variable. Of patients with primary HSV type 2 infection of the genitalia, 95 per cent will have a recurrence with a median time to first recurrence of about 50 days.[3] The median number of recurrences during the first year is four; 40 to 50 per cent of patients have more than six recurrences per year. Since the prevalence of HSV-2 genital infections in the middle class population of the United States is between 20 and 35 per cent, there are millions of recurrences per year. Of patients with primary HSV-1 genital infection, about 50 per cent will recur, but the median time for recurrence is about 1 year, and the disease may not recur for more than

TABLE 3. Differential Diagnosis in HSV Infection

Primary Herpetic Gingivostomatitis:	Erythema multiforme Vincent's infection Streptococcal pharyngitis
Genital Herpes:	Primary syphilis (chancre) Candidiasis Chancroid
Recurrent HSV:	Fixed drug eruption Contact dermatitis Herpes zoster Aphthous stomatitis

450 days. There is no correlation between the severity of the first episode of genital herpes and subsequent recurrence rates. Orolabial herpetic recurrences are usually 2 to 3 times a year, and rarely as often as 12 times a year.

It is beyond the scope of this chapter to discuss all the types of herpetic infections; however, because of their seriousness certain types must be recognized and, therefore, will be discussed briefly here (Table 3). Herpes simplex encephalitis is the most common cause of fatal sporadic encephalitis in the western world, and should be considered in the differential diagnosis of any nonbacterial encephalitis.[4] Treatment with acyclovir, if started early, can be lifesaving in this encephalitis. Neonatal congenital and acquired herpes simplex virus infection should be in the differential diagnosis of any infant failing to thrive, who was delivered of a mother with genital HSV infection at the time of delivery even when no skin lesions were apparent. Early treatment with acyclovir before internal organ involvement occurs will decrease the morbidity and mortality from this disease. To prevent acquired neonatal HSV infection, it is the accepted practice today among obstetricians to perform a cesarean section on any woman with primary genital HSV infection who is actively shedding HSV during labor.[5]

■ KAPOSI'S VARICELLIFORM ERUPTION

Kaposi's varicelliform eruption (eczema herpeticum) is a generalized infection of the skin, and sometimes of internal organs, with HSV. Kaposi's varicelliform eruption appears in people who have atopic dermatitis or some other skin diseases such as Darier's disease, congenital ichthyosiform erythro-derma, pemphigus, or mycosis fungoides. There is a predilection for infants and children, although no age group is exempt. HSV-1 is the usual causative agent, being acquired from others or by reactivation of latent virus. Initially one sees a worsening of the patient's original disorder, followed by the development of multiple 1- to 2-mm vesicles, which usually become umbilicated, enlarge, and become pustular. New lesions often appear in croplike fashion. Secondary bacterial infections with staphylococci and streptococci are common. The disease peaks at 7 to 10 days with prominent crusting; crusts heal over the next 2 weeks, leaving behind hypopigmentation, depigmentation, and occasional superficial scarring. Treatment with acyclovir should be instituted immediately upon suspecting this disease, for the mortality rate can reach up to 10 per cent in untreated cases.[6] In the past, a similar disease was also caused by the vaccinia virus used in smallpox vaccinations (eczema vaccinatum).

■ HSV AND ERYTHEMA MULTIFORME

Herpes simplex virus infections can act to trigger erythema multiforme. Herpes simplex–associated erythema multiforme is the most common etiologic subset of erythema multiforme.[7] The disease presents with polymorphic skin lesions, including targetoid lesions, macules, papules, vesicles, bullae, and wheal-like lesions, usually in a symmetric distribution and sometimes distributed in sun-exposed areas, with a predilection for the elbows, knees, dorsal aspect of the hands and feet, palms, soles, and sometimes the oral mucous membranes. The disorder is characterized by recurrences, usually following an HSV infection by 7 to 14 days. Herpes labialis followed by herpes genitalis is the most common trigger.[7] Not all herpes recurrences are followed by erythema multiforme, and not all episodes of erythema multiforme are preceded by a definite herpes simplex lesion. The erythema multiforme usually lasts 1 to 4 weeks, with the skin lesions resolving with hyperpigmentation. The disease primarily affects young healthy persons, usually in the spring and fall, with a slight tendency to affect men more than women. Viral cultures from the lesions are negative. Prophylactic treatment with acyclovir will prevent the HSV infection from triggering the erythema multiforme. Once the erythema multiforme occurs, standard treatment is used.

HSV OF THE EYE

HSV can infect the eye and cause both primary and recurrent disease. The disease can appear as herpetic conjunctivitis, ulcerative herpetic keratitis, keratouveitis, and even posterior segment disease. In addition to systemic preparations, there are topical ophthalmologic preparations, including trifluridine ophthalmic solution (Viroptic), vidarabine ophthalmic ointment (Vira-A), and idoxuridine eyedrops (Stoxil), to treat these infections.[8]

LABORATORY TESTS

There are many different laboratory tests for diagnosing herpetic infections. The easiest test is the Tzanck smear, in which one obtains the specimen by scraping the base of the lesion onto a slide. Using one of several stains to stain the specimen, one looks through a microscope to find multinucleated giant cells with convoluted nuclei. The Tzanck smear is 70 per cent sensitive in vesicles[9] but less sensitive in erosions. A biopsy can be done, but one will have to wait for about 24 hours for the results. Both direct immunofluorescence on the patient's tissue and indirect immunofluorescence on the patient's serum are good techniques.[10] Serologic testing has only a minor role in the diagnosis of HSV infections. Its use is primarily to document primary infections; antibodies are absent at the onset of the clinical or subclinical infection and appear in rising titers during the course of the infection. The gold standard for the diagnosis of HSV infection is by virus isolation in tissue culture. Viral culture, however, is not 100 per cent sensitive or specific. The virus may not grow in culture for several reasons, including (1) the virus may not survive transport conditions, (2) the sample may have too little virus, or (3) antiviral therapy may have eliminated the virus.[9] Culture results take from 2 to 7 days. Although not yet widely available, some laboratories are able to detect HSV DNA from routinely processed, paraffin-embedded biopsy specimens.[11]

In the majority of patients, the diagnosis of HSV infection may be made clinically. If the disease is not characteristic, and if proof is desired, a Tzanck smear can be done. If the Tzanck smear is negative and this does not agree with the clinical impression, a culture or immunofluorescent studies can be done. A biopsy can be done for the more bizarre lesions. If the Tzanck smear is positive and you want to know whether it is HSV or varicella zoster virus, or whether this is a primary or a secondary infection, culture and serologic studies may be performed.

Management

This decade has brought specific and often effective new therapy for HSV infections. With the advent of acyclovir (Zovirax), first topically and then orally and parenterally, a therapeutic modality has been made available to physicians. Acyclovir is absorbed into cells and prevents viral DNA replication with little effect on normal, uninfected cells' processes and replication. The systemic treatment approach is most important because, by the time the patient sees the physician, several days from the primary inoculation have elapsed, giving ample time for the virus to enter the neural ganglia, which topical therapy would not reach. Systemic therapy is beneficial in infections of the cervix, mucous membrane of the mouth, pharynx, and urethra, where topical application is difficult or impossible. Topical acyclovir can be used in patients who are severely immunosuppressed, not too ill from the HSV infection, and taking multiple drugs, when one wishes not to add another oral medication. We see many AIDS and other immunosuppressed patients who have bizarre, chronic, nonhealing, crusted, ulcerative lesions that are often not recognized by physicians until cytology or culture studies are done. Topical treatment dramatically speeds healing and rapidly decreases viral shedding and pain in these patients.[12]

FIRST EPISODE HSV INFECTION THERAPY

In initial, or first episode, HSV infection (herpes genitalis, oral herpes, and herpetic whitlow) and in nonprimary first episode in-

TABLE 4. Episodic Therapy for Recurrent HSV Infection

Medication	Route	Dose
Acyclovir (Zovirax)	Topical	Apply to affected area at onset of symptoms, every 2–3 hours, up to six times daily for 7–10 days
	Oral	200 mg five times daily, for 5 days
	Intravenous	5 mg/kg every 8 hours, for 7–10 days
Trisodium phosphonoformate* (Foscarnet)	Topical	0.3% cream for men, 1.0% for women; apply every 2 hours for one day, then every 4 hours for 4 days
	Intravenous	50 mg/kg every 8 hours for 7–10 days
Vidarabine (Ara-A, Vira-A)	Intravenous	15 mg/kg daily for 10 days, dose infused over 12–24 hours
Vidarabine ophthalmic ointment 3% (Vira-A)	Topical	One-half inch into lower conjunctival sac, every 3 hours, up to five times daily
Idoxuridine ophthalmic solution (Stoxil)	Topical	One drop every hour during daytime, every 2 hours at night
Trifluridine ophthalmic solution 1% (Viroptic)	Topical	One drop every 2 hours, up to 9 times daily

*Not FDA-approved for this usage.

fection, when the patient has significant constitutional symptoms or life-threatening disease, intravenous acyclovir, 5 mg/kg every 8 hours (pediatric dose of 250 mg/M^2 every 8 hours) for 7 to 10 days is indicated[12] (Table 4). If the patient has only mild disease, oral acyclovir, 200 mg five times a day for 10 days, should be given. With these doses, healing occurs 50 per cent faster, and viral shedding stops 90 per cent sooner. When taken orally, 20 per cent of the drug is absorbed, with serum equilibrium occurring 24 hours later, indicating that oral therapy is almost as effective as intravenous therapy. There was some concern that acyclovir might suppress the body's immune response to the virus, leading to more frequent recurrences after stopping therapy. In studies comparing immunologic and clinical responses of patients with first-episode infections treated with acyclovir and those treated with placebo, acyclovir-treated patients initially showed a decreased rise in neutralizing antibodies and antibodies to several viral glycoproteins compared with placebo-treated patients; however, despite the decrease in the rise of antibodies, at 6 months the recurrence rate was about equal in the two groups.[13] In another study, acyclovir temporarily depressed cell-mediated and antibody responses, but these later returned to normal and there was no effect on recurrence or on the subsequent clinical course of the herpetic infection.[14]

■ RECURRENT HSV INFECTION THERAPY

When a patient returns with an apparent recurrence of the HSV infection of the mouth, genitalia, buttocks, or fingers, one can culture the lesion to confirm the diagnosis. A patient with fewer than six recurrences per year could be given a prescription for acyclovir and be told to take 200 mg orally five times a day for 5 days, beginning at the onset of the symptoms of the recurrence. Other studies have shown that 800 mg orally twice a day is equally effective[15] (Table 5). Because the course of recurrent disease may be diminished by only 1.5 days, some patients feel that it is not worth taking the acyclovir, whereas others prefer taking it. Patients with more than six recurrences per year will require prophylactic acyclovir therapy for at least 6 months. Often, 200 mg orally three

TABLE 5. Prophylactic Therapy for Recurrent HSV Infection

Medication	Route	Dose
If less than six recurrences per year		
Acyclovir (Zovirax)	Oral	200 mg five times daily at onset of symptoms, or 800 mg BID, for 5 days
If more than six recurrences per year		
Acyclovir (Zovirax)	Oral	200 mg TID, or 400 mg BID, for 6 months

times a day or 400 mg two times a day will be enough to prevent 70 per cent of patients from having a recurrence during this treatment. The 30 per cent of patients with recurrences have fewer or less severe episodes. One study showed that in patients receiving 400 mg orally twice a day for 2 years, 29 per cent had no recurrence, while the remainder had 1.4 to 1.9 recurrences per year.[16] Intermittent therapy does not suppress recurrences or reduce the frequency of recurrences, as continuous prophylactic therapy does. Currently, FDA approval is for 6 months of prophylactic therapy only.

Acyclovir Side Effects

Acyclovir ointment shows no increased adverse local, systemic, or laboratory effects when compared with placebo.[17] With oral acyclovir, during short-term use the most frequent side effects are nausea and vomiting; with continuous use one can also see headaches and diarrhea. The most frequent reaction after intravenous acyclovir is inflammation and phlebitis at the injection site, if there is infiltration of the tissues by the drug. Rapid or bolus intravenous, intramuscular, or subcutaneous injections must be avoided, because this can lead to the precipitation of acyclovir in renal tubules when the solubility of acyclovir in intratubular fluid is exceeded. One per cent of patients have encephalopathic changes, with abnormal encephalograms and lethargy, tremors, confusion, and seizures. The drug must be used with caution in patients with neurologic, renal, or hepatic disease and in patients receiving intrathecal drugs, such as methotrexate and interferon.

■ ACYCLOVIR-RESISTANT HSV INFECTION THERAPY

Currently, acyclovir is the only FDA-approved drug for orolabial HSV infection. However, severe mucocutaneous infections caused by acyclovir-resistant herpesvirus infection are now occurring with increasing frequency in patients with the acquired immunodeficiency syndrome (AIDS). An alternative therapy for HSV mucocutaneous infection that fails to resolve with acyclovir therapy is trisodium phosphonoformate (Foscarnet), a pyrophosphate analog that in-

hibits HSV DNA polymerase without activation by viral thymidine kinase. Acyclovir requires activation by thymidine kinase. In one case of a patient with acyclovir-resistant HSV infection, the administration of intravenous trisodium phosphonoformate (50 mg/kg TID) yielded complete healing of lesions by day 16.[18] Trisodium phosphonoformate cream was used in a study on recurrent genital herpes.[19] Men were treated with 0.3 per cent trisodium phosphonoformate cream (Astra Pharmaceutical) and women were treated with 1.0 per cent trisodium phosphonoformate cream. This preparation did not improve statistically the times to healing or the loss of symptoms overall but did result in a higher proportion of symptom-free individuals after one day of treatment.

Another alternative therapy for HSV mucocutaneous infection that fails to resolve with acyclovir therapy is vidarabine (Vira-A), which is activated to the triphosphate form by cellular enzymes, and inhibits HSV DNA polymerase. Vidarabine is FDA approved for HSV neonatal infections and is also used in HSV encephalitis.[20,21] The intravenous dose is 15 mg per kg of body weight per day, at a concentration of no greater than 0.7 mg per ml in standard intravenous IV fluid over a period of 12 hours daily for 10 days. In a study using topical vidarabine applied by using iontophoresis for orolabial HSV infection, vidarabine treatment yielded a decrease in viral titers, as well as a 20 per cent reduction in the time lesions took to heal.[22]

■ Issues and Risks

Management of HSV infection is very frustrating to the physician due to the high frequency of recurrences, even during prophylactic therapy with acyclovir. The nature of the disease, which may entail frequent recurrences, should be explained to patients. Use of condoms or abstinence during periods of viral shedding should be encouraged. Viral culture and sensitivity assays may help delineate which drugs may be more efficacious in treating the disease. However, the patient should be made aware that even with use of the correct drug, there is a high likelihood of recurrence.

REFERENCES

1. Rüdlinger R, Norval M. Herpes simplex virus infections: new concepts in an old disease. Dermatologica 1989; 178:1–5.
2. Wheeler CE. The herpes simplex problem. J Am Acad Dermatol 1988; 18:163–168.
3. Corey L. First-episode, recurrent, and asymptomatic herpes simplex infections. J Am Acad Dermatol 1988; 18:169–172.
4. Whitley RJ. Antiviral treatment of a serious herpes simplex infection: encephalitis. J Am Acad Dermatol 1988; 18:209–211.
5. Arvin AM. Antiviral treatment of herpes simplex infection in neonates and pregnant women. J Am Acad Dermatol 1988; 18:200–203.
6. Niimura M, Nishikawa T. Treatment of eczema herpeticum with oral acyclovir. Am J Med 1988; 85:49–52.
7. Huff JC. Acyclovir for recurrent erythema multiforme caused by herpes simplex. J Am Acad Dermatol 1988; 18:197–199.
8. Falcon MG. Rational acyclovir therapy in herpetic eye disease. Br J Ophthalmol 1987; 71:102–106.
9. Solomon AR. New diagnostic tests for herpes simplex and varicella zoster infections. J Am Acad Dermatol 1988; 18:218–221.
10. Schmidt NJ, Dennis J, Devlin V, Gallo D, Mills J. Comparison of direct immunofluorescence and direct immunoperoxidase procedures for detection of herpes simplex virus antigen in lesion specimens. J Clin Microb 1983; 18:445–448.
11. Cao M, Xiao X, Egbert B, Darragh TM, Yen TSB. Rapid detection of cutaneous herpes simplex virus infection with the polymerase chain reaction. J Invest Dermatol 1989; 82:391–392.
12. Krusinski PA. Treatment of mucocutaneous herpes simplex infections with acyclovir. J Am Acad Dermatol 1988; 18:179–181.
13. Bernstein DI, Lovett MA, Bryson YJ. The effects of acyclovir on antibody response to herpes simplex virus in primary genital herpetic infections. J Infect Dis 1984; 150:7–13.
14. Lafferty WE, Brewer LA, Corey L. Alteration of lymphocyte transformation response to herpes simplex virus by acyclovir therapy. Antimicrob Agents Chemother 1984; 26:887–891.
15. Goldberg LH, Kaufman R, Conant MA, et al. Oral acyclovir for episodic treatment of recurrent genital herpes. J Am Acad Dermatol 1986; 15:256–264.
16. Goldberg LH, Kaufman R, Conant MA, et al. Episodic twice-daily treatment for recurrent genital herpes. Am J Med 1988; 85:10–13.
17. Arndt KA. Adverse reactions to acyclovir: topical, oral, and intravenous. J Am Acad Dermatol 1988; 18:188–190.
18. Chatis PA, Miller CH, Schrager LE, Crumpacker CS. Successful treatment with trisodium phosphonoformate of an acyclovir-resistant mucocutaneous infection with HSV in a patient with AIDS. N Engl J Med 1989; 320:297–300.
19. Sacks SL, Portnoy J, Lawee D, et al. Clinical course of recurrent genital herpes and treatment with trisodium phosphonoformate cream: results of a Canadian multicenter trial. J Infect Dis 1987; 155:178–186.
20. Whitley RJ, Alford CA, Hirsch MS, et al. Vidarabine versus acyclovir therapy in herpes simplex encephalitis. N Engl J Med 1986; 314:144–149.
21. Whitley RJ, Soong S-J, Dolin R, et al. Adenine arabinoside therapy of biopsy-proved herpes simplex encephalitis: National Institute of Allergy and Infectious Diseases Collaborative Antiviral Study. N Engl J Med 1977; 297:289–294.
22. Gangarosa LP, Hill JM, Thompson BL, Leggett C, Rissing JP. Iontophoresis of vidarabine monophosphate for herpes orolabialis. J Infect Dis 1986; 154:930–934.

Human immunodeficiency virus (HIV)-infected patient

Harold Horowitz ■ *Gary P. Wormser*

Medical management of the human immunodeficiency virus (HIV)-infected patient is a challenging problem. In part this is due to lack of a complete understanding of the natural history of the disease. The natural history information is needed to identify when during the course of infection to employ the various prophylactic and treatment modalities now available. Another factor hindering management is the similarity at presentation of the numerous opportunistic infections; this can delay the initiation of specific therapy. Moreover, specific therapies are often incompletely effective or may have to be continued for indefinite periods. Toxicities induced by therapeutic regimens may also complicate the use of these agents. Finally, coordination of the many medical practitioners from multiple specialties that are required for the care of these patients is in itself a formidable task.

■ Background

■ EPIDEMIOLOGY

It is estimated that 5 to 10 million people in the world are infected with the HIV. Of those, more than 1.5 million are in the United States. Over 121,000 cases of acquired immune deficiency syndrome (AIDS) have been reported from the United States and another 95,000 have been officially reported from 153 other countries as of February, 1990.

Infection with HIV is the result of exposure to the virus either sexually, through receipt of contaminated blood products, or neonatally. In this country, the major reservoirs for infection are homosexual or bisexual men and intravenous drug users, the latter being responsible in large measure for HIV spread in the heterosexual community and in children.

■ INITIAL INFECTION

After exposure to the virus, antibodies to HIV may be found as early as 2 weeks later. The majority of infected individuals make antibodies by 3 months. However, there is a subgroup of patients, to date poorly characterized, who may not demonstrate antibodies for several years after infection.[1] Seroconversion may or may not be associated with an acute, transient, flulike illness lasting nearly 2 weeks (5 to 44 days), manifested by fevers, malaise, sore throat, mouth ulcers, rashes, myalgias, arthralgias, meningitis, encephalitis, gastrointestinal symptoms, or lymphadenopathy.[2] The most distinctive feature may be the roseola-like rash on the trunk and extremities that often occurs with initial infection.[2] The incidence of this acute syndrome is unknown, and estimates vary widely. The appearance of such an illness in an individual after possible exposure should alert the physician that the individual may be infected.

■ DIAGNOSIS

Antibody testing for HIV is the primary means of diagnosis. Because of the implications of a positive serologic test, it is essential that the test results be accurate. A screening enzyme-linked immunosorbent assay (ELISA), which is reactive on two tests and validated by a positive Western blot (WB), is required before considering a person infected with HIV. ELISA tests currently marketed have sensitivities and specificities of greater than 99 per cent.[3] In a population at low risk for HIV infection (less than 0.1 per cent prevalence), a reactive ELISA has a positive predictive value of only 10 per cent.[4] Alternatively, in a high-risk population, a strongly reactive enzyme immunoassay (EIA) has a positive predictive value of greater than 97 per cent.[4] False-positive ELISA tests have been reported in patients with systemic lupus erythematosus, rheumatoid arthritis, infectious mononucleosis, candidiasis, alcoholic liver disease, primary biliary cirrhosis, chronic renal disease, HIV-2 infection, hematologic malignancies, cystic fibrosis, and pregnancy. False positivity seems to be related to the cross-reactivity of antibodies produced in various autoimmune and other states when the immune system is activated. Cross-reacting antibodies include those against class II leukocyte antigens (HLA-DR4, DQw3) present on the H9 cells that are used in certain culture systems to grow HIV, or those against mitochondrial, parietal cell, smooth muscle, and nuclear antigens.[5] False-negative EIAs have been noted early in disease prior to seroconversion, and in various conditions associated with profound immunosuppression (e.g., certain malignancies, bone marrow transplantation, B cell abnormalities, immunosuppressive medications), including the later stages of HIV infection.[5]

For a WB to be considered positive, antibody must react with multiple virus-specific antigens. With fewer reactions, the test is considered indeterminate. Only if no bands react is the test considered negative. Recently infected people may show an indeterminate pattern. However, retesting in 6 months will yield a positive pattern in most cases. Sera from patients with advanced HIV-induced immunodeficiency also may reveal indeterminate patterns because of the loss of antibodies to core proteins. False-positive WB tests are extremely rare when strict requirements for reactivity with multiple antigens are met.[5]

Test for viral p24 core antigen may be useful in detecting HIV infection in either very early or in late disease and, in the latter instance, may serve as a poor prognostic marker. This test is now commercially available. Recently, gene amplification techniques have been applied to detect HIV proviral DNA in peripheral blood mononuclear cells using the polymerase chain reaction (PCR). This may prove to be a very sensitive assay for detecting HIV. Presently this technique is laborious and the incidence of false-positive tests not fully determined.

■ NATURAL HISTORY

Factors affecting the rate of progression to AIDS after exposure to HIV are poorly delineated. It is not known whether there is a group of exposed patients who will be spared progressive disease. As yet, poorly defined cofactors, including genetic factors or concomitant infection with HTLV-I, may play a role in determining disease progression.

It is useful to consider HIV as causing a spectrum of disease, from asymptomatic infection to frank AIDS. Progression of disease from the asymptomatic stage represents a deterioration in the patient's immune system. AIDS rarely develops within 2 years of viral exposure. The delay from exposure to frank AIDS may more commonly be in the range of 7 to 10 years.[6] Whereas lymphadenopathy itself does not indicate a poor prognosis, 15 to 35 per cent of those with lymphadenopathy will develop AIDS within 3 years. Prognostic factors indicating a high probability of development of AIDS include thrush, chronic fevers, unexplained weight loss, persistent diarrhea, anemia, neutropenia, elevated erythrocyte sedimentation rate, elevated β_2-microglobulins, elevated serum neopterin levels, detectable HIV p24 antigen in serum, and CD4+ cells (helper T cells) less than $200/mm^3$.[7,8] The most helpful readily available laboratory marker is the number of helper T cells.

■ Management

Management of an HIV-infected individual requires a strategy for the evaluation and treatment of the HIV infection itself as well as for the secondary infectious and noninfectious complications. As a patient progresses from the asymptomatic stage to AIDS, management will change. Depending upon the stage of illness, various prophylactic and treatment regimens may be indicated.

■ INITIAL ASSESSMENT

The majority of HIV-infected people are asymptomatic. It is essential to perform an initial thorough history and physical examination in an effort to find subtle symptoms and physical findings that may require further evaluation. This initial examination will also serve as a baseline with which to compare subsequent examinations. The review of systems should pay particular attention to systemic complaints, visual disturbances, neurologic changes, and gastroenterologic and respiratory problems. Physical examination should include the patient's weight and a thorough skin, mouth, funduscopic, lymphatic, and neurologic examination.

Baseline laboratory tests (Table 1) should be performed in order to pinpoint conditions needing further evaluation or treatment at the onset. Some may also prove helpful in management of complications as they arise at a later date. The need for antiretroviral or chemoprophylactic therapies should be ascertained as well.

***Toxoplasma Gondii* Titers.** A baseline *Toxoplasma gondii* IgG determination will confirm prior exposure to this organism. Most *Toxoplasma* infection in HIV patients represents reactivated infection, and all but

TABLE 1. Baseline Evaluation of HIV-Infected Patients

History and physical examination
Complete blood count with differential, platelets
Chemistry profile, including LDH, CPK, liver
   functions
Erythrocyte sedimentation rate, B_{12}, folate
Antibody titers for syphilis, *Toxoplasma*, hepatitis B
   surface antigen, hepatitis B core antigen
Hepatitis B surface antigen
T-Helper cell count (CD4)
Stool for ova and parasites for selected patients
PPD with controls
Papanicolaou smear for female patients
Chest roentgenogram

3 per cent of HIV-positive individuals who develop central nervous system (CNS) toxoplasmosis have low or moderately elevated IgG titers. Knowledge of the titers will help in the management of the patient who later presents with CNS symptoms and a computed axial tomographic or magnetic resonance image suggestive of toxoplasmosis. In this instance, empiric therapy will more likely be started if the titer is positive. Seronegative individuals should be counseled to avoid raw meat and exposure to cat litter.

Hepatitis B Serology. The majority of HIV infected individuals will have had previous infection with hepatitis B. Serology studies will help identify those who have not had infection and who may warrant vaccination (see later). Hepatitis B surface antigen positivity also serves as a separate concern for health care workers if they are exposed to these patients' blood.

Syphilis Serology. Some estimates note a five times higher incidence of positive serology for syphilis in HIV-infected individuals compared with HIV noninfected people. Individuals with a positive serology test who have never been adequately treated for syphilis should have a lumbar puncture and be treated as recommended (see chapter, "Infections in the AIDS Patient"). Knowledge of baseline syphilis serology also may prove useful in comparison with subsequent tests in individuals who develop meningitis.

PPD with an Anergy Panel. The PPD-positive HIV-infected patient is at high risk of developing active tuberculosis and should be given chemoprophylaxis with isoniazid after active tuberculosis has been excluded (see chapter, "Infections in the AIDS Patient"). Patients who are anergic and have a previous history of a positive PPD that was untreated also should be given prophylaxis. Presently, it is impossible to judge the need for prophylactic treatment in the anergic person without a history of a positive PPD. Demonstration of anergy is also important in and of itself. Anergy places the individual in a poor prognostic category for the further progression of HIV-related disease.

Stool for Ova and Parasites. Homosexual men or persons who have resided in areas endemic for *Strongyloides stercoralis* should have stool examinations. Patients who are infected with *Strongyloides* may be at risk of developing dissemination of this helminthic infection as HIV infection progresses. Gay men also may be infected with *Giardia lamblia*, *Entamoeba histolytica*, and other emerging intestinal parasites such as *Blastocystis hominis* and Microsporida.

Chest Roentgenogram (CXR). CXR will help identify possible foci for reactivated tuberculosis or fungal disease. Perihilar lymphadenopathy also may be noted and followed. Most important, the CXR serves as a baseline for comparison during future episodes of pulmonary infections.

Vitamin B_{12} and Folate Levels. These should be measured and replacement therapy begun if levels are low. Low levels are associated with increased marrow toxicity with the use of azidothymidine or trimethoprim-sulfamethoxazole.

Papanicolaou Smear. Because of the increased incidence of papilloma virus infection and cervical dysplasia among women with HIV infection, a Papanicolaou smear should be performed initially and subsequently repeated at 6- to 12-month intervals.

CD4 Cell Count. This is a most essential element of the initial workup of the HIV-infected patient. CD4 cell counts below 200/ mm^3 have been demonstrated to be the most important single prognostic indicator for the development of opportunistic infections and AIDS.[9] Further management will depend upon these counts. The overall trend of the CD4 count is more important than any single evaluation since variations of up to 100 cells/mm^3 have been noted on testing of single samples.

■ INITIAL MANAGEMENT

Asymptomatic Patients with over 500 CD4 Cells/mm^3. These individuals in general are not at risk for serious opportunistic infections. Patients in this subgroup of HIV-infected individuals are the most likely to develop an immunologic response to vaccines, and appropriate vaccinations should be given (Table 2).

Although it is tempting to initiate 3'-azido-2,3'-dideoxythymidine, also called zidovudine (AZT), in this population with the belief that progression of HIV infection may be slowed, at this time it cannot be recommended. Investigations are currently in progress to determine whether early initiation of AZT is beneficial. Recent reports of HIV resistance to AZT emerging during prolonged drug usage and concerns about the

TABLE 2. Intervention in HIV-Infected Patients

All patients
  Counseling about transmission of HIV
  Pneumococcal vaccine × 1
  Influenza vaccine yearly
  Hepatitis B vaccine if susceptible
  INH if PPD-positive currently or in the past
  Syphilis management if serologic test positive
  Treatment of intestinal protozoa and helminths as
    needed

T-helper cell count > 500
  History, physical examination, CBC, SMA, PAP, CD4
    counts every 4–6 months

T-helper cell count 200–500
  Initiate low-dose AZT therapy
    Work up symptoms as appropriate
  History, physical examination, CBC, SMA, CD4
    counts every 3–4 months

T-helper cell count <200
  History, physical examination, CBC, SMA every 4–6
    weeks
  AZT, 200 mg orally every 4 hours × 1 month, then
    100 mg q 4 hours (check CBC every other week
    until stable, then monthly)
  PCP prophylaxis with trimethoprim-sulfamethoxa-
    zole or inhaled pentamidine

cumulative bone marrow suppressive activity and oncogenicity of AZT raise questions about such early usage.

Patients in this category of HIV disease should be evaluated every 4 to 6 months with repeat interviews and examinations. Repeat complete blood counts and CD4 cell studies should be done at these visits. The CD4 cell count can be expected to fall 85 cells/mm^3 per year on average.[7] However, there is considerable variability.

HIV-Positive with 200-500 CD4 Cells. Evaluations of patients in this category should be performed more frequently than for those in the preceding group. Evaluations and CD4 counts should be done every 3 to 4 months. Recent data have shown that AZT (100 mg five times daily) retards the development of AIDS in these patients. If a patient is symptomatic, workup should be performed as appropriate for the clinical situation.

CD4 Cells less than 200/mm^3. Because of the proven increased incidence of serious opportunistic infections and the efficacy of AZT in this group, AZT should be initiated at a dose of up to 1200 mg daily. The patient should be followed for side effects, and complete blood counts should be done initially every 1 to 2 weeks until they stabilize. At approximately 4- to 6-week intervals, the patient should be thoroughly interviewed and examined, with complete blood counts and blood chemistry studies done. When the blood counts are stabilized, prophylaxis for *Pneumocystis carinii* pneumonia (PCP) should be initiated (see chapter, "Infections in the AIDS Patient"). An alternative approach is to begin anti-PCP prophylaxis first and then start AZT. We prefer not to start the two therapies simultaneously, especially if trimethoprim-sulfamethoxazole is used for PCP prophylaxis, to judge individual drug tolerance better.

■ ANTIRETROVIRAL THERAPY

AZT

Zidovudine (AZT) is the only agent presently FDA-approved for treatment of HIV infection. As a thymidine analog, AZT interferes with HIV reverse transcriptase, thereby interrupting the viral reproductive cycle. AZT has been demonstrated to decrease circulating HIV p24 antigen, improve functional status, reduce the number of opportunistic infections, and improve survival in adults with advanced AIDS-related complex or AIDS.[9] AZT crosses the blood-brain barrier, attaining 50 to 60 per cent of serum levels, and has been shown to improve encephalopathy and other neurologic problems associated with HIV infection.[10] Better outcome is associated with pretherapy Karnofsky scores greater than 90 per cent, hemoglobin levels greater than 12 gm/dl, and CD4 cells greater than 100/mm^3.[11]

In adult patients with less than 200 CD4 cells/mm^3, AZT is given orally at doses of 200 mg every 4 hours for one month, then 100 mg every 4 hours. In patients with more than 200 CD4 cells/mm^3, the AZT dose is 100 mg five times daily. The major side effect is bone marrow suppression. Up to 21 per cent of patients will require multiple blood transfusions, and 16 per cent of AZT recipients develop neutropenia (less than 500 neutrophils/mm^3).[12] Nearly 50 per cent of patients will not tolerate AZT at all or need lower doses. A higher risk of hematologic toxicity has been noted if CD4 cells, vitamin B$_{12}$ levels, or neutrophil counts are low at the initiation of therapy.[12]

High-dose AZT therapy can be continued despite anemia if blood transfusion support is given. Alternatively, in an attempt to decrease the number of transfusions required, the dose of AZT can be lowered. During AZT therapy, the mean corpuscular volume of erythrocytes frequently becomes elevated. Vitamin B_{12} or folate supplementation is not indicated unless these levels are found to be deficient. Recombinant human erythropoietin given subcutaneously in various doses has been shown to decrease significantly the blood transfusion requirements in patients with less than 500 mU/ml of endogenous erythropoietin who are receiving AZT. Presently, trials are in progress to substantiate these findings.

AZT doses should be decreased to approximately half the full dose if neutrophils fall below 1500/mm^3 and should be stopped in patients who develop severe neutropenia with less than 500 granulocytes/mm^3. Both lithium carbonate and granulocyte-macrophage–stimulating factor have been reported to increase the number of circulating neutrophils in patients receiving AZT, thereby allowing for higher doses of AZT to be administered. Studies are ongoing to verify this and to determine the clinical significance of this effect.

Other toxicities of AZT include nausea, myalgia, myopathy, confusion, insomnia, and severe headaches. These side effects may occur early in therapy and may dissuade the patient from continuing with therapy. Since these effects may be transient or relieved by lowering the dose of AZT, attempts should be made to continue the drug with symptomatic treatment of these problems as needed. Lower doses of AZT also may be tried. Seizures and hepatic failure have been reported rarely with the use of AZT, necessitating stopping of the drug. It is notable that AZT appears to have little effect on reducing the platelet count.

AZT toxicity may be increased with drugs such as acetaminophen or aspirin, which can compete with AZT for glucuronidization, and with probenecid because of a reduction in both metabolism and renal excretion. Close attention, particularly to hematologic toxicity, is necessary when patients take these drugs concurrently with AZT.

The lowest effective dose of AZT has not been established. Doses of 500 or 600 mg daily, however, appear to be equally as effective as the previously recommended 1200-mg daily dosage.

AZT is not curative in HIV infection, because it does not affect the latent virus. Opportunistic infection and disease progression have been noted often within 6 months after the initiation of AZT.[13] Moreover, recent reports have noted increased resistance to AZT of HIV-isolates recovered from blood in long-term AZT recipients.[14] Clinical correlation with progressive disease in these instances has not been reported. When discontinuing AZT, the physician must watch for the possibility of a rapid progression of disease, manifested by myelopathy or meningoencephalitis, but this appears to be quite rare.

■ OTHER AGENTS

The search for less toxic and more active antiretroviral agents is an active field of research. Several hundred agents have been shown to limit HIV replication in vitro, many of which are presently undergoing investigational trials. Combination therapies are also avidly being investigated.[15–17] Antiviral agents may be divided into different categories based upon mechanism of action and what step in the life cycle of HIV is in-

TABLE 3. Experimental HIV therapy

Reverse transcriptase inhibitors
  3'-azido-2,3'-dideoxythymidine (AZT)
  2',3'-dideoxycytidine (ddC)
  2',3'-dideoxyinosine (ddI)
  2',3'-dideoxyadenosine (ddA)
  suramin*
  phosphonoformate (Forscarnet)
  rifabutin

Viral attachment and penetration inhibitors
  CD4
  AL 721
  catanospermine
  dextran sulfate
  peptide-T

Post-transcription and translation inhibitors
  ampligen*
  ribavirin*

Viral protein assembly and release inhibitors
  interferons
  granulocyte-macrophage–stimulating factor

Immunomodulators
  interleukin 2
  isoprinosine
  imuthiol
  imreg

Combination therapies
  AZT plus acyclovir
  AZT plus alpha-interferon

*Not proved effective clinically.

terrupted. Some of the drugs and drug combinations presently under trial are listed in Table 3.[15-17]

■ VACCINATION

HIV-infected individuals respond less well than non-HIV-infected people to inactivated vaccines. Response to the plasma-derived hepatitis B, inactivated influenza, and pneumococcal vaccines depends upon the severity of HIV infection at the time of vaccination.[18,19] Asymptomatic HIV-infected individuals respond better than people with AIDS. The theoretic argument that antigenic stimulation of the immune system would lead to increased HIV replication and progression of disease has not been substantiated in vaccine trial studies.

There is little information documenting the duration of response postvaccination. However, it is safe to administer these vaccines to HIV-infected patients. The pneumococcal vaccine should be given to HIV-infected patients once. Recommendations regarding the need for further vaccination are forthcoming. The latest influenza vaccine should be given yearly during the autumn months. Patients who are hepatitis B antigen–negative and core and surface antibody–negative who remain at high risk of exposure to this virus should be given three doses of the hepatitis-B vaccine. Patients should be warned that our understanding of the protective efficacy of these vaccines in this population is not well known. Moreover, the need and timing of booster vaccinations has not been determined. There are a few studies which note that *Haemophilus influenzae* is a common infecting agent in HIV-infected adult patients. Many of the studies have not typed the *Haemophilus* species. If it is found that these individuals are at an increased risk for infection with *H. influenzae* type b, the conjugate Hib vaccine may also be recommended. To date there are few data regarding the response to this vaccine in this patient population.

■ SPECIAL PATIENT GROUPS

Pregnant Women. The great majority of HIV-infected adult women are in their reproductive years and are intravenous drug users or sexual partners of intravenous drug users. The role of HIV infection on the outcome of pregnancy and the role of pregnancy on the progression of HIV infection have not been well defined. Although several women with HIV infection have developed pneumonia during pregnancy,[20] it does not appear that asymptomatic infected women have a significant progression of disease during pregnancy.[21] However, the rate of progression to AIDS after pregnancy seems to be more rapid than in other groups. Although the reported adverse pregnancy outcome frequency (ectopic pregnancy, spontaneous abortion, preterm delivery and low birth weight infants) is high, it has been difficult to show that the rates are higher than those in a cohort of women of similar socioeconomic and drug use patterns who are HIV negative.[21]

HIV-infected women should be counseled regarding the risks to the fetus of HIV infection. Of note is the fact that the frequency of elective abortions and recurrent pregnancies was not affected by HIV status among intravenous drug users in one study.[21] Careful evaluation for concomitant diseases that may be transmitted in utero or perinatally to the neonate, such as syphilis, tuberculosis, herpes simplex virus, *Toxoplasma*, and hepatitis B, should be made during pregnancy and the conditions treated when appropriate. Nonspecific symptoms such as fatigue, weight loss, and anorexia may be attributed to pregnancy and not HIV infection. They should be monitored closely and evaluated judiciously.

The safety of AZT has not been established in pregnancy. In vitro and animal studies have revealed little mutagenicity or teratogenicity of AZT.[22] Presently, AZT cannot be recommended for pregnant HIV-positive women, although studies are ongoing to determine the side effects and efficacy of such therapy.

Preterm and labor care of the HIV-infected pregnant woman is similar to that of noninfected women.[23] It is advisable, however, to use external fetal monitoring when possible to avoid the possibility of increased transmission of HIV to the infant. Present data do not support the notion that operative delivery decreases the transmission of HIV to the neonate. In developed countries, breast-feeding should probably be avoided, since HIV may be transmitted in breast milk.[23]

Infants and Children. Eighty per cent of HIV infection in children is transmitted by transplacental or perinatal exposure of the fetus or infant by infected mothers.[24] The remaining 20 per cent is the result of exposure to blood products or replacement coagulation factors from before 1985. It is estimated that approximately 25 to 40 per cent of infants born to HIV-infected mothers will be infected with HIV. Sixty-five per cent of children born to mothers who have had previous HIV-infected children may be infected. Children of high-risk mothers should be screened for HIV infection if possible. Moreover, the physician must be aware of the clinical and laboratory findings of HIV infection in infants and children, since at the time of birth the infected mother may be undiagnosed as HIV-infected.[25] In children with immunodeficiencies of undetermined origin, HIV infection must also be considered.

A major obstacle to the management of HIV-infected infants is that the diagnosis may be obscured because of transplacental transmission of maternal HIV antibody that may be present as long as 15 months after delivery.[26] Although not widely available at this time, a positive viral culture of the infant's peripheral blood mononuclear cells is the most reliable indicator of infant infection. HIV p24 antigen determinations on sera are often negative in children who are later shown to be HIV-infected. On an experimental level, IgM antibodies to HIV and specific patterns of HIV antibody among IgG subclasses also have proved useful in identifying HIV-infected infants.[27] Most recently, the polymerase chain reaction has been shown to be positive in up to 75 per cent of infected infants. This test is also not commercially available at present. The false-positivity rate for this test is undetermined. In older children, serologic diagnosis for HIV antibody is accurate and is the diagnostic method of choice.[24]

The natural history of HIV infection in children is still uncertain. Initial reports noted a 75 per cent mortality within 2 years of the diagnosis of AIDS in infants. Children who are diagnosed before 1 year of age and those who present with encephalopathy have a particularly poor prognosis. As more experience is being gained with HIV infection in children, it is becoming clear that the incubation period may be as long as 9 years in some instances.[24] However, the median age of diagnosis of AIDS in perinatally infected children is 9 months.

It is recommended that the routine, inactivated childhood vaccinations, including diphtheria, tetanus, pertussis, and Hib, be administered to HIV-infected children in the same schedule as other children. Initially, the Immunization Practices Advisory Committee recommended against the use of live vaccines in HIV-infected children.[28] However, because of several cases of severe measles in unvaccinated children, the live measles, mumps, rubella vaccine is now recommended for HIV-infected children. The enhanced inactivated poliovirus vaccine should be given, rather than the live vaccine, to both the HIV-infected child and any noninfected siblings. Pneumococcal vaccine is recommended at 2 years for all HIV-infected children. Influenza vaccine use also should be considered. Children exposed to the varicella-zoster virus should be given varicella-zoster immune globulin, while those exposed to measles should be given immune globulin, even if they were previously immunized.

Serious bacterial infections may occur more frequently in HIV-infected children and may be the presenting manifestation. Aggressive treatment of these infections is warranted. Some investigators have found that immune globulin infusions at monthly intervals decrease the incidence of bacterial infections.[29] Controlled studies are presently in progress to determine the efficacy of immune globulin for this use. In infants, trimethoprim-sulfamethoxazole may be better tolerated than in adults and should be used for the prevention of PCP in symptomatic HIV-infected children.

The use of AZT in children has not been adequately evaluated, despite the fact that many physicians are choosing to treat their infected patients with this drug. Continuous intravenous infusion of AZT, with doses ranging from 0.9 to 1.4 mg/kg/hr, has been demonstrated to be effective in children, leading to increased appetite and weight, decreased lymphadenopathy, decreased immune globulin levels, and increased CD4 cells. Improvement in the encephalopathy, which is such a prominent and tragic feature of HIV infection in children, also may occur.[30] Toxicities of AZT are primarily hematologic, including anemia and neutropenia.[30] Studies are in progress evaluating intermittent intravenous infusion at doses of

80 to 160 mg/m² every 6 hours and oral therapy with doses of 120 to 220 mg/m² every 6 hours.[24] The pharmacology of oral AZT in children is similar to that in adults. There have also been reports of neurologic and immune function recovery in children receiving AZT orally.[24]

Since many children with HIV infection will fail to thrive and may have chronic debilitating diarrhea, nutritional support, including total parenteral nutrition, is an essential part of their management.

It may be wise to keep young children with immune dysfunction out of the day care center where the risks of acquiring infection are increased. Children without control over oral behavior and body secretions may be a threat to others and probably should not be sent to day care centers or to schools.[31] Children with control of bodily function and without wounds that are uncoverable and actively bleeding should be allowed to go to school. Parents of HIV-infected children and school personnel in general should be educated about the handling of blood and bodily secretions and the import of avoiding blood contact with open wounds.

■ Issues and Risks

■ RISKS TO HEALTH CARE WORKERS

A major concern for physicians and other health care workers is their risk of infection with HIV and other transmissible agents through contact with HIV-infected patients. However, HIV has not been shown to be transmitted through casual contact. Of greater concern is the risk to the health care worker of HIV infection from percutaneous or permucosal exposures with HIV-infected blood by accidental needlestick injuries. Studies have shown a risk of 0.35 per cent per accident in health care workers exposed in this way.[32]

General precautions dictate that physicians assume that all patients are HIV positive, avoid needlestick injuries, and avoid direct skin or mucous membrane contact with blood and body fluids of all patients.[33] Practical implementation of these recommendations depends on the type of exposure. In spite of the HIV-infected patient's

TABLE 4. Infections and Isolation Precautions in Patients with HIV

Potentially Transmissible Infection	Isolation Precautions*
Tuberculosis	Modified respiratory
Salmonellosis	Enteric
Shigellosis	Enteric
Staphylococcal infection	Contact (for other than mild infection)
Varicella zoster	Strict
Herpes simplex	Contact (for severe disease)
Cryptosporidiosis	Enteric
Cytomegalovirus	None
Hepatitis B	None
Non-A non-B hepatitis	None

*In addition to universal precautions necessary for all patients.

relatively high frequency of additional infection with numerous respiratory, blood-borne, and enteric pathogens, spread to health care workers of these agents has been limited. Table 4 lists the recommended isolation precautions for a number of these transmissible agents, the most important of which is *Mycobacterium tuberculosis*.[33]

■ COUNSELING

Because of the extraordinary psychosocial impact that a diagnosis of HIV infection carries with it, and the need for the individual who is being tested to have an understanding of the implications of the test results, HIV counseling is an essential part of the management of the patient. Informed consent must be obtained prior to testing. The purpose and meaning of the test, the testing procedure itself, and the potential issues of discrimination should be explained to the patient.

At the time of communicating the test results, post-test counseling should be made available. This should include a discussion of the coping mechanisms of learning the result, potential discrimination problems from disclosure, behavioral changes that might decrease the transmission of infection, available medical treatments, and the importance of notifying the person's contacts.

It is hoped that through the efforts of counseling the individual will become better educated and will help voluntarily with the process of identifying contacts.

■ CONFIDENTIALITY

Strict confidentiality of the test results should be maintained except if the patient allows (and signs for) his or her release. It is hoped that by ensuring confidentiality efforts to increase voluntary testing among high-risk groups will improve. The individuals or groups who may receive HIV-related information will vary among geographic locations. It is imperative that physicians be acquainted with the laws of the particular state in which they practice.

REFERENCES

1. Imagawa DT, Moon HL, Wolinsky SM, et al. Human immunodeficiency virus type 1 infection in homosexual men who remain seronegative for prolonged periods. N Engl J Med 1989; 320:1458–1462.
2. Gaines H, von Sydow M, Pehrson PO, Lundbergh P. Clinical picture of primary HIV infection presenting as a glandular-fever-like illness. Br Med J 1988; 297:1363–1368.
3. Centers for Disease Control. Update: Serologic testing for antibody to human immunodeficiency virus. MMWR 1988; 36:833–840.
4. Sivak SL, Wormser GP. Predictive value of a screening test for antibodies to HTLV-III. Am J Clin Pathol 1986; 85:700–703.
5. Schleupner CJ. Detection of HIV-1 infection. In Mandell GL, Douglas RG, Jr, Bennett JE (eds). Principles and Practice of Infectious Diseases. 3rd ed. New York: Churchill Livingstone, 1989:1092–1102.
6. Lifson AR, Rutherford GW, Jaffe HW. The natural history of human immunodeficiency virus infection. J Infect Dis 1988; 158:1360–1367.
7. Moss AR, Bacchetti P, Osmond D, et al. Seropositivity for HIV and the development of AIDS or AIDS-related condition: three year follow-up of the San Francisco General Hospital cohort. Br Med J 1988; 296:745–750.
8. Kaslow RA, Phair JP, Friedman HB, et al. Infection with the human immunodeficiency virus: Clinical manifestations and their relationship to immune deficiency. Ann Intern Med 1987; 107:474–480.
9. Fischl MA, Richman DD, Grieco MH, et al. The efficacy of azidothymidine (AZT) in the treatment of patients with AIDS and AIDS-related complex. N Engl J Med 1987; 317:185–191.
10. Yarchoan R, Brouwers P, Spitzer AR, et al. Response of human immunodeficiency virus–associated neurological disease to 3′-azido-3′-deoxythymidine. Lancet 1987; 1:132–135.
11. Creagh-Kirk T, Doi P, Andrews E, et al. Survival experience among patients with AIDS receiving zidovudine. JAMA 1988; 260:3009–3015.
12. Richman DD, Fischl MA, Grieco MH, et al. The toxicity of azidothymidine (AZT) in the treatment of patients with AIDS and AIDS-related complex. N Engl J Med 1987; 317:192–197.
13. Bach MC. Failure of zidovudine to maintain remission in patients with AIDS (letter). N Engl J Med 1989; 320:594–595.
14. Larder BA, Darby G, Richman DD. HIV with reduced sensitivity to zidovudine (AZT) isolated during prolonged therapy. Science 1989; 243:1731–1734.
15. Yarchoan R, Broder S. Pharmacologic treatment of HIV infection. In DeVita VT Jr (ed). AIDS; Etiology, Diagnosis, and Prevention. 2nd ed. New York: JB Lippincott, 1988:277–293.
16. Polsky B, Armstrong D. Other agents in the treatment of AIDS. In De Vita VT Jr (ed). AIDS; Etiology, Diagnosis and Prevention. 2nd ed. New York: JB Lippincott, 1988:295–303.
17. Surbone A, Yarchoan R, McAtee N, et al. Treatment of the acquired immunodeficiency syndrome (AIDS) and AIDS-related complex with a regimen of 3′-azido-2′,3′-dideoxythymidine (azidothymidine or zidovudine) and acyclovir. Ann Intern Med 1988; 108:534–540.
18. Collier AC, Corey L, Murphy VL, Handsfield HH. Antibody to human immunodeficiency virus (HIV) and suboptimal response to hepatitis B vaccination. Ann Intern Med 1988; 109:101–105.
19. Nelson KE, Clements ML, Miotti P, Cohn S, Polk BF. The influence of human immunodeficiency virus (HIV) infection on antibody responses to influenza vaccines. Ann Intern Med 1988; 109:383–388.
20. Koonin LM, Ellerbrock TV, Atrash HK, et al. Pregnancy-associated deaths due to AIDS in the United States. JAMA 1989; 261:1306–1309.
21. Selwyn PA, Schoenbaum EE, Davenny K, et al. Prospective study of human immunodeficiency virus infection and pregnancy outcomes in intravenous drug users. JAMA 1989; 261:1289–1294.
22. Retrovirus Product Information. Research Triangle Park, NC, Burroughs Wellcome Co, 1987.
23. Minkoff HL. Care of pregnant women infected with human immunodeficiency virus. JAMA 1987; 258:2714–2717.
24. Falloon J, Eddy J, Wiener L, Pizzo PA. Human immunodeficiency virus infection in children. J Pediatr 1989; 114:1–30.
25. Pahwa S, Kaplan M, Fikrig S, et al. Spectrum of human T-cell lymphotropic virus type III infection in children. JAMA 1986; 255:2299–2305.
26. Mok JQ, De Rossi A, Ades AE, Giaquinto C, Grosch-Worner I, Peckham CS. Infants born to mothers seropositive for human immunodeficiency virus. Lancet 1987; 1:1164–1168.
27. Pyun KH, Ochs HD, Dufford MTW, Wedgwood RJ. Perinatal infection with human immunodeficiency virus. N Engl J Med 1987; 317:611–614.
28. Centers for Disease Control. Immunization of children infected with human immunodeficiency virus: supplementary ACIP statement. MMWR 1988; 37:181–183.
29. Ochs HD. Intravenous immunoglobulin in the treatment and prevention of acute infections in pediatric acquired immunodeficiency syndrome patients. Pediatr Infect Dis J 1987; 6:509–511.
30. Pizzo PA, Eddy J, Falloon J, et al. Effect of continuous intravenous infusion of zidovudine (AZT) in children with symptomatic HIV infection. N Engl J Med 1988; 319:890–896.
31. American Academy of Pediatrics. School attendance of children and adolescents with human T lymphotropic virus III/lymphadenopathy-associated virus infection. Pediatrics 1986; 77:430–431.
32. Wormser GP. Avoiding AIDS in the physician's office. Postgrad Med 1988; 83:183–191.

Human immunodeficiency virus–related disease

Harold Horowitz ■ *Gary P. Wormser*

Skillful management of the human immunodeficiency virus (HIV)–infected patient involves blending common sense and compassion with information learned from rigorous, large-scale scientific trials and carefully investigated single case studies. Care of HIV-infected patients is constantly changing and improving, which is reflected by objective increases in patient survival. These rapid changes impose additional challenges on the clinician for whom "routine" management often involves combining approved with investigational therapies. Indeed, HIV-infected patients are probably the largest single group of patients in the United States receiving experimental medications. A partial list of newly approved drugs already widely used in the care of HIV-infected patients includes zidovudine (AZT), pentamidine for parenteral administration, inhalational pentamidine, ganciclovir, and interferon alfa-2. Diagnostic procedures and methods are also in flux, constantly being tailored to the specific needs associated with the HIV epidemic.

Newly acquired information on the natural history of HIV infection has indicated the necessity of, and proper timing for, beginning inhalational pentamidine or other prophylaxis for prevention of *Pneumocystis carinii* pneumonia. The writing of this article coincides with the advent of *Pneumocystis* prophylaxis as the accepted standard of practice. This single intervention will in turn have far-reaching consequences on the natural history of HIV infection and on management approaches in the years to come.

We present here clinical perspectives on the HIV-infected patient with fever, pulmonary infiltrates, diarrhea, neurologic disease, malignancy, and many other complications; it is current as of February, 1990.

■ Background

Infection with HIV causes abnormalities in virtually all aspects of the immune system. This results primarily from the virus' ability to bind to the CD4 receptor on the CD4 T lymphocyte and infect these cells. The CD4 helper/inducer lymphocyte plays a pivotal role in the functioning of both the humoral and cellular arms of the immune system, since induction of both T-cell cytotoxic responses and B-cell immunoglobulin production requires CD4 cells.[1] After HIV infection, the mechanisms by which CD4 lymphocytes are depleted are multifactorial and may include direct lysis, lysis of syncytia of CD4 lymphocytes, autoimmune antibody responses, and induction of cytotoxic mechanisms.[1] The end result of their depletion is a patient at risk for a wide variety of opportunistic infections and several specific tumors. HIV also infects macrophages and mononuclear cells. The effect that infection of these cells has on the overall immune suppression in HIV infection is unclear.

It appears that the majority of HIV-infected individuals will have a period ranging from 2 to 8 years after infection during which they are asymptomatic. When the HIV-infected individual becomes symptomatic, almost every organ system may be involved. HIV may cause disease by direct infection of both the central nervous system and the immune system, and possibly also the gastrointestinal tract, kidneys, and heart (and perhaps other organs). Autoimmune phenomena may be triggered by HIV and most commonly cause thrombocytopenia, and occasionally anemia or neutropenia. Defects in host defenses, which are the hallmark of the disease, lead to an array of other infectious complications (opportunistic and nonopportunistic), which may also involve any organ system. HIV-associated tumors, such as Kaposi's sarcoma (KS), primary central nervous system lymphoma, and aggressive non-Hodgkin's lymphomas outside the central nervous system (CNS), must also be considered when evaluating the ill HIV-infected patient.

■ Management

FEVER

The majority of HIV-infected people will have fever at some point in the course of their illness. Low-grade fevers are most common, but high temperatures in the range of 40°C (104°F) may occur, frequently with no apparent clinical compromise or obvious site of localization. Management of the febrile HIV-infected patient is integrally related to establishing an etiology for the fever (Tables 1 and 2). This can be extremely difficult, in part because culture results of some specimen samples that have been in contact with mucous membranes may indicate colonization rather than infection, because multiple infections may be present simultaneously, and because serodiagnostic studies may be ambiguous in this population (see later). Fever may be related to nonopportunistic infections presenting typically or atypically, opportunistic infections, hypersensitivity to drugs, malignancy such as disseminated Kaposi's sarcoma or lymphoma, and HIV infection itself. The latter, however, is a diagnosis of exclusion and is rarely

TABLE 1. General Principles in Management of HIV-Infected Patients

Serious opportunistic infections usually first occur with CD4 cell counts of less than 200/mm³.

Persistent fever indicates opportunistic infection or neoplasia, not HIV.

Multiple opportunistic infections and neoplasia may occur simultaneously, even in the same organ or tissue.

Serodiagnostic studies and the PPD skin test may not be reliable in some patients.

Cultures of some opportunistic organisms, e.g., cytomegalovirus, *Mycobacterium avium intracellulare,* from the urine or sputum may not indicate active infection.

Treatment of opportunistic infections is rarely curative; more commonly, suppressive therapy must be given for an indeterminate duration.

TABLE 2. Evaluation of the Febrile HIV-Infected Patient

Evaluate if patient falls into a group at high risk for serious opportunistic infections, i.e., CD4 cells less than 200/mm³

Direct history to determine possible geographic, ethnic, or lifestyle risk factors for specific infections. Pay particular attention to neurologic, respiratory, dermatologic, visual, and gastrointestinal complaints

Note medication list

Physical examination

Laboratory tests: CBC; chemistry profile, including liver function tests; urine analysis; cultures of blood, urine, and sputum for bacteria and fungi; chest roentgenogram

If initial cultures are negative, culture on multiple occasions blood, urine, sputum, and stool for mycobacteria. Do serum cryptococcal antigen, *Toxoplasma* titer, VDRL. Do PPD with controls unless known to be anergic.

If no source yet identified, consider:

- computed tomography of the abdomen
- examination by ophthalmologist for CMV retinitis
- lymph node biopsy if enlarged node is accessible
- bone marrow biopsy and aspiration (especially if anemic)
- skin lesion biopsy (if present)
- lumbar puncture
- gallium scan
- liver biopsy (if liver function studies are abnormal)

in our experience an explanation for persistent fever (see Table 1). Furthermore, nosocomial infection from intravascular catheters, decubiti, and urinary tract infections must not be overlooked in the hospitalized HIV-infected patient.

It is important at the onset to determine whether the patient fits into a prognostic group that is predisposed to serious opportunistic infections (see preceding chapter on the HIV-infected patient). If not, the physician should direct the evaluation toward the discovery of more common infectious pathogens and conditions—for example, sinusitis and herpes zoster. In patients with less severe immunodeficiency, the presentation tends to be more typical and the process localizing, allowing for a more directed evaluation.

It is also important to note epidemiologic clues that may help in identifying specific infectious risks. For example, Haitians have an increased risk of tuberculosis, and patients from the southwestern United States have an increased risk for disseminated *Coccidioides immitis* infection (see Infections in the AIDS Patient).

In the patient who is predisposed to develop serious opportunistic infections (i.e., those with CD4 cell counts of less than 200/mm³), the initial evaluation should carefully note ophthalmologic, neurologic, gastrointestinal, and respiratory complaints and findings. Initial laboratory evaluation should include a complete blood count with differential count, routine cultures of the blood, urine and sputum (if cough is present), urine analysis, serum chemistry studies including liver function tests, and a chest roentgenogram (CXR). The patient's medications should be reviewed, since several of the drugs commonly used to treat HIV patients, including AZT, rifampin, isoniazid, trimethoprim-sulfamethoxazole, and sulfadiazine, may cause drug fever.

If the source of the fever has not yet been identified, then further diagnostic studies are necessary. Blood cultures for fungi and mycobacteria (using the lysis-centrifugation method if available) should be obtained. Multiple cultures of stool, urine, and sputum for mycobacteria should also be considered. Stool smears and culture for *Mycobacterium avium intracellulare* (MAI) are especially helpful for making the diagnosis of disseminated MAI, since the bowel wall is often involved in disseminated disease. However, single positive cultures from any of these sites (except blood) for nontuberculous mycobacteria may represent contamination or colonization and not indicate true infection. Although cytomegalovirus (CMV) also may be a cause of fever in these patients, positive cultures for CMV from urine, throat, or even blood are so frequent in HIV-infected patients that they cannot be relied on to pinpoint the cause of fever. For the same reasons, serology for CMV is also nondiagnostic. It is of utmost importance to attempt to establish the pathogenicity of an organism that has been cultured, since treatment for some, such as CMV or MAI, may be at best partially effective, toxic, inconvenient (e.g., requires intravenous antibiotic administration), or prolonged.

Additional diagnostic studies should include a test for serum cryptococcal antigen, since it is positive in most patients with disseminated disease, an illness that may present insidiously. Serodiagnosis of *Histoplasma capsulatum* and *Coccidioides immitis* also has proved helpful for selected patients.

Giemsa stain preparations of the buffy coat of peripheral blood also may be helpful in the diagnosis of disseminated histoplasmosis.

A careful funduscopic examination by an ophthalmologist may help establish the diagnosis of disseminated CMV infection in HIV-infected individuals without a known source of fever. Although the patient with CMV retinitis usually reports visual disturbances, this is not uniformly true, particularly in patients with an altered mental status.

Biopsies for culture, special stains, and histologic examination of sites such as bone marrow, lymph nodes, gastrointestinal tract, or skin lesions ultimately may be very helpful in diagnosis of disseminated fungal disease, MAI, *Mycobacterium tuberculosis* (MTb), CMV, lymphoma, or KS when other modalities of diagnosis are either nondiagnostic or negative. It is particularly important to perform a lymph node biopsy in patients who have a single group of lymph nodes that are disproportionally enlarged or in whom a rapid increase in size of the lymph nodes has occurred. Computed tomography (CT) may be used to locate an intra-abdominal tumor or enlarged lymph nodes for biopsy. In patients with an elevated alkaline phosphatase level and fever, a liver biopsy for histologic examination and culture may be useful. However, this procedure is usually not necessary, since other sources of culture material will be diagnostic.

The stable febrile patient need not be started on a course of antibiotics, since these drugs may be toxic, lead to increasingly resistant organisms, or confound the diagnostic evaluation. However, if the patient is clinically unstable or profoundly neutropenic (less than 500 PMN/mm³), broad-spectrum antibiotics must be initiated promptly. Empiric therapy for specific opportunistic infections in the febrile HIV-infected patient is also recommended in a few other clinical settings (Table 3).

■ GASTROENTEROLOGIC MANIFESTATIONS

All areas of the gastrointestinal tract may be affected in patients with HIV infection with multiple, sometimes overlapping entities of infectious and noninfectious origin. The specific symptom complex may help direct

TABLE 3. Organisms for Which Empiric Therapy May Be Appropriate in Febrile HIV-Infected Patients

Staphylococcus aureus, Streptococcus pneumoniae, Haemophilus influenzae, Salmonella, other gram-negative rods if either septic-appearing or profoundly neutropenic (use broad-spectrum antibiotic therapy)

Streptococcus pneumoniae, Haemophilus influenzae, Branhamella catarrhalis, Staphylococcus aureus, Legionella, Klebsiella, Escherichia coli in a patient with lobar pneumonia (e.g., use erythromycin plus third-generation cephalosporin)

Toxoplasma gondii in patients with single or multiple ring enhancing mass lesions on MRI or CT, especially if serum *Toxoplasma* titer positive (e.g., use pyrimethamine plus sulfadiazine)

Pneumocystis carinii in patients with hypoxia and diffuse interstitial lung infiltrates (e.g., use trimethoprim-sulfamethoxazole)

Candida albicans in patients with odynophagia or dysphagia* (e.g., use ketoconazole)

Mycobacterium tuberculosis if an ill patient is at high risk; e.g., positive PPD, history of positive PPD, or a member of a population with known high exposure (of particular importance if diffuse infiltrates are present on CXR and response to PCP therapy is poor, or if hilar adenopathy is present)

**Candida* esophagitis often does not present with fever.

the evaluation toward a particular area of the GI tract. For instance, KS may cause oral lesions, gastric outlet obstruction, malabsorption, or, rarely, massive bleeding. Abdominal pain with severe nausea and vomiting associated with an elevated alkaline phosphatase level may indicate sclerosing cholangitis. Unfortunately, however, the symptom complex is often nonspecific.

Diarrhea. Diarrhea in HIV-infected patients spans the spectrum from watery and profuse to an occasional loose stool. Twenty to thirty per cent of HIV-infected patients will have diarrhea. Severe, disabling diarrhea with weight loss may antedate the diagnosis of AIDS. Careful study has found an infectious etiology in 85 per cent of diarrheal episodes.[2] Multiple infectious agents are frequently discovered simultaneously. For infectious etiologies that are treatable, cure or marked improvement can be expected.[2] The most common infectious agents that cause diarrhea in this population include *Cryptosporidium*, MAI, CMV, *Giardia*, *Salmonella*, and *Campylobacter*.[2,3] Viruses such as rotavirus and adenovirus may also be responsible for diarrhea, especially in HIV-infected homosexual men.[4] HIV infec-

tion itself is thought to cause enteropathy leading to diarrhea. In this last instance, biopsy of the small bowel reveals nonspecific inflammation with partial villous atrophy, crypt hyperplasia, and increased numbers of intraepithelial lymphocytes.[5] KS is rarely responsible for diarrhea in HIV-infected patients.

Evaluation of diarrhea should begin with stool examinations for occult blood, white blood cells, ova and parasites, *Cryptosporidium*, acid-fast bacilli culture and smear, and cultures for *Salmonella, Shigella, Campylobacter* and other routine enteric pathogens. If the patient is taking, or has recently received, antibiotics, tests for *Clostridium difficile* toxin should be obtained. Examination of several stool samples will enhance the chances of detecting many potential enteric pathogens, including *Cryptosporidium, Salmonella* sp., *Giardia lamblia, Blastocystis hominis, Isospora belli*, and *Entamoeba histolytica*. Although enzyme-linked immunosorbent assays (ELISA) are available for the detection of rotavirus antigens in stool, this test is not routinely available in most clinical laboratories. Fecal leukocytes are most commonly seen with *Shigella, Salmonella, Campylobacter*, and *Clostridium difficile* infections. HIV enteropathy and CMV, MAI, and *Cryptosporidium* infections are not in general associated with fecal leukocytes. If diarrhea persists despite negative initial cultures and smears, colonoscopy is warranted for biopsy and cultures. Diagnosis of *Cryptosporidium*, MAI, or CMV colitis may be made with this approach.

If an infectious agent is either not diagnosed or not effectively treated with available antibiotics—e.g., MAI, cryptosporidia, or enteric viruses—antiperistaltic agents such as loperamide may prove beneficial in some patients. Somatostatin analog (SMS-201-995) in doses of 100 to 300 μg three times a day has been successfully used to reduce the diarrhea associated with cryptosporidia[6] and is currently being studied for diarrhea due to HIV enteropathy. Pending the results of these studies, the role of this drug in management is uncertain. Whether AZT will prove useful in AIDS enteropathy is also unknown.

Dysphagia, Odynophagia, and Retrosternal Pain. These symptoms are frequent in HIV-infected patients. During acute HIV infection, esophogeal ulcers of unknown etiology that resolve spontaneously over several weeks may occur. However, these symptoms are more likely found in chronic HIV disease. Dysphagia and odynophagia are most commonly caused by infection with *Candida albicans*. Patients with these symptoms may have alternative diagnoses, such as herpes simplex virus (HSV) or CMV infections of the esophagus. Although it is uncommon for candidal esophagitis to occur in the absence of thrush, it certainly happens, particularly when topical antifungals are given orally. We have not found that a barium swallow is useful in differentiating candidal infection of the esophagus from viral disease. Endoscopy with biopsies for culture and histologic preparations is the preferred diagnostic method. In the absence of a definitive diagnosis, empiric treatment with ketoconazole is usually given. If improvement is not forthcoming within 5 to 7 days, endoscopy should be performed to exclude the presence of HSV, which requires acyclovir therapy; CMV, which requires ganciclovir therapy; or severe unresponsive candidal esophagitis, which may require systemic amphotericin B (see "Infections in the AIDS Patient").

Proctitis. This is particularly a problem in homosexual men with HIV infection. Rectal pain on defecation and intermittent, bloody, small-volume, watery stools are frequent presenting symptoms. Appropriate cultures and stains are required to make a diagnosis. Sigmoidoscopy may be necessary if external disease is not present. Common infecting organisms include HSV (diagnosis suggested by Tzanck test and histology and proved by cultures), *Neisseria gonorrhoeae* (diagnosis made by cultures on Thayer-Martin media), *Treponema pallidum* (diagnosis suggested by a positive syphilis serology), enteric organisms such as *Campylobacter* species (diagnosis made by culture), and CMV (diagnosis made by histology and culture).

Hepatobiliary Disease. Stenotic biliary tract disease is being increasingly recognized in HIV-infected individuals. Patients typically present with fever, periumbilical or right upper quadrant pain, and nausea and vomiting. Laboratory studies reveal a markedly elevated alkaline phosphatase level, with relatively lower bilirubin and hepatocellular enzyme elevations. Dilated intra- or extrahepatobiliary ducts are frequently found on ultrasound or computed tomography (CT). Evidence of papillary stenosis and sclerosing cholangitis may be found together or individually on endoscopic evaluation.[7] CMV and *Cryptosporidium* are often present in bile or on histologic preparations of ampulla of Vater tissue or papillary and peripapillary duodenal tissue. MAI, KS, and lymphoma have also been found in periampullary or biliary ductal tissue. However, 45 per cent of the time, no HIV-related opportunistic infection or tumor has been noted.[7] The role of HIV itself in this entity is not known. Endoscopic sphincterotomy is often useful in relieving the pain. However, the alkaline phosphatase level may continue to rise, suggesting the presence of diffuse hepatic parenchymal disease.[7]

Hepatic parenchymal disease identified by clinical features, biochemical data, or histology has been documented in nearly 90 per cent of AIDS patients.[8] Liver function abnormalities are generally thought to be due to chronic non-A, non-B hepatitis but may occur as a result of disseminated systemic disease with infections such as CMV, MAI, MTb, and fungi, or with tumors, including KS and lymphoma. Medications including antituberculous therapy, ketoconazole, sulfonamides, and AZT also may play an etiologic role in hepatocellular dysfunction and should be reviewed. In most cases, liver biopsy is not needed to establish the diagnosis but may prove helpful in selected patients. It is noteworthy that despite the fact that 5 to 15 per cent of HIV-infected patients are positive for hepatitis B virus surface antigen, the specific histologic diagnosis of chronic active hepatitis is rare in these patients.

Weight Loss and Cachexia. These problems are widespread in the AIDS population. The HIV-related wasting syndrome is now a criterion for the diagnosis of AIDS. Causes of weight loss are multifactorial and possibly include anorexia, malabsorption, diarrhea, systemic infection, elevated cachexin levels, and socioeconomic factors. Weight loss and cachexia may contribute to the immune suppression in AIDS patients owing to the detrimental effects of malnutrition on immune function. AZT at doses of 100 to 200 mg every 4 hours has been shown to lead to weight gain in AIDS patients.[9] Megesterol acetate also has led to increased appetite and weight gain in a small number of AIDS patients evaluated in one uncontrolled trial.[10] The latter results suggest that megesterol should be evaluated further.

Nutritional support must not be overlooked in the care of the AIDS patient. Calorie supplementation may be required if the patient is losing weight. If diarrhea is marked, a diet that is lactose-free should be tried, and caffeine should be avoided.[11] In extreme instances, when widespread small bowel disease and malabsorption are present, total parenteral nutrition (TPN) may be required. The decision whether to use TPN must be made on a case-by-case basis.[11] It may be particularly useful when the underlying cause of the small bowel disease can be at least partially reversed, as in KS or MAI infection, allowing for oral feeding at a later date.

■ HEMATOLOGIC MANIFESTATIONS

Hematologic manifestations of HIV infection include immune thrombocytopenia, thrombotic thrombocytopenic purpura, immune hemolytic anemia, anemia, and neutropenia. Circulating lupus-like anticoagulants also have been found. Many HIV-infected patients have a mild pancytopenia that does not require treatment. Bone marrow examination with cultures and histology is an essential aspect of the evaluation of severe cytopenia. This may help determine whether the problem is one of marrow arrest or failure, or whether the cells in question are being destroyed peripherally. Bone marrow biopsy will help rule out infectious etiologies, such as disseminated MAI or fungal infections—e.g., histoplasmosis—and tumors, such as lymphoma, that may cause myelosuppression due to infiltration. The pathogenesis of most of the hematologic abnormalities in HIV-infected patients is not known.

Neutropenia. This complication of HIV infection may interfere with initiation or continuation of certain myelosuppressive therapeutic modalities, including AZT and ganciclovir. Preliminary studies with recombinant granulocyte-macrophage colony–stimulating factor (rGM-CSF) have shown that in doses of greater than 2×10^3 μg/kg/day, total leukocyte and absolute neutrophil counts are normalized in HIV-infected patients; after discontinuation, however, levels fall to baseline within 3 to 9 days.[12] Data on the clinical significance of this therapy are unavailable. Medications that may contribute to neutropenia should be reduced or stopped if possible.

Autoimmune Thrombocytopenia Purpura (AITP). AITP has been widely reported in HIV-infected patients and may be a presenting manifestation. If the platelet count is over 30,000/mm^3 and no bleeding is documented, treatment is not necessary. Thrombocytopenia remits spontaneously in 50 per cent of these patients. Prednisone in doses of 60 to 100 mg per day will lead to elevations of platelet counts in most patients. However, when discontinued, thrombocytopenia is likely to recur, and steroids may have deleterious effects on immune defenses. AZT in doses of 200 mg every 4 hours has also proved modestly effective in elevating platelet counts in 30 to 50 per cent of cases.[13] Its method of action is unknown, since its effects are too rapid simply to be a result of decreasing viral replication. When both glucocorticoids and AZT fail, splenectomy may lead to prolonged response more than 50 per cent of the time.

Other therapies, including infusion of immunoglobulin or anti-Rh globulin, immunoadsorption of immune complexes using staphylococcal protein A columns, and administration of alpha-interferon, danazol, or vincristine, all have proved to be of transient benefit in some patients. These therapies are under investigation and should be utilized only in the patient who fails to respond to more conventional management.

Thrombotic thrombocytopenia purpura (TTP) has been recently reported in HIV patients.[14] Treatment with plasmapheresis and prednisone, 100 mg per day, was successful in inducing remission in several reported cases. The autoimmune hemolytic anemia associated with HIV infection appears to be very unusual. It has been treated successfully with high-dose steroids in anecdotal cases.

Lupus-Like Anticoagulant. This is found in up to 45 per cent of HIV-infected patients. The anticoagulants are immunoglobulins that interfere with several coagulation assays, including partial thromboplastin time (PTT) and prothrombin time (PT).[15] The majority of patients who have this factor have had prior opportunistic infections. In most instances this factor does not need to be treated and does not cause excessive bleeding unless coagulation factors are also abnormal, or qualitative or quantitative platelet abnormalities exist. Patients with the lupus-like anticoagulant should be carefully questioned about bleeding disorders prior to undergoing invasive procedures, and further coagulation or platelet studies should be performed as required. The anticoagulant also may present a problem in hemophilics, since it may interfere with the monitoring of factor VIII levels during transfusion therapy. The addition of high phospholipid concentrations to the assay will neutralize the inhibition and allow accurate factor VIII determinations.[15] As in patients with systemic lupus erythematosus, thrombotic episodes have been reported in HIV patients with the lupus-like anticoagulant.[15] The relationship of this factor to thrombosis in HIV-infected patients is unclear at present.

■ RENAL MANIFESTATIONS

Clinically apparent renal disease occurs in 10 to 30 per cent of AIDS patients. In HIV-infected populations in whom many patients are intravenous drug users, proteinuria of greater than 0.5 gm per 24 hours occurs in more than 40 per cent of AIDS patients, with nephrotic-range proteinuria occurring in 10 per cent.[16] In nondrug-abusing populations of AIDS patients, the incidence of clinically apparent renal disease appears to be much lower. AIDS patients with renal disease have been divided into three groups based upon the presentation of renal disease and the prognosis.[17]

Group 1 consists of patients who suddenly develop renal failure because of an acute insult to the kidneys, such as dehydration, sepsis, hypotension, hypoxia, or nephrotoxic agents, including nonsteroidal anti-inflammatory agents, pentamidine, trimethoprim-sulfamethoxazole, or radiocontrast dye. In these patients, the creatinine level rarely climbs higher than 6 mg/dl. These patients benefit from dialysis when it is needed. It is essential to recognize and treat renal failure caused by these etiologies in AIDS patients since a good outcome can be expected.[17]

Group 2 of AIDS patients with renal disease have AIDS-associated nephropathy.[17] These patients have nephrotic syndrome and, even in the absence of ischemic or nephrotoxic injury, a rapidly progressive course to uremia. The most common pathologic abnormality seen in these patients is focal and segmental glomerulosclerosis, which is reminiscent of the glomerular lesions seen in patients using drugs intravenously before the AIDS epidemic.[16] The etiology of these lesions is unknown. CD4 receptors have been demonstrated on glomerular cell membranes, suggesting that direct infection of these cells by HIV may be involved. These patients fare poorly on dialysis, with complications of severe cachexia, malnutrition, and opportunistic infections frequently leading to death within 5 months.[17] The role of steroids in this group is being studied.

Group 3 are patients who already have end-stage renal disease (often due to heroin-induced nephropathy) and subsequently develop AIDS.[17] These patients have had a progressive downhill course once the diagnosis of AIDS is made. The majority have died within 3 months, with marked cachexia.[17]

■ NEUROLOGIC MANIFESTATIONS

HIV is neurotropic, and virus has been recovered on culture from both the central and peripheral nervous systems. Nearly 50 per cent of HIV-infected adults at some point will manifest a clinically apparent neurologic disorder, while 80 per cent will show autopsy findings of HIV-induced disease.[18] Central or peripheral nervous system disease may be the initial manifestation of HIV infection. The role of HIV in the pathogenesis of neurologic disease is unclear. However, direct infection seems to play an important role in the CNS manifestations of HIV infection. Complicating the primary neurologic disease process caused by HIV are multiple potential opportunistic infections or the development of lymphoma, both of which may cause diffuse or focal neurologic abnormalities. Effective management requires evaluation for and treatment of the treatable infectious and oncologic entities.

The neurologic history should attempt to ascertain the duration, rapidity of progression, and focality of the disease process.[18] The physical examination should aim to localize the anatomic level of the neurologic problem. Frequently cerebrospinal fluid (CSF) analysis is required. CSF studies should include cell counts and cytology, protein and glucose determinations, VDRL, cultures for bacteria, viruses, fungi and mycobacteria, acid-fast bacilli and Gram stains, and India ink and cryptococcal antigen determinations. If there are no focal findings on the physical examination, the lumbar puncture can be performed prior to radiologic imaging. Computed tomography or magnetic resonance imaging frequently provides useful information in the evaluation of HIV-infected patients who present with focal or nonfocal neurologic complaints or findings.

Nonlocalizing CNS Disease. HIV-related meningitis may occur as part of the acute HIV syndrome (see preceding article), at a later date as an acute illness with headaches and fever, or in a chronic, indolent form with headaches that may last for months. Meningeal signs are frequent in the acute disease but are uncommon with the chronic form. In both types, the sensorium is generally intact. The acute syndrome usually lasts less than 2 weeks but may last as long as a month and resolves without treatment.[19] The CSF in both acute and chronic HIV meningitis shows a lymphocyte-predominant pleocytosis, with protein elevations in more than 50 per cent and normal glucose levels.[20] CSF abnormalities are more marked in the acute disease. Meningitis caused by HIV must be differentiated from cryptococcal, other fungal, tuberculous, syphilitic, and lymphomatous meningitis by CSF culture, stains, antigen studies, VDRL, and cytologic examination.[19] A negative serum *Toxoplasma* titer is strong evidence against *Toxoplasma* meningitis.

Diffuse brain disease without localizing findings is characteristic of AIDS-related dementia. This entity must be differentiated from other causes of nonlocalizing disease, such as metabolic insults including anoxia, renal disease, and hepatic disease; and from encephalitis caused by infectious agents, such as HSV or CMV; or, rarely toxoplasmosis. Consciousness is often altered when metabolic or infectious etiologies are responsible for diffuse brain disease, whereas in AIDS encephalopathy consciousness remains clear until late in the disease process despite marked cognitive dysfunction. Progression of disease is also usually slower in HIV-related encephalopathy than in metabolic or infectious encephalopathy. The CSF formula is nonspecific, with mononuclear pleocytosis and elevated protein levels most commonly found. In AIDS encephalopathy, the most common CT and MRI finding is cerebral atrophy. Although HIV can be cultured from CSF in demented patients, the clinical and pathophysiologic significance of this finding is uncertain, as HIV also may be cultured from asymptomatic patients. Neuropsychiatric tests can be used to follow the disease progression of HIV dementia. AZT has been shown to improve neuropsychiatric testing scores[21] and decrease the level of dementia[22] in uncontrolled studies. AZT should be administered to patients who have this entity.

Focal Brain Disease. Management of focal brain disease depends very much upon the results of neuroradiologic evaluation. If ring-enhancing lesions are noted on CT or MRI, a therapeutic trial of anti-*Toxoplasma* therapy is warranted (see "Infections in the AIDS Patient"). Improvement in the radiologic examination generally occurs within 2 weeks. In over 95 per cent of cases, the serum *Toxoplasma* IgG antibody will be modestly elevated because the CNS disease usually represents reactivation of long-standing latent infection. CNS toxoplasmosis generally progresses rapidly and may be accompanied by alterations in level of consciousness. The major consideration in the differential diagnosis of CNS toxoplasmosis is primary CNS lymphoma. The latter tends to have a more slowly progressive course and demonstrates a more diffuse contrast enhancement on CT. If lesions do not respond to therapy for *Toxoplasma*, a brain biopsy should be performed.

Progressive multifocal leukoencephalopathy (PML), caused by the JC papovavirus, also may cause focal disease, which is frequently manifested by hemiplegia or visual disturbances.[23] The CSF formula is nondiagnostic. The cranial CT is distinctive and reveals hypodense white matter lesions without contrast enhancement.[23] Definitive diagnosis is made by brain biopsy, which reveals papovavirus-like particles on electron microscopy and JC virus when tested using immunofluorescent anti-JC virus antibodies. PML usually progresses more slowly (over weeks) than toxoplasmosis or lymphoma, and there is rarely a decrease in consciousness until late in the course (in contradistinction to toxoplasmosis and lymphoma). No specific therapy is available.

Focal disease caused by tuberculosis, cryptococcosis, and, less commonly, aspergillosis requires culture or pathologic confirmation for diagnosis. When biopsy of a lesion is done, acid-fast bacilli and fungal stains and cultures are essential. Lesions caused by these organisms also may be confused with bacterial abscesses on radiologic imaging. Treatment depends upon the organism isolated.

Transient focal neurologic deficits (an episode lasting less than 24 hours) or cerebral infarction may occur in nearly 1 per cent of HIV-infected patients.[24] It has been estimated that such events occur nearly 30 times more frequently in HIV-infected individuals than in the general population of the same age. Prompt evaluation is essential, since approximately 50 per cent of these episodes will be associated with a treatable infection, including tuberculosis, cryptococcal meningitis, syphilis, toxoplasmosis, and herpes zoster.[24] However, 50 per cent of the time no systemic or CNS disease is apparent. In some of these cases, vasculitis of unknown etiology is noted at autopsy.[24] In patients without an etiology for the neurologic deficit, serial CT scans often show resolution without specific treatment.

A vacuolar myelopathy characterized by vacuolization of the spinal cord white matter that leads to ataxia and spastic paraparesis has been described in HIV-infected patients.[25] It is often associated with dementia. The direct role of HIV in this syndrome is unclear. Vacuolar myelopathy tends to present subacutely, and a well-defined spinal level is not demonstrated on physical examination.[25] This may help differentiate this entity from transverse myelitis caused by epidural lymphoma and varicella zoster virus. The therapeutic role of AZT for this condition is unknown.

Peripheral Neuropathy. Peripheral neuropathies of different types occur in HIV infection and may occur at any stage of disease.[26] Several syndromes are well delineated, although the classification scheme remains tentative at present (Table 4). The syndromes are not mutually exclusive clinically or pathologically. A neurologist's evaluation often will be necessary to determine the extent of the neurologic deficits. Electromyelograms (EMG) and nerve conduction studies also may help delineate the specific areas of neurologic involvement. CSF analysis is nonspecific and may or may not reveal pleocytosis and elevated protein levels.

Treatment approaches are limited and in most instances are based on anecdotal reports. Table 4 lists the more common types of peripheral neuropathies associated with HIV infection and the treatment approaches that have been attempted. It is of note that the mononeuropathies and polyneuropathies associated with acute HIV disease and seroconversion generally resolve without specific therapy.[27] Several of the syndromes, including the acute and chronic inflammatory demyelinating polyneuropathies and sensory multiple mononeuropathies, are similar to syndromes that appear in non-HIV-infected individuals and may be related to immune phenomena.[27] Treatment of these entities is based on drug-induced immune suppression and plasmapheresis, as in the non-HIV-infected population.

The most common peripheral neuropathy that occurs in AIDS patients is a distal axonal motor and sensory neuropathy in which the sensory component predominates. Painful paresthesias manifested as "burning" feet may be severely debilitating. Treatment for this disorder is primarily symptomatic.

Polymyositis. This usually presents subacutely with proximal muscle weakness. Creatine kinase levels are elevated. EMG re-

---

TABLE 4. Peripheral Neuropathies and Radiculopathies Associated with HIV Infection

Syndrome	Management
Acute mono- or polyneuropathy associated with seroconversion	Spontaneous resolution
Acute inflammatory polyneuropathy (Guillain-Barré)	Plasmapheresis
Chronic inflammatory polyneuropathy	Plasmapheresis,* steroids
Mononeuropathy multiplex	
Necrotizing vasculitis	?
Multifocal sensory	Spontaneous resolution, plasmapheresis
Ascending polyneuropathy—cauda equina presentation (? CMV related)	? AZT ? Ganciclovir
Distal symmetric polyneuropathy	Symptomatic relief—various analgesics, tricyclic anti-depressants, anticonvulsants, ? AZT
Autonomic neuropathy	?

*Treatment of choice.

veals myopathy and abnormal membrane irritability. Muscle biopsy is often distinctive. Response to steroids has been noted anecdotally.[28] AZT also may cause a myositis. It should be discontinued if a patient develops myositis after being placed on it.

■ PULMONARY MANIFESTATIONS

In eliciting the history, the physician must try to differentiate the fatigue and weakness that may be reported as shortness of breath from true lung disease. The evaluation and empiric treatment of patients with shortness of breath and cough is influenced by the chest roentgenogram (CXR) appearance. Acutely ill patients who present with cough, fever, and infiltrates on CXR should be evaluated with sputum Gram and acid-fast bacilli stains, and bacterial as well as mycobacterial and fungal sputum cultures. An arterial blood gas analysis (ABG) also should be done. If a lobar infiltrate is present on CXR, the patient should be managed initially like the non-HIV-infected patient with lobar pneumonia. Initial antibiotic coverage should be based upon the sputum Gram stain if a good sample is obtained. If little sputum is being produced or the Gram stain is inconclusive, empiric antibiotic therapy should cover the more common pathogens, including *Streptococcus pneumoniae*, *Haemophilus influenzae*, and *Staphylococcus aureus* (see Table 3). *Legionella* or *Mycoplasma* coverage or both may need to be added, depending upon the epidemiologic risks for these infections. For the severely ill patient with this presentation, one approach to empiric therapy is maximal intravenous doses of erythromycin plus a third-generation cephalosporin.

Most HIV-infected patients with pulmonary symptoms and hypoxia, however, have a diffuse pattern of infiltration on CXR. The majority of these patients have *Pneumocystis carinii* pneumonia (PCP), and empiric therapy for this infection should be started (see "Infections in the AIDS Patient") (see Table 3). An induced sputum for immunofluorescent monoclonal antibody testing for *P. carinii* should be obtained if it is available. Bronchoalveolar lavage (BAL) is also an excellent modality for diagnosing PCP and is the diagnostic method of choice if an induced sputum examination for PCP is not available. BAL is positive in more than 95 per cent of AIDS patients with biopsy-proved PCP. However, its role may be more limited in the diagnosis of invasive fungal or CMV disease, in which case a lung biopsy (bronchoscopic or open thoracotomy) may be required. BAL is not beneficial in the diagnosis of pulmonary KS. It is important to confirm PCP because of its prognostic significance and the continuing need for prophylactic therapy after primary treatment. If the BAL is negative for PCP or is positive but the patient is deteriorating despite maximal PCP therapy, bronchoscopic biopsy specimens may be very helpful for diagnosis of other opportunistic infections. Open lung biopsy is rarely required but may be necessary to establish the diagnosis of KS.

Lymphocytic Interstitial Pneumonitis (LIP). Diffuse pulmonary infiltrates are also seen with LIP. LIP and its nodular variant, pulmonary lymphoid hyperplasia, are noted in up to 50 per cent of children with HIV infection but are rare in adults. This disease must be differentiated from PCP. Based on anecdotal experiences of successful treatment with steroids, their use has been advocated.[29] The potential risks of steroids in this population warrant caution in their use until the results of ongoing controlled studies are reported.

Nonspecific Interstitial Pneumonitis. Nonspecific interstitial pneumonitis also may be associated with diffuse pulmonary infiltrates on CXR. This entity has been described recently in HIV-infected adults.[30] The patients clinically present with cough and fever similar to that of patients with PCP. The CXR is normal, however, 50 per cent of the time, although gallium scan is usually positive. Lung biopsy reveals diffuse alveolar damage without *P. carinii* cysts. The etiology of this process is unknown. Resolution usually occurs without specific treatment. However, many patients subsequently develop disease owing to opportunistic infections such as CMV or PCP (which present as separate clinical episodes) in the months following the diagnosis of nonspecific interstitial pneumonitis.[30] Further studies are needed to define better the cause, natural history, and treatment of this condition. At present, its importance lies in its potential confusion with PCP.

Patients with respiratory complaints and fever also may present with a normal CXR. This occurs in up to 5 to 10 per cent of patients with PCP, in one half of the patients with nonspecific interstitial pneumonitis, and in some patients with pulmonary tuberculosis or CMV infection. In these instances, a gallium scan of the lung is often helpful in determining that an inflammatory process is present. If the gallium scan is positive and sputum is not available for analysis, bronchoalveolar lavage (BAL) should be done. It is important to note that a negative gallium scan does not completely exclude active pulmonary infection.

■ HIV-RELATED TUMORS

Several tumors, including Kaposi's sarcoma, high-grade non-Hodgkin's B-cell lymphoma, and primary lymphoma of the CNS, have been linked to HIV infection. The exact relationship between HIV infection and these "opportunistic" tumors is not clear. However, they are known to occur in other immunocompromised populations. An etiologic role for CMV and Epstein-Barr virus (EBV) in KS and non-Hodgkin's lymphoma, respectively, has been suggested but remains unproved. The benefits of chemotherapy for any of these tumors must be weighed against the potential risk of further immunocompromising the already severely compromised host. Hodgkin's lymphoma has not been epidemiologically linked with HIV infection. However, in HIV-infected patients, Hodgkin's disease may present in a more aggressive fashion and may respond to chemotherapy less well.

Since development of these tumors in HIV-infected patients is sufficient for the diagnosis of AIDS, the use of AZT should be considered. To date, AZT has not been shown to have a direct effect on altering tumor progression.

Kaposi's Sarcoma. Specific treatment of KS depends upon the extent of the disease. Localized disease in patients can be treated expectantly or with local therapy such as electrocautery, surgical excision, or radiotherapy. Focal lesions that are disfiguring, painful, or producing lymphedema may be benefited by radiation therapy.[31]

Patients with KS principally involving the skin (with widespread lesions) or lymph nodes and who have CD4 cells greater than $400/mm^3$ may benefit from immunomodulator therapy, such as interferon alfa-2 (IF-2). Doses greater than 20 million IU per day have led to responses (partial plus complete) 45 per cent of the time in patients with greater than 400 CD4 cells/mm^3.[32] Lower

rates of response are reported with reduced CD4 cell counts. One recommended regimen is gradual dose escalation to 36 million IU daily.[32] This is considered the highest tolerable dose without extreme side effects. Toxicity includes a flulike illness with fatigue, fever, and malaise, gastrointestinal complaints such as anorexia and nausea, and cytopenias (all cell lines).[32] The latter toxicity may limit the concomitant use of AZT. Treatment should continue indefinitely.

Patients who have symptomatic visceral KS and who are in a poor prognostic group, i.e., CD4 cell counts of less than $400/mm^3$, should be treated initially with single-agent chemotherapy with etoposide (VP-16) or vincristine. These are the most active single agents studied to date. Rapidly progressive disease, disease not responding to single agent therapy, and pulmonary disease should be treated with multidrug regimens. Several multidrug combinations, including vincristine plus bleomycin, vincristine plus vinblastine, and daunorubicin plus bleomycin and vincristine, yield response rates greater than 45 per cent. However, response rates are generally short-lived and measured in terms of months.[31] The optimal duration of therapy is not known.

Malignant Lymphoma. Malignant lymphoma often presents with advanced disease (stages III and IV) and with extranodal involvement. Prognosis is poor, with survival rarely greater than 1 year even with intensive chemotherapy.[33,34] The dismal prognosis is multifactorial and often related to concurrent opportunistic infections, limitation of chemotherapy doses because of HIV bone marrow suppression, difficulty in maintaining remission, and high rates of CNS involvement both at the onset and during relapse. Aggressive multidrug chemotherapeutic regimens such as COMET-A (cyclophosphamide, vincristine sulfate, methotrexate, etoposide, cytarabine)[33] and MACOP-B (methotrexate, Adriamycin, cyclophosphamide, vincristine, prednisone, bleomycin)[34] can achieve complete responses in greater than 50 per cent of cases.

Although the mean and median survival rates are higher for those who respond to therapy versus those who either do not respond or do not receive therapy, the median survival rate for those who respond was still only 7 months in one study.[34] Moreover, less intensive chemotherapy regimens may be preferable, since some have been shown to be just as effective in respect to tumor response and patient survival.[33]

Patients with HIV infection but without a previous diagnosis of AIDS should be treated with chemotherapy, since a tumor response is likely in this group. In the setting of previously diagnosed AIDS, however, the risk-to-benefit ratio is higher, and the decision whether to treat the lymphoma must be individualized. Studies using chemotherapy in combination with hematopoietic growth factors to decrease the toxicity of the myelosuppressive drug regimens are in progress.

Primary CNS Lymphoma. Although diagnosis of primary CNS lymphoma is suggested by CT or MRI of the brain, it must be confirmed by biopsy. Controlled trials of various chemotherapeutic regimens with or without radiotherapy are lacking. Whole brain irradiation with 3000 to 6000 cGy has been reported to lead to significant remission in several patients.[35] Even with treatment, survival is on the order of months, most patients dying as a result of respiratory compromise, development of opportunistic infections, or tumor progression.[35]

REFERENCES

1. Seligmann M, Pinching AJ, Rosen FS, et al. Immunology of human immunodeficiency virus infection and the acquired immunodeficiency syndrome. Ann Intern Med 1987; 107:234–242.
2. Smith PD, Lane HC, Gill VJ, et al. Intestinal infections in patients with acquired immunodeficiency syndrome (AIDS). Ann Intern Med 1988; 108:328–333.
3. Rolston KV, Rodriguez S, Hernandez M, Bodey GP. Diarrhea in patients with the human immunodeficiency virus. Am J Med 1989; 86:137–138.
4. Cunningham AL, Grohman GS, Harkness J, et al. Gastrointestinal viral infections in homosexual men who were symptomatic and seropositive for human immunodeficiency virus. J Infect Dis 1988; 158:386–391.
5. Kotler DP, Gaetz HP, Lange M, Klein EB, Holt PR. Enteropathy associated with the acquired immunodeficiency syndrome. Ann Intern Med 1984; 101:421–428.
6. Cook DJ, Kelton JG, Stanisz AM, Collins SM. Somatostatin treatment for cryptosporidial diarrhea in a patient with the acquired immunodeficiency syndrome (AIDS). Ann Intern Med 1988; 108:708–709.
7. Cello JP. Acquired immunodeficiency syndrome cholangiopathy: spectrum of disease. Am J Med 1989; 86:539–546.
8. Schneiderman DJ, Arenson DM, Cello JP, Margaretten W, Weber TE. Hepatic disease in patients with the acquired immune deficiency syndrome (AIDS). Hepatology 1987; 7:925–930.
9. Yarchoan R, Klecker RW, Weinhold KJ. Administration of 3′azido-3′-deoxythymidine, an inhibitor of HTLV-III/LAV replication, to patients with AIDS or AIDS-related complex. Lancet 1986; 1:575–580.
10. Von Roenn JH, Murphy RL, Weber KM, Williams LM, Weitzman SA. Megestrol acetate for treatment of cachexia associated with human immunodeficiency virus (HIV) infection. Ann Intern Med 1988; 108:840–841.
11. Task Force on Nutrition Support in AIDS. Guidelines for nutrition support in AIDS. Nutrition 1989; 5:39–46.
12. Groopman JE, Mitsuyasu RT, DeLeo MJ, Oette DH, Golde DW. Effect of recombinant human granulocyte-macrophage colony-stimulating factor on myelopoiesis in acquired immunodeficiency syndrome (AIDS). N Engl J Med 1987; 317:593–598.
13. Swiss Group for Clinical Studies on Acquired Immunodeficiency Syndrome (AIDS). Zidovudine for the treatment of thrombocytopenia associated with human immunodeficiency virus (HIV). Ann Intern Med 1988; 109:718–721.
14. Ratner L. Human immunodeficiency virus–associated autoimmune thrombocytopenic purpura: a review. Am J Med 1989; 86:194–198.
15. Bloom EJ, Abrams DI, Rodgers G. Lupus anticoagulant in the acquired immunodeficiency syndrome. JAMA 1986; 256:491–493.
16. Pardo V, Aldana M, Colton RM, et al. Glomerular lesions in the acquired immunodeficiency syndrome. Ann Intern Med 1984; 101:429–434.
17. Rao TKS, Friedman EA, Nicastri AD. The types of renal disease in the acquired immunodeficiency syndrome (AIDS). N Engl J Med 1987; 316:1062–1068.
18. Gabuzda DH, Hirsch MS. Neurologic manifestations of infection with human immunodeficiency virus. Ann Intern Med 1987; 107:383–391.
19. Price RW, Brew B. Management of the neurologic complications of HIV infection and AIDS. Infect Dis Clin North Am 1988; 2:359–372.
20. Hollander H, Stringari S. Human immunodeficiency virus–associated meningitis. Am J Med 1987; 83:813–816.
21. Schmitt FA, Bigley JW, McKinnis R, et al. Neuropsychological outcome of zidovudine (AZT) treatment of patients with AIDS and AIDS-related complex. N Engl J Med 1988; 319:1573–1578.
22. Yarchoan R, Brouwers P, Spitzer W, et al. Response of human immunodeficiency virus–associated neurological disease to 3′-azido-3′deoxythymidine. Lancet 1987; 1:132–135.
23. Berger JR, Kaszovitz B, Post JD, Dickinson G. Progressive multifocal leukoencephalopathy associated with human immunodeficiency virus infection. Ann Intern Med 1987; 107:78–87.
24. Engstrom JW, Lowenstein DH, Bredesen DE. Cerebral infarctions and transient neurologic deficits associated with acquired immunodeficiency syndrome. Am J Med 1989; 86:528–532.
25. Petito CK, Navia BA, Cho ES, Jordon BD, George DC, Price RW. Vacuolar myelopathy pathologically resembling subacute combined degeneration in patients with the acquired immunodeficiency syndrome. N Engl J Med 1985; 312:874–879.
26. Parry GJ. Peripheral neuropathies associated with human immunodeficiency virus infection. Ann Neurol 1988; 23(suppl):S49–S53.
27. Cornblath DR. Treatment of the neuromuscular

complications of human immunodeficiency virus infection. Ann Neurol 1988; 23(suppl):S88–S91.

28. Simpson DM, Bender AN. Human immunodeficiency virus–associated myopathy: analysis of 11 patients. Ann Neurol 1988; 24:79–84.

29. Rubinstein A. Pediatric AIDS. Curr Probl Pediatr 1986; 16:361–409.

30. Suffredini AF, Ognibene FP, Lack EE, et al. Nonspecific interstitial pneumonitis: a common cause of pulmonary disease in the acquired immunodeficiency syndrome. Ann Intern Med 1987; 107:7–13.

31. Mitsuyasu RT. Kaposi's sarcoma in the acquired immunodeficiency syndrome. Infect Dis Clin North Am 1988; 2:511–523.

32. Roferon-A product information. Nutley, NJ, Roche Laboratories, 1988.

33. Kaplan LD, Abrams DI, Feigal E, et al. AIDS-associated non-Hodgkin's lymphoma in San Francisco. JAMA 1989; 261:719–724.

34. Bermudez MA, Grant KM, Rodvien R, Mendes F, et al. Non-Hodgkin's lymphoma in a population with or at risk for acquired immunodeficiency syndrome: indications for intensive chemotherapy. Am J Med 1989; 86:71–76.

35. So YT, Beckstead JH, Davis RL. Primary central nervous system lymphoma in acquired immune deficiency syndrome: a clinical and pathological study. Ann Neurol 1986; 20:566–572.

Hypercholesterolemia

Gary Walter Crooks ■ *David Bret Nash*

Hypercholesterolemia, as established by the Expert Panel on Detection, Evaluation and Treatment of High Blood Cholesterol in Adults, is defined as a condition in which a nonfasting total cholesterol level measures greater than 200 mg/dl. Prior to labeling a patient as hypercholesterolemic, the treating physician should confirm the patient's level by a repeat value. If the average of these two determinations is greater than 240 mg/dl, then the patient should undergo lipoprotein electrophoresis after fasting for 12 hours. If the average determination is between 200 and 240 mg/dl (borderline high cholesterol) *and* the patient has definite coronary artery disease (CAD), or has two other risk factors for CAD (as listed in Table 1), lipoprotein analysis also should be performed. If the patient's total cholesterol is borderline high, and he or she is without other risk factors, general dietary counseling should be given and the determination repeated in 1 year.

This article discusses those patients with cholesterol values greater than 240 mg/dl and those patients with values greater than 200 mg/dl with coronary heart disease (CHD) or two other risk factors for CHD. Hypertriglyceridemia as an isolated phenomenon is not thought to be a significant risk factor for CHD and will not be discussed. Causes of secondary hypercholesterolemia, as listed in Table 2, should be excluded prior to directing therapeutic intervention of the elevated blood cholesterol level.

TABLE 1. Risk Factors for Coronary Heart Disease

Male sex
Family history of coronary heart disease (developing at 55 years of age)
Cigarette smoking
Hypertension
Low HDL cholesterol
Diabetes mellitus
Definitive cerebrovascular or peripheral vascular disease
Severe obesity

TABLE 2. Principal Causes of Nonessential Hypercholesterolemia

Hypothyroidism
Nephrotic syndrome
Chronic renal disease
Obstructive liver disease
Multiple myeloma
Dysglobulinemia
Anabolic steroids
Progestational agents
Drugs: thiazides, beta-blockers

■ Background

Most commonly, a patient will be seen who desires to learn his or her blood cholesterol value, or the patient may have had a screening value and wishes to address the finding of a high level. He or she will have no symptoms of CHD. Less frequently, a patient with known CHD will have been taking antianginal medications but will not have had the issue of hypercholesterolemia addressed as a risk factor. Other risk factors, particularly hypertension, diabetes mellitus, and perhaps cigarette smoking and obesity, may have received attention in the course of treating the angina, but until the last 5 years or so, cholesterol may have been ignored.

The average cholesterol level for middle-aged men and women in the United States is 215 mg/dl. Approximately half of American adults over the age of 20 have cholesterol values over 200 mg/dl; 25 per cent have levels over 240 mg/dl. Compared with people who have levels less than 200 mg/dl, those with values over 200 mg/dl have 2.5 times the attributable risk of developing CHD.[1] This must be compared with the attributable risk of other cardiac risk factors, as listed in Table 3.[2]

Cholesterol reduction should not be emphasized at the expense of programs that encourage weight loss, control of diabetes, or smoking cessation. The benefit of reduction in serum cholesterol levels has as yet only been well proved in men aged 20 through 55.[3-5] The benefit of a reduction in serum cholesterol levels in women, particularly those over 65 years of age, has not been proved.[6,7] The most impressive study to date that supports the lowering of serum lipids in patients who have angiographically demonstrated CAD is the Cholesterol-Lowering Atherosclerosis Study (CLAS), in which 16 per cent of drug-treated (diet plus cholestipol and niacin) patients showed a reduction in coronary atherosclerosis in comparison with 2 per cent of controls (less stringent diet and placebo) (P = 0.002).[8]

TABLE 3. Attributable Risk for CAD Death in Middle-Aged White Men

Cholesterol ($\geq$ 240 mg/dl vs. $\leq$ 200 mg/dl)	2.5
Hypertension (BP diastolic $\geq$ 96 vs. $\leq$ 96)	3.0
Smoking (yes vs. never)	3.2
Diabetes mellitus (yes vs. normal blood sugar)	6.4

■ Management

The World Health Organization (WHO) cooperative trial, the Coronary Drug Project (CDP), the Lipid Research Clinic's Coronary Primary Prevention Trial (LRC-CPPT), the Helsinki Heart Study, the National Heart, Lung and Blood Institute's Type II Coronary Intervention Study, and CLAS all have lent support to the concept of the more aggressive approach to the treatment of elevated cholesterol levels. The therapy should be aimed at the prevention of primary and secondary CAD and not at an isolated abnormal blood value. The aforementioned studies also discovered some increase in noncardiovascular morbidity and mortality with several of the proposed therapeutic agents: clofibrate,[3,4] cholestyramine,[6] and gemfibrozil.[7]

A reasonable approach first emphasizes dietary changes, maintenance of ideal body weight, adherence to an exercise program, and drug therapy. If the total cholesterol level is greater than 240 mg/dl or the value is between 200 and 239 mg/dl in the presence of two CHD risk factors or known CHD, a lipoprotein analysis should be performed after a 12-hour fast. Total cholesterol, HDL-cholesterol, and triglycerides should be measured. Estimate of the LDL-cholesterol can be made using the following formula:

$$\text{LDL-cholesterol} = \text{total cholesterol} - \text{HDL-cholesterol} - \frac{(\text{triglycerides})}{5}$$

The LDL-cholesterol should be an average of two to three such calculations taken 1 to 8 weeks apart. If the LDL-cholesterol is greater than or equal to 130 mg/dl, dietary modification for a minimum of 6 months should be undertaken.

■ DIET

Dietary therapy focuses on a two-step approach. The first step is the American Heart Association (AHA) diet as recommended for the general public. Fat should account for less than 30 per cent of daily calories and should be balanced in monounsaturated, polyunsaturated, and saturated fats. Cholesterol intake should be less than 300 mg per day; fiber (as in oat bran, beans, and barley) use is encouraged, as is exercise. Common items to avoid are egg yolks (one yolk contains 250 mg of cholesterol), liver and other organ meats, and processed meats such as hot dogs or bologna. Patients must be taught to read labels to avoid fats commonly used in baked products, such as coconut oil, palm oil, or palm kernel oil. Total cholesterol levels should be checked at 6 and 12 weeks. If the patient's cholesterol has not dropped to the desired range after 3 months, then Step 2 diet therapy should be initiated and a dietitian's help elicited.

Some people do not respond to dietary therapy, particularly those with total cholesterol values greater than 300 mg/dl. For those who do respond, long-term monitoring with biannual checks is indicated. For those who do not respond, lipid-lowering drugs should be added; the importance of continued dietary restrictions should be emphasized.

■ FISH OILS

Fish oil capsules have received a great deal of publicity nationally. Many patients have tried them. Fish oils are only useful in certain patients with isolated hypertriglyceridemia and would require a dosage of 8 to 20 capsules per day to lower LDL levels significantly. Current data cannot support the use of fish oil capsules for those patients with elevated cholesterol levels, and some capsules may contain so much saturated fat that they actually raise LDL-cholesterol levels.[9] Other concerns with their usage are vitamin E deficiency, vitamins A and D toxicity, and the concentration of DDT from the process used to make the capsules.

In 1987, over 90 companies were making fish oil capsules, but many have since abandoned the business,[10] and sales forecasts have been drastically altered.

■ BRAN AND FIBER

Soluble fibers such as oat bran and psyllium (Metamucil or Citrucil), when consumed in quantities of 20 or more grams per day, can lower LDL cholesterol values by 10 to 20 per cent. These fibers are not systemically absorbed and have few side effects. In addition, fiber consumption tends to regulate bowel movements and lessen constipation and may have a protective effect against colon carcinoma.

■ FIRST-LINE DRUGS

The drugs proven to be effective in lowering LDL-cholesterol and shown not to cause an offsetting decrease in HDL-cholesterol are listed in Table 4. The first drug therapy to consider should be that with the fewest side effects, and the bile acid sequestrants fit the

TABLE 4. First-Line Drugs for Lowering LDL-Cholesterol

Drug	Starting Dose	Average Adult Dose Per Day	Side Effects	Cost* (30 Days)
Cholestyramine (Questran)	4 gm BID	16 gm	Constipation; GI discomfort; decreased absorption of digoxin, thyroxine, thiazides, and β-blockers	$57.60
Colestipol (Colestid)	5 gm BID	15 gm	Vitamin K deficiency	41.07
Niacin (generic)	100–250 mg BID–QID	2–3 gm	Flushing, upper GI discomfort, hepatic damage, increased uric acid	7.91
Nicolor				58.82
Nico-400				50.92
Lovastatin (Mevacor)	20 mg/day	20–40 mg	Increased LFTs, alteration in bowel function, headache, fatigue, myalgias, insomnia	41.63

*Cost to pharmacist for 30-day prescription, based on *Drug Topics Red Book* (Cardinale VA: Oradell, NJ. Medical Economics Book Co, 1988).

bill best.[11] Their use has been shown to reduce CHD risk in large-scale studies; long-term safety is known; and they are not absorbed from the gastrointestinal tract, making them particularly suitable for younger patients, especially women of child-bearing age and children. Bile acid sequestrants are contraindicated as primary therapy in patients with triglyceride values greater than 500 mg/dl or in patients who suffer from severe constipation.

Nicotinic acid was found to be effective in the coronary drug project. It was associated with reducing subsequent myocardial infarctions and overall mortality.[5] Niacin has had additional benefit in that it raises HDL-cholesterol. Although the side effects of flushing often have limited its use, starting at a very low dose (100 to 250 mg/day) and increasing by increments of 250 mg per day each week until the desired cholesterol level is reached have improved patient compliance. Flushing also can be decreased by pretreatment with 325 mg of aspirin or the use of a longer-acting NSAID, and by avoiding administration on an empty stomach. Sustained-released preparations also reduce flushing but greatly increase cost. As is shown in Table 4, the generic form of niacin, nicotinic acid, is the least costly of the presently available medications. Hyperuricemia, hyperglycemia, and elevated liver function tests are common adverse side effects, usually with higher doses. Contraindications are pre-existing hyperuricemia, gout, hepatic disease, and peptic ulcer disease.

OTHER AGENTS

Clofibrate (Atromid-S, Abitrate), probucol (Lorelco), and gemfibrozil (Lopid) have been advocated as therapy for hypercholesterolemia. Clofibrate lowers serum triglyceride levels and can result in increased LDL-cholesterol when triglyceride levels decline. More importantly, in the WHO clofibrate study, clofibrate use resulted in increased mortality from malignancy and from gastrointestinal disease. An increased need for cholecystectomy was also found.

Probucol appears to be well tolerated, but in lowering LDL-cholesterol by 10 to 15 per cent, it also lowers HDL-cholesterol by 20 to 30 per cent. This latter effect may be offset if probucol is used in conjunction with colestipol.

Lovastatin is well tolerated and easy to take. Of the aforementioned agents, lovastatin is reported to lower cholesterol by the greatest percentage, from 18 to 34 per cent, depending on the dose. The long-term safety with regard to liver toxicity is as yet unknown. The reduction of serum cholesterol values by lovastatin has not yet been proved to slow or reverse atherosclerosis. For patients unable to tolerate first-line therapy, who have total cholesterol values of 280 mg/dl or greater, and who are at high risk of CHD or CVA, the risk of lovastatin's side effects must be weighed against the probability of early cardiovascular morbidity and mortality.

INVESTIGATIONAL DRUGS

Several new HMG-CoA-reductase inhibitors that will act like lovastatin are being developed. Simvastatin and pravastatin are currently undergoing clinical trials. Also undergoing development are fimbric acid compounds similar to gemfibrozil and clofibrate, but with greater ability to lower LDL-cholesterol.

COMBINATION THERAPY

The cholesterol-lowering ability of the recommended drugs appears to be greatly enhanced by binary and even triple-drug regimens.[12] The side effect profiles do not appear to be increased. Table 5 illustrates some of the cholesterol reductions that have been reported with combination therapy. The toxicity from such combinations and the optimal therapeutic doses for such therapy have yet to be established.

TABLE 5. Per Cent Reduction in Cholesterol Levels with Various Agents

Agent(s)	Range of Total Cholesterol Reduction (%)
Cholestyramine	13.4–25
Colestipol	13.4–25
Niacin	9.6
Lovastatin	18.0–34
Colestipol & lovastatin	52.0–54
Colestipol & lovastatin & niacin	54 –79

■ Issues and Risks

One could argue that the mass media, well aware of our society's obsession with health matters, has provided the lay public with a blow-by-blow description of the unfolding cholesterol saga.[13] Although most physicians accept the lipid hypothesis (the assumption that lowering the serum cholesterol level reduces the risk for the development of ischemic heart disease), recent evidence indicates that the entire picture is still developing. One Harvard-based research group developed a model that estimates the increase in life expectancy to be gained by a reduction in cholesterol for a person initially free of "overt" ischemic heart disease.[14] Their model calculates the increased life expectancy as a function of age, sex, and risk factors for ischemic heart disease such as blood pressure, smoking habits, HDL cholesterol, and total cholesterol. Their surprising analysis revealed that for persons aged 20 to 60 years who are at low risk, a gain in life expectancy of only 3 days to 3 months could be expected from a lifelong program of cholesterol reduction. For persons at high risk, the calculated gain ranges from 18 days to 12 months. Their results also showed that men gained *less* life expectancy than women for a specified set of risk factors and a specified amount of cholesterol reduction.

Commenting on this Harvard project, some observers believe that we need additional studies that compare the cost-effectiveness of alternative cholesterol-lowering programs,[15] as well as their value relative to other types of health-promoting and disease-preventing activities. Major medical groups such as the American Medical Association (AMA) have even taken issue with a panel of experts convened by the National Heart, Lung, and Blood Institute, which recommended that all Americans adopt the "prudent diet" to lower saturated fats promulgated by the American Heart Association. The AMA recommends dietary therapy only for those with serum cholesterol levels above the 90th percentile.[15] Faced with these conflicting recommendations and surprising study findings, how can clinicians help guide the individual patient seeking advice about his or her cholesterol level (no doubt prompted in part by the medical overexposure to this issue)?

Clinicians treat individuals and not populations. Most of the relevant research literature reports relative measures of risk, such as the risk ratio. Clinicians are concerned with the magnitude of risk, or *attributable* risk, the difference in risk in those with highest and lowest serum cholesterol levels.[2] One can take this line of reasoning one step closer to the patient by estimating the practical attributable risk, which is the difference in disease incidence between the patient's current risk and that which is achievable. For example, the clinician may have to counsel a patient that lowering the cholesterol level from the fourth quintal to the third quintal is all that can reasonably be achieved, given the individual risk factors, family life, motivation, and other intangibles. Patients are more apt to respond to an individually tailored cholesterol target than to some specified societal level. Clinicians should remember that "treating hypercholesterolemia to prevent coronary heart disease is more like immunizing to prevent diphtheria than treating pneumococcal pneumonia in terms of the proportion of treated patients who benefit."[12] Patients need and deserve an individualized plan. Therefore, Malenka and colleagues believe that the decision to treat not only must be patient-specific, it also should hinge on consideration of the practical attributable risk, the efficacy of treatment, and patient's preferences concerning the risks and benefits of treatment.[2]

After dutifully considering the aforementioned three-point plan, what happens when a clinician labels a patient as having hypercholesterolemia? The effects of "labeling" a patient (as having hypercholesterolemia) might include increased absenteeism from work, increased physical complaints, poorer self-perceived health status, anxiety, and depression; in more extreme cases, unemployment or even suicide can result.[16] Controlling a high blood cholesterol level will require that physicians and patients spend considerably more time and effort on therapy than may be usually necessary for treating other chronic conditions such as hypertension. Some researchers point out that, after screening for hypercholesterolemia, physicians must be able to offer concrete, behavioral recommendations as to how to act on the new findings.[17]

Beyond the labeling phenomenon, another issue of concern with regard to screening for and treating hypercholesterolemia remains—the accuracy of the tests themselves. In 1986 reports in the lay press[18] and professional literature[19] highlighted the poor quality of some commercial laboratories and the marked differences in what one laboratory called a normal finding vis-a-vis other laboratories. More recently, one group tested four of the most common laboratory instruments used for measuring cholesterol and found very acceptable precision and accuracy scores.[20] The National Cholesterol Education Program (NCEP) recently completed a large survey utilizing regional quality-control data and national proficiency testing results; they report that just about one half of laboratories are using a nationally acceptable reference method for measuring total cholesterol.[20] Because the potential size of the market is so great,[21] and the attendant publicity about cholesterol incessant, it is incumbent upon clinicians to check the quality-control information on file with their local laboratory to assure high levels of precision and accuracy for patients.

■ TESTING AND TREATING CHILDREN

The role of dietary intervention, cholesterol screening, and the prevention of atherosclerosis in children remains controversial. While a detailed discussion is clearly beyond the scope of this chapter, certain key concepts will be reviewed. As Becker reports, one cost-effectiveness analysis of a comprehensive program to prevent heart disease by lowering cholesterol levels in children (from mass media and school-based strategies to targeted interventions for children at high risk) estimated that, using a 10 per cent discount rate, it would cost about $83,000 for boys and $105,000 for girls to obtain one additional year of life.[13] Some clinicians believe that in pediatric practice screening should identify those at high risk—defined as a patient with a serum cholesterol level of more than 200 mg/dl[22] and with a positive family history of CHD. At what age to begin screening for and treating hypercholesterolemia is not well established. Groups such as the American Academy of Pediatrics have suggested that a screening cholesterol level should be ob-

tained beginning at age 2 years only for those children with a positive family history of CHD. In certain tertiary medical centers for children, this has become standard practice, and those children without a positive family history are not screened until 5 years of age. Currently, the treatment of hypercholesterolemia in children focuses on dietary intervention. Most pediatricians use only bile sequestrants such as cholestyramine (Questran) and colestipol (Colestid) when drug therapy is required because of failed dietary therapy. Lovastatin (Mevacor) and other drugs in its class have not yet been approved for use in children.

■ FUTURE CONSIDERATIONS

In 1986, a survey of physicians conducted by the National Heart, Lung, and Blood Institute revealed that cholesterol levels as triggers for initiating therapy often were unacceptably high.[23] Also in this survey, only 59 per cent of physicians felt capable of providing nutrition counseling, and 15 per cent felt they were successful in such counseling. Only 40 per cent indicated that reducing dietary fat would have a large effect on the risk of developing CHD. Clearly, there is a need to educate not only the general public but also clinicians about the risk of hypercholesterolemia.

One potential drawback to appropriate therapy for hypercholesterolemia is the high cost of drug therapy. Kinosian and colleagues looked at several cost-effective alternatives for treating hypercholesterolemia.[24] They simulated a program for lowering cholesterol levels that was similar to that of the Coronary Primary Prevention Trial, and then used the outcomes of the trial to calculate the incremental cost per year of life saved (YOLS) from the perspective of society. Their findings suggest that the cost of YOLS ranges from $117,400 (cholestyramine resin packets) to $70,900 (colestipol packets) down to $17,800 using a soluble fiber like oat bran. Kinosian contends that although the cost of medical therapy to reduce cholesterol levels is substantial, analyzing the more expensive agents has obscured some important policy implications—namely, a broad public health approach to lowered cholesterol levels by using a soluble fiber such as oat bran may be preferred to a medically oriented campaign that focuses on expensive drug therapy.

ically oriented campaign that focuses on expensive drug therapy.

Other innovative therapies for hypercholesterolemia might include the future use of granulocyte-macrophage colony stimulation factor (GM-CSF), which was recently serendipitously discovered[25] to lower total cholesterol during a treatment trial for aplastic anemia. Some pharmaceutical firms are making sweet-tasting candy bars out of cholestyramine in an effort to make it a more palatable drug.[26]

REFERENCES

1. Rose G, Shipley M. Plasma cholesterol concentration and death from coronary heart disease. Ten-year results of the Whitehall study. Br Med J 1986; 293:306–307.
2. Malenka DJ, Baron JA. Cholesterol and coronary heart disease: the importance of patient-specific attributable risk. Arch Intern Med 1988; 148:2247–2252.
3. Oliver MF, Heady JA, Morris JN, Cooper J. A cooperative trial in the primary prevention of ischemic heart disease using clofibrate: report from the committee of principal investigators. Br Heart J 1978; 40:1069–1118.
4. Coronary Drug Research Group. Natural history of myocardial infarction in the coronary drug project: long-term prognostic importance of serum lipid levels. Am J Cardiol 1978; 42:489–498.
5. Canner PL, Berge KG, Wenger NK, et al (for the Coronary Drug Project Research Group). Fifteen year mortality in Coronary Drug Project patients; long-term benefit with niacin. J Am Coll Cardiol 1986; 8:1245–1255.
6. Lipid Research Clinics Program. The Lipid Research Clinics Coronary Primary Prevention Trials Results. II. The relationship of reduction in incidence of coronary heart disease to cholesterol lowering. JAMA 1984; 251:365–374.
7. Frick MH, Elo O, Haapa K, et al. Helsinki Heart Study: primary-prevention trial with gemfibrozil in middle-aged men with dyslipidemia: Safety of treatment, changes in risk factors, and incidence of coronary heart disease. N Engl J Med 1987; 317:1237–1247.
8. Blankenhorn DH, Nessin SA, Johnson RL, Sanmario ME, Azen SP, Cashin-Hempill L. Beneficial effects of combined colestipol-niacin therapy on coronary atherosclerosis and coronary venous bypass grafts. JAMA 1987; 257:3233–3240.
9. Yetiv JZ. Clinical applications of fish oils. JAMA 1988; 260:665–670.
10. Bivens T. Sweet smell of success eludes fish-oil trade. Philadelphia Inquirer 1989; Jan 22:1(Sect E), (col 1).
11. Lipid Research Clinics Program. The Lipid Research Clinics Coronary Primary Prevention Trial Results: I. Reduction in the incidence of coronary heart disease. JAMA 1984; 251:351–364.
12. Malloy MJ, Kane JP, Kunitake ST, Tun P. Complimentarity of colestipol and lovastatin in treatment of severe familial hypercholesterolemia. Ann Intern Med 1987; 107:616–623.
13. Becker MH. The cholesterol saga; whither health promotion (editorial)? Ann Intern Med 1987; 106:623–626.
14. Taylor WC, Pass TM, Shepard DS, Komaroff AL. Cholesterol reduction and life expectancy: a model incorporating multiple risk factors. Ann Intern Med 1987; 106:605–614.
15. Epstein AM, Oster G. Cholesterol reduction and health policy: taking service to patient care (editorial). Ann Intern Med 1987; 106:621–623.
16. Havas S. The challenge of lowering blood cholesterol levels (editorial). Arch Intern Med 1988; 148:1910–1913.
17. Lefebvre RC, Hursey KG, Carledon RA. Labeling of participants in high blood pressure screening programs: regulations for blood cholesterol screenings. Arch Intern Med 1988; 148:1993–1997.
18. Bogdanich W. Inaccuracy in testing cholesterol hampers war on heart disease. Wall Street Journal 1987; Feb 3:1(col 1).
19. Blank DW, Hoeg JM, Droll MH, et al. The method of determination must be considered in interpreting blood cholesterol levels. JAMA 1986; 256:2867–2870.
20. Koch DD, Hassemer DJ, Wiebe DA, Laessing RH. Testing cholesterol accuracy: performance of several common laboratory instruments. JAMA 1988; 260:2552–2557.
21. Waldholz M. Fat chance: the age of cholesterol dawns for marketer, at food, drug makers. Their publicity efforts are a big reason the public is rushing to doctors. Wall Street Journal 1988; June 14:1(col 1), 22(col 1).
22. Jacobson MS. The pediatrician's role in atherosclerosis prevention. J Pediatr 1988; 112:836–841.
23. Schucker B, Wittes J, Cutler J. Changes in physician perspective on cholesterol and heart disease: results from two national surveys. JAMA 1987; 258:3521–3526.
24. Kinosian BP, Eisenberg JM. Cutting into cholesterol: cost-effective alternatives for treating hypercholesterolemia. JAMA 1988; 259:2249–2254.
25. Nimer SD, Chaplin RE, Golde DW. Serum cholesterol-lowering activity of granulocyte-macrophage colony-stimulating factor. JAMA 1988; 260:3287–3300.
26. Waldolz M. Warner-Lambert offers a candy bar to fight cholesterol. Wall Street Journal 1988; Dec. 1:B3.

Hypertension in pregnancy

John W. Saultz ■ *Dean McGinty*

Hypertension is the most common medical complication of pregnancy, affecting 10 to 21 per cent of all pregnant women.[1,2] The importance of this problem lies in the increased risk of maternal and fetal complications with which it is associated. In spite of intensive clinical investigation over the past 30 years, the etiology and pathophysiology of hypertensive disorders in pregnancy are still poorly understood. Fortunately, if identified early and carefully managed, the adverse effects to both mother and fetus from hypertension in pregnancy are largely preventable.

■ Background

In normal pregnant patients, the blood pressure gradually decreases from the late first trimester until the early third trimester. This decrease is followed by a gradual increase during the third trimester, and most women have a blood pressure near the prepregnancy level at the time of term delivery. This normal decrease in the resting blood pressure during the middle trimester often makes it difficult to identify and classify hypertensive disorders in patients who are not seen until after the twelfth week of pregnancy.

Hypertension in pregnancy may be defined by the following criteria:

1. A diastolic blood pressure greater than 110 mm Hg on any single occasion, or
2. A diastolic pressure greater than 90 mm Hg on two consecutive readings, greater than 4 hours apart, or
3. A rise in diastolic blood pressure greater than 15 mm Hg over the nonpregnant baseline on two consecutive readings more than 4 hours apart.

Systolic blood pressure readings generally are not used in the definition of hypertension in pregnancy, because they are less predictive of maternal or fetal risk than the diastolic pressure.

Also important in distinguishing the hypertensive disorders of pregnancy is to determine accurately whether the patient has proteinuria. Proteinuria in pregnancy is defined as greater than 300 mg of protein per 24-hr urine specimen. When prenatal patents are screened for proteinuria in the physician's office with urine dipsticks, it is important to encourage them to obtain true clean-catch specimens to eliminate false positive tests. Patients who have 2+ or greater protein (1 gm/L) on dipstick testing should be further evaluated with a 24-hr urine protein evaluation.

■ Diagnostic Classifications

Because the risk of complications for the mother and baby varies greatly from one category to another, it is important to assign the hypertensive pregnant woman accurately into one of five diagnostic categories. The following criteria are used to make this distinction:

Pregnancy-induced hypertension without proteinuria (PIH). This diagnosis is made using the following criteria:

1. Hypertension that develops after the twentieth week of pregnancy;
2. Absence of proteinuria, as defined earlier;
3. Absence of evidence of chronic hypertension.

Evidence of chronic hypertension may include documented blood pressures in the hypertensive range prior to pregnancy or the presence of complications of chronic hypertension, such as hypertensive retinopathy. The only exception to the cutoff of 20 weeks is pregnancy-induced hypertension associated with hydatidiform mole, which may occur before the twentieth week.

Pregnancy-induced hypertension (PIH) with proteinuria. This diagnostic category has traditionally been termed preeclampsia and consists of the triad of hypertension, proteinuria, and edema that develops after the twentieth week of pregnancy. This syndrome probably presents a greater risk to the patient than PIH and affects 5 to 10 per cent of all pregnancies.[3] It is more likely to occur in women with a family history of preeclampsia, nulliparous women, patients under 18 or over 35 years of age, multiple gestation pregnancies, and in women with a past history of either pregnancy-induced or chronic hypertension. The proteinuria that occurs in this syndrome is one manifestation of a microvascular disease affecting multiple organ systems. It is crucial to identify patients in this category as early as possible in the course of the disease because of the marked increase in risk of morbidity for both the mother and infant. Because preeclampsia is not always easy to separate on clinical grounds from other types of hypertension, researchers have looked for laboratory tests that may be helpful in identifying preeclamptic patients. Commonly used tests are:

1. A rising or elevated uric acid level (nonpregnant: 4.1 $\pm$ 1.2 mg/dl; normotensive: 5.4 $\pm$ 1.2 mg/dl; and preeclampsia: 6.4 $\pm$ 1.0 mg/dl);[4]
2. A rising or elevated blood urea nitrogen (normotensive: 9.2 $\pm$ 2.4 mg/dl versus preeclamptic patients: 12.2 $\pm$ 3.9 mg/dl);[4]
3. Elevated serum liver transaminase levels (AST, ALT) in severe cases;
4. A rising hematocrit (secondary to hemoconcentration);
5. A falling or depressed platelet count;
6. Peripheral smear changes suggesting microvascular hemolysis; and
7. Changes in fibrinogen and fibrin split products consistent with consumptive coagulopathy.

Chronic hypertension. The pregnant patient should be considered to have chronic hypertension under the following conditions:

1. Hypertension discovered prior to the twentieth week in the absence of trophoblastic disease;
2. Hypertension at any stage of pregnancy in patients known previously to have hypertension; and
3. Hypertension that persists for greater than 6 weeks following delivery.

Although the perinatal outcome of patients with chronic hypertension is less favorable than that of the normotensive population, it is now believed that this increase in morbidity and mortality is due almost entirely to an increased incidence of superimposed PIH in patients with chronic hypertension. Hypertensive women whose gestations are not complicated by superimposed PIH are now believed to have an outcome similar to that of normotensive patients.[5] Once the patient has been categorized as having chronic hypertension, the primary task is to observe the patient carefully for worsening hypertension and proteinuria, which may indicate the develop of superimposed PIH.

Chronic hypertension with superimposed pregnancy-induced hypertension. Patients with chronic hypertension have a three- to sevenfold increased risk of developing superimposed PIH. The diagnosis is based on the development of proteinuria, edema, and worsening hypertension after the twentieth week of pregnancy in a patient with chronic hypertension. This condition results in a marked increase in the risk of intrauterine growth retardation, prematurity, and perinatal mortality. Indeed, this syndrome probably presents the greatest risk to both mother and infant of the five diagnostic categories discussed in this chapter.

Unclassifiable hypertension. Often women display elevated blood pressure or proteinuria or both for the first time after the twentieth week of pregnancy and there are no previous data to sort out whether the patient has pregnancy-induced or chronic hypertension. Although laboratory data, as discussed, may be of assistance, it is not always possible to classify patients confidently. Accurate classification is sometimes not possible until the postpartum period, when chronic hypertension will persist past the sixth week after delivery and PIH will not.

■ Management

Several management principles pertain to all the hypertensive disorders of pregnancy. First, because of the importance of early identification, early and regular prenatal care is of great importance. Second, because of the importance of accurate classification, great effort should be made to obtain medical records that contain prepregnancy blood pressure levels and information about complications in previous pregnancies. Third, the greatest risk to both mother and baby is presented by the microvascular complications of PIH and not the hypertension itself. It is more important to assess and treat these complications carefully than to focus excessively on blood pressure control. There is little evidence at this time that these complications can be prevented by control of blood pressure. What follows is discussion of an appropriate management plan once patients have been accurately assigned to the appropriate diagnostic category (Table 1).

■ Pregnancy-Induced Hypertension

The definitive treatment of PIH, with or without proteinuria, is delivery of the fetus. Unfortunately, this syndrome often presents before the fetus is sufficiently mature to be safely delivered. The management of such a patient involves a careful comparison of the risks to mother and fetus of the complications of PIH compared with the risk of early delivery. To the fetus, the risk associated with early delivery is related to fetal maturity. To the mother, the risk of early delivery is the increased chance of requiring cesarean section delivery if labor is induced.

These risks of early delivery must be weighed against a careful assessment of the risk of PIH. To understand this risk, it is useful to separate pregnancy-induced hypertension into mild and severe cases.

Severe pregnancy-induced hypertension. Pregnancy-induced hypertension should be considered severe when one or more of the following are present:

1. Blood pressure elevation greater than 160/110 mm Hg on two occasions at least 6 hours apart while patient is at bed rest;
2. Proteinuria exceeding 5 gm/24 hr;
3. 24-hour urine output less than 400 ml;
4. Pulmonary edema;
5. Marked visual disturbance, headache, or altered consciousness;
6. Thrombocytopenia or coagulopathy; or
7. Abnormal liver function studies.

The fetuses of all women who have severe PIH should be immediately assessed for maturity. If mature, steps should be taken to deliver the infant promptly.

Because of the risks of life-threatening complications, ranging from seizures (eclampsia) to disseminated intravascular coagulation, all patients with severe PIH should be hospitalized. The decision of when to induce labor when patients do not yet have a mature fetus is difficult and multifactorial and is best accomplished by a team of physicians, including the patient's family physician, a perinatologist or other obstetrician who is experienced in managing high-risk pregnancies, and a neonatolo-

TABLE 1. Management Plan for Hypertension in Pregnancy

Diagnostic Category	**Fetus Mature**	**Fetus Premature**
Severe PIH with or without proteinuria	Hospitalize MgSO$_4$ Control BP Deliver infant immediately	Hospitalize Control BP Observe for complications MgSO$_4$ Deliver infant
Mild PIH with or without proteinuria	Hospitalize MgSO$_4$ Deliver infant	Manage at bed rest until fetus matures **OR** PIH worsens **OR** signs of fetal distress develop
Chronic hypertension	Deliver infant	Assess fetal growth and well-being Observe closely for superimposed PIH
Chronic hypertension with superimposed PIH	Same as severe PIH	Same as severe PIH
Unclassified hypertension	Same as chronic HTN	Same as chronic HTN

gist or other pediatrician who is adept in managing premature infants. In general, immediate delivery is recommended if the patient develops pulmonary edema, worsening coagulopathy, evidence of central nervous system dysfunction, seizures, or blood pressure elevations exceeding 200/140 mm Hg in spite of antihypertensive measures. Similarly, if ultrasound and fetal heart monitor assessments indicate deterioration of fetal growth or well-being, immediate delivery is recommended.

In the absence of these ominous signs of impending maternal or fetal complications, delivery may be delayed for a period of days to allow steps, such as the administration of steroids, that may enhance fetal lung maturity. Antihypertensive agents should be used with great care in these patients. Excessive decrease in the blood pressure, even to levels that are usually considered in the normal range, may precipitate a reduction in placental perfusion and impair fetal well-being. Most authorities recommend the institution of agents to lower the blood pressure when the mean arterial pressure rises above 130 mm Hg or the diastolic pressure is consistently greater than 110. The preferred agent is 5 mg of intravenous hydralazine given very slowly. The blood pressure should be recorded at 5- to 10-minute intervals, and additional hydralazine should be given if the blood pressure has not been reduced to an appropriate level within 30 minutes. There is little benefit in instituting oral antihypertensive therapy in patients with severe PIH, and most authorities recommend against attempting to prolong pregnancy by controlling the pressure. Hydraliazine is recommended because of extensive experience with this medication in this clinical setting and data to indicate that placental perfusion actually may increase with this agent. Recently, several other classes of medication have been used, including sodium nitroprusside, angiotensin-converting enzyme inhibitors such as captopril or enalapril, beta-blockers, and diazoxide.

Because of the risk of seizures (eclampsia), and because this complication most often occurs during labor, all laboring patients with PIH should receive prophylactic therapy with magnesium sulfate (MgSO$_4$). This agent has been shown conclusively to decrease the incidence of seizures complicating PIH. Magnesium sulfate can be administered by either an intramuscular or an intravenous route. Intramuscular treatment involves administration of 10 ml of a 50 per cent solution injected deeply into each buttock. This 10-gm loading dose generally causes the serum magnesium level to increase to a concentration of between 3.5 and 6 mEq/L. The serum magnesium level usually returns to the pretreatment level over approximately 6 hours, and thus it is recommended that the doses be repeated at 5 gm every 4 hours. Intravenous magnesium sulfate is usually administered as a 4-gm loading dose followed by an infusion of 2 gm/hr.[6] Patients being treated with magnesium sulfate should be carefully observed for signs of toxicity. These appear at magnesium levels exceeding 7 mEq/L. Clinically, these signs may include disappearance of deep tendon reflexes, followed by respiratory depression and respiratory arrest, therefore careful observation of changes in these reflexes is recommended. Because the risk of seizures extends past the time of delivery, magnesium sulfate should be continued for 24 hours after delivery of the fetus.

Mild pregnancy-induced hypertension. Patients who have PIH with or without proteinuria are considered to have mild PIH if they do not satisfy the aforementioned criteria for severe disease. Again, delivery of the fetus is the treatment of choice if it is mature enough. The management of this clinical situation is sometimes frustrating when the patient's cervix is not favorable for the induction of labor. As long as the patient's PIH continues to be mild, blood pressure declines to an acceptable range at bed rest, and monitoring reveals adequate fetal growth and well-being, these patients may be closely observed to allow time for the cervix to ripen.

Mild PIH that occurs prior to fetal maturity is best managed with careful observation and bed rest. Approximately 80 per cent of such patients will become normotensive at bed rest. Some authorities have recommended low-dose beta-blocker therapy for patients in this group and argue that while bed rest is useful to lower the blood pressure, it is not associated with improvement in outcome of the pregnancy.[2] Because the incidence of adverse outcomes from PIH has decreased to 0.8 per 1000 pregnancies during the past 25 years, any clinical trial to assess improvement in outcome with antihypertensive therapy will require very large numbers of patients in both the treatment and control groups.[1] It is unlikely, therefore, that any definitive information regarding the utility of antihypertensive medication in these patients will be forthcoming in the foreseeable future. The current recommendation is to observe these patients carefully at bed rest until either the fetus reaches maturity or the disease becomes severe.

Chronic Hypertension

The management of chronic hypertension in a pregnant patient also has been a controversial topic. The increased incidence of poor perinatal outcome in these patients appears to depend primarily on the increased susceptibility of this population to superimposed PIH. As many as one third of patients with chronic hypertension will develop superimposed preeclampsia.[7] In the two thirds who do not, the incidence of maternal and fetal complications is not dramatically higher than in normotensive populations.[5] The management of pregnant women with chronic hypertension, therefore, is based on the following four principles:

1. Careful and meticulous observation for the development of superimposed preeclampsia should begin at 20 weeks' gestation.
2. Women who are on medication for the treatment of hypertension at the onset of pregnancy should be maintained on their antihypertensive medication unless their blood pressures fall into a clearly normotensive range and remains there as medications are tapered and stopped.
3. Women with chronic hypertension who are not on medication should be assessed for the need to start therapy. Investigators generally agree that patients with diastolic blood pressures of less than 90 mm Hg do not require antihypertensive therapy and that women with diastolic pressures greater than 110 mm Hg should receive antihypertensive medication. If the diastolic pressure is between 90 and 110 mm Hg, the use of antihypertensive medication is controversial. Most authorities seem to recommend the initiation of medication when blood pressure exceeds 160/100 mm Hg. The

most widely used antihypertensive medications in pregnancy are methyldopa and beta-blockers. Methyldopa has been used the longest and therefore has the most reassuring safety record. Beta-blockers have the advantage of fewer maternal side effects. Both types of medications seem to be effective and safe in pregnancy.[8]

Nifedipine has recently been used in pregnant patients with chronic hypertension, and it appears to be safe and effective. Because the clinical experience with this medication is less extensive, it seems appropriate at present to use this agent as a second choice when more commonly used medications are not effective.

Diuretics have long been controversial in the management of hypertension in pregnancy. Women who are taking thiazide diuretics do not demonstrate the normal amount of volume expansion with the onset of pregnancy. However, pregnancy outcome does not seem to be adversely affected. It is usually recommended to continue diuretic therapy in women who were receiving the medication prior to pregnancy, assuming antihypertensive therapy continues to be necessary. There is no role for the use of diuretics in managing edema in pregnant patients.

4. The fourth principle of managing chronic hypertension in pregnancy is to document evidence of adequate fetal growth and well-being during the third trimester. This can best be accomplished by regular fetal nonstress testing and ultrasound assessment of fetal growth beginning around 32 weeks' gestation. Evidence of poor fetal growth or well-being may be an indication for early delivery even in the absence of superimposed PIH.

Chronic Hypertension with Superimposed Pregnancy-Induced Hypertension

In spite of therapy, there is a three- to sevenfold increase in PIH in patients with chronic hypertension. These patients should be carefully observed, particularly during the second half of pregnancy, for the development of proteinuria, which may be the earliest sign of this condition. The early recognition of this complication requires meticulous attention to prenatal care in these patients. At highest risk are patients who have chronically impaired kidney function. Perinatal mortality may be as high as 40 to 80 per cent, depending on the degree of renal impairment. Severe pregnancy-induced hypertension superimposed on chronic hypertension is also associated with a 70 per cent risk of recurrence in future pregnancies. The risk of adverse maternal and fetal outcome in such patients is so high that some authorities recommend counseling against future pregnancies.[6]

The management of superimposed PIH is essentially the same as the management of severe PIH discussed earlier. The primary difference to the patient lies in the risk of recurrence of PIH in future pregnancies, which is much higher in patients with superimposed disease.

■ Unclassified Hypertension

Patients with hypertension that cannot be classified may be the most difficult to manage, since the assignment of risk depends on differentiating chronic hypertension and PIH. Very careful assessment of these patients during the course of the pregnancy often will allow assignment to another category, but in some situations final differentiation will not be possible until the postpartum period, in which pregnancy-induced hypertension will tend to resolve by the sixth postpartum week.

■ Issues and Risks

■ Anesthesia in the Hypertensive Pregnant Patient

Two primary issues have received attention in the anesthesia literature regarding the management of pregnant patients with hypertension in labor and delivery. Since most investigators suggest that severe PIH is associated with a cesarean section rate approaching 50 per cent,[9] several studies have addressed the appropriate agents to be used for general anesthesia in these patients. A particular concern is the marked elevation of systolic blood pressure during intubation, which may place the patient with severe PIH at risk of intracranial bleeding. Some authorities suggest a supplementation of the usual technique of induction and recommend the use of central venous pressure or arterial lines or both to monitor these patients.[10]

The use of lumbar epidural anesthesia during labor also has been a source of some controversy. Since patients with severe PIH are often volume contracted, the administration of lumbar epidural anesthesia without adequate hydration may precipitate a hypotensive episode. Controlled studies that have examined the use of epidural anesthesia in patients who have been adequately hydrated suggest that the risk of this form of anesthesia is acceptable for these patients.[11,12]

■ Low-Dose Aspirin in Pregnancy-Induced Hypertension

Although the etiology of PIH remains unknown, the potential role of prostaglandins has received much attention.[13] Of particular interest is the ratio of thromboxane A_2 to prostacyclin in normal and preeclampic pregnancies. Several studies have noted that low-dose aspirin (60 to 150 mg/day) affects this ratio in a way that may be favorable. In some studies, low-dose aspirin used early and throughout pregnancy has been shown to decrease the incidence of preeclampsia. While these data are not yet sufficient to warrant preventive therapy in all or most pregnant women, some patients who are at high risk for PIH may warrant treatment with low-dose aspirin, since the risk of treatment appears small.

■ Calcium Supplementation in Preeclampsia

Epidemiologic evidence and some preliminary clinical research suggests an inverse relationship between calcium intake and hypertension in the pregnant and nonpregnant state.[14] Although these data are not sufficient to recommend routine calcium supplementation, they do underscore the importance of adequate dietary calcium and may represent an important area for future research.

REFERENCES

1. Kincaid-Smith P. The management of hypertensive disorders of pregnancy. Aust NZ J Med 1987; 17:187–188.
2. Rubin PC. Hypertension in pregnancy. J HTN 1987; 5(suppl 3):S57–S60.
3. Lindheimer MD, Katz AI. Hypertension in pregnancy. N Engl J Med 1985; 313(11):675–680.
4. Goldkrand JW, Fuentes AM. The relation of angiotensin-converting enzyme to the pregnancy-induced hypertension–preeclampsia syndrome. Am J Obstet Gynecol 1986; 154(4):792–799.
5. Redman CW. Therapy of non-preeclamptic hypertension in pregnancy. Am J Kidney Dis 1987; 9(4):324–327.
6. Worley JR. Pregnancy-induced hypertension. *In* Danforth DW, Scott JR (eds). Obstetrics and Gynecology. 5th ed. Philadelphia: JB Lippincott, 1986:446–466.
7. Mabie WC, Pernoll ML, Biswas MK. Chronic hypertension in pregnancy. Obstet Gynecol 1986; 67(2):197–205.
8. Doany W, Brinkman CR. Antihypertensive drugs in pregnancy. Clin Perinatol 1987; 14(4):783–805.
9. Lawes EG, Downing JW, Duncan PW, Bland B, Lavies N, Gane GA. Fentanyl-droperidol supplementation of rapid sequence induction in the presence of severe pregnancy-induced and pregnancy-aggravated hypertension. Br J Anaesthesiol 1987; 59:1381–1391.
10. Reti LL, Ross A, Kloss M, Paull J, Markman L. The management of severe preeclampsia with intravenous magnesium sulphate, hydralazine and central venous catheterization. Aust NZ J Obstet Gynaecol 1987; 27:102–105.
11. Ramanathan J, Bottorff M, Jeter JN, Khalil M, Sibai BM. The pharmacokinetics and maternal and neonatal effects of epidural lidocaine in preeclampsia. Anesth Analg 1986; 65:120–126.
12. Newsome LR, Bramwell RS, Curling PE. Severe preeclampsia: hemodynamic effects of lumbar epidural anesthesia. Anesth Analg 1986; 65:31–36.
13. Freidman SA. Preeclampsia: a review of the role of prostaglandins. Obstet Gynecol 1988; 71:122–137.
14. Belizan JM, Villar J, Repke J. The relationship between calcium intake and pregnancy-induced hypertension: up-to-date evidence. Am J Obstet Gynecol 1988; 158:898–902.

Hypertension, refractory

Gregory A. Kozeny ■ *Richard F. Afable*

■ Background

Refractory hypertension means different things to different people. Some physicians consider any persistent blood pressure elevation that has not been adequately controlled by the drug or drugs they have prescribed as resistant hypertension. Similarly, many patients are labeled as refractory hypertensive because they have failed to respond or could not tolerate a series of antihypertensive drugs prescribed sequentially as monotherapy. Here we will discuss true resistant hypertension, which has been defined by Gifford[1] as follows:

Provided that adherence to the regimen can be assured, hypertension should be considered resistant if the blood pressure cannot be reduced to < 150/100 mm Hg by a rational triple drug regimen, including a diuretic prescribed in nearly maximal doses and if the pretreatment blood pressure was ≥180/115 mm Hg. If the pretreatment blood pressure was <180/115 mm Hg, resistance should be defined as failure to achieve normotension (<140/90 mm Hg) on a rational triple drug regimen in nearly maximal doses.

For elderly patients with isolated systolic hypertension, resistance in an adherent patient is defined as failure of a rational triple drug regimen to reduce the systolic blood pressure to <170 mm Hg if pretreatment systolic blood pressure was >200 mm Hg or to <160 mm Hg and by at least 10 mm Hg if pretreatment systolic blood pressure was 160 to 200 mm Hg.

This definition is used because it provides guidelines for the appropriateness of workups and referrals and for more precise communication between physicians. This definition of resistant hypertension excludes patients who fail serial monotherapies. It is important to remember that most patients with moderate-to-severe hypertension and up to 30 per cent of patients with mild hypertension are not adequately controlled with single drug therapy.[2] Also, it is empha-

TABLE 1. Questions to Ask in the Management of Refractory Hypertension

1. Does the patient have "true resistant hypertension" only failed to respond to a series of antihypertensive drugs prescribed as monotherapy?
2. Is the patient compliant?
3. Does the patient have pseudohypertension?
4. Does the patient have "office" hypertension?
5. Does the patient have secondary hypertension?
6. Are there any possible drug-drug or drug-lifestyle interactions?
7. Is the present drug regimen rational and are doses adequate?
8. Does the patient have hemodynamic factors that play a role in the refractory nature of the hypertension?

sized that malignant hypertension is not synonymous with resistant hypertension.

In dealing with a patient whose blood pressure is not responding to therapy, the physician must address a number of issues before deciding on alternative therapies. Table 1 lists eight questions that should be asked in all patients with refractory hypertension. The first question simply reminds one of the definition of resistant hypertension and that monotherapy does not work for all hypertensive patients. The following seven questions are more difficult to answer but provide insight into the problem of the refractory hypertensive patient.

■ IS THE PATIENT COMPLIANT?

Noncompliance is a difficult problem to evaluate. Clinical studies have estimated noncompliance as high as 50 per cent in taking medication and 20 to 50 per cent in keeping appointments. Factors most often cited as contributing significantly to noncompliance are (1) the patient-physician relationship, (2) drug side effects, (3) expense of the medication, (4) the number of different drugs as well as how often a drug is to be taken a day, (5) the amount and type of support a patient gets from the environment, and (6) the patient's perception of the severity of the illness.

To deal with noncompliance, a physician first must recognize which patients are noncompliant and why they are noncomplaint.

There are two ways to find out whether a patient is noncompliant. The first is to look for subtle but objective clues. Is the serum uric acid level elevated and the potassium level depressed in patients on thiazide diuretics? Is the pulse rate less than 80 beats/min in patients on a beta-blocker? Does the patient request prescription refills at appropriate time intervals? The second way is to ask the patient, in a nonjudgmental, nonconfrontational way whether he or she has been taking the medication. Using this approach, Haynes and associates reported a 75 per cent agreement rate between self-reported compliance, pill counts, and blood pressure response to therapy.[3] Patient age and the level of health knowledge do not appear to correlate with compliance, although younger patients tend to be more likely to discontinue their medication than are older ones.

It is just as hard to tell why patients do not follow a therapeutic regimen as it is to tell who is the noncompliant patient. Expense is clearly an issue in the poor and elderly patient. Patients cannot be expected to comply with medical therapy, no matter how successful, that they cannot afford. The complexity of antihypertensive therapy also inversely relates to drug compliance. The number of times a day a medication must be taken, as well as the number of different types of drugs prescribed, will affect compliance.

A number of excellent reviews of techniques to improve patient compliance are available.[2] In general, the two most successful features of any program to improve compliance are (1) the level of attention paid to the patient and the family by the physician, and (2) the extent to which compliance is reinforced, rewarded, or encouraged. Kaplan summarized a number of specific techniques that can help improve compliance:[2]

- encouraging family support
- providing feedback of patient's blood pressure response, either directly by home blood pressure monitoring or by the physician
- involving patient in the medical decision-making process
- giving patients verbal as well as written information about their medication, as well as instructions on how often to take it
- attempting to use the fewest daily doses of drugs needed and appropriate use of combination tablets

- keeping the hypertensive care as inexpensive as possible
- anticipating medication side effects and adjusting therapy to ameliorate side effects that do not spontaneously disappear
- educating the patient about the goals of therapy as well as the tangible rewards of lowered blood pressure

Side effects account for 10 to 15 per cent of patients who discontinue drug therapy. Multiple drug regimens should be selected so that side effects are not additive. For instance, the combination of captopril and hydrochlorothiazide significantly blunts the metabolic alterations seen when either drug is used alone.

DOES THE PATIENT HAVE "PSEUDOHYPERTENSION"?

Pseudohypertension occurs primarily in the elderly patient population with systolic hypertension. Medial sclerosis of the brachial arteries leads to spuriously high systolic blood pressure readings when determined with a sphygmomanometer cuff, because the calcified, rigid arteries are very difficult to compress. Patients with pseudohypertension have no signs of organ damage because of sustained elevation of blood pressure. Thus, an elderly patient with chronic systolic blood pressures of greater than 190 mm Hg but without left ventricular hypertrophy on electrocardiogram and the absence of hypertensive retinopathy should be considered to have pseudohypertension. The diagnosis can be suggested on physical examination by performing Osler's maneuver.[4] Osler's maneuver is the ability to palpate the radial artery between heart beats and after a sphygmomanometer cuff has been inflated high enough to compress the brachial artery. In patients with pseudohypertension, the intra-arterial pressure as measured with an intra-arterial cannula connected to a pressure transducer is normal, so no antihypertensive therapy is needed.

DOES THE PATIENT HAVE "WHITE COAT" HYPERTENSION?

Office or white coat hypertension has been recognized as a clinically relevant entity in the past few years.[5,6] Office hypertension applies to a small group of patients who have no evidence of end-organ damage as a consequence of their hypertension and have normal home blood pressure readings but consistently high office blood pressure readings.

The cause of this phenomenon is still unknown. White coat hypertension seems to be more common in women than in men. Anxiety associated with an unfamilar environment and the classic defense reaction involved in the stress of a visit to a physician's office are the most obvious explanations for this syndrome. Some investigators have even postulated that office hypertension is a conditioned response—that in certain individuals the initial blood pressure is high due to anxiety. Telling these individuals that their blood pressure is high and needs to be rechecked reinforces the pressor response for the next visit.

Home blood pressures correlate better with funduscopic changes and with left ventricular hypertrophy than do office blood pressures in this group of patients. Pickering has suggested that all patients with resistant hypertension and absence of target organ damage undergo home blood pressure monitoring.[7] If a discrepancy is found between office and home blood pressure readings, the physician should use the home readings to adjust antihypertensive therapy. If home blood pressure readings are to be used to guide therapy, the physician must check the accuracy of the blood pressure measuring device and the patient's technique for measuring his or her own blood pressure routinely. Ambulatory blood pressure monitoring also should be employed periodically in these patients, to ensure that the patient has been accurately reporting the data.

DOES THE PATIENT HAVE A SECONDARY FORM OF HYPERTENSION?

It is not uncommon for a patient whose blood pressure has been reasonably well controlled to develop resistant hypertension. Acquired resistance to drug therapy suggests the development of a secondary form of hypertension, such as renovascular hypertension. All patients with resistant hypertension should be evaluated for secondary hypertension. Bravo and associates reported that 30 per cent of the patients originally referred to the Cleveland Clinic for resistant hypertension were ultimately found to have a form of secondary hypertension.[8] Patients should be evaluated for renovascular disease, primary aldosteronism, pheochromocytoma, and renal insufficiency. Acquired resistance to a previously successful regimen in patients over the age of 55 years is so often associated with renovascular disease that most, if not all, patients should undergo renal arteriogram. In patients with renal artery stenosis and refractory hypertension, renal revascularization or angioplasty may be the only way to reduce the blood pressure.

Levels of plasma catecholamines and urinary metanephrines, normetanephrine (free catecholamines), and vanillylmandelic acid should be determined to rule out pheochromocytoma. Determinations of serum renin activity and aldosterone level following high- and low-sodium diets or an aldosterone suppression test should be done to exclude primary aldosteronism.

ARE DRUG-DRUG OR DRUG-ENVIRONMENT INTERACTIONS DECREASING DRUG EFFECTIVENESS?

Physicians treating hypertension should be aware of the drugs that interfere with the action of antihypertensive medication. Table 2 lists many of the more common drug interactions that may lead to resistant hypertension.

As will be discussed later, the combination of various antihypertensive drugs without adequate salt restriction and diuretic therapy will lead to excessive volume expansion. This drug-induced sodium retention will present clinically as edema and refractory hypertension.

Besides drug-drug interaction, drug-lifestyle interactions can cause refractory hypertension. Alcohol consumption, cigarette smoking, a high sodium diet, and obesity all can blunt the antihypertensive effect of many drugs.

IS THE PRESENT DRUG REGIMEN RATIONAL AND ARE THE DOSES ADEQUATE?

As discussed earlier, refractory hypertension refers to the inability of triple-drug therapy to normalize blood pressure. The doses of all three medications should be maximal or near-maximal. If the doses are appropriate, one must make sure the antihypertensive agents work synergistically to lower blood pressure. For instance, the use of various vasodilators without a diuretic will lead to increased renal sodium and water reabsorption, volume expansion, and the development of pseudotolerance.

TABLE 2. Common Drugs That Can Adversely Interact with Antihypertensive Agents

Drug	Mechanism of Interaction
Nonsteroidal anti-inflammatory agents	Antagonize effects of all antihypertensive drugs by cyclo-oxygenase inhibition and inducing sodium avidity
Phenylpropanolamine, nasal decongestants, cocaine, chlorpromazine, tricyclic antidepressants	Sympathomimetic (like amphetamine and ephedrine), causes increased systemic vascular resistance, which limits the response to all antihypertensive agents
Cholestyramine	Inhibits gut absorption of thiazides
Rifampin	Induces hepatic enzymes, thus increase propranolol clearance by 2- to 3-fold
Cimetidine	Inhibits hepatic enzymes, so decreases propranolol clearance by 50%
Nicotine (cigarette smoking)	Can induce hepatic enzymes and increase clearance of propranolol
Alcohol	Lessens antihypertensive effect of most drugs
Increased dietary sodium	Causes volume expansion and can blunt action of any antihypertensive drug
Oral contraceptives	Sodium retention, mild volume expansion, may increase sympathetic nervous system activity; may alter renin-angiotensin-aldosterone axis by increasing renin substrate
Corticosteroids	Sodium retention and volume expansion

In general, triple-drug therapy should include initially: (1) a diuretic (use a thiazide diuretic if the serum creatinine level is less than 2.0 mg/dl and a loop diuretic if the serum creatinine level is over 2.0 mg/dl); (2) an angiotensin-converting enzyme (ACE) inhibitor or calcium channel blocker or beta-blocker; and (3) hydralazine or minoxidil or one of the other agents listed earlier.

As can be seen in Table 3, each class of antihypertensive drugs induces a hemodynamic counterregulatory response that tends to negate the drug's effect. Thus combinations of drugs that act synergistically must be used. Successful triple therapies that have been studied and shown to be effective include a diuretic (the equivalent of 50 mg of hydrochlorothiazide if the serum creatinine level is less than 2.0 mg/dl, or furosemide, up to 240 mg/day) plus two of the following agents:

(1) A direct vasodilator (e.g., hydralazine, 300 mg/day or minoxidil, 20 mg/day).
(2) A beta-blocker (equivalent to 100 mg of atenolol/day).
(3) An ACE inhibitor (e.g., captopril, 150 mg daily in divided doses, or enalapril, 40 mg daily).
(4) Calcium channel blockers (e.g., verapamil SR, 240 mg twice a day; nifedipine, 20 mg four times a day; or diltiazem, 120 mg three times a day).
(5) Clonidine, 1 mg daily in divided doses.
(6) An alpha-blocker (e.g., prazosin, 20 mg daily in divided doses).

It is important that drug therapy be started and the doses increased in a stepwise fashion, as indicated by the report of the 1988 Joint National Committee on hypertension.[9]

◼ DOES THE PATIENT HAVE HEMODYNAMIC FACTORS THAT PLAY A ROLE IN RESISTANT HYPERTENSION?

Sodium intake, extracellular fluid volume, renal insufficiency or failure, or alterations in cardiac output or cardiogenic reflexes may perpetuate hypertension. These hemodynamic, renal, and cardiac factors can occur as part of the counterregulatory processes just discussed or as a consequence of a chronic disease. If any of these factors exist in a patient with resistant hypertension, the current drug regimen must be modified or an additional drug added to counteract these factors. Antihypertensive drugs must be selected that negate whatever hemodynamic, cardiac, or renal factors are operative.

The correlation between sodium intake and hypertension is well known. There is considerable evidence to support dietary sodium restriction as an important element in successful treatment of hypertension. Excessive sodium intake can counteract the blood pressure–lowering effects of all antihypertensive agents. Implementation of a low sodium diet may cause a reduction of blood pressure in some patients with resistant hypertension. Beard and associates have shown that the combination of salt restriction and diuretics was superior to either therapy alone.[10]

Closely tied to sodium intake is the size of the extracellular fluid volume as a factor in promoting drug resistance. Chronic administration of many antihypertensive agents, particularly the direct vasodilators, is associated with sodium and water retention, which may lead to drug tolerance. Finnerty has demonstrated that 89 per cent of 73 patients with refractory hypertension who

TABLE 3. Counterregulatory Mechanisms Activated by Antihypertensive Drugs Leading to Decreased Drug Effectiveness

Class	Sympathetic Tone	Peripheral Resistance	Cardiac Output	Angiotensin II	Sodium Avidity
Diuretics	↑	↑	↓	↑	↓
β-Blockers	↓	↑	↓	↓	↑
Central agents	↓	↓	—	↓	↑
ACE inhibitors	—	↓	↑	↓	—
Calcium blockers	—	↓	variable	↑	variable
Alpha-blockers	↓	↓	—	—	—

↑, Increased; ↓, decreased; —, no change.

were on multiple drugs had significant improvement in their blood pressures following a reduction in body weight and extracellular volume.[11,12] These findings were confirmed by Dustan and associates, who showed that intensified diuretic therapy to reduce plasma volume below normal was associated with near-normal blood pressure.[13] These studies emphasize the importance of volume control during antihypertensive therapy. It must be pointed out that these observations do not mean that the extracellular fluid volume is expanded in all patients with refractory hypertension; most patients have normal plasma and extracellular fluid volumes.

Renal insufficiency is commonly associated with the development of hypertension or resistance to antihypertensive regimens. In fact, hypertension is present in almost 100 per cent of patients with renal dysfunction, regardless of the type of renal disease present. Kidney disease can affect blood pressure by (1) expansion of the plasma and extracellular fluid volume; (2) loss of effectiveness of thiazide diuretics as the serum creatinine level rises above 2.0 mg/dl; (3) an increase in cardiac output early in the course of renal parenchymal disease, followed by a rise in peripheral vascular resistance as renal failure progresses; (4) lack of norepinephrine or renin responsiveness induced by uremia; and (5) inappropriate relationship between the renin-angiotensin system and sodium and volume retention. The development of renal dysfunction as a consequence of renovascular hypertension is not uncommon. In one series, renovascular hypertension with renal insufficiency was found in 32 per cent of 76 white patients and 47 per cent of 47 black patients with severe or refractory hypertension.[14]

As mentioned earlier, the blood pressure may not become normal in patients with resistant hypertension who are found to have renal artery stenosis until renal perfusion is improved. Angiotensin-converting enzyme inhibitors, like captopril, may be successful in lowering blood pressure in many patients with renovascular disease. Functional acute renal failure has been reported to occur in 8 per cent of patients with unilateral disease and in as many as 20 per cent of patients with bilateral renovascular disease treated with ACE inhibitors. The risk of reversible renal failure induced by ACE inhibitors can be minimized if the amount of the diuretic used is substantially decreased. Table 4 lists the antihypertensive drugs that have been found to be consistently effective in patients with abnormal renal function.

The heart also may interfere with blood pressure control. Cardiac causes of resistant hypertension are antihypertensive therapy inducing either an increase in cardiac output or initiation of cardiogenic pressor reflexes. High cardiac output associated with a reduction in peripheral resistance (as seen with vasodilator therapy) causes an increased blood pressure only if the change in cardiac output is larger than the fall in afterload. For example, minoxidil causes a reduction in arteriolar resistance without an associated venodilatation. This causes a decreased afterload but an increased preload. The net effect of this selective drop in arteriolar resistance is a reflex stimulation of sympathetic activity leading to a significant rise in cardiac output. This may be large enough to offset the reduction in total peripheral resistance, and so blood pressure remains unchanged. The reflex activation of the sympathetic nervous system also increases the renin-angiotensin-aldosterone system. The addition of a beta-blocker to minoxidil or hydralazine therapy can normalize cardiac output, leading to a dramatic fall in blood pressure.

Many investigators have postulated that the abnormal left ventricular diastolic function found in severe hypertension could be associated with abnormal cardiopulmonary pressor reflexes. Antihypertensive agents that either reduce left ventricular hypertrophy (Table 5) or improve diastolic function (like calcium channel blockers or β-blockers) may be beneficial.

Host-drug factors make one group of drugs more effective in specific patient groups. Patients with chronic renal parenchymal dis-

TABLE 4. Drugs Particularly Useful in Renal Disease–Associated Hypertension

Class	Examples
ACE inhibitors	Captopril
β-Blockers	Propranolol, labetalol
Direct vasodilators	Minoxidil
Central-acting agents	Clonidine
Loop diuretics	Furosemide
Calcium blockers	Nifedipine

TABLE 5. Ability of Antihypertensive Drugs to Reverse Left Ventricular Hypertrophy in Humans

Proven Ability	Questionable Ability	No Ability
All β-blockers	Reserpine	Diuretic
Clonidine	Nifedipine	Minoxidil
Alpha-methyldopa	Verapamil	Hydralazine
Guanabenz	Prazosin	
Captopril		
Enalapril		

ease and creatinine clearances of less than 30 ml/min (serum creatinine level > 2.0 mg/dl) will have a poor response to thiazides but an excellent response to loop diuretics.

Older patients with predominately systolic hypertension tend to be less volume-dependent than younger patients, despite a low plasma renin level. Elderly patients also are more susceptible to orthostatic hypotension and diuretic-induced hyponatremia. A combination of calcium channel blocker, ACE inhibitor, and diuretics may be especially useful in elderly patients.

Young white patients usually are hyperdynamic and hyperadrenergic and have high renin hypertension. Angiotensin-converting enzyme inhibitors or beta-blockers are especially effective in this group. Obese and black hypertensive patients tend to have low renin hypertension and are extremely responsive to diuretics or calcium channel blockers or both. Recently, Williams and Hollenberg have identified a group of sodium-sensitive essential hypertensive patients who they termed "nonmodulators."[15,16] These patients have a defective ability to suppress renin and aldosterone in response to angiotensin II infusion and increased sodium intake. These individuals do not modulate the kidney's and adrenal gland's responsiveness to angiotensin II. As a result of these abnormalities, the nonmodulators fail to suppress renin activity and appropriately excrete a sodium load. The blood pressures of these patients are usually controlled when ACE inhibitors are included in their antihypertensive regimen. Another group of patients who show a unique responsiveness to ACE inhibitors are individuals with connective tissue diseases such as scleroderma.[17,18]

■ Therapy for Resistant Hypertension

After a remediable cause for resistant hypertension has been ruled out, the physician can choose to alter the patient's current antihypertensive regimen, add a fourth agent, or combine both options. Drug regimens proved effective in resistant hypertensive patients include

1. Diuretic, beta-blocker, hydralazine, and clonidine (the use of a beta-blocker and clonidine may cause marked central nervous system side effects);
2. Diuretic, angiotensin-converting enzyme inhibitor, and calcium channel blocker with or without minoxidil (the use of captopril, 25 mg every 6 hours, and nifedipine, 20 mg every 6 hours, in combination with a diuretic and minoxidil is one of the most potent antihypertensive combinations currently available);
3. Diuretic, angiotensin-converting enzyme inhibitor, minoxidil, and beta-blocker.

One must remember that the serum creatinine level is important on deciding which type of diuretic to use. Concomitant illness is an important factor in deciding which drugs to use. Asthmatics or patients with diabetes may not tolerate beta-blockers, whereas beta-blockers will be invaluable in individuals with angina. If at all possible, drug therapy should be chosen that effectively lowers blood pressure, prevents or limits end-organ damage, and has minimal side effects.

■ Conclusion

The most common causes for what appears to be resistant hypertension are poor compliance with diet or drug therapy and inadequate or inappropriate drug regimens. When all the questions asked in this chapter have been answered, and correction of remediable causes is unsuccessful in lowering blood pressure, it is appropriate to modify the antihypertensive therapy as outlined. This must be done after taking into account the patient's clinical status, concurrent illnesses, and any abnormal hemodynamic mechanism that may be operative in maintaining the hypertension. If the preceding measures are followed conscientiously, less than 1 per cent of hypertensive patients will have truly resistant hypertension.

REFERENCES

1. Gifford RW. Resistant hypertension: introduction and definitions. Hypertension 1988; 11(suppl II):1165–1166.
2. Kaplan NM. Treatment of hypertension: drug therapy. In Kaplan NM (ed). Clinical Hypertension. Baltimore: Williams & Wilkins, 1986:180–272.
3. Haynes RB, Taylor D, Sackett DL, Gibson ES, Bernholz CD, Mukherjee J. Can simple clinical measurements detect patient non-compliance? Hypertension 1980; 2:757–764.
4. Messerli FH, Ventura HO, Amodeo C. Osler's maneuver and pseudohypertension. N Engl J Med 1985; 312:1548–1551.
5. Pickering TG, James GD, Boddie C, et al. How common is white coat hypertension? JAMA 1988; 257(2):225–228.
6. Jeter CR, Bush JP, Porter JH. Situational anxiety and blood pressure lability in the physician's office. Clin Exp Hypertens 1988; 10(1):169–185.
7. Pickering TG. Blood pressure monitoring outside the office for the evaluation of patients with resistant hypertension. Hypertension 1988; 11(suppl II):II-96–II-100.
8. Bravo EL, Taraz RC, Dustan HP, et al. The changing spectrum of primary aldosteronism. Am J Med 1983; 74:641–651.
9. The Joint National Committee on the Detection, Evaluation and Treatment of High Blood Pressure. The 1988 report. Arch Intern Med 1988; 148(5):1023–1038.
10. Beard TC, Cooke HM, Gray WR, Barge R. Randomized controlled trial of no added sodium diet for mild hypertension. Lancet 1982; 2:455–458.
11. Finnerty FA. Relationship of extracellular fluid volume to the development of drug resistance in the hypertensive patient. Am Heart J 1971; 81:563–565.
12. Finnerty FA. Resistant hypertension. Compr Ther 1982; 8:53–59.
13. Dustan HP, Tarazi RC, Bravo EL. Dependence of arterial pressure on intravascular volume in treated hypertensive patients. N Engl J Med 1972; 286:861–866.
14. Davis BA, Crook JE, Vestal RE, Oates JA. Prevalence of renovascular hypertension in patients with grade 3 or 4 retinopathy. N Engl J Med 1979; 301:1273–1276.
15. Williams GH, Hollenberg NK. Are non-modulating patients with essential hypertension a distinct subgroup? Implications for therapy. Am J Med 1985; 79(suppl 3c):3–9.
16. Williams GH, Hollenberg NK. Non-modulating essential hypertension. A subset particularly responsive to converting enzyme inhibitors. J Hypertens 1985; 3(suppl 2);581–587.
17. Lopez-Overjero JA, Saal SD, D'Angelo WA, et al. Reversal of vascular and renal crisis of scleroderma by oral angiotensin converting enzyme blockade. N Engl J Med 1979; 300(suppl 25):1417–1419.
18. Becket VL, Donaldio JV, Brennan LA, et al. Use of captopril as early therapy for renal scleroderma: a prospective study. Mayo Clin Proc 1985; 60:763–771.

Hypertensive crisis

Robert A. Phillips ■ *David L. Garbowit* ■ *Lawrence R. Krakoff*

■ Background

A hypertensive crisis exists when elevated blood pressure is either causing or acutely aggravating end-organ damage to the heart, brain, kidneys, or vasculature. The diastolic blood pressure is usually greater than 120 mm Hg, but lower levels can be harmful in a previously normotensive individual whose blood pressure has risen acutely, and lower levels can aggravate heart failure, myocardial infarction, stroke, and subarachnoid hemorrhage. Although the etiology may be obscure, the diagnosis is usually obvious, ascertained from a rapid history, physical examination, and laboratory evaluation. Many drugs can lower severely elevated blood pressure successfully, regardless of the cause. Management is optimal, however, when therapy is based on the affected organs and directed toward alleviating a specific etiology. Therefore, the treating physician must be familiar with the causes, pathophysiology, and manifestations of various disorders that can cause an abrupt rise in blood pressure (Table 1) and must have a working knowledge of the newly available and useful older drugs for the treatment of these disorders.

■ Management

This section will begin with a discussion of the drugs that are currently used for the treatment of hypertensive crisis, followed by discussion of the specific entities responsible for hypertensive crisis. The decision on whether to use a parenteral or oral agent is somewhat arbitrary and is usually determined by the severity of the crisis and whether or not the patient will receive intensive care after initial evaluation. The onset of action of many oral drugs is similar to that of parenteral agents, and, with the exception of nitroprusside, the duration of action of commonly used parenteral drugs is similar to that of the oral agents.

TABLE 1. Clinical Conditions Causing a Hypertensive Crisis

Malignant or Accelerated Hypertension
 Diastolic pressure ≥ 130 mm Hg or evidence of
  rapid, recent increase
 Advanced retinopathy; retinal hypertensive
  hemorrhages and exudates (grade III) with or
  without papilledema (grade IV)
 Progressive renal insufficiency; increasing serum
  urea nitrogen and creatinine levels with
  proteinuria and hematuria

Hypertensive Encephalopathy

Pre-eclampsia/Eclampsia

Adrenergic Excess
 Pheochromocytoma
 Monoamine oxidase inhibitors and tyramine-
  containing foods
 Overdose of "diet pills" (amphetamines or
  phenylpropanolamine)
 Cocaine overdose
 Clonidine or alpha$_2$-receptor agonist withdrawal
  syndrome

**Cardiovascular and Neurologic Emergencies
Complicated by Hypertension**
 Myocardial infarction
 Unstable angina
 Pulmonary edema
 Aortic dissection or expanding abdominal
  aneurysm
 Cerebrovascular accident (hemorrhage or
  thromboembolism)

■ PARENTERAL DRUGS

Nitroprusside. Because of its efficacy, ease of titration, and negligible acute side effects, this direct-acting arteriolar and venodilator is often used in hypertensive crisis.[1] It is usually recommended that an intra-arterial line be placed before treatment begins, but several centers use automatic cuff blood pressure monitoring, with measurements taken every minute. The initial dose is 0.5 to 1.5 μg/kg/min and the maintenance dose is up to 10 μg/kg/min. Peak effects are achieved within minutes, and the duration of action is 3 to 5 minutes. A 20 per cent increase in heart rate is common. Thiocyanate levels of less than 10 mg/dl are well tolerated, but after infusions of 24 to 48 hours the risk of thiocyanate toxicity increases, the treatment of which is hemodialysis. Nitroprusside can be used in virtually all types of hypertensive crisis, and since it does not cause steal phenomena, it can be used when myocardial ischemia is a feature of the syndrome.

Labetalol. Labetalol is a combined alpha- and beta-adrenergic receptor peripheral antagonist, which as an intravenous drug has a reported ratio of 7:1 for beta:alpha antagonism. Labetalol's major advantage over nitroprusside is that it can be used without invasive monitoring, because rapid fluctuations in blood pressure do not usually occur.[2] Administration is by bolus injections starting, at a dose of 20 mg over 2 minutes. If a response is not seen, the dose can be doubled every 10 minutes to a total dose of 300 mg. The onset of action is within minutes, and the effects last for 4 to 6 hours. Labetalol may be particularly useful in patients with angina and in states of adrenergic excess, such as pheochromocytoma, in which combined alpha- and beta-blockade is necessary. Labetalol should be avoided if there is poor systolic left ventricular performance, a history of asthma, significant sinus bradycardia, or heart block greater than first-degree.

Phentolamine. This alpha-blocker is used in suspected pheochromocytoma or other hyperadrenergic state.[3] A test dose of 1 mg is given IV over 2 minutes, and, barring the occurrence of marked hypotension, another 4 mg can be infused over the next 5 minutes. If a hyperadrenergic state is the cause of the crisis, a marked drop in blood pressure should occur within minutes. Effects are short-lived, and blood pressure will begin to rise again within 10 minutes. Control of blood pressure is then achieved either with intermitent boluses or with a continuous drip; a patient with a pheochromocytoma may require 100 mg/hr. Because of reflex tachycardia, a beta-blocker is usually used after full alpha-blockade has been achieved.

Enalaprilat. Enalaprilat, an intravenous angiotensin-converting enzyme (ACE) inhibitor, is the active metabolite of enalapril. Its advantages over oral ACE inhibitors are faster onset of action, complete absorption, lack of sulfhydryl groups, and use in a patient who cannot swallow.[4] Enalaprilat is given as an intravenous infusion over 5 minutes, with onset of action within 5 minutes and peak within 30 minutes, although the peak can be delayed for up to 4 hours. The duration of action is dose dependent and can be up to 12 hours. The starting dose is 1.25 mg (1 ml of a 2 ml vial), increasing to 5 mg and then 10 mg if there is an inadequate response within 20 to 30 minutes. There is no evidence that doses higher than 10 mg are beneficial. Once the patient has responded, the appropriate dose is 10 mg given every 6 hours until the patient can be switched to an oral ACE inhibitor. Hypotension occurs relatively infrequently and can be treated with intravenous fluids. Congestive heart failure and suspected hyperreninemic states are situations in which the drug may be particularly useful, whereas hypotension might be encountered more often with prior diuretic and vasodilator treatment.

Hydralazine. This potent vasodilator acts directly on arterioles to decrease peripheral resistance. It is a second-line drug in the treatment of hypertensive crises, because its antihypertensive effect is mitigated by reflex sympathetic activity resulting in increases in renin, heart rate, and cardiac output.[5] If hydralazine is used, its action will be potentiated by administering it with a beta-blocker and possibly a diuretic. It is used frequently in pre-eclampsia/eclampsia because of lack of toxicity to the fetus. One advantage hydralazine offers is that it can be given intramuscularly, which is helpful if venous access is difficult to obtain. The initial dose is 10 to 20 mg IV (onset of action in 10 minutes) or 10 to 50 mg IM (onset of action in 20 to 30 minutes), with peak effect occurring at 20 to 80 minutes. Because of reflex tachycardia, hydralazine should not be used in patients with evidence of myocar-

dial ischemia. Headache, flushing, and vomiting can occur after initial administration.

Nitroglycerin. Nitroglycerin is primarily a venodilator, and because of this it is not a very effective antihypertensive agent. However, it may be very helpful when myocardial infarction, unstable angina, and pulmonary edema are complicated by hypertension. The dose is 5 to 100 μg/min, and the onset of action is within 2 to 5 minutes.[6]

Nicardipine. This is a promising intravenous dihydropyridine type of calcium entry blocker that has been used successfully in lowering blood pressure in severe hypertension.[7] Experience in the setting of a hypertensive crisis, however, is limited at this time.

ORAL DRUGS

Nifedipine. This calcium channel blocker has become a first-line oral agent in the treatment of hypertensive crises.[8] The advantages of using nifedipine are its fast onset of action, high degree of efficacy regardless of etiology of the crisis, and maintenance or even increased cerebral blood as blood pressure is lowered. A 10-mg nifedipine capsule can be swallowed intact or swallowed after the capsule has been bitten ("bite and swallow"), or the capsule contents can be placed sublingually. The onset of action after "bite and swallow" is within 10 minutes, and peak effect is reached within 30 to 45 minutes. One 10-mg dose will lower diastolic blood pressure to less than 110 mm Hg in almost all patients. If an antihypertensive effect is observed, then 10 mg can be given orally 4 to 6 hours later. If a 10-mg capsule is ineffective, another drug should be used rather than a second dose of nifedipine, since severe hypotension and its consequences may be more common when 20 mg is administered in a brief period. In a hypertensive crisis complicated by unstable angina or an evolving myocardial infarction, nifedipine should be avoided because it may lower perfusion pressure excessively. By contrast, asymptomatic repolarization abnormalities that commonly occur after acute administration of nifedipine do not appear to represent myocardial ischemia.[9] Headache, nausea, tachycardia, and palpitations can occur after acute administration.

Clonidine. This alpha$_2$ central agonist reduces sympathetic outflow and is particularly useful in hypertensive crises secondary to adrenergic excess, such as cocaine toxicity, clonidine withdrawal, MAO inhibitors with tyramine ingestion, and phenylpropanolamine (diet pills). It also does not cause reflex tachycardia and can be used in patients with congestive heart failure (CHF) and myocardial ischemia. Clonidine is given initially in a 0.1- to 0.2-mg dose and, if necessary, can be followed by 0.1 mg every hour to a total dose of 0.6 to 0.7 mg over 6 to 7 hours.[10] The onset of action is within 30 to 60 minutes, and peak effect is not reached until 2 to 4 hours following the initial dose. Due to its slow onset of action, the drug is more useful in hypertensive urgencies rather than true hypertensive emergencies.

A major disadvantage to using clonidine is sedation; therefore it should not be used in patients who have altered CNS status, i.e., hypertensive encephalopathy, stroke, subarachnoid hemorrhage. Clonidine also can cause significant bradycardia and, if stopped abruptly, rebound hypertension.

Captopril. This ACE inhibitor has several features that make it a first-line oral agent in hypertensive crisis:[11] lack of reflex tachycardia or salt retention, maintenance of cerebral blood flow as pressure is lowered (due to a leftward shift of the autoregulatory curve), and particular effectiveness in patients with elevated renin. Thus it is useful in patients with malignant hypertension, CHF, renovascular disease, and cerebrovascular disease. A 25-mg tablet has an onset of action in 15 minutes, and peak effect is reached within 2 to 3 hours. The settings in which precipitous drops in blood pressure can occur are in patients previously treated with diuretics or vasodilators and those with renovascular disease or CHF. Lisinopril and oral enalapril (two other ACE inhibitors available in the United States) have slower onsets of action than captopril and should not be used when rapid reduction of blood pressure is required.

Minoxidil. This potent vasodilator acts directly on arterioles to reduce peripheral vascular resistance.[12] As does hydralazine, it causes a predictable increase in sympathetic activity, which can modify its antihypertensive action. Consequently, it is usually administered with a beta-blocker and a diuretic. The initial dose of minoxidil is 5 mg, with a repeat dose given in 6 hours if necessary. Minoxidil's major advantage is its effectiveness in severe hypertension. How-

ever, it has two important disadvantages with respect to using it in hypertensive crises. It does not cause a rapid reduction in blood pressure, as its onset of action is 30 minutes and the time to peak antihypertensive action can be up to 6 hours. Second, minoxidil should not be used in patients with CHF, myocardial ischemia, or pheochromocytoma because of the reflex increase in sympathetic activity.

■ CLINICAL CONDITIONS CAUSING A HYPERTENSIVE CRISIS

Treatment of severe hypertension occasionally causes serious complications—an acceptable risk when treating a life-threatening situation, but an unacceptable risk when rapid reduction of blood pressure is not necessary. The patient's history, physical examination, and rapidly available laboratory results usually can determine whether a marked elevation in blood pressure is a crisis situation (Table 2). Symptoms that cause a patient with a hypertensive emergency to seek treatment include complaints related to the central nervous system (headache, nausea, confusion, blurred vision), cardiovascular system (chest pain, shortness of breath, palpitations), and adrenergic excess (weight loss, sweating, tremor). Clues from the history are often diagnostic of the mechanism of the blood pressure elevation. Hy-

TABLE 2. Clinical Evidence of a Hypertensive Crisis

Physical Signs	
Neurologic	Confusion, diffuse sensory or motor deficits
Funduscopic	Advanced retinopathy, grade III or IV
Cardiovascular	Orthostatic hypotension, murmur of aortic insufficiency, unequal pulses, left ventricular decompensation
Laboratory Data	
Hematologic	Microangiopathic hemolytic anemia
Serum chemistry	Hypokalemic, hypochloremic alkalosis; elevated creatinine level
ECG	Ischemic changes
Chest radiograph	Widened thoracic aorta
Echocardiography	Wall-motion abnormalities, widened aortic root/intimal flap and false lumen

peradrenergic states are suggested by a history of weight loss, paroxysms of chest pain, palpitations, and headache (pheochromocytoma); the use of cocaine or "diet pills" (amphetamines or phenylpropanolamine) and monoamine oxidase (MAO) inhibitors; and the abrupt cessation of alpha$_2$-agonists. Renal artery stenosis is suggested by uncontrolled blood pressure in a young woman with no family history of hypertension or in an elderly compliant patient whose blood pressure has suddenly elevated. Inadequate dialysis in the patient with renal failure suggests volume overload. A history of collagen vascular disease suggests active glomerular disease, and scleroderma suggests renal vasoconstriction.

The physical examination can help ascertain whether the symptoms are secondary to hypertension and will provide diagnostic clues to the etiology. Vital signs provide the first clues. Though nonspecific, tachycardia suggests adrenergic excess, and orthostatic hypotension with severe hypertension in the supine position suggests a pheochromocytoma. Bilateral papilledema, hemorrhage, or cotton wool spots provide compelling reasons to treat immediately, and their presence may point toward the etiology of the hypertension; a study of patients with these findings showed that one third had renal artery stenosis.[13] Aortic insufficiency in a patient with an acute onset of severe chest pain is highly suggestive of an aortic dissection, as are asymmetric carotid, brachial, or femoral pulses. An abdominal bruit, though nonspecific, suggests renal artery stenosis and stimulation of the renin-angiotensin-aldosterone axis in this setting. A point of caution is that if pheochromocytoma is suspected, then deep palpation of the abdomen should be avoided to prevent acute expression of catecholamines from an adrenal or abdominal mass. Diffusely abnormal neurologic function, as opposed to focal findings, suggests that elevated blood pressure is the cause of the neurologic dysfunction. Focal neurologic findings suggest a thrombotic or hemorrhagic stroke, in which elevation of blood pressure may be a consequence, rather than the cause, of the blood pressure elevation.

Laboratory test results that can be obtained in the first 60 minutes of evaluation not only are helpful in determining whether or not the rise in blood pressure is having acute pathophysiologic consequences, but also they may help make a specific diagnosis. Evidence of microangiopathic hemolytic anemia on blood smear, in the setting of severely elevated blood pressure, is diagnostic of malignant hypertension. Hypokalemic, hypochloremic alkalosis is suggestive of a highly stimulated renin-angiotensin-aldosterone axis, which often accompanies malignant hypertension. A chest x-ray film that shows an abnormally wide aorta in a patient with chest pain suggests an aortic dissection, and this can be rapidly evaluated with two-dimensional echocardiography.

Malignant or Accelerated Hypertension. This disorder is characterized by severely elevated diastolic blood pressure, usually over 130 mm Hg, with advanced retinopathy and renal insufficiency. Once grade III retinal changes are detected the patient should be aggressively treated, since there is no apparent clinical basis for the distinction between malignant and accelerated hypertension based on the degree (grade IV vs. grade III) of retinopathy.

Poorly controlled essential hypertension is the major cause of malignant hypertension (Table 3), and most cases now occur in previously diagnosed but impoverished patients who have discontinued medication.[14] A large number of patients with malignant hypertension smoke, and this may be a risk factor.[15] Essential hypertension enters a malignant phase when the kidney vasculature and other arterial beds develop lesions consisting of necrosis, which is followed by deposition of fibrin (fibrinoid necrosis). This initiates a cascade of renal ischemia and a low-flow state, resulting in renal insufficiency and activation of the renin-angiotensin-aldosterone axis, which aggravates the elevated blood pressure by causing generalized vasoconstriction. Laboratory studies that suggest the diagnosis are an elevated creatinine level; a hypokalemic, hypochlor-

TABLE 3. Most Common Causes of Malignant or Accelerated Hypertension

Essential hypertension
   Poor compliance
   Superimposed renal artery stenosis or renal disease
Renal artery stenosis
Chronic renal disease
Scleroderma/collagen vascular disease

emic alkalosis, since it suggests stimulation of the renin system; and a microangiopathic hemolytic anemia that results from a generalized arteriolitis.[16] Thrombocytopenia due to vascular damage may occur in the absence of anemia, and its presence in conjunction with a severely elevated blood pressure suggests a malignant state.

Because the renin-angiotensin-aldosterone axis is often activated in malignant hypertension, an ACE inhibitor is rational first-line therapy (Table 4). If ACE inhibitors are ineffective, then nifedipine, labetalol, or nitroprusside can be used. ACE inhibitors are extraordinarily effective in treating the "renal crisis" of scleroderma, which is a dangerous form of malignant hypertension.[17] Patients with scleroderma should be treated with ACE inhibitors at the first sign that arterial pressure is rising, without waiting for evidence of renal dysfunction. By contrast, patients with systemic lupus erythematosus who enter a malignant phase of hypertension rarely have activation of the renin-angiotensin system, and therefore other forms of therapy should be used.

Maintenance of renal perfusion and function can be problematic during treatment of malignant hypertension. Patients with malignant hypertension may be volume depleted because of pressure-induced natriuresis, and therefore diuretics usually are not used acutely unless there is evidence of volume overload. In patients with chronic renal disease, a decrease in arterial pressure may be followed by a brief 1- to 2-week period of further impairment before ultimate improvement occurs.

Renal Artery Stenosis. This is a common cause of severe hypertension, which may present as malignant or accelerated hypertension. It occurs secondary to fibromuscular dysplasia, which is predominantly a disease of young women, or atherosclerosis, which may be superimposed upon essential hypertension in elderly patients. Decreased blood flow to the affected kidney causes increased renin release and then generation of angiotensin II and increased aldosterone production. Prompt reduction of blood pressure with an ACE inhibitor supports the diagnosis, whereas its ineffectiveness is strong

TABLE 4. Treatment of Choice for Specific Hypertensive Crisis

Condition	Treatment*	Avoid
Malignant hypertension	ACE inhibitor	
	Nitroprusside	
	Labetalol	
	Nifedipine	
Pre-eclampsia/eclampsia	Hydralazine	Nitroprusside
	Alpha-methyldopa†	
Hypertensive encephalopathy	Nitroprusside	Clonidine
	Labetalol	
	Nifedipine	
	ACE inhibitor	
Adrenergic excess	Phentolamine	
	Labetalol	
	Nitroprusside	
	Clonidine	
Myocardial infarction and	Nitroglycerin	Hydralazine
unstable angina	Nitroprusside	?Nifedipine
	Labetalol	
Pulmonary edema	Nitroprusside	Beta-blockers
	Nitroglycerin	
	Nifedipine	
	Furosemide	
Aortic dissection	Nitroprusside	
	Beta-blockers	
	Labetalol	

*Refer to text for dosages and side effects
†3000 mg in four divided doses of alpha-methyldopa may be given. Drowsiness is the most prominent side effect.

evidence against the diagnosis.[18] The patient may be kept on ACE therapy prior to correction of the stenosis, but renal function must be carefully monitored because reversible renal dysfunction may develop if bilateral renal artery stenosis is present.

Hypertensive Encephalopathy. This syndrome is clinically defined as cerebral dysfunction, usually diffuse, which is reversible when elevated blood pressure is restored to normal. The condition often occurs in the setting of malignant hypertension, but it can be an independent phenomenon. It should be distinguished from a cerebrovascular accident, which usually presents with more focal neurologic deficits; subdural hematoma; brain tumor (especially posterior fossa); encephalitis; and toxic encephalopathy. The pathophysiology is probably a consequence of arterial pressure exceeding the autoregulatory range of cerebral blood flow, resulting in cerebral edema. Cerebral blood flow is normally kept constant over a wide range of arterial pressure, and treatment is directed at lowering the blood pressure into this autoregulatory range. The level to which blood pressure can be lowered before hypoperfusion occurs is variable, but in general chronically hypertensive subjects have an autoregulatory curve that has adapted to a higher level, and reduction of blood pressure below a diastolic reading of 100 mm Hg may be deleterious. By contrast, if the patient was previously normotensive, blood pressure can be reduced to the normal range since the autoregulatory curve is set at lower levels.

All the aforementioned parenteral and oral agents may be effective, but clonidine should be avoided because it might further depress consciousness. With treatment, usually improvement of neurologic function occurs within a few hours, but residual dysfunction may last for as long as 5 to 7 days after blood pressure has been effectively controlled.

Pre-eclampsia/Eclampsia. Hypertension in pregnancy in association with proteinuria and edema constitute the syndrome of pre-eclampsia. The pathogenesis of this disorder is complex but may include reduced secretion of vasodilating prostaglandins. Eclampsia (seizures and coma) usually occurs only when the pre-eclampsia is inadequately controlled. Treatment of pre-eclampsia is delivery if the fetus is viable, and blood pressure is controlled with intravenous hydralazine and alpha-methyldopa. Because of potential cyanide poisoning, nitroprusside should not be used. Magnesium sulfate is used to prevent seizures.

Adrenergic Excess. These crises arise either because of a pheochromocytoma or because of drug-related syndromes. Pheochromocytomas are usually benign adrenal tumors secreting norepinephrine. Severe hypertension is usually due to alpha-receptor–mediated vasoconstriction. There is an extraordinary degree of variability in the pattern of arterial pressure. Some patients are normotensive except under stresses such as surgical anesthesia or invasive procedures, whereas others may have surges of severely elevated pressure in the setting of chronically elevated blood pressure. There is often a history of weight loss, inappropriate sweating, palpitations, headaches, and nervousness. Renal functional impairment, proteinuria, and hematuria are extremely rare in this disease.

When pheochromocytoma is suspected as the cause of severe hypertension, intravenous phentolamine is the drug of choice for immediate treatment. A continuous infusion of phentolamine or oral phenoxybenzamine is then used, and after blood pressure has been well controlled, a beta-blocker can be added to offset the reflex tachycardia from the alpha-blockers. Because intravascular depletion is common, intravenous fluids are usually administered. Since renin is often elevated (suggested by hypokalemic metabolic alkalosis secondary to chronic adrenergic stimulation of receptors in the kidney and because of intravascular depletion), an ACE inhibitor may be useful in controlling blood pressure. Before surgery, the tumor should be localized by imaging techniques and, if time permits, confirmed by identification of increased circulating levels of catecholamines.

MAO-tyramine interactions are treated with intravenous phentolamine. Tyramine is a sympathomimetic amine that causes norepinephrine release from nerve endings. MAO inhibitors block the usual metabolism of tyramine in the intestine and liver. In most cases, intravenous phentolamine restores blood pressure to normal and only needs to be administered long enough for the tyramine effect to wear off—no long-term therapy is required. Hypertensive crises resulting from cocaine, diet pill overdose, and alpha$_2$-agonist withdrawal are also treated with phentolamine.

■ CARDIOVASCULAR AND NEUROLOGIC EMERGENCIES COMPLICATED BY OR RESULTING FROM SEVERE HYPERTENSION

Myocardial Infarction (MI). Although it is unclear whether reduction of severe blood pressure reduces infarct size or improves survival, lowering markedly elevated blood pressure is rarely harmful and is beneficial when pulmonary edema complicates an MI. Intravenous administration of nitroprusside or nitroglycerin at 5 to 100 μg/min is safe, but the latter may not effectively lower blood pressure. Nifedipine has not improved survival when given in acute myocardial infarction and may be deleterious.[19] Severe systemic hypertension at any time during the initial presentation of a myocardial infarction is a relative contraindication for the use of thrombolytic agents, since there is a higher incidence of intracerebral hemorrhage in this setting.

Unstable Angina. One approach is to lower blood pressure with IV nitroglycerin, alone or in combination with labetalol or another beta-blocker. Although calcium antagonists are often the mainstay of therapy for unstable angina when blood pressure is not markedly elevated, their role in unstable angina accompanied by markedly elevated blood pressure is not clear.

Pulmonary Edema. Increased left ventricular (LV) wall stress induced by markedly elevated blood pressure predictably will lower LV ejection fraction, which may lead to pulmonary edema. If elevated blood pressure is the primary cause of pump dysfunction, then marked improvement should occur when pressure is lowered with IV nitroprusside or nitroglycerin or treatment with nifedipine. Furosemide is usually indicated, but it should be used with caution in acute myocardial infarction since, if the patient is euvolemic, diuresis may cause LV filling pressure to fall too low, resulting in decreased cardiac output and hypotension.

Aortic Dissection. Elevated blood pressure often accompanies aortic dissection. Administration of intravenous beta-blockade (to reduce ventricular contractility), followed by nitroprusside to lower blood pressure, is an effective way to stabilize patients with severe hypertension and aortic dissection immediately. Labetalol, which reduces blood pressure and ventricular contractility, is an effective drug. Angiography, computed tomography or magnetic resonance imaging, and transesophageal 2-D echocardiography (which can be performed within 15 minutes) can be used to confirm the diagnosis and identify the origin of the dissection.[20] Surgery for proximal aortic dissections clearly improves survival, whereas most dissections in the distal aorta can be managed medically.

Cerebrovascular Accident. Autoregulation of blood flow is compromised in the zone of a cerebral infarct, making the ischemic area especially vulnerable to the consequences of hypotension. Because of this, therapy of hypertension during acute stroke remains controversial, because clinical trials have not established the rate and the level to which diastolic blood pressure should be lowered. It is generally accepted that diastolic blood pressure should not be treated unless it is severely elevated, as blood pressure will tend to normalize spontaneously in the first few days following a stroke. If the choice is made to treat blood pressure, it should not be lowered below 100 mm Hg over the first 48 hours.

All the agents discussed earlier may be effective in lowering blood pressure, but clonidine should be avoided because of its sedating effects. Since ACE inhibitors may shift the lower limit of autoregulation to lower pressures in the brain, they may prove to be advantageous. Dihydropyridine calcium blockers increase cerebral blood flow and may maintain cerebral perfusion during a stroke. In a recent study, oral nimodipine, a dihydropyridine, administered at 30 mg every 6 hours, improved survival after ischemic stroke, compared with placebo.[21] Blood pressure response was not reported, but the dose at which this improved survival was achieved may have few or no effects on systemic blood pressure.

■ Issues and Risks

Many of the conditions resulting in a hypertensive crisis are unavoidable, but uncontrolled essential hypertension should be preventable. Although the incidence of hypertensive crisis appears to be decreasing, many patients with severe essential hypertension still remain at risk for developing malignant and accelerated hypertension. Often poor and underserved, the majority of patients in this group who develop a hypertensive crisis know they are hypertensive,[14] but for any of a number of reasons they have difficulty taking medication on a regular basis. Strategies directed toward preventing catastrophic hypertensive crisis in this group would be beneficial to the patient and cost-effective for society. Convenient and effective once-a-day medications should improve patient compliance.[22] Directing resources toward improved tracking and frequent evaluation of the severe hypertensive patient, whose chances of developing a complication are significant, may be more rational than efforts to normalize blood pressure in mild hypertensive patients, whose risks of complications are small.

REFERENCES

1. Bhatia SK, Frohlich ED. Hemodynamic comparison of agents useful in hypertensive emergencies. Am Heart J 1973; 85:367–373.
2. Wilson DJ, Wallin JD, Vlachakis ND, et al. Intravenous labetalol in the treatment of severe hypertension and hypertensive emergencies. Am J Med 1983; 75(4A):95–102.
3. Weiner N. Drugs that inhibit adrenergic nerves and block adrenergic receptors. In Goodman AG, Goodman LS, Rall TW, Murad F, (eds). The Pharmacological Basis of Therapeutics. 7th ed. New York: Macmillan, 1985:181–214.
4. Strauss R, Gavras I, Vlahakos D, Gavras H. Enalaprilat in hypertensive emergencies. J Clin Pharmacol 1986; 26:39–43.
5. Koch-Weser J. Hypertensive emergencies. N Engl J Med 1974; 290:211–214.
6. Flaherty JT, Becker LC, Bulkley BH, et. al. A randomized prospective trial of intravenous nitroglycerin in patients with acute myocardial infarction. Circulation 1983; 68:576–588.
7. Wallin JD, Cook ME, Blanski L, et al. Intravenous nicardipine for the treatment of severe hypertension. Am J Med 1988; 85:331–338.
8. Bertel O, Radu EW, Muller J, Lang C, Dubach UC. Nifedipine in hypertensive emergencies. Br Med J 1983; 286:19–21.
9. Phillips RA, Ardeljan M, Eison HB, Goldman ME, Krakoff LR. Left ventricular function during nifedipine administration in hypertensive urgencies (abstract). Am J Hypertens 1988; 1(3, pt 2):7A.
10. Anderson R, Hart GR, Crumpler C, Reed WG, Matthews C: Oral clonidine loading in hypertensive urgencies. JAMA 1981; 246:848–850.
11. Biollaz J, Waeber B, Brunner HR: Hypertensive crisis treated with orally administered captopril. Eur J Clin Pharmacol 1983; 25:145–149.
12. McNeil JJ, Louis WJ. Minoxidil. In Doyle AE (ed). Clinical Pharmacology of Antihypertensive Drugs. (Vol II of Handbook of Hypertension, edited by Birkenhager WH, Reid JL.) New York: Elsevier, 1980:410–423.
13. Davis BA, Crook JE, Vestal RE, et al. Prevalence of renovascular hypertension in patients with grade III or IV hypertensive retinopathy. N Engl J Med 1979; 301:1273–1276.
14. Bennett NM, Shea S. Hypertensive emergency: case criteria, sociodemographic profile, and previous care of 100 cases. Am J Public Health 1988; 78:636–640.
15. Isles C, Brown JJ, Cummings AMM, et al. Excess smoking in malignant-phase hypertension. Br Med J 1979; 1:579–581.
16. Linton AL, Gavras H, Gleadle RI, et al. Microangiopathic haemolytic anaemia and the pathogeneis of malignant hypertension. Lancet 1969; 1:1277–1282.
17. Lopez-Ovejero JA, Saal SD, D'Angelo WA, et al. Reversal of vascular and renal crisis of scleroderma by oral angiotensin converting enzyme blockade. N Engl J Med 1979; 300:1417–1419.
18. Muller FB, Sealey JE, Case DB, et al. The captopril test for identifying renovascular disease in hypertensive patients. Am J Med 1986; 80:633–644.
19. Muller JE, Morrison J, Stone PH, et al. Nifedipine therapy for patients with threatened and acute myocardial infarction: a randomized, double-blind, placebo-controlled comparison. Circulation 1984; 69:740–747.
20. Erbel R, Daniel W, Visser C, Engberding R, et al. Echocardiographic diagnosis of aortic dissection. Lancet 1989; 2:457–460.
21. Gelmers HJ, Gorter K, De Weerdt CJ, Wiezer HJA. A controlled trial of nimodipine in acute ischemic stroke. N Engl J Med 1988; 318:203–207.
22. Phillips RA, Ardeljan M, Goldman ME, Eison HB, Krakoff LR. Cardiac and hemodynamic adjustments to rapid and sustained blood pressure reduction. Am J Hypertens 1989; 2:1965–1995.

Hyponatremia

Marc B. Goldstein

Hyponatremia is one disorder in which the inappropriate management may pose a much greater risk to the patient than the initial abnormality. As the appropriate management is dictated by the cause of the disorder, a substantial portion of this article will be directed at ensuring that the treating physician makes the appropriate diagnosis of the basis of the hyponatremia.

Definition. Hyponatremia is a laboratory diagnosis in which the serum sodium concentration, [Na], is less than 136 mEq/L.

The sodium concentration reflects the ratio of sodium to water in the extracellular fluid and indicates a reduction in the amount of sodium relative to the amount of water. The presence of hyponatremia has no specific implications with respect to total body sodium, which may be increased, decreased, or normal in the hyponatremic patient.

■ Background

Because of the varied etiologies of hyponatremia as well as the varied natural history (acute or chronic disorder), the patient with hyponatremia may be totally asymptomatic and the diagnosis appears unexpectedly when "routine electrolytes" are ordered. On the other hand, the patient with hyponatremia may present with a major central nervous system (CNS) derangement, ranging from mild confusion to seizures and coma. The CNS symptoms result from brain swelling within the restricted volume of the skull. The swelling results from water movement from the extracellular fluid (ECF) to the intracellular fluid (ICF) down the osmotic gradient.

Patients who develop significant hyponatremia acutely (over less than 48 hours) will have little time for defense of ICF volume and therefore generally will have more striking neurologic symptoms at the time of presentation. Conversely, those patients whose hyponatremia has developed chronically may have a paucity of symptoms despite very severe hyponatremia. Patients whose ICF osmoles have changed in order to defend the ICF volume (those with chronic hyponatremia) must have the hyponatremia corrected slowly to avoid serious complications from the therapy.

■ CLASSIFICATION OF PATIENTS WITH HYPONATREMIA

An initial classification can be constructed on the basis of the effective serum osmolality (measured serum osmolality minus contribution by urea and alcohol) (Figure 1):

1. **Normal effective serum osmolality:** pseudohyponatremia.
2. **Increased effective serum osmolality:** hyperglycemia or mannitol administration.
3. **Reduced effective serum osmolality:** water retention syndromes.

Hyponatremia with Normal Effective Serum Osmolality

Pseudohyponatremia is solely a laboratory phenomenon in patients with severe hyperlipidemia or hyperproteinemia.[1] In these patients there is an increase in the nonaqueous component of blood (lipid or protein), and sodium is distributed only in the aqueous component of blood. Therefore, the sodium concentration per total volume of serum is reduced, even though the sodium concentration per aqueous volume of serum is normal. As the sodium concentration in the aqueous volume is normal, the osmolality is also normal. This problem is obviated when ion-specific electrodes, rather than flame photometry, are used to measure the serum sodium concentration.

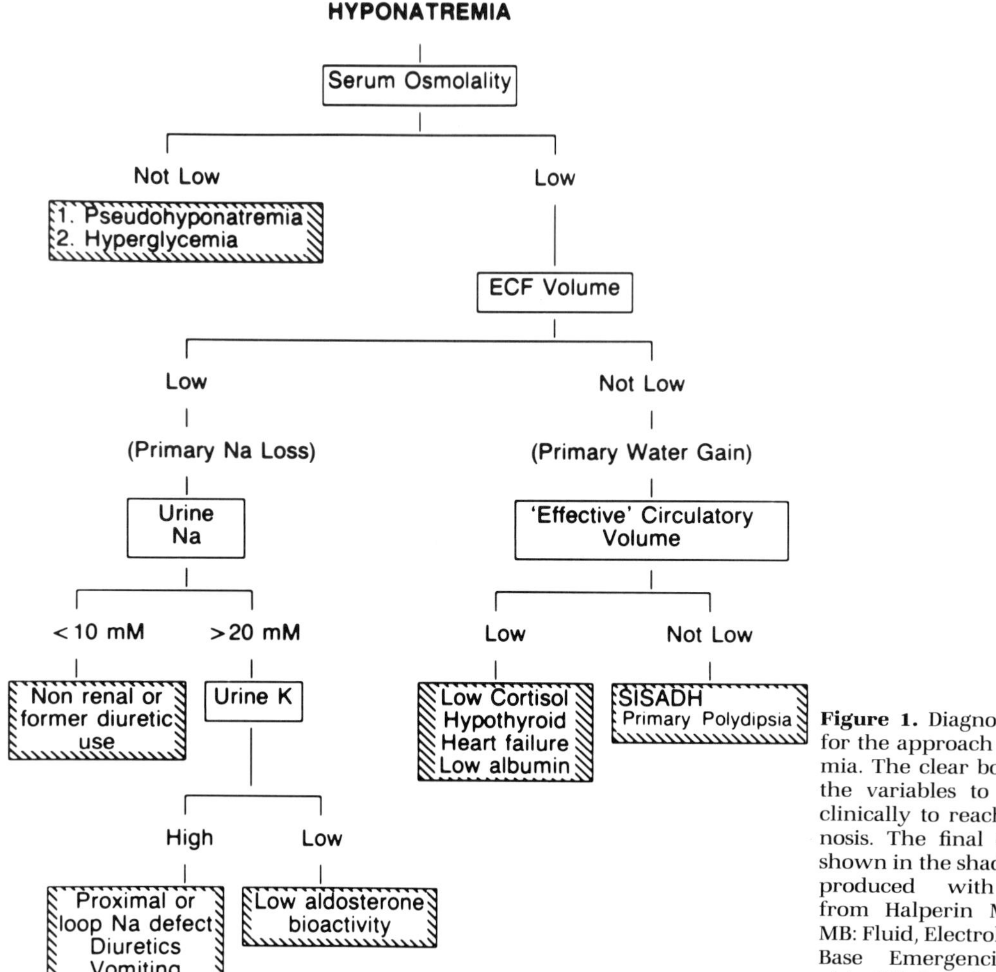

Figure 1. Diagnostic algorithm for the approach to hyponatremia. The clear boxes represent the variables to be evaluated clinically to reach a final diagnosis. The final diagnoses are shown in the shaded boxes. (Reproduced with permission from Halperin ML, Goldstein MB: Fluid, Electrolyte, and Acid-Base Emergencies. Philadelphia, WB Saunders, 1988.)

Hyponatremia with an Increased Effective Serum Osmolality

In these patients with hyponatremia, the serum osmolality is increased, generally because of hyperglycemia, and the glucose is restricted to the ECF, raising the ECF osmolality. This increase causes water to move from the ICF to the ECF, reducing the ECF sodium concentration. The actual contribution to the fall in serum sodium concentration by the blood sugar can be calculated: expect a 1.35 mEq/L fall in sodium concentration for every 100 mg/dl (5.5 mmol/L) increase in blood glucose concentration.[2]

In contrast to the water retention syndromes, these patients do *not* have an increase in the ICF volume of their brain; they do have a reduction in the ICF volume of muscle, which accounts for the major water movement into the ECF. The ICF volume of other organs depends on whether insulin is required for glucose entry into their cells. With respect to the brain, the brain cell volume may well be little affected by hyperglycemia, as glucose enters the brain in the absence of insulin.

Hyponatremia with a Reduced Effective Serum Osmolality

These hyponatremic patients have lost the ability to regulate the serum osmolality by matching renal water excretion to water intake. A very brief review of the physiology of water excretion is appropriate to understand the pathophysiology. Normally, dilute urine is formed in the ascending limb of the loop of Henle and delivered into the distal tubule. If antidiuretic hormone (ADH) is absent, this dilute urine is excreted as long as there is a reasonable flow rate through the collecting duct. On the other hand, if ADH secretion is present, the collecting duct becomes permeable to water. As long as the renal medulla is hypertonic, water is reabsorbed from the collecting duct (rendered permeable to water by ADH), because of the hypertonic medulla, and concentrated urine is excreted.[3] Patients with hypo-osmolar hyponatremia can be divided into two groups: those who are able to dilute their urine and those who cannot.

Patients with Dilute Urine (Osmolality Less Than 100 mOsm/kg). There are two groups in this category:

1. Patients with a huge water intake that exceeds the renal ability to excrete water (the kidney can excrete 12 liters of free water daily). These patients are referred to as psychogenic water drinkers.
2. Those patients with a transient reduction in their ability to excrete free water, who are being assessed at a time when this inability has reversed or has been attenuated (e.g., drug-induced prolongation of ADH action).

Patients with Failure to Dilute the Urine Maximally (Urine Osmolality Greater Than 100 mOsm/kg). The key issue in these patients is to understand why the physiologic action of ADH is present when they have hyponatremia and ADH should be turned off.

These patients can be classified into three groups:

1. Patients with ECF volume contraction (Table 1). These patients have an increased blood urea concentration and low urine sodium concentration (<20 mM) (unless they are receiving diuretics).
2. Patients with ECF volume expansion (edema) (Table 1). These patients have ECF volume expansion but have underfilling of their arterial circulation owing to the presence of cardiac limitation to cardiac output, hepatic disease resulting in hypoalbuminemia, or the nephrotic syndrome. These patients have an increased blood urea concentration (reduced renal perfusion) and low urine so-

dium concentration (<20 mM), unless they are receiving diuretics.
3. No major alteration in ECF volume. These patients have ADH release for any of the reasons outlined in Table 2. These patients have a low blood urea and low

TABLE 1. Causes of "Effective" Circulatory Volume Contraction

ECF Volume Depletion (Na Loss)

Nonrenal Na Loss
Gastrointestinal tract: vomiting, drainage, ileus, diarrhea
Skin: excessive sweating, burns

Renal Na Loss
Diuretics:
    Drugs
    Osmotic (glucose, urea)
Low aldosterone
Tubular disorders
    Proximal (Fanconi syndrome, etc)
    Loop (Bartter's syndrome?)
    Distal (interstitial disease, etc; low aldosterone)

ECF Volume Normal or Increased but Maldistributed
High interstitial and low vascular volume
Low plasma albumin (e.g., liver disease, nephrotic syndrome)
Albumin leaks out of capillaries
Low arterial volume, high venous volume
Primary myocardial, valvular, or pericardial disease

TABLE 2. Origin of the High ADH in Hyponatremia

ADH from Posterior Pituitary Gland
Cardiovascular (low "effective" circulating volume)
Specific diseases
    Pulmonary lesion
    CNS lesion
    Endocrine disorders (e.g., hypothyroidism, hypoadrenalism)
    Metabolic disorders (e.g., acute intermittent porphyria)
    Excessive pain (e.g., during postoperative period) or vomiting
Drug-induced (see Table 3)
Mechanism unclear

ADH from Other Sources
Solid neoplasms (especially oat cell carcinoma of lung)
Possibly granulomas such as tuberculosis
Exogenous administration
    ADH (e.g., treatment for diabetes insipidus)
    Oxytocin for labor induction

Potentiation of Endogenous ADH by Drugs
Adenylate cyclase activation
Phosphodiesterase inhibition
Adenosine receptor antagonists
Prostaglandin inhibitors

uric acid concentrations and high urine sodium concentration (>20 mM), unless their total body sodium is low.

■ Management

The management of hyponatremic patients clearly will be based upon the diagnostic category into which they fall and the severity of their symptoms.

■ PSEUDOHYPONATREMIA

This disorder is only a laboratory phenomenon. The osmolality of the extracellular fluid is normal, and no therapeutic intervention is necessary.

■ HYPEROSMOLAR HYPONATREMIA

A great majority of patients with hyperosmolar hyponatremia also will have hyperglycemia, and the first step in management is to ascertain the basis of the hyperglycemia. In stable diabetic patients, the most important cause for increased insulin needs is sepsis.

Severe ECF volume contraction usually will be present, owing to the hyperglycemia-induced osmotic diuresis. The patient may have the hyperosmolar hyperglycemic non-ketotic coma syndrome. In these patients, the hyponatremia is not as severe as anticipated from calculating how far the sodium concentration should fall due to hyperglycemia-mediated water movement into the ECF. This is a result of the substantial water loss subsequent to the osmotic diuresis. These patients also often have associated hypokalemia and metabolic alkalosis. Often the impaired insulin secretion is in part or entirely due to the profound volume contraction and to the catecholamine release that inhibits insulin secretion.

The priorities in the management of these patients are:

1. Restoration of ECF volume contraction with normal or half-normal saline. The latter is preferred if there is a normal blood pressure and if the calculation of the degree of hyponatremia to be expected from the level of blood sugar is more severe than the value observed, indicating a significant water deficit and the presence of the hyperosmolar syndrome. If the patient is hypotensive due to ECF volume contraction, normal saline should be used until the blood pressure is stable. Begin with 1 liter per hour in the hypotensive patient.
2. Restoration of potassium deficits. Potassium depletion may be profound from a long-standing osmotic diuresis and ECF volume contraction. A severe potassium depletion results, caused by mineralocorticoid-mediated renal potassium excretion. If possible, give some potassium orally. Limit intravenous potassium administration to 60 mEq/hr. Ongoing renal potassium loss may be substantial as ECF volume is restored, and this can be reduced with amiloride. If amiloride is used, watch the serum potassium level hourly and reduce potassium administration as the serum potassium level rises. The need for insulin in the hyperosmolar hyperglycemic nonketotic syndrome is controversial, and in the early stages of treatment insulin may be dangerous. As these patients are generally very potassium-depleted and as insulin causes potassium movement into cells, if insulin is given prior to potassium replacement life-threatening hypokalemia may result. This topic is discussed further in the concluding Issues and Risks section.

In the patient receiving mannitol, there is no need to correct the hyponatremia; however, one should look for signs of sodium depletion (reduced ECF volume) from the osmotic diuresis and correct it with saline administration. Once the mannitol administration is stopped, the hyponatremia will resolve. These patients may also have substantial potassium deficits.

■ SYNDROMES RELATED TO DIMINISHED WATER EXCRETION

Patients with ECF Volume Contraction. These patients have hyponatremia from the loss of sodium and water, but their net deficit of sodium is greater than their net deficit of water, resulting in hyponatremia. These patients have water retention subsequent to ADH release (from ECF volume contraction) and concomitant water intake. Restoration of their ECF volume deficits will result in a reduction in ADH secretion and a return of the ability to dilute the urine. Therefore, the backbone of treatment in such patients is normal saline infusion.

If the patient has been receiving diuretics, clearly these should be discontinued.

One should also identify the basis for the ECF volume contraction, as this may well be associated with other disorders that require attention. For example, the patient may be ECF volume–contracted due to the use of diuretics and have associated potassium depletion, which also requires correction.

Patients with hypothyroidism and hypoadrenalism also may develop hyponatremia, which is attributable to the cardiovascular effects of these hormone deficiencies, resulting in reduced cardiac output and ADH release on that basis. They are thus akin to the ECF volume–contracted patients.

An additional issue, discussed in the section on Issues and Risks, is the role of exogenous antidiuretic hormone in the treatment of these patients to control the degree of water diuresis once ADH secretion has been turned off.

Patients with ECF Volume Expansion. These patients have ADH release due to underfilling of their arterial tree,[4] and therapy takes several routes, depending on the degree of symptomatology.

In all cases, water intake should be limited, as these patients have impairment of water excretion. To be effective, one should limit daily free water intake to less than 600 ml/day.

In hyponatremic patients, the goal is to increase the excretion of free water. By increasing the sodium concentration in the urine in these patients, who often have low urine sodium concentration because of underfilling of the arterial tree, diuretics *reduce* the free water excretion. Therefore, if diuretics are necessary, water intake must be restricted. If the patient is symptomatic and the serum sodium must be reduced acutely, this can be achieved with the use of hypertonic saline combined with a loop diuretic. This issue will be discussed further in the Issues and Risks section.

Patients with No Major Change in ECF Volume. These patients generally have ADH release for reasons other than underfilling of

the arterial circulation or ECF volume contraction. The approach in these patients is to:

- Restrict water intake to less than 600 ml/day.
- Look for drugs contributing to ADH release or action and discontinue them (Table 3).
- Identify specific disease processes associated with inappropriate antidiuretic hormone secretion (see Table 2).
- Antagonize the effects of antidiuretic hormone on the collecting duct. As one cannot turn off ADH secretion in these patients, one tries to antagonize its action. In the near future, ADH antagonists will be commercially available.

Demeclocycline (Declomycin) is an agent capable of interfering with cyclic AMP formation (the second messenger of ADH). This agent can be used safely in patients with chronic ADH release for reasons that cannot be controlled (oat cell carcinoma of the lung).

Another agent with the ability to inhibit cyclic AMP formation is lithium; however, this agent has too many side effects to make it therapeutically useful.

If these patients have serious symptoms from their hyponatremia (significant alterations in cognitive function, seizures, or coma), they should receive therapy with hypertonic saline. If there is any concern that their cardiac state may be compromised by the salt load, the administration of hyper-

TABLE 3. Drugs That May Cause High ADH in Hyponatremia

Central Stimulation of ADH Release
  Nicotine
  Morphine
  Clofibrate
  Tricyclic antidepressants
  Antineoplastic agents, such as vincristine, cyclophosphamide
"ADH-Like" Agents
  Oxytocin
Drugs Promoting ADH Action on the Kidney by Increasing Cyclic AMP
  Oral hypoglycemics (e.g., chlorpropamide)
  Methylxanthines (e.g., caffeine, aminophylline)
  Analgesics that inhibit prostaglandin synthesis (e.g., aspirin, indomethacin)

tonic saline should be accompanied by the administration of a potent diuretic.

■ THE USE OF HYPERTONIC SALINE

Hypertonic saline should be used only in patients with severe symptoms from their hyponatremia, irrespective of the level of sodium concentration. One should use 5 per cent saline as the agent of choice and be aware of the sodium load administered: 500 ml contain 428 mEq of sodium. As hypertonic saline is added to the ECF, the ECF sodium concentration rises, moving water from the ICF to the ECF.

One should calculate the volume of distribution of administered Na as 60 per cent of the body weight and should calculate the rate of sodium administration to be sufficient only to raise the sodium concentration by 0.5 to 1 mEq/L/hr. In a 70-kg man, 42 mEq of sodium will raise the serum sodium by 1 mEq/L. This sodium will expand the ECF volume by close to 300 ml. Thus the impact of this treatment on ECF volume is substantial. If there is clinical evidence of significant ECF volume expansion, salt excretion can be promoted by the administration of diuretics. The impact on the serum sodium concentration will not be negated by the use of diuretics, as hypertonic solutions are being administered and isotonic urine will be excreted, resulting in a net loss of water. The serum sodium concentration should be monitored hourly to ensure that it is not rising more rapidly than desired. Once the patient's symptoms improve, the use of hypertonic saline should be discontinued and more conservative methods of raising the sodium concentration employed (continued water restriction).

■ Issues and Risks

The rate at which one should correct hyponatremia is a controversial issue. One school of thought proposes that serious brain damage may occur from symptomatic hyponatremia unless it is treated quickly.[5] Another school of thought states that the rapid correction of hyponatremia may lead to central pontine myelinolysis.[6] At least part of this controversy relates to the need for a differ-

ent therapeutic approach to the acute as compared with the chronically hyponatremic patient. When patients are symptomatic from hyponatremia, an appropriate approach is to treat aggressively but to limit the rate of rise of the sodium concentration to 1 to 2 mEq/hr. As the patient's symptoms improve, one should slow the rate of rise of sodium concentration toward 0.5 mEq/L/hr until the symptoms have cleared or a sodium concentration of 120 mEq/L is reached.

The patient with chronic hyponatremia (longer than 48 hours) should be treated differently. In these patients, there has been time for the brain cells to become volume-regulated, and generally the symptoms are mild relative to the level of sodium concentration. These patients' hyponatremia should be corrected more slowly, aiming at increasing the serum sodium concentration at a rate of no more than 0.5 mEq/L/hr. If they are totally asymptomatic, it would be reasonable to treat them entirely by water restriction unless the ECF volume is contracted.

Avoidance of a rapid correction in the serum sodium concentration also has relevance to the patient whose ECF volume contraction is the basis of the hyponatremia. In these patients, the stimulus for ADH secretion is turned off as the ECF volume contraction is corrected with saline administration. These patients, therefore, are at risk of suddenly undergoing a water diuresis as the effect of the ADH wears off. The water diuresis may bring about a very rapid increase in serum sodium concentration and put the patient at risk for the development of central pontine myelinolysis. It is therefore reasonable to consider exogenous vasopressin (aqueous vasopressin or DDAVP) for such a patient, once the water diuresis ensues, to minimize the rate at which the serum sodium concentration rises.

The role of insulin therapy in the hyperglycemic hyperosmolar syndrome without ketoacidosis is also controversial.[7] These patients usually have been hyperglycemic for at least several days and therefore are usually ECF volume–depleted and potassium-depleted from the ongoing osmotic diuresis coupled with the mineralocorticoid secretion as a result of ECF volume contraction. As insulin causes potassium movement into cells, it can provoke severe hypokalemia and subsequent arrhythmias. A rapid lowering of the blood sugar due to the action of insulin will also liberate substantial amounts of water from the ECF and allow it to flow into the ICF, worsening the ECF volume contraction and perhaps precipitating hypotension. The only benefit derived from insulin therapy in this setting is to lower the blood glucose concentration, and that benefit can be achieved by restoring the ECF volume contraction with normal saline containing potassium chloride. As the volume contraction is corrected, the glomerular filtration rate increases and enhanced glycosuria ensues, lowering the blood sugar. Therefore I recommend withholding insulin therapy in the initial stages as long as the patients are neither acidemic nor hyperkalemic. As long as the anion gap is not increasing and acidemia is not developing, it is safe to withhold insulin.

Often the blood sugar will return to normal and insulin therapy will never be required. In some cases, however, hyperglycemia persists despite restoration of the ECF volume, and in these cases insulin therapy will be necessary. However, this is usually several days after presentation, at which time the ECF volume and potassium depletion have been corrected. In all cases, water intake should be limited, as these patients have impairment of water excretion. To be effective, free water intake should be limited to less than 600 ml/day.

REFERENCES

1. Weisberg LS. Pseudohyponatremia: a reappraisal. Am J Med 1989; 86:315–318.
2. Roscoe JM, Halperin ML, Rolleston FS, Goldstein MB. Hyperglycemia induced hyponatremia: metabolic considerations in calculation of expected serum sodium depression. Can Med Assoc J 1975; 112:452–453.
3. Halperin ML, Goldstein MB. Sodium and water physiology. In Fluid, Electrolyte, and Acid-Base Emergencies. Philadelphia: WB Saunders, 1988:140–165.
4. Schrier RW. Pathogenesis of sodium and water retention in high output and low output cardiac failure, nephrotic syndrome, cirrhosis and pregnancy (2 parts). N Engl J Med 1988; 319:1065–1072, 1127–1134.
5. Ayus JC, Krothapalli RK, Arief AI. Treatment of symptomatic hyponatremia and its relation to brain damage. N Engl J Med 1987; 317:1190–1195.
6. Sterns RH. Severe symptomatic hyponatremia: treatment and outcome. A study of 64 cases. Ann Intern Med 1987; 107:656–664.
7. Halperin ML, Goldstein MB. Metabolic and physiologic aspects of hyperglycemia and ketoacidosis. In Fluid, Electrolyte, and Acid-Base Emergencies. Philadelphia: WB Saunders, 1988:274–287.

Impotence

Timothy M. Roddy ■ *Irwin Goldstein* ■ *Jocelyne Tessier*

Recent advances made in the study of normal male erectile physiology have contributed to the improved understanding of the pathophysiology of impotence and ultimately to its diagnosis and treatment. It is estimated that 10 million American males suffer from erectile insufficiency.[1,2] This disorder is age-dependent and has a prevalence of 35 to 50 per cent in certain systemic disorders such as diabetes mellitus.[3] Contrary to previous hypotheses, an organic cause for erectile complaints is common and accounts for the majority of the underlying pathophysiology of persistent erectile dysfunction in men. The negative social stigma associated with impotence is diminishing, and men with their partners are actively seeking answers for their problems.

■ Background

■ CLASSIFICATION AND NOMENCLATURE

Erectile potency is defined as the ability to achieve sufficient erectile rigidity to achieve penetration and sustain penetration until ejaculation. This is a subjective term, and erectile potency may be temporary, inconsistent and situational. Erectile potency may still be present with organic pathology in the erectile mechanism. **Erectile insufficiency** describes a consistent change in *all* erections (morning, masturbatory, coital), in terms of rigidity or sustaining capabilities, for greater than 1 year. More than 90 per cent of patients with erectile insufficiency have an organic basis for their complaints. **Erectile failure** is the consistent inability for greater than 1 year to achieve sufficient rigidity to achieve penetration or sustain penetration until ejaculation. Potency usually does not exist at any time with erectile failure.

Failure to initiate erectile dysfunction implies the inhibition of the normal release of endogenous neurotransmitter substances that are responsible for the changes in penile hemodynamics with erection. Failure to initiate erectile dysfunction, therefore, may be secondary to neurologic disorders or lesions that affect the sacral parasympathetic spinal cord or the peripheral efferent autonomic fibers to the corpora cavernosa. Other etiologies include psychogenic stimuli that act at the sacral cord level, inhibiting reflexogenic erections and activation of the parasympathetic vasodilator nerves to the penis. It is possible that hormonal disorders with associated hypogonadism and diminished libido affect erections in the same manner. **Failure to fill** erectile dysfunction implies an arterial occlusion within the hypogastric-cavernous arterial bed, with diminished cavernosal artery perfusion pressure and inflow. Examples of failure to fill dysfunction include atherosclerotic or traumatic arterial occlusive disease. **Failure to store** erectile dysfunction implies that the corporal veno-occlusive mechanism is not functioning normally, and that the venous outflow from the corporal bodies during erection is excessive. Failure to store erectile dysfunction may occur in anxiety states with excessive adrenergic constrictor tone or in cases of poor compliance within the fibroelastic components of the corpora as occurs with aging, hypercholesterolemia, trauma, priapism, and surgery.

■ NORMAL ANATOMY

The penis consists of two paired corpora cavernosa and a corpus spongiosum. In the perineum, the corpora cavernosa are separated to form the crura, which attach bilaterally to the ipsilateral ischium. In the pendulous penis, the corpora cavernosa communicate via a midline septum. Each corpus is surrounded by the tunica albuginea, a thick, fibrous sheath encasing the cavernosal tissue. This tissue consists of multiple communicating vascular spaces, lacunae, lined by vascular endothelium. Surrounding the lacunar spaces are the trabeculae, which consist of vascular smooth muscle, fibroblasts, collagen, and elastin.[4]

The main arterial supply to the penis is usually from the internal pudendal artery, a branch of the internal iliac artery. After passing through the urogenital diaphragm in the pelvis, it gives rise to the common penile artery, which provides origin to four branches: (1) the dorsal artery, which supplies the glans, (2) the cavernosal artery, which supplies the corpora cavernosa, (3) the spongiosal artery, which supplies the spongiosum, and (4) the bulbar artery, which supplies the urethral bulb. Emanating from the cavernosal artery are multiple helicine arteries that open directly into the lacunae. These helicine arteries serve as the major resistance vessels modulating arterial inflow to the lacunar spaces.

Venous drainage is from the periphery of the corpora cavernosa through subtunical venules that drain peripheral lacunar spaces. These venules, which exist in the subtunical space, coalesce to form emissary veins that penetrate the tunica albuginea to enter the systemic venous circulation. Drainage from the mid and distal corpora cavernosa passes via the deep dorsal vein into the preprostatic plexus. The proximal crura are drained separately via the cavernosal and crural emissary veins into the preprostatic plexus and the internal pudendal vein. The corpus spongiosum is drained via the circumflex and urethral veins to the deep dorsal vein and internal pudendal veins. The glans penis empties directly into numerous large and small veins to join the deep and superficial dorsal veins.[5]

The peripheral innervation of the penis includes the thoracolumbar sympathetic, the sacral parasympathetic, and the sacral somatic nerves.[6] The pelvic plexus serves as a relay and integration center within which preganglionic axons make synaptic connections with postganglionic neurons innervating the penis. The autonomic fibers projecting to the penis from the pelvic plexus are known as the cavernosal nerves. These are located within the pelvic fascia and are anatomically located along the dorsolateral aspect of the prostate. The pudendal nerve has fibers innervating the striated muscles of the pelvis and perineum and has sensory fibers to the penis and perineal skin. It branches to become the perineal nerve and the dorsal nerve of the penis. The dorsal nerve forms the afferent limb of the penile erectile reflex by transmitting sensory impulses from the penile skin, prepuce, and glans.[6]

■ PHYSIOLOGY OF ERECTION

The initiation and maintenance of a normal erection require the appropriate balance of psychologic, endocrinologic, neurologic, and vascular (arterial and venous) elements. Erection results following both helicine artery and trabecular smooth muscle relaxation. Vasodilatation of the cavernosal and helicine arteries results in increased arterial inflow and a transmission of systemic arterial perfusion pressures to the lacunae. Relaxation of the trabecular smooth muscle results in engorgement of these spaces with expansion of the trabecular structures against the tunica albuginea. This causes passive compression of subtunical venules, increasing the resistance to venous outflow during erection. The mechanical compression of these subtunical venules is known as the corporal veno-occlusive mechanism. The pressure within the corpora cavernosa during erection is the result of the equilibrium between the perfusion pressure within the cavernosal arteries and the resistance to venous outflow through the compressed subtunical venules.[5,7,8]

Detumescence results following both helicine artery and trabecular smooth muscle contraction. Vasoconstriction of the cavernosal and helicine arteries results in diminished arterial inflow and a gradient between the systemic perfusion pressure and the lacunar space pressure. Constriction of the trabecular smooth muscle results in contraction of the lacunar volume, with return of the trabecular structures and the subtunical space to their baseline states. This results in a lowered resistance to venous outflow through the subtunical venules, returning the corporal body pressure to systemic venous pressure.[5,7,8]

Relaxation of corporal smooth muscle most likely occurs secondary to the release of cholinergic and nonadrenergic, noncholinergic neurotransmitters.[9,10] Smooth muscle relaxation also may result from local vasoactive factors released from intact endothelial cells lining the lacunar spaces.[11] Endothelium-derived relaxing factor, EDRF, is released from lacunar endothelial cells and induces surrounding trabecular smooth muscle relaxation.[9,11] Prostaglandins are also endothelial-derived substances that may affect penile smooth muscle tone.[12] Constriction of corporal smooth muscle is mediated via adrenergic nerves that release norepinephrine to act upon the alpha$_1$-adrenoceptors of smooth muscle.

■ EVALUATION OF THE IMPOTENT MALE

History and Physical Examination

The history and physical examination remain the cornerstone of the impotence evaluation. As much pertinent information as possible is gathered during the initial office visit, and this directs further diagnostic testing.

Key questions pertinent to the history include the duration of erectile dysfunction and whether the onset was acute or gradual. It is important to note whether the patient has had a recent change in his lifestyle (divorce, death of loved one, loss of job, and so on) and whether this change is temporally related to his erectile complaints. Subjective assessment (graded 0 to 100 per cent) of the patient's maximal erectile rigidity in regards to his morning, masturbatory, and coital erections is important. It is also useful to have subjective assessment of his present ability to maintain any erections he achieves. Is he able to achieve better quality erections with different partners or under different circumstances? Has there been a change in his libido? If there is a change in his libido, did this occur before or after the change in his erections? What is the status of his ejaculations in terms of volume, strength, and sensation?

A thorough medical and surgical review is indicated at this time. The history of cryptorchidism, postpubertal mumps orchitis, testicular torsion, or trauma is relevant to identify possible hypogonadal states. Identifiable vascular risk factors for failure to fill and/or store erectile dysfunction include present or past history of cigarette smoking, hypertension, obesity, diabetes mellitus, hypercholesterolemia, and signs of atherosclerosis or other vascular disease.[13,14] A present or past history of alcohol or drug abuse can predispose the patient to peripheral neuropathies and hormonal imbalances. Neurologic disorders, including spinal cord injuries, cerebrovascular accidents, transverse myelitis, multiple sclerosis, and Parkinson's disease, should be ruled out. A careful review of medications is indicated, with special note of antihypertensives, tranquilizers, antidepressants, and antipsychotics. Medications can affect erectile function through alterations in hemodynamic, neurologic, and hormonal mechanisms.[15] A history of trauma should be carefully sought out, especially any pertaining to perineal trauma ("straddle injuries") or pelvic fractures. Such injuries can result in failure to fill and/or store impotence by direct injury to the crura.[16] Along these lines, it is important to document the history of cycling, horseback riding, or motocross riding. A complete list of all prior operations is essential, with emphasis placed on back, bladder, prostate, rectal, penis/urethra, and radical pelvic cancer surgery. Such surgery can result in efferent sympathetic nerve injury. A history of exposure to toxins may increase the risk for a peripheral neuropathy. A history of radiation therapy to the pelvis is important, as this reportedly can cause a radiation-induced vasculitis with arterial insufficiency.[17] In the general review of systems, it is helpful to elicit a detailed voiding history as well as bowel habits, as this will allow preliminary assessment of the sacral roots (S2-4) and may indicate a cystometrogram as part of the workup.

The physical examination should begin with the search for physical signs of hypogonadism, such as eunuchoid features or gynecomastia. A detailed genital examination should be performed, beginning with the penis, noting any obvious dermatologic lesions or palpable plaques (Peyronie's disease). Peyronie's disease is a connective tissue disease of the penis that may cause pain or curvature with erection. It is also commonly associated with complaints of erectile insufficiency, most likely on the basis of corporal veno-occlusive dysfunction.[18] The scrotal contents should be examined and any abnormalities noted. The rectal examination should note whether normal anal sphincter tone is present, the size and consistency of the prostate gland, and the presence or absence of the bulbocavernosal reflex (S2-4). This reflex is noted by sensing a slight increase in anal tone in response to a gentle squeeze of the glans penis. Sensory testing of the perineum and lower extremities and motor testing of the upper and lower extremities may be performed. Absent or hypoactive reflexes suggest segmental abnormalities, and hyperactive reflexes imply suprasegmental corticobulbar lesions. Peripheral pulses (femoral, popliteal, posterior tibial, and dorsalis pedis) should be noted. Patients with peripheral neuropathies secondary to alcoholism or diabetes may have a pain and touch sensory loss in a stocking and glove distribution. Patients with posterior column disease (tabes dorsalis) may have associated pain and position sensory deficits. Occult herniated disc disease may have a loss of sensation in the lateral aspect of the leg (L4-5) or lateral aspect of the foot (S1-2). Although a careful physical examination is indicated in all patients, it will rarely yield a definitive diagnosis as to the cause of the erectile dysfunction.

Noninvasive Diagnostic Studies

During the initial office visit, objective information about the arterial supply of the penis can be obtained by measuring penile artery systolic occlusion pressures in the flaccid state. The integrity of the dorsal nerve sensory pathway can be assessed by measuring vibratory sensation thresholds using a penile biothesiometer. Psychologic assessment can be performed in a 1-hour interview with a psychologist. Nocturnal tumescence monitoring can be evaluated in a hospital or home setting. Finally, laboratory tests can be used to screen for diabetes mellitus, hypercholesterolemia, hyperprolactinemia, thyroid disease, and low serum testosterone.

The measurement of penile blood pressures was introduced as a means of identifying cavernosal arterial insufficiency. Patients undergo measurement of the penile artery systolic occlusion pressure in the flaccid state, using a pediatric blood pressure cuff at the base of the penis and Doppler ultrasound. This value is compared to the brachial artery systolic occlusion pressure defining the penile:brachial index (PBI).[19] If the PBI ratio is less than 0.6 there is evidence for arterial insufficiency; however, a ratio greater than 0.6 does not rule out significant arterial disease.

Penile biothesiometry is a screening test of the afferent dorsal neurologic pathway, and if there is evidence for sensory loss, then neurophysiologic evaluation may be required.[20,21] Such testing may involve the determination of dorsal nerve somatosensory evoked potentials, dorsal nerve conduction velocity, or bulbocavernosus reflex latencies to gain an objective assessment of the peripheral and central afferent nerve pathways. These objective data can distinguish peripheral sensory neuropathies, sacral lesions, and suprasacral lesions based on nerve conduction velocities. Most patients with neurogenic impotence will have known neurologic disease, but there will be some individuals in whom the erectile problems are the first manifestation of a neurologic disease.

Psychologic testing involves a psychologic interview as well as sexual personality or stress factor questionnaires. During the interview, the couples' subjective experience of the sexual problem should be noted. Patterns of sexual avoidance should be identified. Questionnaires used to assess sexual attitudes and function have not been useful in the differentiation of organic versus psychogenic impotence.

Erectile activity during sleep (nocturnal penile tumescence, NPT) is a normal phenomenon unrelated to sexual stimulation.[22,23] It occurs most often, but not exclusively, during REM sleep. NPT testing remains one of the main diagnostic tools to distinguish organic from psychogenic impotence.[24] This is based on the assumption that psychogenic factors do not influence nocturnal erections. However, there are organic conditions that impair sexual erections but do not impair nocturnal erections. NPT recordings should be made for changes in both penile circumference and rigidity. The results may be correlated with simultaneously recorded sleep patterns to avoid the interpretation of abnormal erectile activity secondary to abnormal sleep.

Screening for the hypothalamic-pituitary-gonadal axis will yeild an endocrinologic abnormality in 5 to 15 per cent of patients and is especially considered for those patients with a history of decreased libido; physical signs of hypogonadism, gynecomastia, or galactorrhea; or a documented low serum testosterone.[25] If a single serum testosterone determination is low, pooled serum testosterone and luteinizing hormone, three samples 20 minutes apart in the morning, may be measured.[26] This may avoid the interpretation of a low testosterone value based on a normal trough caused by the normal variation in testosterone secretion.

Serum prolactin assays are made in those men with decreased libido, low testosterone without a concurrent rise in serum luteinizing hormone, and hypogonadism. Hyperprolactinemia can be attributed to medications associated with overproduction of prolactin, chronic renal failure, pituitary adenoma, or laboratory error, or it can be idiopathic.[27–29]

Screening of thyroid function may be performed, as erectile complaints are seen in both the hyper- and hypothyroid states.[30] Hyperthyroid states are associated with higher serum estrogen levels, and an elevated serum testosterone should be considered a biochemical marker for occult hyperthyroidism. Hypothyroid states can be associated with low testosterone secretion and elevated prolactin levels.[31]

Invasive Diagnostic Studies

An office screening test has been recently introduced in which the erectile response is observed following **intracavernosal injection of vasoactive agents** that directly relax the corporal smooth muscle or block adrenergically induced smooth muscle tone.[32] A normal erection should develop within 5 to 10 minutes and last approximately 1 hour following the injection. Such a response in an impotent patient implies normal hemodynamics with neurologic or psychologic dysfunction as likely etiologies. Partial, short-lived or absent erections suggest either hemodynamic impairment or excessive adrenergic constrictive tone secondary to anxiety. To avoid misinterpretation, this test is performed with manual, vibratory, or audiovisual sexual stimulation.

Duplex ultrasound scanning of the dorsal and cavernosal arteries involves sonographic measurements of arterial luminal diameter and blood flow velocity, made before and after the intracavernosal injection of vasoactive agents.[33] Atherosclerotic cavernosal arteries demonstrate minimal changes in luminal diameter and diminished blood flow velocity compared with normals. Sonographic criteria to distinguish patients with normal arterial capacity from those with varying degrees of arterial disease have been established.

Dynamic infusion cavernosometry and cavernosography (DICC) is a dynamic test in which information concerning the interaction of arterial and corporal veno-occlusive hemodynamics can be obtained.[34] The first phase of this study monitors the corporal body pressure response to the intracavernosal injection of vasoactive agents. The dose is calculated to relax corporal smooth muscle maximally and block adrenergic constrictor tone. This phase is similar to the aforementioned office screening study, except that a graphic record of the corporal pressure response is obtained. The equilibrium corporal body pressure response is determined by the perfusion pressure of the cavernosal artery (a value recorded during phase 3 of this study) and by the loss of pressure from venous outflow during the erection. In a normal erection, the corporal body pressure should approximate the mean systemic arterial blood pressure. Impotent patients with this pattern are considered to have failure to initiate erectile dysfunction. The second phase of the study evaluates the corporal veno-occlusive mechanism by infusing heparinized saline to a suprasystolic corporal body pressure and determining the rate of pressure fall following termination of the infusion. In corporal veno-occlusive dysfunction, there is a low resistance to venous outflow and a rapid fall in corporal body pressure. Impotent patients with this pattern are considered to have failure to store erectile dysfunction. During this phase, perineal compression may be applied to the crural bodies to identify any alteration in the rate of pressure fall following termination of the infusion. Impotent patients showing a rapid fall in corporal body pressure that is markedly diminished following perineal compression have a pattern consistent with focal corporal veno-occlusive dysfunction involving the crura. This pattern is commonly seen in young patients with a history of blunt perineal trauma. The third phase of the study records the cavernosal artery systolic occlusion pressure. This is performed by recording cavernosal arterial flow by Doppler ultrasound. The corporal body pressure is increased by saline infusion until the audible arterial flow ceases. The infusion is terminated at this point, and the corporal body pressure is allowed to decrease until the reappearance of pulsatile flow in the cavernosal artery. The corporal body pressure at which flow is re-established is the cavernosal artery systolic occlusion pressure, and it defines the maximal perfusion pressure that can be delivered to the lacunar spaces during erection. An abnormal cavernosal artery systolic occlusion pressure is consistent with a gradient between the cavernosal and brachial artery systolic occlusion pressure. Impotent patients with this gradient are considered to have failure to fill erectile dysfunction. The fourth phase of this study involves cavernosography to visualize any veins draining the corporal bodies during erection. Radiopaque contrast is infused intracavernosally in the erect state, and multiple views are taken. In the presence of normal corporal veno-occlusion, minimal or absent visualization of draining veins is observed.

Selective internal pudendal arteriography is reserved for those patients being considered for arterial reconstructive surgery. The study is performed under local anesthesia using intracavernosal vasoactive agents to allow optimal visualization of the hypogastric-cavernous arterial bed. The internal iliac artery and internal pudendal artery are selectively catheterized via a femoral approach. Anteroposterior and oblique positions allow visualization of the common penile, dorsal, and cavernosal arteries. Results of the arteriogram are interpreted in conjunction with the results of other functional studies (DICC and duplex Doppler scanning).[35,36]

■ Management

An understanding of the patient's goals and expectations will direct therapy to the patient's individual needs.

■ PSYCHOLOGIC THERAPY

Those patients whose evaluation suggests a primary psychogenic origin for their sexual dysfunction are referred to an appropriate therapist. In addition, men with organic disease may have adjustment problems with nonpsychologic treatment and may require counseling to improve sexual relationships.

Behavior-oriented sexual therapy has replaced classic psychotherapy for the treatment of psychogenic impotence.[37,38] The approach in behavior therapy is to minimize performance anxiety using sensate focus exercises.[38,39] Whenever possible, such therapy involves the patient and his sexual partner.

A 35 to 80 per cent success rate has been reported using these techniques.[40] It appears that long-term erectile dysfunction, older age, decreased libido, and psychopathology are negative prognostic indicators.

■ MEDICAL THERAPY

The simplicity of oral and transcutaneous therapy makes these alternatives attractive, and research in these fields is ongoing. Oral therapy is divided into hormonal and nonhormonal manipulation.

Erectile dysfunction secondary to endocrine abnormalities is often suspected clinically after the history and physical examination. The three categories of endocrine dysfunction associated with erectile disturbances are (1) hyperprolactinemia, (2) hypogonadotropic hypogonadism, and (3) hypergonadotropic hypogonadism.

Hyperprolactinemia is associated with impotence and low or low-normal serum testosterone levels.[27-29] Treatment of this disorder is aimed at reducing the serum prolactin, not at testosterone replacement. Those patients with hyperprolactinemia secondary to medications usually respond to appropriate changes in those medications. Patients with pituitary adenomas respond to bromocriptine therapy (usual daily dose: 5 to 7.5 mg).[41] Follow-up consists of serum prolactin levels, visual field examinations, and radiologic examination of the sella turcica. Pituitary adenomas that are large and not responsive to medication require surgical ablation.[41]

In cases of hypogonadism, it would be most desirable to identify and reverse the cause. If the cause cannot be eliminated, then replacement androgen therapy becomes necessary. The preferred route for replacement is intramuscular testosterone enanthate (200 to 300 mg intramuscularly every 2 to 3 weeks).[31,41] Oral testosterone is too unpredictable in terms of its absorption characteristics. The risks of androgen therapy must be considered carefully.[31] These include hepatotoxicity and hepatoma formation, polycythemia, and feminizing side effects secondary to peripheral conversion to estradiol. Liver-related side effects are greater in those patients with some degree of baseline hepatic disease. Androgen therapy risks also include diminished spermatogenesis, increased prostate size (but no increased risk for cancer), weight gain due to sodium retention, acne, and hyperlipidemia.[31] Appropriate screening and follow-up are essential in these patients.

To date, no satisfactory nonhormonal agent has been found that can induce and maintain an erection reliably by either the oral or transcutaneous route.

Yohimbine, an indole alkaloid, is an alpha$_2$-adrenergic receptor antagonist that was regarded initially to have aphrodisiac properties.[42] It has been utilized as an oral therapy for impotence. Earlier studies comparing yohimbine versus placebo in the treatment of organic impotence were unable to establish a statistically significant advantage for yohimbine.[41]

The use of transcutaneous nitroglycerin applied to the penile shaft as a means of relaxing smooth muscle and inducing erection is still at the investigational level and has not been widely implemented clinically. Problems with vaginal absorption of the drug have been reported.[43]

One of the major advances made in the field of impotence therapy has evolved over the last 10 years. Use of intracavernosal vasoactive agents to relax corporal smooth muscle directly and block vasoconstrictor tone has dramatically changed the approach to treatment for erectile dysfunction.[44]

For patients with failure to initiate erectile dysfunction, such as psychogenic impotence unresponsive to counseling and neurogenic impotence, intracavernosal self-injection mimics endogenous physiologic mechanisms. Such patients are ideal candidates for this therapy.[45,46] Since they usually have normal penile hemodynamics, they require very low doses of the medication.

For patients with failure to fill or failure to store erectile dysfunction, the use of intracavernosal vasoactive agents provides pharmacologic-mediated arterial and trabecular smooth muscle relaxation maximizing arterial inflow and corporal veno-occlusion.[47] Such patients with hemodynamic impairment usually require higher doses of intracavernosal therapy.

The combination of **papaverine hydrochloride** and **phentolamine mesylate** can be injected intracavernosally to initiate and maintain erection. Patients can learn proper self-injection techniques in three to four office visits. During these visits, they are given titrated doses of medication to achieve an erection for approximately 45 minutes. Risks with the injection therapy program include ecchymosis at the injection site if compression is not adequate, possible tissue fibrosis at the injection sites and within the corpora, potential infection if aseptic technique is not followed, and priapism (prolonged erection).[48-51] Prolonged erection for more than 4 hours is a urologic emergency and requires prompt presentation to a physician for reversal of this "drug erection." These episodes of priapism can be treated successfully with intracavernosal alpha-agonists that induce smooth muscle contraction and effectively re-establish corporal venous drainage.[52] In some patients, corporal aspiration through large-bore needles will be necessary in addition to corporal irrigation with alpha-agonists. In rare instances when erections have been prolonged for more than 24 to 36 hours and have not subsided with alpha-agonist therapy, surgery will be necessary for detumescence.

Prostaglandin E_1 is another agent that causes smooth muscle relaxation and will induce erection when injected intracavernosally.[53,54] It is not in widespread clinical use yet but, because it is locally metabolized within the penis, there is less risk for prolonged erection episodes.

Long-term follow-up with pharmacologic therapy is still in progress, but to date few serious problems have been noted. One large series reported a 72 per cent success rate using this modality, regardless of the etiology of the impotence, and most failures were in patients over 75 years old or with severe aortoiliac arterial disease.[55] Satisfaction rates with this therapy are excellent.[56] Scarring of the tunica albuginea at the site of repeated injections and smooth muscle cell hypertrophy in the corpora cavernosa have been reported.[56]

Vacuum constriction therapy has been a nonsurgical treatment option for impotence for many years. Since 1917, the United States Patent Office has dealt with inventors of various devices.[57] Until recently the suction devices have not received much attention in the urologic literature, but with improved technology they must now be considered a viable option available to the impotent man. The vacuum constriction device consists of a plastic external cylinder that is placed over the penis in such a fashion as to attain an airtight seal at the penile base. Tubing from the cylinder tip is attached to a hand-held pump that is used to create a vacuum within the cylinder as the air is removed. This negative pressure state within the cylinder draws blood into the pendulous penis, resulting in distal engorgement. When an adequate state of tumescence has been reached, a constricting band is placed around the base of the penis to maintain distal shaft erection. The suction device can be used to produce an erection-like state or to augment patients with partial erections. The constricting band should not be in place for more than 30 minutes.[58,59] Ninety-two per cent of patients reportedly have been able to achieve adequate rigidity for intercourse, and satisfaction rates of 80 per cent have been reported.[58] Complaints with the vacuum devices include penile cyanosis and superficial vein distention secondary to venous obstruction from the constricting band, mild decreases in penile skin temperature, diminished or no ejaculation secondary to the bands, and some erection instability since the penis is erect only distal to the bands and may pivot at the base.[58,60] Reports of initial discomfort using the device diminish with time.

■ SURGICAL THERAPY

The goal of arterial vascular reconstructive surgery is to increase perfusion pressure to the lacunar spaces, bypassing arterial obstruction. Such surgery for the impotent patient is different from revascularization surgery in other vascular beds in that erectile function depends not only on arterial perfusion but also on veno-occlusion.

Revascularization surgery that involves aortoiliac reconstruction has been largely unsuccessful in restoring potency.[61] Such failure is most likely related to the presence of distal arterial disease as well as corporal veno-occlusive dysfunction. Revascularization surgery currently focuses on microscopic vascular bypass procedures. The usual neoarterial inflow source is the inferior epigastric artery. Distal anastomotic sites have included the tunica albuginea, the dorsal artery, the cavernosal artery, and the dorsal vein.[62-64] Although long-term follow-up is unavailable, it appears that the younger patient with focal arterial occlusive disease secondary to blunt perineal or pelvic trauma has a better prognosis for restoration of potency than the older patient with diffuse arterial disease involving the cavernosal artery. Success in selected patients has been reported as high as 80 per cent.[63,65] Patients with diffuse cavernosal arterial disease may consider a venous arterialization procedure in which the inferior epigastric artery is anastomosed to a segment of the deep dorsal vein. In this procedure, retrograde flow of arterial blood passes into the corporal bodies through the emissary veins and subtunical venules. Success rates with the procedure have been reported to vary from 40 to 75 per cent in small series without long-term follow-up.[65,66]

The goal of surgery for corporal veno-occlusive dysfunction is to increase resistance to venous outflow in the erect state. Such surgery was attempted back at the turn of the century with ligation of the deep dorsal vein of the penis.[67,68] The initial successes were short-lived. Present-day operations have included excision of the deep dorsal vein, ligation of the cavernosal veins, crural ligation, crural plication, and spongiolysis.[69-73] It appears that the patient who has cavernosometric documentation of corporal veno-occlusive dysfunction confined to the proximal portion of the corpora cavernosa has a better prognosis for restoration of potency than does the patient with generalized corporal veno-occlusive dysfunction involving the glans or corpus spongiosum.[74]

Some patients will require supplemental self-injection therapy postoperatively to achieve adequate rigidity.

The use of penile prostheses will continue to play a major role in the management of erectile dysfunction, but it should not be considered a first-line therapy for the majority of patients. The physician and patient should explore alternative treatment options before proceeding with a penile prosthesis. The patient and his partner should undergo appropriate counseling prior to penile prosthesis implantation. The aim of the surgery is to restore sexual function by providing sufficient penile rigidity for intercourse. Patient expectations that exceed the realistic capabilities of the devices usually result in dissatisfaction. Patient and partner satisfaction rates approach over 90 per cent with this treatment when it is used in the properly selected patient.[75,76]

Penile implants have been used for at least 50 years; early materials used included cartilage and bone grafts, but success rates were poor.[77,78] The introduction of synthetic penile prostheses in 1952 (acrylic and polyethylene) improved results somewhat, but there were still significant problems with erosion and infection.[79] The use of silicone prostheses placed within the tunica albuginea of the corpora dramatically improved the surgical results. Problems with the earlier implants related to their constant rigidity and poor cosmetic appearance. Today the two types of penile prostheses are the semirigid and inflatable models. The choice of prosthesis is individualized for each patient, based on which model will best serve his clinical situation.

The first inflatable penile prosthesis was introduced in 1973 in an attempt to improve the penile rigidity, girth, and cosmetic appearance that could be obtained with an implant.[80] This device has evolved over the years to improve earlier problems with mechanical failure. This evolution has given rise to models of varying design and simplicity and to more reliable and durable devices.[75,81-86] Infection rates with either the semirigid or inflatable penile prostheses are 2 to 3 per cent.[81]

■ Conclusion

The complaint of impotence by the patient should be followed by a comprehensive investigation to define underlying pathophysiology. Based on the information obtained, patients should be offered the appropriate psychologic, medical, or surgical treatment options available.

REFERENCES

1. Shabsigh R, Fishman IJ, Scott FB. Evaluation of erectile impotence. Urology 1988; 32:83–90.
2. Furlow WL. Prevalence of impotence in the United States. Med Aspects Human Sex 1985; 19:13–16.
3. McCulloch DK, Campbell IW, Wu FC, Prescott RJ, Clarke BF. The prevalence of diabetic impotence. Diabetologia 1980; 18:279–283.
4. Goldstein AMB, Meehan JP, Zakhary R, Buckley PA, Rogers FA. New observations in the microarchitecture of corpora cavernosa in man and possible

relationship to mechanism of erection. Urology 1982; 3:259–266.

5. Lue TF, Tanagho EA. Functional anatomy and mechanism of penile erection. *In* Tanagho EA, Lue TF, McClure RD (eds). Contemporary Management of Impotence and Infertility. Baltimore: Williams & Wilkins, 1988:39–50.

6. de Groat WC, Steers WD. Neuroanatomy and neurophysiology of penile erection. *In* Tanagho EA, Lue TF, McClure RD (eds). Contemporary Management of Impotence and Infertility. Baltimore: Williams & Wilkins, 1988:3–27.

7. Saenz de Tejada I, Goldstein I, Blanco R, Cohen RA, Krane RJ. Smooth muscle of the corpus cavernosa; role in penile erection. Surg Forum 1985; 36:623–624.

8. Lue TF, Tanagho EA. Physiology of erection and pharmacological management of impotence. J Urol 1987; 137:829–836.

9. Saenz de Tejada I, Blanco R, Goldstein I, et al. Cholinergic neurotransmission in human corpora cavernosa. 1. Responses of isolated tissue. Am J Physiol 1988; 254:H459–H467.

10. Blanco R, Saenz de Tejada I, Goldstein I, et al. Cholinergic neurotransmission in human corpora cavernosa. 2. Acetylene synthesis. Am J Physiol 1988; 254:H468–H472.

11. Furchgott RF, Zawadski JV. The obligatory role of endothelial cells in the relaxation of arterial smooth muscle to acetylcholine. Nature 1980; 288:373–376.

12. Van houtte PM, Rubanyi GM, Miller VM, Houston DS. Modulation of vascular smooth muscle contraction by the endothelium. Annu Rev Physiol 1986; 48:307–320.

13. Virag R, Bouilly P, Frydaman D. Is impotence an arterial disorder?—A study of arterial risk factors in 400 impotent men. Lancet 1985; 1:181–184.

14. Michal V. Arterial disease as a cause of impotence. Clin Endocrinol Metab 1982; 11:725–748.

15. Wein AJ, Van Arsdalen KN. Drug-induced male sexual dysfunction. Urol Clin North Am 1988; 15:23–51.

16. Sharlip I. Penile arteriography in impotence after pelvic trauma. J Urol 1981; 126:477–479.

17. Goldstein I, Feldman MI, Deckers PJ, et al. Radiation-associated impotence. A clinical study of its mechanism. JAMA 1984; 251:903–910.

18. Metz P, Ebbehoj J, Uhrenholdt A, Wagner G. Peyronie's disease and erectile failure. J Urol 1983; 130:1103.

19. Mueller SC, Lue TF. Evaluation of vascular impotence. Urol Clin North Am 1988; 15:65–76.

20. Padma-Nathan H. Neurologic evaluation of erectile dysfunction. Urol Clin North Am 1988; 15:77–80.

21. Padma-Nathan H, Goldstein I. Neurologic assessment of the impotent patient. *In* Montague DK (ed). Disorders of Male Sexual Function. Chicago: Year Book Medical Publishers, 1988:86–94.

22. Kessler WO. Nocturnal penile tumescence. Urol Clin North Am 1988; 15:81–86.

23. Fisher C, Gross J, Zuch J. Cycle of penile erections synchronous with dreaming (REM) sleep. Arch Gen Psychiatr 1965; 12:29.

24. Karacan I. Clinical value of nocturnal erection in the prognosis and diagnosis of impotence. Med Aspects Hum Sex 1970; 4:27–34.

25. Spark RF, White RA, Connolly PB. Impotence is not always psychogenic. JAMA 1980; 243:750.

26. Goldzieher JW, Dizier TS, Smith KD, et al. Improving the diagnostic reliability of rapidly fluctuating plasma hormone levels by optimized multiple-sampling techniques. J Clin Endocrinol Metab 1976; 43:824.

27. Franks S, Jacobs HS, Martin N, Nabarro JDN. Hyperprolactinemia and impotence. Clin Endocrinol 1978; 8:277–287.

28. Pogach LM, Vaitukaitis JL. Endocrine disorders associated with erectile dysfunction. *In* Krane RJ, Siroky MB, Goldstein I (eds). Male Sexual Dysfunction. Boston: Little, Brown, 1983:63–76.

29. Perryman RL, Thorner MO. The effects of hyperprolactinemia on sexual and reproductive function in men. J Androl 1981; 5:233.

30. Kidd GS, Glass AR, Vigersky RA. The hypothalamic-pituitary-testicular axis in thyrotoxicosis. J Clin Endocrinol Metab 1983; 57:557.

31. McClure RD. Endocrine evaluation and therapy. *In* Tanagho EA, Lue TF, McClure RD (eds). Contemporary Management of Impotence and Infertility. Baltimore: Williams and Wilkins, 1988:84–94.

32. Abber JC, Lue TF. Evaluation of impotence. *In* deVere White R (ed). Problems in Urology: Sexual Function. Philadelphia: JB Lippincott, 1987:476–486.

33. Lue TF, Hricak H, Marich KW, et al. Vascular impotence evaluated by high resolution ultrasonography and pulsed Doppler spectrum analysis. Radiology 1985; 155:777–781.

34. Padma-Nathan H, Gasior B, Roddy T, Tessier J, Payton T, Goldstein I, Krane RJ. Dynamic infusion cavernosometry and cavernosography (DICC): The interaction of arterial and veno-occlusive function (abstract 207). J Urol 1989; 141:67A.

35. Zorgniotti AW, Padula G, Shaw W. Selective arteriography for vascular impotence. World J Urol 1983; 1:213–217.

36. Bookstein JJ, Valji K, Parsons L, Kessler W. Pharmacoarteriography in the evaluation of impotence. J Urol 1987; 137:333.

37. Smith AD. Psychologic factors in the multidisciplinary evaluation and treatment of erectile dysfunction. Urol Clin North Am 1988; 15:41–51.

38. Golden JS. Behavioral approaches to the treatment of sexual problems. *In* Zales M (ed). Eating, Sleeping and Sexuality: Treatment of Disorders in Basic Life Functions. New York: Brunner-Mazel, 1982:236–257.

39. Masters WH, Johnson VE. Human Sexual Inadequacy. Boston: Little, Brown, 1970.

40. Lopiccolo J, Stock WE. Treatment of sexual dysfunction. J Consult Clin Psychol 1986; 54:158–167.

41. Morales A, Condra MS, Owen JE, Fenemore F, Surridge DH. Oral and transcutaneous pharmacological agents in the treatment of impotence. Urol Clin North Am 1988; 15:87–93.

42. Nickerson M, Collier B. Drugs inhibiting adrenergic nerves and structures innervated by them. *In* Goodman L, Gilman A (eds). The Pharmacological Basis of Therapeutics. 4th ed. New York: Macmillan, 1975:533–564.

43. Talley JD, Crawley IS. Transdermal nitrate, penile erection and spousal headache. Ann Intern Med 1985; 103:804.

44. Junemann KP, Lue TF, Fournier GR, Tanagho EA. Hemodynamics of papaverine- and phentolamine-induced penile erection. J Urol 1986; 136:158–161.

45. Wyndaele JJ, De Meyer JM, et al. Intracavernous injection of vasoactive drugs, an alternative for treating impotence in spinal cord injury patients. Paraplegia 1986; 24:271–275.

46. Kiely EA, Williams G, Goldie L. Assessment of the immediate and long-term effects of pharmacologically-induced penile erections in the treatment of psychogenic and organic impotence. Br J Urol 1987; 59:164–169.

47. Buvat J, Buvat-herbant M, Dehaene JL, Lemaire A. Is intracavernous injection of papaverine a reliable screening test for vascular impotence? J Urol 1986; 135:476.

48. Padma-Nathan H, Goldstein I, Payton T, Krane RJ. Intracavernous pharmacotherapy: the pharmacological erection program. World J Urol 1987; 5:160.

49. Levine SB, Althof SE, Turner LA, et al. Side effects of self administration of intracavernous papaverine and phentolamine for the treatment of impotence. J Urol 1989; 141:54–57.

50. Trapp JD. Pharmacologic erection program for the treatment of male impotence. South Med J 1987; 80:426–427.

51. Zentgraf M, Baccouche M, Junemann KP. Diagnosis and treatment of erectile dysfunction using papaverine and phentolamine. Urol Int 1988; 43:65–75.

52. Broderick GA, Lue TF. Priapism and the physiology of erection. AUA Update Series #29, 1988.

53. Stackl W, Hasun R, Marberger M. Intracavernous injection of prostaglandin E_1 in impotent men. J Urol 1988; 140:66–68.

54. Lee LM, Stevenson RWD, Szasz G. Prostaglandin E_1 versus papaverine/phentolamine for the treatment of erectile impotence: a double blind comparison. J Urol 1989; 141:549–550.

55. Zorgniotti AW. Corpus cavernosum blockade for impotence: practical aspects and results in 250 cases (abstract 208). Part 2. J Urol 1986; 135:306A.

56. Sidi AA, Vasoactive intracavernous pharmacotherapy. Urol Clin North Am 1988; 15: 95–101.

57. Lederer O. Surgical device. U.S. Patent Number 1,225,341, 5/8/17.

58. Witherington R. Suction device therapy in the management of erectile impotence. Urol Clin North Am 1988; 15:123–128.

59. Nadig PW, Ware JC, Blumoff R. Noninvasive device to produce and maintain an erection-like state. Urology 1986; 27:126–131.

60. Witherington R. Vacuum constriction device for management of erectile impotence. J Urol 1989; 141:320–322.

61. Dewar ML, Blundell PE, Lidstone D, Herba MJ, Chiu RC. Effects of abdominal aneurysmectomy, aortoiliac bypass grafting and angioplasty on male sexual potency: a prospective study. Can J Surg 1985; 28:154.

62. Michal V, Kramar R, Pospichal J, Hejhal L. Direct arterial anastomosis on corpora cavernosa penis in therapy of erectile impotence. Rozhl Chir 1983; 52:587–590.

63. Goldstein I. Overview of types and results of vascular surgical procedures for impotence. Cardiovasc Intervent Radiol 1988; 11:240–244.

64. McDougal WS, Jeffrey RF. Microscopic penile revascularization. J Urol 1983; 129:517–521.

65. Sharlip ID. Treatment of arteriogenic impotence by penile revascularization. In Proceedings of the Sixth Biennial International Symposium for Corpus Cavernosum Revascularization and Third Biennial World Meeting on Impotence. Boston, 1988:135.

66. Virag R, Zwang G, Dermange H, Legman M. Vasculogenic impotence: a review of 92 cases with 54 surgical operations. Vasc Surg 1981; 15:9–17.

67. Wooten JS. Ligation of the dorsal vein of the penis as a cure for atonic impotence. Tex Med J 1902; 18:325.

68. Lydston GF. The surgical treatment of impotence. Am J Clin Med 1908; 15:1571.

69. Wespes E, Schulman CC. Venous leakage: surgical treatment of a curable cause of impotence. J Urol 1984; 133:796.

70. Lewis RW, Pauyau FA. Procedures for decreasing venous drainage. Semin Urol 1986; 4:263–272.

71. Lue TF. Treatment of venogenic impotence. In Tanagho EA, Lue TF, McClure RD (eds). Contemporary Management of Impotence and Infertility. Baltimore: Williams & Wilkins, 1988:175–177.

72. Bar-Moshe O, Van dendris M. Treatment of impotence due to perineal venous leakage by ligation of the crura penis. J Urol 1988; 139:1217–1219.

73. Glina S, Puech-leao P, Reis JMSM, Reichelt AC, Choa S. Surgical correction of corpora cavernosa leakage responsive to perineal compression: late results. Proceedings of the Sixth Biennial International Symposium for Corpus Cavernosum Revascularization and Third Biennial World Meeting on Impotence. Boston, 1988:142.

74. Roddy T, Tessier J, Gasior B, Goldstein I. Glans and/or spongiosum leak: a negative prognostic indicator for reconstructive surgery (abstract 478). J Urol 1989; 141:96A.

75. Gregory JG, Purcell MH. Scott's inflatable penile prosthesis: evaluation of mechanical survival in the series 700 model. J Urol 1987; 137:676.

76. Malloy TR, Wein AJ, Carpiniello VL. Reliability of AMS 700 inflatable penile prosthesis. Urology 1986; 27:385.

77. Bogoras NA. Über die volle plastiche überherstellung an einem koitusfähigen Penis (Peniplastica totalis). Zentralbl Chir 1936; 197:2029.

78. Bergman RT, Howard AH, Barnes RW. Plastic reconstruction of the penis. J Urol 1948; 59:1174.

79. Goodwin WE, Scott WW. Phalloplasty. J Urol 1952; 68:903.

80. Scott FB, Bradley WE, Timm GW. Management of erectile impotence: use of implantable inflatable prosthesis. Urology 1973; 12:80.

81. Kabalin JN, Kessler R. Penile prosthesis surgery. Monogr Urol 1989; 10(2):21–32.

82. Merrill DC. Clinical experience with Mentor inflatable penile prosthesis in 206 patients. Urology 1986; 28:185.

83. Mulcahy JJ. Use of CX cylinders in association with AMS 700 CX inflatable penile prosthesis. J Urol 1988; 140:1420–1421.

84. Mulcahy JJ. The hydroflex self-contained inflatable prosthesis: experience with 100 patients. J Urol 1988; 140:1422.

85. Merrill DC. Clinical experience with the Mentor inflatable penile prosthesis in 301 patients. J Urol 1988; 140:1424.

86. Kabalin JN, Kessler R. Five-year followup of the Scott inflatable penile prosthesis and comparison with semirigid penile prosthesis. J Urol 1988; 140:1428.

Infections in the acquired immunodeficiency syndrome patient

Aaron E. Glatt ■ *Bruce D. Agins*

Human immunodeficiency virus (HIV), the retrovirus that induces immune suppression in acquired immunodeficiency syndrome (AIDS) rarely causes death directly. Rather, the underlying disruption of the cell-mediated immune system results in susceptibility to unusual or opportunistic infections. The pathogens encountered in these infections rarely infect normal hosts but are seen in other immunocompromised patients, such as those undergoing surgery or transplant or cancer chemotherapy and those with congenital or other acquired immunodeficiency syndromes. However, many unique features make treatment and management of these infections especially difficult in the patient with HIV disease. (Also see pages 300–312.)

Familiarity with basic underlying principles in HIV infection will aid the clinician in developing a logical approach to the patient.[1] Many infections are caused by low-virulence organisms or parasites that are ubiquitous in nature and in the environment. Major exceptions include tuberculosis and herpes viruses, which affect normal hosts quite easily. These organisms asymptomatically colonize ("infect") healthy patients, at various times throughout their lives, and usually do not cause significant disease. However, in the presence of HIV infection, "latent" organisms can reactivate and cause disease of great severity.

For less ubiquitous organisms, geographic considerations and travel history are extremely important in evaluating the type of pathogens and the range of organisms to which a person may have been exposed and become colonized. For example, in the Southwestern United States, coccidioidomycosis is one of the most common causes of pneumonia in HIV-infected patients, second only to *Pneumocystis*. In the Midwestern United States, however, histoplasmosis ranks number two. Infections with these unusual pathogens would be unlikely in a person who did not have the proper travel exposure. Tuberculosis is extremely prevalent in inner city low socioeconomic centers, in immigrants, and in prisoners. INH-resistant mycobacteria are more frequently seen in certain populations, specifically patients from Haiti and Southeast Asia. These epidemiologic factors must be considered in diagnosis and treatment of patients with HIV-associated infections.

The general Oslerian principle of attributing all symptoms and signs to a single disease process does not apply to most patients with HIV infection. Multiple simultaneous infections are frequent; they are the rule, not the exception. This concept is especially important to remember when a patient does not respond to appropriate therapy. Rather than assume that the diagnosis is incorrect or that treatment has failed, one should search very carefully for additional pathogens that are more likely to be the true cause of the patient's distress.

Furthermore, in contrast to the usual treatment of infection in clinical practice, in which a cure is usually achievable with appropriate antimicrobial therapy, the goal of treatment of many IIIV-associated opportunistic infections is often suppression. Maintenance therapy may be necessary to control the disease and prevent exacerbations, and prophylaxis of primary infection is often essential. Adverse drug reactions are also frequent and can greatly confuse treatment efficacy. Finally, the presentation of many infections is atypical and/or more severe than the identical infection in an immunocompetent host. A bacterial pathogen that causes localized mild pneumonia in a healthy host may cause rampant diffuse disease in an HIV-infected patient. Other examples include disseminated and extrapulmonary tuberculosis, salmonellosis, and herpes infections.

■ Parasites

■ *PNEUMOCYSTIS CARINII* PNEUMONIA

Pneumocystis carinii pneumonia is both the most frequent treatable opportunistic pneumonia in patients with AIDS and the most common cause of death in these patients. The great majority (over 80 to 85 per cent) of patients with AIDS will acquire *Pneumocystis carinii* pneumonia (PCP) at some point during the course of their disease. Because the organism is already present in the lungs of most people, there is no known way to prevent acquisition of the organism. Therefore, therapeutic management must aim at preventing and treating the disease, not the "infection." Clinical manifestations of *Pneumocystis carinii* infection can be quite varied.[1,2] The classic clinical picture is that of a patient with an indolent, subacute infection with nonproductive cough, mild shortness of breath, low-grade intermittent fever, sweats, and malaise. However, a more fulminant course resembling acute bacterial pneumonia with rapid progression to adult respiratory distress syndrome (ARDS) may also occur. Any new pulmonary symptom, no matter how mild, mandates aggressive investigation and diagnostic testing in a patient with AIDS or HIV infection. The initial chest radiograph may be perfectly normal, and physical examination may not provide any specific clues as to the underlying disease process. An arterial blood gas determination should be obtained. Hypoxemia and an arteriolar-alveolar gradient increase will usually (but not always) be present.

Evaluation of sputum can confirm the diagnosis and obviate further workup. An adequate specimen is best obtained via induction with saline solution. In expert hands this technique has a diagnostic yield of between 50 and 80 per cent and is both noninvasive and relatively inexpensive.[1,2] Should induced sputum not be possible, or fail to reveal a pathogen, bronchoalveolar lavage will establish a definitive diagnosis.[1,2] Treatment of PCP may be initiated prior to the confirmation of diagnosis and does not significantly lower the yield. Transbronchial biopsy or lung biopsy is rarely necessary to establish the diagnosis of *Pneumocystis carinii* pneumonia and these usually are reserved for patients in whom other diagnoses or co-infection is likely. Gallium scans will be abnormal in nearly all patients with *Pneumocystis carinii* pneumonia but are not specific. They are not necessary if a strong clinical suspicion of *Pneumocystis* exists.

Two equally efficacious therapeutic regimens exist to treat *Pneumocystis carinii* pneumonia.[1-3] (The use of both regimens simultaneously is potentially dangerous.) Treatment may be initiated with trimethoprim/sulfamethoxazole (TMP/SMX) (with the trimethoprim component given at 15 to 20 mg/kg/day) in either three or four divided doses. Intravenous administration is preferred for very ill patients. However, in mild to moderately severe disease, when absorption and distribution are not compromised, the oral route is equally efficacious and less expensive. If adequate supervision is available, outpatient therapy offers personal and financial benefit.

Alternatively, pentamidine isoethionate (4 mg/kg of body weight/day), given intravenously via slow infusion (1 to 1.5 hours) is an equally effective therapy. Intramuscular pentamidine, once previously the route of choice, is associated with significant complications, especially sterile abscesses, and is no longer recommended routinely. Treatment (with either regimen) is usually given for three weeks, depending on clinical response. Clinical success is achieved in 60 to 90 per cent of first episodes of *Pneumocystis carinii* pneumonia. Unfortunately, recurrent episodes are common, and therapeutic efficacy for these episodes may not be as good. Inhaled pentamidine, currently not approved for treatment of *Pneumocystis carinii* pneumonia, may be an effective, noninvasive, inexpensive method for treating mild to moderate disease.[1,4,5] Alternative regimens, not yet well-tested, include dapsone, 100 mg/day, plus trimethoprim, 15 to 20 mg/kg/day; trimetrexate; and eflornithine. The latter two are available only via compassionate release or study protocols.[1]

Major and minor adverse reactions occur with great frequency with either pentamidine or TMP/SMX. The most frequent adverse reactions associated with TMP/SMX are rashes, fever, abnormal serum aminotransferase levels, and, most importantly, leukopenia. Mild hyponatremia is frequent but rarely severe enough to require cessation of therapy. Pentamidine has been associated with renal insufficiency, hypoglycemia (usually not related to administration of the drug and may be fatal), and fatal arrhythmias. If the rate of infusion is too rapid, significant hypotension may occur. Hyperglycemia may occur weeks to months *after* therapy has been completed and is probably related to the total cumulative dose received. Pancreatitis may also occur, as well as elevated serum transaminase levels. Leukopenia is also an extremely important and limiting toxicity in the usage of pentamidine.

The toxicity of dapsone/trimethoprim is similar to that of TMP/SMX. Dapsone is also associated with hemolytic anemia, especially in the presence of G6PD deficiency. However, patients who are allergic to sulfamethoxazole may be able to take dapsone, since cross-allergy is not frequent. Regular monitoring of hematologic parameters, renal function, and liver enzymes is necessary to discover early toxicity.

Both primary prophylaxis of PCP (for the initial episode in high-risk patients, i.e., those with less than 200 CD4 cells) and secondary prophylaxis (for recurrent episodes) are useful in patients with HIV disease. With the advent of zidovudine (AZT), the role of prophylaxis is still under investigation. Preliminary studies suggest that patients on AZT will have fewer and milder episodes of PCP than untreated patients, although possibly for a limited time period.[1] TMP/SMX has been proved efficacious in various patient groups and is a fine choice, if tolerated. The optimal dosage has not been determined; some experts suggest a double-strength tablet (160/800 mg) twice daily.[6] Inhaled pentamidine monthly also appears very promising as a nontoxic and noninvasive means of prophylaxis.[2,7] Potential problems that need further investigation are the incidence of extrapulmonary pneumocystosis, which is uncommon but would not be prevented using an inhalational method, and atypical upper lobe recurrent pulmonary pneumocystosis. Preliminary investigation suggests that dapsone is also effective in the prevention of primary *Pneumocystis carinii* pneumonia.[1]

■ TOXOPLASMOSIS

The protozoan *Toxoplasma gondii* is the major treatable cause of central nervous system mass lesions in patients with HIV disease.[8-10] Clinical manifestations depend on the size and location of the brain mass(es). The spectrum of clinical disease ranges from a chronic, indolent course to a more subacute or even fulminant presentation. Symptoms may include mild to severe headache, acute focal neurologic deficits, subtle or drastic mental status changes, and even coma. Clinical disease is mainly limited to the central nervous system, unlike other patients with toxoplasmosis.

The diagnosis of cerebral toxoplasmosis in an AIDS patient is usually established clinically. Although brain biopsy is the definitive way to make the diagnosis, it is usually not performed. History and physical findings with computed tomagraphy (CT) scanning or magnetic resonance imaging (MRI) abnormalities offer sufficient evidence to warrant an empiric trial of therapy. For patients with toxoplasmosis, serology actually is not very helpful: titers are nearly always present, yet the height of the titer is of little clinical significance because of HIV-induced immune dysfunction. The presence of multiple central nervous system (CNS) lesions that may or may not "ring enhance" with contrast in a patient with HIV disease suggests toxoplasmosis. However, single lesions are very common, and nonenhancing lesions may occur occasionally. The CT scan may even be normal. MRI and "double contrast" CT scanning are more useful and sensitive alternatives and should be performed in high-risk patients when toxoplasmosis is strongly suspected and the CT scan is negative. Also, other diagnostic possibilities in a patient with a single CNS mass lesion should be considered and merit evaluation even if presumptive toxoplasmosis therapy is begun. In certain patients, empiric therapy also may be warranted for bacterial brain abscesses, central nervous system tuberculosis, or herpes simplex encephalitis, pending definitive studies.

Therapy of toxoplasmosis is relatively straightforward.[1,9-11] Standard regimens include sulfadiazine given orally, 6 to 8 gm/day in four divided doses, and pyrimethamine. The optimal dose of pyrimethamine has yet to be determined. Initial studies used an oral dose of 25 mg/day, but more recent evidence suggests that doses ranging from 50 to 100 mg may be more efficacious without adding significant toxicity.[9] The major toxicity of pyrimethamine is bone marrow suppression; significant leukopenia is an extremely important hazard of therapy and often requires discontinuation of the drug. The toxicities of sulfadiazine are similar to those of sulfamethoxazole. For patients allergic to sulfa drugs, optimal therapy has not been determined. Experimental regimens under investigation include spiramycin and clindamycin, both macrolide antibiotics. Central nervous system penetration with these drugs is not good. Further investigation is necessary before either of these two agents can be recommended routinely.

The optimal duration of therapy also has not been determined. A minimum of 3 to 6 months of therapy is required; many experts recommend continuing therapy for the remainder of the patient's life because of the frequency of relapses. A maintenance regimen of pyrimethamine and sulfadiazine three to five times weekly may be acceptable. No data are available to assess the benefits of prophylactic antibiotics in preventing the occurrence of clinical toxoplasmosis in HIV-infected patients with positive *Toxoplasma* serology.

■ CRYPTOSPORIDIOSIS

Cryptosporidium is a protozoan parasite that rarely causes acute, self-limiting diarrhea in the competent host. In patients with HIV infection, however, persistent, severe, watery diarrhea may occur, as well as acalculous cholecystitis. Diagnosis is established via microscopic examination of stool (or biliary) specimens by modified acid-fast staining or by using monoclonal stains.[1] Treatment for cryptosporidiosis is mainly supportive. Preliminary reports suggest that the macrolide antibiotic spiramycin is of limited benefit.[1,11]

■ *ISOSPORA BELLI* INFECTION

Isospora belli is another protozoan that has been associated with diarrhea in AIDS patients. As in cryptosporidial infection, the clinical presentation is of severe debilitating diarrhea. Diagnosis is established by examination of stool specimens with modified acid-fast staining, similar to that for crypto-

sporidiosis. The *Isospora* are football-shaped and much larger than the *Cryptosporidium* and are readily distinguished by nonexperts. Therapy with TMP/SMX has been successful in certain studies, at a dose of 160 mg/800 mg two to four times a day for at least 10 days.[1,11]

■ Mycobacterial Disease

Clinically important mycobacterial disease can be divided into tuberculosis and nontuberculous mycobacterial infection. *Mycobacterium avium* complex (*M. avium* and *M. intracellulare*) is the most common mycobacterial pathogen in HIV-infected patients, occurring in 30 to 50 per cent of patients in different clinical and autopsy series.[1,12,13] *M. tuberculosis* infection occurs in up to 10 per cent of all patients with AIDS, with particularly high frequency in people from areas where the disease is endemic (especially intravenous drug users, prisoners, and Haitians).

Diagnosis of mycobacterial disease requires a high degree of suspicion—extrapulmonary manifestations are present in the majority of patients. The clinician must look for acid-fast bacilli (AFB) in all tested specimens—sputum, stool, blood, bone marrow, and tissue biopsies—as the clinical presentation of tuberculosis in HIV-infected patients is usually atypical.[1,14] When the lung is involved, parenchymal infiltrates with mediastinal lymphadenopathy are more common than in the classic apical cavitary disease. Disseminated or extrapulmonary disease occurs frequently and may include central nervous system disease.

■ TUBERCULOSIS

Tuberculin skin testing should be performed, although absence of a reaction *does not* exclude the diagnosis, since most patients with AIDS are anergic. The major indication for skin testing, actually, is to determine the need for prophylaxis. Any HIV-infected patient who has a positive test should receive prophylactic isoniazid for at least 1 year after active tuberculosis has been adequately excluded.[15]

When AFB are found, or even strongly suspected, antimycobacterial therapy should be initiated after appropriate cultures are obtained. At minimum, this regimen should include three effective antituberculosis drugs initially. If a patient is from an area of multiple drug resistance, more will be necessary. Hepatic or hematologic abnormalities do not contraindicate the use of the best available agents. The duration of therapy and the selection of specific agents will depend on speciation and drug susceptibility testing of the organism, hence the need for adequate cultures prior to therapy.

Initial treatment of active tuberculosis should include oral isoniazid (INH), 300 mg/day; rifampin, 600 mg/day; and usually also pyrazinamide (PZA), 25 to 35 mg/kg/day. Ethambutol, 15 to 25 mg/kg/day may be added (or substituted for PZA) in selected situations. Whenever INH resistance is documented or suspected, at least two additional agents (i.e., rifampin and PZA) must be used to prevent further resistance from occurring. Other currently available antituberculosis agents acceptable for chemotherapy if necessary include streptomycin, 0.75 to 1.0 gm/day, plus second-line agents such as ethionamide and capreomycin. Therapy should be continued for a minimum of 9 months, including at least 6 months after conversion to sterile cultures. Current available data do not suggest that continued INH therapy for prophylaxis of recurrent infection is necessary. All cases of tuberculosis should be reported to local public health officials for routine contact investigation. Hospitalized patients with suspected pulmonary tuberculosis should be placed on standard airborne isolation precautions. Directed observed therapy (minimum twice weekly) is essential in suspected or proved cases of noncompliance to prevent disastrous resistance problems.

■ *M. AVIUM* COMPLEX INFECTION

Clinical symptoms and signs associated with disseminated *M. avium* complex infection are nonspecific and may include fever, weight loss, sweats, cachexia, malaise, weakness, diarrhea, lymphadenopathy, and hepatosplenomegaly.[1,13] Anemia is often present and may be severe, and the serum alkaline phosphatase and gamma-glutamyl transpeptidase (GGTP) levels may be elevated. Sites likely to yield *M. avium* complex from noninvasive procedures include

sputum, stool, and blood.[1,12] Isolation of organisms from the respiratory tract and feces often precedes disseminated disease. The clinical significance of those isolates remains to be determined. More invasive procedures, such as bone marrow and liver biopsies, may be indicated in the further evaluation of nonspecific symptoms. Although currently no treatment improves overall survival, multidrug chemotherapy may result in clinical improvement and reduction of mycobacteremia and is suggested for refractory symptoms.[16] Regimens may include oral rifabutin (ansamycin), 300 mg/day (obtained from the Centers for Disease Control); clofazimine, 100 mg/day; ethambutol, 15 to 25 mg/kg/day; ciprofloxacin, 750 mg twice a day; and isoniazid, 300 mg/day. Intravenous/intramuscular amikacin has also been tried. The duration of therapy is unknown; lifelong treatment is probably necessary to suppress clinical symptoms.

Other mycobacterial species, such as *M. kansasii* and *M. xenopi*, occasionally cause infection in patients with HIV.

■ **Fungi**

■ *CANDIDA ALBICANS* INFECTION

The fungal pathogen encountered most often in patients with AIDS is *Candida albicans*. Common manifestations of this infection are oral candidiasis, or thrush, and esophageal candidiasis. Thrush appears as white patches in the oropharynx. Diagnosis is usually made by clinical examination, although it may be confirmed by culture or scrapings of the lesions. Therapy with oral agents such as clotrimazole troches, nystatin pastilles, or nystatin oral suspension is often successful. In severe cases, oral ketoconazole at doses of 200 to 400 mg/day may be necessary.

Although oral and vaginal *Candida* infections may occur in the normal host, esophageal invasion with *Candida albicans* indicates the cell-mediated immune dysfunction that is characteristic of AIDS.[1] Typically, patients present with dysphagia and odynophagia and retrosternal pain upon swallowing. Empiric treatment with ketoconazole at doses of from 200 to 400 mg/day may resolve the clinical picture and establish a presumptive diagnosis. Although esophagram or barium swallow may show evidence of esophagitis, it will not prove the diagnosis, since the radiographic findings may represent herpes simplex or cytomegalovirus esophagitis. Definitive diagnosis then must be made by endoscopic examination.

If patients do not respond to ketoconazole therapy, consideration should be given to the presence of AIDS gastropathy.[17] This condition has been described recently and is characterized by the absence of acid production in the stomach. When this occurs, ketoconazole cannot be absorbed properly. Therapy with oral glutamic acid (4 capsules given simultaneously with ketoconazole) may facilitate absorption. Drug interactions with ketoconazole may pose problems for the clinician. Simultaneous administration of H_2 blockers and antacids may prevent absorption of ketoconazole. In addition, rifampin also may block absorption of the drug, necessitating administration of these two antibiotics 12 hours apart. Ketoconazole is generally very well tolerated, although at high doses of 600 to 800 mg/day, chemical hepatitis with hepatic necrosis has been reported, as well as disruption of adrenal function.

■ CRYPTOCOCCAL MENINGITIS

The most common cause of meningitis in patients with HIV infection is the fungus *Cryptococcus neoformans*.[1,18] Presentation may be similar to that of typical acute bacterial meningitis (i.e., high temperatures, photophobia, meningismus, and severe headache). Alternatively, patients may present with a more chronic, "subacute meningitis" picture, with mild headaches over a period of time. Non-CNS manifestations rarely occur and should be sought diligently.

The diagnosis of cryptococcal meningitis may be established readily. Serum and cerebrospinal fluid (CSF) cryptococcal antigens are present in nearly all HIV patients with cryptococcal disease. False-positives almost never occur.[1,18] False-negative results are rarely seen, are attributed to a "prozone phenomenon," and are corrected with dilution.

Cryptococci may be visualized in the CSF using an India ink preparation, which is a quick, simple, inexpensive, and easy stain to perform. In contrast to non-HIV-infected patients with cryptococcal disease, the India ink preparation is positive in the majority of patients with HIV disease.[1] Classically, a nonspecific CSF pleocytosis is present, with a normal or low glucose level and a normal or elevated protein value. Cultures are usually positive within several days. Thus a negative India ink preparation, negative cryptococcal antigen, and negative culture exclude this diagnosis.

Amphotericin B is currently the mainstay of therapy.[1,18] After administration of a test dose (usually 1 mg given over 1 to 2 hours), doses are increased over the next several days till the desired dose (approximately 0.5 mg/kg/day) is achieved. Premedication a half hour prior to the infusion and 3.5 hours into the amphotericin infusion, using antihistamines and antipyretics, is usually given to prevent pyrexia, severe rigors, and general malaise. Additional agents, such as meperidine or corticosteroids, sometimes are necessary to control these immediate reactions. Even those patients initially intolerant of amphotericin are often able to receive large doses as time passes.

The optimal duration of amphotericin therapy is unknown. Most authorities recommend a total dose of at least 1.5 to 2 gm and look for serial improvement in CSF antigen titers and pleocytosis. Longer courses of therapy may be necessary, based on clinical and laboratory findings. In patients not infected with HIV, the addition of 5-fluorocytosine (5-FC) is beneficial and permits lower total doses of amphotericin B. The benefit of this drug in patients with HIV infection has not been proved. 5-FC is a marrow-suppressive agent and should be used only for refractory cases. The major side effects of amphotericin B include renal insufficiency, which is usually reversible and responds to cessation or lowering of the dose; electrolyte (i.e., potassium and magnesium) imbalances; normochromic normocytic anemia; and the aforementioned infusion-related adverse effects. Although not readily available, liposomal formulations of amphotericin may reduce the incidence of side effects dramatically without compromising, and possibly even improving, treatment. Currently, no data support the use of intrathecal amphotericin, unlike the case in other fungal diseases, such as coccidioidomycosis.

An investigational drug, fluconazole, related to ketoconazole, appears extremely promising as an efficacious oral agent against systemic fungal disease.[1,18,19] Limited anecdotal reports suggest that fluconazole may be at least as effective as, if not superior to, amphotericin B. Major trials are currently investigating fluconazole therapy for primary cryptococcal meningitis and prophylaxis of recurrent disease.

Recurrent cryptococcal disease is quite common in patients infected with HIV, mandating suppressive therapy.[1,18] The optimal regimen, however, has not been determined. Some authorities recommend weekly, twice weekly, or thrice weekly amphotericin to prevent recurrence. Others have used high-dose oral ketoconazole or itroconazole; CFS penetration by these agents is poor, and results to date are equivocal. Oral fluconazole, with its superior CSF penetration, offers much promise as an effective, safe, nontoxic alternative.

■ HISTOPLASMOSIS

The fungus *Histoplasma capsulatum* is a major pathogen in HIV-infected patients from endemic areas such as the Ohio River Basin.[1,20] Although a high percentage of patients living in these endemic areas have serologic evidence of exposure to *Histoplasma*, only a small minority acquire clinical disease. Of those, a much smaller group acquires disseminated histoplasmosis. Patients infected with HIV are more prone to develop dissemination.

The key factor in making the diagnosis of histoplasmosis is to think of the diagnosis. A very careful travel history, encompassing the entire lifetime of the patient, must be taken. One need not have visited an endemic area recently to be at risk to reactivate the disease. Patients may present with primarily pulmonary disease: shortness of breath, cough, productive sputum, or they may have a nonspecific systemic illness composed of malaise, fevers, weight loss, and cutaneous lesions. Diagnosis is made by stain and culture of infected tissue specimens or secretions; rarely, the diagnosis can be made by examining a peripheral smear or buffy coat.

Therapy of disseminated histoplasmosis in a patient with HIV infection is similar to that of cryptococcal disease.[1,20] Amphotericin B is currently the only available agent, as opposed to non-HIV-infected patients in

whom high-dose ketoconazole or itraconazole is equally effective. The role of fluconazole remains to be determined. As with cryptococcal disease, recurrence is common, therefore suppressive therapy is necessary. Here too, the benefit of high-dose ketoconazole, fluconazole, or amphotericin is not yet known.

■ COCCIDIOIDOMYCOSIS

As with histoplasmosis, the fungus *Coccidioides immitis* is a major pathogen in HIV-infected patients from endemic areas, specifically the San Joaquin Valley in Western United States.[1,21] In these areas, coccidioidomycosis ranks with *Pneumocystis carinii* as the most frequent lung pathogen. Both diffuse nodular pulmonary disease and systemic dissemination are common. Early evidence suggests that coccidioidal antigens are usually present, despite the immune dysfunction of HIV. Prolonged (probably lifelong) amphotericin B therapy is required. In preliminary reports, fluconazole looks promising for coccidioidomycosis and may be able to replace amphotericin.

■ Bacteria

In addition to the well-described abnormalities in T cell function seen in patients with HIV infection, major deficits in B cell function have been recognized as well, which predispose patients with HIV disease to certain bacterial infections. Although the clinical presentation of these bacterial infections is similar in normal hosts and in HIV-infected patients, a higher incidence of bacteremia and more severe illness occur in HIV-infected patients, especially with *Streptococcus pneumoniae*, *Salmonella* species, *Haemophilus influenzae*, *Listeria*, and *Staphylococcus aureus*.[1,22,23] Enterobacteriaciae and *Pseudomonas* infections, however, remain quite unusual.

In general, treatment of these bacterial infections is identical in immunocompetent and HIV-infected hosts. The dosage and duration of therapy should be geared to clinical and laboratory evidence of response. Relapse is usually not a problem if adequate initial therapy is given. Special mention must be made of two organisms, *Salmonella* and the spirochete *Treponema pallidum*, the causative agent of syphilis. Persistent *Salmonella* bacteremia and disease is a major problem in HIV-infected patients.[1] Patients may present with predominantly gastrointestinal symptoms, pneumonia, or more diffuse disease. Unless patients are from an area known to have certain resistance patterns, ampicillin, TMP/SMX, and chloramphenicol remain acceptable choices for treating salmonellosis. The newer fluorinated quinolones, such as norfloxacin or ciprofloxacin, and the third-generation cephalosporins appear to be equally efficacious alternatives. The least toxic and least expensive agent should be selected for maintenance therapy, once sensitivity patterns are known. Suppressive therapy is warranted to eradicate the organism from the body.

Syphilis, still a major sexually transmitted disease in the United States, has acquired new significance in the era of HIV disease. Disseminated spirochetemia is quite common, even in the early stages of syphilis, and single-dose intramuscular regimens may not be effective therapy to eradicate CNS foci of disease. Since all patients with syphilis are at high risk of having acquired HIV infection, these findings are of major public health importance. Recent studies suggest that the current Centers for Disease Control guidelines for the routine treatment of syphilis may be ineffective for HIV-infected patients.[1,24] Pending further guidelines from the Centers for Disease Control, it appears prudent to suspect all HIV-infected patients with any stage of syphilis of having central nervous system involvement. For patients without CSF abnormalities and with primary or secondary lues, intramuscular benzathine penicillin, 2.4 million units, should be adequate. With CSF abnormalities, a 10-day course of intravenous aqueous penicillin (24 million units/day) followed by a 3-week regimen of intramuscular benzathine penicillin may be necessary. Whether a third-generation cephalosporin such as ceftriaxone offers superior efficacy remains to be determined. It is important to remember that false-negative syphilis tests can occur. A high index of suspicion and low threshold for therapy should be maintained at all response times, especially in patients with cutaneous and central nervous system manifestations. Close follow-up is necessary to ensure adequacy of treatment.

■ Viruses

■ CYTOMEGALOVIRUS

Clinical cytomegalovirus infection occurs in up to 25 per cent of AIDS patients and represents reactivation of the latent virus. The eye, gastrointestinal tract, lungs, central nervous system, and adrenal glands are infected most frequently, but other organ systems may become involved as well.

Retinitis usually begins unilaterally and may present with blurred vision, scotoma, flashing lights, or black spots in front of the eye. As a result of viremia, disease often spreads to the contralateral eye. The diagnosis should be confirmed by an ophthalmologist, with visualization of the typical lesions, described as large, white exudates with associated perivascular hemorrhages, "cottage cheese and tomato ketchup" in appearance.

Although the diagnosis of CMV is established clinically, standard practice includes determining the presence of the virus elsewhere in the host by obtaining cultures of urine and blood. Serologic titers are of little help since they are uniformly elevated in HIV-infected patients.

When infection is diagnosed at an early stage, therapy with ganciclovir has been shown to be successful in preventing complete blindness and spread to the other eye. Ganciclovir is given intravenously, with an induction regimen of 10 to 15 mg/kg/day for 14 days. Patients frequently relapse, necessitating a chronic intravenous maintenance regimen (optimal dose remains undetermined). The major toxicity from ganciclovir is neutropenia, which is severe and frequent enough to recommend extreme caution in using concomitant zidovudine (AZT) therapy.[1,25] Recently, resistance to ganciclovir has been reported,[26] which is of great potential concern. Newer investigational agents such as foscarnet are being studied.

Cytomegalovirus infection in the gastrointestinal tract may take three different forms: colitis, esophagitis, and gastritis.[1,25] The most common manifestation of CMV infection is colitis, which may present with combinations of diarrhea, abdominal pain, weight loss, anorexia, and fever. If standard cultures for bacteria and mycobacteria and stains for ova and parasites do not yield pathogens, then sigmoidoscopy or colonoscopy with diagnostic biopsy and culture is advised. The appearance of the bowel is usually one of erythema, submucosal hemorrhage, and diffuse ulcerations. Biopsy will show a vasculitis with neutrophilic infiltration and typical CMV inclusions in the infected cells. Ganciclovir therapy for colitis has been reported to be successful in up to 50 per cent of patients, and a maintenance regimen is usually not required.

CMV esophagitis occurs in AIDS patients as well, although less frequently than esophageal infection with *Candida albicans* or herpes simplex virus. When suspected clinically, diagnosis must be confirmed by biopsy and culture via endoscopy. Gastritis may also occur, presenting with severe epigastric pain and ulcers in the gastric mucosa. Endoscopic biopsy is also necessary to establish this diagnosis.

CMV pneumonitis occurs often in AIDS patients. While virus may be isolated from bronchial secretions or tissue biopsy specimens, this does not necessarily indicate true pathogenicity. Usually, cytomegalovirus is a co-pathogen with other organisms such as *Pneumocystis carinii,* and most likely adds little clinical morbidity itself. When true CMV pneumonitis does occur, it presents as interstitial pneumonitis with a dry cough and progressive dyspnea. Lung examination may yield minimal findings. Diagnosis is established either by culturing bronchoalveolar lavage specimens, or by biopsy, the specimen of which may be analyzed by immunofluorescent staining or DNA probes as well as traditional histopathologic methods. The role of ganciclovir therapy for this manifestation of CMV infection remains controversial.[1,25]

CMV hepatitis may occur in HIV-infected individuals, although it generally has minimal clinical significance. Central nervous system infection is characterized clinically by fever, altered mental status, personality changes, headache, confusion, and somnolence. Since diagnosis must be established by biopsy of the brain, this infection is usually proved only at autopsy. CMV also may involve the adrenal glands, producing a typical picture of adrenal insufficiency, and

may also invade pancreatic tissue where its role is not yet defined.[1,25]

■ HERPES SIMPLEX VIRUSES

Both herpes simplex types I and II frequently cause recurrent, painful oral, genital, and perianal ulcerations in AIDS patients. The esophagus may also be involved; central nervous system involvement is less frequent. Diagnosis of herpes infection may be confirmed easily by Tzanck preparation, viral culture, or fluorescent antibody stains. However, since patients with herpes infection are usually very uncomfortable, empiric treatment with oral acyclovir (200 mg five times a day) may be warranted until the results of cultures are available. If ulcerations are extensive, particularly in the perirectal region, then intravenous acyclovir therapy (15.0 mg/kg/day in three divided doses) may be necessary. Patients with severe recurrent disease will require suppressive therapy with oral acyclovir, 200 mg three (or rarely five) times daily.[1] Alternative therapies for acyclovir-resistant organisms have not been well established.[27] Acyclovir toxicity is usually mild, although mild elevations of serum creatinine and miscellaneous neurologic symptoms have been reported, especially with intravenous therapy and higher doses.

■ HERPES ZOSTER

Herpes zoster or varicella zoster virus infection usually presents as shingles in HIV-infected patients prior to the development of CDC-confirmed AIDS.[28] Although shingles is the most common manifestation of this infection, chickenpox also may occur in the previously unexposed host. Retinitis has been described as well. Generally, the diagnosis is clinical, although the virus can be isolated from blister fluid or by biopsy. Most often therapy is not indicated for shingles since the disease is usually self-limiting. In severe cases, oral (4 to 5 gm/day in five divided doses) or intravenous acyclovir (30 to 45 mg/kg/day in three divided doses) may be warranted.[1] Care must be taken in the hospital setting to avoid spread of this virus to nonimmune hospital employees and unexposed immunocompromised patients. Strict isolation must be maintained.

■ OTHER VIRUSES

Although clinical Epstein-Barr virus infection has not been described frequently in AIDS patients, recent data have suggested the association of this virus with oral hairy leukoplakia, which is typically seen as a serpiginous raised white area on the lateral side of the tongue. This condition usually responds well when acyclovir therapy is given. Progressive multifocal leukoencephalopathy is a white matter CNS lesion caused by a papovavirus.[1] No effective therapy is available.

REFERENCES

1. Glatt AE, Chirgwin K, Landesman SH. Treatment of infections associated with human immunodeficiency virus. N Engl J Med 1988; 318:1439–1448.
2. Hopewell PC. *Pneumocystis carinii* pneumonia: diagnosis. J Infect Dis 1988; 157:1115–1119.
3. Wharton JM, Coleman DL, Wofsy CB, et al. Trimethoprim-sulfamethoxazole or pentamidine for *Pneumocystis carinii* pneumonia in the acquired immunodeficiency syndrome. Ann Intern Med 1986; 105:37–44.
4. Golden JA, Hollander H, Conte JE Jr. Inhaled pentamidine or low dose intravenous pentamidine as novel therapy for *Pneumocystis carinii* pneumonia (PCP) in the acquired immunodeficiency syndrome (abstract). Am Rev Respir Dis 1987; 135:Suppl:A168.
5. Montgomery AB, Debs RJ, Luce JM, et al. Aerosolised pentamidine as sole therapy for *Pneumocystis carinii* pneumonia in patients with acquired immunodeficiency syndrome. Lancet 1987; 2:480–483.
6. Fischl MA, Dickinson GM, LaVoie L. Safety and efficacy of sulfamethoxazole and trimethoprim chemoprophylaxis for *Pneumocystis carinii* pneumonia in AIDS. JAMA 1988; 259:1185–1189.
7. Conte JE, Chernoff D, Feigal D, Hollander HH. Once monthly inhaled pentamidine for the prevention of PCP. Fourth International Conference on AIDS, Stockholm, 1988, p 7165.I.
8. Luft BJ, Remington JS. Toxoplasmic encephalitis. J Infect Dis 1988; 157:1–6.
9. Navia BA, Petito CK, Gold JWM, Cho ES, Jordan BD, Price RW. Cerebral toxoplasmosis complicating the acquired immune deficiency syndrome: clinical and neuropathological findings in 27 patients. Ann Neurol 1986; 19:224–238.
10. Wanke C, Tuazon CU, Kovacs A, et al. *Toxoplasma* encephalitis in patients with acquired immune deficiency syndrome: diagnosis and response to therapy. Am J Trop Med Hyg 1987; 36:509–516.
11. Soave R, Johnson WD. *Cryptosporidium* and *Isospora belli* infections. J Infect Dis 1988; 157:225–229.
12. Hawkins CC, Gold JWM, Whimbey E, et al. *Mycobacterium avium* complex infections in patients with the acquired immunodeficiency syndrome. Ann Intern Med 1986; 105:184–188.
13. Young LS. *Mycobacterium avium* complex infection. J Infect Dis 1988; 157:863–867.
14. Sunderam G, McDonald RJ, Maniatis T, Oleske J, Kapila R, Reichman LB. Tuberculosis as a manifestation of the acquired immunodeficiency syndrome (AIDS). JAMA 1986; 256:362–366.
15. Centers for Disease Control, Department of Health and Human Services. Diagnosis and management of mycobacterial infection and disease in persons with human immunodeficiency virus infection. Ann Intern Med 1987; 106:254–256.
16. Agins BD, Berman D, Spicehandler D, El-Sadr WE, Simberkoff MS, Rahal JJ. Effect of combined therapy with ansamycin, clofazimine, ethambutol and isoniazid for *Mycobacterium avium* infection in patients with AIDS. J Infect Dis 1989; 184:784–785.
17. Lake-Bakaar G, Winston T, Lake-Bakaar D, et al. Gastropathy and ketoconazole absorption in AIDS. Ann Intern Med 1988; 109:471–473.
18. Dismukes WE. Cryptococcal meningitis in patients with AIDS. J Infect Dis 1988; 157:624–628.
19. Stern JJ, Hartmen BJ, Sharkey P, et al. Oral fluconazole therapy for patients with acquired immunodeficiency syndrome and cryptococcosis: experience with 22 patients. Am J Med 1988; 85:477–480.
20. Wheat LJ, Slama TG, Zeckel ML. Histoplasmosis in the acquired immune deficiency syndrome. Am J Med 1985; 78:203–210.
21. Bronnimann DA, Adam RD, Galgiani JN, et al. Coccidioidomycosis in the acquired immunodeficiency syndrome. Ann Intern Med 1987; 106:372–379.
22. Whimbey E, Gold JWM, Polsky B, et al. Bacteremia and fungemia in patients with the acquired immunodeficiency syndrome. Ann Intern Med 1986; 104:511–514.
23. Jacobson MA, Gellerman H, Chamberg H. *Staphylococcus aureus* bacteremia and recurrent staphylococcal infection in patients with the acquired immunodeficiency syndrome and AIDS-related complex. Am J Med 1988; 85:172–176.
24. Lukehart SA, Hook EW, Baker-Zander SA, Collier AC, Critchlow CW, Handsfield HH. Invasion of the central nervous system by *Treponema pallidum*: implications for diagnosis and treatment. Ann Intern Med 1988; 109:855–861.
25. Drew WL. Cytomegalovirus infection in patients with AIDS. J Infect Dis 1988; 158:449–456.
26. Erice A, Chou S, Biron KK, Stanat SC, Balfour HH, Jordan MC. Progressive disease due to ganciclovir-resistant cytomegalovirus in immunocompromised patients. N Engl J Med 1989; 320:289–293.
27. Erlich KS, Mills J, Chatis P, et al. Acyclovir-resistant herpes simplex virus infections in patients with the acquired immunodeficiency syndrome. N Engl J Med 1989; 320:293–296.
28. Friedman-Kien AE, Lafleur FL, Gendler E, et al. Herpes zoster: a possible early clinical sign for development of AIDS in high-risk individuals. J Am Acad Dermatol 1986; 14:1023–1028.

Infections in the diabetic patient

Francisco L. Sapico ■ *Camilo A. Leslie* ■ *Alice N. Bessman*

It is a common belief among clinicians that infections occur with increased frequency among patients with infections in diabetes mellitus. Questions have been raised, however, as to whether these infections (with the exception of bacteriuria in diabetic women) have been proved to be statistically more common in comparison with infections in nondiabetics.[1] The medical literature demonstrates convincingly that diabetic patients are overrepresented in certain specific infections. For example, diabetics constitute approximately 90 per cent of the reported cases of invasive (or malignant) external otitis.[2] At least 75 per cent of patients with rhinocerebral mucormycosis have been diabetic patients in ketoacidosis.[3,4] Approximately 35 per cent of reported cases of emphysematous cholecystitis have been described in diabetics.[5,6] Diabetes mellitus has been documented in almost 90 per cent of patients with emphysematous pyelonephritis, in over 50 per cent of those with renal papillary necrosis, and in 30 per cent of patients with perinephric abscesses.[7,8] Diabetics represent 50 to 70 per cent of all patients who undergo nontraumatic foot or leg amputation (most of which are secondary to infectious problems).[9]

■ Background

Three basic abnormalities have become implicated in the diabetic patient's predisposition to infection: immunocompromise, neuropathy, and peripheral vascular disease.

Defective ability of the white blood cell to function in chemotaxis, diapedesis, adherence, phagocytosis, and microbicidal activity has been described in diabetics.[10–13] Impaired granuloma formation and poor healing have been seen in diabetic mice,[14] and impaired T lymphocyte–mediated function has been described in diabetic patients.[15] Poor metabolic control usually has been associated with these abnormal white cell functions.

Peripheral neuropathy can result in loss of sensation, muscle imbalance resulting in foot deformities, autonomic dysfunction with subsequent reduced sweating, and loss of vasomotor response. All these factors can contribute to subsequent foot infections. The development of a neurogenic bladder with resultant increased urinary bladder residual volume can lead to complicated urinary tract infections.

Peripheral vascular disease in the diabetic patient is manifested by accelerated atherosclerosis. Subsequent vascular compromise may result in foot gangrene and impaired diffusion of humoral and cellular immune factors, as well as of antibiotics (when needed). Microangiopathy results in retinopathy with resultant diminished vision and impaired ability to detect small, infected lesions.

■ Management

Metabolic control of the diabetic state is essential in the management of infections in diabetics. The stress of infections is well recognized for causing instability and poor control of the diabetic patient. In the insulin-dependent (Type I) diabetic patient, the stress of severe infection can precipitate diabetic ketoacidosis. The catabolic state of diabetes out of control with hyperglycemia has been shown to interfere with various aspects of white cell function and other facets of immune resistance. Rapid and aggressive control of diabetes is indicated to maximize immune system functions and healing potential.

If a diabetic patient presents with an infection and "diabetes out of control" and is taking oral hypoglycemic agents as current treatment of the diabetes, therapy should be changed immediately to insulin. The temptation to raise the dose of the oral agent in hope that a larger dose may effect better control can waste valuable time.

If a patient is already taking insulin, aggressive therapy, to be described, should be initiated. Such therapy can restore metabolic control within 24 to 48 hours.

There are three major insulin regimens from which to choose:

- 1. Continuous intravenous regular (CZI) insulin therapy
- 2. Intensive insulin therapy with frequent (every 4 to 6 hours) injections of subcutaneous short-acting regular insulin
- 3. A combination of intermediate-acting insulin (NPH or Lente) twice a day, combined with regular insulin.

In all but the most serious infections accompanied by diabetic ketoacidosis, the second or third choice is appropriate. With frequent bedside glucose monitoring, dosages can be rapidly adjusted.

For method 1, continuous intravenous infusion of regular insulin for diabetic ketoacidosis has been well described; a commonly accepted regimen uses an initial infusion rate of 5 to 7 units per hour.

Using method 2, subcutaneous injection of regular insulin can be ordered on a "sliding scale." Since subcutaneous insulin usually has peak action 2 to 3 hours after injection, an example of an initial sliding scale is: 6 to 10 units for a blood glucose level of 180 to 250 mg/dl, 10 to 14 units for a glucose level of over 250; fingerstick blood glucose values are to be measured 3 hours after the injection of insulin; and the next dose of insulin is to be given 4 hours after the previous dose. The dose of insulin is adjusted according to the patient's response.

With method 3, using the intermediate-acting/short-acting insulin combination, the effect of the morning dose can be gauged by the 4 P.M. glucose determination, and the effect of the evening dose by the fasting blood glucose level.

Prelunch and bedtime blood glucose levels reflect the effect of morning and evening short-acting insulin, respectively. Appropriate adjustments are made on the basis of these parameters.

For patients about to undergo surgery it is imperative that metabolic control (including correction of severe hyperglycemia and dehydration) be achieved *prior* to the surgical procedure. Any of the aforementioned methods can be used. If a patient is not eating, calories must be furnished by the intravenous route with concomitant insulin therapy to maintain a blood glucose level of around 200 mg/dl.

■ MUCORMYCOSIS

The mycoses falling under this category are caused by fungi belonging to the order Mucorales which, in turn, encompasses the genera *Absidia*, *Mucor*, *Rhizomucor*, and *Rhizopus*. The major forms of mucormycosis include rhinocerebral, pulmonary, disseminated, gastrointestinal, and cutaneous. Of these, the rhinocerebral form is the most strongly associated with poorly controlled diabetes mellitus, especially in association with the ketoacidosis.

Surgical extirpation of diseased tissue is generally felt to be essential in the treatment of rhinocerebral mucormycosis. The extent of the disease process can be evaluated by the use of computed tomography (CT) or by magnetic resonance imaging (MRI). Infected sinuses and focal abscesses must be drained and necrotic tissue or bone removed surgically. Early diagnosis and treatment may obviate the need for more drastic surgical procedures, such as orbital exenteration.

Amphotericin B is the antifungal agent of choice and is the only drug with demonstrated clinical efficacy. If the patient tolerates the test dose of 1 mg intravenously, 15 mg of the drug can be given on the same day intravenously over 2 to 4 hours. Subsequent doses can be raised by 5 mg per day until a dose of 1.0 mg/kg/day is reached. Adverse drug reactions, such as chills, fever, nausea, and vomiting may be controlled by premedication with aspirin, antihistamines, antiemetics, and small doses of corticosteroids. Severe febrile reactions sometimes may be controlled with small doses of meperidine hydrochloride. Some patients tolerate every other day administration of amphotericin B at about 1.5 mg/kg/day better than daily administration. Serum electrolytes, the CBC and differential, platelet counts, serum calcium, magnesium, and creatinine levels, and urinalysis should be followed serially while the patient is on amphotericin B. If the serum creatinine rises to levels of 3.0 to 3.5 mg/dl, use of the drug can be suspended and the creatinine levels allowed to drop to near-normal levels, then the amphotericin B can be restarted at half the original dose and again slowly increased. The total dose of the amphotericin B required varies according to the severity of the disease, but total doses of 3 or 4 grams may be necessary in most cases.

With early diagnosis and proper therapy, survival rates of 50 to 85 per cent can be achieved. Extensive reconstructive surgery may be necessary in some survivors.

■ INVASIVE ("MALIGNANT") EXTERNAL OTITIS

This disease is almost always caused by *Pseudomonas aeruginosa* and is locally invasive, penetrating the epithelial barrier of the external auditory canal to involve surrounding subcutaneous tissue. The infection frequently advances along the cleft between the cartilaginous and bony portion of the canal, and granulomatous polyps are frequently present in this region. Local invasion may lead to involvement of the temporomandibular joint, the parotid gland, the mastoid sinuses, the temporal bone, the base of the skull, the cervical vertebrae, the venous sinuses of the brain, the meninges, and the brain tissue itself. Cranial nerves IX to XII may be involved. Involvement of these cranial nerves (with the possible exception of CN VII), generally implies a poorer prognosis. The extent of local involvement can be assessed by using CT scans.

Therapy consists of appropriate surgical debridement, frequent cleaning of the ear canal, and about 4 weeks of intravenous antibiotics directed against *P. aeruginosa*. The combination of an antipseudomonal beta-lactam agent such as ticarcillin, together with an aminoglycoside such as tobramycin or gentamicin, is the most frequently employed. More clinical experience with monotherapy using antipseudomonal agents such as ceftazidime or aztreonam is needed. The choice of antimicrobial agents will have to be guided by antimicrobial susceptibility test results. There are preliminary reports of good results with intensive antimicrobial therapy and less aggressive surgical debridement. The role of oral antipseudomonas agents, such as ciprofloxacin and other quinolones is still unclear and has to be evaluated.

■ BACTERIAL PNEUMONIA

There is no evidence that the incidence of pneumococcal pneumonia in diabetics is any higher than in nondiabetics. However, diabetics appear to be overrepresented in bacterial pneumonias when *Staphylococcus aureus*, *Klebsiella pneumoniae*, and *Escherichia coli* are the etiologic agents.[15,16] The management of pneumonia in diabetic patients is similar to the management in nondiabetics. Due to the severity and necrotizing propensity of the pathogens, parenteral therapy is generally required, at least in the first 2 weeks of therapy. Often a total of 4 weeks therapy is necessary, and some authorities recommend two synergistic antibiotics for pneumonia due to *Klebsiella* (e.g., cephalosporin plus aminoglycoside). However, we feel that, as long as good clinical response is achieved with combination therapy, the aminoglycoside may be discontinued after 1 or 2 weeks. We have also observed good response to single-drug therapy of *Klebsiella* pneumonia with some of the newer beta-lactams, such as the third-generation cephalosporins.

■ TUBERCULOSIS

The incidence of tuberculosis in diabetes has decreased dramatically in the last few decades. However, most clinicians still feel that diabetes mellitus still may predispose to reactivation of latent tuberculosis and also to potentially more severe diseases.[17] It is still recommended, therefore, that tuberculin skin test–positive diabetic patients should receive prophylactic isoniazid therapy. Treatment of active tuberculosis is similar to that for nondiabetic patients.

■ EMPHYSEMATOUS CHOLECYSTITIS

This disease is characterized by a highly virulent course, the presence of gas in or around the gallbladder, its predominance in men (70 per cent), a high rate of gallbladder gangrene (74 per cent) and perforation (21 per cent), and a high mortality rate (15 to 25 per cent). All diabetic patients with a clinical picture of cholecystitis, therefore, should have serial abdominal radiographs for at least 4 days to detect the presence of gas in or around the gallbladder or biliary tree. The infection is frequently polymicrobial, with *Clostridium* spp. and gram-negative bacilli (*E. coli, Klebsiella,* and so on) being common pathogens. High-dose parenteral antibiotic therapy directed at these organisms should be instituted promptly, but definitive therapy consists of cholecystectomy, which should be performed within 48 hours of diagnosis.

■ URINARY TRACT INFECTION (UTI)

Diabetic women have been shown to have a two- to fourfold higher incidence of bacteriuria compared with nondiabetics.[18] Diabetic patients are also more likely to develop nosocomial UTI. The treatment of cystitis in diabetic patients may not necessarily be different from that of nondiabetic patients. However, the presence of a neurogenic bladder may make single-dose antibiotic treatment less efficacious. The presence of a neurogenic bladder can be demonstrated by bladder cystometric studies. Relapse or failure to respond may call for a longer course (i.e., 5 to 7 days) of treatment.

Diabetic patients appear to be predisposed to develop upper UTI from a previous urinary bladder infection.[19] A particularly severe and life-threatening form of renal infection seen in diabetic patients is emphysematous pyelonephritis.[7] Diagnosis is usually made by showing gas mottling of the involved kidney on plain radiographs or on CT scanning. The gas tends to spread to surrounding areas, including subcutaneous tissue. This disease entity often requires nephrectomy (it is usually unilateral), together with parenteral high-dose antibiotic therapy using agents to which the causative organism is susceptible. The survival rate with antibiotic therapy alone is much lower than when antibiotic therapy is combined with surgical drainage or nephrectomy. Antibiotic therapy of 2 or more weeks' duration is often necessary.

Renal papillary necrosis often presents with flank pain, fever, microscopic or macroscopic hematuria, and pyuria. Fifteen per cent of patients may develop renal failure. Some patients, however, may be relatively asymptomatic, with passage of the sloughed papillary tissue in the urine as the only clinical manifestation. Ureteral colic may be the result of obstruction, which can be confirmed by retrograde pyelography. Surgical removal of the obstruction is indicated, and this usually can be done through a cystoscope with ureteral instrumentation. Antibiotic therapy should be given simultaneously, as in pyelonephritis.

Patients with perinephric abscess often appear to have pyelonephritis, but response to antibiotics is invariably poor. Renal ultrasound or CT scanning will reveal the diagnosis. Surgical drainage of the abscess is mandatory, in conjunction with parenteral antibiotic therapy. Some patients have responded to drainage of the abscess performed through a percutaneous catheter.

■ FUNGAL INFECTIONS

Candida mucocutaneous colonization is more common in diabetic patients than in nondiabetic and is more common in women than in men.[20] *Candida* infections of the skin and mucous membranes are also felt to be more common in diabetic patients. Diabetics also appear to be overrepresented in fungal infections caused by such dimorphic fungi as *Cryptococcus, Histoplasma, Coccidioides,* and *Blastomyses.*[1] The management of fungal infections in diabetic patients is no different from that in nondiabetics, except for the need for aggressive metabolic control in diabetics. Local infections, such as *Candida vaginitis,* are managed with topical antifungal therapy. *Candida* esophagitis sometimes may respond to mystatin pastilles, but refractory cases may require oral ketoconazole or intravenous amphotericin B therapy.

■ SKIN AND SOFT TISSUE INFECTIONS

Diabetic patients are more likely to carry *Staphylococcus aureus* in their skin and nasopharynx, compared with nondiabetics. However, it has not been proved conclusively that diabetic patients are more predisposed to staphylococcal skin infections.

On the other hand, diabetics appear to be clearly overrepresented among patients with necrotizing infections, such as synergistic necrotizing fasciitis or synergistic necrotizing cellulitis.[21,22] The latter entity is now usually called nonclostridial anaerobic myonecrosis. These infections can involve the anterior abdominal wall (i.e., after abdominal surgery or penetrating trauma), the perineum (often following surgery, instrumentation, or local infections), and, most commonly, the lower extremities. Other body sites are much less commonly involved.

Aggressive parenteral antibiotic therapy is mandatory for patients with necrotizing soft tissue infections. Since these infections are most commonly polymicrobial, initial antibiotic therapy prior to culture results should cover microorganisms such as *Staphylococcus aureus*, gram-negative enteric bacilli such as *E. coli*, *Proteus* spp., *P. aeruginosa*, *Bacteroides fragilis* and other anaerobes, and *Enterococcus* spp. The choice of antibiotics can be altered depending on subsequent culture and susceptibility results.

Surgical drainage of abscesses and debridement of necrotic tissue are of paramount importance in the management of patients. These treatments should be done aggressively and repeatedly, as necessary. "Filleting" the area and leaving it open for irrigation and subsequent debridement is often done. In nonclostridial anaerobic myonecrosis, necrotic muscle tissue has to be completely removed.

DIABETIC FOOT GANGRENE

Like necrotizing soft tissue infections, moderate-to-severe diabetic foot gangrene is usually polymicrobial in etiology,[23,24] especially when necrotic or gangrenous tissue is present and when associated with a fetid smell. Aerobes, as well as anaerobes, are usually present. Depending on the severity of the soft tissue infection, on involvement of bone, and on the adequacy of the blood flow to the involved area, limited amputation often may be necessary (i.e., toe, ray, transmetatarsal, through the ankle, or below the knee). Antimicrobial therapy is similar to that of necrotizing soft tissue infections. The presence of osteomyelitis may be demonstrated by a sequential technetium bone and gallium scan or by nuclear magnetic resonance imaging. Bone involvement may necessitate debridement or resection or a trial of long-term antibiotic therapy (i.e., 1 month of parenteral therapy, or about 2 weeks of parenteral therapy followed by several weeks of appropriate oral therapy).[25]

Nonhealing, long-standing foot ulcers associated with peripheral neuropathy and with no associated tissue necrosis or gangrene often will respond to conservative measures such as local debridement, bed rest without wearing offending footwear, and topical wet-to-dry dressings with normal saline or mild antiseptics. Cultures of these lesions often yield one or few organisms. *Staphylococcus* spp. and *Enterococcus* spp. are the most commonly isolated organisms, and anaerobes are distinctly much less frequently seen.[26] The presence of surrounding cellulitis prompts a 2-week course of appropriate antibiotic therapy, but the role of antibiotics in lesions that are not obviously infected is unclear. If these lesions are associated with significant vascular insufficiency, as demonstrated by Doppler ultrasound and by arteriography, vascular reconstruction may result in accelerated healing of the lesion. Contrast arteriography should not be done routinely in the diabetic patient unless vascular reconstruction is planned, in view of the perceived predisposition of the diabetic patient to develop contrast-induced acute renal failure.

■ Issues and Risks

Good metabolic control of the diabetic state is essential in the management of infections in the diabetic patient. Since infection, per se, aggravates the diabetic state, simultaneous control of the infection is necessary. The infected diabetic patient can develop a variety of complications, including septic shock, disseminated intravascular coagulation, respiratory distress syndrome, metastatic dissemination of infection associated with bacteremia, renal failure, electrolyte imbalance, including the hyperosmolar syndrome, and ketoacidosis. Prompt therapy of the infection and the hyperglycemia may help avoid these complications.

Thorough surgical removal of dead tissue is generally felt to be an absolute necessity. This holds true regardless of whether one is dealing with necrotizing soft tissue infection, mucormycosis, or emphysematous pyelonephritis. When polymicrobial infection is likely or has been established to be present, antimicrobial therapy should be directed at the various microorganisms that are present or likely to be present. Since diabetic patients often have pre-existent renal dysfunction, many clinicians are loathe to use aminoglycosides in the antibiotic therapy of these patients. Fortunately, our choice of antimicrobial agents has been broadened by the advent of newer beta-lactam antibiotics, such as the third-generation cephalosporins, imipenem/cilastatin, ampicillin / sulbactam, ticarcillin / clavulanate, aztreonam, and the quinolone ciprofloxacin. Septic and severely ill patients should receive antibiotics that adequately cover commonly isolated organisms, such as *S. aureus, B. fragilis, E. coli, P. mirabilis, P. aeruginosa,* enterococci, and anaerobic streptococci. This would generally mandate a combination of antimicrobial agents. Monoantibiotic therapy, using agents such as imipenem/cilastin, ticarcillin/clavulanate, or ampicillin/sulbactam, may be employed in less serious infections pending the results of culture and sensitivity studies.

REFERENCES

1. Wheat LJ. Infection and diabetes mellitus. Diabetes Care 1980; 3:187–197.
2. Doroghazi RM, Nadol JB, Hyslop NE, Baker AN, Axelrod L. Invasive external otitis: report of 21 cases and review of the literature. AM J Med 1981; 71:603–614.
3. Abramson E, Wilson D, Arky RA. Rhinocerebral phycomycosis in association with diabetic ketoacidosis. Ann Intern Med 1967; 66:735–742.
4. Pillsbury HC, Fischer ND. Rhinocerebral mucormycosis. Arch Otolaryngol 1977; 103:600–604.
5. Mentzer RM Jr, Golden GT, Chandler JG, Horsley JS III. A comparative appraisal of emphysematous cholecystitis. Am J Surg 1975; 129:10–15.
6. Abengowe CU, McManamon PJM. Acute emphysematous cholecystitis. Can Med Assoc J 1974; 111:1112–1114.
7. Michaeli J, Mozle P, Perlberg S, Heiman S, Caine M. Emphysematous pyelonephritis. J Urol 1984; 131:203–208.
8. Thorley JD, Jones SR, Sanford JP. Perinephric abscess. Medicine 1974; 53:441–445.
9. Gibbons GW, Eliopoulos GM. Infection of the diabetic feet. *In* Kozak GP, Noar CS Jr. Rowbotham JL, et al (eds). Management of Diabetic Foot Problems. Philadelphia: WB Saunders, 1984:97–102.
10. Bagdade JD, Root RK, Bulger RJ. Impaired leukocyte function in patients with poorly controlled diabetes. Diabetes 1974; 23:9–15.
11. Molinar DM, Palumbo PH, Wilson WR, Ritts RE. Leukocyte chemotaxis in diabetic patients and their first degree relatives. Diabetes (Suppl 2)1976; 25:880–883.
12. Repine JE, Clawson CC, Goetz FE. Bactericidal function of neutrophils from patients with acute bacterial infections and from diabetics. J Infect Dis 1980; 142:869–875.
13. Katz S, Klein B, Elian I, Fishman P, Djaldetti M. Phagocytic activity of monocytes from diabetic patients. Diabetic Care 1983; 6:479–482.
14. Mahmoud AAF, Rodman HN, Mandel MA, Warren KS. Induced and spontaneous diabetes mellitus and suppression of cell-mediated immunologic responses: granuloma formation, delayed dermal reactivity, and allograft rejection. J Clin Invest 1976; 57:362–367.
15. Coopan R. Infection and diabetes. *In* Marble A, Krall LP, Bradley RF, Christlieb AR, Soeldner JS (eds). Joslin's Diabetes Mellitus. 12th ed. Philadelphia: Lea and Febiger, 1985:737–747.
16. Fekety R Jr, Caldwell J, Gump D, et al. Bacteria, viruses, and mycoplasms in acute pneumonia in adults. Am Rev Respir Dis 1971; 104:499–507.
17. Root HF. The association of diabetes and tuberculosis: epidemiology, pathology, treatment and prognosis. N Engl J Med 1934; 210:1–13.
18. Hansen RO. Bacteriuria in diabetic and non-diabetic outpatients. Acta Med Scand 1964; 176:721–730.
19. Farland M, Thomas V, Shelokov A. Urinary tract infections in patients with diabetes mellitus. JAMA 1977; 238:1924–1926.
20. Barlow AJE, Chattaway FW. Observations on the carriage of *Candida albicans* in man. Br J Dermatol 1969; 81:103–106.
21. Stone HH, Martin JD Jr. Synergistic necrotizing cellulitis. Ann Surg 1972; 175:702–710.
22. Rea WJ, Wyrick WJ Jr. Necrotizing fasciitis. Ann Surg 1978; 172:957–964.
23. Sapico FL, Canawati HN, Witte JL, et al. Quantitative aerobic and anaerobic bacteriology of infected diabetic feet. J Clin Microbiol 1980; 12:413–420.
24. Sapico FL, Witte JL, Canawati HN, Montgomerie JZ, Bessman AN. The infected foot of the diabetic patient: quantitative microbiology and analysis of clinical features. Rev Infect Dis 1984(suppl); 6:S171–S176.
25. Bamberger DM, Daus GP, Gerding DN. Osteomyelitis in the feet of diabetic patients. Am J Med 1987; 83:653–660.
26. Leslie CA, Sapico FL, Ginunas VJ, Adkins RH. Randomized clinical trial of hyperbaric oxygen for treatment of diabetic foot ulcers. Diabetes Care 1988; 11:111–115.

Inflammatory bowel disease

V. Alin Botoman ■ *Richard A. Kozarek*

■ Background

Crohn's disease and chronic ulcerative colitis (CUC) are chronic, relapsing, inflammatory conditions of unknown etiology. The prevalence of inflammatory bowel disease (IBD) is estimated at 90 to 300 cases per 100,000 people, with over 600,000 patients affected in the United States alone.[1] The peak age of onset is between 15 and 30 years for Crohn's disease and between 30 and 60 years for chronic ulcerative colitis.

The cause of both ulcerative colitis and Crohn's disease is not known. Infectious agents, autoimmune host factors, dietary factors, or combinations of these have been implicated. To date, no conclusive etiology has been established, nor do any data allow a separation between the two disorders on the basis of etiologic factors.

Both Crohn's disease and chronic ulcerative colitis cause episodic diarrhea, rectal bleeding, abdominal pain, fever, weight loss, and malnutrition. Crohn's disease typically causes a segmental inflammatory process with "skip areas" of normal intervening mucosa. It can involve the gastrointestinal tract at any point from the mouth to the anus, with the most common areas of involvement being the terminal ileum and colon. CUC is confined to the colon and produces a more continuous inflammatory response that begins at the rectum. Differential diagnostic features are noted in Table 1. In addition, a number of conditions can mimic inflammatory bowel disease and need to be excluded with appropriate studies (Table 2).

Proctosigmoidoscopy, barium enema, and small bowel radiographs have been the mainstay of diagnosis for patients with inflammatory bowel disease. Biopsies are essential in the diagnosis. However, in approximately 10 per cent of patients mucosal biopsy, radiologic studies, and other diagnostic studies cannot reliably distinguish between Crohn's disease and CUC.

Colonoscopy has improved the diagnostic sensitivity and increases the yield by 20 per cent over conventional radiologic studies in determining disease extent.[2] In particular, shallow ulcerations may not be seen on barium enema. Colonoscopy allows one to obtain tissue from the colon and terminal ileum, thus allowing accurate evaluation of colonic strictures and also accurate evaluation prior to consideration of a surgical resection.

TABLE 1. Differences Between Chronic Ulcerative Colitis (CUC) and Crohn's Disease

	Crohn's	*CUC*
History/Physical Examination		
Diarrhea	+++	+++
Rectal bleeding	±	+++
Fever	++	++
Abdominal pain	+	+
Anal fissure	+	−
Perianal fistulas	+	−
Other fistulas: enterovesical, enterocutaneous	+	−
Barium Studies/Colonoscopy/Flexible Sigmoidoscopy		
Proctitis	±	+
Rectal sparing	+	−
Aphthous "ulceration"	+	−
Cobblestoning/deep ulceration	++	±
Diffuse ulceration/ friability	+	+++
Pseudopolyps	++	++
Colonic stricture	++	+
Small bowel stricture ("string sign")	+	−
Ileitis	+	+
Small bowel/duodenal involvement	+	−
Pathology		
Patchy involvement	+	−
Transmural involvement	+++	−
Crypt abscess	+	++
Granuloma	+	−

(Adapted from Donaldson M Jr. Crohn's disease. *In* Sleisenger MH, Fordtran JS (eds). Gastrointestinal Disease; Pathophysiology, Diagnosis, Management. 4th ed. Philadelphia: WB Saunders, 1989:1328.)

TABLE 2. Disorders That May Mimic Inflammatory Bowel Disease

Crohn's-Like	Either	CUC-Like
Segmental ischemia (ischemic colitis, birth control pills)	Salmonella infection	*Shigella* infection
	Amebiasis	*Campylobacter* infection
	Lymphogranuloma venereum proctitis	Toxigenic *Escherichia coli*
	CMV colitis (immunosuppressed patients)	Gonococcal proctitis
Behçet's syndrome		Syphilitic proctitis
Ileocarcinoma	Fungal infections	Collagen vascular disease
Appendicitis	Pseudomembranous (*C. difficile*) colitis	
Yersinia infection	Schistosomiasis	
Tuberculosis	Radiation proctocolitis	
Lymphoma	Drug-induced colitis	
Diverticulitis		
Cancer of colon		
Duodenal ulcer		

(Adapted from Itzkowitz SH. Conditions that mimic inflammatory bowel disease. Diagnostic clues and potential pitfalls. Postgrad Med 1986; 80:219–231.)

Both Crohn's disease and CUC are characterized by their relapsing course in 70 to 80 per cent of patients. Approximately 5 to 10 per cent of patients can have a very fulminant downhill course, whereas another 5 to 10 per cent may have one flare and then no symptoms subsequently. The presence of diarrhea, rectal bleeding, fever, abdominal pain, nausea, vomiting, or a palpable abdominal mass can all be signs of active inflammatory bowel disease that can be readily elicited on history and physical examination. The presence of these symptoms determines whether medical therapy should be started or altered.

In assessing disease activity, the aforementioned diagnostic studies can be employed. In addition, for following patients, a number of noninvasive laboratory studies have been proposed. The erythrocyte sedimentation rate (ESR) is time honored but has low sensitivity and specificity. In a few patients it can correlate and can be used to follow the course of inflammatory bowel disease, particularly its response to treatment. A number of radionuclide-labeled blood cell scanning techniques have been employed.[3] They are noninvasive and can be used both for diagnosis and follow-up of disease activity. In our experience, these techniques have a limited role at present and still are considered investigational at this time. For most patients, disease activity is best determined by history and physical examination, with confirmation by laboratory studies, radiologic examination, or endoscopic studies that include proctosigmoidoscopy, flexible sigmoidoscopy, or colonoscopy.

A note of caution, however, should be given for patients who have severe disease. Both barium studies and colonoscopy should be avoided since they may further increase disease activity or precipitate toxic megacolon (see article on Toxic Megacolon in Inflammatory Bowel Disease). Proctosigmoidoscopy or flexible sigmoidoscopy without preparation can be done with little risk to the patient and, together with a kidney, ureter, and bladder radiograph, can be quite helpful in assessing disease activity and making a diagnosis in this situation.

■ Management

Because of their chronic relapsing course, both CUC and Crohn's disease remain a difficult problem and a significant challenge. Potentially toxic medications need to be used, sometimes for prolonged periods of time, to control the disease. The toxicity of the therapy needs to be balanced against the severity of the illness. Meyers and Janowitz have pointed out, in a review of placebo-controlled Crohn's disease trials, that up to 50 per cent of patients with a mild flare respond to "placebo"—that is, time and general supportive measures.[4] In most patients, however, more intensive medical therapy needs to be undertaken.

■ NUTRITIONAL THERAPY

Dietary therapy and nutritional recommendations have a long tradition in the treatment of inflammatory bowel disease, despite the paucity of controlled data defining efficacy. Lactose intolerance can be present in up to 30 per cent of patients with Crohn's disease and in some patients with CUC. In such patients lactose restriction can help improve symptoms of diarrhea, bloating, and abdominal cramps. Lactose restriction has no effect on the activity of IBD, and lactose malabsorption does not interfere with the absorption of dietary calcium. Thus, indiscriminate restrictions of lactose should not be undertaken, and confirmatory testing for intolerance is recommended.

Low-fiber diets traditionally have been advocated. Controlled studies have shown no benefit;[5] however, a low-fiber diet can be quite helpful in managing patients with partially obstructive symptoms from strictures.

In patients with symptoms refractory to oral outpatient therapy, complete bowel rest with hospitalization and concomitant intravenous fluids or hyperalimentation have been advocated. Although 30 to 80 per cent of patients improve on such a regimen, recent controlled studies suggest that bowel rest per se, may have a limited role in patients with uncomplicated IBD. Thus, Greenberg and associates recently randomized three groups of patients with steriod-refractory Crohn's disease; one group received full parenteral nutrition and nothing by mouth, a second group received a defined formula diet by nasogastric tube, and a third group, partial parenteral nutrition and unlimited oral intake.[6] At the end of a 3-week period, clinical remission occurred in 58 to 72 per cent of the patients without any statistically significant differences in outcome. The 1-year remission rates were also similar. Similar data are available for patients with CUC. However, these studies demonstrate that adjunctive nutritional therapy, whether intravenous or oral, clearly appears to help put 50 to 70 per cent of patients with refractory symptoms in remission. Bowel rest in addition is clearly indicated in patients with obstruction or internal fistula.

What is the role of total parenteral nutrition (TPN) in inflammatory bowel disease? TPN is useful in patients who are severely malnourished with protein/calorie malnutrition and fluid depletion. If bowel obstruction or fistula has complicated the course of IBD, TPN can help restore nutritional parameters. In malnourished patients, surgical intervention carries an increased risk, par-

ticularly of infection, and preoperative TPN may also be of benefit.[7] In patients with short bowel syndrome from repeated resections, home TPN can allow a normal lifestyle and avoidance of hospitalization. We also have used home TPN in a few selected patients with Crohn's disease with recurrences or fistula refractory to all other therapy. However, we caution against the indiscriminate and widespread use of TPN in treating patients with refractory IBD. TPN is expensive and, due to catheter sepsis and thromboembolic complications, not without risks.

Elemental diets have been advocated as a means of providing "partial bowel rest" and therapy for inflammatory bowel disease. A number of studies from Europe, particularly in patients with Crohn's disease, suggested that such therapy is effective and may be as efficacious as corticosteroids. However, a recent prospective randomized study comparing corticosteroids and elemental diets in the treatment of Crohn's disease found corticosteroids to be superior.[8] Elemental diets (e.g., Vivonex) are unpalatable and difficult to take for a prolonged period of time, and their value is as yet unproved.

Nutritional deficiencies can complicate the course of inflammatory bowel disease and need to be sought and treated diligently. Vitamin B_{12} deficiency can occur with severe ileal Crohn's disease or following resection of the terminal ileum and can be prevented with appropriate supplementation. A Schilling test is diagnostic. Folate deficiency can result from poor oral intake or from interference of folate absorption by sulfasalazine. Iron deficiency can be seen from chronic gastrointestinal bleeding in patients with refractory IBD or from malabsorption in patients with gastroduodenal Crohn's disease. Calcium malabsorption is also common and can result in metabolic bone disease or hyperoxaluria with oxalate stones. Other trace minerals also can become depleted in patients with severe refractory IBD. Zinc deficiency is particularly common in patients with profuse drainage from fistulas and can result in poor wound healing, anosmia, and rarely a peculiar skin disorder, acrodermatitis enteropathica. Oral replacement therapy is the method of choice for mild mineral and trace element deficiencies, whereas intravenous or intramuscular therapy may be required for patients with more severe abnormalities.

SULFASALAZINE

Sulfasalazine (SAS) has been found to be effective in treating inflammatory bowel disease since the 1950s. Colonic flora deconjugate the drug, releasing sulfapyridine, a sulfa antibiotic moiety that is systemically absorbed and therapeutically inactive, and 5-aminosalicylic acid (5-ASA), which binds to inflamed mucosa and is therapeutically active.[9]

In patients with CUC the drug is superior to placebo in patients with mild-to-moderate disease, but it has not been studied in patients with severe disease. A major use of SAS in chronic ulcerative colitis is in maintaining remission. Patients who are maintained on 2 gm of SAS daily have a fourfold decrease in relapse. Both therapeutic and prophylactic activity increase as the dosage increases from 2 to 4 gm daily. However, side effects are also more common as the dosage increases, and up to one third of patients may not tolerate a 4-gm per day dose.

In patients with Crohn's disease, SAS is superior to placebo in patients with Crohn's colitis but not in patients with small bowel Crohn's.[10] We have found it effective in patients with ileocolonic disease, presumably due to bacterial overgrowth and deconjugation of the drug in the terminal ileum. Again, a dose-response relationship has been demonstrated, with higher response rates at higher doses. SAS has a limited role in patients with refractory Crohn's disease. Specifically, adding SAS for patients with disease refractory to corticosteroids provides no therapeutic benefit, whereas adding corticosteroids to patients initially treated with SAS produces further improvement.[10] Unlike CUC, SAS has not been demonstrated to be effective in preventing relapses of Crohn's disease. Some physicians continue to use it for prophylaxis in patients with Crohn's relapses, with anecdotal benefit.

The side effects of SAS are primarily due to the sulfapyridine moiety. The more common effects are nausea and headache, which are dose-dependent. The nausea can be decreased by beginning the dosage slowly, with gradual increase over several days to one week. More serious side effects of the drug include hemolytic or aplastic anemia, leukopenia, hepatitis, Stevens-Johnson syndrome, or pulmonary hypersensitivity. These require prompt discontinuation of the drug. A reversible effect on sperm motility and thus male fertility also has been reported. In patients with drug-induced rash, desensitization can be carried out successfully by using small, gradually increasing doses of the drug.[11] Desensitization is contraindicated in patients who have had hepatitis, leukopenia, hemolytic anemia, or other significant side effects.

5-AMINOSALICYLIC ACID (5-ASA) DERIVATIVES

Although 5-ASA is the therapeutically active moiety in sulfasalazine, if given alone it is absorbed in the proximal small intestine and is thus of little therapeutic benefit. A number of 5-ASA preparations have been developed that can deliver the active drug to the distal small bowel and colon. These include 5-ASA enemas and preparations that use either a diazo bond or various types of enteric coatings to deliver the active drug.

5-ASA melsalamine enemas (Rowasa) now have been approved for treatment of distal ulcerative proctitis. They are superior to corticosteroid enemas and probably superior to sulfasalazine and steroids in the treatment of that disorder. The recommended dosage is one enema nightly for 3 to 6 weeks. In patients with relapses when the drug is discontinued, a prophylactic enema every 2 to 3 days can be used. 5-ASA suppositories also have been shown to be effective, as have para-aminosalicylic acid (PAS) enemas and suppositories.

The most promising preparations use either a pH-dependent coating to release 5-ASA in the distal small bowel and colon (Asacol, Pentasa) or link two 5-ASA molecules with a diazo bond that is cleaved by colonic bacteria (olsalazine-Dipentum).

The therapeutic benefit of 5-ASA derives from the absence of a sulfa moiety and thus sulfa-related side effects, and also because one can give a higher dose of 5-ASA compound than could be tolerated with equivalent doses of SAS. Thus, 4.8 gm of Asacol allows delivery of therapeutic drug equivalent to 12 gm of SAS. One study of patients with mild to moderately active CUC showed that 4.8 gm of Asacol was superior to placebo, with 24 per cent of the patients showing a complete response at 6 weeks and 50 per cent, a partial response.[12] The dose of 1.6 gm per day (equivalent to 4 gm of SAS) was not as effective. Olsalazine also has been demonstrated to be superior to placebo in the treatment of CUC, as have a number of studies showing that oral 5-ASA compounds can be equal to or superior to sulfasalazine in maintaining remission in CUC patients.

The 5-ASA compounds also have been studied in the treatment of Crohn's disease. They are effective drugs in a manner and potency similar to that of SAS.[13]

The side effects of 5-ASA compounds include alopecia, which is infrequently reported with melsalamine, and diarrhea, which appears to be particularly common with olsalazine, in which the diazo bond 5-ASA entity, if not deconjugated, may produce secretory changes in the small intestine and diarrhea in 5 to 13 per cent of patients. 5-ASA compounds are potentially nephrotoxic, and urinary sediment abnormalities have been reported in patients on high-dose Asacol. Careful monitoring of renal function and the urinary sediment to look for early nephrotoxicity should be carried out in patients treated with such drugs. The potential for systemic absorption also exists with topical enemas. However, the amounts absorbed are much less, and thus the potential for toxicity is decreased. Skin rashes and hypersensitivity also have been reported rarely with 5-ASA compounds.

■ SYSTEMIC CORTICOSTEROIDS

Since the initial work by Truelove in 1955, demonstrating the superiority of oral cortisone over placebo in chronic ulcerative colitis, corticosteroids have been the mainstay of therapy, particularly in patients with severe inflammatory bowel disease.

In patients with mild disease, we use sulfasalazine as the initial therapy in patients with CUC that extends past the rectum and in patients with Crohn's colitis or ileocolitis. We add corticosteroids only if such patients do not respond to SAS.

In patients with moderate or severe IBD not requiring hospitalization, oral corticosteroids are the drugs of choice. We use a dosage of 40 to 60 mg given as a single morning dose; although some practitioners prefer a divided dose regimen, the latter can cause more adrenal suppression. Once a clinical response has been achieved, we decrease the dosage by 10 mg every 1 to 2 weeks until a dosage of 20 mg is reached, and then by 5 mg every 1 to 2 weeks. In some patients, a flare of symptoms can occur with dosage below 20 mg, and a slower prednisone taper of 2.5 to 5 mg every 2 to 4 weeks may be required.

Patients with severe inflammatory bowel disease, manifested by anemia, significant rectal bleeding, hypoalbuminemia, intractable diarrhea, and systemic symptoms such as fever, who do not respond to oral therapy, generally require hospitalization. In such patients we prefer intravenous hydrocortisone, 300 mg per day administered either as three 100-mg doses or as a continuous drip. Some investigators have preferred ACTH in this setting. One controlled study showed a superiority of ACTH in patients who had not received steroids prior to admission and a superiority of hydrocortisone over ACTH in patients with prior steroid therapy.[14]

The overall remission rates for patients with CUC treated with an intensive intravenous steroid regimen are 50 to 70 per cent.[15] Responses will occur by 5 or at the latest 10 days, and longer courses of intravenous corticosteroids or changing from hydrocortisone to ACTH is of little or no benefit. In patients who do respond to intravenous corticosteroids, a transition to oral therapy is made with a gradual outpatient taper. The remission rate with intravenous steroids depends on the severity of symptoms and the extent of the disease. CUC patients with mild and primarily distal colitis have a remission rate of over 90 per cent, whereas patients with pancolitis and more severe disease have a remission rate of 40 to 50 per cent.[15] Fifty per cent of patients with pancolitis in this study[15] required surgery within 3 weeks. Furthermore, 48 per cent of patients with pancolitis who went into initial remission relapsed within 1 year and required subsequent surgery. These investigators also looked at the role of intravenous steroids in conjunction with bowel rest and TPN in a small group of patients with chronic continuous symptoms unresponsive to oral therapy. None of the patients with pancolitis responded, but half of those with less extensive disease did go into remission.

In contrast to their use in CUC, similar systemic corticosteroid regimens have been used for patients with intractable Crohn's disease. The best-controlled studies in Crohn's disease, however, have been in patients requiring oral steroid therapy.[10,16]

A number of studies have addressed the

use of corticosteroids to maintain remission in patients with refractory relapsing inflammatory bowel disease. Prednisone (15 mg daily) is no better than placebo for CUC prophylaxis. On the other hand, sulfasalazine in doses of 2 to 4 gm per day maintains remission in up to 75 per cent of patients with CUC. The National Crohn's Cooperative Study [10] showed that neither corticosteroids nor sulfasalazine was superior to placebo for prophylaxis. Our anecdotal experience, however, is that a subset of patients with Crohn's disease remains in remission on low doses of steroids, with prompt relapse when these are decreased or discontinued. A recent European study supports that view. [16]

The long-term morbidity and side effect profile of corticosteroids is considerable and has been well described in the literature. In addition to the predictable adrenal suppression and cushingoid facies, seen particularly with doses larger than 20 mg per day, other side effects such as diabetes, glaucoma, immunosuppression, and aseptic necrosis of long bones can occur. This latter condition is of particular concern, since its time of onset is unpredictable, either with regard to duration of therapy or dose. Every-other-day corticosteroid therapy is associated with a reduced incidence of side effects and has less adrenal suppression. This strategy, however, may be effective in controlling symptoms in only 25 per cent of patients with IBD. We strongly consider "steroid-sparing" agents, such as 6-mercaptopurine (6-MP), azathioprine, or methotrexate, in any patient with CUC or Crohn's disease who requires continuous steroids for prolonged periods of time or has multiple steroid-requiring relapses.

◼ TOPICAL STEROIDS

Topical steroids have been shown to be superior to placebo in patients with distal ulcerative colitis, particularly proctosigmoiditis. Hydrocortisone suspension or a foam preparation can extend as far up as the splenic flexure and produce a 50 to 70 per cent clinical and sigmoidoscopic response rate by 3 to 6 weeks. [17] Relapse rates, however, can be high, and a tapering every other or every third day regimen may help. As discussed previously, topical 5-ASA preparations such as mesalamine (Rowasa) are ef-

fective in patients with distal proctitis who do not respond to steroid enemas. In patients with anorectal Crohn's disease, topical steroid use is ineffective and limited by the high prevalence of anal fissures, skin tags, and fistulas that make insertion difficult.

Although the systemic absorption of topical steroids is low, adrenal suppression, immunosuppression, osteonecrosis, and other steroid-related side effects have been reported, particularly with prolonged use.

Two as yet unmarketed nonabsorbable steroids, tixocortal pivolate and beclomethasone, are effective in CUC and hold promise of avoiding these side effects. [18]

◼ ANTIBIOTICS

The medical literature is replete with anecdotal reports of improvement of refractory IBD with systemic antibiotics, including tetracycline, ampicillin, metronidazole, trimethoprim-sulfa, and so on. Few, if any, controlled reports are available.

In patients with Crohn's disease, most of the controlled data have been on the use of metronidazole. Initial reports from Sweden suggested significant benefit, particularly in children and adolescents with anorectal disease. Bernstein and associates showed a similar benefit in 70 per cent of patients with refractory perianal fistulas and fissures. The dosage used was high (1.5 to 2.0 gm/day) and was limited by side effects, particularly paresthesias and metallic taste, in one third of the patients. [19] The relapse rate was very high upon medication cessation, requiring long-term therapy. This is of particular concern in patients with paresthesias, in whom irreversible neuropathy has been reported. A controlled trial comparing sulfasalazine (3 gm/day) to metronidazole (800 mg/day) in patients with mild-to-moderate Crohn's disease found metronidazole to be slightly superior. [20] In our experience, the high doses of metronidazole required for therapeutic benefit and its side effect profile limit its use in patients with refractory Crohn's disease.

Metronidazole is not superior to placebo in patients with active CUC. The role of metronidazole as an adjunct in patients with refractory IBD requiring corticosteroids has not been studied. Our own experience is that it is of little benefit. We prefer other agents in this setting.

■ 6-MERCAPTOPURINE (6-MP) AND AZATHIOPRINE

The side effect profile of long-term corticosteroids for patients with refractory inflammatory bowel disease stimulated an interest in agents with "steroid-sparing" effect that would help control bowel inflammation and lead to a concomitant reduction in corticosteroid dosage. Early anecdotal reports in the 1970s regarding the benefits of both azathioprine and its active metabolite, 6-MP, resulted in two controlled trials looking at its effect in Crohn's disease. The first, The National Crohn's Cooperative Study, looked at relatively low doses of azathioprine for a relatively short period of time (4 months).[10] No benefit over placebo could be demonstrated. Both the dosage and duration of treatments were criticized as shortcomings of that trial. A subsequent placebo-controlled cross-over trial by Present and associates showed improvement in 67 per cent of 6-MP courses versus 8 per cent of placebo courses in the 83 patients studied.[21] A reduction of steroid dosage could be accomplished in 75 per cent of the patients treated with the active drug versus 36 per cent treated with placebo. The onset of response to the medication took longer than 3 months in 32 per cent of the patients and longer than 4 months in 19 per cent. If the drug were discontinued, 81 per cent relapsed with 90 per cent of those patients responding to reintroduction of the drug and remaining in remission.

The same group has reported their experience in 34 patients with Crohn's disease fistulas.[22] Whereas in their initial controlled study most of the patients were on corticosteroids and 6-MP was used as the corticosteroid-"sparing" drug, in this later uncontrolled study only 12 patients were on steroids. Corticosteroid use did not seem to predict a response or lack of improvement for 6-MP. Thirty-nine per cent of the patients had complete fistula closures, and 26 per cent showed marked improvement. These investigators suggest that in patients with refractory IBD, particularly those who are steroid-dependent and those with fistulous complications, adjunctive 6-MP may be a good agent. The current dosage of the Mt. Sinai group is 50 mg of 6-MP per day, increasing after several weeks, if tolerated, to 75 mg per day.

A major disadvantage of this class of drugs is their delay in onset of benefit; often 2 to 6 months is required for improvement. In addition, potential serious side effects have been reported with these agents, particularly a 3 per cent incidence of pancreatitis within 6 weeks of institution of therapy, dose-dependent leukopenia, and, at times, allergic reactions. These drugs also may increase one's incidence of secondary hematopoietic neoplasms, similar to other alkylating agents. This incidence is currently estimated by the Mt. Sinai group to be at 1 in 400 patient years. These drugs are teratogenic and contraindicated in pregnancy. Nevertheless, inadvertent pregnancies while the patient was taking the drug have occurred, with only one case report of von Gierke's disease in twins. Despite these concerns, the track record for these agents is reasonable, and their side effect profile is less than that of long-term corticosteroids.

There are many fewer data for azathioprine or 6-MP in CUC, and three controlled trials reported so far give contradictory results. A recent uncontrolled report, the largest to date, of 60 patients with refractory CUC suggested benefit, with a 43 per cent complete remission rate, and a 30 per cent moderate improvement rate.[23]

■ METHOTREXATE

Patients with symptoms that are refractory to conventional therapy with corticosteroids have been traditionally treated with immunosuppressive agents such as 6-MP and azathioprine (discussed earlier). An average 2- to 6-month delay in onset of action of these agents, as well as potential side effects, limits their use. This has prompted us to investigate methotrexate in the treatment of inflammatory bowel disease. In low doses, this drug is anti-inflammatory and not immunosuppressive. It has been quite effective in a number of other refractory inflammatory conditions, particularly psoriasis and rheumatoid arthritis. A recent placebo-controlled study from our institution showed it to be a very effective drug in patients with steroid-dependent asthma.[24]

In our preliminary open label study, a total of 21 patients were enrolled, 14 with Crohn's disease and 7 with chronic ulcerative colitis.[25] All had refractory inflammatory bowel disease, defined as unresponsive to medical therapy with steroid-dependence for at least 2 months in 17 of the 21 patients, dependence on home TPN in 3 patients, and failure of azathioprine therapy for 3 to 6 months in 10 patients. Five patients with Crohn's disease had had previous small bowel or colon resections. Fourteen of the twenty-one patients were also taking concomitant sulfasalazine or metronidazole. Baseline evaluation included CBC, ESR, chemistry profile, urinalysis, and either colonoscopy or flexible sigmoidoscopy plus biopsies. Most patients also had prior colon radiographs and small bowel radiographs, which were repeated as needed to assess disease activity. We treated the patients for a total of 12 weeks, measuring disease activity with modified Crohn's disease activity index, and a similar clinical activity index for patients with CUC. Both activity indices ranged from 0 (no active disease) to 15 (fulminant disease). The responders were continued on long-term oral therapy.

Treatment consisted of 25 mg of methotrexate intramuscularly weekly for 12 weeks. The patients who were responders were then changed to an oral regimen of 15 mg per week with a gradual taper to 7.5 mg per week. Laboratory studies were monitored weekly for the first 3 months and every 4 to 6 weeks thereafter for the responders. Twenty-four-hour methotrexate levels were obtained at week 8, and all patients had repeat endoscopic and histologic studies at week 12.

Sixteen of the twenty-one patients had significant clinical improvement, with a fall in the Crohn's disease activity index from 13.3 to 5.4 and in the CUC activity index from 13.3 to 6.3. Five of the fourteen Crohn's disease patients had complete endoscopic remission, with four of the five showing normal histology on biopsy. Five of the seven patients with CUC improved; however, none had histologic or endoscopic remission. Corticosteroid dosage fell from a mean of 27 mg at the onset of the study to 8.5 mg by 12 weeks; corticosteroids could be tapered in 15 of 18 patients and withdrawn in 5. Two of the three patients on long-term home parenteral TPN could be weaned off in the course of this study. Five patients were withdrawn from therapy by week 12 because of lack of response. Two additional patients had an excellent response on parenteral therapy but relapsed on oral therapy after week 12 and were withdrawn from the study. One additional patient with Crohn's disease also relapsed on oral therapy but responded to repeat parenteral therapy.

Side effects were infrequent, with one patient developing transient leukopenia and two patients, showing mild, transient SGOT increases. Two patients experienced nausea and diarrhea 24 hours postinjection, and a fifth patient developed atypical pneumonia that was, in fact, associated with an obstructive endobronchial neoplasm. No other complications were noted. Twenty-four-hour methotrexate levels ranged from 0.010 to 0.27 but did not correlate with clinical response. We chose the parenteral delivery route for the drug because of its unpredictable bioavailability in patients with gastrointestinal tract disease.

A traditional concern with methotrexate use has been development of hepatic fibrosis, at times with full-blown cirrhosis, in patients treated with prolonged daily therapy for psoriasis. More recently, a number of studies have demonstrated that the risk of hepatotoxicity is minimized in patients with rheumatoid arthritis treated with once a week low-dose methotrexate therapy.[26] It is not clear whether this is simply due to the low dosage used or the once weekly regimen or, most likely, both. A cumulative dosage of 2 to 3 gm of the drug is needed before hepatotoxicity has been noted with this regimen. Hepatic toxicity is more common in patients who are massively obese and who have a heavy alcohol history; the drug should be avoided in both those situations. In contradistinction to 6-MP and azathioprine, methotrexate does not appear to carry an increased risk of secondary neoplasia, i.e., leukemia and lymphoma. However, the drug is teratogenic, and patients need to be on birth control while on the drug.

Our study has many limitations, including a relatively short duration of therapy in disorders with a variable course. However, in this group of patients who had been refractory to virtually anything else tried, we were impressed with the dramatic and relatively rapid improvement at 2 to 8 weeks.

Many questions remain to be answered, particularly regarding the duration of a therapeutic trial of methotrexate, whether an oral dose is as effective as a parenteral dose, and what minimum drug dose is needed to maintain remission. We are in the process of setting up a double-blind, placebo-controlled, long-term trial of methotrexate. As with the previous study, in addition to the clinical disease activity indices traditionally used we feel it is important that therapy also be followed endoscopically.

Although methotrexate shows quite a bit of promise in inflammatory bowel disease, this drug is considered investigational for these disorders. It should not be used without careful monitoring and informed consent, and it is advocated primarily in the setting of a prospective trial.

■ OTHER AGENTS

A number of other medications have been reported, mostly in anecdotal fashion, to be of benefit in inflammatory bowel disease. Thus, in chronic ulcerative colitis, in which eosinophils can be seen on biopsy, a mast cell–stabilizing agent, disodium chromoglycate, has been claimed to be efficacious. Subsequent controlled studies have been contradictory. This agent is of no benefit in Crohn's disease.

Cyclosporine has been tried in inflammatory bowel disease with preliminary reports of benefit.[27] The renal and central nervous system toxicity of the drug, however, limits its use. There are similar reports for antimycobacterial agents in Crohn's disease.[28] This is based on the premise that cell-defective mycobacteria may be involved in its pathophysiology. However, we note controlled studies showing that these mycobacteria are as prevalent in patients with Crohn's disease as in patients with CUC and in normal controls. T lymphocyte apheresis is also claimed to be of benefit in patients with severe Crohn's disease.[29] It carries significant expense and potential risk liability. For all these agents, no placebo-controlled data substantiate effectiveness.

■ SURGICAL THERAPY

In the patient with chronic ulcerative colitis, surgery is indicated for intractable disease, development of persistent high-grade dysplasia and carcinoma, toxic megacolon, hemorrhage, and perforation. A Brooke ileostomy with total proctocolectomy is the time-honored operation. In CUC, this cures the patient. Unfortunately, the need for a continuous ileostomy appliance is associated with emotional difficulties and problems in approximately 20 per cent of patients. Stenosis of the ileostomy also can occur rarely and requires revision. Thus, alternative surgical approaches have been used in young patients with CUC, in whom an appliance presents particular difficulty. The two major alternative surgical techniques employed include a Koch pouch and ileoanal anastomosis.

The Koch pouch is a continent ileostomy that is fashioned from small bowel mucosa with an intussuscepted small bowel "nipple valve."[30] A catheter is left in the pouch for 3 weeks postoperatively. When successful, this procedure results in a completely continent ileostomy without the need for an appliance. The patient intubates the ileostomy daily to empty it out. Unfortunately, the learning curve is steep for a surgeon beginning this procedure, with a high incidence of complications in the first 50 to 75 patients. The most common problem is nipple valve dysfunction, which may require revisions in 10 to 40 per cent of patients. Seven per cent of the patients ultimately require conversion to a standard ileostomy. Pouchitis, an inflammatory process secondary to anaerobic bacteriostasis, has been reported in 10 to 40 per cent of patients. They generally respond to broad-spectrum antibiotics, particularly metronidazole. The Koch pouch is relatively contraindicated in patients with Crohn's disease. However, if inadvertently done, it is often tolerated in this setting.

Because of problems with the Koch pouch, another approach in the patient with CUC has been an ileoanal pull-through procedure with a proximal pouch.[31] After total proctocolectomy, a small portion of rectum is stripped of its overlying mucosa, with the rectal musculature left intact; an S-, J-, or H-shaped proximal small bowel pouch is formed; and then the small bowel is anastomosed to the anus. A diverting ileostomy is required for several months to allow healing, and then intestinal continuity is re-established. The major drawback of this procedure is diarrhea, with an average of 10 bowel movements daily for the first 6 to 10 months postoperatively. In most patients, however, bowel movements will decrease with time to 3 to 5 per day without any nocturnal soiling and with concomitant high patient acceptance. Potentially serious complications of perianal sepsis and anastomosis breakdown have been reported in 5 to 8 per cent of cases. Intestinal obstruction occurs in 10 per cent. Anorectal manometry, defecography, and scintigraphic study of pouch emptying can be used postoperatively to influence the outcome more favorably and to study pouch function. Pouchitis also can complicate this procedure and is typically treated with metronidazole with good response. This operation is contraindicated in Crohn's disease and will lead to perianal problems in that setting. The absence of rectal bleeding and the presence of perianal fistulas in someone with a diagnosis of chronic ulcerative colitis should serve as a "red flag" and make one very cautious in employing this procedure.

In contrast, an operation that may be encountered occasionally in patients with CUC is an ileorectal anastomosis. This was widely done in the 1960s in this country and is still practiced in Europe. Because of concerns, particularly about dysplasia and carcinoma of the rectal stump, this operation is not widely performed in this country currently.

Crohn's disease presents a much more difficult surgical problem because of inability to cure the disease by complete removal of involved intestinal segments. Early attempts of "cure" with extensive surgical resections often resulted in short bowel syndrome and a high postoperative recurrence rate. This resulted in a subsequent reluctance to refer patients for surgery. More recently, however, the pendulum has swung to favor relatively early, but limited, resections in patients who have severe intractable disease or who do not tolerate medical therapy. Despite the postoperative recurrence rate, which by life-table analysis averages 60 to 90 per cent by 25 years, such surgery may provide many years of a reasonable lifestyle off medications for many patients.[32] Only gross disease need be removed, and microscopic involvement at the anastomosis margin does not seem to affect outcome or recurrence. Patients with extensive colonic disease and rectal sparing may be candidates for an ileoproctostomy. If only segmental colonic involvement is present, a limited resection and colonic reanastomosis can be employed. In patients who have intractable disease with rectal involvement, total proctocolectomy and ileostomy can be done with an acceptable 20 per cent recurrence rate.

Two special situations need to be mentioned. Patients with perianal disease, extensive fissues, and fistulas are a problem.

Surgical therapy should be limited to symptomatic disease, and an extensive surgical procedure should be avoided in asymptomatic patients since it may lead to morbidity. Therapy should consist primarily of incision and drainage of any abscess collections or unroofing of superficial fistulas. Some have advocated an internal sphincterotomy: very small incisions allow drainage of the fistulous tracts through the internal sphincter from which they arise; results are good. Patients with Crohn's disease commonly develop large hypertrophic tags that can be mistaken for hemorrhoids. Hemorrhoidectomy or removal of these tags should be avoided in these patients, since these procedures may lead to considerable morbidity.

A second unusual situation is that of patients with multiple small bowel strictures, particularly those who have had surgery previously. A recent novel approach for this has been the use of a stricturoplasty of the involved segment. A group from England and groups from Cleveland and the Mayo Clinic have reported good results, despite the stricturoplasty's leaving active disease in place. This operation should be considered in patients who have recurrent bouts of obstruction or bacterial overgrowth caused by multiple tight strictures. It is best done at a center with considerable expertise in handling IBD.

The incidence of postoperative Crohn's disease recurrence depends on one's definition. Asymptomatic, colonoscopically documented aphthous ulcerations near the anastomosis can be demonstrated in over 90 per cent of the patients undergoing an ileocolonic anastomosis. The clinical recurrence rate, however, is much lower and typically will follow these aphthous ulcerations by 1 to 3 years. As stated, corticosteroids and sulfasalazine have been shown to have no benefit in preventing postoperative recurrences. However, they are quite effective in patients who have recurrence of symptoms in the postoperative period. We do not treat patients who have colonoscopic ulcerations without symptoms. Immunosuppressive agents, such as 6-MP, may be of benefit in selected patients for prevention of postoperative recurrence; however, its use in this setting has not been studied nor proved.

Enterovesical and enterocutaneous fistulas are also a problem in Crohn's disease. Enterovesical fistulas present typically with recurrent urinary tract infections or pneumaturia. Although some reports have suggested closing such fistulas with 6-MP,[22] most patients require surgery. The fistulas usually resolve with sharp dissection and resection of them and the intestine involved. Rectovaginal fistulas are often difficult to manage with primary surgical closure. Diverting procedures may be the only recourse, even though they may not be satisfactory at times.

In summary, surgical procedures are curative in chronic ulcerative colitis. Particularly in young patients, the emphasis has been on the ileoanal pull-through as an alternative to ileostomy, which may be more acceptable to the patients. We emphasize, however, a steep learning curve for the surgeon in this procedure, as well as anticipation of the 6 to 12 months of diarrhea that will follow. For Crohn's disease, the trend is toward earlier and limited surgical resection in patients who fail medical therapy or who have complicating obstruction or fistulous disease. In very selected patients, stricturoplasties of involved bowel appear to be safely tolerated and, in fact, quite successful in maintaining lumen patency. Surgical therapy for perianal disease remains difficult and unsatisfactory, should be performed only if there are sufficient symptoms, and should be limited in its scope. Postoperative recurrences in Crohn's disease can be treated medically in most patients, but 50 to 60 per cent of patients may require a second operation in the next 10 years.

■ Issues and Risks

■ TOXIC MEGACOLON

Toxic megacolon is a rare but potentially life-threatening complication of IBD. Its management is discussed in the article entitled "Toxic Megacolon in Inflammatory Bowel Disease."

■ PREGNANCY

In the past, pregnancy in a patient with active inflammatory bowel disease was thought to be an indication for abortion. Our thinking now has changed, and most pregnant patients can be managed medically. In fact, the outcome of such pregnancies appears to be no different in patients with IBD, whether active or quiescent, than in normal controls.[33] In approximately 50 per cent of pregnant patients with either Crohn's disease or ulcerative colitis, the disease either relapses or increases in activity, whereas in the other 50 per cent its activity will decrease or become quiescent. Hormonal influences may play a role.

Radiologic procedures cannot be performed during pregnancy. Limited proctosigmoidoscopy can be done safely but should be avoided, particularly in the first trimester of pregnancy. Colonoscopy also should be avoided, although it can be done if needed.

Sulfasalazine can be used safely in pregnant patients, despite theoretic concerns of kernicterus from sulfa excretion in breast milk. Prednisone also can be used at any stage in the pregnancy and appears not to affect outcome. Not treating active IBD, however, can carry risks both to the mother and the fetus.

Immunosuppressive agents are contraindicated during pregnancy. If a patient on immunosuppressive drugs becomes pregnant, these drugs should be stopped, immediately if possible. We note, however, that the Mt. Sinai group has reported a number of pregnancies in patients taking 6-MP without apparent increase of risk to the fetus. Metronidazole also may be teratogenic and should not be used.

In most patients with active IBD, full-term pregnancy and vaginal delivery occur in an uneventful fashion. In a few patients with severe perianal Crohn's disease, a cesarean section may be worthwhile. Both the patient and family need to be reassured that pregnancy is possible and that medications are generally quite safe during the gestation period.

■ DYSPLASIA AND CARCINOMA

Patients with chronic ulcerative colitis experience a significantly increased risk of colon cancer over control populations. This begins after 8 to 10 years of disease. Estimates of the risk are widely disparate but approximate 0.5 to 1 per cent per year. Patients with extensive CUC or pancolitis have the highest risk, whereas the risk is negligible in patients who have proctosigmoiditis or proctitis alone. The increased risk of colon cancer is present, even in patients who have long-standing *quiescent* disease. This has led to unfortunate delays of diagnosis in some patients and the misconception that the colon cancer of CUC is more aggressive than other colon cancers.

These figures have led to recommendations for screening for dysplasia in patients with extensive CUC of greater than 7 to 10 years' duration.[34] The premise of these screening programs is that dysplasia is present in virtually all cases of colonic carcinoma and that 50 to 80 per cent of patients with persistent high-grade dysplasia may have an associated carcinoma. Such changes are detected only through multiple colonoscopic biopsies from all parts of the colon. Macroscopic and mass-type lesions usually are not seen, but, if encountered, they should undergo additional biopsies.[34] This type of examination is best performed on a patient whose disease is in remission, since the presence of colonic inflammation can make interpretation of dysplasia very difficult.

If the initial screening colonoscopy is normal and no dysplasia is seen, the examination is repeated every 1 to 3 years. If dysplasia is encountered, colonoscopy is repeated within a short period of time. Colectomy is recommended for patients with persistent, particularly high-grade dysplasia. More frequent surveillance intervals are recommended with increasingly long-standing disease. Although early colon carcinoma can be clearly detected with this type of program, it is intensive and expensive, and its efficacy has been questioned by some.[35] It is not yet clear whether it is cost-effective. We practice this approach in our institution.

Not so commonly appreciated is the fact that Crohn's colitis also carries an increased risk of colon cancer. There is also associated dysplasia. Of particular note is the fact that most such cancers are within the reach of the flexible sigmoidoscope.[36] The small bowel carcinoma incidence is also increased in Crohn's. However, because of its rarity, the overall prevalence remains extremely low.[36] Bypassed small bowel intestinal segments are of particular concern, since there development of carcinoma may go undetected until quite late. Periodic surveillance

colonoscopy is not recommended for most patients with Crohn's disease. In selective cases with very long-standing involvement, however, it may have some benefit.

REFERENCES

1. Mayberry JF, Rhodes J. Epidemiologic aspects of Crohn's disease: a review of the literature. Gut 1984; 25:886–899.
2. Meuwissen SGM, Pape KSSB, Agenant D, Oushoorn HH, Tytgat GJ: Crohn's disease of the colon: analysis of the diagnostic value of radiology, endoscopy, and histology. Am J Dig Dis 1976; 21:81–88.
3. Pullman WE, Sullivan PJ, Barratt PJ, Lising J, Booth JA, Doe WF. Assessment of inflammatory bowel disease activity by technetium^{99m} phagocyte scanning. Gastroenterology 1988; 95:989–996.
4. Meyers S, Janowitz HD. "Natural history" of Crohn's disease. An analytic review of the placebo lesson. Gastroenterology 1984; 87:1189–1192.
5. Levenstein A, Prantera C, Luzi C, D'Ubaldi A. Low residue or normal diet in Crohn's disease: a prospective controlled study in Italian patients. Gut 1985; 26:989–993.
6. Greenberg GR, Fleming CR, Jeejeebhoy KN, Rosenberg IH, Sales D, Tremaine WJ. Controlled trial of bowel rest and nutritional support in the management of Crohn's disease. Gut 1988; 29:1309–1315.
7. Kushner RF, Craig RM. Intense nutritional support in inflammatory bowel disease: a review. J Clin Gastroenterol 1982; 4:511–520.
8. Lochs H, Steinhardt HJ, Klaus-Wenz B, Bauer P, Malchow H. Enteral nutrition versus drug treatment for the acute phase of Crohn's disease: results of the European Cooperative Crohn's Disease Study IV (abstract). Gastroenterology 1988; 94:A267.
9. Peppercorn MA. Sulfasalazine. Pharmacology, clinical use, toxicity, and related new drug development. Ann Intern Med 1984; 101:377–386.
10. Summers RW, Switz DM, Sessions JT Jr, et al. National Cooperative Crohn's Disease Study: results of drug treatment. Gastroenterology 1979; 77:847–869.
11. Taffet SL, Das KM. Sulfasalazine. Adverse effects and desensitization. Dig Dis Sci 1983; 28:833–842.
12. Schroeder KW, Tremaine WJ, Ilstrup DM. Coated oral 5-aminosalicylic acid therapy for mildly to moderately active ulcerative colitis. N Engl J Med 1987; 317:1625–1629.
13. Rasmussen SN, Binder V, Maier K, et al. Treatment of Crohn's disease with peroral 5-aminosalicylic acid. Gastroenterology 1983; 85:1350–1353.
14. Meyers S, Sachar DB, Goldberg JD, Janowitz HD. Corticotropin versus hydrocortisone in the intravenous treatment of ulcerative colitis. A prospective, randomized, double-blind clinical trial. Gastroenterology 1983; 85:351–357.
15. Jarnerot G, Rolny P, Sandberg-Gertzén H. Intensive intravenous treatment of ulcerative colitis. Gastroenterology 1985; 89:1005–1013.
16. Malchow H, Ewe K, Brandes JW, et al. European Cooperative Crohn's Disease Study (ECCDS): results of drug treatment. Gastroenterology 1984; 86:249–266.
17. Jay M, Digenis GA, Foster TS, Antonow DR. Retrograde spreading of hydrocortisone enema in inflammatory bowel disease. Dig Dis Sci 1986; 31:139–144.

18. Bansky G, Bühler H, Stamm B, Hacki WH, Buchmann P, Müller J. Treatment of distal ulcerative colitis with beclomethasone enemas. High therapeutic efficacy without endocrine side effects. A prospective, randomized, double-blind trial. Dis Col Rec 1987; 30:288–292.

19. Bernstein LH, Frank MS, Brandt LJ, Boley SJ. Healing of perineal Crohn's disease with metronidazole. Gastroenterology 1980; 79:357–365.

20. Ursing B, Alm T, Barany F, et al. A comparative study of metronidazole and sulfasalazine for active Crohn's disease: the Cooperative Crohn's Disease Study in Sweden. Gastroenterology 1982; 83:550–562.

21. Present DH, Korelitz BI, Wisch N, Glass JL, Sachar DB, Pasternack BS. Treatment of Crohn's disease with 6-mercaptopurine. A long-term randomized, double-blind study. N Engl J Med 1980; 302:981–987.

22. Korelitz BI, Present DH. Favorable effect of 6-mercaptopurine on fistulae of Crohn's disease. Dig Dis Sci 1985; 30:58–64.

23. Present DH, Chapman ML, Rubin PH. Efficacy of 6-mercaptopurine (6MP) in refractory ulcerative colitis (abstract). Gastroenterology 1988; 94:A359.

24. Mullarkey MF, Blumenstein BA, Andrade WP, Bailey GA, Olason I, Wetzel CE. Methotrexate in the treatment of corticosteroid-dependent asthma. A double blind crossover study. N Engl J Med 1988; 318:603–607.

25. Kozarek RA, Patterson DJ, Gelfand MD, Botoman VA, Ball TJ, Wilske KR. Methotrexate induces clinical and histologic remission in patients with refractory inflammatory bowel disease. Ann Intern Med 1989; 110:353–356.

26. Lewis JH, Schiff E. Methotrexate-induced chronic liver injury: guidelines for detection and prevention. Am J Gastroenterol 1988; 88:1337–1345.

27. Brynskov J, Binder V, Riis P, et al. Cyclosporine in inflammatory bowel disease (abstract). Transplant Proc 1988; 20(3 Supp 4):309.

28. Hampson SJ, Parker MC, Saverymuttu SH, McFadden JJ, Hermon-Taylor J. Results of quadruple antimicrobial chemotherapy in 17 Crohn's disease patients completing six months' treatment (abstract). Gastroenterology 1988; 94:A170.

29. Bicks RO, Groshart KD, Luther RW. Total parenteral nutrition (TPN) plus T-lymphocyte apheresis (TLA) in the treatment of severe chronic active Crohn's disease (abstract). Gastroenterology 1988; 94:A34.

30. Cohen Z. Current status of the continent ileostomy. Can J Surg 1987; 30:357–358.

31. Pemberton JH, Kelly KA, Beart RW Jr, Dozois RR, Wolff BG, Ilstrup DM. Ileal pouch anal anastomosis for chronic ulcerative colitis. Long-term results. Ann Surg 1987; 206:504–513.

32. Wolff BG. Crohn's disease. The role of surgical treatment. Mayo Clin Proc 1986; 61:292–295.

33. Vender RJ, Spiro HM. Inflammatory bowel disease and pregnancy. J Clin Gastroenterol 1982; 4:231–249.

34. Rosenstock E, Farmer RG, Petras R, Sivak MV, Rankin GB, Sullivan BH. Surveillance for colonic carcinoma in ulcerative colitis. Gastroenterology 1985; 89:1342–1346.

35. Collins RH, Feldman M, Fordtran JS. Colon cancer, dysplasia, and surveillance in patients with ulcerative colitis. A critical review. N Engl J Med 1987; 316:1654–1658.

36. Petras RE, Mir-Madylessi SH, Farmer RG. Crohn's disease and intestinal carcinoma. A report of 11 cases with emphasis on associated epithelial dysplasia. Gastroenterology 1987; 93:1307–1314.

Laryngotracheobronchitis, bacterial tracheitis, and epiglottitis in children

Larry G. McLain

Acute infection and inflammation of the airway in young children are always a great concern for the physician. The young child, with a small airway, is predisposed to critical narrowing and possibly eventual obstruction with the same degree of infection and inflammation that an adult might have. The disease entities discussed here are (1) laryngotracheobronchitis, (2) bacterial tracheitis, and (3) epiglottitis. These entities are difficult medical management problems because of confusion in diagnosis, occasional

TABLE 1. Clinical Characteristics of Croup, Bacterial Tracheitis, and Epiglottitis

	Croup	Bacterial Tracheitis	Epiglottitis
Incidence	Common	Uncommon	Uncommon
Etiology	Viral	Bacterial: *Staphylococcus aureus*	*Haemophilus influenzae,* type b
Age	6 months–3 years	Infancy to adolescence	2–6 years
Clinical Features	Gradual onset, preceding URI, barking cough, hoarse voice	Preceding URI, harsh cough, develop airway obstruction, poor response to standard LTB therapy	Rapid onset, fever, drooling, dysphagia
Physical Examination	Respiratory distress, inspiratory stridor, low-grade temperature, will lie quietly	Inspiratory stridor, moderate-to-high temperatures, toxic looking	Toxic looking, anxious, muffled voice, chin forward, drooling, high temperature common
Laboratory Findings	WBC usually below 10,000, lymphocytosis; x-ray film—narrowing at subglottic region	Indecisive WBC; x-ray film—subglottic narrowing and thick, purulent secretions	WBC often greater than 10,000 with bands increased; x-ray film—swollen epiglottis

delays in beginning therapy, and controversial therapeutic regimes. Their clinical characteristics are listed in Table 1.

■ Background

■ LARYNGOTRACHEOBRONCHITIS

Laryngotracheobronchitis is also known as LTB, croup, or acute viral croup. It is from 100 to 1000 times as common as epiglottitis and is more frequently seen than is bacterial tracheitis. Although seen in children of all ages, it occurs most frequently in children 3 months to 3 years of age, with a peak during the second year of life.[1,2] Laryngotracheobronchitis is more common in the late fall and early winter months.[3] In most instances it is a viral infection. Parainfluenza virus is the organism most frequently isolated.[4] Young children are particularly susceptible to this type of life-threatening upper airway obstruction for several reasons: the child's laryngeal airway is smaller in diameter and surface area than in an adult, the glottis is small, and the mucous membrane is more loosely attached, with greater vascularity.[3] Also, the subglottic region is a rigidly confined space in the airway, encircled by the cricoid cartilage.

The illness has a gradual onset, often beginning as a mild upper respiratory infection. Epiglottitis, in contrast, has sudden onset. The upper respiratory infection is usually followed by a mild cough progressing to a brash, harsh cough. Inspiratory stridor occurs next, followed by mild dyspnea. The temperature may be as high as 39.5°C but is often 38 to 38.5°C. The symptoms are frequently worse at night. Clinical characteristics are listed in Table 1.

Physical examination of the child with laryngotracheobronchitis reveals a child in mild-to-moderate respiratory distress. Inspection of the pharynx is usually normal, and nothing is to be gained by attempting to visualize the larynx. Suprasternal and intercostal retractions may be noticeable. Breath sounds are slightly diminished, but auscultation of the lungs usually reveals clear breath sounds.

The diagnosis of laryngotracheobronchitis is primarily made on a clinical basis. There are no definitive laboratory tests, only supportive ones. The white blood cell count often is within normal limits or shows a mild lymphocytosis. Throat cultures, blood cultures, and viral studies are of little help. Radiographs may be helpful in confirming the diagnosis of laryngotracheobronchitis. An A-P view of the chest may show a narrowing of the trachea in the subglottic area,

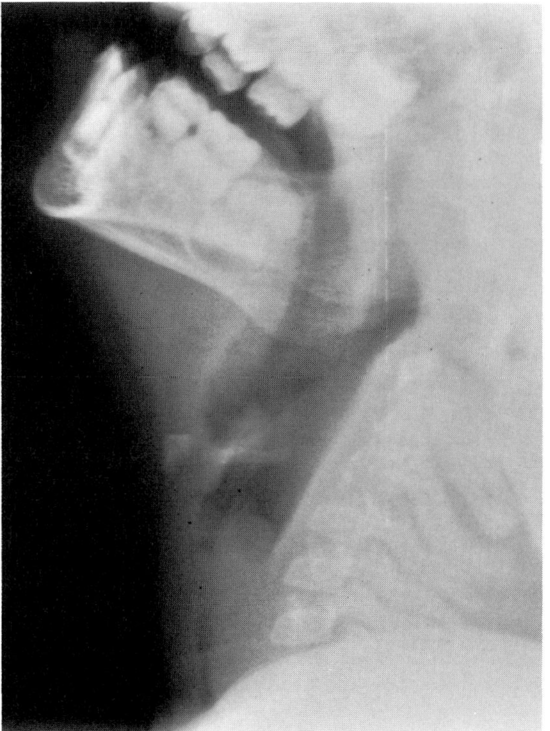

Figure 1. Lateral neck radiograph showing narrowing of the subglottic portion of the trachea.

the so-called "wine-bottle" contour. A lateral neck film also may show the narrowing of the subglottic portion of the trachea (Fig. 1). Any child with suspected severe airway obstruction should not be sent to the Radiology Department of a hospital. If radiographs are needed, portable films must be taken in the Emergency Department. Only a small percentage of children with laryngotracheobronchitis will need mechanical relief of the obstruction.[5]

■ BACTERIAL TRACHEITIS

Bacterial tracheitis, also referred to as membranous laryngotracheobronchitis, is an acute infectious disease affecting the upper airway. The pathology in this illness has been shown to be subglottic edema and purulent tracheal secretions.[6,7] It has been described in children aged 3 weeks to 12 years.[6,8] *Staphylococcus aureus* is the organism most commonly cultured, with *Haemophilus influenzae*, type b, occasionally present, and in some children this may represent a bacterial infection superimposed on viral laryngotracheobronchitis. Although it

is seen much less often than laryngotracheobronchitis, in one study it was seen more frequently than epiglottitis.[6]

The children present with symptoms similar to those seen in laryngotracheobronchitis—i.e., upper respiratory infection followed by a harsh, stridulous cough. Within a short period of time, however, they develop severe upper airway obstruction and temperatures greater than 39°C and look quite toxic. Physical examination reveals an acutely ill child with inspiratory stridor and retractions. Characteristics of the disease are listed in Table 1.

Lateral neck films usually will reveal the subglottic narrowing typically seen in laryngotracheobronchitis, as well as shadows in the trachea that may be mistaken for a foreign body (Fig. 2). These shadows are created by thick mucopurulent secretions that may represent a partially deteached membrane. *Staphylococcus aureus* is cultured from these secretions 65 per cent of the time. A chest film usually is not helpful.

■ EPIGLOTTITIS

Epiglottitis is a serious, life-threatening illness. The organism isolated in most cases is *Haemophilus influenzae*, type b. Other or-

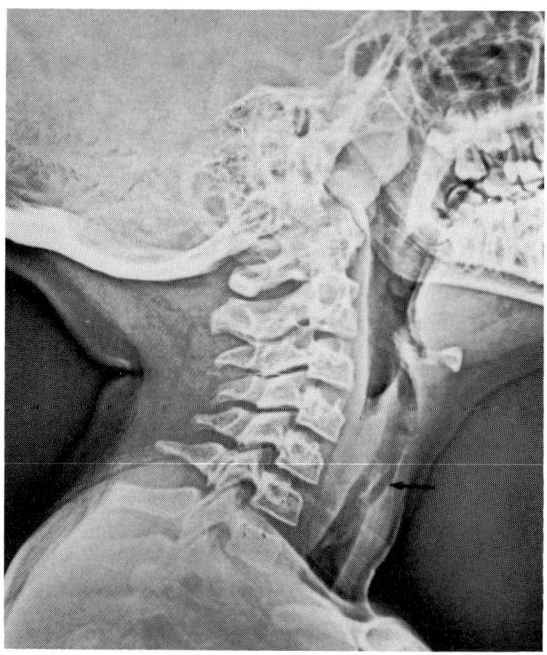

Figure 2. Sugblottic narrowing that might be mistaken for a foreign body.

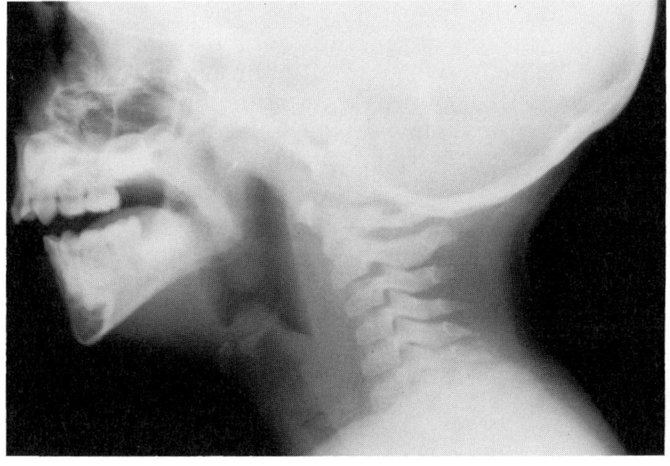
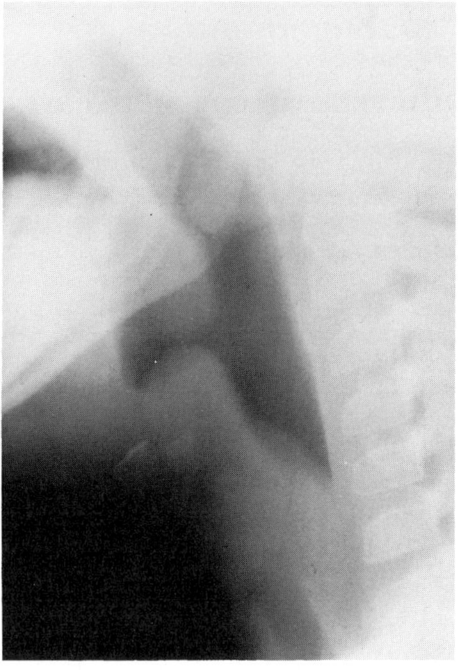

Figure 3. *A,* Enlarged epiglottis. *B,* Markedly swollen epiglottis.

ganisms occasionally seen are *Streptococcus* and *Staphylococcus.* The disease is most commonly seen in children aged 2 to 6, but it also is seen in older children and adults. The pathology in this illness is usually well defined as an acute inflammatory edema occurring in the supraglottic area of the larynx.

The onset of the illness is often abrupt; most children are seen in the Emergency Department within 16 hours of developing their first symptoms.[9] They will complain of a sore throat and difficulty in swallowing. The temperature usually is 30°C or higher. The child may have a muffled pattern of speech and may be unable to swallow secretions, causing excessive drooling. Drooling is one of the cardinal signs of epiglottitis and, if present, should immediately alert the examiner. Cough, when present, is inspiratory and stridulous. Clinical characteristics are listed in Table 1.

Physical examination reveals a toxic-looking, apprehensive child sitting quietly. The child prefers sitting upright, with the jaw protruding forward. Drooling may be excessive. The child may have significant pallor and, although looking toxic, may not be crying or struggling. Retractions may be seen in an occasional child; auscultation of the lungs rarely reveals significant findings.

The diagnosis of epiglottitis is based pri-marily on clinical findings. The complete blood count may reveal a leukocytosis with an increase in bands. Blood for tests, including cultures, may be drawn, but often this upsets the child and should be delayed. The child should *not* be sent to the Radiology Department unless accompanied by professional personnel skilled at intubation. Ideally, the child should remain in the Emergency Department, and portable films should be ordered. Children with epiglottitis will exhibit the "thumb sign"; that is, their epiglottis is the size of an adult's thumb.[10,11] Figure 3*A* shows an enlarged epiglottis, and Figure 3*B* is an enlarged photograph showing the markedly swollen epiglottis.

The top of a markedly swollen epiglottis in a young child may be seen by merely having the child open the mouth and shining a light into the oropharynx. If the physician is unable to visualize the epiglottis adequately in this fashion, further attempts should not be made. Depression of the base of the tongue may cause laryngeal spasm.[3,12] A recent article suggested that it may be safe to directly visualize the epiglottis in the Emergency Department.[13] However, there is little consensus for this approach; if inspection of the epiglottis is necessary to confirm the diagnosis, it should be done in the operating room where the airway can be controlled.

■ Management

■ LARYNGOTRACHEOBRONCHITIS

Most children seen in the Emergency Department with laryngotracheobronchitis respond well to therapy and can be safely managed at home. There is general consensus that proper humidification is of benefit.[3] This can be provided at home from a hot shower or bath or from a vaporizer or nebulizer. Parents should be instructed that "cold steam" is as effective as hot steam and is safer. Antibiotics are of no benefit. Sedation is never indicated. These children should be left undisturbed as much as possible, but they must be closely observed and monitored.

Although the use of racemic epinephrine for laryngotracheobronchitis has resulted in a decrease in the incidence of tracheostomies,[14,15] a recent study has somewhat tempered the initial enthusiasm.[16] The use of racemic epinephrine is based on its topical vasoconstrictive effect when applied to inflamed swollen mucosa. It is given as an aerosol, 0.5 ml of 2.25 per cent racemic epinephrine in 2 ml of normal saline over 15 minutes, administered by a face mask with nebulization. Most children will show clinical improvement immediately after therapy.[1] The clinical improvement is often transient, however, and within 1 to 2 hours the children often will revert to their original clinical presentation. Children who receive two or more treatments often develop acute tolerance to racemic epinephrine.[1] Because of this, children who are treated with racemic epinephrine should be admitted to the hospital so they can be monitored.[16]

The use of corticosteroids in the treatment of laryngotracheobronchitis is controversial. Numerous reports of clinical trials of corticosteroid therapy have yielded widely divergent results, partially because of the different methodologies used in many of the studies. A recent study reviewed 10 published reports and concluded that the use of steroids in children hospitalized with laryngotracheobronchitis resulted in significant clinical improvement and a reduced incidence of endotracheal intubation.[17] Those patients with severe laryngotracheobronchitis may benefit from dexamethasone, 1 to 2 mg/kg day.

Five to 10 per cent of children presenting to the Emergency Department with laryngotracheobronchitis will need admission.[18] One to two per cent of hospitalized children with laryngotracheobronchitis will require an artificial airway—either a nasotracheal tube or a tracheostomy.[19] If there is ongoing airway obstruction that is not responding to therapy, airway intervention may be indicated. The child with a pulse greater than 150 per minute, a rising respiratory rate, a rising Pco (greater than 45 mg Hg), worsening stridor, or progressive fatigue will be a prime candidate for the establishment of an artificial airway. (The details of establishing an airway will be discussed in the section on epiglottitis.)

■ BACTERIAL TRACHEITIS

Because this disease is often not recognized early in the course of the illness, many children are treated as though they have laryngotracheobronchitis and fail to respond to the usual therapy. The most important aspect of therapy is to establish a clear airway. Ideal treatment includes endoscopy performed in the operating room, with tracheal suctioning done with direct airway visualization. Most children also will require endotracheal intubation; in one study, three of seven children also required tracheostomy.[8] Humidification and oxygen are also beneficial. In addition to repeated suctioning, intravenous nafcillin (Nafcil, Unipen), 150 mg/kg/day, should be given as soon as possible. Because a small number of children may grow *Haemophilus influenzae*, type b, cefuroxime (Zinacef), 100 to 150 mg/kg/day, may be added.

This disease has a high mortality rate and the children should be carefully monitored in an intensive care unit. It is unclear whether this is a new disease or a re-emergence of an older disease. Whatever the case, prompt recognition and appropriate therapy are necessary if these children are to survive.

■ EPIGLOTTITIS

Therapeutic measures for epiglottitis are well established. The child must be constantly observed but not disturbed unnecessarily. Most affected children are more comfortable in the upright position and should not be forced to lie down. Blood for cultures should be drawn and an intravenous catheter should be inserted if it can be done without disturbing the child. Antibiotic therapy should begin as soon as possible. Ampicillin, 200 mg/kg/day, was used in the past, but it is no longer acceptable to use this antimicrobial alone, for up to 25 per cent of *Haemophilus influenzae*, type b, may be resistant to ampicillin. Chloramphenicol, 50 to 75 mg/kg/day, should be added to the therapeutic regime. It may be discontinued in 2 to 3 days if the organism is shown to be sensitive to ampicillin. Cefuroxime, 100 to 150 mg/kg/day, is also effective. These antibiotics are given intravenously. Racemic epinephrine has not been proved to be effective in children with epiglottitis and may have adverse effects. The use of steroids in epiglottitis remains controversial. It may help reduce the amount of swelling, but conclusive studies of its efficacy do not exist.

The physician's primary concern is the establishment of an adequate airway once the diagnosis of epiglottitis is made. Historically, this meant early tracheostomy.[20,21] Over the last decade, however, the trend has been toward tracheal intubation, and nasotracheal intubation appears to be safe and highly efficient.[22–24]

The management of this disease requires a team effort. Ideally, the child should be taken to the operating room where proper anesthesia can be given and an otolaryngologist can visualize and then intubate the airway. Children aged 6 months to 2 years require a size 3.5 tube (inside diameter); those aged 2 to 5 years, a size 4.0 tube; and those over age five years, a size 4.5. The duration of intubation in children with epiglottitis is usually 24 to 48 hours—significantly less than the 3 to 5 days needed by children intubated for laryngotracheobronchitis. A shorter period of intubation is aided by daily laryngeal inspection in the intensive care unit.[25]

■ Issues and Risks

Laryngotracheobronchitis is the most common of the airway disorders discussed here, which is fortunate, for it is rarely fatal. If the correct diagnosis has been made, the management is usually straightforward. Physicians must be aware, however, that

occasionally a child with laryngotracheobronchitis will have a potential life-threatening outcome. In general, it is reasonable to suggest that all children who require racemic epinephrine should be admitted for observation and further therapy. If a child's condition deteriorates, a trial of steroids is indicated. If that fails, the child will need intubation.

Bacterial tracheitis is seen much less frequently than laryngotracheobronchitis, and because of this it presents a difficult management problem. The physician must have a high index of suspicion for this entity in the following sitaution: a child is admitted with the diagnosis of laryngotracheobronchitis, is treated appropriately, and gets progressively worse. Bacterial tracheitis must be suspected in this situation, and direct visualization of the airway is indicated. It is critical to make the earliest possible diagnosis, for this condition carries a much higher mortality rate than laryngotracheobronchitis.

Epiglottitis is a true emergency and physicians must be aware that this devastating illness also occurs in adults. The onset is explosive, and deterioration occurs quickly. The diagnosis of epiglottitis must be thought of in any febrile child with inspiratory stridor. If the diagnosis is suspected, optimal management requires direct visualization of the airway by skilled personnel in the operating room. Early diagnosis is critical, as delaying therapy may result in the death of the child.

REFERENCES

1. Lockhardt CH, Battaglia JD. Croup (laryngotracheal bronchitis) and epiglottitis. Pediatr Ann 1977; 6:262–269.
2. Cramblett HG. Croup (epiglottitis; laryngitis; laryngotracheobronchitis). *In* Kendig EL (ed): Disorders of the Respiratory Tract in Children. 3rd ed. Philadelphia: WB Saunders, 1977:353–360.
3. Fried MP. Controversies in the management of supraglottitis and croup. Pediatr Clin North Am 1979; 26:931–942.
4. Denny FW, Murphy TF, Clyde WA, Collier AM, Henderson FW. Croup: an 11 year study in a pediatric practice. Pediatrics 1983; 71:871–876.
5. Milner AD, Buffin JT. Upper airway obstruction. *In* Black JA (ed). Pediatric Emergencies. London: Butterworth, 1979:217–223.
6. Jones A, Santos JI, Overall JC. Bacterial tracheitis. JAMA 1979; 242:721–726.
7. Denneny JC 3d, Handler SD. Membranous laryngotracheobronchitis. Pediatrics 1982; 70:705–707.

8. Henry RL, Mellis CM, Benjamin B. Pseudomembranous croup. Arch Dis Child 1983; 58:180–183.
9. Lewis JK, Gartner JC, Galvis AG. A protocol for management of acute epiglottitis. Clin Pediatr 1978; 17:494–496.
10. Rapkin RH. The diagnosis of epiglottitis: simplicity and reliability of radiographs of the neck in the differential diagnosis of the croup syndrome. J Pediatr 1972; 80:96–98.
11. Pedgore JK, Bass JW. The "thumb sign" and "little finger sign" in acute epiglottitis. J Pediatr 1976; 88:154–155.
12. Rapkin RH. Acute epiglottitis: pitfalls in diagnosis and management. Clin Pediatr 1971; 10:312–324.
13. Mauro RD, Poole SR, Lockhardt CH. Differentiation of epiglottitis from laryngotracheitis in the child with stridor. Am J Dis Child 1988; 142:679–681.
14. Singer OP, Wilson WJ. Laryngotracheobronchitis: two years' experience with racemic epinephrine. Can Med Assoc J 1976; 115:132–134.
15. Jordan WS, Graves CL, Elwyn RA. New therapy for post-intubation laryngeal edema and tracheitis in children. JAMA 1970; 121:585–588.
16. Westley CR, Cotton EK, Brooks JG. Nebulized racemic epinephrine by IPPB for the treatment of croup. Am J Dis Child 1978; 132:484–487.
17. Kairys SW, Olmstead EM, O'Connor GT. Steroid treatment of laryngotracheitis: a meta-analysis of the evidence from randomized trials. Pediatrics 1989; 83:683–693.
18. Levison H, Tabachnik E, Newth C. Wheezing in infancy; croup and epiglottitis. Curr Prob Pediatr 1982; 12.
19. Proctor DF. The air passages. In Cooke RE (ed). The Biologic Basis of Pediatric Practice. New York: McGraw-Hill, 1968:281–282.
20. Bass JW, Steele RW, Wiebe RA. Acute epiglottitis, a surgical emergency. JAMA 1974; 229:671–675.
21. Margolis CZ, Ingram DL, Meyer JH. Routine tracheotomy in *Hemophilus influenzae* type b epiglottitis. J Pediatr 1972; 81:1150–1152.
22. Battaglia JD, Lockhardt CH. Management of acute epiglottitis by nasotracheal intubation. Am J Dis Child 1975; 129:334–336.
23. Faden HS. Treatment of *Haemophilus influenzae* type b epiglottitis. Pediatrics 1979; 63:402–407.
24. Cantrell RW, Bell RA, Morioka WT. Acute epiglottitis: intubation versus tracheostomy. Laryngoscope 1978; 88:994–1005.
25. Gonzalez C, Reilly JS, Kenna MA, Thompson ME. Duration of intubation in children with acute epiglottitis. Otol Head Neck Surg 1986; 95:477–481.

Malabsorption

Ingram M. Roberts

■ Background

The workup of the patient with malabsorption follows a logical sequence of screening and diagnostic testing that usually reveals the correct etiology for the patient's condition. Commonly, the classic history and physical findings suggestive of malabsorption are not found. The clinician must therefore suspect the presence of malabsorption and determine objectively whether evidence for malabsorption exists.

As a myriad of conditions can cause malabsorption, therapy should not be "shotgunned"; the exact diagnosis should be sought before the proper medical management can be instituted. Steatorrhea (the presence of excess fat in the stool) is the hallmark of malabsorption. The most widely used test for malabsorption is the Sudan stain for stool fat, as described by Drummey and associates.[1] The qualitative fecal fat determination with the Sudan stain has been found to be 100 per cent sensitive and 96 per cent specific as a screening test for steatorrhea.[2] Other tests lack the proper sensitivity and specificity for routine use.

The definitive "gold standard" test for the diagnosis of malabsorption is the 72-hour quantitative stool collection for fecal fat, as described by van de Kamer and associates.[3] In several situations, fecal fat excretion is increased under physiologic conditions: (1) in the presence of high-fiber diets (100 gm of fiber per day),[4] (2) when dietary fat is given in a form such as whole peanuts,[5] and (3) in the neonatal period when intraluminal levels of pancreatic lipase and bile salts are low.[6] If none of these uncommon circumstances exists, the finding of a coefficient of fat absorption less than 93 per cent indicates steatorrhea secondary to malabsorption.

Once the presence of steatorrhea is confirmed, one should determine whether malabsorption is caused by disease of the intestinal mucosa or by abnormalities of intraluminal digestion. To distinguish between these possibilities, the workup follows a simple nomogram (Fig. 1) at this juncture. An upper gastrointestinal series and small bowel follow-through (UGI/SBFT) may demonstrate anatomic abnormalities, such as jejunal diverticula; show the abnormal mucosal pattern (thickening of the folds, dilatation, segmentation) seen in association with many malabsorption syndromes; or show the characteristic narrowing seen with Crohn's disease ("string sign"). The abdominal flat plate may show pancreatic calcifications, which are diagnostic for chronic pancreatitis.

The most useful way to examine the absorptive integrity of the intestinal mucosa is the D-xylose test. D-Xylose is a pentose that is absorbed from the small bowel via the same transport mechanism as glucose and excreted unchanged in the urine. The usual dose is 25 gm, administered orally after an overnight fast, with urine collection for 5 hours; a normal urinary excretion should be more than 5 gm. Haeney and associates have shown that measuring the serum D-xylose 1 hour after oral ingestion yields a higher sensitivity and specificity than the 5-hour urine collection;[7] a normal serum level is more than 20 mg/dl. Low values for D-xylose are commonly found in diseases of the intestinal mucosa and in bacterial overgrowth (owing to ingestion of xylose by the bacteria), whereas normal values are consistent with pancreatic insufficiency.

The radioimmunoassay (RIA) for serum trypsinogen is extremely specific for the diagnosis of chronic pancreatitis if the trypsinogen value is below 10 ng/ml. Other nonpancreatic causes for malabsorption almost always yield a normal serum trypsinogen value (10 to 75 ng/ml).[8] Therefore, if steatorrhea and a low serum trypsinogen level are found, the diagnosis of chronic pancreatitis is likely.

If the D-xylose test and UGI/SBFT are abnormal, a small bowel biopsy should be obtained for histologic diagnosis. Recent evidence suggests that grasp forceps biopsy specimens obtained from the distal duodenum via the endoscope may be oriented properly for diagnostic interpretation, in similar fashion to the larger biopsy specimens obtained with a Quinton-Rubin tube.[9] Small bowel biopsy is diagnostic in conditions such as Whipple's disease, abetalipoproteinemia, lymphoma, lymphangiectasia, parasitic infections, eosinophilic enteritis,

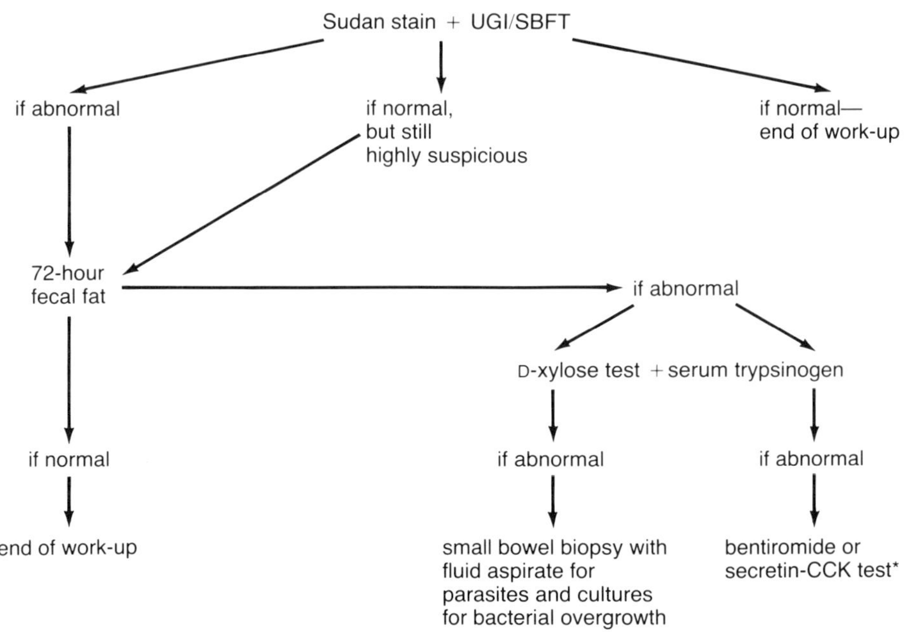

Figure 1. Decision tree for suspected malabsorption.

amyloidosis, immunodeficiency syndromes, mastocytosis, and Crohn's disease, and is helpful in suggesting the diagnosis of celiac sprue, tropical sprue, bacterial overgrowth, and radiation enteritis. The small bowel biopsy is normal in conditions such as pancreatic insufficiency and postgastrectomy malabsorption that do not involve the intestinal mucosa.

A normal D-xylose test and a low serum trypsinogen level strongly suggest the diagnosis of chronic pancreatitis. The presence of pancreatic calcifications on abdominal flat plate secures the diagnosis and no further studies need be performed. If no calcifications exist, the bentiromide test, a "tubeless" test of pancreatic function, or a direct pancreatic stimulation test with secretin or secretin-cholecystokinin (CCK) should be performed. Bentiromide is N-benzoyl-L-tyrosyl-para-aminobenzoic acid; pancreatic chymotrypsin cleaves this tripeptide in the intestinal lumen, liberating para-aminobenzoic acid (PABA). PABA is absorbed from the intestine, conjugated by the liver, and excreted in the urine. The usual orally administered dose is 500 mg followed by a urine collection for 5 hours in similar fashion to the D-xylose test. Drugs such as thiazides, chloramphenicol, sulfonamides, acetaminophen, phenacetin, sunscreens, and "caine" anesthetics may cause false-negative tests.

Pancreatic stimulation testing with intravenous administration of CCK and secretin, or secretin alone given at pharmacologic doses, are the most sensitive tests for diagnosing chronic pancreatitis. Because these tests require duodenal intubation, collection of intestinal contents, and detailed analysis for bicarbonate and enzymes (trypsin, lipase or amylase), they have not achieved widespread popularity. Bicarbonate concentrations of less than 70 mEq/liter and a secretion volume of less than 2 ml/kg body weight/hr are considered abnormal.

Occasionally, patients have malabsorption associated with disorders of intestinal motility (scleroderma, intestinal pseudo-obstruction, and so on), intestinal surgery, or anatomic abnormalities (small intestinal diverticula), in which case the diagnosis of bacterial overgrowth should be considered. Patients with overgrowth (more than 10^6 organisms per ml of intestinal content) may have positive D-xylose tests secondary to ingestion of the sugar by bacteria, and the small bowel biopsy is often nonspecifically abnormal (partially blunted villi, increased inflammatory cells in the lamina propria); tests of pancreatic function are normal in these patients. Tests for bacterial overgrowth include culture of intestinal content for aerobic and anaerobic bacteria, the Schilling test, the bile acid breath test, the ^{14}C-xylose breath test, the lactulose breath hydrogen test, and the fasting breath hydrogen determination. The Schilling test, performed before and repeated after administration of antibiotics, is universally available and is the most useful adjunct to culture of intestinal fluid for aerobes and anaerobes. The bile acid and ^{14}C-xylose breath tests measure $^{14}CO_2$ excreted in breath as a result of bacterial deconjugation of cholyl-glycine-1-^{14}C and metabolism of ^{14}C-xylose, respectively. Although these breath tests have been shown by several groups of investigators to be highly sensitive and specific for the diagnosis of bacterial overgrowth,[10,11] they are routinely available at only a few selected institutions.

■ Management

After the etiology of the malabsorptive process has been established, the appropriate treatment regimen can be instituted.

■ SPECIFIC DIETARY MANIPULATIONS

Gluten-Free Diet for Celiac Disease. A gluten-free diet is the mainstay of therapy in those who suffer from celiac disease (Table 1). The Celiac Society can help newly diagnosed patients adjust to instituting a gluten-free diet. Should a patient with celiac disease worsen clinically, noncompliance with the gluten-free diet should be suspect. If this is not shown to be the case, the development of refractory sprue, collagenous sprue, or lymphoma needs to be ruled out.

Low-Oxalate Diet. Patients with Crohn's disease may develop calcium oxalate renal stones if they have ileal disease plus an intact colon. It is often prudent to suggest a low-oxalate diet, which excludes foods such as beets, carrots, greens, spinach, green pepper, yams, sweet potato, plums, berries, rhubarb, tea, cocoa, and chocolate.

TABLE 1. Gluten-Free Diet

Beverages	Milk, coffee, tea, carbonated drinks
Breads	Breads made from rice, corn, soybean, and potato flours
Cereals	Cornflakes, rice cereals
Fats, meats, eggs, vegetables, fruits	No restrictions unless prepared with wheat flour or bread crumbs
Desserts	Gelatin, sherbet, tapioca, rice pudding, custard
Miscellaneous	Honey, sugar, corn syrup, nuts

Low-Fat Diet for Short Bowel and Intestinal Lymphangiectasia. Patients may benefit from a reduced fat diet (50 gm/day) that will help alleviate steatorrhea. Typical foods that should be excluded from the diet to reduce fat content are listed in Table 2. This diet may be supplemented with medium-chain triglycerides to add increased easily digestible calories (discussed later).

Enteral Liquid Diets. Some selected patients with Crohn's disease, short bowel syndrome, and so on, may respond to enteral diets given either orally or with a nasoenteral feeding tube. In those patients treated with tube feedings, No. 5 to 10 French silicone feeding tubes are often more comfortable than conventional No. 16 to 18 French Levin nasogastric tubes. Liquid diets may need to be initially diluted two- to fivefold, with their concentration gradually increased to full strength over the first week of therapy. This may help avoid a hyperosmolar load and "dumping" syndrome. This therapy may be administered during sleeping hours, using a pump for constant infusion.[12,13] Often preparations like Ensure or Vivonex are utilized.

Parenteral Alimentation for Severe Malabsorption. A major advantage of total parenteral nutrition is that solutions with 1800 mOsm/L or higher can be administered, in the subclavian or jugular vein, as the solution is rapidly diluted by the high central blood flow. Patients with short bowel syndrome and insufficient absorptive surface (usually less than 60 to 100 cm of jejunum) often require permanent total parenteral nutrition.

Some evidence suggests that those patients who absorb less than 60 per cent of the energy content by bomb calorimetry after a liquid test meal will require total parenteral nutrition indefinitely.[14] Many patients with short bowel syndrome can be trained to self-administer parenteral nutrition under sterile conditions and are able to be managed at home with indwelling Broviac or Hickman catheters. Other patients with severe mucosal disorders, such as Crohn's disease and celiac sprue, also may occasionally need a course of inpatient parenteral nutrition until their disease process remits to the degree that oral feeding can be reinstituted. A typical parenteral nutrition prescription is given in Table 3. Note that essential vitamins and trace elements are given in the solutions, along with the appropriate amounts of fat, glucose, and amino acids.

Medium-Chain Triglycerides. These triglycerides (composed of fatty acid chains from 6 to 12 carbons in length) are transported into enterocytes by simple diffusion and do not require lipase digestion for absorption. Therefore, they are absorbed directly into the portal venous system without the need for re-esterification. The dose is usually 15 ml (1 tablespoon, 115 kcal) TID orally and serves as a good supplemental energy source in addition to decreasing steatorrhea. Unfortunately, medium-chain triglycerides cannot totally replace the need

TABLE 2. Fifty-Gram Low-Fat Diet

Beverages	Coffee, tea, skim milk, carbonated beverages allowed; no whole milk products
Breads	White, rye, whole grain allowed; no pancakes, waffles, or doughnuts
Cereals	No granola or 100% bran; all others allowed
Fats	Exclude bacon; margarine allowed
Soups	Only bouillon and fat-free broth allowed
Meat	5 oz daily allowed: must be broiled, boiled, or baked
Cheese	Cottage cheese allowed
Eggs	1 daily allowed, but no fried or creamed eggs
Vegetables	No creamed, escalloped, or fried vegetables allowed
Potatoes	Creamed, fried, and escalloped potatoes excluded; no egg noodles or potato chips allowed
Fruits	All allowed except avocado
Desserts and sweets	No pastries, pies, cake, ice cream, ice milk, chocolate, or coconut allowed
Miscellaneous	No cream sauces or gravies, no nuts, no olives, no buttered popcorn, no cocoa

TABLE 3. Typical Daily Requirements for Parenteral Nutrition

Calories (kcal/kg body weight)	30–45
Fat (% total calories)	20–40
Glucose (% total calories)	50–60
Amino acids (% total calories; gm/kg)	10–20; 1–4
Water (liters)	2–4
Vitamins	
D (IU)	100
E (mg)	50
A (IU)	2500
K (mg)	1
Water-soluble (thiamine, folate, etc.)	1 amp of MVI
Trace elements	
Cu (mg)	1.6
Cr (μg)	2
Se (μg)	120
Fe (mg)	2
Mn (mg)	2
Zn (mg)	3
Electrolytes (approximate mEq/day)	
K	55–90
Na	100–200
Ca	25–30
Mg	20–30
Cl	120–250
HPO_4	17–40
HCO_3	22–40

IU = International Units;
MVI = multivitamins.

for long-chain triglycerides, which still need to be administered to prevent essential fatty acid deficiency.

■ ANTIBIOTIC THERAPY

Whipple's Disease. The usual initial therapy for Whipple's disease consists of parenteral antibiotics. Procaine penicillin, 1.2 million units, and streptomycin, 1 gm daily for 2 weeks, are the drugs of choice for most patients with Whipple's disease. Trimethoprim-sulfamethoxazole, double strength, given twice daily orally, is suggested as follow-up therapy for 1 year.[15]

Bacterial Overgrowth. Patients with bacterial overgrowth should undergo surgery if a discrete anatomic cause of overgrowth is felt to be the etiology of the problem—e.g., jejunal diverticula, postsurgical fistula, and so on. In those patients without obvious anatomic abnormalities, a course of either tetracycline, 250 mg, or ampicillin, 250 mg; erythromycin, 250 mg; or metronidazole,

250 mg, is indicated QID for 10 to 14 days. If patients undergo a clinical response with diminished steatorrhea, periodic therapy with antibiotics may be used to treat relapses.

Giardiasis and Other Parasites. Therapy for *Giardia* usually consists of a course of quinacrine hydrochloride, 100 mg TID, or metronidazole, 250 mg QID, given for 7 to 10 days. Other parasitic infestations that less commonly cause malabsorption include ascariasis, strongyloidiasis, and capillariasis. Treatment usually consists of a course of an antihelminthic, such as thiabendazole or mebendazole.

■ PANCREATIC ENZYME REPLACEMENT

In many patients, conventional enzyme replacement for pancreatic insufficiency will reduce steatorrhea but rarely eliminates fat malabsorption altogether. All pancreatic enzymes are sensitive to acidic pH, but lipase is especially labile, being irreversibly denatured at pH 4 or below. The major advantage to enteric-coated preparations is that they do not dissolve until alkaline pH is reached. This presumably protects the enzymes during transit through the stomach. In Europe, some patients have been treated with enzyme preparations from fungi that have stability over a broader range (pH 2 to 8) than do pancreatic enzymes. These preparations appear to have comparable efficacy to enteric-coated pancreatic enzymes[16] but are currently not available in this country. In the future, other acid-stable lipases, such as lingual or gastric lipase, may be produced through recombinant DNA techniques as both these genes have been cloned by investigators.[17] H_2-blockers, bicarbonate, or antacids may be administered as adjuncts in selected patients taking conventional pancreatic enzyme therapy. These medications aid in stabilizing lipase in the intragastric environment, allowing for the delivery of more active lipase to the small intestinal lumen.

There is also evidence that diets high in protein or fat content preserve lipase activity in the small intestinal lumen better than the high-carbohydrate diets that are often prescribed for patients with pancreatic insufficiency.[18] It might be prudent to suggest that patients whose steatorrhea is difficult to correct by enzyme therapy avoid high-carbohydrate diets. In addition to malabsorption, patients with chronic pancreatitis often suffer from abdominal pain. Pancreatic proteases may help reduce pain in such patients[19] and should be offered prior to considering nerve blocks or pancreatic surgical therapy.

■ COMMON VITAMIN AND MINERAL DEFICIENCIES

Vitamin B_{12}. Vitamin B_{12} may be replaced in doses of 100 μg intramuscularly every month. Vitamin B_{12} deficiency is most commonly associated with diseases of the terminal ileum, such as Crohn's disease, ileal resection, or bacterial overgrowth.

Folate. Folic acid is usually given in a dose of 1 mg orally QD in patients with malabsorption due to celiac disease or tropical sprue. It is interesting that patients with bacterial overgrowth are often not folate deficient as the bacteria produce copious amounts of folate derivatives.

Iron. Iron is absorbed in the proximal small bowel (duodenum and jejunum). Patients with severe proximal disease, such as celiac sprue, occasionally require intramuscular iron, but often short bowel syndrome patients require iron supplementation in their parenteral nutrition solutions.

■ Issues and Risks

Enteral alimentation may be complicated by pulmonary aspiration, the "dumping" syndrome, or tube obstruction. Although parenteral hyperalimentation is a beneficial and at times life-saving therapy, several complications may develop. The catheter may become infected and lead to sepsis (the most common organism is *Staphylococcus epidermidis*), and pneumothorax or subclavian or vena caval thrombosis may complicate catheter placement. Air embolism may occur if the intravenous infusion tubing is accidentally disconnected from the catheter. Electrolyte disturbances, such as hypokalemia and hypophosphatemia, can lead to cardiac arrhythmias and hemolytic anemia, as well as abnormalities in glucose metabolism, such as hyperosmolar coma and dehydration secondary to the hypertonic sugar

loads given in the parenteral nutrition formulas. Monitoring urine specific gravity may help in adjusting infusion requirements. Abruptly stopping parenteral nutrition may lead to hypoglycemia as a consequence of high endogenous insulin output; TPN should be tapered slowly. Essential fatty acids and trace elements need to be administered in TPN solutions to prevent deficiency states. Finally, the costs of parenteral nutrition remain problematic; conservative estimates place the costs to the patient at from $100 to $300/day on either an inpatient or outpatient basis.

REFERENCES

1. Drummey GD, Benson JA Jr, Jones CM. Microscopic examination of the stool for steatorrhea. N Engl J Med 1961; 264:85–87.
2. Luk GD. Qualitative fecal fat by light microscopy: a sensitive and specific screening test for steatorrhea and pancreatic insufficiency (abstract). Gastroenterology 1979; 76:1189.
3. van de Kamer JH, ten bokkel Huinink H, Weyers HA. Rapid method for the determination of fat in feces. J Biol Chem 1949; 177:347–355.
4. Levine AS, Silvis SE. Steatorrhea due to high dietary fiber (abstract). Gastroenterology 1979; 76:1183.
5. Levine AS, Silvis SE. Absorption of whole peanuts, peanut oil and peanut butter. N Engl J Med 1980; 303:917–918.
6. Finley AJ, Davidson M. Bile acid excretion and patterns of fatty acid absorption in formula-fed premature infants. Pediatrics 1980; 65:132–138.
7. Haeney MR, Culank LS, Montgomery RD, Sammons HG. Evaluation of xylose absorption as measured in blood and urine: a one-hour blood xylose screening test in malabsorption. Gastroenterology 1978; 75:393–400.
8. Jacobson DG, Currington C, Connery K, Toskes PP. Trypsin-like immunoreactivity as a test for pancreatic insufficiency. N Engl J Med 1985; 310:1307–1309.
9. Achkar EA, Carey WD, Petras R, Sivak MV, Revta R. Comparison of suction capsule and endoscopic biopsy of small bowel mucosa. Gastrointest Endosc 1986; 32:278–281.
10. Farivar S, Fromm H, Schindler D, Schmidt F. Sensitivity of bile acid breath test in the diagnosis of bacterial overgrowth in the small intestine with and without the stagnant (blind) loop syndrome. Dig Dis Sci 1979; 24:33–40.
11. King CE, Toskes PP. Comparison of the 1-gram [^{14}C] xylose, 10-gram lactulose-H_2, and 80-gram glucose-H_2 breath tests in patients with small intestinal bacterial overgrowth. Gastroenterology 1986; 91:1447–1451.
12. Heymsfield SB, Bethel RA, Ansley JD, Nixon DW, Rudman D. Enteral hyperalimentation: an alternative to central venous hyperalimentation. Ann Intern Med 1979; 90:63–71.
13. Heymsfield SB, Smith-Andrews JL, Hersh T. Home nasoenteral feeding for malabsorption and weight

loss refractory to conventional therapy. Ann Intern Med 1983; 98:168–170.
14. Rodrigues CA, Lennard-Jones JE, Thompson DG, Farthing MJG. Energy absorption as a measure of intestinal failure in the short bowel syndrome. Gut 1989; 30:176–183.
15. Fleming JL, Wiesner RH, Shorter RG. Whipple's disease: clinical, biochemical, and histopathologic features and assessment of treatment in 29 patients. Mayo Clin Proc 1988; 63:539–551.
16. Schneider MU, Knoll-Ruzicka ML, Domschke S, Heptner G, Domschke W. Pancreatic enzyme replacement therapy: comparative effects of conventional and enteric-coated microspheric protein and acid-stable fungal enzyme preparations on steator-

rhea in chronic pancreatitis. Hepato-gastroenterology 1985; 32:97–102.
17. Bodmer M, Angal S, Yarranton G, Harris T, Lyons A, King D, Pieroni G, Riviere C, Verger R, Lowe P: Molecular cloning of a human gastric lipase and expression of the enzyme in yeast. Biochim Biophys Acta 1987; 909:237–244.
18. Kelly DG, Sandberg RJ, Bentley KJ, Zinsmeister AR, DiMagno EP. Protection of lipolytic activity (L) by nutrients in simulated pancreatic insufficiency (abstract). Pancreas 1988; 3:601.
19. Slaff J, Jacobson D, Tillman CR, Curington C, Toskes PP. Protease-specific suppression of pancreatic exocrine secretion. Gastroenterology 1984; 87:44–45.

Malignant melanoma

Dougald C. MacGillivray ■ *Bimal C. Ghosh*

Cutaneous malignant melanoma is one of the most challenging health care problems that physicians will encounter as we enter the next decade. Malignant melanoma was once a rare disease. It now comprises 3 per cent of all malignancies diagnosed in the United States each year.[1] The disease that once was labeled "the black death" has had a startling increase over the past decade, which shows no evidence of abating. Figures from the National Cancer Institute's Surveillance, Epidemiology, and End Result (SEER) program show that from the years 1950 to 1985 there has been a 242 per cent increase (from 2.8 cases per 100,000 population to 11.1 cases per 100,000 population) in the incidence of, and a 150 per cent increase in mortality from, malignant melanoma in the United States.[2,3] This rate of increase is greater than that of all other cancers except lung cancer in women, and, unlike most other malignancies, it has occurred in all age groups.[2,3]

It is estimated that in 1987 there will be 25,800 new cases of malignant melanoma of the skin in the United States and 7800 deaths.[2] Fortunately, approximately 80 per cent of patients have early, localized melanoma at the time of presentation.[1] Patients with early, thin melanomas that are promptly treated with appropriate surgical excision can be expected to have 5-year survival rates of 89 per cent.[1] Therapy for advanced melanoma is still ineffective, and the prognosis is generally poor, with only 39 per cent of patients surviving 5 years.[1] Because melanoma can be cured if it is diagnosed and treated at an early stage, physicians must have a clear understanding of the increasing incidence of melanoma, its risk factors, and the proper steps needed to ensure its prompt recognition and treatment.

■ Background

Melanocytes are neural crest derivatives that migrate during embryogenesis to sites in the skin, eyes, gastrointestinal mucosal surfaces, and nervous system. Malignant melanoma can develop in any of these sites; however, over 90 per cent of melanomas develop from melanocytes located in the basal layer of the epidermis.

The events that lead to the malignant transformation of melanocytes into melanoma are still poorly understood. There is clearly an ethnic predilection toward white-skinned races, especially those of northern European descent, that burn from the sun rather than tan. In the United States, 98 per cent of all melanomas occur in whites. Only 1 per cent of melanomas occur in Asians or Hispanics, and less than 1 per cent occur in blacks.[4]

Exposure to solar radiation seems to be a major factor in the development of melanoma. The incidence of melanoma in whites increases steadily as latitude approaches the equator, and the cutaneous distribution of melanoma is greatest on sun-exposed areas.[5] Intense sun exposure early in life may increase the risk of developing melanoma two to three times.[6]

A familial form of malignant melanoma has been recognized. Familial melanoma is expressed as an autosomal dominant trait and is responsible for as many as 6 per cent of all melanomas.[7] Melanomas in these families occur in association with the familial dysplastic nevus syndrome, formerly referred to as the B-K mole syndrome.[8] Members of these families have several hundred times the risk of developing melanoma than the general population. These individuals tend to develop melanomas at a younger age and are more likely to develop multiple melanomas.[7,8]

Dysplastic nevi also may be present in individuals without the inherited dysplastic nevus syndrome. These people are also at greater risk for developing melanoma.[8] Dysplastic nevi are acquired lesions that are different from the more common pigmented nevi, which are not associated with the development of melanoma.

Most cutaneous melanomas develop in individuals without dysplastic nevi or a family history of melanoma. They occur in adults of all ages, with the median age being 48 years, and with an equal sex distribution. Melanoma is exceedingly rare in children.

■ HISTOPATHOLOGY

Melanoma can be characterized into four different groups; superficial spreading melanoma, nodular melanoma, lentigo maligna melanoma, and acral lentiginous melanoma.[9–11] Each of these lesions has a unique histologic appearance, and a behavior that is reflected in its local growth characteristics and metastatic potential.

Melanoma evolves through two different growth phases: the radial growth phase, in which the lesion is still confined to the epidermis and superficial papillary dermis; and the vertical growth phase, in which there is an intralesional transformaton of the melanocytes that enables them to invade the deeper layers of the papillary and reticular dermis. During the vertical growth phase, most metastasis from melanoma occurs.[9,10] These unique differences are important to recognize because they predict prognosis and influence the extent of surgical resection.

Superficial Spreading Melanoma (SSM)
(Fig. 1)

This is the most common form of melanoma (60 to 80 per cent), and it occurs predominantly in whites aged 30 to 50 years, with an equal sex ratio. Superficial spreading melanoma occurs most often on the trunk in both sexes. It is frequently found on the neck and head in men and on the extremities, especially the lower extremity, in women. These lesions are generally sharply demarcated, with a notched or arched appearance, and are slightly elevated and nodular. Their most distinctive characteristic is a variegated color, with a mixutre of brown, black, purple, blue, pink, and even gray or white pigmentation. SSM may develop over a long period of time, remaining in the radial growth phase for years before entering the vertical growth phase.

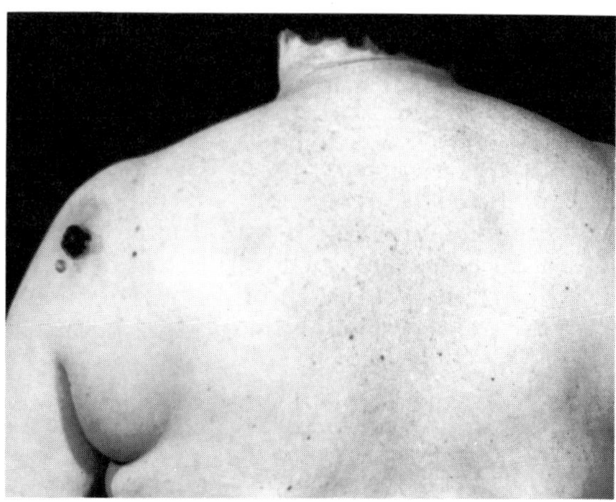

Figure 1. Superficial spreading malignant melanoma with satellite lesions.

Nodular Melanoma (NM)

Nodular melanoma is the most aggressive and malignant form of melanoma. It accounts for about 15 to 30 per cent of all melanomas, is twice as common in men as in women, and is usually found on the back, neck, and head. These lesions are mostly uniform in color—dark black or blue-black—and are raised and nodular. The virulence of this tumor is due to its lack of a radial growth phase. It is in a vertical growth phase from the onset.

Lentigo Maligna Melanoma (LMM)

Lentigo maligna melanomas comprise approximately 10 to 15 per cent of all melanomas. These tumors usually arise in a large melanotic freckle ("Hutchinson's freckle") on the face, neck, and hands of elderly individuals. They may be very large—up to 5 to 10 cm—and are flat with irregular borders and variegated pigmentation. These tumors have a very long radial growth phase that may last 10 to 20 years.

Acral Lentiginous Malignant Melanoma (ALMM)
(Fig. 2)

This lesion accounts for about 5 per cent of all melanomas. These are the most common melanomas in blacks. They have an equal sex distribution and occur on the palms, soles and subungual and periungual areas. These tumors have a long radial growth phase but are usually recognized late, after they have entered the vertical growth phase.

Melanoma-in-Situ

Melanoma-in-situ, also termed atypical melanocytic hyperplasia, or Clark Level 1 melanoma, has been recognized with increasing frequency. It is a noninvasive precursor to melanoma. These lesions have no risk of metastasis and should not be considered, or treated as, malignant melanomas.

■ LEVEL OF INVASION (MICROSTAGING)

The recognition that the metastatic potential of melanomas could be predicted based

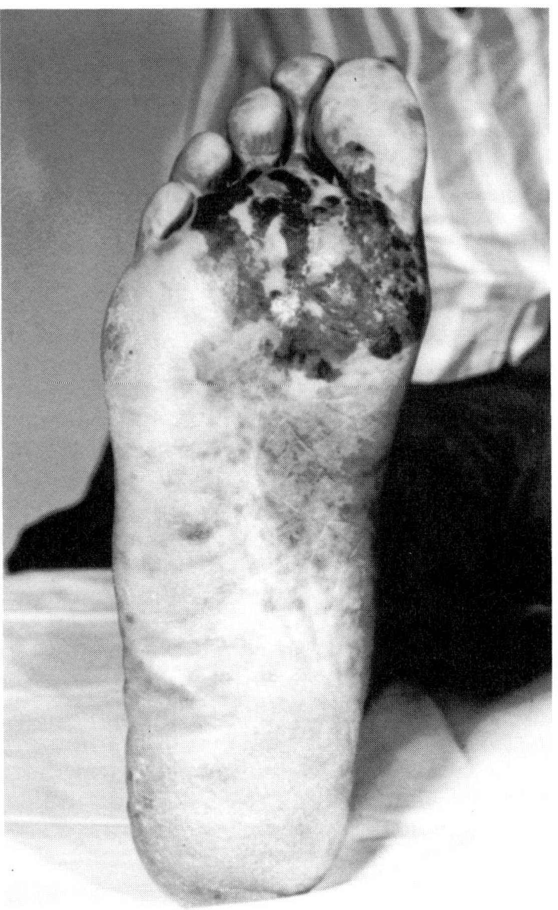

Figure 2. Acral lentiginous malignant melanoma.

on the level of invasion of the primary lesion was one of the most important advances in understanding the biologic behavior of these tumors. By studying the patterns of growth and metastasis of melanomas, Clark developed a microstaging classification that predicted prognosis based on four levels (Levels II to V) of histologic invasion of the tumor (see Table 1).[9,10]

Breslow further refined this concept by identifying that the metastatic risk of melanoma was directly related to tumor thickness and not just the depth of invasion of the lesion.[12]

The Breslow microstaging technique uses an ocular micrometer to measure tumor thickness precisely and classifies melanomas as those that are less than 0.76 mm, 0.76 to 1.5 mm, 1.5 to 4.0, and more than 4.0 mm thick. As tumor thickness increases, so does the risk of metastasis (see Table 1).

TABLE 1. Prognosis of Patients with Clinical Stage 1 Melanoma Based on Microstaging[17,29]

Level of Invasion	Thickness (mm)	10-Year Survival (%)
II Papillary Dermis	< 0.76	95–98
	0.76–1.49	85–90
III Papillary-Reticular Dermis Junction	< 0.76	80–90
	0.76–1.49	70–80
	1.5+3.99	50–60
	> 4.0	30–50
IV Reticular Dermis	< 0.76	75–85
	0.76–1.49	65–75
	1.5–3.99	40–60
	> 4.0	20–30
V Subcutaneous Fat	< 3.99	30–50
	> 4.0	16–28

All melanomas should be microstaged. Both the Clark and Breslow methods offer useful prognostic information, and they should be used to supplement each other. However, the Breslow classification is now accepted as the preferred microstaging technique. It gives the most reliable predictions of prognosis because it allows for the wide range of tumor thicknesses that can occur in Level III and greater lesions, and it is a more accurate and reproducible measurement.

In addition to microstaging, patients with melanoma should be staged on the presence or absence of metastasis into these groups:

- Stage I: localized disease without lymph node metastasis
- State II: metastasis limited to regional lymph nodes
- State III: distant metastasis

■ Management

A complete history and examination of the skin should be part of every physical examination. Patients should be questioned about sun exposure, family history of melanoma, appearance of new skin lesions, and changes in the color, size, and texture of existing skin lesions. In a survey conducted by the American College of Surgeons, 81 per cent of 4545 patients with melanoma had noticed a change in the appearance of a skin mole: a change in the size, color, or nodularity of a mole was noticed most often.[4] Itching, scaling, ulceration, bleeding, and discharge from a mole are less common but should alert the clinician to the possible presence of melanoma.

The patient should be completely undressed to ensure examination of all the skin, including the scalp, palms, soles, and subungual areas. If needed, a magnifying lens should be used. Good lighting is a must. Patients with multiple skin moles or a family or personal history of melanoma should have photographs made of skin areas at risk for developing melanoma. These photographs should be referred to on all subsequent examinations so that any subtle change in the appearance of a mole may be appreciated.

Any unusual or suspicious skin lesion and every mole that has changed must be biopsied. The technique used to obtain the biopsy is very important and should be done only by physicians who are trained and competent in doing this procedure. The standard procedure is total excisional biopsy, with a scalpel, using a elliptical incision, of the entire lesion with a small rim of surrounding skin (1 to 2 mm), including the underlying subcutaneous fat. The biopsy must be carefully planned and the incision oriented in such a way that, if melanoma is present, a wide excision of the biopsy area will not be compromised. This method of biopsy ensures that an adequate specimen will be available and allows examination of the entire lesion for the presence of melanoma. Should melanoma be present, accurate microstaging will be possible without distortion or destruction of the specimen.

Incisional biopsy or punch biopsy is acceptable only when the lesion is extremely large, or is located in an area, such as the face, where complete excision would be disfiguring, or could not be closed primarily. In these situations, the most suspicious areas should be biopsied and must include the subcutaneous fat. Tangential excisions, shave biopsies, curettage, and electro- and cryodesiccation of suspicious skin lesions should never be done.

The entire specimen should be submitted for permanent fixation and pathologic examination. Experienced pathologists can diagnose melanoma on frozen section examination of the specimen. This technique, however, is not as accurate as examination of fixed, paraffin-imbedded tissue and can lead to errors in microstaging the lesion.

■ MANAGEMENT OF THE PRIMARY LESION

The diagnosis of melanoma must be confirmed by biopsy before definitive therapy is undertaken. Even experienced clinicians are mistaken in approximately 30 per cent of cases when the diagnosis of melanoma is made on the gross appearance of the skin lesion.[12]

Surgery—wide local excision of the site of the primary lesion—is the standard and only effective treatment of melanoma. Wide excision of the biopsy site, including satellite lesions, with a rim of normal skin and all underlying subcutaneous fat should be done in all cases as soon as the diagnosis of melanoma is confirmed.

The extent of excision required to treat melanoma adequately has been modified in recent years. Standard surgical teaching for years stressed that proper treatment of melanoma required excision of the lesion with a 5-cm margin of normal skin on all sides and placement of a skin graft in virtually every case. Recent evidence has shown that these wide margins are not necessary.[13] The extent of resection should be individualized, based on the type of melanoma, its location, and, most importantly, its level of invasion based on microstaging.

Melanoma-in-situ has a tendency to recur after excisional biopsy alone. These lesions should be re-excised with 0.5 to 1.0-cm margins. Patients with melanomas less than 1 mm in thickness can be treated safely with margins of 1 to 2 cm. Lesions between 1 and 3 mm should be resected with margins of 2 to 3 cm. Melanomas that are greater than 3-mm thick, are ulcerated, or have satellite lesions are at greatest risk for local recurrence. These tumors should be resected with 3-cm margins.[13] Using these guidelines, most patients with thin melanomas can have curative resection of the lesion and primary closure of the wound with a good cosmetic result.

■ MANAGEMENT OF REGIONAL LYMPH NODES

Regional lymph nodes are the most common site of metastasis of melanoma. The risk of

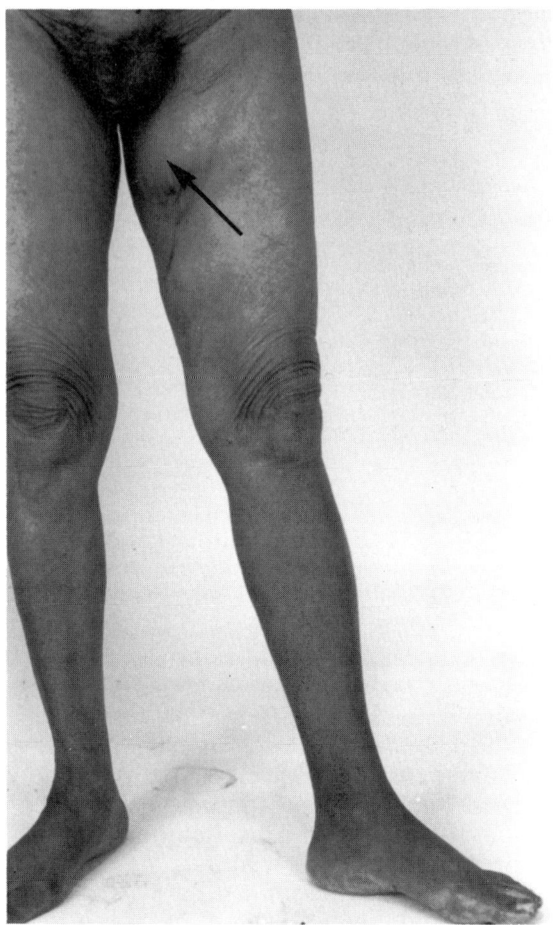

Figure 3. Large metastatic lymph nodes in the groin—previously resected cutaneous melanoma.

lymph node metastasis is directly related to the type of melanoma, the thickness of the lesion, the presence of ulceration, the anatomic site of the lesion, and the sex of the patient.[14] Lymph node metastases may be present as enlarged, firm palpable nodes (Fig. 3) or as occult microscopic disease that does not become clinically evident for months to years after excision of the primary lesion.

For all melanomas, the risk of lymph node metastasis correlates best with the thickness of the lesion. Lesions less than 0.76 mm thick have less than a 5 per cent chance of having lymph node metastasis. Regional lymph node metastasis will occur in approximately 10 to 25 per cent of patients with lesions 0.76 to 1.5 mm thick and in about 20 to 55 per cent of patients with lesions 1.5 to 4.0 mm thick. At least 60 per cent of patients with lesions thicker than 4 mm will develop regional lymph node metastasis.[14] Lentigo maligna melanomas, especially those on the face in older individuals, have a very low risk of metastasis. Nodular melanomas, on the other hand, have the highest risk of lymph node metastasis. Melanomas in men, lesions that are ulcerated, and those arising on the trunk are all more prone to metastasize to regional lymph nodes.[14]

Considerable controversy exists regarding the efficacy of lymph node dissection in patients with melanoma. The crux of this controversy centers on the perceived morbidity associated with radical lymph node dissection and the lack of prospective randomized studies that show a survival advantage in patients with melanoma who have lymph node dissections. Adding to the confusion is the extremely variable biologic behavior of melanoma that is dependent on its histologic type, thickness, location, and the sex of the patient. Most studies of melanoma have not examined these variables independently.

There is general agreement that patients with clinically suspicious or proven lymph node metastasis should undergo therapeutic lymph node dissection. Lymphadenectomy in these patients provides important staging and prognostic information, is the most effective treatment for the control of the nodal metastasis, and offers the best chance for long-term survival and cure. Five-year survival rates of 20 to 37 per cent are possible for patients undergoing therapeutic radical lymphadenectomy.[15]

A small number of patients with melanoma, approximately 5 per cent, present with lymph node metastasis from an unknown primary site.[16] These patients have the same prognosis and should have the same treatment, radical lymphadenectomy, as patients with metastasis from a known primary site.[16]

The role of elective lymph node dissection (ELND) in the management of patients with clinical stage 1 melanoma is still unclear. Data conflict on whether or not resection of clinically negative but histologically involved lymph nodes confers a survival advantage over patients who have lymph node dissection only after nodal disease becomes clinically evident. Two prospective randomized studies, conducted by the World Health Organization Melanoma Group and the Mayo Clinic, failed to show survival benefit in those patients who had ELND. However, the design of these studies has been criticized, and their results are not uniformly accepted.[14]

The results of several large retrospective studies and a prospective but not randomized study have demonstrated a prolonged disease-free interval and survival benefit in selected groups of patients undergoing ELND.[14,17,18] The groups of patients who benefited from ELND had melanomas 1.5 to 4.0 mm thick. For lesions less than 1.5 mm thick, there was no advantage in adding ELND to wide excision of the lesion.

Currently there is no accepted consensus regarding the efficacy of ELND in the management of melanoma, except that it may be of benefit in selected cases.

■ ADJUVANT THERAPY

There is no evidence that adjuvant therapy, immunotherapy, chemotherapy, or chemoimmunotherapy improves survival in patients with melanoma.[19] Patients should not be offered adjuvant therapy unless it is as part of an approved, controlled research protocol.

■ ISOLATED LIMB PERFUSION

A number of centers are using isolated limb perfusion as adjuvant therapy and as treatment of advanced or recurrent disease in patients with melanoma of the extremity. This procedure involves surgical isolation and cannulation of the major vessels to the extremity to be perfused. Venous blood is collected, pumped through an oxygenator, and returned to the limb via the arterial catheter. Most protocols involve hyperthermic perfusion of the limb at a temperature of 42°C, with L-phenylalanine mustard (Melphalan), for between 45 and 120 minutes.

There is a trend toward improved local control and 5-year survival for all stages of melanoma in patients receiving isolated limb perfusion as adjuvant therapy, compared with surgery alone. In patients with localized melanoma, 5-year survival may be increased by 10 to 15 per cent.[20] However, not enough firm data exist demonstrating a significant survival advantage with limb perfusion to advocate its routine use.[20]

Isolated limb perfusion has been proved to be very effective in providing palliation to patients with locally advanced or recurrent melanoma of the extremity, especially those who would otherwise require amputation. In these cases, hyperthermic limb perfusion can provide prolonged locoregional control of the disease in 70 to 80 per cent of cases.[20,21]

■ MANAGEMENT OF DISTANT METASTASIS

Melanoma has shown the ability to metastasize to virtually every organ system. The most common sites of distant metastases are the skin, subcutaneous tissues, and distant lymph nodes (60 per cent), lung (36 per cent), liver (20 per cent), brain (20 per cent), and bone (17 per cent). Median survival of patients with distant metastases is only 5 to 8 months, regardless of therapy.[22] Complete surgical resection of isolated metastasis, particularly subcutaneous and pulmonary lesions, in carefully selected patients can improve median and long-term survival, with 20 per cent of patients surviving 5 or more years.[23,24] Surgery is the most effective therapy in providing palliation and improving the quality of life in patients with symptomatic metastasis to the subcutaneous tissues, alimentary tract, and lung.[23-25]

Melanomas have been considered to be relatively radioresistant tumors. Higher-dose fractions of radiation have proved to be more effective in some trials than conventional radiation doses in providing palliation, especially for soft tissue, bone, and brain metastases.[26]

Chemotherapy has been very disappointing in the treatment of melanoma. The most active agent currently in use is dimethyl-tri-azeno-imidazole-carboxamide (DTIC). Trials using DTIC, either alone or in combination with other agents, have shown an objective remission rate of less than 20 per cent.[27]

Immunotherapy studies are now underway, but it is too soon to report on the results of these trials.

■ METASTATIC EVALUATION AND FOLLOW-UP

The metastatic evaluation of patients with recently diagnosed melanoma must include a careful examination of regional and distant lymph nodes. Chest radiograph and liver function tests are the only routine screening studies that are needed. Unless the patient has signs or symptoms suggestive of metastasis, there is no need for routine liver, brain, or bone imaging studies.

All patients who have had melanoma are at risk for developing recurrent or metastatic disease. Even patients with thin melanomas (less than 0.76 mm) have a 1 to 5 per cent risk of developing metastasis, usually more than 2 years after treatment of the primary lesion.[28,29] In addition, once a person has had melanoma there is a 7 per cent chance that he or she will develop a second primary lesion.[18] Patients who have had melanoma must have frequent and careful follow-up for the remainder of their lives.

A recommended schedule for following these patients is routine examination every 3 to 4 months for the first 2 years, every 6 months until year 5, and then once every year. The routine evaluation must include a complete history and physical examination, with particular attention to the skin and lymph nodes, a chest radiograph, alkaline phosphatase determination, and liver function tests.

■ Issues and Risks

Melanoma is a disease that is evolving in its presentation and in our understanding of its behavior and variability. The increasing incidence of melanoma has been greater than the increase in its mortality. This is reflected in improved survival rates of patients with all stages of melanoma.[2] Part of the improvement in survival is probably due to increased patient and physician awareness and education regarding melanoma. There is now a clearer understanding of the appearance of melanoma and its precursor lesions, leading to earlier detection and treatment. Patients are now presenting with thinner, less invasive, and more curable lesions.[2,4]

Therapy of melanoma has not changed appreciably. Surgery is still the only effective treatment. Recognition of thickness as the most important variable in predicting the behavior of melanoma has allowed the extent of surgical margins to be modified. The majority of melanomas can be excised and closed primarily with good cosmetic results.

The increase in the incidence of melanoma can be correlated with increased exposure to ultraviolet solar irradiation. This parallels the increase in outdoor leisure activities and changes in clothing patterns in Western societies.[5] Sunburning in early life seems to place one at higher risk for developing melanoma.[6]

Our understanding of the pathophysiology of malignant melanoma is far from complete, though much has been learned about its evolution and natural history. Educational programs, such as the Queensland Melanoma Project, have alerted the public and physicians of the increased incidence of melanoma and the appearance of skin lesions at risk of being a melanoma. More patients with melanoma are being recognized and treated at an early stage, when they have thin, curable lesions. However, increasing the public's awareness of the dangers of intense sun exposure and stressing the importance of sunscreens and sunblocks may be the most effective measure in controlling this disease.

REFERENCES

1. Cancer Facts and Figures 1987. New York: American Cancer Society, 1987.
2. National Cancer Institute's Surveillance, Epidemiology, and End Result Program: Annual Cancer Statistics Review. Washington, DC, US Department of Health and Human Services, Public Health Service, National Institutes of Health, 1988:61.
3. Devesa SS, Silverman DT, Young JL, et al. Cancer incidence and mortality trends among whites in the United States, 1947–84. 1987; 79:701–770.
4. Balch CM, Karakousis C, Mettlin C, et al. Management of cutaneous melanoma in the United States. Surg Gynecol Obstet 1984; 158:311–318.
5. Elwood JM, Lee JAH. Recent data on the epidemiology of malignant melanoma. Semin Oncol 1975; 2:149–154.
6. Holman DA, Armstrong BK. Cutaneous melanoma and the indicators of total accumulated exposure to the sun: an analysis separating histologic types. JNCI 1984; 73:75–82.
7. Koph AW, Hellman LJ, Rogers GS, et al. Familial malignant melanoma. JAMA 1986; 256:1915–1919.
8. Greene MH, Clark WH, Tucker MA, et al. Acquired precursors of cutaneous malignant melanoma. The familial dysplastic nevus syndrome. N Engl J Med 1985; 312:91–97.
9. Clark WH, Lynn F, Bernardino EA, Mihm MC. The histogenesis and biologic behavior of primary human malignant melanomas of the skin. Cancer Res 1969; 29:705–726.
10. Clark WH, Ainsworth AM, Bernardino EA, Yang CH, Mihm MC, Reed RJ. The developmental biology of primary human malignant melanomas. Semin Oncol 1975; 2:83–103.
11. Wade TR, White CR. The histology of malignant melanoma. Med Clin North Am 1986; 70:57–70.
12. Breslow A. Thickness, cross-sectional area and depth of invasion in the prognosis of cutaneous melanoma. Ann Surg 1970; 172:902–908.
13. Urist MW, Balch CM, Soong SJ, Shaw HM, Milton GW, Maddox WA. The influence of surgical margins and prognostic factors predicting the risk of local recurrence in 3445 patients with primary cutaneous melanoma. Cancer 1985; 55:1398–1402.
14. Balch CM. The role of elective lymph node dissection in melanoma: rationale, results, and controversies. J Clin Oncol 1988; 6:163–172.
15. Karakousis CP, Emrich LJ, Rao U. Groin dissection in malignant melanoma. Am J Surg 1986; 152:491–495.
16. Wong JH, Cagle LA, Morton DL. Surgical treatment of lymph nodes with metastatic melanoma from unknown primary site. Arch Surg 1987; 122:1380–1383.
17. McCarthy WH, Shaw HM, Milton GW. Efficacy of elective lymph node dissection in 2347 patients with clinical stage I malignant melanoma. Surg Gynecol Obstet 1985; 161:505–508.
18. McCarthy WH, Shaw HM, Thompson JF, Milton GW. Time and frequency of recurrence of cutaneous stage I malignant melanoma with guidelines for follow-up study. Surg Gynecol Obstet 1988; 166:497–502.
19. Koh HK, Sober AJ, Harmon DC, Lew RA, Carey RW. Adjuvant therapy of cutaneous malignant melanoma: a critical review. Med Pediatr Oncol 1985; 13:244–260.
20. Cumberlin R, DeMoss E, Lassus M, Friedman M. Isolation perfusion for malignant melanoma of the extremity: a review. J Clin Oncol 1985; 3:1022–1030.
21. Storm FK, Morton DL. Value of therapeutic hyperthermic limb perfusion in advanced recurrent melanoma of the lower extremity. Am J Surg 1985; 150:32–35.
22. Nambisan RN, Alexiou G, Reese PA, Karakousis CP. Early metastatic patterns and survival in malignant melanoma. J Surg Oncol 1987; 34:248–252.
23. Overett TK, Shiu MH. Surgical treatment of distant metastatic melanoma. Indications and results. Cancer 1985; 56:1222–1230.
24. Hena MH, Emrich LJ, Nambisan RN, Karakousis CP. Effect of surgical treatment on stage IV melanoma. Am J Surg 1987; 153:270–275.
25. Wornom IL, Soong SJ, Urist MM, Smith JW, McElvein R, Balch CM. Surgery as palliative treatment for distant metastasis of melanoma. Ann Surg 1986; 204:181–185.
26. Conefal JB, Emani B, Pilepich MV. Analysis of dose fractionation in the palliation of metastasis from malignant melanoma. Cancer 1988; 61:243–246.
27. Kleeberg UR. Clinical trials in disseminated malignant melanoma. Antica Res 1987; 7:423–428.
28. Singluff CL, Vollmer RT, Reintgen DS, Seigler HF. Lethal "thin" malignant melanoma. Identifying patients at risk. Ann Surg 1988; 208:150–161.
29. Balch CM, Soong SJ, Milton GW, et al. A comparison of prognostic factors and surgical results in 1786 patients with localized (stage I) melanoma treated in Alabama, USA and New South Wales, Australia. Ann Surg 1982; 196:667–684.

Meniere's disease

Sidney N. Busis

It has been estimated that 7 million Americans have Meniere's disease and that 100,000 new cases develop each year.[1] Although Meniere's disease is sometimes used as a "wastebasket" diagnosis for any patient complaining of dizziness, it is a distinct clinical entity. Its characteristic symptoms are vertigo, hearing loss, tinnitus, and a sensation of fullness or pressure in the affected ear.

■ Background

Meniere's disease is named for Prosper Meniere, a French physician, who in 1861 first described this symptom complex. The pathology—endolymphatic hydrops with distention of the endolymphatic system—is better understood today,[2] but the etiology and the exact pathophysiology of Meniere's disease are still unknown.[3] It occurs at all ages, but the mean age is the fourth decade.[3] It rarely occurs in childhood. Meniere's disease is most often unilateral but may become bilateral in 30 to 50 percent of the patients.[2-4]

The characteristic attack of vertigo, called the definitive attack, consists of an illusion of motion with a sensation of spatial disorientation. This is most often a feeling of rotation but may be in any plane or direction. Occasionally preceded by an aura, such as a change in the character of the tinnitus or the ear pressure, the definitive attacks occur suddenly and may be violent and prostrating, frequently accompanied by nausea and vomiting. The definitive spell may last for minutes to hours. There is no loss of consciousness. The patient must have had more than one attack before the diagnosis of Meniere's disease can be made.

Between the discrete spells, patients may have adjunctive symptoms of dysequilibrium, such as occasionally bumping into walls or door frames. However, there are no neurologic sequelae. The hearing loss of Meniere's disease is a flat sensorineural hearing loss accompanied by diplacusis (different pitch in each ear) and paracusis (distorted hearing in the affected ear). The associated tinnitus is characteristically low-pitched and roaring, frequently described as sounding like the ocean.

In the natural course of the disease there may be long periods of remission of vertiginous episodes, and the spells usually become less severe. However, some patients never improve and become disabled because of vertigo. Although hearing loss fluctuates at the beginning, it frequently gets progressively worse as time goes on.

■ Management

■ MEDICAL TREATMENT

All patients should be treated medically first. If this fails and the patient has incapacitating vertiginous symptoms, surgical treatment may be considered.[3]

Acute Spells. An acute attack of vertigo with a violent spinning sensation accompanied by nausea and vomiting is a terrifying experience that requires immediate attention. The patient should be put to bed at home or in the hospital. Acute vertigo is accompanied by horizonto-rotary nystagmus that beats (fast phase) toward one side. The patient will be more comfortable lying on the side toward which the nystagmus (fast phase) is beating. This encourages the patient to look in the opposite direction, toward the slow phase of the nystagmus, the direction of gaze that will suppress the nystagmus, the vertigo, and the nausea and vomiting. The patient should lie quietly because head movement, which stimulates the vestibular end-organ, will activate more dizziness and more nausea and vomiting.[5]

If the patient is dehydrated, intravenous

fluids should be started. Medication is best given by intramuscular injection or by rectal suppository.[5] Prochlorperazine (Compazine), 5 to 10 mg intramuscularly or in a suppository of 25 mg, or a chlorpromazine (Thorazine) suppository of 25 to 50 mg is effective for controlling nausea and vomiting as well as the vertigo. The chlorpromazine (Thorazine) suppository is usually very effective and can be the first choice. Dimenhydrinate (Dramamine), 50 mg intramuscularly, may control dizziness and can be repeated if needed. Atropine, 0.5 to 1 mg intramuscularly, may be effective in some patients, and diazepam (Valium), 5 to 10 mg intramuscularly or intravenously, is preferred by some physicians. For the hospitalized patient, the combination of fentanyl (Sublimaze), 0.05 mg/ml, and droperidol, 2.5 mg/ml (Innovar), may be useful. This is a mixture of a potent opioid analgesic (fentanyl) and a tranquilizer (droperidol), given intravenously, and should be administered only by an anesthesiologist. The dose is one ampule (2 ml) or less, as determined by the patient's response. Acute vertiginous episodes from Meniere's disease are unusual in children and rarely require drug therapy. However, if medication is necessary, the only drug recommended is dimenhydrinate (Dramamine). For children 8 to 12 years of age, the dose is 1.25 mg/kg of body weight. The total daily dose should not exceed 300 mg.

Long-Term Care. Acute attacks subside. The challenge is the long-term management of the Meniere's disease patient. Understandably, most patients are anxious and fear the recurrence of attacks of disabling vertigo. So the first aspect of treatment is reassuring the patient that there is no life-threatening disease and that the symptoms should be controllable. However, before offering this reassurance the physician must be reasonably certain that the diagnosis of Meniere's disease is correct, and that there is no evidence of an acoustic tumor or other central nervous system disease. The physician should be certain that the patient has had a proper history and physical examination and appropriate auditory and vestibular tests. If there is uncertainty about the diagnosis, a computed tomography (CT) scan or magnetic resonance imaging (MRI) should be performed.

After reassurance, it can be explained to the patient that there is increased fluid pressure in the inner ear, and, when the pressure changes, symptoms occur. The aim of treatment is to lower inner ear fluid pressure and to maintain it at a normal level. It is believed that anxiety and stress through the autonomic nervous system can impair inner ear function. In some Meniere's disease patients there may be a psychosomatic element. But the symptoms of Meniere's disease can cause great stress, so there also may be what has been called a "somatopsychic" component.[6] This possibility should also be recognized; the stress may be alleviated by treatment. The physician and the patient should work together to achieve a state of equanimity; a good physician-patient relationship is important for successful management.[3]

Treatment of Associated Systemic Disorders. It should be ascertained whether any systemic medical abnormalities are present, such as glucose intolerance, hyperlipidemia, lues, vascular disease, thyroid dysfunction, or autoimmune disease, that might afflict inner ear structures such as the stria vascularis or the endolymphatic duct or sac. Treatment of certain systemic disorders may alleviate the symptoms of Meniere's disease.

Spencer was among the first to recognize that there is a distinct relationship between hyperlipoproteinemia and inner ear disease.[7] He reported a series of over 1400 patients and summarizes that "most patients seen by otolaryngologists because of Meniere's disease come from that same large population group who are prone to obesity, maturity-onset diabetes, coronary artery disease, and atherosclerosis." He noted that these patients are unable to handle refined carbohydrates well and have been found to have hyperinsulinism. He recommends a diet of complex carbohydrates with increased fiber. Lehrer and associates identified a group of patients, common to specialists in internal medicine and otology, who are overweight and have elevated triglyceride levels, abnormal glucose tolerance, and/or insulin response patterns.[8] These patients appear to be at greater risk for heart and ear disease. Dietary management alleviated vertigo in a significant number of these patients. Linthicum and El-Rahman demonstrated histopathologically endolymphatic hydrops caused by obliteration of the endolymphatic duct by luetic microgumma.[9] Syphilis should be considered early in the evaluation, because hearing loss due to lues may respond to treatment with penicillin, and the improved hearing may be maintained with prednisone. In 1979, McCabe first reported autoimmune disease as a treatable cause of sensorineural hearing loss.[10] Later, Hughes and associates found autoimmune disease in Meniere's disease patients.[11] Autoimmune disease affecting the inner ear can be treated with prednisone. Cyclophosphamide (Cytoxan) also has been suggested for treatment.[10] This should be administered in consultation with an oncologist. Caffeine, alcohol, and tobacco are considered to be toxic to the inner ear and are to be avoided.

Body Fluid Control. All patients with Meniere's disease should be placed on a low-salt diet and a diuretic. In a landmark paper published in 1934, Furstenberg and colleagues, after a study of "water balance," proposed that retention of sodium was a main causative factor in the development of Meniere's disease.[12] He then successfully treated patients with low-salt diet and a diuretic.[13] Over the years, the "Furstenberg diet" has been prescribed with various modifications, such as specifying a diet of 1500 to 2000 mg of salt per day.[3] Patients are advised to avoid salt, not to add any to their food, and not to cook with it. They are instructed not to eat packaged foods, especially those wrapped in plastic film, because these are usually highly salted to make them tasty. The preferred diuretics are hydrochlorothiazide (HydroDIURIL), 25 mg daily or triamterene and hydrochlorothiazide (Dyazide, Maxzide, Maxzide-25 MG), one daily. Blood electrolytes are checked periodically.

Exercise Programs. The brain has the property of plasticity, which means that it can adapt itself to change, whether it be change due to destruction of cells by a stroke or change due to a training program that challenges a brain function. The latter capacity is particularly true of the vestibular system.[14] This vestibular system plasticity is evident when a person who never before wore a pair of ice skates learns to skate and even to spin on them, a skill that would be impossible without the accommodation of the vestibular system. Meniere's disease patients who have persistent poor balance are encouraged to carry out a general body exercise program, and then they are given a set of balance exercises to perform twice a day at home (Table 1). Exercises that are performed regularly promote vestibular compensation.

Drug Therapy. Since the cause of Meniere's disease is unknown, there is no specific drug for treatment of the disease process. Certain drugs, described earlier, are effective for the control of an acute attack of vertigo. In the management of less severe exacerbations of dizziness or continuing poor balance, the aim of drug treatment is to afford symptomatic relief.[5] The choice of drug depends on the physician's experience and the patient's response.[5]

As a class, antihistamines have been most widely used. They are usually effective for controlling dizziness but may cause drowsiness. The most frequently prescribed antihistamine is meclizine (Antivert, Bonine). It is often the drug of first choice. For recurrent vertigo, dosage starts at 25 mg four times a day and then is reduced as symptoms subside or if too much drowsiness occurs.

Another antihistamine that has been effective is buclizine (Bucladin-S Softab), 50 mg, which may be taken without water twice a day to start, then once a day. Cyclizine (Marezine) is useful in a dosage of 50 mg three to four times a day.

One of the earliest drugs developed for control of motion sickness and dizziness, dimenhydrinate (Dramamine), is effective in a dosage of 50 mg three or four times a day. As noted earlier, it is the only antivertigo drug recommended for children.

Diphenidol (Vontrol), an antivertigo drug that acts directly on the vestibular system and is not related to the antihistamines, phenothiazines, or barbiturates, has been effecacious in controlling dizziness.[15] However, it can have side effects of disorientation, confusion, and hallucinations and therefore should only be used under close supervision. Patients are told about its possible side effects and advised to discontinue the drug if any sign of them occurs. The dosage is 25 mg three times a day.

Scopolamine (Transderm-Scōp), with its transdermal delivery system, has been helpful in some patients. However, it may have unpleasant side effects of dryness of the mouth and blurred vision.

Histamine has been considered to be an autonomic nervous system regulator that has an anticholinergic action, and it is also thought to have a beneficial effect as a vasodilator[16] on the vasculature of the stria

TABLE 1. Balance Exercises

Start out doing one or two exercises at a time. Gradually increase the number until you do them all. Perform the complete set of exercises twice a day for at least 30 minutes. Once you are feeling better, you can perform them only once a day.

Eyes	Look up and down as far as you can without moving your head, at first slowly and then quickly, for 20 times. Look as far as you can to one side and then to the other side without moving your head, at first slowly and then quickly, for 20 times. Focus on your index finger at arm's length and then move your finger in and out, at first slowly and then quickly, for 20 times. Repeat with the other hand.
Head	Bend your head forward then backward with your eyes open, at first slowly and then quickly, for 20 times. Turn your head from side to side as far as you can, at first slowly and then quickly, for 20 times. When you feel comfortable with these exercises, start doing them with your eyes closed.
Sitting	Shrug your shoulders up and down as far as you can, 20 times. Then turn your shoulders as far as you can to the right and then to the left for 20 times. While sitting in a chair, bend over and pick something up off the floor, at first slowly and then quickly, for 20 times. Repeat this exercise, putting the object first to the right of the chair and then to the left of the chair. While sitting, extend one foot and then the other alternately as far as you can, at first slowly and then quickly, for 20 times.
Standing	Stand up from a chair, at first slowly and then quickly, for 20 times with your eyes open. As you feel more comfortable doing this, do the exercise with your eyes closed. Toss a ball from one hand to the other below eye level, at first slowly and then quickly, for 20 times; and then above eye level, at first slowly and then quickly, for 20 times. Toss a ball from one hand to the other under one knee for 20 times and then repeat on the opposite side.
Walking	Walk across the room with your eyes open, make a sudden turn and then walk back to where you started, at first slowly and then quickly, for 20 times. If you feel comfortable doing this exercise, try it with your eyes closed. Walk up and down at least 4 steps, holding onto a railing with your eyes open. Walk up and down 10 times. As you feel more comfortable, repeat the exercise while holding onto the railing with your eyes closed. With someone walking beside you for help if needed, try these exercises without holding onto the railing. *Do not do the walking exercises* if you think they are too strenuous for you or if you are afraid you are going to fall. As your dizziness improves, you will be able to do these more comfortably.

vascularis.[3] It can be prescribed sublingually, in a dilution of 1:10,000, five drops under the tongue twice daily; intramuscularly in titrated doses starting at a dilution of 1:100,000; or intravenously, 2.75 mg of histamine phosphate in 250 ml of normal saline.[16]

Diazepam (Valium), 2 to 5 mg alone or in combination with promethazine hydrochloride (Phenergan), 25 mg, is the first choice of some physicians for the management of recurrent dizziness that is difficult to control.

Some physicians consider vasodilators such as nylidrin hydrochloride (Arlidin) to be useful.[3] The dose is 3 to 12 mg three to four times a day.

Streptomycin sulfate is toxic to the vestibular hair cells and eventually causes their destruction. For treatment of disabling symptoms in patients with bilateral Meniere's disease or with unilateral Meniere's disease in the only hearing ear, this toxicity

has been utilized to perform what may be called a "chemical labyrinthectomy."[17] The dose of the drug is titrated according to the patient's response. The total dose may vary from 10 gm to 60 gm over a period of days. In a series of 20 patients, Graham and Kemink reported improved equilibrium in 18 and poorer equilibrium in 2. None of the patients had poorer hearing after treatment and about one third had improved hearing.[17]

Allergy. If there is a history of untreated allergy or suspicion that there is an allergic disorder, a formal allergy study can be performed. In some patients, treatment for allergy may relieve the chronic vertiginous symptoms of Meniere's disease.[3]

Hearing Aids. Increasing hearing loss, either unilateral or bilateral, may become a problem to patients and their families. In these cases a trial period with a hearing aid is recommended. Fitting Meniere's disease patients with hearing aids is difficult because the hearing loss fluctuates, there is usually poor speech discrimination ability, and there is a narrow dynamic range of hearing. This means that sound is frequently perceived as either too soft to be heard or so loud that it is uncomfortable. However, successful fitting can be accomplished by incorporating special circuits.[18] The patient is given a 30-day trial period to decide whether the aid is helpful before commitment to purchase the aid.

■ SURGICAL TREATMENT

Surgical treatment is reserved for patients who have not responded to medical management and who are essentially disabled because of recurrent bouts of dizziness. Hearing loss and tinnitus are rarely indications for surgery, although occasionally these symptoms may be somewhat ameliorated following surgery for dizziness.

Rationale

There are two distinct rationales for surgery. The first one is based on the presumption that the cause of the symptoms of Meniere's disease is endolymphatic hydrops, and the aim of surgery is to relieve endolymphatic pressure. These are classified as conservative procedures. The second rationale is directed at neural fibers, and the goal of surgery is to sever the connections between the vestibular labyrinth and the brain, either by destroying the vestibular hair cells in the labyrinth or by transecting the nerve trunk. These are destructive procedures.

Conservative Procedures. Almost all operations designed to relieve endolymphatic pressure are called "sac" operations, because the procedure in some way involves the endolymphatic sac that is located on the posterior fossa wall of the temporal bone and contains endolymph.[2] After a mastoidectomy, the endolymphatic sac may be decompressed by removing the overlying bone only or by removing the bone and opening the sac to allow endolymph to drain into the mastoid cavity.[3] To maintain patency of the endolymphatic sac and duct, a plastic capillary tube or Silastic sheeting may be placed into the sac as a shunt. Arenberg has developed an inner ear valve to insert into the endolymphatic sac and duct to maintain proper endolymphatic pressure.[19] Drainage

may be established into the subarachnoid space by inserting a shunt tube from the sac to the subarachnoid space. All these procedures are reported to afford significant relief of vertigo in 70 to 80 percent of patients.[4]

In 1981, Thomsen reported the results of a double-blind, placebo-controlled study on endolymphatic sac shunt surgery.[20] He found only minor differences between the two groups of patients: those who had a Silastic sheeting shunt procedure and those who had a sham operation. Both groups had improved significantly. He was "of the opinion that the impact of surgery on the symptoms of Meniere's disease is completely nonspecific and unrelated to the actual shunt procedure." There has been continuing controversy over this report and rebuttals and compelling challenges to the statistical analysis and to the conclusions have been made.[4] It is safe to say that the otologic consensus today is that sac surgery is effective in a significant number of patients as a conservative surgical procedure, with low risk of increased hearing loss or other complications, such as facial paralysis or cerebrospinal fluid leak.[3,4]

Operations have been designed to relieve endolymphatic pressure in the vestibule by puncturing the distended saccule or by creating a fistula into the membranous labyrinth. These include the sacculotomy, the Cody tack, and the cochlear endolymphatic shunt.[2] These operations are seldom performed today. Another conservative procedure, cryosurgery, has been reported to successfully relieve vertigo in over 70 percent of patients.[21] Hearing was unaffected. In another approach, Møller has reported some success in treating patients with classic symptoms of Meniere's disease by microvascular decompression of the eighth nerve.[22] This requires neurosurgical entry and manipulation in the posterior cranial fossa, with their attendant risks. All the patients had abnormal brain stem auditory evoked potentials, suggesting an eighth nerve or brain stem etiology for their symptoms.

Destructive Procedures. The intent of the vestibular nerve section operation, a destructive procedure, is to disconnect the vestibular labyrinth from the brain while avoiding the cochlear nerve fibers so that hearing may be preserved. The nerve section can be performed through a mastoidectomy by dissecting behind the labyrinth (retrolabyrinthine), through the posterior fossa behind the sigmoid venous sinus (restrosigmoid), or by approaching the nerve in the middle fossa.[3] These operations carry a higher risk of cerebrospinal fluid leak and facial paralysis than the conservative procedures.

If the patient has no usable hearing, a labyrinthectomy can be performed either through the mastoid process or through the middle ear. The postauricular route allows complete dissection of the mastoid process and the bony labyrinth, so that all neural tissue in the semicircular canals and the vestibule can be exenterated.[3] In the transcanal middle ear approach, there is limited access to the vestibule and the ampullated ends of the semicircular canals where vestibular hair cells are located, so that there is the possibility that all neural tissue will not be removed and vertiginous symptoms will persist.

When a patient has uncontrollable, disabling vertigo and surgery is being considered, a decision as to what procedure might be performed depends on a full explanation to the patient about the benefits and risks of the various operation choices and on the experience and skill of the surgeon. All patients who have a destructive procedure performed on the labyrinth experience an immediate postoperative increase in vertigo accompanied by nystagmus, because of an increase in the imbalance of the vestibular activity of the two labyrinths. Vertigo subsides as vestibular compensation takes place. The older the patient, the longer the time for compensation. Some elderly patients never fully compensate and some dizziness lingers. This possibility should be discussed with the patient preoperatively.

■ Issues and Risks

"Meniere's disease is capricious both in its behavior and its response to treatment. Criteria for diagnosis may vary greatly. Its puzzling periodicity with characteristic remissions and exacerbations make evaluation of treatment methods difficult and frustrating. A uniform set of criteria for diagnosis and judging and reporting the results of treatment is needed to facilitate and validate clinical studies of this disease."

This introduction to the guidelines for the reporting of treatment results, established in 1972 by the Committee on Hearing and Equilibrium of the American Academy of Ophthalmology and Otolaryngology,[23] summarizes the dilemma facing treating physicians and Meniere's disease patients today. The main problem confronting us is the unknown etiology and thus the lack of a specific medical or surgical treatment modality.

Is Meniere's disease truly an independent disease entity? Is it a local manifestation of a recognized systemic disease? Is it an emotional disorder mediated through the autonomic nervous system? Should the physician probe more into the patient's personal life? Basic research in pathology and pathophysiology continues in many centers throughout the world.[1,24] Clinical treatment today is empiric, based on the individual physician's training and personal experience. Evaluation and standardization of medical and surgical treatment methods require the cooperation of all treating physicians.

In response to many comments and suggestions concerning the 1972 guidelines, the Committee on Hearing and Equilibrium of the American Academy of Otolaryngology–Head and Neck Surgery updated the guidelines for reporting treatment results in 1985.[25]

The effect of treatment on vertigo, the most disabling symptom, is measured by comparing the average number of definitive spells per month in the 24-month period after treatment to the average number of definitive spells per month in the 6-month period prior to therapy. The effect of treatment on hearing is measured by comparing the average pure tone loss and the speech discrimination scores in these same time periods. The degree of disability is judged by the patient as improved, unchanged, or worse. Although tinnitus, unsteadiness, and fullness in the ear can be very annoying, these symptoms are too subjective to be quantified meaningfully. Interested physicians and other investigators should refer to the detailed 1985 reporting system.[25]

REFERENCES

1. Harris JP. What's new in surgery for 1989: Otorhinolaryngology. Bull Coll Surg 1989; 74:23–27.
2. Schuknecht HF. Endolymphatic hydrops: can it be controlled? Ann Otol Rhinol Laryngol 1986; 95:36–39.
3. Glasscock ME III, Gulya AJ, Pensak ML, Black JN Jr.

Medical and surgical management of Meniere's disease Am J Otol 1984; 5:536–542.

4. Smith WC, Pillsbury HC. Surgical treatment of Meniere's disease since Thomsen. Am J Otol 1988; 9:39–43.
5. Baloh RW. The dizzy patient: symptomatic treatment of vertigo. Postgrad Med 1983; 73:317–324.
6. Wexler M, Crary WG. Meniere's disease: the psychosomatic hypothesis. Am J Otol 1986; 7:93–96.
7. Spencer JT. Hyperlipoproteinemia, hyperinsulinism, and Meniere's disease. South Med J 1981; 74:1194–1200.
8. Lehrer JF, Poole DC, Seaman M, Restivo D, Hartman K. Identification and treatment of metabolic abnormalities in patients with vertigo. Arch Intern Med 1986; 146:1497–1500.
9. Linthicum FH, Jr, El-Rahman AGA. Hydrops due to syphilitic endolymphatic duct obliteration. Laryngoscope 1987; 97:568–574.
10. McCabe BF. Autoimmune sensorineural hearing loss. Ann Otol 1979; 88:585–589.
11. Hughes GB, Barna BP, Calabrese LH, Kinney SE, Nalepa NJ. Clinical diagnosis of inner-ear disease. Laryngoscope 1988; 98:251–253.
12. Furstenberg AC, Lashmet FH, Lathrop F. Meniere's symptom complex: medical treatment. Ann Otol Rhinol Laryngol 1934; 43:1035–1046.
13. Furstenberg AC, Richardson G, Lathrop FD. Meniere's disease: addenda to medical therapy. Arch Otolaryngol 1941; 34:1083–1092.
14. Rudge P. Clinical Neurology and Neurosurgery Monographs: Clinical Neuro-Otology. Vol 4. New York: Churchill Livingstone, 1983:174–186.
15. Futaki T, Kitahara M, Morimoto M. Meniere's disease and diphenidol. Acta Otolaryngol 1975; (Suppl) 330:120–128.
16. Sheehy JL, Robinson JV, Bush JE. Intravenous histamine in otologic practice. Arch Otolaryngol 1980; 106:159–160.
17. Graham MD, Kemink JL. Titration streptomycin therapy for bilateral Meniere's disease: a progress report. Am J Otol 1984; 5:534–535.
18. Johnson EW, House J. Meniere's disease: clinical course, auditory findings, and hearing aid fitting. J Am Auditory Soc 1979; 5:76–83.
19. Arenberg IK. Results of endolymphatic sac to mastoid shunt surgery for Meniere's disease refractory to medical therapy. Am J Otol 1987; 8:335–344.
20. Thomsen J, Bretlau P, Tos M, Johnsen NJ. Placebo effect in surgery for Meniere's disease. Arch Otolaryngol 1981; 107:271–277.
21. Wolfson RJ. Labyrinthine cryosurgery for Meniere's disease—present status. Otolaryngol Head Neck Surg 1984; 92:221–224.
22. Møller MB. Controversy in Meniere's disease: results of microvascular decompression of the eighth nerve. Am J Otol 1988; 9:60–63.
23. Alford BR. Criteria for diagnosis and evaluation of therapy for reporting. Trans Am Acad Ophthalmol Otolaryngol 1972; 76:1462–1464.
24. Abstracts of the Second International Symposium on Meniere's Disease: Pathogenesis, Pathophysiology, Diagnosis, and Treatment. Cambridge, MA: Harvard University, June 20–22, 1988.
25. Pearson BW, Brackmann DE. Editorial: Committee on Hearing and Equilibrium Guidelines for reporting treatment results in Meniere's disease (editorial). Otolaryngol Head Neck Surg 1985; 93:579–581.

Meningitis and encephalitis

Kent Crossley ■ *Keith Henry* ■ *Joseph Thurn*

The occurrence of fever and a changing mental status or neurologic examination suggest that infection involving the central nervous system (CNS) may be present. Although these same findings may be due to other causes (e.g., pneumonia in a patient with metabolic encephalopathy), any patient with fever and changes on neurologic or mental examination must be assumed to have an intracranial infection until proved otherwise. Careful diagnostic evaluation and prompt initiation of correct therapy are often keys to a favorable outcome. Human immunodeficiency virus (HIV)–infected patients pose their own particularly difficult management problems when there is evidence of CNS infection.

■ Background

Intracranial infection must be considered at least briefly in any patient who presents with changes in mental status or in neurologic function even in the absence of fever. Although most patients are febrile, those who are at the extremes of life or who are immunocompromised may have significant intracranial infection but muted physiologic responses (i.e., fever, leukocytosis, and so on).[1]

The key to the optimal management of intracranial infection is a correct diagnosis.[2] Most manifestations of central nervous system infection may result from a variety of different etiologies. Thus, a septic embolus in a patient with endocarditis, brain abscess, viral meningoencephalitis, extension into the brain of a sinus or otic infection, bacterial meningitis, or viral encephalitis all could produce identical localizing neurologic findings associated with fever.

Although the causes of bacterial meningitis are known to most physicians, the etiologies of viral meningoencephalitis are less well known organisms, and the process of defining a diagnosis is often very difficult (Table 1).

A large number of viral agents may cause encephalitis.[3] The most common cause of sporadic fatal encephalitis is herpes simplex virus (HSV). This organism may cause infection at any age and in both sexes and does not have a seasonality.[4-6] Cases typically occur in previously healthy patients who do not have antecedent or concurrent skin lesions. About a third of cases may be associated with primary HSV infection. The electroencephalogram (EEG) is the most useful diagnostic aid and shows a characteristic picture of a temporal focus with spikes and slow waves. Technetium and computed tomographic (CT) scans and magnetic resonance imaging (MRI) all have shown utility in diagnosis.[7,8] The cerebrospinal fluid (CSF) examination may be helpful, but some patients lack the characteristic presence of red blood cells or elevated protein levels. Culturing and antibody tests are not useful, and brain biopsy remains the definitive technique for a diagnosis.

Arrival at the correct diagnosis in a patient with intracranial infection requires that a variety of different types of information be considered.[9] A patient's age, past medical history, and the time of year are helpful in including or excluding certain eti-

TABLE 1. Etiology and Differential Diagnosis of Encephalitis (After Ref. 3)

Infections

  Bacterial
    Borrelia burgdorferi
    Brucella
    Leptospira species
    Listeria monocytogenes
    Mycobacterium tuberculosis
    Mycoplasma pneumoniae
    Rickettsia rickettsii
    Treponema pallidum

  Fungal
    Cryptococcus neoformans
    Coccidioides immitis

  Protozoal
    Toxoplasma gondii
    Naegleria fowleri
    Acanthamoeba species

  Viruses
    "Arboviruses"* (California [LaCrosse], eastern and western equine encephalitis viruses)
    Herpes viruses (herpes simplex, varicella-zoster, cytomegalovirus, Epstein-Barr virus)
    Enteroviruses (Coxsackie viruses, ECHO viruses)
    Rabies virus
    Adenovirus

Etiologies that may mimic encephalitis

  Noninfectious
    Collagen vascular diseases (lupus cerebritis)
    Toxic and metabolic encephalopathies
    Cerebrovascular hemorrhage
    Malignancy (lymphoma, leukemia, carcinomatosis)

  Infections
    Brain abscess
    Parameningeal infection

*Arbovirus is a common term for RNA viruses that are transmitted by arthropod vectors.

ologies. A history of travel (coccidioidomycosis), rash (erythema chronicum migrans in Lyme disease), or underlying disease (*Listeria* meningitis is most common in patients with alcoholism and malignancies) may be helpful, and some activities such as diving in brackish water (amebic meningoencephalitis) also may suggest an etiology. Contact with pets or exposure to insects may be important.

Clinical findings are also helpful because seizures, visual changes, and paralysis imply involvement of the brain and thus suggest brain abscess or viral encephalitis. Almost inevitably, patients with these types of findings require CT scanning. CT may demonstrate an unsuspected intracranial abscess but is also useful to exclude evidence of a mass lesion or ventricular enlargement that would require careful reassessment of the need for lumbar puncture.

Lumbar puncture and examination of CSF are keys to determining the likely etiology in a patient with meningitis or encephalitis. Although initial findings are often helpful in arriving at a tentative diagnosis (with a polymorphonuclear leukocytosis suggesting bacterial infection and a lymphocytic one suggesting viruses or fungi), culturing of fluid for bacteria, mycobacteria, viruses, and fungi (as appropriate) is often the route by which CNS infections are defined. Unfortunately, in up to three fourths of cases of viral meningoencephalitis, the etiology remains undetermined. It must be stressed again that prompt, careful identification of the likely etiology of CNS infection is absolutely crucial to selecting appropriate therapy.

■ Management

■ MENINGITIS

Major changes have occurred in the antibiotic therapy of bacterial meningitis in recent years.[9-12] Treatment of bacterial meningitis may be initiated depending on the age or other characteristics of the patient (Table 2). The recommended therapy is closely tied to the likely pathogen in each age group: gram-negative bacteria in neonates, *Haemophilus influenzae* in children, and meningococci or pneumococci in older children and adults. In patients thought to have pneumococcal and meningococcal infection and who are allergic to penicillin, chloramphenicol is the recommended alternative agent. In immunocompromised patients, a broad-spectrum third-generation cephalosporin along with ampicillin (for *Listeria monocytogenes*) is recommended.

The broad-spectrum cephalosporins have become important in both the management of community-acquired and of nosocomial meningitis. Thus, for an organism like *Pseudomonas aeruginosa*, use of parenteral therapy with a drug such as ceftazidime (Fortaz, Tazicef, Tazidime) dramatically simplifies therapy when compared with using agents such as the aminoglycosides, which must be administered by the intrathecal route.

Some concerns have developed about the use of broad-spectrum cephalosporins in the treatment of community-acquired meningitis caused by *Haemophilus* or *Streptococcus pneumoniae*. Recently published studies of ceftriaxone (Rocephin) and cefuroxime (Zinacef) have demonstrated delayed CSF sterilization.[13,14] Whereas delayed sterilization also has been noted with ampicillin and chloramphenicol, it has been reported more frequently with the cephalosporins. (It is interesting that apparently it has not been reported with cefotaxime [Claforan].) We recommend proceeding with caution before choosing to use ceftriaxone or cefuroxime as single agents in the treatment of *Haemophilus* meningitis.

■ PROPHYLAXIS

A particularly vexatious issue that often faces the physician treating a patient with meningitis is the need for prophylactic treatment of contacts. For intimate contacts of patients with meningococcal meningitis, rifampin (Rifadin), 10 mg/kg (not over 600 mg/dose) BID for 2 days is recommended.[15] Among household (and perhaps day-care center) contacts of patients with *Haemophilus influenzae* meningitis, prophylaxis is recommended if the contacts have been exposed to the index case during the week prior to onset of meningitis. The index case, as well, should be treated prophylactically with rifampin, in a single dose of 20 mg/kg (not over 600 mg/dose) once daily for 4 days, in addition to appropriate therapeutic medication.[16] Recent data suggest that, if a patient is intolerant of rifampin, ceftriaxone may be the preferred agent for eradication of

TABLE 2. Therapy of Bacterial Meningitis (after Henry and Crossley[9])

Known Cause

Pneumoccal and meningococcal meningitis
  Penicillin G, 200,000 units/kg/day (given q 6 hr) for neonates; 18–24 × 10^6 units/day for adults. Penicillin-allergic: chloramphenicol (Chloromycetin). Alternative agents: third-generation cephalosporins.* Test pneumococci for penicillin susceptibility
Haemophilus meningitis
  Ampicillin plus chloramphenicol or a second- or third- generation cephalosporin
Gram-negative meningitis
  Uncomplicated: third-generation cephalosporin. Complicated: consider addition of an intrathecal aminoglycoside
Listeria monocytogenes meningitis
  Ampicillin or trimethoprim-sulfamethoxazole. (Note: cephalosporins are not active against *Listeria*)

Initial Empiric Therapy of Presumed Meningitis

Neonate (<2 mo)
  Ampicillin, 200 mg/kg/day IV (given q 8 hr) plus gentamicin, 7.5 mg/kg/day (given q 8–12 hr) or a third-generation cephalosporin
Child (<6 yr)
  Ampicillin, 200 mg/kg/day IV (given q 6 hr) plus chloramphenicol, 100 mg/kg IV/day (given q 6 hr) or a third-generation cephalosporin
Child or adult (>6 yr)
  Penicillin G, 200,000–300,000 units/kg/day IV (given q 4–6 hr) plus a third-generation cephalosporin
Immunocompromised patient
  Third-generation cephalosporin plus ampicillin (for *Listeria*)
Nosocomial or post-traumatic meningitis
  Third-generation cephalosporin plus an intrathecal aminoglycoside

---

*Appropriate third-generation cephalosporins for meningitis include cefotaxime (Claforan), ceftriaxone (Rocephin), and ceftazidime (Fortaz, Tazidime, Tazicef).

---

the carrier state.[17] A detailed discussion of some of the controversy surrounding prophylaxis can be found in Peter, Georges (editor), Report of the Committee on Infectious Diseases, 21st edition, American Academy of Pediatrics, Elk Grove Village, Illinois, 1988.

■ ENCEPHALITIS

It is beyond the scope of this chapter to deal with management of all the potential causes of encephalitis. For herpes simplex encephalitis (HSE), acyclovir (Zovirax) is the treatment of choice and has been shown to be superior to vidarabine (Vira-A).[18] When given in a dose of 10 mg/kg every 8 hours for 10 days, acyclovir has reduced the mortality of HSE to 20 per cent, with 40 per cent of survivors having no or only minimal neurologic impairment. Survival depends on age (mortality in those over 30 years of age still approaches 70 per cent, duration of disease before therapy, and level of consciousness.

The side effects of acyclovir include irritation and phlebitis at the administration sites and rarely rash and nausea. There have been some reports of CNS toxicity. The major adverse effect is renal dysfunction, with reversible elevations in serum creatinine. Renal toxicity from acyclovir is more common in the presence of dehydration, pre-existing renal insufficiency, and high-dose bolus infusion. It is therefore imperative that the drug be given by slow infusion over 1 hour, that renal function be monitored, and that adequate hydration and urine output be monitored.

■ Issues and Risks

■ MENINGITIS

Considerable controversy has surrounded the use of corticosteroids in the management of patients with bacterial meningitis. A significant amount of data has accumulated in the last 2 years to suggest that these drugs may be very appropriate. Administration of dexamethasone (Decadron) (which appears in animal models to be more effective than methylprednisolone) has been associated with more rapid cytologic resolution of inflammation and appears also to be associated with less severe or protracted neurologic sequelae. This applies particularly to hearing loss. The recommended dosage of dexamethasone is 0.15 mg/kg every 6 hours each day for the first 4 days of therapy. It is not surprising that patients who receive corticosteroids as part of the therapy of meningitis appear to have an increased frequency of gastrointestinal hemorrhage.[19]

■ ENCEPHALITIS

Controversies in the management of HSE include the need for brain biopsy and, more recently, the duration of therapy. Standard therapy has been 10 days of intravenous acyclovir for biopsy-proved cases, but two cases of recurrence after this regimen led to the suggestion of a 21-day course of therapy.[20]

The brain biopsy controversy has been long-standing and is less likely to be easily resolved.[21] Those who argue against routine brain biopsy suggest that it is not justified because of its associated risks of morbidity and mortality, the low toxicity of acyclovir, and the small chance of finding another specifically treatable disease. We suggest that the decision for brain biopsy be made on an individual basis. Biopsy may be beneficial for select groups of patients. It has been found useful, for instance, in patients with a low initial CSF glucose level for whom other treatable conditions are more often found. We also would recommend brain biopsy for any patients who do not present with typical symptoms and signs associated with "classic" findings on EEG or neurologic imaging.

■ HIV-ASSOCIATED CNS INFECTIONS

As clinical experience with human immunodeficiency virus infection (HIV) has broadened, a wide range of neurologic manifestations of both primary and secondary infections has been reported.[22] A number of meningeal/encephalopathic conditions are associated with HIV and need to be considered in the differential diagnosis of persons presenting with CNS processes. With 100,000 cases of AIDS already diagnosed in the United States and over 1,000,000 Americans estimated to be infected, CNS problems related to HIV will be increasingly encountered by physicians. The diagnosis of HIV-related CNS disease cannot be made unless the possibility of HIV infection is considered.

CNS manifestations of HIV infection can be divided into primary manifestations due directly to HIV and secondary manifestations caused by opportunistic pathogens or tumors. It is beyond the scope of this brief review to detail the burgeoning CNS syndromes due to HIV. Entire textbooks on the subject are available for the reader seeking more details.[23] Table 3 provides an overview of neurologic syndromes due to HIV. CNS involvement can encompass all areas of the nervous system, including diffuse encephalopathies, focal brain disease, myelopathies, peripheral neuropathies, and radiculopathies. The most striking CNS syndromes are aseptic meningitis and the AIDS-dementia complex (ADC). HIV-associated aseptic meningitis is seen in all stages of HIV disease, including primary HIV infection. ADC has been characterized by Price and Brew to entail early symptoms of forgetfulness, poor concentration, loss of interest in work, blunted affect, and psychomotor retardation, whereas late signs include confusion, seizures, mutism, dementia, coma, and gait disturbances.[24] Administration of zidovudine (Retrovir) may result in some clinical benefit for ADC.

TABLE 3. Central Nervous System Infections in Patients with HIV Infection (after Price and Brew[24])

CNS Syndrome Attributable to HIV
Diffuse brain disease
    Acute HIV encephalitis (with depression of alertness)
    AIDS dementia complex (preservation of consciousness)
Aseptic meningitis
Vacuolar myelopathy

Secondary CNS Problems Due to HIV-Associated Infections and Tumors
Diffuse brain disease with depression of alertness
    Toxoplasmosis
    Cytomegalovirus (CMV) encephalitis
    Herpes simplex encephalitis
Focal brain disease
    Cerebral toxoplasmosis
    Primary CNS lymphoma
    Progressive multifocal leukoencephalopathy
    Cryptococcoma
    Varicella-zoster virus (VZV) encephalitis
    Herpes simplex encephalitis
Meningitis
    Mycobacterium tuberculosis
    Cryptococcus neoformans
Transverse myelitis owing to VZV, CMV, tumors

Table 3 summarizes the spectrum of HIV-related CNS syndromes caused by opportunistic infections or tumors. Again, all regions of the CNS can be affected. The most significant of the AIDS-related CNS infections are cryptococcal meningitis and toxoplasmosis. Those infections can be treated successfully but require maintenance therapy to prevent relapse.[25]

REFERENCES

1. Lukes SA, Posner JB, Nielsen S, Armstrong D. Bacterial infections of the CNS in neutropenic patients. Neurology 1984; 34:269–275.
2. Benson CA, Harris AA. Acute neurologic infections. Med Clin North Am 1986; 70:987–1011.
3. Ho DD, Hirsch MS. Acute viral encephalitis. Med Clin North Am 1985; 69:415–429.
4. Kohl S. Herpes simplex virus encephalitis in children. Pediatr Clin North Am 1988; 35:465–483.
5. Whitley RJ, Soong S-J, Linneman C Jr, et al. Herpes simplex encephalitis. Clinical assessment. JAMA 1982; 247:317–320.
6. Whitley RJ. Herpes simplex virus infections of the central nervous system. Am J Med 1988; 85(Suppl 2A):61–67.
7. Kaufman DM, Zimmerman RD, Leeds NE. Computed tomography in herpes simplex encephalitis. Neurology 1979; 29:1392–1396.
8. Schroth G, Gawehn J, Thron A, Vallbracht A, Voigt K. Early diagnosis of herpes simplex encephalitis by MRI. Neurology 1987; 37:179–183.
9. Henry K, Crossley K. Meningitis. Principles of diagnosis; advances in treatment. Postgrad Med 1986; 80:59–71.
10. Klein JO, Feigin RD, McCracken GH Jr. Report of the task force on diagnosis and management of meningitis. Pediatrics 1986; 78(Suppl):959–982.
11. Roos KL, Scheld WM. The management of fulminant meningitis in the intensive care unit. Infect Dis Clin North Am 1989; 3:137–154.
12. Kaplan SL. Recent advances in bacterial meningitis. Adv Pediatr Infect Dis 1989; 4:83–110.
13. Jacobs RF, Wright MW, Deskin RL, Bradsher RW. Delayed sterilization of *Haemophilus influenzae* type b meningitis with twice-daily ceftriaxone. JAMA 1988; 259:392–394.
14. Marks WA, Stutman HR, Marks MI, Abramson JS, et al. Cefuroxime versus ampicillin plus chloramphenicol in childhood bacterial meningitis: a multicenter randomized controlled trial. J Pediatr 1986; 109:123–130.
15. Shapiro ED. Prophylaxis for bacterial meningitis. Med Clin North Am 1985; 69:269–280.
16. American Academy of Pediatrics Committee on Infectious Diseases. Revision of recommendation for use of rifampin prophylaxis of contacts of patients with *Haemophilus influenzae* infection. Pediatrics 1984; 74:301–302.
17. Schwartz B, Al-Tobaiqi A, Al-Ruwais A, et al. Comparative efficacy of ceftriaxone and rifampicin in eradicating pharyngeal carriage of group A *Neisseria meningitidis*. Lancet 1988; 1:1239–1242.
18. Dorsky DI, Crumpacker CS. Drugs five years later: acyclovir. Ann Intern Med 1987; 107:859–874.
19. Lebel MH, Freij BJ, Syrogiannopoulos GA, et al. Dexamethasone therapy for bacterial meningitis. Results of two double-blind, placebo-controlled trials. N Engl J Med 1988; 319:964–971.
20. VanLandingham KE, Marsteller HB, Ross GW, Hayden FG. Relapse of herpes simplex encephalitis after conventional acyclovir therapy. JAMA 1988; 259:1051–1053.
21. Wasiewski WW, Fishman MA. Herpes simplex encephalitis: the brain biopsy controversy. J Pediatr 1988; 113:575–578.
22. Gabuzda DH, Hirsch MS. Neurologic manifestations of infection with human immunodeficiency virus. Clinical features and pathogenesis. Ann Intern Med 1987; 107:383–391.
23. Rosenblum JL, Levy RM, Bredesen DE (eds). AIDS and the Nervous System. New York: Raven Press, 1988.
24. Price RW, Brew B. Management of the neurologic complications of HIV infection and AIDS. Infect Dis Clin North Am 1988; 2:359–372.
25. Glatt AE, Chirgwin K, Landesman SH. Treatment of infections associated with human immunodeficiency virus. N Engl J Med 1988; 318:1439–1448.

Multiple sclerosis

Jack C. Sipe

■ Background

Multiple sclerosis (MS) is the most common demyelinating disease of the central nervous system (CNS) in North America and in most temperate climates of the world.[1] This disease is characterized by multifocal destruction of normally formed myelin sheaths of the nerve fibers and relative preservation of CNS axons.[2] Estimates of the MS prevalence rate in the United States are about 60/100,000, compared with 500/100,000 for seizure disorders, 200/100,000 for Parkinson's disease, and 60/100,000 for cerebral palsy.[3] Women are affected more frequently than men, in a ratio of about 1.8 to 1.

At least three clinical forms of the disease are generally recognized. Most often MS is characterized by recurrent exacerbations and remissions of neurologic symptoms, known as the exacerbating/remitting (E/R) form. A more malignant form, manifested by recurrent exacerbations without significant recovery and a progressive downhill course, has been termed the exacerbating/progressive (E/P) form. There is also a relatively benign type with gradual, at times almost imperceptible, worsening that may result in slow accumulation of neurologic symptoms, termed the chronic progressive (CP) form. Some patients may exhibit features of more than one of these clinical forms, and a single patient may evolve from the E/R to CP types over several years of active disease. Benign forms of MS are encountered, in which few mild attacks or exacerbations are widely separated in time, with little or no accumulated disability.

Specific neurologic symptoms are clearly related to the location, size, number, and severity of MS lesions in the CNS. The initial symptoms may vary considerably from one person to another and even from one exacerbation to another in the same patient. The most frequent initial symptoms include visual loss due to optic neuritis, sensory loss, ataxia, diplopia, weakness, clumsiness, slurred speech, and bladder dysfunction. More chronic symptoms are extreme fatigue, spasticity, extremity spasms, disorders of mood and thought, pain syndromes, infrequent seizures, and impairment of autonomic activity, including sexual function. The transient and occasionally bizarre nature of the neurologic symptoms may be mistaken for a psychiatric disorder.

Despite persistent activity, MS rarely leads to a premature death. However, the physical and emotional problems associated with MS are substantial. This is largely a result of onset of disease during the most productive adult years—the twenties or thirties—and the tendency for accumulated neurologic symptoms to result in disability, despair, and depression. The clinical course of any MS patient is completely unpredictable, and there is presently no curative treatment. In the following sections we shall review briefly the current knowledge of the basic mechanisms of MS and the scientific rationale for the management of this difficult medical problem.

■ EPIDEMIOLOGY AND GENETIC FACTORS

Decades of epidemiologic study and contemporary genetic studies of MS have revealed some consistent features.[4,5] In general, the prevalence of MS increases with progression to more Northern and Southern latitudes. Thus, the prevalance rate of MS in the Southern United States is about 15/100,000 and rises to over 100/100,000 in the Northern tier of states. In Canada, the MS prevalence reaches 130/100,000. The lowest risk areas of the world are generally located within 40 degrees of the Equator, such as Central America, Israel, Africa, and Northern Australia. Evidence from migration studies suggests that MS may begin in childhood or adolescence, remain quiescent, and then appear in early to mid-adulthood. This can be seen in persons who migrate from high prevalence zones to low prevalence regions after the age of 15 years. The emigrants may retain the high prevalence of MS typically seen in their region of birth. Migration in childhood from a low to a high prevalence area may be followed by an increased risk of developing MS. These observations have been interpreted as suggesting an environmental agent or cause for MS.

It is also clear that genetic susceptibility to MS can be found in a number of racial or ethnic groups, some of which have a very low incidence of the disease, as contrasted with the high incidence in the white Northern European population and its descendants. In the past decade, studies searching for genetic markers of MS have demonstrated certain patterns of human lymphocyte antigens (HLA) that are distinctly different in persons free from MS. Patients with MS have a higher than normal presence of HLA A3, B7, and Dw2 (DR2).[6] Because the prevalence of Dw2 antigen is about 70 per cent in MS patients versus 16 per cent in the normal population, the gene for susceptibility to MS may reside close to the Dw2 gene locus.[3] Familial instances of MS are not frequent but occur significantly often enough to determine that siblings of MS patients may have a 10 to 15 times greater risk of developing MS than the general population. Taken together, the genetic observations and epidemiologic data suggest an inherited susceptibility to MS, possibly triggered by exposure to an environmental agent or factor.

■ PATHOPHYSIOLOGY OF MS

The neuropathology of MS was described in 1835 by the prominent French neurologist Charcot. He termed the multiple scarred focal lesions in the brain and spinal cord *"sclerose en plaques,"* from which multiple sclerosis derives its name. Despite over 150 years of research, the pathogenesis of MS remains unknown. However, contemporary studies have revealed several important features of the disease.[7] The earliest feature of the MS lesion is focal perivascular inflammation and demyelination, termed *plaques.*

Inflammation results from transvascular migration of activated lymphocytes, typically T4 helper cells, and produces perivascular mononuclear cell infiltration and edema. Subsequent active myelin breakdown is produced by macrophages that strip the leaves of myelin from the CNS axons, resulting in phagocytosis of myelin debris. Lesions may progress to active remyelination by oligodendrocytes after disappearance of inflammation or may evolve to proliferation of astrocytes and scarring in zones of more persistent or repeated demyelination.[8]

CNS conduction failure or inhibition may occur as a result of edema and segmental demyelination of otherwise functional axons. Axonal destruction may occur in larger lesions with severe or persistent inflammation. Other factors impairing conduction may include myelin basic protein released during demyelination, the presence of lymphokines released by activated T cells, antibodies against ion channels, and elevated body temperature that can lower the "safety factor" for saltatory conduction.[3]

■ DIAGNOSIS OF MS

The clinical history, examination, and documentation of neurologic abnormalities remain the basis for the diagnosis of MS, since there is no specific laboratory indicator of disease activity.[9] Poser and associates[10] proposed the following generally accepted diagnostic criteria for MS:

A. Clinically Definite MS (CDMS)
   1. Two attacks and clinical evidence of two separate lesions, or
   2. Two attacks; clinical evidence of one lesion and paraclinical (laboratory tests, i.e., evoked responses, imaging studies) evidence of another separate lesion.
B. Laboratory-Supported Definite MS (LSDMS). The demonstration of spinal fluid IgG oligoclonal bands (OB) or of increased CNS synthesis of IgG. OB must not be present in patient serum, and the serum IgG level must be normal. Other diseases causing CSF changes must be excluded (i.e., syphilis, subacute sclerosing panencephalitis, sarcoid, collagen vascular diseases, Lyme disease, and others).

1. Two attacks; either clinical or paraclinical evidence of two separate lesions and CSF IgG oligoclonal bands.

C. Clinically Probable MS (CPMS)
   1. Two attacks and clinical evidence of one lesion.
   2. One attack and clinical evidence of two separate lesions.
   3. One attack, clinical evidence of one lesion, and paraclinical evidence of another separate lesion.

According to these criteria, the diagnosis of MS cannot be made on the basis of a single attack or on the basis of historical information and subjective complaints alone. Care must be taken to investigate thoroughly each patient suspected of having MS and to exclude other neurologic diseases that may mimic MS. Although the clinical criteria continue to be the generally accepted basis for the diagnosis of MS, recent application of magnetic resonance imaging (MRI) to the problem has improved both the accuracy and the specificity of neurodiagnostic testing.[11] MRI is quite sensitive for visualization of the CNS lesions of MS, and it has become the primary imaging procedure. Serial studies of immune function in a small group of MS patients have shown that changes in immune function correlate with disease activity as demonstrated by MRI.[12] By utilizing gadolinium intravenous contrast enhancement, it appears possible to distinguish between active or acute CNS plaques and chronic or quiescent plaques.[13] MRI is particularly useful in establishing paraclinical evidence of multiple separate lesions, thereby confirming probable or definite MS and excluding other conditions that may simulate MS. Aside from excluding some diseases that may mimic MS, computed tomographic (CT) brain scans appear to be of limited usefulness in the evaluation of patients suspected of having this disease.

Other neurodiagnostic studies are helpful in supporting or confirming the clinical diagnosis of MS. Evoked-response studies are sensitive, noninvasive diagnostic procedures for evaluating the visual system (visual evoked-response, or VER), brain stem auditory system (brain stem auditory evoked-response, or BAER), and somatosensory system (somatosensory evoked-response, or SER). Approximately 80 to 90 per cent of patients with clinically definite MS will have at least one abnormal evoked-response if all three tests are performed.[14] The cerebrospinal fluid examination is often useful, although the abnormalities typically seen in MS are not specific for the disease but rather are complementary and provide laboratory support for the diagnosis. The CSF in MS may demonstrate a modest increase in mononuclear cells and generally normal total protein, but elevated levels of IgG synthesized within the brain and IgG oligoclonal bands on electrophoresis of concentrated CSF. The CSF abnormalities may be present in up to 80 to 85 per cent of clinically definite MS patients.

The differential diagnosis of MS must be considered in every patient suspected of having the disease. The most common conditions that may simulate MS include systemic lupus erythematosus (SLE); cervical spondylosis with cervical cord compression; syringomyelia; neoplasms of the brain and spinal cord; cobalamin (vitamin B_{12}) deficiency; infectious, postinfectious, or postvaccinal encephalomyelitis; meningovascular syphilis; CNS Lyme disease; Behçet's syndrome; familial ataxias and paraplegias; subacute sclerosing panencephalitis (SSPE); progressive multifocal leukoencephalopathy (PML); and human immunodeficiency virus (HIV) infection. Patients suspected of having MS should be referred to a neurologist early in the course of the symptoms for diagnostic evaluation and confirmation of the diagnosis.

■ SCIENTIFIC BASIS FOR THERAPY

The scientific basis for many of the treatments currently under trial in MS is provided by basic research in the neuropathology of the CNS lesions and the factors that seem to contribute to the development of these lesions. Four important elements lend themselves to therapeutic intervention in MS: (1) transvascular migration of activated lymphocytes and the development of perivascular mononuclear cell inflammation and edema; (2) destruction of myelin and occasionally of other tissue elements by infiltrating macrophages; (3) astrocyte proliferation and scarring after repeated or prolonged tissue damage; and (4) impaired conduction of CNS impulses resulting from demyelination, edema, and scar formation.[15]

A reproducible experimental model of CNS demyelination has been developed in the form of chronic relapsing experimental autoimmune encephalomyelitis (EAE), but there is no spontaneously occurring disease resembling MS in experimental animals. EAE produces lesions with most of the features regarded as pathognomonic for MS and can be induced in genetically susceptible animals by immunization with myelin components.[16] This disorder is linked to immune-response genes and appears to involve a failure of immune regulation at the level of the suppressor T lymphocytes.

Current research studies in humans indicate that MS is an immunologically mediated disease.[17,18] Susceptibility appears linked to genes in the D (DR) region of the major histocompatibility complex (MHC) in which T cell–mediated regulation of immune responses is encoded.[6] Patients with active MS have low levels of suppressor T-cell function and numbers of T cells, as measured by functional assays and monoclonal antibodies. There is evidence of polyclonal B-cell stimulation with intrablood-brain barrier synthesis of immunoglobulins and the appearance of IgG oligoclonal bands in the spinal fluid. It is thought that the chronic character of MS may result from a genetically determined abnormality of T-cell regulatory function, perhaps a failure of suppressor T cells to turn off the immune response directed against CNS myelin antigens.[18] The critical difference, therefore, between MS and other CNS demyelinating diseases is its chronic character, often progressive, determined by immune dysregulation. Much of the current thinking today holds that MS will likely prove to be an autoimmune disorder, possibly triggered by an infectious event.

Despite decades of research, the molecular or biochemical basis for MS remains unknown. In the absence of a basic understanding of the disease, a rational therapy cannot be devised. At present, the treatments available are necessarily nonspecific and are directed against the immune response that seems to mediate or produce the disease.

■ Management

Therapeutic efforts in multiple sclerosis may be separated into three categories: (1) treatment designed to modify the disease course; (2) symptomatic treatment of MS and management of medical complications; and (3) management of associated personal and psychosocial problems.

■ TREATMENT OF THE DISEASE COURSE IN MS

Currently no effective, scientifically established treatment can alter the disease course satisfactorily or be safely administered over the long term to prevent disease progression. In other words, there is no curative treatment. However, several treatments have shown some degree of promise and are under investigation or in clinical use.

Anti-inflammatory Drugs. The best-known and best-studied drug in this category is adrenocorticotropic hormone (ACTH). ACTH (Table 1) has been used in doses of 80 to 100 IU daily for 7 to 10 days, given by the intravenous or intramuscular route, but the bioactivity of ACTH may be somewhat unpredictable.[19] ACTH has been found to hasten the return of vision in patients with optic neuritis and may be particularly effective in the treatment of MS exacerbations.[20]

Synthetic adrenocorticosteroids, such as prednisone, methylprednisolone, and dexamethasone have been used to treat ambulatory patients during MS exacerbations (Table 1). Prednisone is typically given in a dose of 60 to 120 mg/day in four divided doses for 2 to 6 weeks for clinically definite acute exacerbations.[21] Dexamethasone has been advocated in a dose of 16 mg/day in four divided doses for 2 to 6 weeks.[22] Some investigators report that oral corticosteroids are less beneficial than ACTH, but oral preparations are more convenient in ambulatory patients. Because of the high frequency of corticosteroid side effects, each MS patient should have a pretreatment examination to screen for tuberculosis, diabetes, hypertension, peptic ulcer disease, and electrolyte disturbances, which may be contraindications to therapy. During treatment, weight, blood pressure, and fluid retention should be evaluated regularly. A high-potassium, low-sodium diet is advised. The most frequent limiting side effects include exacerbation of pre-existent euphoria or depression, emotional lability, insomnia, and occasional frank psychosis or mania. High-dose methylprednisolone, 0.5 gm given as an

TABLE 1. Suggested Drug Therapy of Acute MS Exacerbations

Generic Drug	Brand Name	Dose	Precautions	Preparation
ACTH (aqueous)	ACTHAR	80–120 U/day for 7–10 days	Edema, hypokalemia, hypertension, gastric irritation/hemorrhage, anxiety/depression. Taper to zero	Intravenous
ACTH (gel)	ACTHAR Gel	80 U/day for 2–6 weeks	Same as ACTH	Intramuscular
Prednisone	Prednisone	60–120 mg/day for 2–6 weeks	Same as ACTH	Oral
Methylprednisolone sodium succinate	Solu-Medrol	0.5 gm/day for 5–7 days	Same as ACTH	Intravenous
Dexamethasone	Decadron	16 mg/day for 2–6 weeks	Same as ACTH	Oral

intravenous solution over 1 hour daily for 5 days, was effective in improving disability scores in a recent double-blind placebo-controlled trial.[23] Primary side effects of methylprednisolone are facial flushing, transient ankle edema, and a metallic taste in the mouth.[24] With all forms of adrenocorticosteroids, the risk of major complications such as perforating ulcer or avascular bone necrosis appears to be related to the duration of treatment rather than to the dose.[25] Thus, many neurologists recommend only short-term (2 to 6 weeks) intravenous or oral corticosteroid treatment for clinically definite or disabling exacerbations. The risks of intraspinal injection of methylprednisolone acetate (Depo-Medrol) have recently been reviewed,[26] and this mode of therapy currently is not being advised.

Immunosuppressive Treatments. The immunotherapy of MS has been extensively reviewed,[27,28] and Supplement 2 to *Neurol-*ogy, Volume 38, Number 7, 1988, contains the rationale for current immunomodulating therapies in MS. In general, ACTH and corticosteroids are used by clinicians to treat acute MS exacerbations.

Several treatments have been proposed recently in an attempt to halt the progressive phase of MS. These treatments include nonspecific or pan-immunosuppression (Table 2), removal of T helper/inducer cells, manipulation of activated T cells, alteration of lymphocyte traffic into the CNS, removal by plasma exchange of serum factors or cells, and manipulation of antigen-specific cells.[27,28]

Immunosuppression by azathioprine, a purine antagonist, has been tested in several clinical trials either alone or in combination with other drugs.[29–31] Controlled trials of azathioprine have suggested some benefit in progressive MS, but the effect is not dramatic and does not appear to influence the

TABLE 2. Possible Immunosuppressive Regimens for Progressive MS

Generic Drug	Brand Name	Dose	Precautions	Preparation
Cyclophosphamide	Cytoxan	0.5 gm IV/day in 4 doses. May use with ACTH (see Table 1)	Discontinue when WBC falls to 4000/mm³, or if hematuria, major infection	Intravenous
Azathioprine	Imuran	50–200 mg/day	Lower WBC, below 4000/mm³. Discontinue if leukopenia below 2000/mm³, thrombocytopenia, or hepatotoxicity	Oral
Cyclosporine A	Sandimmune	2.5–5 mg/kg/day	Discontinue if creatinine clearance falls below 80% of normal or if marrow suppression	Oral

long-term course of the disease. Cyclophosphamide, an alkylating agent, has been reported to be of benefit in reducing both the severity of symptoms and arresting progression in MS for up to 6 months.[32-34] However, relapses occurred in all patients treated with cyclophosphamide within 24 months of therapy, and the drug has produced significant undesirable side effects in some patients receiving chemotherapy. The long-term risks for the development of secondary neoplasms in patients treated with immunosuppression are unknown. Total lymphoid irradiation[35] has been said to arrest progression in MS for 1 year or more, but again the long-term risks are unknown. Cyclosporine, a metabolite isolated from fungi, has been used for immunosuppression in organ transplantation and recently in progressive MS.[36,37] But cyclosporine has a low therapeutic index, so that low doses are not effective, and therapeutic doses are associated with significant toxicity.[38] In addition, the disease may relapse when cyclosporine is stopped.

Plasmapheresis and lymphocytapheresis have been carried out in MS patients but to date there is no clear evidence of sustained clinical benefit.[39,40] Monoclonal antibodies directed against specific T-cell subsets has been tried in MS,[41] but the primary obstacle to long-term treatment has been the development of human antimonoclonal antibodies.[42]

Interferon. The rationale for the use of interferon in MS relates to its effect against viruses and natural killer cell activity. Clinical trials of interferon, especially alpha-interferon, have been reviewed.[43] Patients with the strictly exacerbating-remitting type of MS showed a reduction in the frequency and severity of exacerbations with systemic natural alpha-inferon, but those with progressive MS did not benefit.[44] Gamma-interferon treatment has been reported to cause a worsening of MS symptoms and is not currently advocated.[45]

Myelin Antigens and Vaccines. Myelin basic protein (MBP) has been used to treat MS based on effects against EAE in experimental animals, but in one careful clinical trial, MBP failed to alter the disease course.[46] Copolymer I is a synthetic amino acid polymer resembling the structure of MBP. In a small controlled trial of exacerbating-remitting MS, a decrease in the exacerbation frequency and progression were reported,[47] but

confirmation must await further clinical trials. Treatments with proteolipid protein of CNS myelin and T-cell vaccines are being considered for future clinical studies.

Other Therapeutic Claims. A number of proposed treatments have been advanced in the past quarter century, but most of them have met with little or no success. They have included various diets, megavitamin and ascorbic acid (vitamin C) treatment, vitamin B_{12} injections, and various calcium compounds. No scientific evidence has been marshalled to support the use of antifungal agents in MS, such as nystatin or broad-spectrum antibotics. Feeding of immune bovine colostrum has been advocated, but clinical trials were not placebo-controlled. Various circulatory agents, such as heparin, dicumarol, Hydergine, histamine, and clofibrate, are unproved, and vascular surgery for straightening the vertebral arteries is of doubtful benefit in MS. Some recent proposed treatments for which there is no clear scientific proof include hyperbaric oxygen therapy. dimethylsulfoxide (DMSO), snake venom, superoxide dismutase, removal of mercury-based dental fillings and transcutaneous neurostimulation.

For each MS patient, the treatment regimen, dose, duration, and follow-up should be selected only after a complete medical evaluation, usually in consultation with a neurologist. Factors such as age, general health, associated medical conditions, drug allergies and sensitivities, and response to previous treatment need to be considered before recommending a specific therapy. MS patients should be educated about the significant risks and side effects of the anti-inflammatory and immunosuppressive treatments as well as their benefits and the alternatives.

■ SYMPTOMATIC TREATMENT OF MS AND MANAGEMENT OF COMPLICATIONS

The quality of daily life for the MS patient can be significantly improved by effective management of symptoms and complications (Fig. 1). The following is a brief overview of presently available treatments.

Bladder Dysfunction. This is a common and disabling symptom that may present as urinary retention, incontinence, or a combination of both. Simple time-contingent

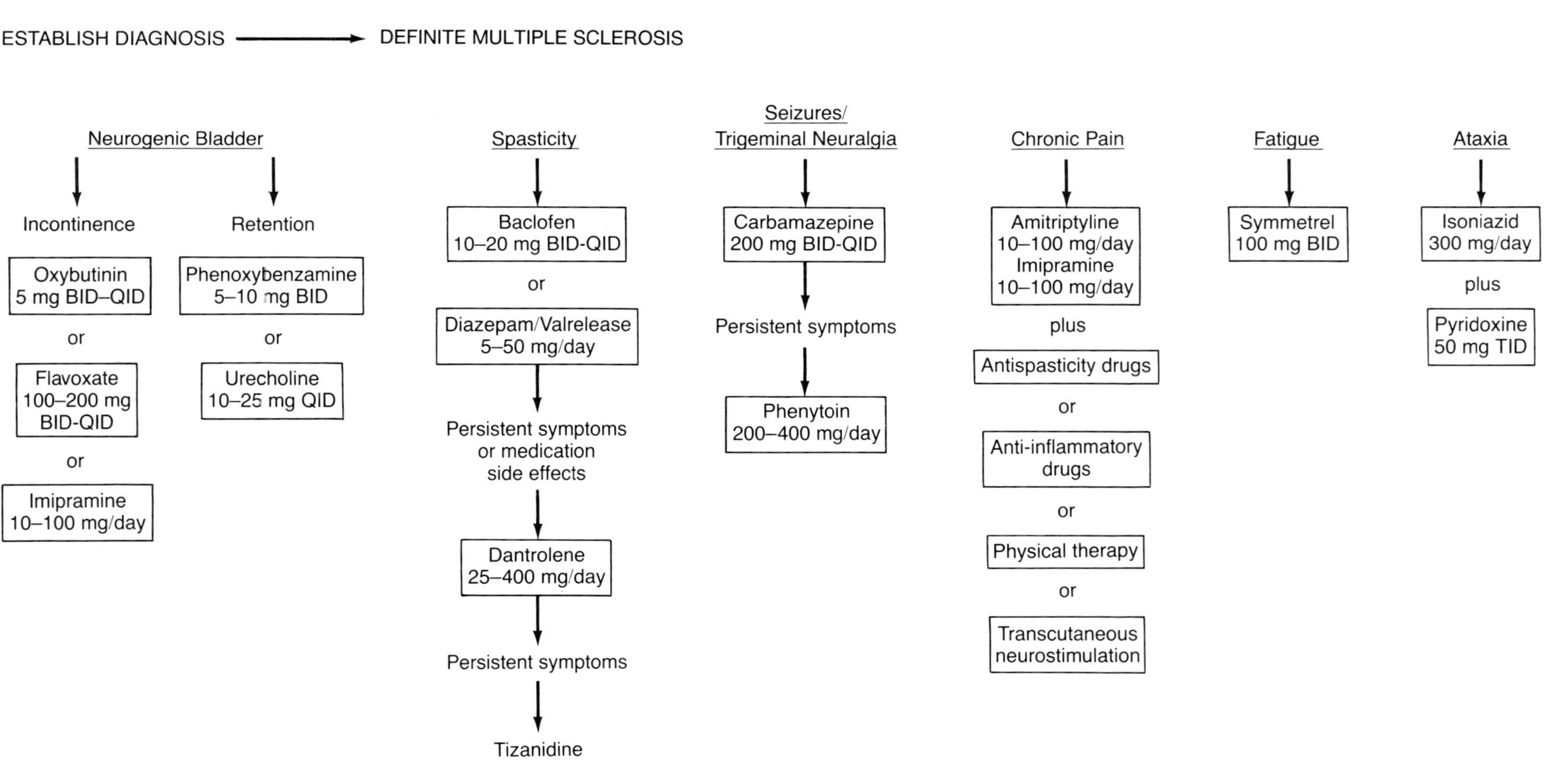

Figure 1. Management of MS symptoms and complications.

voiding, for example voiding every 2 hours, may be effective management for urinary urgency and occasional accidental incontinence. Fluid restriction and small doses of oxybutinin chloride (Ditropan) or flavoxate hydrochloride (Urispas) may relieve urgency, dysuria, frequency, and incontinence. In patients with functional obstruction at the bladder neck and incomplete emptying of the bladder, phenoxybenzamine (Dibenzyline, 5 to 10 mg BID) may be of value, and weak detrusor contractions may be augmented with bethanechol (Urecholine, 10 to 25 mg QID). Urologic evaluation may be required in cases of persistent incontinence, recurrent infections, or urinary retention. Indwelling catheters should be avoided because of the nearly inevitable complicating infections. Intermittent self-catheterization combined with drugs such as oxybutinin can be managed by patients with preserved strength and coordination in the hands.

Spasticity. Painful involuntary spasms and chronic spasticity can be alleviated in most cases with drug therapy. Baclofen (Lioresal) given 30 to 100 mg/day in divided doses, may be beneficial in reducing spasticity. Dantrolene sodium (Dantrium) is an alternative drug that has potential hepatotoxicity and offers no clear advantage over baclofen. A new drug, tizanidine, has recently been studied in clinical trials.[48] Diazepam, including the sustained release preparation (Valrelease), is useful in some patients who do not tolerate other antispasticity drugs, but unacceptable sedation is the major limiting side effect. Given at bedtime, diazepam may be helpful in preventing painful nocturnal flexor spasms of the extremities. Thyrotropin-releasing hormone (TRH) is being investigated as a potential antispasticity agent. It should be borne in mind that reducing spasticity, especially in the lower extremities, may be accompanied by increased weakness and difficulty in walking, since some patients unconsciously rely on increased muscular tone and spasticity to support the body weight. A marked increase in weakness or loss of ambulation may necessitate lowering the dose or discontinuing the antispasticity drug.

Ataxia. Isonicotinic acid hydrazide (INH) has been reported to be of limited benefit for disabling incoordination and ataxia. Clonazepam may be useful but has not been tested in a controlled trial.

Gait Difficulty. This can be the result of combined weakness, ataxia, and spasticity. In some instances, customized light-weight plastic leg braces may be beneficial in assisting the ability to walk, especially in the presence of footdrop. Crutches and canes are often used by patients with progressive ambulation difficulty.

Pain. Pain syndromes are more common in MS than previously thought, and treatment strategies for dealing with both acute and chronic pain syndromes have recently been reviewed.[49] Acute pain in MS may be related to active demyelination; syndromes such as trigeminal neuralgia, Lhermitte symptoms, or tonic seizures have been found to respond well to carbamazepine (Tegretol) in therapeutic doses. Chronic pain in MS is a difficult problem and has been managed with tricyclic antidepressant drugs, nonsteroidal anti-inflammatory drugs, physical therapy, antispasticity drugs and transcutaneous neurostimulation.

Fatigue. Extreme fatigue and energy loss are quite common in MS and may reflect the malaise of chronically active autoimmune disease. Amantadine (Symmetrel, 100 mg BID), an antiviral drug, has been claimed to be effective in improving fatigue and lassitude. Tricyclic antidepressant drugs and the newer fluoxetine (Prozac) may be used to treat associated depression and loss of energy.

Potential Complications. Every effort should be made to prevent major medical complications in the course of MS. These may include infections of the urinary tract or pulmonary system, limb contractures, and decubitus ulcers. Patients who are bedridden or wheelchair-bound need a daily program to prevent pressure sores and contractures. This usually involves physical therapy exercises, changing position every 2 to 3 hours, and maintenance of cleanliness and hygiene. At the first sign of a decubitus ulcer, specific treatment should be instituted and nursing efforts intensified.

■ MANAGEMENT OF ASSOCIATED PROBLEMS

A wide spectrum of psychosocial and personal difficulties may occur as a result of MS. These include marital, financial, occupational, legal, psychosexual, and disability problems. Most physicians will require the assistance of other professionals, such as social workers, psychologists, marriage counselors, vocational rehabilitation counselors, and lawyers; other MS patients in the form of support groups also may be helpful. The National Multiple Sclerosis Society provides broad-based support in the areas of research, dissemination of information, and psychosocial services to combat some of the many problems related to MS.

Issues and Risks

DIFFICULTIES IN EVALUATING MS TREATMENTS

Several factors combine to make assessment of treatments difficult in MS. Because there are no easily recognized treatments that completely arrest exacerbations and progression, the less pronounced effects of treatment can be ascertained only by carefully controlled clinical studies using adequate numbers of MS patients. In this disease, there is a well-known tendency for patients to improve with any treatment, even placebo treatments. The strong placebo effect means that clinical studies of MS need to be double-blind and placebo-controlled, preferably with a cross-over design, so that all partcipants may be evaluated on both placebo and treatment modalities. Unfortunately, few of the proposed treatments in the past quarter century have been so rigorously tested. In evaluating potential new treatments, care should be taken to assure that the studies are scientifically sound and controlled for observer and patient bias.

WHEN TO TREAT MS

Assuming the presence of some forms of therapy that are scientifically proved to be beneficial, the decision about when to treat an individual MS patient becomes important. Clearly this needs to be a joint patient and physician decision, with the patient well-informed of the potential benefits, risks, side effects, and alternative forms of treatment. The patient should know that along with the characteristic exacerbations often come spontaneous remissions, and in some patients remissions are maintained for relatively long periods of time. In general, most MS patients decide to take some form of corticosteroid treatment during clear-cut acute exacerbations in an attempt to shorten the duration, hasten recovery, and prevent long-term complications. For patients with the progressive forms of MS, the decision to begin treatment with one of the immunosuppressive drugs is a calculated risk and may be taken in cases of rapid deterioration of neurologic function. Pregnancy for women of child-bearing age is also a risk factor in MS. The risk of exacerbation during pregnancy is not significantly higher than that of nonpregnancy, but one study found a significantly higher exacerbation rate in the first 6 months to 1 year postpartum.[50] This fact, coupled with a potentially progressive neurologic disease during the years of motherhood, should be carefully considered by any woman with MS who contemplates pregnancy.

RISKS OF IMMUNOSUPPRESSIVE TREATMENT

Long-term treatment (more than 6 weeks) with corticosteroids has not been proved effective and is almost always attended by the potential for major side effects, including aseptic necrosis of the femoral or humeral heads, peptic ulcer disease, cataracts, osteopenia, opportunistic infections, and adrenal insufficiency. Experience with other forms of immunosuppressive therapy has shown similar long-term risks. Cyclophosphamide may produce nausea, vomiting, hemorrhagic cystitis, increased susceptibility to infection, and temporary alopecia. The appearance of tumors and sterility have been reported in some patients whose neoplasms have been treated with cyclophosphamide, but the long-term risks in MS are unknown. Azathioprine has been associated with marrow suppression, hepatotoxicity, and the risk of neoplasia with long-term treatment. In the case of cyclosporine, nephrotoxicity is a potentially serious problem, and other reversible effects may include hypertension, seizures, gum hypertrophy, arthralgias, and anemia. Plasmapheresis is costly and may be attended by volume depletion, hypocalcemia, and occasional bleeding.

■ WHEN TO INFORM THE PATIENT ABOUT A DIAGNOSIS OF MS

Most patients with MS suspect the correct diagnosis, but it is important to make a complete neurologic evaluation to exclude diseases that may simulate MS. In some instances of suspected MS, the extreme anxiety produced by a discussion of the disease may need to be avoided until the diagnosis is clinically proved and supported by laboratory studies. Since MS is a fluctuating disease, time and repeated clinical examinations may be required to finalize the diagnosis. When MS is clearly present and the diagnosis can be established with certainty, every effort should be made to educate the patient and family about the disease.

Finally, it should be said that the approach and attitude of the physician will have a powerful effect on the MS patient and family. An excessively negative or pessimistic view is unwarranted in view of the many possibilities available today for the management of MS and its symptoms. A positive, realistic approach tempered with kindness and hopefulness can greatly improve a patient's sense of well-being and avoid needless despair. Many patients are driven to popular or unproved treatments by negative attitudes of their physicians. Helplessness should be discouraged and cooperation between MS patients and physicians encouraged, since this partnership holds the promise of developing more effective treatments for the disease in the future.

REFERENCES

1. McAlpine D, Lumsden CE, Acheson ED. Multiple Sclerosis, A Reappraisal. Baltimore: Williams and Wilkins, 1972.
2. Adams RD, Victor M. Principles of Neurology. New York: McGraw-Hill, 1981:647.
3. Waksman BH, Reingold SC, Reynolds WE. Research on Multiple Sclerosis. New York: Demos Publications, 1987.
4. Kurtzke JF. Epidemiology of multiple sclerosis. In Hallpike JF, Adams CWM, Tourtellote WW (eds). Multiple Sclerosis. London: Chapman and Hall, 1983:47–95.
5. Stewart GJ, Kirk RL. The genetics of multiple sclerosis: the HLA system and other genetic markers. In Hallpike JF, Adams CWM, Tourtellote WW (eds). Multiple Sclerosis. London: Chapman and Hall, 1983:97–128.
6. Hauser SL, Fleischnick E, Weiner HL, et al. Extended major histocompatibility complex haplo-
types in patients with multiple sclerosis. Neurology 1989; 39:275–277.
7. Ebers GC. Multiple sclerosis and other demyelinating diseases. In Asbry AK, McKhann GM, McDonald WI (eds). Diseases of the Nervous System. Philadelphia: WB Saunders, 1986:1268–1281.
8. Waksman BH. Pathogenetic mechanisms in multiple sclerosis. Ann NY Acad Sci 1984; 436:125–129.
9. Poser CM, Alter M, Sibley WA, Scheinberg LC. Multiple sclerosis. In Rowland LP (ed). Merritt's Textbook of Neurology. Philadelphia: Lea and Febiger, 1984:593–611.
10. Poser CM, Paty DW, Scheinberg L, et al. New diagnostic criteria for multiple sclerosis: guidelines for research protocols. Ann Neurol 1983; 13:227–231.
11. Fazekas F, Offenbacher H, Fuch S, et al. Criteria for an increased specificity of MRI interpretation in elderly subjects with suspected multiple sclerosis. Neurology 1988; 38:1822–1825.
12. Oger J, Kostrukoff LF, Li DKB, Paty DW. Multiple sclerosis: in relapsing patients immune functions vary with disease activity as assessed by MRI. Neurology 1988; 38:1739–1744.
13. Grossman RI, Gonzalez-Scarano F, Atlas SW, Galetta S, Silberberg DH. Multiple sclerosis: gadolinium enhancement in MR imaging. Radiology 1986; 161:721–725.
14. Romine JS. Demyelinating disorders. In Wiederholt WD (ed). Neurology for Non-Neurologists. New York: Academic Press, 1982:205–217.
15. Waksman BH, Rationales of current therapies for multiple sclerosis. Arch Neurol 1983; 40:671–672.
16. Raine CS, Traugott U. Experimental autoimmune demyelination: chronic relapsing models and their therapeutic implications for multiple sclerosis. Ann NY Acad Sci 1984; 436:33–51.
17. Lisak RP. Overview of the rationale for immunomodulating therapies in multiple sclerosis. Neurology 1988; 38(Suppl 2):5–8.
18. Arnason BGW, Antel JP, Reder AT. Immunoregulation in multiple sclerosis. Ann NY Acad Sci 1984; 436:133–139.
19. Maider L, Summer K. Differing responses to synthetic ACTH. Neurology 1979; 22:1943.
20. Rose AS, Kuzma JW, Kurtzke JF, et al. Cooperative study in the evaluation of therapy in multiple sclerosis: ACTH vs. placebo. Final report. Neurology 1970; 20(No 5–Part 2):1–59.
21. Eadie JM, Tyrer JH. Neurological Clinical Pharmacology. Lancaster, England: MTP Press Ltd., International Medical Publishers, 1980.
22. Tourtellotte WW, Baumhefner RW, Potvin AR, et al. Multiple sclerosis; de novo CNS IgG synthesis: effect of ACTH and corticosteroids. Neurology 1980; 30:1155–1162.
23. Milligan NM, Newcombe R, Compston DAS. A double-blind controlled trial of high dose intravenous methylprednisolone in patients with multiple sclerosis. I. Clinical effects. J Neurol Neurosurg Psychiatry 1987; 50:511–516.
24. Lyons PR, Newman PK, Sanders M. Methylprednisolone therapy in multiple sclerosis: a profile of adverse effects. J Neurol Neurosurg Psychiatry 1988; 51:285–287.
25. Felson DT, Anderson JJ. A cross-study evaluation of association between steroid dose and bolus steroids and avascular necrosis of bone. Lancet 1987; 1:902–905.
26. Nelson DA. Dangers from methylprednisolone ace-

tate therapy by intraspinal injection. Arch Neurol 1988; 45:804–806.

27. Weiner HL, Hafler DA. Immunotherapy of multiple sclerosis. Ann Neurol 1988; 23:211–222.
28. Sipe JC. Immunotherapy in multiple sclerosis. West J Med 1987; 146:351–352.
29. Ellison GW, Myers LW, Mickey MC, Graves MC, Tourtellotte WW, Nuwer MR. Clinical experience with azathioprine: the pros. Neurology 1988; 38(Suppl 2):20–23.
30. Rosen JA. Prolonged azathioprine treatment of non-remitting multiple sclerosis. J Neurol Neurosurg Psychiatry 1979; 42:338–344.
31. Patzold U, Hecker H, Pocklington P. Azathioprine in the treatment of multiple sclerosis. J Neurol Sci 1982; 54:377–394.
32. Weiner HL, Hauser SL, Hafler DA, Fallis RJ, Lehrich JR, Dawson DM. The use of cyclophosphamide in the treatment of multiple sclerosis. Ann NY Acad Sci 1984; 436:373–381.
33. Carter JL, Hafler DA, Dawson DM, Orav J, Weiner HL. Immunosuppression with high-dose IV cyclophosphamide and ACTH in progressive multiple sclerosis: cumulative 6 year experience in 164 patients. Neurology 1988; 38(Suppl 2):9–14.
34. Goodkin DE, Plencer S, Palmer-Saxerud J, Teetzen M, Hertsgaard D. Cyclophosphamide in chronic progressive multiple sclerosis, maintenance vs. nonmaintenance therapy. Arch Neurol 1987; 44:823–827.
35. Cook SD, Troiano R, Zito G, et al. Effect of total lymphoid irradiation in chronic progressive multiple sclerosis. Lancet 1986; 1:1405–1409.
36. Dommasch D. Comparative clinical trial of cyclosporine in multiple sclerosis: The pros. Neurology 1988; 38(Suppl 2):28–29.
37. Kappos L, et al. Cyclosporine versus azathioprine in the long-term treatment of multiple sclerosis. Ann Neurol 1988; 23:56–63.
38. Rudge P. Cyclosporine and multiple sclerosis: The cons. Neurology 1988; 38(Suppl 2):29–30.
39. Tindall R. A closer look at plasmapheresis in multiple sclerosis: The cons. Neurology 1988; 38(Suppl 2):53–56.
40. Hauser SL, Fosburg M, Kevy SV, Weiner HL. Lymphocytapheresis in chronic progressive multiple sclerosis: immunological and clinical effects. Neurology 1984; 34:922–926.
41. Hafler DA, Weiner HL. Immunosuppression with monoclonal antibodies in multiple sclerosis. Neurology 1988; 38(Suppl 2):42–47.
42. Champlin RE. Treating multiple sclerosis with monoclonal antibodies: the cons. Neurology 1988; 38(Suppl 2): 47–49.
43. Knobler RL. Systemic interferon therapy of multiple sclerosis: the pros. Neurology 1988; 38(Suppl 2):58–61.
44. Knobler RL, Panitch HS, Braheny SL, Sipe JC, et al. Controlled trial of systemic alpha interferon in multiple sclerosis. Neurology 1984; 34:1273–1279.
45. Panitch HS, Hirsh RL, Haley AS, Johnson KP. Exacerbations of multiple sclerosis in patients treated with gamma interferon. Lancet 1987; 1:893–895.
46. Romine JS, Salk J. A study of myelin basic protein as a therapeutic probe in patients with multiple sclerosis. In Halpike JF, Adams CWM, Tourtellote WW (eds). Multiple Sclerosis. Baltimore: Williams and Wilkins, 1983:621–630.
47. Bornstein MB, Miller A, Slagle S, et al. A pilot trial of Cop 1 in exacerbating-remitting multiple sclerosis. N Engl J Med 1987; 317:408–414.
48. Bass B, Weinshenker B, Rice GPA, et al. Tizanidine versus baclofen in the treatment of spasticity in patients with multiple sclerosis. Can J Neurol Sci 1988; 15:15–19.
49. Moulin DE, Foley KM, Ebers GC. Pain syndrome in multiple sclerosis. Neurology 1988; 38:1830–1833.
50. Korn-Lubetzki I, Kahana E, Cooper G, Abramsiky O. Activity of multiple sclerosis during pregnancy and puerperium. Ann Neurol 1984; 16:229–231.

Myasthenia gravis

Laird Patterson ■ *John Ravits*

Myasthenia gravis is the most common disorder characterized by impaired transmission across the neuromuscular junction. In myasthenia, the impairment is caused by autoimmune destruction of the postsynaptic membrane and results in defective depolarization of the muscle fibers. There is now a detailed understanding of the pathophysiology of the disease, and its management generally reflects that understanding. There are two main categories of treatment: (1) enhancement of neuromuscular transmission utilizing cholinesterase inhibitors (ChI), and (2) immune system modulation by thymectomy, plasmapheresis, steroids, and nonsteroidal immunosuppressants.[1,2] Occasionally, myasthenic symptoms worsen precipitously, a state referred to as myasthenic crisis, and this requires special therapeutic considerations.

■ Background

The clinical manifestation of myasthenia gravis is muscle weakness. This involves any of the skeletal muscle groups: ocular (diplopia and ptosis), bulbar (dysarthria and dysphagia), respiratory (dyspnea), or limb muscles (proximal weakness). Myasthenic weakness has two unique characteristics. First, it is fatigable, meaning a true decrement of muscle power occurs with repeated effort. Second, there may be a marked variability in the degree of weakness; patients may have weeks or months during which they are relatively symptom-free, followed by equally long symptomatic periods. This variability may confuse the unwary physician and lead to mistakes in diagnosis.

Ten per cent of myasthenic patients are children, and the remainder are adults who tend to be young women or elderly men. Initial symptoms are ocular in 40 per cent, bulbar in 10 per cent, appendicular in 10 per cent, and generalized in 40 per cent of patients. Of those patients with initial isolated ocular involvement, the majority develop generalized disease, usually within the first year. Within the first 3 years, the patients progress to maximal weakness; half of all deaths occur in this time period. The prognosis of myasthenia has steadily improved as a result of better medical management. For example, between 1940 and 1960 the mortality from myasthenic crisis was 30 per cent, as compared with a more recent figure from 1980 to 3 per cent. With current treatment strategies, nearly 90 per cent of patients will either improve or stabilize.[3]

As mentioned, the fundamental abnormality in myasthenia gravis is autoimmune-mediated damage at the postsynaptic region of the neuromuscular junction. The exact immunopathogenesis of this attack is unknown, but clearly it involves the thymus gland and both humoral and cell-mediated immunity. In normal neuromuscular transmission, depolarization of the presynaptic nerve terminal releases acetylcholine into the neuromuscular junction. Acetylcholine diffuses across the junction and interacts with the acetylcholine receptor, which is embedded in a region of postsynaptic muscle fiber membrane called the end-plate zone. This interaction depolarizes the end-plate zone, propagating an action potential along the muscle fiber. In myasthenia gravis, damage to the acetylcholine receptor and end-plate zone compromises end-plate depolarization. If sufficient muscle fibers are not depolarized, muscle contractions will become weaker.

The diagnosis of myasthenia gravis ultimately is clinical. However, pharmacologic, serologic, and electrophysiologic testing has advanced to where the diagnosis can be established with certainty in the majority of patients. The short-acting ChI agent edrophonium (Tensilon) transiently increases junctional acetylcholine levels and thereby improves neuromuscular transmission. Since it may precipitate a crisis or produce nonspecific results, it is often not used or is used cautiously. The acetylcholine receptor antibody serology test is positive in the majority of patients with generalized myasthenia and roughly parallels the extent but not the degree of weakness. Since the antibody titer does not clearly reflect the clinical state, it should be used only as an ancillary measure when following response to therapy. The antistriated muscle antibody test is a less sensitive test for myasthenia than the acetylcholine receptor antibody test, but a positive result may indicate the presence of a thymoma. The electrophysiologic findings include a decremental response to repetitive motor nerve stimulation and abnormalities detected using a specialized technique known as single-fiber electromyography.

■ Management

■ ENHANCEMENT OF NEUROMUSCULAR TRANSMISSION

Therapy is often initiated with ChI medications in symptomatic patients.[2] These drugs inhibit hydrolysis of acetylcholine at the neuromuscular junction and increase its concentration at the synaptic cleft. Pyridostigmine (Mestinon) is the most commonly used drug. It has a short half-life of 2 to 4 hours and is given orally in doses of 30 to 90 mg every 4 to 6 hours, or more frequently if necessary. The dose and schedule are titrated according to the patient's response. Occasionally, higher doses are needed, but they may cause the side effects of increased salivation, abdominal cramping, and diarrhea. These muscarinic symptoms can be controlled with oral atropine, 0.2 to 0.4 mg three or four times a day. Large doses of ChI drugs also cause neuromuscular blockade and may aggravate rather than improve myasthenic symptoms. Long-acting preparations of pyridostigmine are available, and 90 to 180 mg at bedtime will often allow patients a comfortable night's sleep.

A parenteral preparation of pyridostigmine can be used if patients are unable to swallow or are not absorbing the drug. One milligram of the intramuscular or intravenous preparation is equivalent to 30 milligrams of the oral. Other ChI agents include neostigmine and ambenonium (Mytelase). These drugs are infrequently used, since pyridostigmine is a safer and more reliable medication.

It is important to recognize that ChI medications may have a differential effect on certain muscle groups. Ocular symptoms, for example, may be particularly refractory to treatment. Some patients experience excessive weakness due to relative overdosage of the drug in certain muscle groups, whereas other muscles remain relatively refractory, causing some confusion in determining the dosage for a particular individual.

■ IMMUNE SYSTEM MODULATION

Thymectomy

Total removal of the thymus gland has been demonstrated to be effective treatment for myasthenia gravis, and the procedure is now performed with negligible morbidity and mortality rates.[4,5] The sternotomy approach is generally employed. Patients between the ages of 10 and 60 years, or in some cases even those outside this range, who are in relatively good general health should be considered for surgery as soon as practical after the diagnosis of myasthenia gravis has been made. Plasmapheresis, ChI, and prednisone may be needed to stabilize patients preoperatively and to provide relief of symptoms in the postoperative period.

If thymectomy is used as primary treatment for generalized myasthenia, 80 to 90 per cent of the patients may improve, and 40 to 50 per cent will ultimately achieve remission over a 2- to 10-year period.[4] The best chance of remission is in young women, but all groups, even the elderly, show some benefit. A favorable response to thymectomy obviates other treatment regimens that may require more toxic medications. In addition, 10 to 15 per cent of myasthenic patients harbor a thymoma, and it is generally agreed that these should be removed.[4,5] Furthermore, once the diagnosis of myasthenia has been made, there is a future risk of developing a thymoma if thymectomy is not done.

The role of thymectomy for purely ocular myasthenia is still debated. Considering the safe nature of the procedure and the known potential for later progression of ocular myasthenia to generalized myasthenia, thymectomy is advocated as treatment for some cases of ocular myasthenia as well.[6]

Plasmapheresis

The efficacy of plasmapheresis as palliative therapy for severe myasthenia gravis is now recognized.[7] The mechanism of the beneficial effect of plasmapheresis is unknown, though removal of the acetylcholine receptor antibody is probably a factor. Acetylcholine receptor antibodies are noted to fall dramatically after plasmapheresis but often rebound to even higher levels in the following weeks.[7]

The exchange of 2 to 3 liters three times a week for five or six treatments will often relieve acute symptoms, accelerate weaning from a respirator, or help prepare selected patients for thymectomy. The duration of the plasmapheresis effect is only 3 to 6 weeks in most instances, but the concomitant use of prednisone and other immunosuppressants may sustain improvement.

Plasmapheresis is usually reserved for severely affected patients, including those with marked bulbar or respiratory symptoms before or after thymectomy, myasthenic patients in crisis, or those refractory to other forms of treatment. Intermittent or maintenance plasmapheresis in mild-to-moderately affected patients is rarely utilized because of the cost (approximately $1000 per treatment) and the potential, though infrequent, for complications of hypotension, bleeding, embolism, sepsis, and hypocalcemia.[7]

Corticosteroids

Prednisone is the most commonly used corticosteroid for treating myasthenia gravis.[8,9] It often benefits patients who fail to respond to pyridostigmine and thymectomy. Prednisone also can be used to supplement plasmapheresis or to maintain patients who for reasons of age or concomitant disease are not thymectomy candidates. In some instances, it may be used to help prepare patients for thymectomy if ChI medications or plasmapheresis is not effective.

Patients can be started on a daily high single dose of prednisone, 80 to 100 mg, which is maintained until improvement begins, usually within 3 to 9 months.[8] The patient is then gradually switched over to an alternate-day program, and the dose is slowly tapered to a maintenance level of 5 to 30 mg daily over a period of 4 to 6 months. Eighty per cent of myasthenic patients may achieve improvement, and 28 per cent of that group may enter a state of remission, although this often occurs when prednisone is used in combination with other medications or with thymectomy.[8] About 10 to 15 per cent of patients are nonresponders and will require other modes of therapy.[10] It is important to be aware that ChI requirements may decrease during steroid therapy, necessitating a reduction in dose or discontinuation.

Initial high doses of prednisone may precipitate rapid and marked worsening of myasthenic symptoms during the first 1 or 2 weeks of treatment. Because of this paradoxic response, induction of high-dose prednisone therapy should take place in a hospital setting.[10] The large doses are used in severe cases when a rapid response is desired, since most patients begin improvement within 1 to 4 weeks after starting treatment.[8,9]

An alternative regimen may be used in patients who do not require rapidly acting therapy, since it avoids the initial worsening seen with high-dose therapy. The low-dose program begins with 15 to 20 mg on a daily or alternate-day schedule and is increased by 5 to 10 mg every 2 or 3 doses. The ultimate dose requirement is determined by patient response, and it is only rarely that doses as high as 100 mg daily are necessary.

The medication is then tapered once a maximal response occurs.

Another regimen that avoids the potential exacerbation of symptoms during initiation of high-dose oral prednisone is pulse therapy with intravenous prednisolone. Two grams of prednisolone in 250 ml of normal saline is infused over 12 hours to minimize adverse reactions.[11] The infusion is repeated every 5 days for two more doses if there is no significant improvement.[11] Patients who respond are then managed on an alternate-day prednisone program. The rapidity of response of this program is equivalent to that of high-dose daily prednisone without the risk of worsening symptoms.

Chronic steroid therapy is associated with significant side effects. These have been reported in 35 per cent of myasthenic patients.[9] Complications, in addition to a cushingoid appearance and weight gain, include diabetes, hypertension, cataracts, steroid myopathy, compression fractures, and aseptic necrosis of the femur.[9] Alternate-day therapy usually decreases the incidence of side effects; fortunately, most patients can be switched to an alternate-day maintenance program or are eventually able to discontinue the drug.

Nonsteroidal Immunosuppressants

The only nonsteroidal medication that has received extensive use is azathioprine (Imuran). It has been used in Europe for many years and has become accepted as an adjunctive or alternative medication.[12,13] Azathioprine is often used in combination with thymectomy, prednisone, or plasmapheresis. An advantage of azathioprine is that it can be used in place of steroids. Some advocate use of the drug early in the course of myasthenia rather than as a last resort.

Azathioprine is given in doses of 1 to 3 mg/kg/day. The onset of improvement is slow in comparison with prednisone. Most patients show an initial therapeutic response after 3 to 12 months, with a continued improvement up to 24 or even 36 months.[12] Azathioprine will ameliorate symptoms in 80 to 90 per cent of patients and may induce a remission in as many as 40 per cent of patients, although most of these are likely to have had a thymectomy, steroid treatment, or both.[12,13]

Side effects occur in 35 per cent of those treated and may lead to discontinuation of therapy. The most serious of the adverse reactions are hematologic (18 per cent), gastrointestinal (13 per cent), and infectious (13 per cent).[14] Malignant tumors also have been reported during treatment with azathioprine, but a causal relationship has not been firmly established.[14]

The only other nonsteroidal immunosuppressant in use is cyclophosphamide (Cytoxan), but experience with it has been limited.[15] Doses of 1 to 2 mg/kg/day are used, and improvement rates of approximately 80 per cent compare favorably with other forms of treatment.[15] Side effects, however, are more common with cyclosphosphamide and limit its use. It does represent an alternative treatment for patients who fail to respond to or cannot tolerate other treatment modalities.

■ CRISIS

Marked, rapid exacerbation of myasthenic symptoms, including generalized weakness with bulbar and respiratory failure, is termed *crisis*. It can occur as the result of intercurrent infections, surgery, response to medications, or with either the induction or withdrawal of steroid treatment. Cholinergic crisis is equally serious and is precipitated by the overuse of ChI therapy.

Management begins with intubation to provide adequate ventilation, if necessary. Identification and treatment of possible precipitating factors can then proceed. ChI drugs should be withheld until their role in the crisis is clarified. Steroid therapy, if recently begun, should be continued as the patient usually will improve, even though the initial crisis may have been precipitated by the steroid therapy.

Plasmapheresis usually provides the most reliable treatment in crisis, and responses are often favorable after three or four exchanges. Some patients require as many as a dozen exchanges, however, before improvement begins. ChI therapy should be instituted or resumed cautiously, using 1- to 2-mg doses of intravenous pyridostigmine every 3 to 4 hours while respiratory and bulbar function are carefully monitored.

■ Issues and Risks

Myasthenia remains an enigmatic disease despite advances in the understanding of its pathophysiology. It has a relapsing-remitting natural history, making response to treatment sometimes difficult to evaluate. Clearly, treatment that produces the fewest long-term side effects and that may lead to remission is preferable. Currently, the use of ChI medications, plasmapheresis, and early thymectomy is the preferred treatment program. Prednisone and other nonsteroidal immunosuppressants should be used if other measures fail but for as short a period as possible to minimize adverse effects.

Certain drugs should be avoided in patients with myasthenia gravis, since they may complicate treatment or precipitate a crisis.[16] Penicillamine may cause a myasthenic syndrome and should not be used in patients with overt disease. Quinine, quinidine, procainamide, and beta-blockers are known to aggravate myasthenic weakness. Certain antibiotics, such as the aminoglycosides, may cause neuromuscular blockade, as can the muscle relaxants curare and succinylcholine. Hypnotics and sedatives should be used cautiously in symptomatic patients as they may further depress respiratory and bulbar function. Psychotropic agents, including lithium, tricyclic antidepressants, and phenothiazines, have been reported to unmask or aggravate myasthenic symptoms.

The physician must educate the myasthenic patient to anticipate possible exacerbation during periods of intense stress, with viral infections, or as a result of surgery or injury. If patients and physicians are aware of the potential for worsening of the myasthenic condition under these circumstances, crisis or severe and prolonged relapse may be avoided.

REFERENCES

1. Drachman DB. Present and future treatment of myasthenia gravis. N Engl J Med 1987; 316:743–745.
2. Dosterhuis HJGH. Long-term effects of treatment in 374 patients with myasthenia gravis. Monogr Allergy 1988; 15:75–85.

3. Grob D, Brunner NG, Namba T. The natural course of myasthenia gravis and effect of therapeutic measures. Ann NY Acad Sci 1981; 377:652.
4. Olanow CS, Wechsler AS, Sirotkin-Roses M, Stajich J, Roses AD. Thymectomy as primary therapy in myasthenia gravis. Ann NY Acad Sci 1987; 505:595–606.
5. Fischer JE, Grinvalski HT, Nussbaum MS, Sayers HJ, Cole RE, Samaha FJ. Aggressive surgical approach for drug-free remission from myasthenia gravis. Ann Surg 1987; 205:496–503.
6. Schumm F, Wiethölter H, Fateh-Moghadam A, Dichgans J. Thymectomy with pure ocular symptoms. J Neurol Neurosurg Psychiatry 1985; 48:332–337.
7. Seybold ME. Plasmapheresis in myasthenia gravis. Ann NY Acad Sci 1987; 505:584–587.
8. Johns TR. Long-term corticosteroid treatment of myasthenia gravis. Ann NY Acad Sci 1987; 505:568–583.
9. Sghirlanzoni A, Peluchetti D, Mantegazza R, Fiacchino F, Cornelio F. Myasthenia gravis: prolonged treatment with steroids. Neurology 1984; 34:170–174.
10. Pacuzzi RM, Coscett HB, Johns TR. Long-term corticosteroid treatment of myasthenia gravis: a report of 116 patients. Ann Neurol 1984; 15:291–298.
11. Arsura E, Brunner NG, Namba T, Grob D. High-dose intravenous methylprednisolone in myasthenia gravis. Arch Neurol 1985; 42:1149–1153.
12. Chatell G. Immunosuppressive drugs: azathioprine in the treatment of myasthenia gravis. Ann NY Acad Sci 1987; 505:588–594.
13. Witte AS, Cornblath DR, Parry GJ, Lisak RP, Shatz NS. Azathioprine in the treatment of myasthenia gravis. Ann Neurol 1984; 15:602–605.
14. Hohlfeld R, Michels M, Heininger K, Besinger U, Toyka KV. Azathioprine toxicity during long-term immunosuppression of generalized myasthenia gravis. Neurology 1988; 38:258–261.
15. Niakan E, Harati Y, Rolak LA. Immunosuppressive drug therapy in myasthenia gravis. Arch Neurol 1986; 43:155–156.
16. Argov Z, Mastaguia FL. Disorders of neuromuscular transmission caused by drugs. N Engl J Med 1979; 301:409–413.

Myocardial infarction, acute

Daniel L. Kulick ■ *Shahbudin H. Rahimtoola*

■ Background

Acute myocardial infarction (AMI) results in over 700,000 hospital admissions annually in the United States.[1] The in-hospital mortality in patients with AMI prior to the advent of thrombolytic therapy ranged up to 20 per cent, and an additional 10 per cent of hospital survivors died of cardiac causes in the first year following discharge.[2] Most patients with AMI have an occlusive thrombus at the site of a preexisting atherosclerotic narrowing in a coronary artery; approximately two thirds of patients have associated multivessel coronary artery disease. Management strategies in AMI include attempts to limit myocardial infarct size, stabilization of the patient in the hospital, identification of patients at increased risk for subsequent mortality following hospital discharge and efforts at secondary prevention of further cardiac events.

■ Management

■ LIMITATION OF MYOCARDIAL INFARCT SIZE

The primary goal when a patient presents with AMI is to minimize the extent of infarction and preserve the maximal amount of left ventricular myocardium. In the absence of a well-developed collateral circulation, myocardial necrosis is virtually complete *within 3 to 6 hours* following total coronary artery occlusion;[3] any efforts to limit myocardial infarct size, therefore, must be initiated *promptly*. Although many interventions aimed at limitation of infarct size have been studied, the only ones of proven efficacy and practicality are acute reperfusion therapy and the early administration of intravenous beta-adrenergic blocking agents.

Reperfusion Therapy

Following the demonstration that AMI is pathophysiologically associated with an occlusive coronary arterial thrombus in most cases,[4] the past decade has seen the emergence of thrombolytic therapy as a major advance in the management of AMI. Lysis of an occlusive thrombus and restoration of flow in the infarct-related coronary artery can be achieved in approximately 75 per cent of patients and have resulted in reduction of myocardial infarct size and reduced mortality following AMI.[5-8] Initial studies were performed with intracoronary administration of thrombolytic agents, most commonly streptokinase. While a favorable effect can be demonstrated,[9] the time delay and resources required for cardiac catheterization of these patients prior to the initiation of treatment make this, in general, a somewhat impractical form of therapy, and one not available at all facilities.

With demonstration of the efficacy of the intravenous administration of thrombolytic agents in establishing coronary arterial patency, therapy could now be administered rapidly, within the accepted 4 to 6 hour window of maximal therapeutic effect; importantly, this demonstrated that intravenous thrombolytic therapy can be administered in virtually any hospital setting, independent of the capability of performing cardiac catheterization.

Available data from large randomized trials clearly demonstrate a reduction in mortality and preservation of left ventricular function following the administration of intravenous thrombolytic treatment within the first 4 to 6 hours of an AMI.[5-8] Several thrombolytic agents are currently available or under investigation, but the two most commonly employed in the United States at this writing are streptokinase and recombinant tissue plasminogen activator (rt-PA); newer thrombolytic agents may prove to be equally or more efficacious. Details of drug administration are outlined in Table 1. Full heparin anticoagulation should be maintained following thrombolytic therapy, to decrease the likelihood of reocclusion of successfully recanalized arteries, which is still observed in about 15 per cent of patients. Prophylactic administration of lidocaine is advised in these patients, owing to the frequent occurrence of ventricular arrhythmias following successful reperfusion.

TABLE 1. Administration of Intravenous Thrombolytic Therapy in Acute Myocardial Infarction

Streptokinase	1.5 million units intravenously over 1 hour Premedication with 100 mg of intravenous hydrocortisone and 50 mg of intravenous diphenhydramine
Recombinant Tissue Plasminogen Activator (rt-PA)	100 mg intravenously over 3 hours, as follows: 60 mg (or 1 mg/kg, up to 80 mg) in first hour, with 10% as an initial loading dose Remaining balance of 100 mg (or 1.25 mg/kg) infused over next 2 hours
Adjunctive Therapy for Both Agents	1) Continuous lidocaine infusion, initiated prior to treatment 2) Heparin, 5000-unit intravenous bolus, followed by maintenance heparin infusion initiated after infusion of thrombolytic agent

Although prediction of successful thrombolysis may be suggested by certain bedside findings (rapid resolution of chest pain, improvement in ST-segment elevation on the surface electrocardiogram (ECG), absence of pathologic Q-waves on the surface ECG and appearance of "reperfusion" ventricular arrhythmias), none of these findings are of sufficient sensitivity or specificity to predict arterial patency reliably; the only certain method of confirming successful thrombolysis is coronary arteriography.[10]

Thrombolytic treatment is generally indicated for most patients with AMI who meet the following requirements: (1) Chest pain suggestive of myocardial infarction *persisting for less than 4 to 6 hours* and unrelieved with sublingual nitroglycerin; (2) associated ECG changes of acute myocardial injury (ST segment elevation in two contiguous ECG leads; the presence of Q-waves should *not* preclude therapy, as they may not reflect irreversibly damaged myocardial tissue); and (3) absence of specific contraindications to therapy (Table 2). Controversy exists regarding the role of thrombolytic therapy in patients with inferior myocardial infarction, as these infarctions generally are associated with less extensive loss of left ventricular myocardium and lower hospital mortality.

TABLE 2. Contraindications to Thrombolytic Therapy

Absolute	Active internal bleeding
	History of intracerebral pathology (cerebrovascular disease, mass lesion, etc.)
Relative	Recent (10–21 days) surgery, major trauma, biopsy of internal organ, puncture of noncompressible vessel
	Uncontrolled systemic hypertension (>180/110 mm Hg)
	Prolonged (>30–60 sec) cardiopulmonary resuscitation
	History of gastrointestinal bleeding
	Age >70 years

Nonetheless, benefit from thrombolytic therapy can be demonstrated for patients with inferior myocardial infarction as well, and in the absence of specific contraindications, this form of therapy should be considered for patients with inferior infarction, particularly those with ECG changes suggestive of a large infarction (posterior and/or lateral changes, in addition to changes in the inferior leads).[11,12] The need for *prompt* initiation of therapy cannot be overemphasized. Whereas myocardial salvage can be demonstrated with thrombolytic therapy administered within 3 to 6 hours of the onset of symptoms, still greater benefit can be derived in the first 1 or 2 hours. The aim is to administer therapy as *rapidly as possible*; there is no role for a leisurely approach to patients presenting with AMI in the present era.

The major risk associated with thrombolytic therapy is bleeding; this risk seems to be comparable for all available thrombolytic agents. The majority of bleeding complications occur at sites of vascular access (cardiac catheterization puncture sites, sites of venous and arterial cannulation); for this reason, invasive procedures should be kept to the necessary minimum in these patients and performed only by skilled personnel. Most vascular access site bleeding can be controlled by direct compression, although blood transfusion occasionally may be necessary. Spontaneous internal bleeding (gastrointestinal, genitourinary, retroperitoneal) also may occur infrequently. Intracranial hemorrhage is observed in up to 0.5 per cent of patients and remains the most feared complication of thrombolytic therapy,

owing to its associated severe morbidity and mortality. This complication occurs with greatest frequency in patients with a history of severe hypertension and in elderly patients (>70 years of age). It is possible, however, that this incidence of cerebrovascular accidents (0.5 per cent) is similar to that observed in patients with AMI not receiving thrombolytic agents. Streptokinase is uniquely associated with infrequent allergic reactions, manifested by fever and hypotension. These often can be avoided by pretreatment with antihistamines and corticosteroids. Two conditions that may present as acute chest pain syndromes are acute pericarditis and aortic dissection; administration of systemic thrombolytic therapy in either of these conditions may be devastating. A careful history and physical examination directed at excluding these entities is mandatory prior to administration of thrombolytic therapy; if doubt remains, M-mode and two-dimensional echocardiography can be performed rapidly at the bedside.

Management of patients following administration of thrombolytic therapy remains controversial. As the majority of patients with AMI have a residual high-grade coronary artery stenosis in the infarct-related artery following successful thrombolysis, prompt cardiac catheterization and coronary angiography, followed by percutaneous transluminal coronary angioplasty (PTCA), if technically feasible, was advocated initially in all patients following thrombolytic therapy. This approach requires urgent transfer of the patient to a facility with these capabilities and mandates a significant commitment of resources. Large multicenter randomized trials have demonstrated that this approach may not be necessary in most patients following thrombolytic therapy;[13,14] in the stable patient without ongoing or recurrent myocardial ischemia, deferred cardiac catheterization (3 to 7 days), with revascularization if clinically indicated, is equally efficacious in preventing adverse cardiac events (recurrent myocardial infarction, mortality) and may in fact be safer. Further investigation is ongoing to determine whether angiography is mandatory in all these patients or only in those with recurrent myocardial ischemia or other forms of clinical or hemodynamic instability who clearly require urgent angiography.

An alternative reperfusion strategy in AMI is primary PTCA, without preceding thrombolysis. PTCA is a definitive method of establishing arterial patency, is effective in 85 to 90 per cent of patients, does not leave patients with a high-grade residual coronary arterial stenosis, and is not associated with the bleeding complications of thrombolytic therapy.[15] However, acute PTCA is not available in most institutions, and the time required for transfer of the patient to the cardiac catheterization laboratory and initiating the procedure generally outweighs the potential advantages of this approach in most patients; this delay will generally result in *at least* an additional hour of ongoing arterial occlusion and myocardial necrosis prior to reperfusion, as compared with administration of intravenous thrombolysis. The widespread availability and ease of rapid initiation of intravenous thrombolysis make it the reperfusion strategy of choice in the majority of patients with AMI who are suitable for reperfusion therapy. Emergency PTCA has an important role and is indicated in the following groups of patients with AMI: (1) those with continuing myocardial ischemia following thrombolytic therapy; (2) those with contraindications to thrombolytic therapy; and (3) those with acute cardiogenic shock, in whom successful PTCA can have a favorable impact on the grave prognosis associated with this condition.[16]

Beta-Adrenergic Blockade

In the absence of significant heart failure, bradyarrhythmias, or conduction disturbances on admission to the coronary care unit, administration of intravenous beta-adrenergic blocking agents within the first several hours following the onset of symptoms may result in a significant reduction in myocardial infarct size.[17] This therapy may be particularly beneficial in the hyperadrenergic patient with tachycardia and hypertension, in whom beta-adrenergic blockade can reduce myocardial oxygen demand markedly. One must be very cautious when administering beta-adrenergic blocking agents to patients with signs of heart failure or a large anterior infarction; in these patients, such therapy should be administered only during continuous hemodynamic monitoring or following confirmation of adequate left ventricular systolic function by echocardiography. The agents most commonly employed are metoprolol and propranolol, although use of the short-acting beta-adrenergic blocking agent, esmolol, may provide a greater margin of safety. Guidelines for administration of this therapy are given in Table 3. Acute beta-adrenergic blocking agent administration may be combined with reperfusion therapy in appropriate patients to maximize potential salvage of left ventricular myocardium.

■ PAIN CONTROL

The chest discomfort associated with AMI results from a combination of necrotic myocardial tissue and ongoing myocardial ischemia. The administration of supplemental oxygen (1 to 3 liters per minute by nasal cannula) and narcotic analgesics represent appropriate initial management, but all further efforts at pain control should be directed toward the control of myocardial ischemia. Organic nitrates represent a mainstay of anti-ischemic therapy in AMI. Although nitrates may be administered in many forms, intravenous nitroglycerin infusion repre-

TABLE 3. Intravenous Beta-Adrenergic Blocking Agents in Acute Myocardial Infarction

Indications	First 3–6 hours to decrease myocardial oxygen demand and limit infarct size
Precautions	Heart failure, bradyarrhythmias, AV conduction disturbances, large anterior MI, obstructive airway disease
Agents	
Metoprolol	5 mg intravenous bolus q 2–3 minutes × 3 doses (total 15 mg) 50 mg orally q 6 hours × 48 hours, then 50–100 mg orally BID
Propranolol	0.1 mg/kg intravenous (1 mg q 3–5 min) 20–80 mg orally QID
Esmolol	500 μg/kg over 1 minute, then 50 μg/kg/min infusion If no response, repeat loading dose and increase infusion in increments of 50 μg/kg/min q 5–10 min—maximal recommended infusion rate 200 μg/kg/min

sents the safest and most controllable form of nitrate therapy in the acute setting; therapy is initiated at 0.25 μg/kg/min and titrated upward as needed. Further pharmacologic control of ischemia may be attained with the use of beta-adrenergic blocking agents and calcium channel antagonists.

If pharmacologic measures fail to rapidly control ischemic pain following AMI, bedside hemodynamic monitoring should be initiated, and coronary angiography should be emergently performed; the patient should undergo prompt revascularization (with coronary bypass surgery or PTCA) if suitable coronary artery anatomy is present. During this phase, supportive treatment with intra-aortic balloon counterpulsation can improve myocardial perfusion dramatically and decrease myocardial oxygen demand. Prior to embarking on this ambitious and aggressive approach, it is critical for the physician to be certain that ongoing symptoms are in fact related to myocardial ischemia, as certain other conditions associated with AMI also may result in chest discomfort in the coronary care unit (e.g., acute pericarditis, pulmonary embolism). Anginal pain quality, particularly with associated reversible ST and T wave changes on electrocardiography, is most suggestive of ischemia.

■ ARRHYTHMIA MANAGEMENT

Premature ventricular complexes (PVCs) are common in the early phase of AMI, as is the sudden occurrence of ventricular tachycardia (VT) and ventricular fibrillation (VF). These arrhythmias are most likely to occur in the first 24 to 48 hours following hospital admission and are often not preceded by "warning" PVCs. For this reason, prophylactic administration of intravenous lidocaine therapy for the first 24 to 48 hours following AMI is generally recommended; lidocaine prophylaxis has been demonstrated to reduce the incidence of VT and VF in patients with AMI.[18] Lidocaine therapy is generally initiated as a bolus of 1 to 2 mg/kg, followed by a maintenance infusion of 2 mg/min, with a second bolus of 0.5 to 1 mg/kg administered 20 minutes after the initial bolus. Caution should be exercised in those at increased risk of lidocaine toxicity (elderly patients, patients with hypoperfusion states,

and those with hepatic dysfunction); these patients should receive either decreased lidocaine doses or careful arrhythmia monitoring without prophylactic therapy.

Another common ventricular arrhythmia in the setting of AMI is accelerated idioventricular rhythm (AIVR). This rhythm initially may be misinterpreted as VT, but the rate is slower (60 to 100 beats per minute) and is generally not associated with hemodynamic compromise. Recognition is important, as specific therapy is not necessary and may be deleterious.

Sinus bradycardia is observed occasionally in the setting of AMI, particularly with inferior infarction; this may be related to heightened vagal tone and/or ischemia of the sinus node. If the patient is hemodynamically stable, no specific therapy is necessary. If the patient is hypotensive or has an unstable escape rhythm, intravenous atropine is generally successful in accelerating the sinus rate; temporary transvenous pacemaker insertion at times may be necessary.

Atrioventricular block (AVB) also may be observed in the setting of AMI. As a general rule, AVB associated with inferior myocardial infarction is self-limited and, again, related to heightened vagal tone or ischemia of the AV node or both; first- and second-degree (Mobitz I) AVB are relatively common and require no specific therapy. Temporary pacing is indicated for the development of third-degree AVB, particularly if associated with hemodynamic compromise; permanent pacemaker insertion is necessary only very rarely. Conversely, AVB associated with anterior myocardial infarction is most often due to necrosis of the conduction system and may be permanent. The setting is often one of a large infarction associated with a very poor prognosis. Third-degree AVB may occur quite suddenly in anterior infarction. Temporary pacing is indicated at the first sign of either second-degree (often Mobitz II) or third-degree AVB; if the patient survives and the AVB persists for more than 7 to 10 days, permanent pacemaker insertion should be considered. The appearance of new, bilateral, or alternating bundle branch block in the setting of AMI, particularly with concomitant first-degree AVB, is associated with an increased incidence of progression to complete heart block and is generally an indication for temporary pacemaker insertion.

HEMODYNAMIC INSTABILITY COMPLICATING AMI

Patients with AMI who develop hemodynamic instability are at increased risk for myocardial infarct extension and clinical deterioration; prompt and accurate management is essential. Hemodynamic monitoring with a bedside balloon flotation pulmonary artery catheter aids the clinician in reaching an accurate diagnosis of the patient's clinical status and monitoring the response to therapy.[19] When performed by a skilled and experienced operator, the procedure is safe and relatively free of significant complications.

In the patient with findings suggestive of pulmonary congestion (rales at the lung bases, arterial hypoxemia, pulmonary infiltrates on chest film), potential causes may include elevated cardiac filling pressures secondary to left ventricular dysfunction (i.e., "CHF") or noncardiac etiologies. Bedside pulmonary artery catheterization can be invaluable in this setting. It allows accurate diagnosis of the cause of abnormal pulmonary findings. Empiric use of diuretics in patients with presumed "heart failure" associated with AMI can have deleterious consequences if left ventricular filling pressures are not markedly elevated; patients with AMI are very dependent on an adequate left ventricular filling pressure for maintenance of cardiac output, and overzealous use of diuretics can result in a marked fall in cardiac output.

Causes of elevated left ventricular filling pressures in patients with AMI may include (1) loss of left ventricular myocardium secondary to the infarct, with resultant systolic left ventricular dysfunction; (2) severe diastolic left ventricular dysfunction secondary to a large mass of ischemic, noncompliant myocardium; (3) mitral regurgitation due either to transient papillary muscle ischemia or to rupture of a necrotic papillary muscle; and (4) acute ventricular septal defect. Bedside hemodynamics are essential in arriving at the correct diagnosis (Table 4). An important group of patients with pulmonary congestion are those with so-called "flash" pulmonary edema. These patients have transient pulmonary edema due either to transient ischemic dysfunction of a large proportion of the left ventricular myocardium or to transient papillary muscle dysfunction; only a small amount of myocardium is infarcted, with a potentially large amount remaining at risk of further ischemic insult. Bedside hemodynamics may be nearly normal, despite recent acute cardiogenic pulmonary edema. Such patients are candidates for very early coronary arteriography and revascularization if feasible.

Sinus tachycardia may be observed in patients with AMI. It may be due to a wide variety of etiologies, including: (1) compensation for reduced left ventricular stroke volume; (2) hyperadrenergic state; (3) acute pulmonary edema; (4) hypovolemia; (5) fever; (6) infection; (7) anemia; and (8) occult hyperthyroidism. Tachycardia increases myocardial oxygen demand and may extend myocardial infarct size; therefore, treatment of the tachycardia is important but must be directed at the underlying cause and not at the rhythm itself. As the causes of sinus tachycardia in AMI are quite diverse, the treatments are correspondingly diverse; inappropriate therapy can have disastrous consequences (e.g., beta-adrenergic blocking agents to slow sinus rate in a patient with compensatory tachycardia that is serving to maintain cardiac output in the setting of oc-

TABLE 4. Hypotension in Acute Myocardial Infarction

Etiology	Associated Hemodynamics	Therapy
Hypovolemia	↓ RA, ↓ PAWP, ↓ CO	Fluid
LV pump failure	↑ PAWP, ↓ CO	Pressors, inotropes, vasodilators, IABP, urgent cardiac catheterization
RV infarction	↑ RA, RA ≥0.8 (PAWP), ↓ CO	Fluid; inotropes ± vasodilators
Acute MR/PMR	↑ PAWP with large V-waves	IABP; urgent surgery
VSD	O_2 step-up in RV	IABP; urgent surgery
Cardiac rupture	↑ RA, ↑ PAWP, RA = PAWP, ↓ CO	Survival rare; surgery if patient is alive

CO, cardiac output; IABP, intra-aortic balloon pump; LV, left ventricular; MR, mitral regurgitation; PAWP, pulmonary artery wedge pressure; PMR, papillary muscle rupture; RA, right atrial pressure; RV, right ventricle; VSD, ventricular septal defect.

cult left ventricular dysfunction). Bedside pulmonary artery catheterization is useful in helping establish an accurate diagnosis.

Systemic hypotension, with or without associated clinical shock, may be observed with AMI and can result from a variety of causes (Table 4); bedside pulmonary artery catheterization is mandatory in this setting to clarify the etiology of hypotension and monitor the response to therapy. One of the more common causes of systemic hypotension in AMI is hypovolemia, which may result from spontaneous diaphoresis and emesis, from morphine-induced emesis and venous pooling, or from rapid administration of potent diuretics and preload reducing agents (e.g., nitrates). This may produce profound falls in left ventricular filling pressure and cardiac output. Documentation of a low pulmonary artery wedge pressure with bedside pulmonary artery catheterization can prevent the administration of potentially deleterious vasopressor and inotropic agents.

Clinically evident right ventricular myocardial infarction is observed in up to 15 per cent of patients with inferior myocardial infarction[20] and may result in systemic hypotension. This condition may first become manifest following administration of nitrate therapy, which lowers right ventricular filling pressure and results in a fall in cardiac output. Diagnosis of right ventricular infarction is made in the setting of inferior infarction associated with physical findings of elevated right-sided cardiac filling pressures, right-sided precordial ECG leads demonstrating acute ST elevation, and bedside hemodynamics demonstrating elevated right atrial pressures. Physical findings (hypotension and neck vein distention) may mimic cardiac tamponade. Bedside echocardiography can confirm the absence of tamponade, as well as demonstrate right ventricular dilatation and dysfunction. In the absence of signs of peripheral hypoperfusion (altered sensorium, oliguria, cool extremities), no specific therapy is indicated. In the presence of clinical hypoperfusion, isotonic fluid administration to maintain a pulmonary artery wedge pressure of 15 to 18 mm Hg is an appropriate first line of therapy, although inotropic and/or vasodilator therapy is often required. The course of right ventricular infarction is most often self-limited, with hemodynamics gradually stabilizing over several days in most patients.

The presence of cardiogenic shock in AMI due to left ventricular pump dysfunction is generally associated with a net loss of approximately 40 per cent of the left ventricular myocardium and carries a grave prognosis. With conventional medical therapy (inotropic agents, vasopressors, vasodilators, intra-aortic balloon counterpulsation), the hospital mortality ranges from 80 to 100 per cent; the performance of emergency PTCA in these patients, with the aim of salvaging any potentially viable myocardium, has resulted in 50 per cent or more of patients surviving to hospital discharge following successful reperfusion.[16] Patients with hypotension due to acute mechanical complications of AMI (ventricular septal defect, papillary muscle rupture) require emergency stabilization with intra-aortic balloon counterpulsation, followed by emergency cardiac catheterization and early surgical correction. Patients who suffer acute cardiac tamponade following cardiac rupture generally present in a moribund state and rarely survive; the only reasonable treatment is immediate surgical intervention.

■ MANAGEMENT OF HOSPITAL SURVIVORS OF AMI

Of patients surviving to hospital discharge following AMI, approximately 10 per cent will die of cardiac causes (recurrent myocardial infarction, sudden cardiac death) in the first year. Certain clinical characteristics in the first several days following AMI identify a high-risk population, with a 1-year mortality rate of up to 50 per cent.[2] These characteristics include the occurrence of spontaneous myocardial ischemia, the presence of transient or persistent congestive heart failure, the presence of complex ventricular arrhythmias or frequent PVCs after the first 48 to 72 hours, or a history of prior myocardial infarction. The high mortality associated with these conditions mandates an aggressive approach to these patients, generally including cardiac catheterization and angiography. In appropriate patients, revascularization therapy (coronary bypass surgery or PTCA) may enhance survival markedly. Selected patients may benefit from electrophysiologic testing as well.

The majority of patients surviving AMI do not have any of the aforementioned complications, and their 1-year mortality rate is

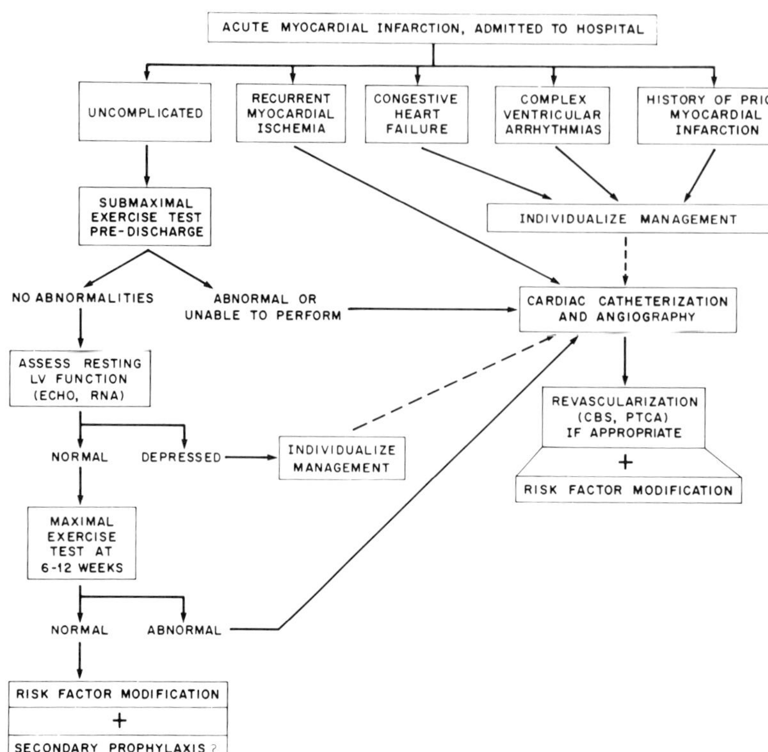

Figure 1. Approach to management of hospital survivors of acute myocardial infarction. CBS, coronary artery bypass surgery; ECHO, two-dimensional echocardiography; LV, left ventricular; PTCA, percutaneous transluminal coronary angioplasty; RNA, radionuclide angiography.

significantly lower. However, within this group of patients with "uncomplicated" AMI, subgroups exist with a truly low mortality risk ($\leq$1 per cent) and those with a somewhat higher risk. Prior to hospital discharge, it is *mandatory* to identify those patients at increased risk and then to take steps to reduce that risk. Numerous clinical studies have demonstrated the safety of pre-discharge submaximal exercise testing following AMI; abnormalities during submaximal exercise testing can identify patients at increased risk for recurrent ischemic events or mortality in the year following hospital discharge.[21] If submaximal exercise testing reveals no abnormalities, maximal exercise testing 6 to 12 weeks later is recommended. If abnormalities suggestive of myocardial ischemia or dysfunction are documented on either test, cardiac catheterization and angiography are appropriate. In patients with no demonstrable ischemia following AMI, noninvasive assessment of left ventricular function by radionuclide angiography or two-dimensional echocardiography is necessary to detect those patients with occult left ventricular dysfunction, in whom the late mortality risk is increased, and who

might benefit from further investigation. In all patients, rigorous modification of risk factors is mandatory (see next section). A suggested scheme for management of hospital survivors of AMI is shown in Figure 1.

■ Issues and Risks

■ NON–Q WAVE MYOCARDIAL INFARCTION

Approximately 25 per cent of AMI are of the non-Q wave variety; this incidence may be increasing with the greater use of reperfusion therapy to limit myocardial infarct size. Although the early, in-hospital mortality associated with non–Q wave AMI is lower than that observed in Q wave AMI, the late (1 to 3 year) mortality observed in non–Q wave AMI is equal to that of Q wave AMI; this suggests that the postdischarge mortality following non–Q wave AMI is in fact higher than that following Q wave AMI.[22] The increased late mortality observed in patients with non–Q wave AMI reflects the increased incidence of recurrent myocardial ischemia observed in these patients.[23] Patients with non–Q wave AMI should be observed carefully for signs of myocardial ischemia, either spontaneous or during submaximal exercise testing, and should undergo coronary arteriography if myocardial ischemia is documented or if the resting ECG suggests a large area of myocardium at risk. Prophylactic adminstration of diltiazem in patients with non–Q wave AMI may reduce significantly the short-term incidence of recurrent myocardial ischemia and reinfarction.[23]

■ SECONDARY PROPHYLAXIS

Aggressive control of risk factors is mandatory in all patients following an AMI in an effort to halt the progression of atherosclerotic disease and prevent recurrent myocardial infarction. These measures should include (1) abrupt and complete cessation of tobacco use; (2) control of systemic hypertension; (3) vigorous efforts to reduce elevated serum lipid levels to an acceptable range; and (4) weight reduction and dietary modification.

Recent randomized trials have demonstrated prophylactic administration of beta-adrenergic blocking agents to reduce mortality for several years following AMI.[24] The mechanism of this benefit remains uncertain, but it may be related to the antiarrhythmic and anti-ischemic properties of these agents. The major part of this benefit, however, appears to occur in patients classified as moderate and high risk following AMI; these patients may derive greater benefit from coronary revascularization, if appropriate, than from pharmacologic prophylaxis. Patients identified as being at very low risk following AMI may have very little further benefit to gain from beta-adrenergic blockade.

Antiplatelet therapy following AMI may reduce the incidence of recurrent myocardial infarction and death.[25] Administration of aspirin in doses as low as 80 mg per day may be sufficient to afford this protection.

REFERENCES

1. The TIMI Research Group. Immediate vs. delayed catheterization and angioplasty following thrombolytic therapy for acute myocardial infarction: TIMI II-A results. JAMA 1988; 260:2849–2858.

2. Moss AJ. Prognosis after myocardial infarction. Am J Cardiol 1983; 52:667–669.

3. Reimer KA, Lowe JE, Rasmussen MM, Jennings RB. The wavefront phenomenon of ischemic cell death. I. Myocardial infarct size vs. duration of coronary occlusion in dogs. Circulation 1977; 56:786–794.

4. DeWood MA, Spores J, Notske R, Mouser LT, Burroughs R, Golden MS, Lang HT. Prevalence of total coronary occlusion during the early hours of transmural myocardial infarction. N Engl J Med 1980; 303:897–902.

5. Gruppo Italiano per lo Studio Della Streptochinasi nell'Infarto Miocardico (GISSI). Effectiveness of intravenous thrombolytic treatment in acute myocardial infarction. Lancet 1986; 1:397–402.

6. Second International Study of Infarct Survival Collaborative Group (ISIS-2). Randomized trial of intravenous streptokinase and aspirin, both or neither, among 17,187 cases of suspected acute myocardial infarction: ISIS-2. Lancet 1988; 2:349–360.

7. Van de Werf F, Arnold AER, European Cooperative Study Group for Recombinant Tissue-Type Plasminogen Activator (rt-PA). Intravenous tissue plasminogen activator and size of infarct, left ventricular function, and survival in acute myocardial infarction. Br Med J 1988; 297:2374–2379.

8. Wasserman AG, Ross AM. Coronary thrombolysis. Curr Probl Cardiol 1989; 14:1–54.

9. Simoons ML, Serruys PW, Van Den Brand M, Res J, Verheught FWA, Krauss XH, Remme WJ, Bar F, De Zwann C, Van Der Laarse A, Vermeer F, Lubsen J. Early thrombolysis in acute myocardial infarction: limitation of infarct size and improved survival. J Am Coll Cardiol 1986; 7:717–728.

10. Califf RM, O'Neill W, Stack RS, Aronson L, Mark DB, Mantell S, George BS, Candela RJ, Kereiakes DJ, Abbottsmith C, Topol EJ, TAMI Study Group. Failure of simple clinical measurements to predict perfusion status after intravenous thrombolysis. Ann Intern Med 1988; 108:658–662.

11. Bates ER. Reperfusion therapy in inferior myocardial infarction. J Am Coll Cardiol 1988; 12(No 6, Suppl A):44A–51A.

12. White HD, Norris RM, Brown MA, Takayama M, Maslowski A, Bass NM, Ormiston JA, Whitlock J. Effect of intravenous streptokinase on left ventricular function and early survival after acute myocardial infarction. N Engl J Med 1987; 317:850–855.

13. Topol EJ, Califf RM, George BS, Kereiakes DJ, Abbottsmith CW, Candela RJ, Lee KL, Pitt B, Stack RS, O'Neill WW, Thrombolysis and Angioplasty in Myocardial Infarction Study Group. A randomized trial of immediate versus delayed elective angioplasty after intravenous tissue plasminogen activator in acute myocardial infarction. N Engl J Med 1987; 317:581–588.

14. Simoons ML, Arnold AE, Betriu A, de Bono DP, Col J, von Essen R, Dougherty FL, for the European Cooperative Study Group for Recombinant Tissue-Type Plasminogen Activator (rt-PA). Thrombolysis with tissue plasminogen activator in acute myocardial infarction: no additional benefit from immediate percutaneous coronary angioplasty. Lancet 1988; 1:197–202.

15. Rothbaum DA, Linnemeier TJ, Landin RJ, Steinmetz EF, Hillis JS, Hallam CC, Noble RJ, See MR. Emergency percutaneous transluminal coronary angioplasty in acute myocardial infarction: a 3-year experience. J Am Coll Cardiol 1987; 10:264–272.

16. Lee L, Bates ER, Pitt B, Walton JA, Laufer N, O'Neill WW. Percutaneous transluminal coronary angioplasty improves survival in acute myocardial infarction complicated by cardiogenic shock. Circulation 1988; 78:1345–1351.

17. Herlitz J, Elmfeldt D, Hjalmarson A, Holmberg S, Malek I, Nyberg G, Ryden L, Swedberg K, Vedin A, Waagstein F, Waldenstrom A, Waldenstrom J, Wedel H, Wilhelmsen L, Wilhelmsson C. Effect of metoprolol on indirect signs of the size and severity of acute myocardial infarction. Am J Cardiol 1983; 51:1282–1288.

18. Lie KI, Wellens HJ, Van Capelle FJ, Durrer N. Lidocaine in the prevention of primary ventricular fibrillation. N Engl J Med 1974; 291:1324–1326.

19. Forrester JS, Diamond G, Chatterjee K, Swan HJC. Medical therapy of acute myocardial infarction by application of hemodynamic subjects. N Engl J Med 1976; 295:1356–1362, 1404–1413.

20. Dell'Italia LJ, Starling MR. Right ventricular infarction: an important clinical entity. Curr Probl Cardiol 1984; 9:1–72.

21. Froelicher VF, Perdue ST, Atwood JE, Des Pois P, Sivarajan ES. Exercise testing of patients recovering from myocardial infarction. Curr Probl Cardiol 1986; 11:369–444.

22. Gibson RS. Non-Q wave myocardial infarction: diagnosis, prognosis, and management. Curr Probl Cardiol 1988; 13:1–72.

23. Gibson RS, Boden WE, Theroux P, Strauss HD, Pratt CM, Gheorghiade M, Capone RJ, Crawford MH, Schlant RC, Kleiger RE, Young PM, Schechtman K, Perryman B, Roberts R, Diltiazem Reinfarction Study Group. Diltiazem and reinfarction in patients with non-Q wave myocardial infarction: results of a double-blind, randomized multicenter trial. N Engl J Med 1986; 315:423–429.

24. Yusuf S, Peto R, Lewis J, Collins R, Sleight P. Beta blockade during and after myocardial infarction: an overview of the randomized trials. Prog Cardiovasc Dis 1985; 27:335–371.

25. Klimt CR, Knatterud GL, Stamler J, Meier P. Persantine-Aspirin Reinfarction Study. Part II: Secondary coronary prevention with persantine and aspirin. J Am Coll Cardiol 1986; 7:251–269.

Narcolepsy

Stephen W. Jennings, M.D. ■ *Martin B. Scharf* ■ *Kathleen A. Fletcher*

Narcolepsy is an incurable illness that is thought to affect between 2 and 10 of every 10,000 Americans.[1] Though recognized notoriously for manifesting as inappropriate "attacks" of daytime sleepiness, it also may involve auxiliary symptoms such as cataplexy, sleep paralysis, and hypnagogic hallucinations. Narcolepsy is sometimes referred to as narcolepsy-cataplexy syndrome.

Probably at least 100,000 individuals in the United States have this disorder. Although the growth of the field of sleep disorders medicine and a recent increase in the number of sleep disorders laboratory facilities have likely begun to change the trend, it has historically been true that individuals with narcolepsy endure an average of 15 years between the onset of the illness and the clinical confirmation of the diagnosis.[2] Many narcoleptic patients spend decades without a proper diagnosis; often their symptoms are mistakenly presumed by one or more clinicians to be attributable to such conditions as obesity, "metabolic problems," cerebrovascular disease, seizure disorder, and a variety of psychiatric problems. As many as 75 per cent of the first-degree relatives of patients with narcolepsy can develop narcolepsy or some other hypersomnolence disorder.[3]

Narcolepsy presents the clinician with problems both in diagnosis and in treatment, although clinical awareness and a high index of suspicion, along with proper consultation with specialists in the field of sleep disorders medicine, facilitate diagnosis.[2–5] Treatment, on the other hand, presents a variety of clinical challenges. The foremost challenges include the abuse potential and tolerance induction associated with the use of stimulant medications; medication side effects; risk versus benefits issues related to prescribing medications in the setting of concomitant conditions like hypertension, cerebrovascular and cardiovascular disease, and prostatic hypertrophy; maintenance medication(s) in women of child-bearing age; teaching and reinforcing necessary patient lifestyle changes; and the refractoriness of some narcoleptic symptoms to conventional therapeutic measures.

■ Background

The classic "narcoleptic tetrad" of symptoms includes excessive daytime sleepiness, cataplexy, sleep paralysis, and hypnagogic hallucinations, although not all symptoms are manifested in all narcoleptic patients, and the full presentation of symptoms may take several years to emerge.[2-4] In all individuals with narcolepsy, excessive sleepiness is the common and cardinal complaint. This sleepiness takes the form of repeated oppressive and at times nearly irresistible sleep urges that can be satiated by naps of between a few minutes and an hour, after which the individual emerges alert and refreshed for a few hours.[6] In spite of the restorative potential of periodic naps, many narcoleptic patients still experience a mild, constant drowsiness and decreased level of alertness. Also, in spite of daytime sleepiness and periodic naps, narcoleptic patients often experience significant nocturnal sleep fragmentation. In fact, individuals with narcolepsy usually do not average an excessive total number of hours of sleep in a 24-hour period.

Cataplexy occurs in about 60 per cent of narcoleptics and may manifest as either discrete, focal, almost imperceptible episodes of muscle weakness or as much more obvious and generalized episodes, even to the extent of total flaccid paralysis. Cataplectic episodes may resolve in a few seconds or may last for a few minutes. Although cataplexy is typically triggered by an emotional display or by anticipation or anxiety, many narcoleptic patients are plagued by unpredictable, spontaneous episodes.[7]

Sleep paralysis may occur upon awakening during the night, upon final awakening in the morning, or during daytime naps. It is often a very frightening experience, occasionally involving a vivid hallucination, and may last anywhere from a few seconds to a few minutes.[8] Brief, bizarre hallucinations most often occur at sleep onset (hypnagogic) at night, when falling back to sleep after a nocturnal awakening, or at the beginning of

a nap, but they can also occur upon awakening (hypnopompic).[9]

In addition to cataplexy, sleep paralysis, and hypnagogic hallucinations, individuals with narcolepsy may experience automatisms of speech and behavior, sensations of extracorporeal experiences (although these phenomena may actually be types of hypnagogic hallucinations), and signs and symptoms of depression.[4]

The age of onset ranges from childhood to the fifth decade, with a peak incidence in the teens. Narcolepsy occurs slightly more frequently in men than in women.[1,4] Controversy persists over the etiology of this disorder. Many human and animal studies have suggested a multifactorial mode of genetic transmission, and there have been further speculations that narcolepsy may represent a point on a continuum of inherited hypersomnolence disorders.[2,4] The very high prevalence of the HLA-DR2 histocompatibility antigen within the genome of narcoleptics, compared with its prevalence in the normal population at large, suggests a role of the immune system in the etiology of narcolepsy.[3,10]

The differential diagnosis of individuals with excessive daytime sleepiness involves a variety of possibilities, including most commonly sleep apnea syndrome, depression, hypothyroidism, nocturnal myoclonus, sustained use of CNS depressants, chronic obstructive pulmonary disease (COPD), idiopathic hypersomnolence syndrome, habitual allotment of insufficient hours for sleep, and a variety of cardiovascular and cerebrovascular disorders. Although many of these possibilities can be eliminated purely on the basis of careful medical and sleep histories and a physical examination, along with appropriate diagnostic studies, narcolepsy must be diagnosed from the history and the findings of a nocturnal polysomnographic evaluation, followed by a multiple sleep latency test. Decisions in equivocal cases may be influenced by the determination of the presence or absence of the HLA-DR2 antigen.

Whenever narcolepsy coexists with another sleep-disruptive disorder, such as sleep apnea or myoclonus—especially sleep apnea of a moderate or severe degree, then that disorder must be initially and adequately treated before the diagnosis of narcolepsy can be made with certainty and before treatment of narcolepsy can be undertaken. Prevalence data do indeed suggest that obstructive sleep apnea and nocturnal myoclonus are each more common in the narcoleptic population than in the population at large.[4] Only after the sleep disruption and the secondary daytime sleepiness and possible other symptoms are eliminated can the full spectrum of presenting narcoleptic symptoms and their severity be subjectively and objectively evaluated and addressed.

■ Management

Although resolving daytime sleepiness is the first consideration in the management of narcolepsy, therapy often must be directed to three fronts. The treatment of the hypersomnolence and the treatment of the auxiliary symptoms involve different approaches and different types of medications, and the treatment of sleep fragmentation may facilitate the treatment of these other symptoms. The primary goal in the treatment of narcolepsy, however, is the restoration of the affected individual to as normal a lifestyle as possible. In the process, it is often the case that the individual's morbidity and mortality risks are markedly reduced.

■ TREATMENT OF SLEEPINESS

Many patients with narcolepsy seem to find it annoying, if not perplexing, that they still experience episodes of daytime sleepiness in spite of what kind or how much of a stimulant medication they take. It is rarely possible to completely alleviate sleepiness with medication alone,[3] and medication has never been proved to be superior to periodic napping in maintaining daytime alertness.[4] Therefore, at the outset it is important to stress to the narcoleptic patient that he or she will need to plan to take daily "therapeutic" naps as an adjunctive "treatment" to whatever medication is prescribed. Beyond this, the narcoleptic patient must be convinced to adhere to as regular a sleep/wake schedule as possible and to allot an adequate number of hours for nighttime sleep. It is best to have the patient keep a daily log of his or her sleep/wake schedule, including the times of episodes of sleepiness and of naps. These logs should be frequently reviewed with the patient early in the course of treatment and periodically or as needed thereafter, to ensure that behavioral modification is employed (e.g., incorporating another daily nap at an appropriate time, or more rigid adherence to a proper bedtime) before a medication adjustment or change is prematurely, and inappropriately, made.

Over 50 years ago, amphetamine was the first medication employed to treat hypersomnolence in narcoleptic patients.[11] Since then, it has remained one of the drugs of choice, although dextroamphetamine is the currently utilized form. Our approach is to prescribe dextroamphetamine only after other medications have been demonstrated to be ineffective or after their efficacy has been exhausted.

Pemoline (Cylert) and methylphenidate (Ritalin) are the first two stimulant medications that we prescribe to treat sleepiness. Pemoline (Schedule IV) is generally the best tolerated although least efficacious of the most commonly used stimulants. Its gradual onset of action and its long half-life (12 hours) make it less likely to produce a "rush" or other hyperstimulation effects. It is usually advisable to begin with a dose of 18.75 mg in the morning and gradually increase as needed to a maximum daily dose of 112.5 mg, initially either by increasing the morning dose to 37.5 mg or by adding a second dose at midday or early in the afternoon. Because of its long half-life, pemoline, if taken too late in the day, may cause difficulty in falling asleep at bedtime. Although this stimulant does not generally impose a significant physiologic stress upon the cardiovascular system, it does have the demonstrated potential to precipitate motor and phonic tics and Tourette's syndrome in individuals genetically predisposed to these disorders.

Methylphenidate (Schedule II) has a more rapid onset of action than does pemoline, but it is still less likely than is dextroamphetamine to cause symptoms of hyperstimulation and is generally well tolerated. The customary therapeutic dosage range is between 5 and 60 mg per day, in divided doses. The half-life of methylphenidate may necessitate dosing it on a TID basis, although many narcoleptic patients do very well on 10 to 20 mg BID, especially if the sustained-release formulation of this medication is employed. In fact, switching to the sustained-release form of methylphenidate occasionally has enabled some patients to function satisfactorily on a smaller total daily dose of the medication than when they were on the conventional tablets.

The total daily dose of dextroamphetamine (Schedule II) generally should not exceed 60 mg.[3] This medication usually has a rather rapid onset of action and reaches maximal effectiveness approximately 3 hours after administration. Its duration of action may be relatively short in some individuals, compared with that of either pemoline or methylphenidate, thus necessitating dosing schedules of 5 to 10 mg four or five times per day. Most patients do well on a once or twice daily dose, though. A long-acting formulation of dextroamphetamine is available and, as in the case of the sustained-release form of methylphenidate, may effectively reduce the total daily dosage requirements in many patients, when compared with the total dosage of standard 5 mg tablets required to achieve satisfactory resolution of sleepiness. Amphetamines have a very high abuse potential because of the euphoria they can induce and because of their capacity to increase alertness and work performance. Tolerance to the stimulant effects of dextroamphetamine can develop after several weeks of sustained use. Administration to patients with concomitant hypertension or cardiovascular disease is contraindicated because of the increases in pulse rate and blood pressure that occur with this medication.

Mazindol (Mazanor, Sanorex) (Schedule IV), an anorectic medication structurally similar to the tricyclic antidepressants but with pharmacologic activity similar to that of the amphetamines, has been reported to treat sleepiness effectively in some patients in a dosage range of 3 to 8 mg per day.[12]

Protriptyline (Vivactil) is a tricyclic antidepressant medication that has the unique property, compared with the other tricyclics, of being nonsedating in many individuals. Although primarily employed in narcolepsy for its efficacy in treating the auxiliary symptoms, it has nevertheless been utilized as a stimulant in some patients, although its primary efficacy in treating hypersomnolence seems to be as an "adjunctive" medication along with a conventional stimulant.[13]

Two rather unconventional medications have been found, under serendipitous circumstances, to behave as stimulants in some narcoleptic patients. Codeine has been determined to render, rather paradoxically, a very satisfactory level of alertness in a few patients, when taken at a dose of 30 mg every 3 to 4 hours during the day.[14] It appears worthy of trial in cases refractory to conventional therapy or when the development of tolerance to conventional stimulants necessitates temporary withdrawal from these medications. Codeine may have abuse potential, and it can cause a variety of unwanted side effects, including respiratory depression, nausea, vomiting, and constipation. Propranolol (Inderal) also may very effectively alleviate hypersomnolence in some narcoleptic patients but only at significant doses of 240 to 480 mg per day.[15] If the coexistence of hypertension makes the treatment of narcolepsy difficult because of the possible adverse effects of the conventional stimulants on the cardiovascular system, then a trial of propranolol is warranted, as long as there are no contraindications to trying a beta-blocker and as long as the medication is tolerated by the patient. Propranolol's onset of action is relatively fast, and its half-life is approximately 4 to 6 hours. Caution must be exercised with this medication because of its potential to induce bradycardia and hypotension, bowel disturbances, depression, insomnia, nightmares, and peripheral vasoconstriction, as well as its capability of masking the signs and symptoms of hypoglycemia. Furthermore, its abrupt withdrawal, especially in patients taking high doses, can precipitate arrhythmias, angina, or myocardial infarction.

■ TREATMENT OF AUXILIARY SYMPTOMS

Inasmuch as cataplexy, sleep paralysis, and hypnagogic hallucinations are abnormal presentations of phenomena normal to REM stage sleep (i.e., muscle inhibition and dreaming), agents that suppress REM sleep have been found useful in treating the auxiliary symptoms of narcolepsy. Cataplexy is frequently severe enough to warrant aggressive therapy, since it can manifest with such a frequency and magnitude as to render an individual virtually totally disabled. On the other hand, cataplexy is often so mild and infrequent that it needs no specific therapy, as is often the case with the other auxiliary symptoms.

As a class of medications, the tricyclic antidepressants are potent suppressors of REM sleep. Imipramine (Tofranil), in total daily doses of up to 200 mg, and protriptyline, in total daily doses of 20 mg or higher, have proved most efficacious and best-tolerated. Contrary to their gradual effectiveness when these medications are employed for their antidepressant qualities, their effects on cataplexy and the other auxiliary symptoms are usually recognizable within the first several hours of administration. The use of these or any of the other tricyclics is often limited by their side effects (most commonly dry mouth, blurred vision, urinary hesitancy or retention, constipation, and sexual dysfunction). However, even when well-tolerated and efficacious, tolerance eventually can develop to the effects of imipramine and protriptyline.

The most potent REM-suppressant agents that have been utilized in the treatment of narcolepsy are the monoamine oxidase (MAO) inhibitors, but their marked potential for drug interactions and the need for patients to avoid foods rich in tyramine limit their usefulness.[2] Patients on MAO inhibitor therapy must be warned very clearly not to self-medicate with such seemingly innocuous over-the-counter drugs as nasal decongestant preparations containing phenylephrine or phenylpropanolamine lest they precipitate an adrenergic crisis, as well as following specific food restrictions.

Clonidine (Catapres), also a potent suppressor of REM, has been demonstrated to work in a small number of cases, but, again, it is a medication of limited usefulness because of its side effects (sedation and dry mouth).[16] Clonidine may induce hypotension, and acute discontinuation of clonidine may be accompanied by hypertensive "overshoot."

Recently viloxazine hydrochloride, an experimental beta-blocker compound, has been found to be not only effective in treating cataplexy but also well-tolerated.[17] Although headache and nausea are potential side effects, especially in elderly patients, it appears that the gradual escalation of the daily dosage from 100 mg to a maximum of 300 mg tends to minimize or avoid these discomforts.

Fluoxetine hydrochloride (Prozac), a unique antidepressant medication by virtue of its potential to block serotonin reuptake, has been demonstrated to help control cataplexy.[18] Although proven to be relatively free of side effects, it may induce anxiety and insomnia.

Gamma-hydroxybutyrate (GHB) is an endogenous CNS substance. Currently available in the United States only as an experimental compound, GHB has been shown to be remarkably effective in controlling cataplexy and the other auxiliary symptoms of narcolepsy and has been purported to decrease daytime sleepiness.[19] It has none of the anticholinergic effects, hence none of the REM-suppressant effects, of the tricyclic drugs. GHB is quite sedating and not only consolidates the nocturnal sleep of narcoleptics but also directly reduces the frequency and severity of cataplexy. The improved sleep consolidation may result secondarily in a reduced amount of stimulant medication needed to maintain daytime alertness.

As might be inferred as a possible effect of a medication that increases slow wave sleep, the compound may cause somnambulism in a few patients, but gamma-hydroxybutyrate is otherwise essentially devoid of side effects.

■ TREATMENT OF SLEEP FRAGMENTATION

It is extremely important not to focus on the hypersomnolence and other daytime symptoms of narcoleptic patients while ignoring their nocturnal sleep disruption. As long as it can be clearly determined that nocturnal sleep disruption is not due to carry-over effects of daytime stimulant dosing, it may indeed be necessary to administer a bedtime dose of a hypnotic medication, such as the benzodiazepines temazepam (Restoril), 15 to 30 mg, or triazolam (Halcion), 0.125 to 0.25 mg. In cases in which symptomatic nocturnal myoclonus coexists with narcolepsy, the utilization of one of these medications is a rational therapeutic decision, since one of the treatments of choice for disruptive myoclonus is a short-acting or an intermediate-acting benzodiazapine. However, myoclonus may be caused by the administration of tricyclics. In patients with coexisting obstructive sleep apnea of a subclinical or mild degree, benzodiazepines may worsen the condition.

■ Issues and Risks

Narcolepsy is a lifelong illness that requires most of those who suffer from it to be dependent upon medication in order to experience a relatively normal lifestyle and be productive in society. Accordingly, and by virtue of the nature of many of the stimulant medications that must be employed to treat hypersomnolence, the potential for abusive dependency on these medications is high in this disorder. Moreover, by the time many narcoleptic patients are properly diagnosed, they already have suffered financial hardships, school or employment problems, marital disruption, and significant degrees of depression and anxiety because of their inability to stay awake and because of the auxiliary phenomenology.

From the outset, the clinician must endeavor to recognize and assess any significant emotional problems in the narcoleptic patient and initiate psychotherapy or refer the patient for appropriate intervention. Sometimes effective restoration of daytime alertness and function will unmask an underlying behavioral or emotional problem, so the clinician must remain vigilant for this situation.[3] Many of a patient's worries, questions, and concerns about his or her condition, as well as those of the patient's family, friends, teachers, and employers, can be capably addressed by putting the patient and those individuals in touch with the American Narcolepsy Association (ANA); many cities and communities have local ANA chapters.

Tolerance to the effects of medications is an issue that is practically inevitable in the course of the treatment of narcolepsy. However, by judicious use of the minimally effective dose of a medication, strategic insertion of drug-free periods ("drug holidays") into the calendar,[3] the incorporation of regular "therapeutic napping" into the daily treatment regimen, and the occasional rotation of medications, the development of drug dependence can be significantly delayed.

Many individuals are capable of taking a drug holiday every weekend, when they are able to satiate their sleep urges by napping as needed, thus refraining from their stimulant medication. This regular 2-day break may suffice, but still it may eventually become necessary to withdraw any narcoleptic patient from medication for a period of 2 to 4 weeks before resuming treatment. Naturally, this can impose significant difficulties temporarily for those in the work force or for those who have child care or other such responsibilities at home.

Extreme caution must be exercised whenever a patient is withdrawn from medication, whether it is from the Schedule II, III, and IV stimulants or from the medications administered for the auxiliary symptoms of narcolepsy. Acute withdrawal from stimulants, especially when tolerance to high doses has developed, can precipitate not only profound hypersomnolence but also marked depressive symptomatology. Unless a gradual and closely monitored withdrawal from anticataplectic therapy is undertaken, there is a significant risk of "rebound cataplexy"[20] of a frequency and severity worse than what existed prior to therapy, even to the extent of temporary status cataplecticus. Cataplectic "rebound" may place the patient's life, health, and safety in considerable jeopardy, especially since some of the cataplexies are not only more severe but also may be spontaneously evoked. Abrupt discontinuation of a nighttime benzodiazepine that has been taken on a chronic basis can precipitate a marked temporary rebound insomnia, which in turn is likely to cause daytime sleepiness to increase significantly until normal or acceptable nighttime sleep is restored. Therefore, narcoleptic patients and those individuals caring for narcoleptic children must be warned never to abruptly discontinue their prescribed medication under any circumstances, make an unauthorized adjustment in their medication dosage(s), or undertake a self-imposed withdrawal from medication without first checking with their treating physician or another qualified clinician.

Individuals with narcolepsy must be clearly and carefully informed about the nature of their illness and the potential problems attendant upon some of the conventional therapies. The risk of acute, overwhelming episodes of sleepiness, in spite of appropriate therapy, must be discussed, and each patient must understand the implications of the hypersomnolence, as well as the implications of cataplexy episodes, on their safety and the safety of others when driving a car, when working with potentially hazardous equipment and machinery both at home and on the job, and during certain recreational activities such as swimming. The nature of drug tolerance and the potential for intentional or unintentional misuse of stimulant medications must be confronted candidly. It is always advisable to offer to communicate with the patient's employer or school officials to explain the nature of the patient's narcoleptic condition, to explain the therapeutic approach and its rationale (especially the concept of therapeutic napping), and to reinforce the fact that the patient retains certain functional capabilities. It is certainly most important to discuss these issues also with the patient's immediate family members or with his or her significant other(s). Local laws in some areas require clinicians to report the names and diagnoses of individuals with narcolepsy and certain other disorders that may significantly impair functional capacity and ability to perform and behave in a safe manner.[3]

REFERENCES

1. Dement WC, Carskadon M, Ley R. The prevalence of narcolepsy. Sleep Res II 1973; 147.
2. Scharf MB, Fletcher K, Jennings SW. Current pharmacologic management of narcolepsy. Am Fam Phys 1988; 38(1):143–148.
3. Mitler MM, Nelson S, Hajdukovic R. Narcolepsy: diagnosis, treatment, and management. Psychiatr Clin North Am 1987; 10(4):593–606.
4. Guilleminault C. Narcolepsy syndrome. In Kryger MH, Roth T, Dement WC (eds). Principles and Practice of Sleep Medicine. Philadelphia: WB Saunders, 1989:338–346.
5. Mitler MM, Van den Hoed J, Carskadon MA. REM sleep episodes during the Multiple Sleep Latency Test in narcoleptic patients. Electroencephalogr Clin Neurophysiol 1979; 46:479–481.
6. Dement WC. Daytime sleepiness and sleep "attacks." In Guilleminault C, Dement WC, Passount P (eds). Narcolepsy. New York: Spectrum, 1976:17–41.
7. Guilleminault C. Cataplexy. In Guilieminault C, Dement WC, Passount P (eds). Narcolepsy. New York: Spectrum, 1976:125–143.
8. Hishikawa Y. Sleep paralysis. In Guilleminault C, Dement WC, Passount P (eds). Narcolepsy. New York: Spectrum, 1976:97–123.
9. Ribstein M. Hypnagogic hallucinations. In Guilleminault C, Dement WC, Passount P (eds). Narcolepsy. New York: Spectrum, 1976:145–159.
10. Juji T, Satake M, Honda Y, Doi Y. HLA antigens in Japanese patients with narcolepsy. All the patients were DR2 positive. Tissue Antigens 1984; 24:316–319.
11. Yoss RE, Daly DD. On the treatment of narcolepsy. Med Clin North Am 1968; 52:781–787.
12. Parkes JD, Schacter M. Mazindol in the treatment of narcolepsy. Acta Neurol Scand 1979; 60:250–254.
13. Mitler MM, Shafor R, Hajdukovich R, Timms RM, Browman CP. Treatment of narcolepsy: objective studies on methylphenidate, pemoline, and protriptyline. Sleep 1986; 9(1:Pt 2):260–264.
14. Fry JM, Pressman MR, DiPhillipo MA, Forst-Paulus M. Treatment of narcolepsy with codeine. Sleep 1986; 9(1:Pt 2):269–274.
15. Kales A, Soldatos CR, Cadieus R, Bixler EO, Tan TL, Scharf MB. Propranolol in the treatment of narcolepsy. Ann Intern Med 1979; 91:741–743.
16. Salin-Pascual R, de la Fuente JR, Fernandez-Guardiola A. Effects of clonidine in narcolepsy. J Clin Psychiatr 1985; 46:528–531.
17. Guilleminault C, Mancuso J, Quera Salva MA. Viloxazine hydrochloride in narcolepsy. Sleep 1986; 9:275–279.
18. Langdon N, Bandak S, Shindler J, Parkes JD. Fluoxetine in the treatment of cataplexy. Sleep 1986; 9:371–372.
19. Scharf MB, Brown D, Woods M, Brown L, Hirschowitz J. The effects and effectiveness of gamma-hydroxybutyrate in patients with narcolepsy. J Clin Psychiatr 1985; 46:222–225.
20. Scharf MB, Fletcher K. Rebound cataplexy: a complication of drug withdrawal in narcolepsy. Sleep Res 1988; 17:246.

Near-drowning

Harold T. Pruessner   *Nancy K. Hansel*

Drowning is the third leading cause of accidental deaths in the United States and is second to motor vehicle accidents as the most common cause of death in persons under 45 years of age.[1] Those at highest risk for drowning are the elderly, infants and children, those with seizure disorders, and users of alcohol and drugs. Management of the near-drowning victim can be difficult owing to the critical nature of procedures undertaken at the scene, in the emergency room, and during hospitalization. Survival and good neurologic outcome rely upon the success of immediate management, followed by careful evaluation and observation.

■ Background

■ TYPES OF DROWNING

Drowning is defined as death from suffocation by submersion in water and near-drowning as survival, at least temporarily, after suffocation by submersion in water.[2] Both drowning and near-drowning can be further classed as "wet," which involves aspiration of water into the victim's lungs and accounts for 80 to 90 per cent of all incidents, and "dry," which does not involve aspiration and occurs when the victim becomes hypoxic from laryngospasm or breath-holding. Delayed death subsequent to near-drowning, termed secondary drowning, is caused by the adult respiratory distress syndrome and constitutes approximately 10 to 25 per cent of deaths following near-drowning.[3] The immersion syndrome is a form of drowning in which cardiac arrest or ventricular fibrillation is precipitated by sudden exposure to cold water.

■ PATHOPHYSIOLOGY OF NEAR-DROWNING

Aspirated Fluids. Significant electrolyte changes occur when at least 22 ml of water per kg of body weight has been aspirated. At least 11 ml per kg is necessary to produce changes in blood volume. Autopsy studies, however, reveal that only 15 per cent of drowning victims aspirate this volume of fluid; near-drowning victims are unlikely to have aspirated more than 4 ml per kg of body weight.[4] For this reason, electrolyte and volume disturbances are rarely clinically significant in near-drowning victims, regardless of whether fresh or salt water has been aspirated.

Pulmonary Responses. Marked disturbance of gas exchange is the most important consequence of near-drowning. Aspiration of as little as 1 to 3 ml of fluid per kg of body weight results in profound impairment of gas exchange.[4,5] In 15 per cent of near-drowning victims, asphyxia results from laryngospasm without apparent fluid aspiration.[6] Recovery from asphyxia is rapid in this situation, if the victim is successfully resuscitated before cardiovascular or neurologic damage occurs.

Aspirated fresh water is absorbed in the circulation rapidly enough to cause transient hypervolemia.[4,5] Fresh water aspiration causes instability of the alveoli from loss of surfactant, resulting in unventilated or poorly ventilated alveoli. The alveoli remain perfused, which leads to increased pulmonary shunting and hypoxia. Salt water is hypertonic and draws fluid from the plasma into the alveoli, increasing the intrapulmonary shunting.

Cardiovascular Derangements. Bradycardia and peripheral vasoconstriction may be secondary to the mammalian diving reflex and subsequently secondary to hypothermia or to a sharp increase in the level of circulating catecholamines. Asystole may occur. Cardiovascular function is affected by changes in blood volume, blood gas levels, serum electrolyte concentrations, and acid-base balance. Electrolyte disturbances and significant changes in blood volume generally occur only when more than 22 ml of fluid per kg of body weight has been aspirated.[4] Central venous pressure increases immediately after aspiration of a small amount of water but rapidly returns to normal.[7] With aspiration of a larger quantity, up to 60 minutes may be required before the central venous pressure returns to normal. Transient hypervolemia may result from freshwater aspiration, but the fluid rapidly redistributes. Fluid may leak from the intravascular space into the lung, rendering the patient hypovolemic.[8]

Central Nervous System Dysfunction. Cerebral edema can develop unexpectedly in some near-drowning victims, including those fully conscious in the emergency room. This usually occurs during the first 24 hours of recovery. Intracranial pressure is often elevated due to the hypoxic insult.[7] Pyrexia, from any cause, is accompanied by an increase in the cerebral metabolic rate and oxygen consumption, adding to the cerebral damage. Hypothermia inhibits oxygen and glucose consumption in the brain.[5] In addition to this protective effect of hypothermia, hypoxemia itself seems to confer protection by producing a barbiturate-like effect, thereby decreasing both active and residual basal metabolism of neurons. Once cerebral ischemia becomes severe, however, basal metabolism can no longer be supported and membrane failure occurs.

Renal Effects. Renal dysfunction is a rare complication of near-drowning. Albuminuria, hemoglobinuria, oliguria, and anuria commonly occur during the postimmersion period. The effects of near-drowning on coagulation vary among individuals. Prothrombin (PT), partial thromboplastin time (PTT), and platelet counts should be determined in the unconscious near-drowning victim; if results prove abnormal, fibrinogen, fibrin, split products, and euglobulin lysis time should be determined.[9]

■ Management

The prevention of irreversible hypoxia with immediate cardiopulmonary resuscitation (CPR) at the scene is the single most important factor influencing long-term survival. Cardiorespiratory status and brain perfusion should be managed as specified by the Advanced Cardiac Life Support (ACLS) standards. Steps in immediate management include (1) implementation of precautions for possible cervical injury, (2) assessment of breathing status, (3) removal of airway-obstructing materials, (4) brief drainage of the lungs, (5) support of respiration by ventilation, (6) closed-chest cardiac massage, and (7) prevention of further heat loss.

Patient management is optimally followed through a system of classifications. (See Table 1.)

■ GROUP 1: CONSCIOUS AND ALERT VICTIMS

Patients in Group 1 are conscious and alert at presentation in the emergency depart-

TABLE 1. Categories of Near-Drowning Victims and Management Guidelines

	Group 1	Group 2	Group 3	Group 4
Presentation	Conscious and alert	Most common group Respiratory distress Conscious or semiconscious with temperatures from 32–35° C (89.6–95.0° F)	Inadequate ventilation	Appear to have suffered cardiac arrest
Management	Admission to hospital for 24 hours of observation Blood gas analysis Temperature measurement Chest film	Admission to ICU and observation for 48 hours Early blood gas analysis Ventilation Appropriate, immediate intravenous infusion Intravenous steroids Intravenous antibiotics Chest film Respiratory therapy	Intubation and ventilation Admission to ICU after tracheal intubation and suction; ventilation with 100% oxygen during transfer PEEP CVP Warmed isotonic peritoneal dialysis fluid Intravenous steroids Intravenous antibiotics Chest film Respiratory therapy	Immediate CPR Intubation and ventilation Cardiac massage Mechanical ventilation Defibrillation Aspirate and ventilate lungs Warmed intravenous fluids Raise body temperature to 31° C (87.8° F) through such measures as peritoneal dialysis, warmed nasogastric fluid, heated and humidified inspired gas mixture
Laboratory Tests	Hemoglobin counts Packed cell volume Blood glucose Blood urea nitrogen Serum electrolytes	Hemoglobin counts Packed cell volume Blood urea nitrogen Serum electrolytes Blood glucose	Blood glucose Acid-base status Hemoglobin counts Packed cell volume Serum electrolytes	Blood glucose Acid-base status Hemoglobin counts Packed cell volume Serum electrolytes Blood urea nitrogen
Possible Complications	Mild hypothermia Onset of pulmonary or cerebral edema	Hypothermia Septicemia Pulmonary or cerebral edema Wheezing respiration Serum electrolyte abnormalities	Hypothermia Rising serum sodium and chloride levels Rising hemoglobin and packed cell volume Septicemia Wheezing respiration	Inability to resuscitate Metabolic acidosis Electrolyte impairment Severe hypothermia

(From Pruessner HT, Zenner GO, Hansel NK: Management of the near-drowning victim. Am Fam Physician 1988; 37:251–260.

ment. These patients should remain in the hospital for at least 24 hours and should be monitored for the development of late-onset pulmonary or cerebral edema. Patients in this category should be managed in the following manner:

Blood Gas Analysis. Although these patients may appear clinically normal, blood gas analysis often reveals metabolic acidosis, which can be severe even when aspiration has not occurred. The degree of hypothermia seems to correlate with the degree of acidosis. If the arterial pH is under 7.2, intravenous sodium bicarbonate should be given.

Temperature. Patients in this group are usually only mildly hypothermic. Treatment of hypothermia is required if the rectal temperature falls to 35°C (95°F) or below. Covering the patient with wool blankets or with a heated water blanket, if available, is usually sufficient.

Chest Radiographs. A chest film is useful primarily as a safeguard in these patients. Even small amounts of water in the lung can be detected on auscultation.

Other Laboratory Tests. Necessary laboratory studies in this group include blood urea nitrogen, electrolyte determination, blood glucose, hemoglobin, and packed cell volume. The results of these tests are usually normal in this group of patients. Blood coagulation studies usually are not required.

■ GROUP 2: RESPIRATORY DISTRESS

Patients in Group 2 are the most frequently encountered near-drowning victims. They often have respiratory distress and cyanosis, with painful wheezing respirations. When possible, these patients should be admitted to an intensive care unit for close monitoring and should be hospitalized for at least 48 hours or until the lungs are radiologically and clinically clear. These patients should be managed in the following manner:

Oxygenation. Oxygen should be administered by mask during transfer from the scene of the accident. The progress of ventilation must be monitored closely by blood gas analysis and clinical examination; Pao_2 is maintained at 60 mm Hg, with an inspired oxygen concentration of no greater than 50 per cent. Young children may require an oxygen tent.

Respiratory Therapy. Respiratory distress in these patients may be characterized by severe retrosternal pain and wheezing respirations. When the patient is able to cooperate with a respiratory therapist, inhaled water should be removed through coughing and deep breathing.

Hypothermia Correction. The majority of patients in this group are semiconscious or fully conscious and have temperatures ranging from 32 to 35° C (89.6 to 95.0° F). Hypothermia can be corrected by covering the patient with wool blankets and administering warmed intravenous fluids if the patient is clinically and hemodynamically stable.

Metabolic Acidosis. As in Group 1 patients, early analysis of acid-base status is required; the pH should be maintained above 7.2 with intravenous sodium bicarbonate.

Intravenous Fluids. All patients in this group should receive intravenous fluids immediately on admission to the intensive care unit. For freshwater near-drowning, normal saline is given, and for saltwater near-drowning, 5 per cent dextrose is administered. All intravenous fluids should be sent through a blood warmer.

Intravenous Antibiotics. Aspiration of water, whether from ocean, river, lake or swimming pool, is highly conducive to pulmonary infection and septicemia. Any near-drowning victim with evidence of aspiration should receive high-dose broad-spectrum antibiotic therapy prophylactically. Although routine use of antibiotics in near-drowning victims is controversial, Simcock demonstrated that prophylactic antibiotic therapy was not associated with complications such as fibrosis, abscess formation, bronchiectasis, or pulmonary infection.[10]

Steroids. For patients who show clinical or radiologic evidence of aspiration, corticosteroids can inhibit late-onset crisis. The most relevant function of steroid use in this situation is inhibition of the inflammatory response. If the decision is made to use steroids, therapy should be started as soon as possible. Intravenous methylprednisolone, 30 mg per kg, is given over a 30-minute period, with the dose repeated 8 hours later. The effects of corticosteroids are well known and numerous. These drugs endow the organism with the capacity to resist many types of noxious stimuli and environmental change.[11] The apparently innocuous character of a single administration of corticosteroids in an amount within the conventional therapeutic range justifies its use. This step is appropriate in near-drowning victims, even if a life-threatening crisis is not imminent. (See Issues and Risks.)

Chest Radiographs. Radiographs usually confirm the clinical impression. The chest film initially shows extensive pulmonary shadowing but usually returns to normal rapidly.

Laboratory Tests. Hemoglobin, packed cell volume, blood urea nitrogen, electrolytes, and blood glucose should be monitored until the patient recovers. Usually, electrolyte abnormalities are minor and consist of small rises in sodium and chloride levels in victims of saltwater near-drowning.

■ GROUP 3: INADEQUATE VENTILATION

Group 3 patients have suffered aspiration and present with inadequate ventilation. They usually have poor peripheral perfusion, and a central venous pressure line should be utilized. In victims of saltwater immersion, occasional abnormal findings include rapidly rising serum sodium and chloride levels, accompanied by a rise in the hemoglobin level and packed cell volume. Rewarming by means of peritoneal dialysis may be required if the ventilatory and cardiovascular status is unstable. Intravenous steroids and respiratory therapy are necessary in these patients.

■ GROUP 4: CARDIAC ARREST

Group 4 patients present without ventilatory function and cardiac output. Near-drowning victims in this category are the most difficult to evaluate and treat. If hypothermia is present, treatment should be initiated even if the heart is in asystole or fibrillating. Adherence to the maxim, "A patient is never dead until he is warm and dead," is advised. Routine resuscitation with 100 per cent oxygen should be used in these patients. If the electrocardiogram reveals asystole, cardiac massage is indicated. Resuscitation should never be abandoned until the body temperature has been raised to 31° C (87.8° F). Ventricular fibrillation is immediately treated by direct current defibrillation. Metabolic acidosis, hypothermia, and electrolyte imbalance may be severe in these victims.

■ Issues and Risks

■ THE USE OF STEROIDS

The use of steroids in the management of near-drowning remains controversial. The prophylactic administration of corticosteroids has been recommended when they are administered intravenously within 5 minutes of the aspiration insult.[12] Others recommend administration of 30 ml per kg on admission and 8 hours later.[10] No response in immersion accident victims with the use of steroids has been cited,[13,14] but those reporting recognize that further, tightly controlled series should be undertaken.

The physiologic and pharmacologic effects of corticosteroids are summarized as follows:

"The effects of corticosteroids are numerous and widespread. They influence carbohydrate, protein, and lipid metabolism; electrolyte and water balance; and the functions of the cardiovascular system, the kidney, skeletal muscle, the nervous system, and other organs and tissues. Furthermore, the corticosteroids endow the organism with the capacity to resist many types of noxious stimuli and environmental change. Cortisol and the synthetic analogs of cortisol have the capacity to prevent or suppress the development of the local heat, redness, swelling, and tenderness by which inflammation is recognized."[11]

Of therapeutic relevance to the physician is that corticosteroids inhibit the inflammatory response whether the inciting agent is radiant, mechanical, chemical, infectious, or immunologic. It is the suppression of inflammation and its consequences that has made the corticosteroids such valuable therapeutic agents—at times lifesaving. If a decision is made to use steroids, avoid the three "toos:" (1) too little (a nontherapeutic dose); (2) too late (onset of action takes 6 to 8 hours); and (3) too long (the cause of all major side effects).

■ PREVENTION: THE PHYSICIAN'S ROLE

Most immersion accidents are preventable, and the role of the physician in preventing premature death from this form of accident cannot be overestimated. The nation's health objectives, established in 1979,[15] state that by 1990, the rate of deaths from drowning should be reduced to no more than 1.5/ 100,000 persons. The rate in 1984 was 2.3/ 100,000, down from 3.2/100,000 in 1978. The 1990 objective is not expected to be reached, however, mainly because of the increased participation of individuals in recreational activities involving bodies of water, particularly boating. The physician should be well informed and should remind patients and families of factors that contribute to morbidity and mortality related to near-drowning and drowning.

Eighty-five per cent of all deaths from drowning are among males, with a maximal incidence in the 10 to 19 year old age group. The death rate for females is highest at age 1, then decreases and does not rise again. The adjusted death rate is also three times greater for blacks than for whites.

The majority of drownings in children less than 4 years of age are caused by falls into swimming pools or natural bodies of water. Physicians should recommend that barriers be erected around pools and other bodies of water, with fences at least 6 feet in height and secure locks. Such structures are known to reduce deaths among children aged 0 to 14 years by as much as 80 per cent when mandated by law. Bathtubs are also a major hazard, and accidents occur among infants and small children who are left unattended. Child neglect or abuse is estimated to account for 6 per cent of all drownings, and murder and suicide are suspected to be disguised as drownings in some cases. The physician should encourage swimming and water safety instruction for children, with the caveat that even after instruction no child should be left unsupervised when near water.

Two thirds of near-drownings and drownings occur in fresh water—commonly in swimming pools, open bodies of water, and containers of water and various fluids. Rates of immersion accidents and deaths are higher among residents of rural areas than those living in urban locations. Other factors play a role in incidence; for example, in Alaska, the heavy exposure to fishing and other recreational and occupational activities, along with very low water temperatures, contributes to a high incidence of drowning deaths (10/100,000). In Louisiana and Florida, where the incidence is also high, the warm climate accounts for an abundance of swimming pools and the extended use of aquatic facilities.[1]

Drownings have a high degree of temporal variation. More than any other type of injury, immersion accidents occur on weekends. Drowning is also seasonal in occurrence, with two thirds of all nonboat drownings, and one half of those involving boats, occurring between May and August.

The physician should educate patients about the strong link between alcohol ingestion and immersion accidents. Evidence suggests that alcohol is a factor in 20 to 80 per cent of drownings, with young men averaging 47 per cent.[16] The mechanisms are multifactorial and can involve postexercise carbohydrate depletion with a subsequent alcohol-induced decrease in blood glucose levels. These conditions can produce weakness and confusion and can disrupt the body's normal temperature-regulating mechanisms, causing rapid hypothermia.

Drug usage is also believed responsible for a large percentage of immersion accidents, and the inability to swim, including overestimation of ability, is a major risk factor. Physicians should advise that seizures, exhaustion, hyperventilation, trauma, unsupervised persons with handicaps, and the elderly who sustain falls are important risk indicators in drowning accidents.

REFERENCES

1. National Safety Council. Accident facts. Chicago, 1985.
2. Modell JH. Drown versus near-drown: a discussion of definitions (editorial). Crit Care Med 1981; 9:351–352.
3. Neal JM. Near-drowning. J Emerg Med 1985; 3:41–52.
4. Modell JH, Moya F. Effects of volume of aspirated fluid during chlorinated fresh water drowning. Anesthesiology 1966; 27:662–672.
5. Modell JH, Moya F, Newby EJ, Ruiz BC, Showers AV. The effects of fluid volume in seawater drowning. Ann Intern Med 1967; 67:68–80.
6. Gilbert J, Puckett J, Smith RB. Near-drowning—current concepts of management. Respir Care 1985; 30:108–120.
7. Sarnaik AP, Vohra MP. Near-drowning: fresh, salt and cold water immersion. Clin Sports Med 1986; 5:33–46.
8. Levin DL. Near-drowning. Crit Care Med 1980; 8:590–595.
9. Modell JH, Graves SA, Ketover A. Clinical course of 91 consecutive near-drowning victims. Chest 1976; 70:231–238.
10. Simcock AD. Treatment of near-drowning—a review of 130 cases. Anesthesia 1986; 41:643–648.
11. Gilman AG, Goodman LS. ACTH: adrenocortical steroids: inhibitors of biosynthesis. *In* Gilman AG, et

al (eds). Goodman and Gilman's The Pharmacological Basis of Therapeutics. 7th ed. New York: Macmillan, 1985:1464–1480.

12. Chokshi SK, Asper RF, Khandheria BK. Aspiration pneumonia: a review. Am Fam Phys 1986; 33(3):195–202.

13. Pearn JH. Secondary drowning in children. Br Med J 1980; 281:1103–1105.

14. Massey DG, Lumeng J. Aspiration pneumonia: a medical emergency. Hawaii Med J 1983; 42(2):48–50.

15. Centers for Disease Control. Progress toward achieving the national 1990 objectives for injury prevention and control. MMWR 1988; 37(9):139.

16. Stanley RJ, Siegal GP. Death by drowning. Minn Med 1981; (1):295–297.

Nutritional support of the acutely and chronically ill patient

Rebecca A. Roubenoff ■ *Ronenn Roubenoff*

No organ system in the human body functions better under conditions of starvation than when fed. Furthermore, the ability of the body to withstand physiologic stress is undercut when it must also contend with limitation of energy, protein, and other essential substrates needed to mount an effective response to a stress, be it infection, burn, surgery, or inflammatory disease. Over the past 20 years, our understanding of the metabolic response to acute illness has developed remarkably. At the same time, technologic advances in enteral and parenteral feeding techniques and formulas have made nutritional and metabolic support of the acutely ill patient possible. In contrast, little is known about the metabolic costs of chronic inflammatory, infectious, and degenerative diseases or the effects of nutritional intervention on the outcome of such diseases. Here we review the current understanding of the optimal metabolic support of acutely and chronically ill patients.

■ Background: The Metabolic Stress Response

Understanding nutrition intervention in the critically ill patient is predicated on an understanding of how the metabolic response to physiologic stress[1,2] acts to inhibit the normal adaptation to starvation that would occur in the nonstressed individual. The metabolic machinery invoked by simple starvation (starvation-induced malnutrition) is radically different from that activated by acute illness (disease-induced malnutrition). Failure to understand this concept leads to iatrogenic malnutrition in hospitalized patients.[3]

Available energy stores in a *healthy* 70-kg man total about 225 gm of glycogen (liver and muscle), 6000 gm of protein, and 15,000 gm of fat.[4] When a person starves, the liver glycogen stores are depleted first as glycogenolysis acts to sustain blood glucose in the absence of exogenous substrate. Liver glycogen reserves supply about 300 calories and are usually exhausted in 15 to 20 hours. If fasting continues, protein from skeletal muscle is mobilized and serves as the primary gluconeogenic substrate to maintain the energy-requiring functions of the body. The use of protein as an energy substrate is very costly to the body—an individual cannot sustain a loss of total body protein greater than 2 kg without compromising normal organ function.[5] In the nonstressed person, the blood glucose and blood insulin levels drop, allowing increased mobilization of fat reserves over 3 to 4 days. Ketoadapta-

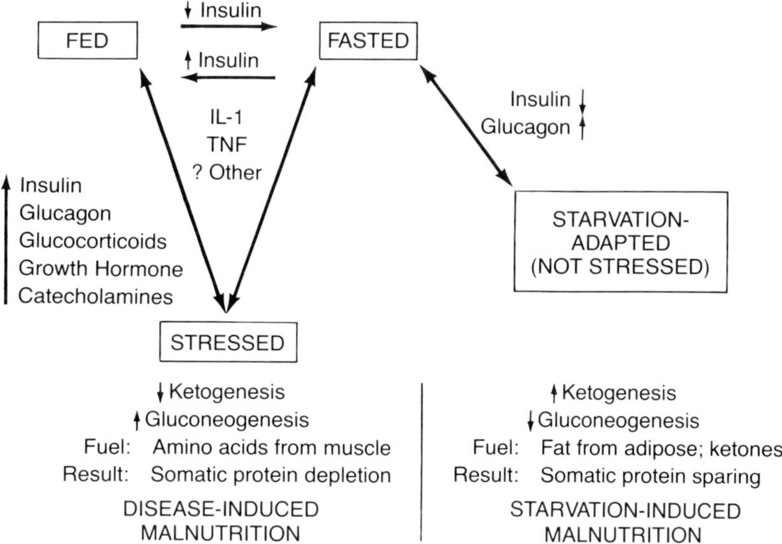

Figure 1. Simplified schema of the metabolic states of humans, their hormonal and cytokine-mediated regulation, and some of their nutritional consequences. During fasting, insulin levels are low; insulin acts as the "fed" signal, moving the body from the fed to the fasted state daily. Prolonged fasting, with low insulin levels and elevated glucagon, leads to starvation adaptation. In the presence of interleukin-1 (IL-1), tumor necrosis factor (TNF), and perhaps other cytokines, transition to the stressed state occurs. High levels of insulin and counterinsulin hormones prevent ketogenesis and starvation adaptation under stress. Note that visceral protein wasting generally accompanies somatic protein wasting.

tion ensues as fat is metabolized to ketone bodies, which are an alternative fuel for the brain and most other tissues. In this way nitrogen losses are attenuated (Fig. 1).

However, in the physiologically stressed patient, hyperglycemia and hyperinsulinemia, promoted by the release of glucagon, glucocorticoids, and catecholamines, impair this ketoadaptation and lead to obligate negative nitrogen balance (Fig. 1). The different hormonal milieu of disease-induced malnutrition is thought to be caused by the direct effect of the cytokines interleukin-1 (IL-1) and tumor necrosis factor (TNF)/cachectin.[6,7] In addition, IL-1 may have direct catabolic effects on skeletal muscle.[8] If left unfed, the patient will continue to cannibalize vital protein tissue for energy and amino acids essential to synthesize body proteins, with important clinical consequences (Table 1).[5,9,10]

■ Management

■ GOALS OF NUTRITION SUPPORT

The goals of nutrition support in acutely ill patients are to (1) maintain immune competence to prevent nosocomial infection; (2) facilitate management of fluid and electrolyte balance when the patient is hemodynamically stable; (3) prevent respiratory in-

TABLE 1. Clinical Impact of Substrate Deprivation on Organ Mass and Function[5,9,10]

Brain
increased lethargy
decreased mental alertness
increased confusion

Respiratory System
deterioration in vital capacity, respiratory rate, and tidal volume
decreased sensitivity of oxygen receptors to hypoxic stimuli
marked blunting of respiratory response to hypercapnia
animals: decreased tissue elasticity of the lung and increased air space

Gastrointestinal System
atrophy and thinning of gastrointestinal tract
blunting of mucosal villi with loss of absorptive surface and brush border enzyme activity
decreased peristalsis
malabsorption
achlorhydria

Liver
decreased liver mass
altered drug metabolism
impaired protein synthesis

Cardiovascular System
cardiac mass depletion proportional to body weight loss
potential for congestive heart failure with refeeding and rebound increase in basal metabolic rate
cardiac arrhythmias

Renal System
decreased ability to excrete titratable acid
decreased renal concentrating capacity and consequent diuresis

sufficiency and muscle weakness secondary to diaphragmatic muscle wasting; (4) maintain skin integrity to prevent decubiti and impairment of surface immunity; and (5) minimize exacerbation of the stress response (hyperglycemia, hyperinsulinemia, enhanced gluconeogenesis and protein catabolism) by providing *optimal,* yet *not excessive* amounts of nutrients.

To meet these goals, five conditions generally must be met. First, sufficient nonprotein calories (NPC) must be provided to satisfy increased metabolic demands and spare nitrogen for its protein-synthetic roles. In general, at least 100 to 130 nonprotein calories per gm of nitrogen are advocated, depending on renal and hepatic status. Second, the nonprotein calories should be distributed so as to prevent the deleterious effects of excessive carbohydrate (hyperglycemia, hyperinsulinemia, enhanced gluconeogenesis and hypercarbia) or excessive fat (possible immunosuppression and hyperlipidemia).[11] Third, the protein delivered should be of high quality and appropriate form to meet the needs of increased catabolism despite any impairment of absorption (again, with consideration of renal and hepatic function). Fourth, vitamins and minerals must be provided in amounts that will compensate for the altered absorption, excretion, and metabolism created by stress, drug-nutrient interactions, and diuretic therapy. Finally, free water should be provided in accordance with the clinical needs of the patient.

In chronic illness, the goals of nutritional therapy depend on the clinical situation and should be in harmony with the goal of the entire care plan. If aggressive medical or surgical measures are called for, then nutritional intervention should be commensurately aggressive. In terminal illness, when comfort is the goal of treatment, this should also be the goal of nutritional therapy.

Nutritional management is the mainstay of many chronic diseases. Dietary intervention in diabetes, hypercholesterolemia, and hypertension is appropriate before any pharmacologic measures are tried in the majority of patients. However, little is known about nutritional requirements in chronic inflammatory diseases, such as rheumatoid arthritis. In such patients, the goal must be to ensure that patients receive sufficient protein, calories, essential fatty acids, vitamins, and minerals to maintain or regain normal body weight and lean body mass. As with acute illnesses, the assistance of a registered dietitian in evaluating the nutritional status and needs of patients with chronic diseases is vital to appropriate management.

■ BASELINE NUTRITIONAL ASSESSMENT—WHO IS AT RISK?

Acutely ill patients generally are of two types in terms of baseline nutritional status. The first category encompasses previously healthy individuals with adequate fat, somatic, and visceral protein stores who suffer an acute illness. If their premorbid intake of macronutrients was sufficient to maintain weight and visceral proteins, then the assumption can be made that intake of essential vitamins and minerals was adequate (possible exceptions are iron and vitamin A). The second category includes individuals whose intake of nutrients or ability to absorb or utilize nutrients has been altered by social conditions (elderly patients living alone or in nursing homes), chronic disease (cancer with anorexia, stroke with cranial nerve deficits, malabsorption), or drugs (polypharmacy, alcohol abuse). This latter group usually will present with depleted fat, somatic, and visceral protein stores, along with vitamin and mineral deficits requiring prompt attention.

Beyond this categorization, only a few of the standard nutritional assessment parameters maintain their validity in critically ill patients.[12] *Per cent usual body weight (% UBW = actual weight/"usual weight" × 100)* is useful, since an involuntary loss of 10 per cent of UBW in the 6 months prior to admission signals an important depletion of fat, protein, and vitamin and mineral reserves. It is desirable to obtain a *documented* "usual weight" from an old medical record, family physician, or family member, since the patient's memory may be impaired. *Anthropometric measurements,* such as skinfold thickness or arm muscle circumference, to assess quantitative changes in body fat and protein are not valid in the acute care settings secondary to fluid retention that masks the true fat-muscle interface. *Visceral status* usually refers to the adequacy of the serum transport proteins synthesized by the liver (albumin, transferrin, retinol-binding protein). Serum albumin or transferrin levels obtained before the administration of intravenous fluids on the day of admission are helpful in assessing baseline visceral status. Although all facets of host resistance are altered in malnutrition (cell-mediated, humoral, and nonspecific resistance), the use of a total lymphocyte count or delayed cutaneous hypersensitivity to known recall antigens is of little benefit in assessing nutritional status in the acute setting, since steroids, infection, uremia, malignancy, and surgery all alter these immune responses.

Since most nutritional indices cannot reliably be used in assessing the critically ill patient, the decision of when to begin nutritional support is one of clinical judgment. The physician should not wait for malnutrition to occur, but rather attempt to predict the course of the disease and its impact on nutrient intake, needs, and utilization, keeping a mental tally of each day's caloric, protein, vitamin, and mineral deficits. It is incorrect to believe that acutely ill patients, especially those in an ICU setting, will be able to satisfy their caloric or protein needs with oral intake. In our experience, calorie counts in the ICU document that this ad lib intake averages 800 to 1000 calories and 40 grams of protein daily. In contrast, a typical 70-kg ICU patient needs about 2500 calories and 100 grams of protein per day, in the absence of renal or hepatic impairment. Vitamin and mineral deficits parallel caloric and protein (nitrogen) deficits (Fig. 2). The longer nutritional deficits are allowed to persist, the more protracted the nutritional rehabilitation phase will be.

CALORIC AND PROTEIN NEEDS

Patients suffering from acute events, such as sepsis, trauma, head injury, or surgical emergencies, are hypermetabolic (increased energy expenditure) and hypercatabolic (increased protein degradation evidenced by high urinary urea nitrogen excretion). The length of the hypermetabolic, hypercatabolic phase parallels the severity of the insult. Infectious complications, steroid administration, persistent tachycardia, or uncontrolled seizure activity can protract this hypermetabolic, hypercatabolic state (Fig. 3). Conversely, lower than predicted energy expenditures have been reported for sedated patients or those with spinal cord injury.

Ideally, energy requirements should be determined by indirect calorimetry, but in many hospitals this is not available. In this case, prudent estimates of needs should be based on the literature consensus and established nutritional guidelines for metabolically stressed patients (Table 2).[13] These estimates will be altered by clinical factors such as mechanical ventilation, fever, and tachycardia. Both overfeeding and underfeeding should be avoided. The best way to avoid underfeeding is to make nutrition a component of rounds, reviewing the nutritional status of the patient with housestaff, nurses, and dietitians on a daily basis.

The most common mistakes that result in overfeeding are (1) approximating caloric needs for an underweight patient based on

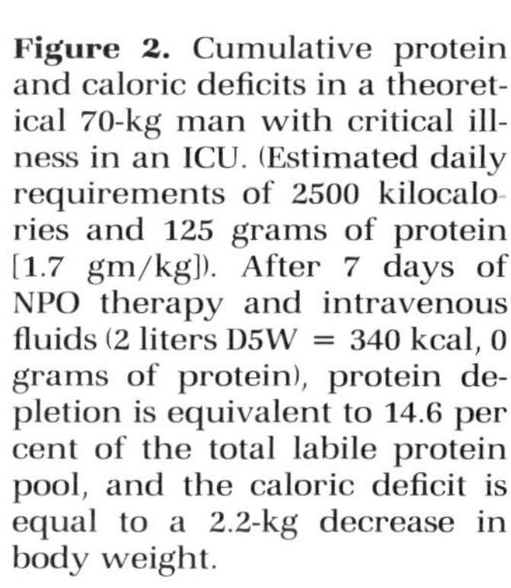

Figure 2. Cumulative protein and caloric deficits in a theoretical 70-kg man with critical illness in an ICU. (Estimated daily requirements of 2500 kilocalories and 125 grams of protein [1.7 gm/kg]). After 7 days of NPO therapy and intravenous fluids (2 liters D5W = 340 kcal, 0 grams of protein), protein depletion is equivalent to 14.6 per cent of the total labile protein pool, and the caloric deficit is equal to a 2.2-kg decrease in body weight.

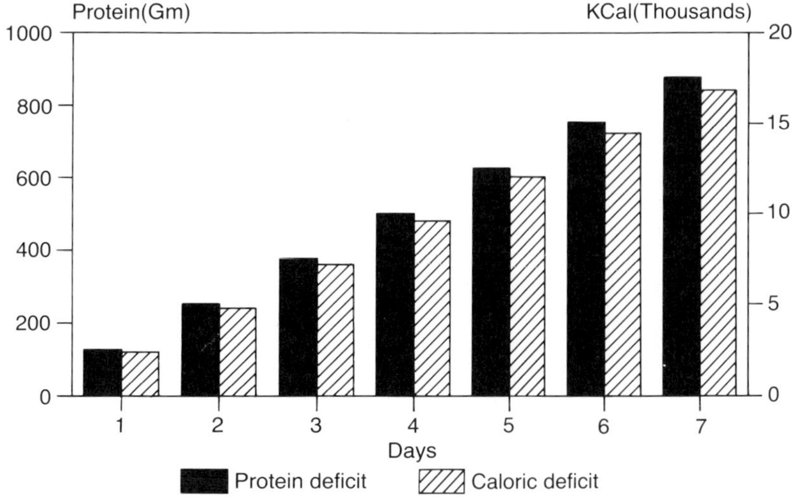

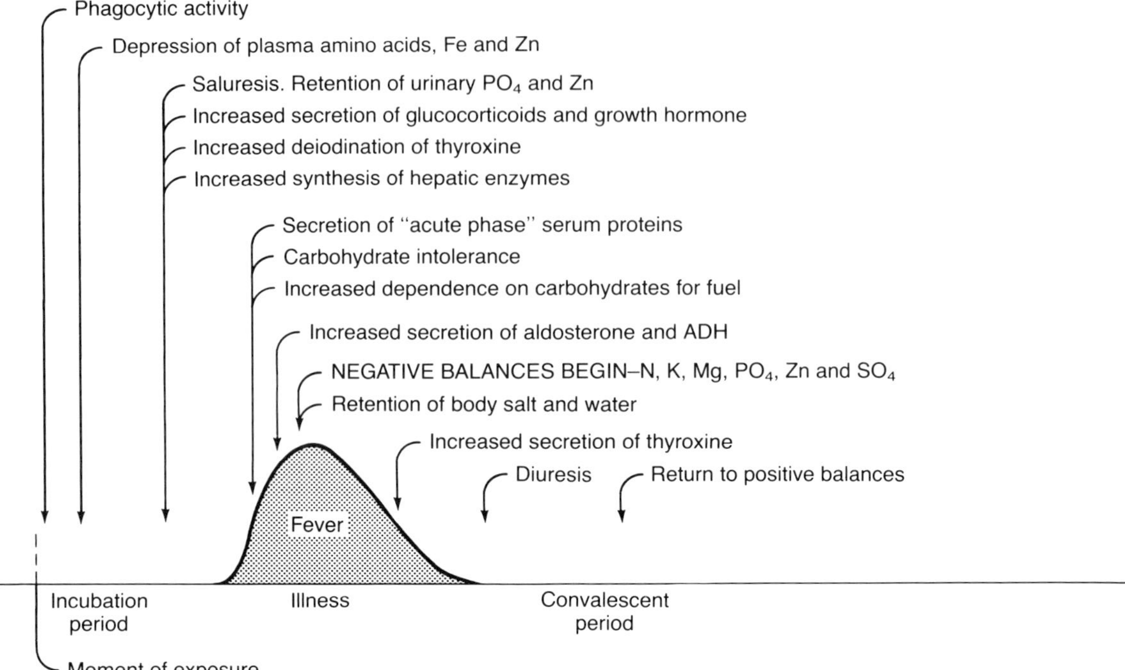

Figure 3. The sequence and relative time of onset of various components of the metabolic stress response to a brief febrile infectious disease. (Reprinted with permission from Beisel WR: Magnitude of the host nutritional responses to infection. Am J Clin Nutr 30:1236–1247, 1977. © American Society for Clinical Nutrition.)

an "ideal weight" from standard reference tables, instead of using actual weight, and (2) use of actual weight to estimate needs in an overweight patient instead of "adjusted" weight (see Table 2). It is also important to

TABLE 2. Estimated *Total* Daily Caloric Requirements in Lieu of Indirect Calorimetry

Situation	Caloric Requirement*
Burn	May exceed BEE × 2.0
Head injury, polytrauma	BEE × 1.6–1.9
Elective surgery	BEE × 1.3–1.6
Sepsis/infection	BEE × 1.5–1.6

*BEE = basal energy expenditure, based on the Harris-Benedict equation:

BEE (male) = (kcal/24 hr) = 66.473 + 13.752(W) + 5.003(H) − 6.755(A)

BEE (female) = (kcal/24 hr) = 655.096 + 9.563(W) + 1.85(H) − 4.676(A)

NOTE: W = weight in kilograms (kg). If patient is at or below ideal body weight (IBW), as determined from standard tables, use actual weight since the regression equations are optimally predictive the closer one gets to lean body mass. If a patient is overweight, use adjusted weight = IBW + 0.25 (actual weight − IBW) to account for metabolically inactive adipose tissue.

H = height in centimeters; A = age in years.

ensure that nonprotein calories are not disproportionately administered as carbohydrate. This may occur in the case of parenteral nutrition without concurrent lipid infusion, or in certain elemental feedings that do not satisfy essential fatty acid (EFA) requirements. When the feeding provides less than 25 per cent of the total calories as fat, at least 3 per cent of total calories should come from essential fatty acids (EFA).[14]

Protein needs for depleted, metabolically stressed patients should total approximately 16 to 20 per cent of the calories provided. An accurate estimate of protein needs can be determined only by conducting a carefully controlled nitrogen balance study. However, if inadequate NPC are provided, the body will simply metabolize dietary protein to energy via gluconeogenesis. Nitrogen balance studies conducted in the face of inadequate NPC will be negative due to the use of protein as an energy substrate and not because of insufficient protein per se. On the other hand, if high protein loads are provided (1.5 to 2.0 gm/kg), then the urinary nitrogen excretion may be driven by excessive nitrogen intake. Also, renal status should be stable during the collection period, since changes in blood urea nitrogen obviously reflect altered excretion. Nitrogen balance studies should not be used to assess protein needs or anabolism/catabolism, unless the clinician is familiar with the subtleties and caveats of the balance technique.[15]

Initially, when caloric needs are high, protein needs will range from 1.5 to 2.0 gm of protein per kg, decreasing to a range of 1.2 to 1.5 gm per kg *provided* hypermetabolism abates. In the beginning, it may be possible only to attenuate nitrogen losses rather than to achieve positive nitrogen balance (anabolism). Determination of protein requirements is always modulated by the patient's hepatic and renal function. Both hepatic and renal insufficiency require a decrease in protein intake. Enteral and parenteral formulations can be modified to provide adequate calories, essential fatty acids, vitamins, and minerals, with a reduced amount of protein.

VITAMIN AND MINERAL CONSIDERATIONS

Vitamin and mineral considerations primarily relate to the drugs commonly prescribed in acute illness and the consequent drug-nutrient interactions, superimposed on altered requirements in stress and infection.[16] Pharmacologic agents often disrupt one or more of the steps of nutrient intake, digestion, absorption, binding, activation, catabolism, or elimination and may precipitate deficiency. Drug-nutrient interactions should be evaluated routinely to prevent deficiencies from arising. Readers are referred to one of several excellent references on this subject.[17]

Further, it is important in the setting of acute illness to interpret low plasma values of certain minerals carefully. In infections or inflammatory conditions, both zinc and iron undergo a dramatic, physiologically controlled redistribution, with sequestration in the liver and reticuloendothelial system. It is hypothesized that this may serve a useful purpose in host defense. If iron is therapeutically administered in persistent infection to attempt reversal of anemia or low serum iron values, this may actually harm host defense by providing needed substrate for bacterial metabolism.[18] One must assess individually whether the enteral or parenteral formulas meet the increased vitamin and mineral needs.

Issues and Risks

CHOICE OF FEEDING ROUTE

Enteral feedings are the first choice for administration of nutrition support in all patients because of their many advantages over parenteral alimentation. Primarily, enteral feeding maintains the integrity and immunologic role of the intestine, which is now regarded as paramount in preventing gram-negative infectious complications in acutely ill patients.[19] When the gut is deprived of nutrients, it atrophies, thins, and becomes more permeable to enteric bacteria. This situation is not improved by intravenous feedings. In addition, enteral feedings provide prophylaxis against stress ulceration, have far lower costs (approximately $20 per day vs. up to $200 per day for parenteral support), and make fluid and nutrient intake manipulation easier in patients with renal/hepatic dysfunction.

Like any medical technology, nasoenteric feeding tubes have certain strengths and limitations that must be recognized. Nasoenteric feeding tubes decrease the risk of sepsis and pneumothorax associated with parenteral nutrition. However, care must be taken in inserting these tubes in patients who are intubated or have a depressed level of consciousness. In such patients, pneumothorax is not uncommon and generally goes unrecognized until a complication, such as bronchopleural fistula or intrapulmonary feeding, occurs. We have recently described a technique for use in such patients that we feel is safe, effective, and inexpensive.[20] The commonest risk associated with enteral feeding is aspiration, which can be greatly reduced with good nursing care, continuous rather than bolus feeding, judicious use of agents that improve gastric emptying (i.e., metoclopramide), strict enforcement of standard aspiration precautions, and/or postpyloric feeding tube placement.

A more subtle risk is that diluted ("quarter- or half-strength") hypocaloric enteral formulas will be delivered for a protracted period, giving the illusion of satisfying a patient's needs although they do not. When delivering nutrients into the stomach, formulas should be started full strength unless there is delayed gastric emptying (despite metoclopramide), unless the feeding is a transition from a prolonged course of NPO and parenteral nutrition, or unless the patient presents with severe protein-calorie malnutrition. In these situations, isotonic concentrations of formulas (which are often hypocaloric for the patient's needs) must be tolerated. The feeding should be advanced expeditiously to full rate, full strength with a specific caloric and protein goal in mind. Postpyloric nutrient delivery is best accomplished with fiber-containing formulas at full strength or other formulas at isotonic strength advancing to full strength as tolerated; the choice will depend on the patient's baseline nutritional status and clinical condition.

In general, central alimentation should be used only when the gut is not functional. For example, central venous nutritional support is indicated in patients with protracted ileus or in uncontrolled seizures with concomitant vomiting and increased aspiration risk. Even then, enteral feedings should be resumed as soon as possible. The additional cost of parenteral nutrition, as well as its decreased efficiency with regard to nutrient delivery to the liver, do not seem to justify its use in the presence of a working gastrointestinal tract.[21] The lack of bowel sounds is not a contraindication to enteral feeding with *isotonic strength predigested formulas*, if the abdominal examination is benign and the patient does not display high gastric residuals upon feeding.

■ MANAGEMENT OF ENTERAL FEEDING COMPLICATIONS

The most frequently observed complications that impair adequate delivery of nutrients enterally are delayed gastric emptying, ileus, and diarrhea. Gastric emptying will be optimal if enteral formulas are isotonic and relatively low in fat. Concurrent administration of metoclopramide and minimization of sedatives also will stimulate gastric emptying. In partial ileus, delivery of a predigested formula postpylorus eliminates the need for digestion and ensures absorption in the upper small intestine, leaving minimal residue. This often obviates the need for parenteral nutrition in partial ileus associated with severe pneumonia, spinal cord injury, or pancreatitis. In pancreatitis, nasojejunal feeding is preferred in order to bypass duodenal stasis.

Enteral tube feeding is *rarely* the etiologic agent for diarrhea. More likely culprits are boluses of hyperosmolar substances like KCl (osmolarity more than 3000 mOsm), broad-spectrum antibiotics, and phosphorus and magnesium supplements (especially magnesium containing antacids). Distribution of about 20 mEq of KCl in 500 ml of tube feeding generally will prevent diarrhea associated with hyperosmolar boluses of potassium. Distributed doses of phosphorus and magnesium are also better tolerated. If patients are transitioning off antibiotics, it is sometimes helpful to attempt recolonization of the large bowel with lactobacillus preparations. Otherwise, the use of a predigested formula with attention to adequate vitamin and mineral supplementation should diminish antibiotic-induced diarrhea. In all cases, an infection or impaction should be ruled out, and bulking agents such as Metamucil should be used before antimotility agents are instituted.

■ FLUID MANAGEMENT: DISORDERS OF SODIUM AND WATER BALANCE

When additional fluid is needed, the rate of parenteral or enteral nutrition often will be increased inappropriately. These fluids represent nutrient fluids with a substantial solute load and cannot act as a substitute for free water. The result is overfeeding and subsequent hyperglycemia, increased blood urea nitrogen, and hypercapnia. Conversely, enteral and parenteral formulations can be modified to meet nutritional needs within the confines of a fluid restriction (i.e., using 2 kcal/ml formulas); merely turning down the rate of a less concentrated solution will result in caloric, protein, vitamin, and mineral deficits. It is also important to remember that all enteral feeding formulas are hyponatremic fluids—nonelemental formulas provide about 20 to 40 mEq Na/liter whereas elemental, predigested, or modular formulas are usually as low as 20 mEq Na/liter. If sodium depletion is documented or risk of seizure secondary to low serum sodium is important, additional sodium can be added to the enteral feeding (1 gm NaCl = 17 mEq Na).

■ APPROACH TO THE ACUTELY ILL PATIENT: THE ABCs

The hypermetabolic, hypercatabolic state of acutely ill patients may lead to significant deterioration in nutritional status in a short period of time if their nutritional requirements remain unsatisfied. Their catabolic status generally presents as a simple weight loss rather than as clinically evident cachexia, and initial routine laboratory tests may reveal only mild hypoalbuminemia, hyponatremia, and hypophosphatemia. The provision of essential nutrients can be an important adjunct to the management of the primary disease, particularly if done in a timely and appropriate fashion. There is evidence that the outcome of acute illness is altered by nutritional therapy.[22] Table 3 shows what we have called the ABCs of nutritional support, which when followed will optimize nutrition in acute illness.

■ APPROACH TO THE CHRONICALLY ILL PATIENT

Two recent studies, one by the Surgeon General[23] and one by the National Research Council,[24] have exhaustively documented the interactions of nutrition and chronic diseases. The evidence for nutritional influence in disease development is strongest for hypertension, atherosclerosis, and obesity. In addition, there is also evidence for the impact of diet on the incidence of cancer, osteoporosis, diabetes, hepatobiliary diseases, and dental caries.

It is important to discriminate between the diseases associated with nutrient excess and chronic wasting illnesses, such as rheumatoid arthritis, emphysema, AIDS, and many cancers. Until better information is available, much of what we have discussed about acute illness pertains to these latter diseases as well (see Table 3). Careful assessment of patients' nutritional status by a registered dietitian and intervention to maintain or attain ideal body weight must be the cornerstone of therapy. In all cases, the burden of proof is on anyone who would claim that the human body functions better when starved than when fed.

TABLE 3. Approach to the Nutritional and Metabolic Support Needs of the Acutely Ill Patient

Assess nutritional status at admission and throughout hospital course. A good baseline nutritional status can deteriorate rapidly in the face of hypermetabolism and hypercatabolism.

Begin feeding as soon as the patient is hemodynamically stable.

Consider enteral nutrition first.

Diets (weight reduction) are for healthy people. Normal starvation adaptation is not possible in the hormonal milieu of acute illness.

End-organ damage affects nutritional needs and alternatives.

Facts are your best ally—consult a nutritionist early and often as to the adequacy of a patient's nutritional intake.

REFERENCES

1. Negro F, Cerra FB. Nutritional monitoring in the ICU: rational and practical application. Crit Care Clin 1988; 4:559–572.
2. Black PR, Wilmore DW. Hormone-substrate interactions. *In* Rombeau JL, Caldwell MD (eds). Enteral and Tube Feeding. Philadelphia: WB Saunders, 1984:60–72.
3. Roubenoff R, Roubenoff RA, Preto J, Balke CW. Malnutrition among hospitalized patients: a problem of physician awareness. Arch Intern Med 1987; 147:1462–1465.
4. Cahill GF. Starvation in man. N Engl J Med 1970; 282:669–675.
5. Aoki TT, Finley RJ. The metabolic response to fasting. *In* Rombeau JL, Caldwell MD (eds). Parenteral Nutrition. Philadelphia: WB Saunders, 1986:15.
6. Pomposelli JJ, Flores EA, Bistrian BR. Role of biochemical mediators in clinical nutrition and surgical metabolism. J Parenter Enter Nutr 1988; 12:212–218.
7. Neta R, Oppenheim JJ. Why should internists be interested in interleukin-1? Ann Intern Med 1988; 109:1–3.
8. Baracos V, Rodeman HP, Dinarello CA, Goldberg AL. Stimulation of muscle protein degradation and prostaglandin E_2 release by leukocytic pyrogen (interleukin-1). A mechanism for the increased degradation of muscle proteins during fever. N Engl J Med 1983; 308:553–558.
9. Grant JP. Clinical impact of protein malnutrition on organ mass and function. *In* Blackburn GL, Grant JP, Young VR (eds). Amino Acid Metabolism and Medical Applications. Boston: Wright, PSG, 1983:347–358.
10. Bryan-Brown CW, Savitz MH, Elwyn DH, Shoemaker WC. Cerebral edema unresponsive to conventional therapy in neurosurgical patients with unsuspected nutritional failure. Crit Care Med 1973; 1:125–129.
11. Sobrado J, Moldawer LL, Pomposelli JJ, et al. Lipid emulsions and reticuloendothelial system function in healthy and burned guinea pigs. Am J Clin Nutr 1985; 42:855–863.

12. Baker JP, Lemoyne M. Nutritional support in the critically ill patient: if, when, how and what. Crit Care Clin 1987; 3:97–113.
13. Long CL, Schaffel N, Geiger JW, et al. Metabolic response to injury and illness: estimation of energy and protein needs from indirect calorimetry and nitrogen balance. J Parenter Enter Nutr 1979; 3:452–456.
14. Krause MV, Mahan LK. Lipids. In Krause MV, Mahan LK (eds). Food, Nutrition and Diet Therapy. Philadelphia: WB Saunders, 1984:50.
15. Kopple JD. Uses and limitations of the balance technique. J Parenter Enter Nutr 1987; 11(Suppl):79S–85S.
16. Roe DA. Concurrent interactions of drugs and nutrients. In Linder MC (ed). Nutritional Biochemistry and Metabolism with Clinical Applications. New York: Elsevier, 1985:411–421.
17. Roe DA. Diet and Drug Interactions. New York: Van Nostrand Reinhold, 1989.
18. Karp JE, Merz WG. Association of reduced TIBC and fungal infections in leukemic granulocytopenic patients. J Clin Oncol 1986; 4:216–220.
19. Wilmore DW, Smith RJ, O'Dwyer ST, Jacobs DO, Ziegler TR, Wang X-D. The gut: a central organ after surgical stress. Surgery 1988; 104:917–923.
20. Roubenoff R, Ravich WJ. Pneumothorax due to nasogastric feeding tubes: report of four cases, review of the literature, and recommendations for prevention. Arch Intern Med 1989; 149:184–188.
21. Heymsfield SB, Bethel RA, Ansley JD, Nixon DW, Rudman D. Enteral hyperalimentation: an alternative to central venous hyperalimentation. Ann Intern Med 1979; 90:639–711.
22. Cerra FB. Influence of nutrition on the outcome of septic patients. In New Aspects of Clinical Nutrition. Basel: Karger, 1983:136–145.
23. The Surgeon General's report on nutrition and health. US DHHS (PHS) Publ 88–50210. Washington, DC: Office of the Surgeon General, 1988.
24. Committee on Diet and Health, Food and Nutrition Board, National Research Council. Diet and Health: Implications for Reducing Chronic Disease Risk. Washington, DC: National Academy Press, 1989.

Obesity in the diabetic patient

Christopher D. Saudek ■ *Adrian S. Dobs*

■ Background

Noninsulin-dependent diabetes mellitus (NIDDM), Type II, is by far the most common form of diabetes, and the majority of people with NIDDM are obese. By virtually any measure, obesity and NIDDM are tightly linked clinical entities. Epidemiologically, the prevalence of diabetes in a nation varies directly with the average body weight of the population.[1] Individually, the risk of developing NIDDM is enormously increased in the setting of obesity. In populations as diverse as the Pima tribe of Native Americans,[2] Norwegians,[3] and residents of Framingham Massachusetts,[4] obesity is an independent risk factor for NIDDM.

The association between diabetes and obesity is particularly important for American minorities. Blacks, native Americans, and Hispanics all have an increased prevalence of NIDDM that is associated with obesity.[5]

But even though obesity and NIDDM are among the most common clinical associations seen by practicing physicians, the problem is neither well understood pathophysiologically nor readily managed clinically. And it is certainly not to be taken lightly. Obesity itself, in the total absence of other comorbidities, may not be an independent risk factor for coronary heart disease at all;[6] but the point is largely academic, since obesity is so often associated with other serious risk factors in addition to diabetes. Hypertension, hypertriglyceridemia, low concentrations of high-density lipoprotein (HDL) cholesterol, and hyperinsulinism are each statistically associated with diabetes, and each increases the risk of cardiovascular disease.

Nor is all obesity alike. It has been well

demonstrated in prospective studies that abdominal obesity, in particular, is a risk factor for glucose intolerance, NIDDM, and atherosclerosis.[7] In managing the obese person with diabetes, the clinician must identify and treat not only the diabetes but also the associated cardiovascular risk factors.

The underlying pathophysiology of diabetes in obesity is peripheral insulin resistance, with inadequate insulin secretion to overcome this resistance. The liver is also resistant to insulin, and hepatic glucose production continues in spite of elevated insulin levels. Some evidence now implicates this insulin resistance as a direct cause of hypertension,[8] although the point remains controversial.

Most obese people who do *not* have diabetes compensate for their obesity-related insulin resistance by secreting large amounts of endogenous insulin. As long as the obese person can continue to maintain unusually high basal and postprandial insulin concentrations, normal glucose tolerance is maintained; but if pancreatic insulin reserve is limited and the insulin resistance becomes more severe than the pancreas can "keep up with," then glucose tolerance deteriorates.

Plasma insulin levels in the obese diabetic patient, therefore, are highly variable and not particularly informative clinically. In general, venous immunoreactive insulin concentrations are elevated when the diabetes is mild, falling into the normal or low range as diabetes worsens and the fasting blood glucose level rises.[9]

Although peripheral insulin resistance in obesity has been recognized essentially since the development of the radioimmunoassay for insulin, its underlying mechanisms are not well understood. Adipose tissue, like other insulin-responsive cells, has insulin receptors on the cell surface. Hyperinsulinism will itself "down-regulate" the number of receptors, but intracellular events—the protein kinase–mediated second messages and the recruitment of glucose transport proteins to the cell surface, for example—appear to have more to do with insulin resistance in obesity.

There is also evidence that pancreatic insulin secretion, although present, is not normal. "First-phase" insulin secretion, that occurring in the first few minutes after stimulation, is blunted, and beta-cell sensitivity to hyperglycemia is blunted. But controversy still exists as to which comes first, the pancreatic secretory abnormalities or the peripheral insulin resistance.

Major alterations in basal metabolic rate (BMR) have not been demonstrated in the obese patient with NIDDM, compared with either the nonobese diabetic or nondiabetic patient. In general, obese individuals have an increased BMR that correlates with their increased lean body mass.

■ Management

■ INITIAL EVALUATION

Diagnosis

Accurately diagnosing diabetes mellitus and obesity is usually, but not always, simple. To begin with, they are separate diagnoses.

No single definition of obesity is universally accepted, but a useful calculation is the body mass index (BMI): Body mass index = weight (kg)/height^2 (m). The ideal BMI for a man is about 22.9 and about 22.6 for a woman. Risk increases above 25, and obesity (over 120 per cent of ideal body weight) corresponds to a BMI of more than about 27.5 for men, 27.1 for women. Based on weight alone, moderate, severe and morbid obesities are defined as 20 per cent, 40 per cent, and over 100 per cent, respectively.[10]

Criteria for the diagnosis of diabetes mellitus are well established (Table 1).[11] Most often, the diagnosis is made by documenting a high random plasma glucose level (over 200 mg/dl) in the setting of classic symptoms of hyperglycemia (polyuria, polydipsia, weight loss). If this criterion is not met, a fasting plasma glucose level greater than 140 mg/dl on two occasions will establish the diagnosis. In the setting of obesity, though, the clinical suspicion may be high enough to warrant oral glucose tolerance testing.

The oral glucose tolerance test (OGTT) (70 gm of oral glucose, with plasma glucose drawn at 0, 30, 60, 90, and 120 min) is needed only when the other criteria are not met, and specifically *not* when frank hyperglycemia has already made the diagnosis. Diabetes is diagnosed, in an OGTT, if the 2-hour glucose level and one other glucose level between 0 and 2 hours are greater than 200 mg/dl.

But there are several more subtleties to in-

TABLE 1. Diagnostic Criteria for Diabetes Mellitus, Impaired Glucose Tolerance, and Gestational Diabetes

Nonpregnant Adults

Criteria for the diagnosis of diabetes mellitus. Nonpregnant adults should have one of the following:

- Random plasma glucose level of 200 mg/dl or greater, plus classic signs and symptoms of diabetes mellitus, including polydipsia, polyuria, polyphagia, and weight loss;
- Fasting plasma glucose level of 140 mg/dl or greater on at least 2 occasions; or
- Fasting plasma glucose level less than 140 mg/dl, plus sustained elevated plasma glucose levels during at least two oral glucose tolerance tests. The 2-hour sample and at least one other between 0 and 2 hours after a 75-gram glucose dose should be 200 mg/dl or greater. Oral glucose tolerance testing is not necessary if the patient has a fasting plasma glucose level of 140 mg/dl or greater.

Criteria for the diagnosis of impaired glucose tolerance. Nonpregnant adults should have all of the following:

- A fasting plasma glucose level of less than 140 mg/dl;
- A 2-hour oral glucose tolerance test plasma glucose level of between 140 and 200 mg/dl; and
- An intervening oral glucose tolerance test plasma glucose level of 200 mg/dl or greater.

Pregnant Women

Criteria for the diagnosis of gestational diabetes: Two plasma glucose values (mg/dl) equal to or exceeding these values after an oral glucose load of 100 gm:

Fasting	1 Hour	2 Hour	3 Hour
105	190	165	145

(Adapted from Lebovitz HE (ed). Physician's Guide to Non-Insulin-Dependent (Type II) Diabetes: Diagnosis and Treatment. 2nd ed. Alexandria, VA: American Diabetes Association, Inc., 1988.)

terpretation of glucose tolerance testing. First, a result may not quite meet the criteria for diabetes but not be normal, either. One value between 0 and 2 hours of more than 200 mg/dl, with the 2-hour reading between 140 and 200 mg/dl, is called "impaired glucose tolerance" (IGT). There are also formal definitions for borderline tests and inconclusive results that do not meet the criteria for IGT, and these tests should be repeated. Terms such as *chemical diabetes*, *borderline diabetes*, and *prediabetes* should be abandoned, since they convey the message of diabetes, with all its social impact and all its employment and insurance implications, when diabetes is not in fact present. About 75 per cent of people with IGT apparently never do go on to develop frank diabetes, although the risk is higher in certain populations.[12,13]

Particularly when associated with obesity, pregnancy is a common time for the first presentation of diabetes. All pregnant women should have glucose tolerance screening in midpregnancy, and if the screen is positive, a 40-gram OGTT should be done. The plasma glucose criteria for gestational diabetes differ from those accepted for the nongravid state (Table 1).

Classification of Diabetes

After the diagnosis of diabetes mellitus is made, the next issue is classification (Table 2). Usually, but not always, diabetes associated with obesity turns out to be Type II NIDDM, the disease that used to be called maturity-onset diabetes. But while age (over

TABLE 2. Classification of Diabetes and Glucose Intolerance

Diabetes mellitus
    Type I: insulin-dependent
    Type II: noninsulin-dependent
    Other types:
        Hormonal
        Drug or chemically induced
        Pancreatic disease
        Insulin receptor abnormalities
        Certain genetic syndromes
        Other types

Impaired glucose tolerance (IGT)

Gestational diabetes (GDM)

Statistical risk classes
    Previous abnormality of glucose tolerance
    Potential abnormality of glucose tolerance

(Adapted from Harvey AM, Johns RJ, McKusick VA, Owens AH Jr, Ross RS (eds). The Principles and Practice of Medicine. 22nd ed. East Norwalk, CT: Appleton and Lange, 1988.)

40 years old) and increased body weight, responsiveness to oral hypoglycemic agents, and a stable metabolic course are strongly suggestive of NIDDM, the true definition of NIDDM is diabetes that does not cause ketoacidosis in the absence of exogenous insulin treatment.[11]

Maturity-onset diabetes of youth (MODY) is a form of NIDDM seen in childhood but is otherwise typical of NIDDM, especially in its association with obesity. An overweight diabetic child with a strong family history of diabetes and relatively stable glycemia, particularly a black child,[14] may in fact have NIDDM rather than the typical insulin-dependent diabetes more often seen in children.

■ HISTORY, PHYSICAL, AND LABORATORY BASELINE

Once an accurate diagnosis is established, baseline history, physical examination, and laboratory tests should be done. Since NIDDM often has a gradual onset, long-term complications may be present when the disease is diagnosed and should be carefully sought.

Risk factor assessment is especially important in the obese diabetic patient. High blood pressure is both a sign and a cause of nephropathy and should be treated diligently. Pressures greater than 140/85 mm Hg should be addressed. Hyperlipidemia, especially hypertriglyceridemia with decreased HDL-cholesterol, is common and requires treatment. The National Cholesterol Education Program has listed diabetes and obesity as risk factors requiring more aggressive treatment. A low-density lipoprotein (LDL) level of less than 130 mg/dl should be the goal for these patients.[15] In addition, smoking has been clearly shown to increase the risk of peripheral vascular and other macrovascular diseases, as well as diabetic retinopathy.

■ OVERALL TREATMENT GOALS

The goals of treating diabetes when combined with obesity are not different from those of treating diabetes alone, although the approaches do differ in many respects. The objective is to control the blood glucose to as close to normal as feasible, and to avoid or treat secondary complications of diabetes and obesity. These goals are approached with the understanding that normoglycemia is not achievable in most people with diabetes, any more than normal body weight is achievable in most obese people. The clinician must be aware of avoiding side effects of treatment, especially serious hypoglycemia or the dangers of faddish weight-loss programs.

Controlling blood glucose, to begin with, will eliminate the acute symptoms and the acute complications of diabetes. Polyuria, thirst, and chronic vaginal yeast infections, for example, are indicators of poor glycemic control. Adequate treatment, by definition, also will avoid hospitalization for diabetic control or for a hyperosmolar nonketotic state. But it does *not* follow that avoidance of acute symptoms and hospitalization for acute loss of control are adequate standards of care.

What, then, is "adequate" or "acceptable" blood glucose control? There is no single answer. Goal setting with the patient, judging when the goal is not met, and moving to the next level of therapy are individualized clinical judgments. Nevertheless, the ideal can be stated: the normal plasma glucose fasting level is less than 115 mg/dl and the postprandial level is less than about 140 mg/dl. In general, a fasting plasma glucose level over 200 mg/dl or postprandial glycemia of greater than 235 mg/dl is *not* good.[16]

The weight of evidence strongly suggests that long-term complications—particularly microvascular complications—are lessened by good diabetic control over the years, although the evidence is confounded by a great many variables. Glycemia is by no means the only, or even the most important, factor in predisposing to certain long-term complications. Blood pressure, plasma lipids, and family history may be more important, for example, in predisposing to atherosclerosis. And there is no reason to think that a control-complications relationship is linear: there may be a threshold below which few complications exist, or a plateau above which no further damage is done. Certainly, individual susceptibility and hereditary factors play a role. But available evidence justifies maintaining good glycemic control while taking care to minimize side effects of therapy.

■ DIABETES EDUCATION

The starting point in establishing good diabetic control is thorough, professional diabetes education. Indeed, a whole new profession as certified diabetes educator has sprung up in the last decade. Large voluntary organizations such as the American Diabetes Association and the American Association of Diabetes Educators may be consulted for available programs in most areas of the country. Practitioners of medicine and their clinical assistants rarely have either the time or the specific expertise to educate patients about diabetes. Formal courses or consultations for diabetic patients are therefore strongly recommended.

■ DIET AND WEIGHT CONTROL

It is reasonable to start most people with NIDDM and obesity on dietary therapy alone. The key, of course, is weight reduction, and the means is reduced total caloric intake. Exercise, while contributory (see later), by itself is usually ineffective. It is interesting, and encouraging to dieting patients, to note that abrupt caloric restriction has a virtually immediate effect on fasting blood glucose levels, and that this effect is largely due to reduced hepatic glucose output. However, improving peripheral insulin resistance, noted earlier as the cardinal pathophysiologic feature of NIDDM with obesity, requires significantly reduced body weight, which is clearly a longer-term proposition.

An understanding of the merits and risks of various approaches to weight control will help the physician oversee a safe and effective program.

Intensive Approaches to Weight Reduction

The benefits of aggressive weight reduction are impressive, at least in the short term, with proven reductions in glycohemoglobin and fasting blood sugars and evidence of improved insulin secretion in response to glucose.[17] Intensive diet strategies can be classified as fasting, very low-calorie, or low-calorie diets. Fasting for up to 1 week under close supervision has been found safe in as many as 10,000 patients.[18] Blood sugars can become normal quickly. Long-term safety, patient acceptability, and weight loss maintenance, however, are the clear problems. In one series of fasters, five deaths were reported (two patients with cardiac arrests, one patient with acute volvulus, one patient with hyperuricemia nephritis, and one patient with an unclear cause).[19] Unless patients are hospitalized under the care of an experienced physician, therapeutic fasting of more than a week's duration is not recommended.

Very low-calorie formula diets are better accepted now that poor-quality protein diets have been replaced by high-quality protein diets. The former had been used in the late 1970s, when 60 deaths were reported among 100,000 people who had no pre-existing disease. The deaths were attributed to ventricular tachycardia, with prolongation of the QT interval in 32 patients.[20]

High-quality protein diets appear more promising, without evidence of causing arrhythmias or increased insulin secretion.[21] These diets are usually commercially prepared and distributed as part of a combined program with social supports and education (e.g., Optifast, Medibase). They offer simplicity and follow-up, and, in close coordination with an internist or a diabetologist, they may be safe. But patients must be aware of the paucity of research using these diets in diabetes and must agree to close supervision. Insulin requirements may change quickly.

Similar to other weight loss programs, the long-term recidivism rate using very low-calorie diets is high, and the transition to a maintenance diet is difficult. In addition, they are costly. Investigations are needed to determine which, if any, obese diabetic patients could benefit from these programs.

Balanced low-calorie food diets are more familiar to doctors and their patients. Their advantage is that, if well planned, they may involve relatively little variation from the patient's usual diet. But without personal tailoring, or if too complicated or lacking in personalized follow-up, these, too, may result in long-term recidivism to obesity.

Multidisciplinary programs, including nutrition counseling, exercise, behavior modification, and physician contacts, have been advocated.[22] Programs such as Weight Watchers and Overeaters Anonymous employ peer support and pressure. These are safe in diabetics and may suit some individuals. However, the attrition rate in some has been 50 per cent at 6 weeks and 70 per cent at 12 weeks.[23]

In conclusion, the initial weight reduction diet must be individualized, be simple, have a social support system, be incorporated within an exercise regimen suitable to the insulin dose and cardiac status, and have reasonable goals for weight reduction and later weight maintenace.

Surgical Treatment of Obesity

Surgical treatment is based on the belief that a short bowel will produce malabsorption of ingested calories or that a small stomach reservoir will reduce caloric intake. Procedures that shorten the bowel are end-to-end or end-to-side connections of the jejunum to the ileum. These methods have been largely abandoned because of resulting electrolyte imbalance, hepatic toxicity, and poly-arthritis.

Gastric bypass procedures include tran-section, stapling, or vertical banding of the stomach, creating a 20- to 60-ml reservoir. Although they are better tolerated than in-testinal procedures, anastomotic leaks and obstructions can be a problem. In addition, diabetic patients can be prone to intra-ab-dominal abscesses and wound infections. Long-term weight loss is generally poor, sec-ondary to the use of high-density liquid or semisolid food that can pass through the stoma easily. Similarly, jaw-wiring and in-tragastric balloons are associated with rapid weight regain. Lipectomy and suction lipec-tomy are new procedures used to treat local, unsightly adiposity cosmetically.

None of these studies have specifically fo-cused on use in the diabetic. Patient selec-tion for any of these procedures should be quite stringent and reserved for those with morbid obesity (more than 100 per cent above ideal body weight).[24]

Weight Maintenance Diet

Whatever the approach to losing weight, pa-tients eventually must be on a weight main-tenance diet if they are not to regain the weight. In establishing a weight mainte-nance diet, distribution of calories is an area of controversy.

Protein is not the issue, though, being rel-atively fixed in most American diets at 12 to 20 per cent of calories. Although there is some indication that reducing dietary pro-tein may reduce the chance of diabetic ne-phropathy, the evidence is far from defini-tive. A common problem in estimating dietary protein intake is to overestimate the protein and underestimate the fat content of a food. A 3-oz hamburger, for example, may have 135 calories as fat and only 84 calories of protein.

If 12 to 20 per cent of the diet is protein, the remaining 80 to 88 per cent of nonpro-tein calories is distributed between fat and carbohydrate. The consensus is that people with diabetes should *not* restrict carbohy-drate intake, but in fact should consume 50 to 60 per cent of their daily calories as car-bohydrate.[16] This approach has several ad-vantages: high-carbohydrate diets actually improve insulin sensitivity and glycemic control in NIDDM; carbohydrates are less "densely packaged" calories (about 4 calo-ries/gm in comparison to fat's 9 calories/ gm), so that, for example, eating an extra 50 gm of carbohydrate represents about 200 calories, whereas 50 gm of fat is about 450 calories; and high-carbohydrate diets will have more fiber than high-fat diets.

All carbohydrates, though, are not equal. Starches are complex carbohydrates that re-quire digestion to simple monosaccharides or disaccharides before they are absorbed. Even among the complex carbohydrates, there is considerable variability in absorp-tion rate—the so-called "glycemic index" compares the amount of blood glucose rise to a standard of white bread. Usually, the dif-ferences in glycemic responses are not re-producible within or between individuals, and thus the clinical use of the index is im-practical.

High-fiber diets have been advocated lately. Soluble fibers (oat, gums, pectin) have the capability of delaying gastric emptying, prolonging absorption of carbohydrates, and enhancing satiety. They are effective in flat-tening the glucose response in both diabetics and nondiabetics. Clinical trials, however, have demonstrated only a modest improve-ment in diabetic control. In addition, soluble fiber is effective in lowering serum choles-terol by binding bile acids in the gut.[25]

Patient acceptance of a 25- to 30-gm high-fiber diet can be a problem due to the gastro-intestinal side effects. However, with reas-surance and gradual increases in quantity, patients usually adapt. Of greater concern is the caloric intake. A bran muffin is approx-imately 500 calories. It is imperative that fiber *replace* calories rather than simply adding fiber to the usual low-fiber American diet.

Simple sugars in the diet, as "concentrated sweets," are absorbed more quickly than complex carbohydrates, since they do not require digestion in the gut. More important, though, is the fact that they are usually eaten in entirely unregulated, unknown amounts. How does a patient compare the sugar content of a candy bar with that of ice cream, a nondiet soda, or a doughnut? For these reasons, it is better for the person with diabetes (and the family) to avoid concentrated sweets, although up to 5 per cent of calories may be incorporated into the diet if avoidance of sweets is regarded as a major sacrifice.

Finally, up to about 30 per cent of calories is taken as fat. More important than the amount of fat consumed, though, is the type of fat. Saturated fats have long been known to increase serum cholesterol. When a person has diabetes, a major independent cardiovascular risk factor, it is all the more important to avoid saturated fats in order not to add another risk factor. The recommendation, therefore, is for not more than 10 per cent of total calories to be taken as saturated fats (mainly animal source), up to 10 to 15 per cent as monounsaturated fats (mainly olive oil), and less than 10 per cent as polyunsaturated fats (mainly vegetable oils and margarine).

Cholesterol intake is a separate issue, but, again, an important one in determining risk of cardiovascular disease. Individuals vary markedly in how responsive their serum cholesterol is to changes in dietary cholesterol, but people with diabetes should try to hold their cholesterol intake down to about 300 mg per day. In the American diet, cholesterol is found largely in eggs. With over 200 mg of cholesterol in the average egg, the "traditional" American diet of bacon and eggs has obvious risks. Cereal and fruit are far preferable on a routine basis.

Finally, sweeteners: The only noncaloric sweetener now available in the United States is saccharin, and it may be ingested essentially without limit. Aspartame (NutriSweet) has minimal calories (4 per teaspoon) and is also an acceptable sweetener. Fructose and sorbitol are each hexoses with the same caloric content as sucrose (16 cal/tsp), but they raise the blood glucose more slowly as they are metabolized gradually to glucose.

Summarizing the weight-maintaining diet: flexibility exists, particularly in the distribution of carbohydrates versus fat; concentrated sweets should be minimized; saturated fats should be avoided; and noncaloric sweeteners may be used as desired. It is beyond the expertise of most physicians to fit these dietary recommendations into a personalized, palatable, and balanced diet. For this reason, professional consultation with a registered dietician is highly recommended.

■ EXERCISE

While a prudent approach to exercise is particularly important when diabetes is associated with obesity, exercise remains a mainstay of treatment. The benefits of exercise—those specific to obesity and diabetes, as well as general health and psychic benefits—are real, but so are the risks.

Exercise is well known to promote insulin action, particularly in glucose uptake by muscle. This suggests that it may be specifically beneficial for the person with insulin resistance, i.e., most obese diabetics. Glycemic control is usually markedly improved by regular exercise, presumably by overcoming insulin resistance. Exercise is also an important adjunct to diet in weight control. Although it is difficult to lose weight by exercise alone, the combination of increased caloric expenditure and reduced dietary intake is more effective than either alone.

Exercise also has been well shown to lower blood pressure and to improve plasma lipid status. Finally, the sense of well-being established by participating in regular exercise, although difficult to quantify, is also hard to dispute.

What, then, are the risks of exercise for the obese diabetic? To begin with, there is the risk of excessive cardiovascular strain if an individual has poor cardiovascular fitness. Orthopedic complications (for instance, knee damage and back pain) are more prevalent in obesity and may be exacerbated by exercise. Three dangers are pertinent specifically to the diabetic: foot care, eye care, and neuropathy. Good foot care is particularly important in the obese diabetic patient. Properly fitting, high-quality footwear, frequent examination to avoid blisters, and other aspects of good foot care are especially important in the overweight person with diabetes. There may be times when unstable retinopathy makes it best to avoid jarring exercise. Neuropathy can cause two problems with exercise: neuropathic numbness of the feet may predispose to undetected injury or blisters, and autonomic neuropathy may mask the pain of myocardial ischemia (angina).

The answer is not to avoid exercise but to institute a carefully planned, gradually increasing exercise program suited to the individual. Cardiovascular status, as well as complications such as peripheral neuropathy and peripheral vascular disease, is to be evaluated in advance and considered carefully in exercise recommendations.

■ ORAL HYPOGLYCEMIC AGENTS

Oral hypoglycemic agents usually provide a reasonable approach to blood glucose control after diet and exercise have been tried to the maximum. They are rarely indicated until after an adequate trial of diet and exercise, and they never replace diet and exercise. Furthermore, if glycemic control of oral agents is optimal, dosage should be reduced; the oral agents should be stopped if glycemia does not deteriorate. Keeping these

caveats in mind, physicians will find that oral hypoglycemic agents will benefit many obese patients.

All oral hypoglycemic agents available in the United States today are sulfonylureas, and all act through similar, if not identical, mechanisms. Their effect is essentially twofold: they stimulate pancreatic insulin secretion, and they enhance insulin's effect in the peripheral tissues. The pancreatic effect is central; there is no benefit if endogenous insulin is absent (as in insulin-dependent diabetes).

Sulfonylureas are often divided into "first generation" and "second generation," based on their introduction into the American market in the 1950s and the 1980s, respectively (Table 3). The major difference is that first-generation agents are used in doses of 250 mg to 1.5 gm, whereas the newer agents require only 1 to 40 mg. The dosage difference is clinically inconsequential, except that the gradations of dosing are finer in the second-generation products. There may be some lessening of drug-drug interactions when second-generation agents are used; but no major clinical differences exist between the two types.

Chlorpropamide does have unique properties, however. Being excreted unaltered by the kidney, it is the longest-acting agent, lasting as long as 36 hours. While this may be an advantage, it also has two potential

TABLE 3. Characteristics of Sulfonylurea Agents

Generic Name	Brand Name	Daily Dosage Range (*mg*)	Duration of Action (*hr*)	Comments
Chlorpropamide	Diabinese	100–500	60	Metabolized by liver (about 70%) to less active metabolites and excreted intact (about 30%) by kidneys; can potentiate ADH action; given once per day
Tolbutamide	Orinase	500–3000	6–12	Metabolized by liver to an inactive product; given 2 to 3 times per day
Acetohexamide	Dymelor	250–1500	12–18	Metabolized by liver to active metabolite; given 1 to 2 times per day
Tolazamide	Tolinase	100–1000	12–24	Metabolized by liver to both active and inactive products; given 1 to 2 times per day
Glyburide	Diabeta Micronase	2.5–20	16–24	Metabolized by liver to mostly inert products; given 1 to 2 times per day
Glipizide	Glucatrol	5–40	12–24	Metabolized by liver to inert products; given 1 to 2 times per day

(Adapted from Lebovitz HE (ed). Physician's Guide to Noninsulin-Dependent (Type II) Diabetes: Diagnosis and Treatment. 2nd ed. Alexandria, VA: American Diabetes Association, 1988.)

drawbacks: it causes a facial flush in about 30 per cent of people when mixed with alcohol; and it may lower serum sodium, even to the point of full-blown hyponatremia.

Allergic reactions, gastrointestinal side effects, and occasional hematologic reactions to sulfonylureas are unusual but well documented.

Throughout most of the world, the biguanides phenformin and metformin are available as nonsulfonylurea oral hypoglycemic agents. They apparently act by different mechanisms from the sulfonylureas and offer a backup approach to sulfonylurea failures. They may be especially useful in treating the obese diabetic patient, since a number of studies have shown that the biguanides promote weight loss. As a class, though, the biguanides were banned in the United States, because of the incidence of lactic acidosis caused by phenformin. (Metformin apparently did not cause this). Given the favorable worldwide experience with metformin, it is possible that it will again become available in the United States.

At present, if the obese diabetic patient has inadequate glycemic control on diet and exercise, progression to sulfonylurea therapy is indicated. About two thirds of patients will show a satisfactory response initially, but it can be anticipated that over the years more and more people will fail on oral agents. This appears to be due to progressive pancreatic failure rather than to resistance to the medication itself, although worsening obesity also can play a role. Whatever the cause, if glycemic control deteriorates with use of oral agents, insulin treatment is the next step.

■ INSULIN TREATMENT

Insulin therapy is not as often recommended for the obese diabetic patient as for the normal weight NIDDM patient or, of course, the insulin-dependent diabetic patient. First, the central problem in NIDDM with obesity is not failure of insulin secretion, but resistance to insulin. Second, given the insulin resistance, large doses of insulin usually are required in treating the obese diabetic patient. Third, these large doses tend to cause weight gain, both by stimulating appetite and by reducing glucosuria. And finally, of course, the patient is never happy with the need to take insulin by injection.

On the positive side, insulin in adequate doses can control the blood glucose of virtually all obese diabetic patients, and the person with overtly poor control will reap marked clinical benefit. Also, since some degree of endogenous insulin secretion is retained in NIDDM, insulin treatment tends to be more quickly successful in NIDDM than in IDDM. There is less need for mixing short- and long-acting doses or splitting doses in NIDDM. Some advocate transient insulin therapy to control blood glucose for periods of several weeks before returning to oral hypoglycemic agents. Good glycemic control does indeed abruptly reduce insulin resistance; but starting and stopping insulin treatment also has disadvantages and is not a generally accepted approach.

Usually, in the obese diabetic patient, the starting insulin dose may be as much as 15 to 20 units of intermediate-acting insulin in the morning. The dose may be raised every 2 to 7 days, seeking a break in the daytime glycemia. If the dose rises above 30 to 40 units, it is usually split to BID dosage. If fasting hyperglycemia continues, the second dose should be NPH or Lente at bedtime; if bedtime glycemia is the worst, add a short-acting insulin (regular or Semilente) before supper.

It is not unusual for the obese diabetic patient to require more than 100 units of insulin daily. Some clinicians prefer to combine insulin with an oral hypoglycemic agent, on the theory that stimulating endogenous insulin and enhancing insulin's peripheral effect (the sulfonylureas' mechanisms of action) will contribute to the effect of exogenous insulin. However, studies thus far have not shown that this combined therapy is better than insulin alone.

■ Follow-Up Management

■ MONITORING DIABETIC CONTROL

Self-monitoring of blood glucose has been widely accepted by patients and is virtually the only way to discern the blood glucose fluctuations in daily living. Using newer equipment, the finger stick to obtain a drop of blood causes minimal or no pain. In the relatively stable Type II diabetic patient with obesity, the blood glucose test may be done only once daily, but the time should be rotated to discover the blood glucose for each of the three daily meals and at bedtime. The fasting blood glucose level does not necessarily reflect daytime glycemia.

Use of the glycosylated hemoglobin (or hemoglobin A_{1c}) assay can help the clinician monitor chronic, as opposed to immediate, diabetic control. When used regularly in office visits, it provides another measure of adequacy of treatment. The important thing is to know the upper limit of normal for the laboratory used. If the result is more than about one and a half times normal (e.g., 9 per cent when the upper limit of normal is 6 per cent), then glycemic control over the previous 3 months has not been good. Urine glucose testing is not optimal, but if the patient will not consider blood glucose testing, it may be the only acceptable monitoring approach. Only general patterns of control (when the blood glucose is highest, when lowest) and general indications of glycemia can be inferred from urine testing.

Finally, plasma glucose determinations should be determined on routine office visits, to derive some indication of glycemic control and to test the accuracy of the patient's meter. The fasting glucose or random plasma glucose level, though, is not a reliable index of chronic glycemia.

■ MONITORING FOR DIABETIC COMPLICATIONS

Diabetes is now the cause for about 30 per cent of all patients undergoing chronic renal dialysis, and the majority of diabetic patients on dialysis have NIDDM. Diabetic nephropathy, therefore, is by no means a disease confined to insulin-dependent diabetes. With onset after a mean of about 15 years, proteinuria is usually the first clinical evidence of nephropathy. Urine dip-stick testing is a crude indication of proteinuria, but one that should be used on all diabetic patients with 10 or more years of disease. More sensitive tests are the tablet test that detects "microalbuminuria" (small quantitites of albumin in the urine) and a 24-hour urine protein test. The blood urea nitrogen and serum creatinine levels increase only in late-stage disease. Creatinine clearance is ordinarily *greater* than normal (120 to 150 ml/min) in people with early diabetes; therefore, a "normal" creatinine clearance

may in fact indicate that the GFR is reduced by nephropathy.

The key to the diagnosis and treatment of diabetic retinopathy is regular dilated fundus examination by an experienced physician, usually an ophthalmologist. The availability of laser therapy to treat proliferative and, in some cases, preproliferative retinopathy makes it essential that the eye disease be correctly diagnosed at the treatable stages. Symptoms of visual impairment are unusual except in advanced retinopathy. General physicians and optometrists are rarely skilled in the diagnosis of early retinopathy and the determination of when laser therapy should be instituted.

The risk of peripheral vascular, cerebrovascular, and coronary artery disease is markedly increased in NIDDM with obesity. There are no unique features of monitoring for these macrovascular complications, however. It is good practice to note carefully the presence or absence of peripheral pulses and to elicit by a careful history the symptoms of coronary artery and cerebrovascular disease.

Sequencing/Progressing Treatment

The adequacy of glycemic control is a clinical judgment to be made by the physician after full consideration of individual circumstances. Four examples may be instructive:

1. An obese 50 year old diabetic patient, sticking with a good diet, has a fasting plasma glucose level in the 150 mg/dl range, random glycemia in the 250 mg/dl range, and glycohemoglobin of 10 per cent. **Treatment:** start oral agents, since diet has been tried and control can be improved relatively simply.
2. An overweight 72 year old has only begun to work on diet, with glycemia similar to the first case. **Treatment:** work further on diet, since it has not been optimized; glycemic goals may be less stringent in older people; and adding medications in this age range can be dangerous.
3. An obese 48 year old woman has never lost weight despite good dietary advice, has a fasting plasma glucose level of less than 250 mg/dl and glycohemoglobin over 12 per cent, and is polydipsic and polyuric with yeast vaginitis. **Treatment:**

advance therapy, both to relieve the symptoms of hyperglycemia and to avoid decompensation if, for instance, acute illness were superimposed on such hyperglycemia. Try oral agents first, but if unsuccessful initiate insulin.

4. An obese 50 year old person with documented diabetes has a fasting plasma glucose level of about 130 mg/dl and random glucose up to about 170 mg/dl; the patient is on a good diet, with no symptoms or complications; glycohemoglobin is 8.2 per cent (upper limit of normal is 7.5 per cent). **Treatment:** a judgment call; this degree of glycemia is close enough to normal that risks of tighter control must be weighed against benefits.

■ TREATMENT OF ACUTE COMPLICATIONS

Acute complications are those due directly and immediately to poor metabolic control—symptoms of hyperglycemia, vaginitis, blurred vision, and, in the case of NIDDM, hyperosmolar nonketotic coma. Prevention, of course, involves maintaining at least adequate diabetic control. Detailed descriptions of how to treat the acute complications of NIDDM are covered elsewhere. We will note here that when treating hyperosmolar nonketotic coma, it is important to reduce the plasma glucose concentration relatively slowly, preferably over 12 to 24 hours, and to be careful to reduce the insulin dose or stop it altogether when the plasma glucose level falls to less than 250 mg/dl.

Occasionally, frank diabetic ketoacidosis (DKA) will occur when the patient with NIDDM is stressed. Although DKA is ordinarily the hallmark of IDDM, obese patients on reduced caloric intake may have mild ketonemia, which, if lipolysis is activated by acute stress, can precipitate DKA.

■ Summary

Obesity is a major contributing factor in the pathogenesis of NIDDM and needs to be treated along with, and as a part of, the attempt to reach euglycemia. Individualized approaches to weight reduction must be pushed to the maximum, working toward an acceptable body weight that can then be maintained. If inadequate glycemic control is achieved with diet alone, treatment is advanced to oral agents and then to insulin. The restoration of an ideal body weight in conjunction with glucose control and aggressive treatment of coexisting risk factors such as high blood pressure, hyperlipidemia, and smoking will reduce the risk of acute and long-term complications of diabetes.

REFERENCES

1. West KM, Kalbfleisch JM. Influence of nutritional factors on prevalence of diabetes. Diabetes 1971; 20:99–108.
2. Hamman RF, Bennett PH, Miller M. Incidence of diabetes among Pima Indians. Adv Metab Disord 1978; 9:49–63.
3. Westlund K, Nicolaysen JM. Ten-year mortality and morbidity related to serum cholesterol: A follow-up of 3.751 men aged 40–49. Scand J Clin Lab Invest 1972; 30:1–24.
4. Wilson PW, McGee DL, Kannel WB. Obesity, very low density lipoproteins, and glucose intolerance over fourteen years: The Framingham study. Am J Epidemiol 1981; 114:697–704.
5. Stegmayer P, Lovrien FC, Smith M, Keller T, Gohdes DM. Designing a diabetes nutrition education program for a Native American community. Diabetes Educ 1988; 14(1):64–66.
6. Keys A, et al. Coronary heart disease: overweight and obesity as risk factors. Ann Intern Med 1972; 77:15–27.
7. Kissebah AH, Peiris AN, Evans DJ. Mechanisms associating body fat distribution to glucose intolerance and diabetes mellitus: window with a view. Acta Med Scand 1988; 723(suppl):79–89.
8. Reaven GM. Banting Lecture 1988: Role of insulin resistance in human disease. Diabetes 1988; 37:1595–1607.
9. Fraze E, Donner CC, Swislocki ALM, Chiou Y-AM, Chen Y-DI, Reaven GM. Ambient plasma free fatty acid concentrations in non-insulin-dependent diabetes mellitus: evidence for insulin resistance. J Clin Endocrinol Metab 1985; 61:807–811.
10. Pozefsky T, Margolis S. Obesity. In Harvey AM, Johns RJ, McKusick VA, Owens AH, Ross RS, eds. The Principles and Practice of Medicine. 22nd ed. East Norwalk, CT: Appleton and Lange, 1988:998.
11. National Diabetes Data Group: Classification and diagnosis of diabetes mellitus and other categories of glucose intolerance. Diabetes 1979; 28:1039–1057.
12. Keen H, Jarrett RJ, McCartney P. The ten-year follow-up of the Bedford survey (1962–1972): glucose tolerance and diabetes. Diabetologia 1982; 22:73–78.
13. Saad MF, Knowler WC, Pettitt DJ, Nelson RG, Mott DM, Bennett PH. The natural history of impaired glucose tolerance in the Pima Indians. N Engl J Med 1988; 319:1500–1506.
14. Fajans SS, Floyd JC, Tattersall RB, Williamson JR, Peks R, Taylor CI. The various faces of diabetes in the young: changing concepts. Arch Intern Med 1976; 136(12):194–202.

15. Report of the National Cholesterol Education Program expert panel on detection, evaluation and treatment of high blood cholesterol in adults. Arch Intern Med 1988; 148:36–69.
16. Lebovitz HE (ed). Physician's Guide to Noninsulin-Dependent (Type II) Diabetes: Diagnosis and Treatment. 2nd ed. Alexandria, VA: American Diabetes Association, Inc., 1988.
17. Hjøllund E, Pedersen O, Richelsen B, Beck-Nielsen H, Sørensen NS. Increased insulin binding to adipocytes and monocytes and increased insulin sensitivity of glucose transport and metabolism in adipocytes from non-insulin-dependent diabetics after a low-fat/high-starch/high-fiber diet. Metabolism 1983; 32:1067–1075.
18. Drenick EJ. Weight reduction by prolonged fasting. In Bray GA (ed). Obesity in Perspective. DHEW publication NO. (NIH) 75-708:341–360. Washington, DC: Government Printing Office, 1975.
19. Spencer IOB. Death during therapeutic starvation for obesity. Lancet 1968; 1:1288–1290.
20. Isner JM, Sours HE, Paris AL, Ferrans VJ, Roberts WC. Sudden unexpected deaths in avid dieters using the liquid-protein–modified fast diet: observations in 17 patients and the role of prolonged QT interval. Circulation 1979; 60:1401–1412.
21. Savage PJ, Knowler WC. Diet therapy for type II (non-insulin–dependent) diabetes mellitus: can new approaches improve therapeutic results? Nutr Abstr Rev Clin Nutr 1984; 54(2–3):69–87.
22. Wing RR. Behavioral strategy weight reduction in obese type II diabetic patients. Diabetes Care 1989; 12:139–144.
23. Volkmar FR, Stunkard AJ, Woolston J, et al. High attrition rates in commercial weight reduction programs. Arch Intern Med 1981; 141:426–428.
24. Grace DM. Patient selection for obesity surgery. Gastroenterol Clin North Am 1987; 16:399–413.
25. Anderson JW. Fiber and health: an overview. Am J Gastroenterol 1986; 81:892–901.

Osteoporosis

Angelo A. Licata

Clinical osteoporosis is a common problem of the aged population, which has staggering effects on health care resources. Direct costs in 1986 were more than 5 billion dollars, and these costs are purportedly increasing as the medical needs and longevity of the population grow.[1] Over 70 per cent of the hospitalizations for this disorder occur in women 75 years and older who comprise only 19 per cent of the total number of women over the age of 45 years.[1] The challenge that these patients pose to physicians is the handling of persistent back pain and generalized skeletal fragility. This article presents some personal views about treating these problems of established osteoporosis. Readers are referred to recent medical reviews for more information on the general topic of osteoporosis.[2,3]

■ Background

Idiopathic or primary osteoporosis presents with two pathologic pictures. An early form (type I) arises in the postmenopausal woman from loss of estrogen and other factors that include nutritional inadequacies, limited physical activity, and small skeletal mass.[2] Spinal and distal forearm fractures predominate, owing to the rapid loss of estrogen-sensitive trabecular bone.[2] A late form of osteoporosis (type II) occurs in women as well as men, resulting from aging-related biochemical changes in both sexes and to the aforementioned factors in women. Paramount abnormalities are changes in calcium absorption, vitamin D metabolism, and parathyroid hormone secretion.[2] Deterioration of trabecular and cortical bone causes fractures of the hip and appendicular skeleton as well as the spine.

Secondary causes of osteoporosis are well outlined in textbooks. These forms of the disease account for a small fraction of the total picture. Most cases of osteoporosis develop in later life, when the incidence of idiopathic disease predominates. Accordingly, minimal effort is expended to search for a secondary cause.

Laboratory tests show no specific abnormality in primary osteoporosis. Changes in biochemical values, however, may indicate an underlying cause. Skeletal biopsies show no unique histologic change but may help rule out subclinical osteomalacia. Radiographic data show generalized osteopenia, anterior vertebral wedging, compression deformities of the end plates of the spine, and overt compression fractures.

The use of densitometry to diagnose skeletal loss and predict future fracture risk is controversial.[4] Diagnostic use of densitometry is superfluous in patients with clinical and radiologic evidence of the problem. However, densitometry is critical to monitor the efficacy of treatment to stimulate new growth of bone. In a pure diagnostic mode, densitometry is appropriately used to detect early mineral loss in the perimenopausal or early postmenopausal woman who is at risk for the disease and has no radiologic or clinical findings.

■ Management

In managing patients, problems arise from the acute or chronic effects of the disorder. During the acute stage, pain from spinal fractures is a major concern, whereas problems of skeletal fragility and persistent back pain arise during the chronic stage.

■ ACUTE PROBLEMS

Pain is a major problem of spinal fractures in the acute stage, because these bones cannot be immobilized as in other fractures. Bed rest may be needed initially for a few days while analgesia becomes effective. On the other hand, some clinicians feel that immediate mobilization is needed. The dictating factor in this regard is the general debility of the patient. Once pain is controlled and the patient is ambulatory, short periods of supine rest daily help to relieve stress on the collapsed vertebrae and diminish discomfort. Five or ten minutes of bed rest every hour help relieve the intensification of discomfort that arises after a person is in the erect posture. A soft back brace provides some limited immobilization when patients are ambulatory. Bulky full-length spinal braces are expensive and more often than

not discarded because of the discomfort and inconvenience.

Rapid control of pain is appropriate. The quicker this can be achieved, the less frightened the patient becomes and the faster mobilization and physical therapy can begin. Narcotic drugs are helpful. Codeine alone, or with aspirin or acetaminophen, is useful initial medication. In using the stronger narcotics, starting with smaller doses helps avoid unpleasant side effects that discourage compliance. Drugs should be given throughout the 24-hour period to ensure continuous analgesia and, eventually, earlier mobilization. Addiction is an exaggerated concern in the acute setting.

Calcitonin is an injectable hormone that has analgesic properties apart from its known uses in Paget's disease of the bone, hypercalcemia, and osteoporosis.[5] Doses of 50 to 100 units daily, every other day, or three times weekly are helpful. Side effects may include nausea, flushing, and less often, increased bowel motility and mild diuresis. The major advantage of this medication is that it does not produce the typical narcotic side effects of sedation or lightheadedness that are so troublesome to older patients.

■ CHRONIC PROBLEMS

The chronic problems of pain and skeletal fragility are the most frustrating because there are no unequivocal treatments.

Causes of Chronic Back Pain

Microfractures, anatomic malalignment, and degenerative joint disease are probably the most common causes of persistent back pain. Postmortem studies reveal callus-like formations around broken trabeculae that suggest healing microscopic fractures of the vertebrae.[6] Such changes precede the ultimate macroscopic compression fracture and may be a source of pain in a vertebra long before it collapses.[6]

Degenerative joint disease is another source of pain. It develops in weight-bearing joints and cervical and distal phalangeal joints, is usually aggravated by movement, and causes stiffness after periods of inactivity. It also causes low back or paraspinal pain, as does osteoporosis, but osteoporotic pain develops during upright or sitting posture and remits with the supine posture.

Anatomic malalignment occurs in some patients. Pre-existing or postspinal fracture scoliosis, spondylolisthesis, and kyphosis are readily identified. Often the kyphotic patient notes dramatic relief when posture is straightened. Hip fractures and any attendant leg shortening may distort gait and cause mechanical lower back pain.

Pain Control

Control of chronic pain may become a multidisciplinary problem that requires use of physical therapy, medications, pain center management, and bracing.

Although some physicians express negative sentiments about using back support, a patient with posture-induced pain experiences relief when using some support in the back. Temporary usage is the key, not total reliance. Physical therapy will tone and strengthen the muscle groups of the abdomen and back and help prevent total reliance upon bracing.

The use of analgesics in the chronic setting is fraught with the danger of addiction. Differentiation of physical pain from physical dependence is difficult. Depression often compounds the problem. Referral to appropriate pain management programs may be needed. Personal experience shows that calcitonin and female hormones may blunt and sometimes eradicate some pain in the older patient.

The usefulness of calcitonin to control chronic pain is empirically determined, since there is no way to identify responders beforehand. Pain relief usually develops within 2 to 4 weeks when the aforementioned doses are used. Patients more often than not try to discontinue the drug after several months since cost, inconvenience of administration, and, in some cases, side effects may limit use. A nasal spray dosimeter of the medicine is now under study.

For unclear reasons, estrogen in combination with progestin can relieve pain in some patients. The daily dosages of estrogen are 0.625 mg of conjugated estrogen or 1 to 2 mg of estradiol. The dosage of progestin is 5 mg of medroxyprogesterone or its equivalent. This drug is used in the woman with a uterus. Dosage regimens have included (1) daily concomitant usage of estrogen and progestin, (2) daily use of estrogen with administration of progestin the first 15 days of the month, and (3) a 25-day monthly cycle of es-

trogen, combined with progestin the last 10 to 13 days of the cycle. The combination of hormones reduces endometrial hyperplasia and the secondary risk of endometrial cancer. Resumption of menstrual flow is an unpleasant side effect. Adjusting the hormones, however, may reduce this to an acceptable level. In some women, menses may eventually cease or diminish to an acceptable level within a matter of months even though hormonal dosage remains the same.

Estrogen-containing skin patches are available in two sizes that deliver 0.05 mg or 0.1 mg of estradiol daily. Biweekly applications provide serum levels of estradiol comparable to the oral medication. Progestin is given as noted. Fewer estrogenic effects on liver function are a distinct advantage. Preliminary information suggests a positive benefit to the skeleton also.

Estrogen has a beneficial effect on cardiovascular risk, but when combined with progestin, this benefit may be negated. The dilemma is to provide enough progestin to reduce the risk of endometrial cancer, but not too much to negate the protective effect on arterial disease. Controversy still exists over this issue. Medroxyprogesterone may be the least likely progestin to affect lipid levels.

Nonsteroidal anti-inflammatory drugs may reduce pain from degenerative joint or disc disease. The long-acting forms are especially useful to ensure compliance in the older patient, since dosages need to be taken once or twice per day [i.e., sulindac (Clinoril), piroxicam (Feldene), and diflunisal (Dolobid)]. Short-acting agents like ketoprofen, ibuprofen, naproxen, and tolmetin are also useful. A new agent, diclofenic (Voltaren), has fewer intestinal side effects. Aspirin should not be considered *passé* since some patients may experience very good relief with it.

Stabilize and Strengthen Skeleton

With pain in control, the next hurdle to overcome is strengthening and stabilizing the skeleton. This process entails use of proper nutrition, exercise, and drugs.

Nutrition. Proper nutrition is essential for the daily intake of calcium. Recommended allowances are 1000 mg for premenopausal women and 1500 mg for the postmenopausal woman. Dairy products are the major source of calcium. High-calcium-fortified fruit juices are substitutes for milk in patients who have lactose intolerance or a general dislike for dairy products. When the total diet contains less than the recommended allowances, supplements of calcium are usually used. Many forms are available. Calcium carbonate is inexpensive, contains more calcium per tablet, and is best given with food since better absorption occurs in an acid environment.[7] Some patients complain of intestinal side effects like bloating and constipation. Preparations of calcium phosphate have fewer intestinal side effects than the carbonate preparations. Calcium citrate may be absorbed better than other forms of calcium.[8] Even with the use of recommended daily allowances, there is no assurance that calcium is adequately absorbed. Significant impairment may be present in healthy, middle-aged women.[9] Measurement of a 24-hour urinary calcium level, though imprecise, may help assess absorption. As long as urinary calcium is above 100 mg per day and rises 40 to 50 mg with the use of supplemental calcium, absorption should be adequate. In the absence of these urinary changes, daily doses of 400 to 1000 units of vitamin D should be tried. Sometimes, calcitriol may be needed.

Since calcitriol (Rocaltrol) is a potent agent, doses of 0.25 μg daily should be used initially. Periodic checks of 24-hour urinary calcium for hypercalciuria are essential to reduce the risk of toxicity.

Activity. Exercise helps maximize stress on the skeleton, strengthen bone, and maintain physical well-being overall. Although patients insist on knowing what exercise to perform, it is preferable to allow them the choice of activity. Any activity that they enjoy will be complied with better. Biking, walking, and mild calisthenics are frequently performed. Prescribed exercise programs often are not adhered to. Swimming may be a very useful exercise in subsets of patients, even though it is not considered nonweight-bearing.[10] Activity that requires flexion of the spine (i.e., rowing, sit-ups) may provoke spinal compression fractures. Any movement that is uncomfortable must be stopped, since this may indicate the beginning of a new fracture.

Medication. When skeletal density falls below a certain level known as the fracture threshold, the risk of atraumatic fracture rises. At this stage, two therapeutic modalities are available. One form stabilizes skeletal density (i.e., antiresorptive), and the other form increases density (i.e., growth promoting) above the fracture threshold and theoretically produces a stronger bone. In the past, all treatment programs that were used stabilized the skeleton. Although new studies show that estrogen, calcitonin, and androgens increase skeletal density, these reported increments have not been of sufficient magnitude to raise levels above the theoretic fracture-threshold.[11–13] Increases occur within the first 2 years and reach a plateau thereafter. It is unclear what effect these changes have on the rate of fractures.

Calcium may be efficacious in retarding further bone loss in the elderly patient with established disease, but it is not as effective as estrogen in preventing early menopausal bone loss.[14] In the past, large doses of vitamin D (i.e., 50,000 units biweekly) were prescribed to facilitate absorption of calcium. Problems of hypercalciuria and hypercalcemia necessitate lower doses (i.e., 400 to 1000 units daily). The use of vitamin D as primary treatment for osteoporosis is controversial. The latest evidence suggests that it has no beneficial effect.[15]

Though unapproved by the FDA, sodium fluoride is used to stimulate osteoblastic activity and promote bone growth. Doses are 1 mg of sodium fluoride per kg body weight daily (40 to 80 mg). A combination of calcium, estrogen, and sodium fluoride is reported to decrease fracture incidence.[16] Improved fluoride preparations are being studied but are not yet available commercially. Intermittent usage also may be advantageous.[17] Gastritis, anemia, synovitis, and stress fractures occur with prolonged usage. Acute side effects are dyspepsia and nausea. Using sodium fluoride with food reduces some of the intestinal side effects. Enteric-coated and slow-release forms have a lower incidence of gastrointestinal side effects but are not yet available.[18] Commercially available preparations that are used for dental prophylaxis contain small amounts of sodium fluoride per tablet (i.e., 2 to 3 mg). Local pharmacists must prepare larger dose formulations. A health food supplement containing sodium fluoride and calcium (Florical) is available. Each capsule contains 8.3 mg sodium fluoride and 364 mg calcium carbonate. The amount of fluoride absorbed may be reduced due to the calcium content.

Monitoring efficacy and toxicity is critical, since fluoride must be administered for at least 1 to 2 years before an effect is noted. Some experts recommend that the treatment be continued for 5 years, but this is still an unsettled issue, since there is a concern that cortical bone may be compromised. Serum fluoride should be kept within a therapeutic range of 95 to 190 ng/ml (5 to 10 micromoles per liter).[17] There is no guarantee, however, that maintenance of this level will be efficacious. Twenty to thirty per cent of patients do not respond to treatment. Densitometry of the spine is the preferred monitoring technique, because it will detect small changes in bone growth faster than will typical radiographs.

Experimental programs show that the bisphosphonates, which are antiosteoclastic drugs, increase skeletal density to a small degree. Etidronate disodium (Didronel) increases density 6 to 8 per cent above that achieved by placebo drugs at 14 to 21 months.[19] The program has been a repeating cycle of 400 mg of etidronate sodium daily for 2 weeks, followed by 13 weeks of calcium and 400 units of vitamin D daily.

A variation on this technique is known as coherence therapy. The principle is to first employ a drug that stimulates bone metabolism (i.e., formation and resorption), then to use an agent to depress the resorptive component and thereby free the formation process to deposit a quantum of bone. Since more bone is deposited than lost, there is a net gain over many months of repetition of the cycle. Experimental regimens used phosphate as the stimulator at doses of 1.5 to 2.0 gm per day for 3 days, bisphosphonates (Didronel, 400 mg per day) for 14 days, and calcium for the remaining 90 days. Calcitonin theoretically may substitute for the bisphosphonates. Uncontrolled studies show increased mean trabecular thickness.[20] An alternative approach employs parathyroid hormone, calcitriol, and calcium.[21]

■ OSTEOPOROSIS IN MEN

In men, treatment of osteoporosis is not satisfactory. Removal of the underlying cause (i.e., alcoholism or excessive steroid usage) may prevent further deterioration, but restoration of lost bone is limited. Sodium fluoride may be the agent of choice. Androgens may help if hypogonadism is present. The utility of the newer therapies has yet to be determined.

■ Issues and Risks

No treatment has been able as yet to restore the riddled three-dimensional network of trabecular bone in the osteoporotic patient. All therapies claiming to increase skeletal density do so by increasing the thickness of the existing trabecular framework. None regrow the missing trabeculae. If the residual architecture is of poor quality, adding new bone may do no more than increase the density of this poor quality of bone and, accordingly, not alter fracture rate. If the architecture is more structurally intact, new bone grown upon the residual structures actually may strengthen them and prevent further fractures. This notion is an important issue, because it challenges the present medical wisdom of treatment. Should patients be treated with these regimens earlier in the course of the disease, when there is more structurally intact bone? Although it is a meritorious question, it poses a problem because it implies that asymptomatic individuals may be the appropriate group of patients in whom to use these newer treatments. The challenge to physicians is to detect the problem and treat the patient before significant destruction develops in the three-dimensional framework. In other words, prevention of the disease still should be everybody's concern and major activity.

REFERENCES

1. Phillips S, Fox N, Jacobs J, Wright WE. The direct medical costs of osteoporosis for American women aged 45 and older, 1986. Bone 1988; 9:271–279.
2. Riggs LB, Melton LJ. Involuticnal osteoporosis. N Engl J Med 1986; 314:1676–1686.
3. Cummings SR, Kelsey JL, Nevitt MC, O'Dowd KJ. Epidemiology of osteoporosis and osteoporotic fractures. Epidemiol Rev 1985; 7:178–207.
4. Health and Public Policy Committee, American College of Physicians. Bone mineral densitometry. Ann Intern Med 1987; 107:932–936.
5. Szanto J, Jozsef S, Rado J, Juhos E, Hindy I, Eckhardt S. Pain killing with calcitonin in patients with malignant tumors. Oncology 1986; 43:69–72.

6. Vernon-Roberts B, Piric CJ. Healing trabecular microfractures in the bodies of lumbar vertebraes. Ann Rheum Dis 1973; 32:406–412.
7. Recker RR. Calcium absorption and achlorhydria. N Engl J Med 1985; 313:70–73.
8. Pak CYC, Harvey JA, Hsu MC. Enhanced calcium bioavailability from a solubilized form of calcium citrate. J Clin Endocrinol Metab 1987; 65:801–805.
9. Heaney RP, Recker RR. Distribution of calcium absorption in middle-aged women. Am J Clin Nutr 1986; 43:299–305.
10. Orwol ER, Ferar J, Oviatt K, Huntington K, McClung MR. Swimming exercise and bone mass. *In* Christiansen CR, Johansen JS, Riis BJ (eds). Proceedings of the International Symposium on Osteoporosis. Aalborg, Denmark, 1987:494–497.
11. Need AG, Horowitz M, Bridges A, Morris HA, Christopher BEC. Effects of nandrolone decanoate and anti-resorptive therapy on vertebral density in osteoporotic postmenopausal women. Arch Intern Med 1989; 149:57–60.
12. Gruber HE, Ivey JL, Baylink DJ, Matthews M, et al. Long-term calcitonin therapy in postmenopausal osteoporosis. Metabolism 1984; 34:295–303.
13. Munk-Jensen N, Nielsen SP, Obel EB, Eriksen PB. Reversal of postmenopausal vertebral bone loss by oestrogen and progestogen: a double-blind placebo-controlled study. Br Med J 1988; 296:1150–1152.
14. Riis B, Thomsen K, Christiansen C. Does calcium supplementation prevent postmenopausal bone loss? A double-blind controlled clinical study. N Engl J Med 1987; 316:173–177.
15. Ott SM, Chestnut CH. Calcitriol treatment is not effective in postmenopausal osteoporosis. Ann Intern Med 1989; 110:267–274.
16. Riggs BL, Seeman E, Hodgson SF, Taves DR, O'Fallon WM. Effect of fluoride/calcium regimen on vertebral fracture occurrence in postmenopausal osteoporosis: comparison with conventional therapy. N Engl J Med 1982; 306:446–450.
17. Pak CYC, Sakhaee K, Zerwekh JE, Parcel C, Peterson R, Johnson K. Safe and effective treatment of osteoporosis with intermittent slow release sodium fluoride: augmentation of vertebral bone mass and inhibition of fractures. J Clin Endocrinol Metab 1989; 68:150–159.
18. Pak CYC, Sakhaee K, Gallagher C, Parcel C, Peterson R, Zerwekh JE, Lemke M, Britton F, Hsen M-C, Adams B. Attainment of therapeutic fluoride levels in serum without major side effects using a slow-release preparation of sodium fluoride in postmenopausal osteoporosis. J Bone Mineral Res 1986; 1(6):563–571.
19. Genant HK, Harris ST, Steiger P, Davey PF, Block JE. The effect of etidronate therapy in postmenopausal osteoporotic women: preliminary results. *In* Christiansen C, Johansen JS, Riis BJ, et al: Proceedings of the International Symposium on Osteoporosis. Aalborg, Denmark, 1987:1177–1181.
20. Anderson C, Cope RDT, Crilly RG, Hodsman AB, Wolfe BMJ. Preliminary observations of a form of coherence therapy for osteoporosis. Calc Tissue Int 1984; 36:341–343.
21. Slovik DM, Rosenthal DI, Doppelt SH, Potts JT Jr, Daly MA, Campbell JA, Neer RM. Restoration of spinal bone in osteoporotic men by treatment with human parathyroid hormone (1-34) and 1,25-dihydroxyvitamin D. J Bone Mineral Res 1986; 1:377–381.

Pain management in the terminally ill patient

Frederick J. Meyers ■ *Mary Kennedy* ■ *Frederick H. Meyers*

■ Background

The management of a terminally ill patient is, of course, emotionally and technically demanding but also can be rewarding. The control of pain is the primary demand on the physician, and appropriate treatment demonstrates the commitment of the physician to provide continuing care as well as to relieve suffering.

These efforts alleviate some of the cancer patient's fears, which frequently center not on dying but on being abandoned to suffer severe, uncontrollable pain. In addition, the patient who is receiving appropriate symptomatic relief is more likely to resist the appeal of charlatans who offer cures for cancer and other diseases that cause disabling pain.

Analgesic drugs and procedures are usually adequate if the doctor responsible for them remembers that the goal is relief of pain with as minimal an alteration of consciousness and daily functioning as is possible; side effects are treated and the issue of addiction ignored.

■ THE EVALUATION OF CLAIMS FOR NEW DRUGS AND PROCEDURES

A problem in pain management is the need to select—or more often reject—those that deserve a trial, from among new drugs, techniques and procedures, and new laboratory research and associated theories. Judgment is difficult because of the subjective nature of pain and its modification by situational and individual factors. In addition, the narcotics act on the perception of pain rather than on some easily quantifiable function, as do the local anesthetics or sedatives, for example.

As a result, animal models or experimental pain in humans is not useful; analgesic agents or techniques can be evaluated only in people who are experiencing pain in an actual clinical situation.

A person's response to a painful stimulus is modified by subjective factors, such as the meaning of the pain and the degree of anxiety associated with the situation. For example, a person who sustains a fracture of the leg in an automobile accident usually requires more analgesia than a soldier who sustains equivalent trauma on the battlefield.[1] The civilian situation is unexpected and is perceived as more threatening than the "ticket home" that a nonlethal injury might provide to the soldier.

Whereas pain is highly subjective, analgesia can be evaluated precisely in double-blind, placebo-controlled clinical trials.[2] The effect of small increments in dosage of a given drug, the differences in effectiveness among drugs, and the biologic rather than the chemical duration of effect can all be quantified.

Nonspecific or placebo effects can induce patients to accept a new drug even though they might be skeptical of an older drug of the same class. However, these effects are short-lived. The placebo response is not a property of the drug; rather, it is a reflection of the fact that 40 per cent of a random group of subjects will respond favorably to any form of therapy, although the response will be brief.[3] The placebo response is important

and must be controlled in drug research, but it is generally not useful as such in patient management.

Parenthetically, the practitioner should be reminded that the need for controlled clinical trials applies not only to drugs but also to new procedures, techniques, and theories. When relevant research in the form of controlled trials is lacking, one must depend regretfully on empiric clinical experience. Mere experience often will mislead, but it is a better guide than vapid theorizing by a scientist seeking to add a specious aura of relevance to otherwise admirable work.

■ Which Agent(s) Should Be Chosen?

Important factors in the evaluation of drug studies and in the day-to-day management of pain are the severity of the pain being treated and the concept that the potency of an analgesic is measured not in milligrams needed but by the severity of the pain that a given agent can relieve.

Mild pain will be controlled by nonsteroidal analgesics as well as by morphine. More severe pain regularly requires more potent analgesics (Table 1). A stepped increase to more potent drugs should be used. The superior effectiveness of morphine-like drugs over aspirin is regularly demonstrated in the management of pain in the terminally ill patient. The fallacy of contrary claims is discussed later.

Aspirin or other nonsteroidal anti-inflammatory drugs (NSAID) probably should be the first agent tried for pain control, but often they will not be adequate. Codeine and related drugs may be potent enough to relieve the pain of a patient with early parenchymal cancer but will be inadequate in a patient suffering from disseminated disease. Morphine and other narcotics of the highest potency usually will control the pain of even widespread bony metastases or of a serious complication such as a pathologic fracture. Oxycodone and related drugs constitute an intermediate group.

The least potent agent that provides sufficient relief should be selected, but the dose of a low-potency narcotic should not be increased beyond the amount that gives maximal effect, such as 100 mg of codeine per

TABLE 1. Use of Analgesics Based on Severity of Pain Relieved

	Route	*Dosage*	*Comments*
Non-Narcotic Analgesics			Available with narcotic analgesics in fixed combinations. Should be used with most potent narcotic analgesics as adjuvants. Cost, patient variability, and GI/platelet dysfunction are major determinants of choice
Aspirin/acetaminophen	Oral	Maximum dose	
Other NSAIDs	Oral	as recommended	
Least Potent Narcotic Analgesics			Ceiling on dose of 8 tablets per day. Do not supplement individually with non-narcotic analgesics
Codeine	Oral	1–2 tabs q 4–6 hr	
Tylenol with codeine	Oral		
Hydrocodone (Vicodin)	Oral		
Intermediate Potency Narcotic Analgesics			Ceiling on dose of 8–10 tablets per day
Oxycodone		1–2 tabs q 4–6 hr	
Percocet/Tylox	Oral		
Percodan	Oral		
Meperidine	Oral	Not recommended	Prominent CNS stimulant toxicity
	IM/IV	50–150 mg q 3 hr	Rarely useful except in the patient allergic to morphine. Shorter half-life than other agents
Most Potent Narcotic Analgesics			
Hydromorphone			
Dilaudid	Oral	2–12 mg q 4 hr	Increase to pain control. Least expensive agent
	IV/SC		More concentrated volume for infusion use
	Rectal	4 mg	Short-term use for patients who cannot continue with oral route. Numorphan suppository as an alternative
Morphine sulfate			Poor oral absorption of all MS preparations. May necessitate large (>100 mg) dose every 4 hours
Elixir, 2 mg/ml	Oral	5–40 mg q 4 hr	
Roxinol, 20 mg/ml	Oral		
MS Contin	Oral	q 12 hr	Dose established from stable dose of short acting drug, e.g., Percocet or Dilaudid
MS solution	IV/SC	Continuous infusion, 2–15 mg/hr or higher	Titrate to control
Methadone	Oral	5 or 10 mg q 6 hr	

dose. Increasing the dose in the hope of controlling severe pain merely increases side effects.

Oral Administration. Narcotics differ in their suitability for oral administration. Hydromorphone (Dilaudid), oxycodone (Percodan), and codeine are widely used because they are well absorbed orally. Morphine (MS) is poorly absorbed and is rapidly conjugated in the intestinal wall and the liver; thus, only a fraction of an oral dose (20 to 30 per cent) survives the portal circulation. This property of morphine may mislead some therapists into believing that they are using large doses orally because of the comparison with parenteral doses.

Rectal Administration. Many patients who have a brief life expectancy wish to remain at home but are unable to take adequate oral fluids and tablets or capsules. Rectal administration is convenient for these patients. Oxymorphone (Numorphan) is one of several analgesics available in suppository form.

Sublingual Administration. The sublingual route of administration is also convenient.[4] Morphine elixir 20 mg/ml, or tablet triturates (hypo tabs) are suitable dosage forms.

■ How Should Dosing Be Established?

■ PATIENT EDUCATION

Prompt control of pain establishes a commitment to the patient for long-term symptom control. The danger of respiratory depression is negligible with oral administration of narcotics. Similarly, the compulsive abuse potential of oral analgesics is slight. These concepts need to be explicitly communicated to patients with pain, or noncompliance with any regimen will be common. Then sufficient doses should be used to achieve pain relief. Patient-controlled dosing is useful; within certain limits the patient is allowed to use more medicine without consulting the caregivers.

A cancer patient with a limited life expectancy should not be denied analgesic drugs because the physician fears the development of compulsive use or the regulatory agencies or regards the therapeutic use of narcotics in the same light as the layman views the street use of narcotics like heroin.

There are important reasons why the therapeutic situation should be considered separately from intravenous abuse. First, narcotics that are administered orally or subcutaneously have a limited potential for addiction. Patients experience insulation from stimuli, and some may seek repetition of the experience; thus, compulsive abuse is possible. However, this late effect is a small pharmacologic reward compared with the total body orgasm or "rush" that is the immediate effect sought by intravenous users of heroin, methamphetamine, or cocaine. Thus, habituation to an orally or subcutaneously administered narcotic is a minor therapeutic problem.

Constipation is an invariable side effect that needs to be anticipated in patients using narcotic analgesics. These patients must use laxatives daily. A stool softener (e.g., dioctyl sodium sulfosuccinate (DSS), 250 mg, 1 to 2 capsules twice a day) should be supplemented with an irritant laxative, e.g., milk of magnesia, Senokot, lactulose.

■ DURATION OF ACTION

Duration of action is unimportant in the selection of an agent. Azotemia reduces excretion and should alert the physician to alter the dose or the interval as renal function worsens.[5] Meperidine and analogs are somewhat shorter-acting than the other narcotics. Narcotic analgesics should be given on a four-hour schedule because of a short half-life. If pain relief is inadequate, the dose should be increased, not the frequency of administration. Methadone (Dolophine) is only marginally longer-acting than morphine. The impression that the drug has a long duration of action is based on a misinterpretation of its use in maintenance programs for heroin users. In that situation, tolerant subjects are given large doses so that they need the medication only once a day. The 24-hour interval between doses represents tolerance and deferral of withdrawal, rather than prolonged duration of analgesic action.

Many caregivers for cancer patients emphasize that opiates must be given on a rigorous schedule, i.e., every 4 hours, without waiting for pain to reappear or the patient to request the drug. Without question, this policy is rational and is demanded in some patients. However, there are several cautions. It must be established that the pain is severe and unremitting and that medication, therefore, must be continuously or prophylactically used. Many patients prefer fewer, larger doses that permit them to be mobile and to continue their normal functioning to a degree.

Slow-release morphine tablets (e.g., MS Contin, Roxinol SR) add convenience because of their every-12-hour scheduling. For example, patients who are taking Dilaudid, 4-mg tablets, one to two orally every 4 hours, can be converted to MS Contin, 30-mg tablets, four to six every 12 hours. More may be necessary because of the erratic systemic absorption of morphine. Patients should be counseled to use the short-acting analgesics, e.g., Dilaudid, for "breakthrough" pain before the fixed time of administration of Contin. After 1 to 2 days, the Contin dose should be increased, based on breakthrough pain needs. Sustained-release preparations are not good initial analgesics because of the difficulty of titration to pain relief, but they are a reasonable alternative for the patient on a routine around-the-clock schedule. No cost savings are realized.

What Drugs Should Be Avoided?

MIXED AGONISTS-ANTAGONISTS

The mixed agonist-antagonist drugs, such as pentazocine (Talwin), nalbuphine (Nubain), and butorphanol (Stadol), cause distorted perception and are often poorly tolerated, especially if the dosage must be increased or if other drugs are also used. They induce narcotic withdrawal in the unsuspecting patient who uses this class of drug concomitant with pure analgesics, e.g., morphine sulfate. These agents have found their way into medical practice mostly because their prescription is less regulated.

ANALGESICS WITH PROMINENT CNS STIMULANT EFFECTS

Narcotics have depressant effects that can be reversed by antagonists such as naloxone (Narcan). Narcan and equipment for the support of respiration allow narcotics to be started cautiously in virtually every patient who requires pain relief. However, narcotics also have stimulant effects, such as tremulousness and convulsions, to which tolerance does not develop and which are not reversed by the antagonists.

The central nervous system (CNS) stimulant effects are especially marked in patients using codeine and meperidine (Demerol). The terminally ill patient, especially older patients, may complain of anxiety and tremulousness, or they may even develop psychosis or convulsions while receiving large doses of analgesics.[6] These symptoms of drug toxicity need to be distinguished from similar symptoms arising from situational anxiety and depression. The CNS stimulant effects are not reversed by narcotic antagonists.

Patients with mild renal failure or who are taking meperidine for long periods (e.g., continuous infusion or supplemental dosing) are at particular risk for convulsions or psychosis. This, combined with poor oral absorption, excludes meperidine from use in the care of the patient with cancer.

Propoxyphene (Darvon, Darvon-N) is the synthetic analog of the naturally occurring opiate alkaloid thebaine, a pure stimulant that is very similar to morphine in its chemical structure. The paradox presented by propoxyphene is explained by its stimulant effect. Propoxyphene has never been shown in an acceptable clinical trial to have an analgesic effect, yet it is active enough to be lethal in an overdose, due to refractory seizures. It continues to be widely used and abused because of its pleasurable, if mild, stimulant effect.[7]

The stimulant effect of codeine is perceived as unpleasant by some patients. Others continue to use codeine for its stimulant effect after they develop tolerance to the drug's depressant and analgesic effects. This is one cause of codeine abuse.

How Should the Physician Respond to the Patient with Worsening Pain?

First, another detailed pain history should be taken. Often, a new complication of cancer will aggravate established pain. For example, the patient with widespread bony metastases is at constant risk of spinal cord compression. Pain, particularly radicular in nature and centered over a vertebral body, is an indication for an imaging procedure (myelogram or magnetic resonance imaging). Radiation therapy reliably provides pain relief and prevents progression to paralysis.

Second, be aware that family or social disruption or other situational anxiety will be converted to heightened pain.

Third, change the analgesic regimen to a more potent combination, e.g., codeine to oxycodone or to hydromorphone.

Fourth, if pain is unremitting or severe, the patient should be hospitalized and a continuous intravenous infusion of morphine administered. In this situation, the constant level of medication establishes control over the pain while other maneuvers are considered. An IV bolus of 5 to 15 mg should be immediately followed by an initial infusion of 2 to 15 mg/hr. The orders should be written to allow qualified nursing personnel a range of dose adjustment. A stable dose can be converted to oral morphine, remembering that three to four times the IV dose will be needed for an equianalgesic effect. Another choice is to establish continuous infusion morphine by the subcutaneous route at home.

Finally, using drugs from other classes concomitant with analgesics will enhance pain relief and minimize narcotic toxicity. These other drugs are discussed next.

■ Adjuvant Drugs and Combinations

The development of tolerance generates many of the difficult problems associated with the use of narcotics. Increasingly larger doses of the drug must be given or a more potent agent must be used to maintain an analgesic effect. Occasionally, a startlingly large and expensive dosage cannot be avoided. Usually, however, the physician and the patient can arrive at a stable routine using reasonable amounts of drugs.

If patients are to cooperate in minimizing analgesic use, they must believe that the physician's stinginess in prescribing narcotics is based on a fear of losing the analgesic effect and a wish to avoid analgesic toxicity, not on a fear of patient addiction or of being disciplined for overprescribing narcotics. Drugs of several classes are useful in reducing the amount of narcotic needed. Other drugs, such as the stimulants, are not analgesics but produce a pleasant euphoria that may be perceived by the patient as an increased tolerance or acceptance of pain.

■ SEDATIVES

The opiates are usually very effective anxiolytic agents, altering perception and insulating patients from or reducing the concern about any continuing stimulus, such as pain or the fear inherent in some situation. Some patients still manifest anxiety and benefit from additional sedation. In others, the need for opiates may be deferred or reduced by daytime or bedtime sedation.

A long-acting sedative, such as phenobarbital or chlordiazepoxide (Librium), may be given to achieve mild daylong sedation. An intermediate-acting sedative-hypnotic, such as diazepam (Valium), may be given with the bedtime dose of narcotic to achieve a narcotic-free interval during the night.

Sedatives are not without some analgesic effect of their own; indeed, the initial effect of their action is the first stage of anesthesia, which is called the stage of analgesia. All antianxiety agents given in amounts sufficient to induce the second stage of anesthesia cause excitement and a drunken, uncontrolled response to stimuli such as pain. The excited response is sometimes called paradoxic or antianalgesic; this disinhibiting effect of a sedative is a frequent cause of unrecognized toxicity. Sedatives add to the depressant effects on respiration that narcotics have. Therefore, sedatives should not be used until the patient's response to the narcotic has been established.

■ ANTIPSYCHOTICS/ TRANQUILIZERS

Antipsychotic drugs of the substituted phenothiazine or other chemical type induce a subjectively unpleasant type of sedation or lassitude and no respiratory depression. A narcotic of intermediate or highest potency in therapeutic amounts causes minimal sedation and respiratory depression that is demonstrable only if the response to increasing concentrations of inhaled carbon dioxide is measured. However, when fractions of the usual doses of a narcotic and chlorpromazine are given together, the resulting sedative effect is much more than additive, but the degree of respiratory depression is only that of the small dose of narcotic.

Analgesia is not potentiated by combining an antipsychotic with a narcotic, but the injected or oral mixture may allow a smaller dose of narcotic, particularly at bedtime. For example, oral administration of 20 mg of morphine and 25 mg of chlorpromazine will provide sedation of a degree that would be undesirable during the day. The duration of action of the neuroleptic or tricyclic antidepressant is many times that of the narcotics. Even without further narcotics, the patient will experience lassitude, sleepiness, and depressed mood for perhaps 18 hours, an unpleasant effect for a patient who otherwise could function. The patient receiving this combination must be protected against postural hypotension caused by vasodilation and the possibility of unrecognized syncope.

■ ANTIDEPRESSANTS

The tricyclic antidepressants, such as amitriptyline (Elavil), are pharmacologically equivalent to the antipsychotics; when given in combination with a narcotic, they may augment sedation. They contribute only subjectively unpleasant sedation; that is, they do not elevate mood. Nevertheless, the antidepressants continue to be widely used, because the presence of pain and the knowledge that one has a lethal or untreatable disease are sources of extreme anxiety, which may manifest as depression.

Until the nosology was hopelessly complicated by advertisements for "antidepressant" drugs, this form of depression was called "agitated depression" and was treated with sedatives. The usefulness of the antidepressants was established in the treatment of an entirely different entity—major, psychotic, or endogenous depression.

The antidepressants apparently do have a weakly beneficial effect on the kinds of pain relieved by sympathetic block. Like the antipsychotics, the antidepressants have multiple action, including a sympatholytic effect. In our experience, the effect is more regularly achieved with propranolol (Inderal).

■ NON-NARCOTIC ANALGESICS

Aspirin and related antipyretic and weakly anti-inflammatory drugs pose fewer problems for the physician and the patient than the narcotics do. These non-narcotic analgesics often provide sufficient relief when given alone. In addition, control of severe pain with narcotic analgesics may unmask mild aches and pain. These pains should be controlled with non-narcotic analgesics rather than using more potent analgesics. The aspirin-like drugs are imputed to control bone pain preferentially by inhibiting prostaglandin (PG) synthesis. Although some cancers do produce prostaglandins and enhance bone resorption, PG synthesis is not invariable. Until controlled trials are completed, all patients should be tried on NSAIDs regardless of PG levels. The non-narcotic analgesics do not act on the central nervous system to alter the perception of pain. Rather, they act peripherally at the site of injury or inflammation to modify minor pain.

The subclasses of non-narcotic analgesics are (1) aspirin and other organic acids or nonsteroidal anti-inflammatory drugs (NSAIDs), and (2) acetaminophen. Acetaminophen has the same limited analgesic potency as aspirin. However, it lacks the anti-inflammatory effect that aspirin and the other NSAIDs have if they are given in large doses. Acetaminophen causes no gastrointestinal irritation, inhibition of platelet function, or other chronic toxicity. Single large doses may cause hepatocellular necrosis.

The newer aspirin-like drugs, the NSAIDs, can be divided into two major categories: derivatives of propionic acid and derivatives of acetic acid (Table 2). The propionic acid derivatives are equivalent to aspirin and may be used interchangeably with aspirin. The acetic acid derivatives, typified by indomethacin (Indocin), are much more likely to cause side effects but are reputedly more effective than aspirin. A recent controlled study does not verify the impression.[8] Piroxicam (Feldene) and meclofenamate (Meclomen) are pharmacologically equivalent to aspirin. Piroxicam has a much longer duration of action than aspirin.

In interpreting claims about the analgesic effectiveness of the NSAIDs and in making comparisons between drugs, the concept of potency (as defined earlier) must be rigorously applied. If analgesic drugs are tested

TABLE 2. Nonsteroidal Anti-Inflammatory Agents

Salicylic acid
Propionic acid derivatives 　ibuprofen (Advil, Motrin) 　fenoprofen (Nalfon) 　ketoprofen (Orudis) 　naproxen (Naprosyn)
Acetic acid derivatives 　indomethacin (Indocin) 　tolmetin (Tolectin) 　sulindac (Clinoril)
Other acid derivatives 　piroxicam (Feldene) 　meclofenamate (Meclomen)

against mild pain, all will be found effective. In patients with more intense pain, the greater potency of the narcotics will become apparent.

One study concluded that oral doses of the NSAID zomepirac (no longer marketed) were as effective as small intramuscular doses of morphine.[9] Although the study purported to test the efficacy of the two drugs against moderately severe postoperative pain, the patients did not require analgesia until an average of 21.4 hours after surgery. The conclusion that under similar conditions aspirin and morphine are equally effective was disproved in an earlier report,[2] which emphasized that potency is defined by the severity of pain.

Why are the NSAIDs used so widely? First, patient variability is such that some patients tolerate one of the newer NSAIDs better than they tolerate aspirin, whereas the reverse is true of other patients. Second, aspirin is a nonprescription drug, and patients may show greater acceptance of an NSAID given by prescription.

■ CORTICOSTEROIDS

The use of steroids in patients with advanced cancer decreases analgesic consumption and improves appetite and daily function.[10] The response is useful but short-lived.

TABLE 3. Special Techniques for Pain Control

Clinical Situation	Solution/Technique
Refractory generalized pain	Hospitalize for continuous infusion MS
Severe pain/inability to use or tolerate oral analgesics	Continuous subcutaneous infusion of MS at home
Pain from refractory, localized visceral (pancreatic or pelvic) malignancy	Intrathecal (epidural or subarachnoid) administration of MS
Disseminated bone metastases	Trans-sphenoidal hypophysectomy
Focal pain, e.g., isolated bone metastasis	Radiation therapy with or without orthopedic fixation
Nerve root pain, e.g., brachial plexus infiltration, post zoster neuralgia	"Vasoactive" drugs— propranolol, imipramine, phenytoin
Refractory head and neck pain	Intraventricular morphine

■ Special Techniques for the Relief of Pain

Some patients will be intolerant of large doses of oral narcotic analgesics or will not achieve adequate relief of pain. In others, pain is focal and can be palliated by directed measures. A hospice team can provide unique supportive resources that, when combined with physician expertise, result in superb control of pain with minimal patient disability (Table 3).

■ HOME CONTINUOUS SUBCUTANEOUS MORPHINE INFUSION

Occasionally, the physician will encounter patients whose pain cannot be managed with oral narcotics administered on a regular basis. Some patients require parenteral administation of narcotics because of difficulty in swallowing, nausea and vomiting, or breakthrough pain between times of drug administration. Continuous subcutaneous infusion of narcotics is a reliable solution for these patients. Clinical trials indicate that continuous narcotic infusions produce more even pain control than does oral medication and lessen the problems related to high peak drug concentrations.[11,12]

Subcutaneous infusions have many advantages over peripheral intravenous infusions. The problems of starting and maintaining venous lines in a population that has received multiple treatments with sclerosing agents are eliminated. The patients have full use of their limbs since subcutaneous sites are usually located in the subclavicular region or the abdominal wall. The expensive and complicated discharge to their homes of patients with intravenous infusions is simplified by the use of the subcutaneous route.

Most patients receive either morphine or hydromorphone subcutaneously via a small portable pump. The outpatient infusions are easily manageable for long periods of time. In some cases, the patient or the family, with instructions, will be able to program the pump, exchange narcotic cassettes or bags, and initiate their own subcutaneous needle sites.

The side effects of subcutaneous continuous infusion are acceptable. Rarely is there significant sedation or local erythema of the skin at the injection site, and nausea does not develop as a new side effect.

The major advantage to subcutaneous infusion is significant lifestyle improvement. Many patients regain mobility that was lost to other forms of administration. Some pumps will allow the patient to receive extra doses of medication on an as-needed basis. Patients can increase their dose during periods of activity and decrease the dosage during the night. Ultimately, the patient's 24-hour dose might be less than if set at a constant rate, regardless of needs.

WHAT IS AVAILABLE FOR THE PATIENT WITH SEVERE PAIN DUE TO ABDOMINAL-PELVIC MALIGNANCY?

The biologic behavior of certain malignancies is to invade locally without distant metastases. Patients may survive for many months. Aggressive control of pain from infiltration of nerve structures is important. Spinal administration is an ideal approach, particularly in patients in whom systemic opiate use has been proven effective initially.

The opiates have well-studied effects on spinal cord reflexes and the opiate receptors in the spinal cord. Small doses of morphine applied to the spinal nerves in the epidural or subarachnoid spaces have been shown to produce sustained analgesia. Epidural or subarachnoid administration of 2 to 10 mg of morphine produces analgesia by a local effect and reduces the toxicity caused by systemic use. Totally implantable, continuous infusion MS is an alternative to twice daily reservoir puncture.[13] To control pain in such situations as recurrent carcinoma of the cervix, bladder, or rectum, a catheter can be placed surgically, and morphine can be infused from an external or subcutaneous reservoir. Even pain from pancreatic carcinoma can be controlled with a catheter placed at the appropriate vertebral level. Rare respiratory depression is seen from intercostal muscle paralysis. The ease of this technique should replace celiac plexus block as the approach of choice.

BONE METASTASES

Focal bone metastases causing pain can be effectively palliated with radiation therapy. Radiation does not stabilize bone. Thus, metastases to bone causing a pathologic fracture or impending fracture should be dealt with by orthopedic fixation whenever possible. Pain relief will be superior and functional lifestyle maintained. Many uncontrolled trials confirm that 60 to 80 per cent of patients with adenocarcinoma of the breast or prostate with disseminated bone metastases will experience significant relief with transsphenoidal pituitary ablation.[14] The mechanism of efficacy is unsettled, but it is not a classic hormonal maneuver as relief can be nearly instantaneous.

HEAD AND NECK CANCER

Recurrent squamous cancer of the head and neck and brachial plexus infiltration have been reported to respond to the injection of morphine (Duramorph) into a lateral cerebral ventricle.[15] Further reports are needed; as with hypophysectomy, adequate neurosurgical skill is a requisite.

THE ROLE OF HOSPICE

Hospice is a service offered in the patient's home or another residence that offers counsel, information, and medical and other care to terminal patients.

The hospice philosophy affirms life and neither hastens nor postpones death, existing in the hope and belief that with information, care, and symptom control, patients and families can achieve a tolerable, even satisfactory, degree of mental and spiritual acceptance of and preparation for death.

The hospice team of patient, family, and experienced physicians, nurses, social workers, clergy, and volunteers evaluates the determinants or components of pain. The interdisciplinary team meets formally and plans interventions based on the sum of all the contributions. The response is optimistic, loving, and promising of continuing support.

When should referral to hospice be made? A national standard suggests referral when life expectancy is less than 6 months, but a practical guideline is to consider referral as soon as the physician determines that there are no interventions that can possibly cure or induce remission. Too long an interval between such determination of the terminal state and referral may lead to doctor and treatment shopping, together with psychosomatic complaints and poor compliance.

REFERENCES

1. Beecher HK. Measurement of subjective responses; quantitative effects of drugs. New York: Oxford University Press, 1959.
2. Houde RW, Wallenstein SL, Rogers A. Clinical pharmacology of analgesics: a method of assaying analgesic effect. Clin Pharmacol Ther 1959; 1:163–174.
3. Shall I please? (editorial). Lancet 1983; 2:1465–1466.
4. Bell MD, Murray GR, Mishra P, Calvey TN, Weldon BD, Williams NE. Buccal morphine—a new route for analgesia? Lancet 1985; 1:71–73.
5. Szeto HH, Inturrisi CE, Houde R, Saal S, Cheigh J, Reidenberg MM. Accumulation of normeperidine in patients with renal failure or cancer. Ann Intern Med 1977; 86:738–741.
6. Kaiko RF, Foley KM, Grabinski PY, et al. Central nervous system excitatory effects of meperidine in cancer patients. Ann Neurol 1983; 13:180–185.
7. Meyers FH. Pharmacology and toxicology. *In* The Investigational Use of Propoxyphene in the Treatment of Narcotic Dependency. Proceedings of a Symposium sponsored by the Research Advisory Panel, San Francisco, 1975:7–18.
8. Gotzsche PC. Patients' preference in indomethacin trials: an overview. Lancet 1989; 1:88–91.
9. Forrest WH Jr. Orally administered zomepirac and parenterally administered morphine. Comparison for the treatment of postoperative pain. JAMA 1980; 244:2298–2302.
10. Bruera E, Roca E, Cedaro L, Carraro S, Chacon R. Action of oral methylprednisolone in terminal cancer patients: a prospective randomized double-blind study. Cancer Treat Rep 1985; 69:751–754.
11. Bruera E, Brennels C, MacDonald RN. Continuous SC infusion of narcotics for the treatment of cancer pain: an update. Cancer Treat Rep 1987; 71:953–958.
12. Kerr IG, Sone M, DeAngelis C, Iscoe N, MacKenzie R, Schuller T. Continuous narcotic infusion with patient-controlled analgesia for chronic cancer pain in outpatients. Ann Intern Med 1988; 108:554–557.
13. Coombs DW, Maurer LH, Saunders RL, Gaylor M. Outcomes and complications of continuous intraspinal narcotic analgesia for cancer pain control. J Clin Oncol 1984; 2:1414–1420.
14. Levin AB, Ramirez LL. Treatment of cancer pain with hypophysectomy: surgical and chemical. Adv Pain Res Ther 1984; 7:631–645.
15. Lobato RD, Madrid JL, Fatela LV, Rivas JJ, Reig E, Lamas E. Intraventricular morphine for control of pain in terminal cancer patients. J Neurosurg 1983; 59:627–633.

Pancreatitis, chronic

I. David Shocket ■ *Stuart Jon Spechler*

Chronic pancreatitis is a clinical syndrome characterized by recurrent or persistent attacks of abdominal pain associated with endocrine or exocrine insufficiency of the pancreas. Diabetes mellitus is the primary clinical manifestation of pancreatic endocrine insufficiency, whereas exocrine insufficiency (inadequate secretion of pancreatic lipases and proteases) causes the malabsorption of fat and protein, which may result in severe nutritional deficiencies. The syndrome is the result of repeated or continuous inflammation of the pancreas, usually induced by alcohol, that leads to destruction of the pancreatic islet and acinar cells. On histologic examination, fibrosis and atrophy of the pancreas are apparent.[1] In practice, however, histologic confirmation of the diagnosis is obtained rarely. In most cases, the diagnosis of chronic pancreatitis is based on clinical, rather than on histologic, criteria. For some patients, pain is the overwhelming feature of the disease; for others, pancreatic endocrine or exocrine insufficiency predominates. For the clinician, chronic pancreatitis can be a difficult management problem. It is uncommon to establish the diagnosis before the pancreas has sustained irreversible structural and functional damage, and hence the treatment usually is aimed at alleviating symptoms rather than at correcting the underlying pancreatic disorder.

■ Background

■ ETIOLOGY

Chronic alcohol ingestion is the most common cause of chronic pancreatitis in the

United States. In developing countries, chronic pancreatic disease often is the result of severe protein-calorie malnutrition. Abdominal trauma or pancreatic cancer can cause obstruction of the pancreatic duct, which may be accompanied by chronic pancreatic inflammation. Other disorders associated with chronic pancreatitis include a rare hereditary form of pancreatitis and, perhaps, hyperparathyroidism. For some patients, there is no obvious cause, and the chronic pancreatitis is deemed idiopathic. Although gallstones are a common cause of acute pancreatitis, they rarely, if ever, cause chronic pancreatitis.

ALCOHOL AND PANCREATITIS

Alcohol-induced chronic pancreatitis usually takes 10 to 20 years to develop, although acute attacks can occur much earlier. The disease has a male predominance, reflecting the pattern of alcohol use in this country. It is not surprising that alcoholic liver disease frequently accompanies chronic pancreatitis.[2]

Alcohol administered chronically to rats results in the formation of protein plugs within the pancreatic ducts. These protein plugs lead to ductal obstruction, followed by pancreatic fibrosis.[3] It is not clear whether a similar process occurs in humans. Despite intensive investigation, the precise pathogenetic events by which alcholism leads to chronic pancreatitis remain to be elucidated.

NATURAL HISTORY

The natural history of chronic pancreatitis has been studied extensively. Typically, patients begin heavy alcohol consumption in their early twenties. The first attack of acute pancreatitis ensues several years later. Pancreatic calcifications and mild diabetes develop after approximately 10 years, followed some 5 years later by the appearance of steatorrhea and overt diabetes.

A recent study found that the mortality rate approaches 50 per cent in patients with chronic pancreatitis over a 20-year period. Age-matched controls have a mortality rate of 23 per cent over the same period of time. Alcohol and tobacco abuse are common findings in patients with chronic pancreati-

tis; patients often die of diseases other than pancreatitis. Liver disease, cancer, and complications of pancreatic surgery are the main causes of death. Factors that have been found to correlate with increased mortality include male gender, diabetes mellitus, pancreatic surgery, alcoholic liver disease, and the absence of acute attacks of pancreatitis.[4]

SYMPTOMS

Most patients seek medical attention because of recurrent attacks of abdominal pain. The pain is located deep in the epigastrium and often radiates to the back. Nausea and vomiting often accompany the pain. Alcohol and large, fatty meals may exacerbate the pain, which typically lasts for days. Patients may assume a fetal position in an attempt to relieve the pain. The pain associated with chronic pancreatitis is often difficult to differentiate from the pain associated with an attack of acute pancreatitis.

Diabetes, weight loss, and steatorrhea may be present. Rarely, patients present with other complications of chronic pancreatitis, such as ascites or jaundice. Ascites may result from rupture of the pancreatic duct or of a pseudocyst into the peritoneal cavity. Jaundice results from a stricture of the common bile duct where it passes through the diseased pancreas, or from a pseudocyst compressing the common bile duct.

DIAGNOSIS

The diagnosis of chronic pancreatitis usually is based on empiric clinical data. The diagnosis is established easily in the alcoholic patient who presents with recurrent attacks of typical abdominal pain, and who has diabetes, steatorrhea, and pancreatic calcifications. The diagnosis may be difficult to ascertain for patients with milder or atypical manifestations of the disease.

Pancreatic calcifications strongly support the diagnosis, as they are virtually pathognomonic for chronic pancreatitis. These calcifications are a common finding in alcohol-induced disease, with approximately 80 per cent of patients showing calcifications on abdominal radiographs. In contrast, calcifications occur in only 20 to 30 per cent of patients with nonalcohol-related pancreatitis. Pancreatic calcifications may regress with time in up to one third of patients; regression correlates with the duration of pancreatic dysfunction and occurs frequently after pancreatic surgery.[5]

Measurement of fecal fat is neither a specific nor a sensitive test for pancreatic insufficiency. Overt steatorrhea develops in only 33 per cent of patients, and stains for fecal fat may be normal in mild cases. With advanced disease, however, steatorrhea may be severe, with fecal fat excretion as high as 60 to 80 gm of fat per day (normal is less than 7 gm/day). Fecal fat collections may be spuriously low if the patient is not consuming an adequate amount of dietary fat.

The serum amylase and lipase estimations are unreliable tests for chronic pancreatitis, as the serum levels of these enzymes frequently are normal. Ultrasonography, computed tomography of the abdomen, and endoscopic retrograde cholangiopancreatography (ERCP) may reveal structural abnormalities of the pancreas but do not provide an assessment of pancreatic function. Furthermore, these tests may reveal no apparent abnormality, even in patients with severe symptoms of chronic pancreatitis.

Approximately 90 per cent of the pancreas must be destroyed before patients manifest evidence of exocrine insufficiency. In equivocal cases, tests of pancreatic function can be used to establish the presence of exocrine insufficiency. The secretin test is the most sensitive test for measurement of pancreatic function and may be the only abnormal test early in the course of the disease before overt steatorrhea develops. To perform the secretin test, a catheter is passed into the second portion of the duodenum under fluoroscopic guidance for collection of pancreatic secretions. After a basal collection, secretin (1 unit/kg body weight) is given intravenously, and fluid is collected over four 15-minute periods. The total volume of the secretions and the concentration of bicarbonate are measured. The bicarbonate concentration must be below 80 mEq/L in all four collection periods after secretin injection for the test to be considered abnormal.

Other tests for pancreatic exocrine insufficiency have been developed in an attempt to avoid the duodenal intubation required for the secretin test. For example, the bentiromide test is noninvasive and requires only a 6-hour urine collection. A 500-mg dose of bentiromide is given orally. The para-aminobenzoic acid (PABA) moiety of bentiromide is released by the action of the pancreatic protease chymotrypsin. The free PABA is absorbed in the small intestine, conjugated by the liver, and excreted in the urine, where its concentration can be measured. The finding of less than 50 per cent excretion in 6 hours confirms pancreatic exocrine insufficiency.

The standard Schilling test is abnormal in approximately 50 per cent of patients with chronic pancreatitis. A modified version of the Schilling test has been developed to distinguish chronic pancreatic disease from other causes of vitamin B_{12} malabsorption. The test involves the administration of radiolabeled cobalamin (B_{12}) attached to R proteins. Pancreatic proteases are required to hydrolyze R proteins to release the attached cobalamin. Patients with pancreatic exocrine insufficiency are unable to hydrolyze the R proteins and therefore do not absorb and excrete the radiolabeled cobalamin in the urine.[6]

■ Management

■ MANAGEMENT OF MALABSORPTION

Pancreatic enzyme preparations are used to treat the malabsorption caused by pancreatic exocrine insufficiency, which is manifested clinically by nutritional deficiencies, weight loss, and diarrhea. The enzyme replacements, which are taken with meals and snacks, are prepared from purified hog pancreas. Although these preparations contain lipase, amylase, and protease, their efficacy is based primarily on lipase content, which varies considerably with different preparations, ranging from 10 to 3600 units of lipase per tablet or capsule. The patient should be given approximately 9000 to 10,000 lipase units with each meal. Therefore, patients taking pancrelipase (Pancrease), which contains 2000 units of lipase per capsule, may require four or five capsules with each meal; for patients taking pancreatin (Viokase), which contains 1600 lipase units per tablet, six tablets may be required with each meal. The dose can be adjusted according to the response to therapy. Enteric-coated microsphere formulations theoretically protect the lipase from degradation by gastric acid and thus may allow more functional enzyme to reach the duodenum.

Quantitation of fecal fat in stool collected for 72 hours is the most sensitive way to determine the response to therapy. Even with dramatic improvement in fat absorption, however, steatorrhea is rarely eliminated. The response to therapy depends on the dosage and bioavailability of the enzyme preparation used. Meal composition (e.g., high-fat versus low-fat content), the degree of pancreatic insufficiency, and the level of gastric secretion are also important factors in determining response to treatment. If the patient does not respond to enzyme replacement, acid-reducing therapy with H_2-receptor antagonists (e.g., cimetidine, ranitidine, and famotidine) or sodium bicarbonate tablets should be added to decrease lipase degradation by gastric acid and thus improve the response to pancreatic enzymes. Antacids that contain magnesium–aluminum hydroxide or calcium carbonate should not be used in an attempt to reduce gastric acidity, however, since these preparations actually may make steatorrhea worse.[7] Lipase acts in the duodenum to cleave fatty acids from triglycerides. The liberated fatty acids can combine with the magnesium and calcium in the antacid preparations to form inabsorbable soaps.

In patients who continue to lose weight or complain of diarrhea on enzyme replacement therapy despite acid reduction therapy, a low-fat diet containing 40 to 50 grams of fat per day should be tried. Because these patients are often malnourished, a high-carbohydrate, high-protein diet also is recommended. If necessary, additional fat may be obtained in the form of medium-chain triglycerides. Medium-chain triglycerides are more easily broken down by gastric and duodenal lipases, and, because they are water-soluble, medium-chain triglycerides can be absorbed directly without hydrolysis by lipase.

Patients with severe steatorrhea may be deficient in the fat-soluble vitamins A, D, E, and K. Supplementation of these vitamins may be necessary. Uncommonly, vitamin B_{12} supplementation also may be required.

▪ MANAGEMENT OF DIABETES

Management of diabetes in chronic pancreatitis should begin with attempts to improve nutritional status and to decrease malabsorption. Oral hypoglycemic agents may be effective early in chronic pancreatitis when some beta-cell function is preserved, but many patients eventually will require insulin. Glucose levels may be difficult to regulate in patients with chronic pancreatitis, and episodes of hypoglycemia are common. The proposed mechanisms for hypoglycemia in this disorder include deficient glucagon secretion, poor glucose intake (especially during attacks of pain), and possibly hypersensitivity to insulin.[8] Coma and death may result from hypoglycemia. Ketoacidosis and the microvascular complications of diabetes are uncommon unless the patient is insulin-dependent. Peripheral neuropathy, if present, is related to concomitant alcohol use more often than to diabetes. (Also see article on Peripheral Neuropathy.)

▪ MANAGEMENT OF PAIN

Pain is both the most disabling symptom in patients with chronic pancreatitis and the most difficult symptom to manage. The mechanism is not known, and pain does not correlate well either with structural abnormalities of the ducts or with the level of pressure in the ductal system.

The first goal of medical therapy is to relieve pain, ideally without the use of narcotics. In patients with alcohol-induced chronic pancreatitis, total abstinence from alcohol is essential, as even small amounts may exacerbate the pain. Also, patients should be advised that small, frequent feedings may be less likely to provoke pain than large meals. When these measures are ineffective in relieving pain, aspirin, acetaminophen, or other nonsteroidal anti-inflammatory agents should be tried.

Pancreatic enzymes have been shown to provide pain relief in some patients with idiopathic chronic pancreatitis.[9] The proposed mechanism is feedback inhibition of pancreatic secretions, induced by the presence of pancreatic proteases in the duodenum. Although the hormone cholecystokinin has been proposed as the mediator of this feedback inhibition, recent evidence suggests that the inhibition may be neurally mediated.[10] If the patient is not already being treated with enzyme replacement therapy for pancreatic insufficiency, then a trial of pancreatic enzymes to control pain is warranted.

Unfortunately, non-narcotic agents frequently do not offer adequate pain relief for patients with chronic pancreatitis. Although the risk of narcotic addiction in this disorder is substantial, the physician should not withhold narcotics when these agents are truly necessary for the patient debilitated by excruciating pain.

In patients who fail to respond to medical therapy, other alternatives are considered. Alcohol injection to obliterate nerves in the celiac plexus that carry pancreatic pain fibers has been tried in small groups of patients. Unfortunately, this procedure may lead to complications, has not been shown to provide long-term pain relief, and is not recommended.[11]

Surgery is considered for patients whose pain is refractory to medical therapy. The goal of surgery is to relieve pain, ideally with preservation of as much functioning pancreatic tissue as possible.[12] The operations for relief of pain include duct drainage procedures, sphincteroplasty, Whipple procedure, and other resections of the pancreas.

Many factors enter into the decision regarding surgery for the patient with chronic pancreatitis. The clinician should consider the patient's overall condition, the likelihood of prolonged abstinence from alcohol, and the ability of the patient to manage the endocrine and exocrine insufficiency that may be exacerbated by surgery. Sphincteroplasty and drainage procedures are more likely to preserve pancreatic function, whereas pancreatic resections often lead to pancreatic insufficiency.[13]

A preoperative endoscopic retrograde pancreatogram is performed to define the ductal anatomy. The information obtained from this test and the extent of disease are used to select the appropriate surgical procedure. For example, ductular disease confined to the tail of the pancreas may be treated effectively by distal pancreatectomy, whereas drainage procedures (e.g., Puestow procedure) may provide the best pain relief for patients with diffusely dilated pancreatic ducts.

Approximately 70 to 80 per cent of patients who undergo surgery will achieve short-term relief; only 50 per cent remain pain-free after 5 years.[13] Controversy exists as to whether relief of pain is related to the surgical procedure or to the natural history of the disease as the pancreas "burns out." Pain relief appears to correlate with the duration of disease, pancreatic dysfunction, and pancreatic calcifications.[14] Factors unrelated to pancreatic surgery or pancreatic insufficiency also may play a role in the relief of pain. Abstinence from alcohol is probably one of the most important factors. For these reasons, the decision to use surgery should be made cautiously, especially in patients who continue to consume alcohol.

■ MANAGEMENT OF COMPLICATIONS

Complications of chronic pancreatitis include thrombosis of the splenic, portal, and mesenteric veins; biliary and duodenal obstruction; pancreatic pseudocysts; pleural and pericardial effusions; and pancreatic ascites. Surgical intervention is often required for management of these complications.

■ Summary

The treatment of chronic pancreatitis remains a challenge for the primary care physician, the gastroenterologist, and the surgeon. Once the diagnosis is established, a team approach is desirable to obtain maximal benefits from therapy. The goals of therapy are to deal effectively with the symptoms of chronic pancreatitis, to prevent further complications of the disease, and to manage expeditiously any complications that do arise. When surgery is necessary for management of pain or a complication of chronic pancreatitis, the surgeon should attempt to preserve as much functioning pancreatic tissue as possible. Advances in endoscopic therapy and in techniques for the transplantation of pancreatic tissue may render this disease more amenable to treatment in the near future.

REFERENCES

1. Sarles H. Revised classification of pancreatitis—Marseille 1984. Dig Dis Sci 1985; 30:573–574.
2. Dutta S, Mobrahan S, Iber F. Associated liver disease in alcoholic pancreatitis. Dig Dis Sci 1978; 23:618–622.
3. Sarles H, Lebrevil G, Tasso F. et al. A comparison of alcoholic pancreatitis in rat and man. Gut 1971; 12:377–388.
4. Levy P, Milan C, Pignon JP, Baetz A, Bernades P. Mortality factors associated with chronic pancreatitis. Unidimensional and multidimensional analysis

of a medical-surgical series of 240 patients. Gastroenterology 1989; 96:1165–1172.

5. Ammann RW, Muench R, Otto R, Buehler H, Freiburghaus AU, Siegenthaler W. Evolution and regression of pancreatic calcification in chronic pancreatitis. Gastroenterology 1988; 95:1018–1028.

6. Brugge WR, Goff JS, Allen NC, Podell ER, Allen RH. Development of a dual label Schilling test for pancreatic exocrine function based on the differential absorption of cobalamin bound to intrinsic factor and R protein. Gastroenterology 1980; 78:937–949.

7. Graham DY, Sackman JW. Mechanism of increase in steatorrhea with calcium and magnesium in exocrine pancreatic insufficiency: an animal model. Gastroenterology 1982; 83:638.

8. Botha JL, Vinik AI, Black HCH, Jackson WPU. Kinetics of insulin secretion in chronic pancreatitis and mild maturity onset diabetes (evidence of 'gut hormone' action beyond glucoreceptor and cyclic adenine monophosphate mediated insulin release). Eur Clin Invest 1976; 6:365–372.

9. Slaff J, Jacobson D, Tillman CR, Curington C, Toskes P. Protease-specific suppression of pancreatic exocrine secretion. Gastroenterology 1984; 87:44.

10. Adler G, Reinshagen M, Koop I, et al. Differential effects of atropine and a cholecystokinin receptor antagonist on pancreatic secretion. Gastroenterology 1989; 96:1158–1164.

11. Leung JW, Aveling W, Bowen-Wright M. Coeliac plexus block for pain control in pancreatic cancer and chronic pancreatitis. Gut 1982; 23:A451.

12. Mannell A, Adson MA, McIlrath DC, Ilstrup DM. Surgical management of chronic pancreatitis: long-term results in 141 patients. Br J Surg 1988; 75:467–472.

13. Moossa AR. Surgical treatment of chronic pancreatitis: an overview. Br J Surg 1987; 74:661–667.

14. Ammann RW, Akovbiantz A, Largiader F, Schueler G. Course and outcome of chronic pancreatitis: longitudinal study of a mixed medical-surgical series of 245 patients. Gastroenterology 1984; 86:820–828.

Panic disorder and agoraphobia

Frederick C. Bittikofer ■ *Michael F. Hoyt*

In recent years, *panic disorder and agoraphobia*, two types of *anxiety disorders*, have become subjects of increasing clinical and research interest. Occurring in up to 5 per cent of the population (with women affected twice as often as men), they often present a confusing picture to the clinician and result in much morbidity and suffering among those afflicted.[1] They merit discussion because of their high incidence, their multisystem symptomatology, and their effective, though complicated, treatment.

■ Background

The essential features of panic disorder are recurrent episodes of intense anxiety, fear, or discomfort, usually lasting 5 to 10 minutes (though occasionally several hours), which rapidly escalate to peak intensity and are accompanied by at least four and usually more of the following symptoms: dyspnea, unsteady feelings or faintness, numbness or tingling sensations (paresthesias), hot flashes (flushes) or chills, nausea or abdominal distress, sweating, trembling, derealization or depersonalization experiences, and a fear of dying, going crazy, or doing something uncontrolled during an attack.[2]

The feeling of panic itself is hard to define. Patients characterize it as distinct from simple fear and often describe it as weird, eerie, or strangely and dreadfully awesome. As opposed to simple phobias (in which a given stimulus produces a characteristic response pattern), the unexpected occurrence of a panic attack is a key feature of this disorder, although as the disorder progresses certain situations such as driving, crossing bridges, going shopping, standing in lines, or being in crowds may become associated with the attacks.[2] The patient becomes afraid of having an attack and is uncertain about when it may occur or if it will occur at all. This condition may remain unchanged in its severity for years or wax and wane for no apparent reason.[3] Some persons may even become housebound and never seek treatment or come to attention only when forced to seek medical help for another, unrelated medical problem. Increased public awareness, via television and print media, of anxiety disorders and their prospect for successful treatment may result in more patients being seen.

After a person begins to have recurrent panic attacks, several patterns may develop. In *panic disorder without agoraphobia*, attacks may occur at any time, including during sleep, but without any discernible pattern. Because of their unpredictable nature, the patient may be disabled during the attack but reasonably problem-free between episodes.[4] More frequently, however, the patient begins to associate specific events or circumstances with the panic attacks and develops elaborate hierarchies of feared situations and various coping strategies, resulting in the condition termed *panic disorder with agoraphobia*. These strategies include avoidance, work absenteeism, encountering phobic areas and activities only with friends or family members ("safe" persons), and ritualistic behavior, e.g., traveling certain routes or shopping at certain times. Indeed, the term *agoraphobia*, from the Greek meaning "fear of the marketplace," refers to the terrible anxiety such patients may experience at the prospect of venturing away from the security of home.

Agoraphobia without panic disorder occurs much less frequently. Here there is no or a limited history of panic attacks per se, but the patient is afraid of having a panic attack (or a limited symptom attack), generally in situations when escape might be difficult or embarrassing. It is unclear whether agoraphobia without history of panic disorder or limited symptom attacks is related to panic disorder with agoraphobia.

Although historical descriptions of agoraphobia and panic disorder date back to Hippocrates, with Westphal introducing the term *agoraphobia* in a paper published in 1871, scientific investigation began only in this century and has proceeded haltingly.[5] Panic disorder has a bimodal age of onset, with one peak occurring between the ages of 15 and 20 years and the second peak between the ages of 30 and 40 years.[5] There is controversy regarding the relative impor-

tance of biologic versus psychologic factors in the etiology of panic disorder. A higher concordance rate in monozygotic than dizygotic twins; increased familial rates of suicide, substance abuse, and major depression (of which panic disorder may be a variant); the high incidence of mitral valve prolapse in these patients; and results of brain imaging, panic provocation, and basal physiology all implicate a biologic component.[6]

Whether this reflects some form of autonomic vulnerability (the catecholamine hypersensitivity syndrome) or faulty biologic mechanisms is unclear. The idea that panic disorder is a biologically based, genetically transmitted illness is a significant departure from earlier theories emphasizing psychodynamic etiologies and mechanisms focusing on heightened sensitivities to normal somatic fluctuations, fears of psychologic change, and rapid conditioning leading to symptom formation.[7,8] It remains true, however, that these psychologic factors can have a significant effect on the time of onset, course, and treatment response.

Afflicted patients often do report a greater number of childhood fears, recall being anxious as children, and have a higher rate of grossly disturbed childhood environments and separation anxiety.[9] As adults, their personality style is marked by increased dependency, avoidance, isolation, interpersonal sensitivity, self-criticism, lowered self-esteem, demoralization, and depression.[9] Klein hypothesized that anxiety attacks represented a discrete biologic alarm mechanism that is evoked when the individual is threatened with separation, and both Katon and Uhde reported significant separation events as precipitants to panic disorder.[1] The cause of panic disorder remains unknown, with genetic vulnerability, hormonal flux, separation experiences, and other as yet unidentified stresses playing a role.[4] The frequent lack of an identifiable precipitant or instigator suggests a strong biologic or endogenous component, although psychologic or biologic factors, or both, may be etiologic in specific cases.[10] Disorders involving anxiety could arise from maladaptive learning, whatever its cause, that activates the anxiety system, or from faulty functioning of the system itself.[11]

Many medical conditions present with panic-like symptoms. An exhaustive differential diagnosis is beyond the scope of this discussion, but it is important to consider the following in initial evaluations: cardiac arrhythmias, asthma, thyroid/parathyroid disease, electrolyte imbalance, hypoglycemia, pheochromocytoma, carcinoid syndrome, premenstrual syndrome and menopause, partial complex seizures, stimulant abuse (including caffeinism), drug withdrawal, major or atypical depression with agitation, and severe generalized anxiety. In addition to a good history and physical examination, baseline laboratory studies should include a complete blood count, thyroid indices, serum calcium level, urinalysis, hepatic and renal function studies, fasting blood sugar, and an electrocardiogram.

■ Management

Because their many and varied symptoms affect almost every major organ system and mimic many medical illnesses, panic disorder patients have usually visited a variety of specialists, endured costly medical workups and consultations (in one study 70 per cent of patients had seen more than ten physicians[12]), received a variety of ineffective treatments, and often feel ashamed, guilty, and demoralized.[13] It is important to reassure patients that anticipatory anxiety and avoidance behavior are normal reactions to panic and that once the attacks are blocked, other aspects of the syndrome can be more easily overcome.[4]

Tricyclic antidepressants (TCAs), monoamine oxidase inhibitors (MAOIs), and the triazolebenzodiazepine alprazolam (Xanax) have all been proved effective in treating panic disorder, and the use of a particular agent should reflect the clinician's experience and the patient's unique needs. TCAs are older and well-studied agents, can be given on a once-daily basis, are available in generic forms, and have antidepressant as well as antipanic effects. Their disadvantages include a delayed onset of action, anticholinergic side effects (especially dry mouth, constipation, and urinary hesitancy), orthostatic hypotension, weight gain, and impotence. Imipramine (Tofranil) is the most studied and commonly used TCA for panic disorder, although clinical experience and anecdotal reports suggest that a variety of others are effective, including desipramine (Norpramin, Pertofrane), amitriptyline

(Elavil, Endep), nortriptyline (Pamelor), doxepin (Adapin, Sinequan), and possibly the newer agents trazadone (Desyrel), maprotiline (Ludiomil), and amoxapine (Asendin).[13] An initial test dose of 10 or 25 mg of imipramine given orally at bedtime will clarify any idiosyncratic responses, and the daily dosage can then be increased by 10 mg per day, or at the patient's own discretion, until persistent side effects that do not bother the patient occur. This dosage level is usually between 50 and 150 mg per day (occasionally given in the morning if the medication interferes with sleep or has an energizing effect), but it may exceed 300 mg.

The most common cause of treatment failure is too small a dose for too short a time. A *maximal* tolerated dose for 4 weeks is an adequate trial. If results are unsatisfactory, one can try a second TCA, especially if one specific side effect has limited the amount tolerated, by stopping the first agent over 2 to 3 days and starting the second, again in small amounts followed by gradual increases. The value of TCA serum levels in the treatment of panic disorder has not been established.

If TCAs prove unsatisfactory in blocking the panic attacks, an MAOI should be tried after a 2-week drug-free washout period. MAOIs, too, have both antidepressant as well as antipanic properties. Although they usually have a lower overall incidence of unwanted side effects, a low-tyramine diet is necessary, and therapeutic doses commonly cause mild-to-moderate orthostatic hypotension [fludrocortisone (Florinef), 0.1 mg orally daily, can help minimize this if needed]. Phenelzine (Nardil) is the most effective (perhaps even more so than imipramine) and best studied, but tranylcypromine (Parnate) and isocarboxazid (Marplan) are probably effective.[14] A test dose of 15 mg orally is followed by 15-mg increases every 2 to 3 days to a maximal tolerated dose of 45 to 90 mg/day, usually in a TID or QID regimen. Again, a maximal dose for 4 weeks is generally an adequate trial, with further time indicated if the patient shows continued improvement. Many patients on TCAs and MAOIs continue to improve over many months, and one needs to avoid premature termination of their medication because of early and bothersome side effects or too slow improvement. The combined use of TCAs and MAOIs is problematic and has not been shown to be of superior efficacy in panic disorder.

Long-term benzodiazepine use is controversial. Until the advent of alprazolam (Xanax), and possibly clonazepam (Klonopin), benzodiazepines were not indicated in the treatment of panic disorder. Alprazolam has been shown to be an effective antipanic medication in both the short-term and long-term.[14]

Although primarily an anxiolytic, alprazolam does have some mild-to-moderate antidepressant effects when used in higher doses. It has a rapid onset of action and can be used as an adjunct to TCAs and MAOIs (in doses of 0.25 mg orally two to four times a day) or by itself. When used alone, its short half-life necessitates a TID or QID regimen, with daily doses ranging from 1 to 4 mg (the initial dose should be 0.25 or 0.5 mg orally TID), although doses ranging from 8 to 12 mg per day are needed occasionally. During the initial weeks of treatment, patients may pass through several dosage plateaus before reaching an ideal dose, but the fear of endless tolerance and ever-increasing dosages has not been borne out clinically.[14] The dosage should be adjusted until there are no panic attacks and only mild side effects (usually slight sedation). The potential for abuse, habituation, and withdrawal seizures must be weighed against its marked clinical effectiveness, either by itself or in conjunction with other agents and therapies.

There is no clinical evidence that other benzodiazepines or beta-selective adrenoreceptor blocking agents, such as propranolol (Inderal) or atenolol (Tenormin), are of particular or unique use in the treatment of panic disorder. They provide some symptom amelioration, but their safe and effective long-term use has not been demonstrated.

With all these agents, the therapeutic dose should block any panic attacks completely, and it usually causes some mild and persistent side effects. If breakthrough panic occurs, incremental dose increases are needed. Once the patient is symptom-free, the medication should be continued for a minimum of 90 days, followed by a *very* gradual tapering over 1 to 6 months. If panic recurs, one should raise the dose to therapeutic levels for an additional 6 to 12 months. Often patients need to be maintained on medication for years, if not indef-

initely, especially when symptoms recur when medications are tapered or stopped.[1] The successful treatment rate is 90 to 95 per cent, but relapse rates range from 30 to 75 per cent, often necessitating several courses of treatment.[15]

For some patients, simply blocking their panic attacks will allow them to resume a normal life. For most, however, there have been months or years of disturbed functioning, and many problem areas remain after they are panic-free. These patients will need a formal psychotherapeutic desensitization program to treat their residual phobic avoidance behavior. A treatment group, as opposed to individual therapy, is a better way to help break through the isolation and feelings of uniquely having this problem. Such a group allows patients to correct (cognitive restructuring) false beliefs (cognitive distortions) that underlie their fears of dying, going crazy, or losing control. A group, which may be conducted by trained paraprofessionals, provides encouragement, support, protection, guidance, focus, accurate criticism, and new information.[5] Patients develop their own hierarchy of phobic situations, from least to most frightening or disabling, and encounter them at a progressively greater frequency and depth until they no longer fear the circumstance or situation. Practicing the feared behavior, changing negative expectations, doing relaxation exercises when anxiety is too high, and diverting thoughts to more neutral subjects (attention refocusing) help minimize residual fears. Working together and keeping diaries help maximize progress.[16] Anticipatory anxiety and setbacks are endemic to the process, and it often takes many months to become symptom-free.

■ Issues and Risks

Many patients with panic disorder require further psychotherapy after successful treatment of their panic attacks. They often have a long history of marginal functioning and poor interpersonal relations, in addition to a specific psychosocial stressor that brought them to treatment. Individual, marital, or family therapy is often indicated. Physicians often find the treatment of panic disorder patients quite challenging and labor-intensive. Patients require frequent reassurance and much emotional support. Their acute anxiety attacks and symptoms may lead them to demand or plead for increased amounts of medication; while such increases may be appropriate if panic symptoms are not well controlled, it is important not to reinforce unnecessary drug-seeking behavior. A clear patient-physician understanding that one provider will monitor all medications can be essential, along with an agreement to avoid unnecessary emergency room visits.

Selected patients may benefit from reading about anxiety attacks, phobias, and panic disorder, as this provides further information about their problem and additional strategies and techniques in dealing with it. Recommended books include Anxiety and Panic Attacks: Their Cause and Cure;[17] Don't Panic: Taking Control of Anxiety Attacks;[18] Stop Running Scared!;[19] and Not To Worry![20]

The relative merits of behavioral versus medication therapy are of great interest and controversy. Behavioral treatments can eliminate the need for medications and may lead to lower relapse rates, but they require highly motivated patients and, while helping patients overcome their phobias, may leave the panic attacks unchanged.[4] Medication treatment is limited by the current inability to predict which patient would benefit most from a specific agent, the morbidity involved with using the medications, and the possibility of drug dependence, if not habituation. It appears clear that combined use of medication and behavioral treatment results in greater, more rapid, and sustained improvement. Future panic disorder treatment may well be a multimodal approach based on adequate and repeated multisystem assessment.[21]

REFERENCES

1. Katon W. Panic disorder: epidemiology, diagnosis, and treatment in primary care. J Clin Psychiatry 1986; 47:21–27.
2. Diagnostic and Statistical Manual of Mental Disorders. 3rd ed. Washington, DC: American Psychiatric Association, 1980:236.
3. Agras S. Panic. New York: WH Freeman, 1985:3.
4. Liebowitz M. Imipramine in the treatment of panic disorder and its complications. *In* Curtis G, Thyer B, Rainey J (eds). Symposium on Anxiety Disorders. Psychiatr Clin North Am 8(1), March 1985.
5. Chambless DL, Goldstein AJ (eds). Agoraphobia. New York: John Wiley, 1982:1, 2.
6. Klein DF, Gorman JM. Panic disorders and mitral valve prolapse. J Clin Psychiatry 1984; 2:14–17.
7. Rapee RM, Barlow DH. Panic disorder: cognitive-behavioral treatment. Psychiatr Ann 1988; 18:473–477.
8. Roy-Byrne PP, Cowley DS. Panic disorder: biological perspectives. Psychiatr Ann 1988; 18:457–463.
9. Cowley DS, Roy-Byrne PP. Panic disorder: psychosocial aspects. Psychiatr Ann 1988; 18:464–467.
10. Sheehan D. Current concepts in psychiatry. N Engl J Med 1982; 307:156–158.
11. Baumbacher GD. Signal anxiety and panic attacks. Psychotherapy 1989; 26:75–80.
12. Ashok R, Sheehan D. Medical evaluation of panic attacks. J Clin Psychiatry 1987; 48:309–313.
13. Lydiard B. Panic disorder: pharmacological treatment. Psychiatr Ann 1988;18:468–472.
14. Sheehan D. Monoamine oxidase inhibitors and alprazolam in the treatment of panic disorder and agoraphobia. *In* Curtis G, Thyer B, Rainey J (eds). Symposium on Anxiety Disorders., Psychiatr Clin North Am 8(1), March 1985.
15. Bittikofer F, Kane C. Panic disorder. West J Med 1987;146:355–357.
16. DuPord RL (ed). Phobia. New York: Brunner/Mazel, 1982.
17. Handly R, Neff P. Anxiety and Panic Attacks: Their Cause and Cure. New York: Fawcett Crest, 1985.
18. Wilson RR. Don't Panic: Taking Control of Anxiety Attacks. New York: Harper & Row, 1986.
19. Fensterheim H, Boer J. Stop Running Scared! New York: Dell, 1977.
20. Goulding M, Goulding R. Not to Worry! New York: William Morrow, 1988.
21. Mavissakalian M, Barlow D (eds). Phobia. New York: Guilford Press, 1981.

Parkinson's disease

Heidi M. Shale ■ *Stanley Fahn*

■ Background

Parkinsonism is a neurologic disorder diagnosed by the presence of at least two of the following cardinal signs: tremor at rest (in hands, legs, tongue, and lower face), rigidity, bradykinesia, and loss of postural reflexes. In addition, a variety of other signs are present, such as decreased facial expression (hypomimia) with lid retraction and decreased blink rate, abnormal speech (either hypophonia and slow, monotone voice or palilalia with abnormally rapid speech), and loss of automatic movements (decreased arm swing, reduced swallowing with sialorrhea).

The most common cause of parkinsonism is Parkinson's disease, a neurodegenerative disorder of unknown etiology. Pathologically, there is a loss of pigmented neurons in multiple areas of the brain, most importantly the dopaminergic neurons in the substantia nigra. Noradrenergic and serotonergic neurons are also affected. The loss of cholinergic neurons in the forebrain may explain the frequent association of cognitive impairment in Parkinson's disease.

Many other etiologies of parkinsonism exist (Table 1). The most frequently observed is in patients receiving dopamine receptor blocking agents, such as the antidepressant amoxapine (Ascendin), gastrointestinal agents (e.g., prochlorperazine, metoclopramide), and neuroleptics used as antipsychotic medication (e.g., haloperidol, thioridazine). The parkinsonism induced by these agents is reversible, although this may take months.

Other neurodegenerative diseases often have parkinsonian features among their symptomatology. These include progressive supranuclear palsy, Wilson's disease, juvenile Huntington's disease, Shy-Drager disease, olivopontocerebellar atrophy, neuroacanthocytosis, Hallervorden-Spatz disease, and cortical-basal ganglionic degeneration. These are referred to as Parkinson's Plus syndromes. Features that suggest that a patient does not have idiopathic Parkinson's disease and that further workup is needed are listed in Table 2.

Although patients with early Parkinson's disease may not need medical treatment, most patients will require medication eventually because of continued degeneration of dopaminergic neurons. However, effective treatment becomes increasingly difficult, because of decreasing response to medication as well as the frequent occurrence of drug-induced side effects.

■ Management

As there is currently no cure for Parkinson's disease, treatment consists of medications to alleviate its symptoms. The aim is to keep an individual functional and independent for as long as possible. This includes recommendations for regular exercise, although there is no evidence that formalized physical or occupational therapy is beneficial. Treatment should be individualized to each patient and will depend on the age, the family, and the social and employment situation. If symptoms are only a minor annoyance, no treatment is necessary. Tremor is rarely debilitating, although it may be a source of embarrassment to some patients.

The evaluation of a patient with Parkinson's disease includes measures of blood pressure and pulse rate in both supine and standing positions, since orthostatic hypotension is a common side effect of some antiparkinsonian medications. Another common side effect is anorexia, and patients should be weighed at each visit. Patients should be questioned as to possible cognitive symptoms (depression, memory impairment, vivid dreams, hallucinations) and also about their ability to perform various activities of daily living, including washing, dressing, and feeding. The physical examination should assess speech, tremor at rest

497

TABLE 1. Major Types of Parkinsonism

Primary (Parkinson's Disease)

Secondary
   Drugs: neuroleptics, reserpine, lithium
   Toxins: manganese, carbon monoxide, cyanide, methanol, carbon disulfide, 1-methyl-4-phenyl-1,2,3,6-
      tetrahydropyridine (MPTP)
   Infectious and parainfectious: postencephalitic Parkinson's, AIDS, Jakob-Creuzfeldt disease
   Vascular infarcts
   Metabolic: hypoparathyroidism with basal ganglia calcification, chronic hepatocerebral degeneration

Parkinson's Plus Syndromes
   Sporadic: progressive supranuclear palsy, Shy-Drager syndrome, striatonigral degeneration, Parkinson's–
      amyotrophic lateral sclerosis, cortical-basal ganglionic degeneration, olivopontocerebellar atrophy
   Inherited: Huntington's disease, olivopontocerebellar atrophy, Hallervorden-Spatz disease,
      neuroacanthocytosis, Wilson's disease

and with action, bradykinesia, ability to perform rapid alternating movements, gait, and postural stability.

The frequency of patient follow-up depends upon the severity of the illness and how often medication changes are made. However, as the disease progresses, the patient's response to medications can become extremely variable throughout the day, and observation during a 1-hour office visit may be inadequate to decide what medication adjustments are needed. In this case, it is useful to have the patient or the family maintain a diary documenting response to medications throughout the day for at least 1 week, to see whether any pattern of response emerges. Patients should record whether they are "on" (i.e., medication is working and patient is responding), "on with dyskinesias," or "off" (i.e., medication has transiently stopped working; patient is parkinsonian) for every hour of the day. If they are incapable of doing this, hospitalization may be required to evaluate the patient multiple times in the course of the day.

It is important to be aware of the high incidence of depression in patients with Par-

TABLE 2. Neurologic Signs in Parkinson's Plus Syndromes

Corticospinal tract signs
Amyotrophy (muscle atrophy, fasciculations, loss of
   tendon reflexes)
Postural hypotension (unless drug-induced) and other
   autonomic features
Cerebellar signs
Ocular palsies (except limited upgaze)
Profound dementia, particularly early in disease
   course
Early, prominent loss of postural reflexes
Poor or no response to levodopa

kinson's disease (one third to one half). This may antedate the clinical appearance of Parkinson's disease or occur concomitantly. The depression does not always correlate with the severity of the Parkinson's disease, and successful treatment of the motor symptoms does not necessarily alleviate the depression. The signs of the two may overlap (bradykinesia, masked facies) and, unless depression is treated, it may be difficult to tell whether the parkinsonian symptoms are adequately treated.

Some depressed patients with Parkinson's disease have low levels of 5-hydroxyindoleacetic acid (5HIAA), a serotonin metabolite, in their spinal fluid, and their depression has been successfully treated with 5-hydroxytryptophan (5HTP), a precursor of serotonin.[1] When this is not available, commercially available antidepressants should be used. Although tricyclic antidepressants with high anticholinergic activity might improve some of the parkinsonian symptoms, the central cognitive and psychiatric side effects, as well as the hypotensive effects, might be detrimental. The monoamine oxidase inhibitors (MAOIs) available in America block the type A MAO enzyme that deaminates serotonin and norepinephrine, as well as the type B enzyme that deaminates dopamine. Blocking MAO-A in a patient receiving levodopa causes marked swings in blood pressure. Therefore, nonselective MAOIs are contraindicated in patients taking levodopa. Recently, selegiline (Deprenyl, Eldepryl, Jumex), a selective MAO-B inhibitor, has become available and may be safely used with levodopa.

In refractory cases of depression, electroconvulsive therapy (ECT) can be given. This might improve the signs of Parkinson's disease temporarily, as well as treat the depression.[2] If medication is necessary to control parkinsonian symptoms, first-line therapy usually will consist of anticholinergics or amantadine or both in the patient who is only mildly impaired.

ANTICHOLINERGICS

With loss of dopaminergic activity in the striatum, there is a relative increase in activity of cholinergic interneurons secondary to disinhibition. Anticholinergics counter this. They are primarily useful for treatment of tremor and less so for the other features of Parkinson's disease. They may also benefit such autonomic features as sialorrhea and excess sweating. Their main drawback is cognitive side effects, particularly impairment of short-term memory; hallucinations and confusion also can occur. These are more apt to arise in elderly patients, particularly if impairment of cognitive ability is already present due to the primary disease. Anticholinergics should be avoided or used with caution in anyone over 70 years of age.

Other side effects, resulting from peripheral parasympathetic blockade, are dry mouth, blurring of near vision due to decreased pupillary accommodation, constipation, urinary retention, and aggravation of narrow angle glaucoma.

The most commonly used anticholinergics are:

- Trihexyphenidyl (Artane): 2-mg and 5-mg tablets. The usual maintenance dose is 6 to 15 mg daily.
- Ethopropazine (Parsidol): 50-mg tablets. The usual maintenance dose is 200 mg daily.
- Benztropine mesylate (Cogentin): 0.5-mg, 1-mg, and 2-mg tablets. The maintenance dose is 2 to 6 mg daily.

Other anticholinergics used less often are procyclidine (Kemadrin) and biperiden (Akineton). The antihistamines diphenhydramine (Benadryl) and orphenadrine (Disipal) have anticholinergic activities and are also useful.

All anticholinergics should be started with the smallest possible dose (one-half tablet) and increased gradually every 4 to 7 days. They are taken three to four times a day.

AMANTADINE (SYMMETREL)

Amantadine is an antiviral agent that combines anticholinergic activity with enhancement of release of dopamine and inhibition of dopamine reuptake at striatal nerve terminals. The onset of benefit is relatively rapid (approximately 2 days to 1 week), although benefit may be lost after several months. However, reintroduction at a later date may result in renewed benefit. Amantadine is often used in conjunction with other antiparkinsonian agents, although it might be tried alone in mild cases.

Amantadine is available in 100-mg capsules. The starting dose is 100 mg twice daily. The maintenance dose is 200 to 300 mg a day.

The main side effects of amantadine are cognitive (confusion, hallucinations, delirium). Other side effects are lower extremity edema and livedo reticularis, a purplish-red, meshlike pattern on the skin of the legs.

LEVODOPA

Levodopa ameliorates the symptoms of Parkinson's disease by replacement of dopamine lost when nigrostriatal dopaminergic neurons degenerate. Dopamine itself does not cross the blood-brain barrier, but its precursor levodopa does. Levodopa is converted to dopamine by the enzyme aromatic acid decarboxylase. When used without a decarboxylase inhibitor, most of the drug is metabolized to dopamine peripherally, which increases the peripheral side effects of levodopa (anorexia, nausea, vomiting, postural hypotension, and, occasionally, cardiac arrhythmias). To minimize these side effects, levodopa is commonly combined with a peripheral decarboxylase inhibitor. This allows for an 80 per cent reduction in the dose of levodopa needed.

The two inhibitors available are carbidopa combined with levodopa (Sinemet) in a 1:10 (10/100 or 25/250) ratio or 1:4 ratio (25/100) or benserazide combined in a 1:4 ratio with levodopa (Madopar, Prolopa). Only Sinemet is available in the United States. The onset of action of levodopa is in 20 to 30 minutes, and the effect usually lasts long enough (6 to 8 hours) to produce a smooth response between doses, at least in the first few years of treatment.

When anticholinergics or amantadine are

inadequate for controlling parkinsonism, Sinemet should be added, usually with one half of a 25/100 tablet three times a day. Dose increases are made by one-half to one tablet every 4 to 7 days (the rate of increase depending on the patient's disability), both to minimize side effects and to establish the lowest possible dose that will improve symptoms effectively. A total daily dose of 75 to 80 mg of carbidopa is usually adequate to block most peripheral side effects.[3] Once this level is reached, further dose increases can be made with 10/100 tablets.

The most common side effects of levodopa are orthostatic hypotension, gastrointestinal symptoms, and cognitive disturbances. The hypotension is a dose-related phenomenon due to impairment of baroreceptor reflexes by dopamine. If increasing the dose of carbidopa is inadequate, use of thigh-high elastic stockings, elevation of the head of the bed at night to increase plasma renin and decrease nocturnal diuresis, increasing dietary salt intake, and fludrocortisone, a mineralocorticoid (0.1 to 0.3 mg), may be tried. Severe, refractory hypotension, particularly if it predates drug treatment and is accompanied by other signs of autonomic dysfunction (pupillary abnormalities, incontinence, laryngeal stridor) suggests Shy-Drager syndrome or striatonigral degeneration.

Anorexia, nausea, and vomiting occur early in treatment with levodopa, when the dose of carbidopa is still low, and usually will alleviate as the carbidopa is increased. If these symptoms persist, and further increases in levodopa are not required, additional carbidopa (Lodosyn) alone can be administered, although this must be obtained from the drug company (Merck, Sharp and Dohme). Domperidone (Motilium), an experimental medication that blocks dopamine receptors in the gut, as well as those in the brain stem chemoreceptor trigger zone for vomiting (the area postrema), has been used successfully to treat levodopa-induced nausea.[4] Although administration of levodopa with meals might delay its onset of action or decrease the degree of benefit, this also may help alleviate the nausea.[5]

Any type of psychiatric disturbance may occur with levodopa and is more common in patients who are elderly or demented. Disturbances can include vivid dreams, nightmares, hallucinations, mania, and hypersexuality. If the patient is taking other medications with potential psychoactive side effects, such as amantadine or anticholinergics, they should be eliminated first. If the symptoms persist, the levodopa should be reduced slowly. (Levodopa should never be discontinued abruptly, as this has been reported to induce a condition resembling the neuroleptic malignant syndrome).[6] Some patients develop psychiatric side effects when they take doses of levodopa that are adequate to produce an "on" state but have debilitating "offs" when the medication is reduced. Use of antipsychotic agents might improve the psychosis but worsen the parkinsonism owing to dopamine receptor blockade. Currently, an experimental agent, clozapine, which primarily blocks mesolimbic and mesocortical dopamine receptors but has only weak effects on striatal dopamine receptors, is being investigated in patients with Parkinson's disease who have psychotic symptoms when treated with antiparkinsonian medications.[7]

Other side effects caused by levodopa are insomnia, myoclonus, episodic excess sweating and hot flashes, skin rash (with the 25/100 pill, presumably due to the yellow dye), and darkening of urine, sweat, and saliva. Levodopa is also a precursor to skin melanin, and some are concerned that it may produce a recurrence in patients with melanoma. To date no causal relationship has been established, but in patients with melanomas, it might be cautious to avoid using levodopa.

■ DOPAMINE RECEPTOR AGONISTS

These agents act by directly stimulating dopamine receptors and are not dependent on surviving dopaminergic neurons for conversion to dopamine or storage, as levodopa is. Theoretically, they would therefore be more useful in patients with Parkinson's disease of longer duration. The two known dopamine receptors are D1, which when stimulated increase cyclic adenosine monophosphate (cAMP), and D2, which do not affect cAMP. The D2 receptor is more important in alleviating the motor symptoms of parkinsonism, but stimulation of the D1 receptor may produce additional benefit.[8] Two dopamine receptor agonists are available in the United States. Bromocriptine (Parlodel) activates only the D2 receptor, and pergolide (Permax) activates both D1 and D2 receptors. Pergolide may be a more powerful antiparkinsonian agent and have a longer duration of action than bromocriptine.

The agonists by themselves have only mild antiparkinsonian effects, and most patients will be able to be maintained on agonists alone for no longer than a year.[9] However, when they are used in combination with levodopa, the effects are additive. Moreover, the combination may prevent some of the long-term complications of levodopa therapy (see Issues and Risks).

Bromocriptine is available in 2.5-mg tablets and 5.0-mg capsules, and pergolide in 0.05-mg, 0.25-mg, and 1.0-mg tablets. Since postural hypotension may occur early in the treatment with the agonists, patients are instructed to begin with the lowest possible dose, taken immediately before retiring at night, for several days. After this time, doses can be taken during the day and can be increased by 2.5 mg of bromocriptine or 0.25 mg of pergolide every 5 to 7 days. The maintenance dose is 10 to 40 mg of bromocriptine or 1 to 4 mg of pergolide daily, in three or four divided doses (but in more advanced cases, a dose may be taken each time the patient takes levodopa).

In addition to orthostatic hypotension, other side effects of the agonists are psychiatric (which occur more frequently than with levodopa) and, less frequently, hypersexuality, pulmonary infiltrates and pleural effusions, nasal stuffiness, and elevated liver function tests. These will resolve upon discontinuation of the medication.

◼ Issues and Risks

◼ PHARMACOKINETIC PROBLEMS OCCURRING WITH LEVODOPA THERAPY

When levodopa treatment is begun, patients often experience a "honeymoon" period during which they are relatively symptom-free. However, after 5 years of treatment, at least 50 per cent of patients will experience troublesome fluctuations in their response to medications, and by 10 years, the figure may be as high as 85 per cent.

Initially, a patient will have a predictably smooth response to each dose of medication and will function at the same high level throughout the day. However, after several years of treatment, the patient begins to experience a return of parkinsonian symptoms (the "off" phase) some time prior to taking the next dose of medication. This deterioration occurs gradually (over many minutes) and the "on" state does not resume until levodopa is taken again.

"Wearing-off" correlates with falling plasma levels of levodopa.[11] Patients with early Parkinson's disease have sufficient endogenous reserves of dopamine to sustain them until the next dose of medication, even while plasma levels of levodopa are dropping. This reserve is lost as the disease progresses, with increasing death of cells in the substantia nigra, as well as loss of storage capacity of dopamine in nerve terminals.

Various therapeutic options exist to treat "wearing-off." The dosing intervals of levodopa can be moved closer together. This will provide only temporary benefit, however, and if the total daily dose is increased, the likelihood of other dopa-related side effects (dyskinesias, orthostatic hypotension, and psychiatric manifestations) will increase. Each individual dose of levodopa can then be reduced, but in patients with advanced disease, this may produce an inadequate "on" state.

Another approach is to add a dopamine agonist, since their duration of action is longer than that of levodopa. Agonists also allow for some reduction (approximately 25 per cent) in the amount of levodopa given.[12] Dopamine agonists may be more effective in the later stages, as they do not depend on intact dopaminergic terminals to synthesize and store dopamine.

Selegiline (Deprenyl), the aforementioned MAO-B inhibitor that decreases the rate of dopamine breakdown, also may prolong the duration of action of levodopa.

With progression of Parkinson's disease and longer levodopa treatment, patients may note a lesser degree of improvement of symptoms after taking medication. A dose that formerly provided them with a normal or near-normal level of functioning may no longer do so. In addition, the onset of action may be prolonged, and instead of an "on" state occurring within one-half hour, it may take an hour or longer to note an effect. Finally, some doses will not produce any beneficial response at all.

There are several reasons for this. Dopamine receptors exist in the stomach, and levodopa is known to delay gastric emptying. In this case, the tablets remain in the stomach. Since levodopa is absorbed only from the small intestine, levodopa may be catabolized before it can be absorbed. The patient may find that the pills taken at mealtimes fail to have the desired effect. High-protein meals, containing neutral amino acids, compete with levodopa for transportation across the duodenal mucosa into the plasma and also across the blood-brain barrier.[13] A possible solution is to dissolve the tablets in water and take them on an empty stomach, 15 to 30 minutes prior to meals. However, in some patients this causes intolerably high peak plasma levels of levodopa. Some patients try to limit their protein intake during the day and consume their daily protein with dinner at the end of the day.

Initially, as the level of dopamine decreases with the death of nigral cells, dopamine turnover increases and postsynaptic receptors become hypersensitive as a compensatory mechanism in order to maximally respond to the limited amount of dopamine present. This actually may mask symptoms of Parkinson's disease for a time, until dopamine falls below a critical level. Continuous bombardment of the hypersensitive receptors with exogenous dopamine, however, causes a "down regulation" of the receptors, undermining the brain's attempts to compensate for decreasing dopamine. Drug holidays have been used to try to counter this problem. These consist of 1 to several weeks during which levodopa is withheld, with the hope that this will "resensitize" receptors, so that when levodopa is resumed, lower dosages will be required, with a better response and fewer side effects. However, drug holidays have not proved to have long-term benefit on the response to levodopa or reduction of drug-related side effects.[14] The risks of medical complication (deep venous thrombosis, pulmonary embolism, myocardial infarction, pneumonia, and malnutrition) from increased parkinsonism during a drug holiday make it a risky method of treatment, considering the lack of sustained benefit obtained.

Abnormal choreic movements (dyskinesias) caused by levodopa can involve any body part. They may be severe enough to be ballistic or can be sustained (dystonic). The dyskinesias can be seen when the patient is at rest, but they are exacerbated by action, as well as by emotional stress. Initially, dyskinesias occur as a peak dose phenomenon correlating with high plasma levels of dopa and presumably too much dopamine in the striatum in the presence of a hypersensitive receptor. As time passes, the patient may go directly from an "off" state into a dyskinetic one and then go "off" again, without ever having a functional "on" period. Also, a poorly explained pattern of diphasic dyskinesias (D-I-D, or dyskinesia-improvement-dyskinesia) is seen in some patients. This consists of dyskinesias as the plasma levels are rising, best motor performance without abnormal movement at peak levels, and reappearance of dyskinesias as the effects of the drug "wear off," prior to going "off."[15]

If dyskinesias are troublesome because of pain or impairment of motor control, an attempt should be made to reduce the total dose of levodopa. Some patients will find that taking their medication on an empty stomach will result in dyskinesias, but will not if medication is taken with food. If this results in an unacceptable increase in parkinsonism, a dopamine agonist should be added to the regimen.

"Freezing," consisting of an inability to initiate a movement (usually walking), is a feature of advanced Parkinson's disease. Initially, it may begin as start-hesitation, when a patient has to begin walking, and also when an obstacle (stairs, doorway, elevator) is reached. If severe, it can preclude walking because of frequent and transient inability to move, as well as frequent falls. Freezing can be seen in both the "on" and "off" phases. Certain "tricks" may be employed to overcome freezing. Walking should be started by marching in place before moving forward and when an obstacle is reached. A turn should be made by making a wide arc. Visual cues, such as stepping on a row of markers, also can help overcome freezing. In some patients, auditory cues (such as listening to marching music on a portable cassette tape) will help "unstick" them. The cause of freezing is unknown. Although levodopa may help with "off" freezing, excessive levodopa sometimes exacerbates the problem.

It is still debated whether the fluctuations seen in Parkinson's disease are due to progression of the disease itself or to prolonged and early treatment with levodopa.[16] A recent study compared patients treated with levodopa alone and levodopa combined with bromocriptine. The patients on a combined regimen received a significantly lower dose of levodopa. After 5 years, the group on both drugs had fewer peak dose dyskinesias and "wearing-off" than the group that received levodopa alone.[9]

We currently recommend forestalling treatment with levodopa for as long as possible, using anticholinergics, amantadine, and dopamine agonists first. If these agents are inadequate for treating the parkinsonian symptoms, levodopa is added. Once started, the dose of levodopa should be kept as low as possible. It is preferable to keep the patient mildly parkinsonian on a lower dose of levodopa than to aim for a totally normal state and risk the occurrence of fluctuations, which, once begun, are difficult to treat. Obviously, this course of treatment will depend on the patient's needs and lifestyle.

■ TRENDS IN MANAGEMENT

There are three new approaches to treating patients with Parkinson's disease, particularly those with intractable drug-related fluctuations. The first involves experimental medications with unique modes of delivery, such as transcutaneous (+) 4-propyl-9-hydroxynaphthoxazine (PHNO), a D2 receptor agonist, or subcutaneous lisuride (another D2 agonist), which are delivered via an infusion pump. The aim is to avoid fluctuations by maintaining steady plasma and brain levels of medication. A sustained-release form of Sinemet has been developed. Levodopa has also been administered via the intraduodenal route to bypass the problem of delayed gastric emptying.

The second approach is surgical treatment. Thalamotomy had been developed prior to the availability of antiparkinsonian drugs. Current use of computed tomography–assisted stereotaxic techniques enables more precise localization of the ventrolateral thalamus. This surgical procedure is reserved for patients whose main problem is with rigidity or tremor or both and who are insufficiently controlled with medicines or unable to tolerate medications in adequate doses owing to side effects.[17]

Recently, multiple centers in the United States, Mexico, Latin America, China, and Europe have performed transplants of autologous adrenal medullary tissues into the striatum.[18,19] Thus far, the patients who improved after surgery have shown an increase in "on" time, with fewer dyskinesias. Most patients have not shown marked improvement. More recently, transplants of fetal mesencephalon to the striatum are being carried out. More time is needed to determine the role of this technique.

The third recent development in the treatment of Parkinson's disease involves a hypothesis of the etiology of the condition and what might be done to prevent its progression. The theory under investigation is that metabolism of dopamine by oxidation produces build-up of toxic free radicals, which in susceptible invidual (e.g., those who already have sustained damage to their substantia nigra, perhaps from an environmental toxin) causes destruction of dopaminergic neurons.[20] When 80 per cent of the neurons are lost, parkinsonian symptoms appear. Two antioxidants, selegiline and tocopherol (vitamin E), are being administered in a multicenter trial to patients with early Parkinson's disease to see whether their disease will progress slower than that of patients who receive placebos.

REFERENCES

1. Mayeux R, Stern Y, Cote L, Williams JB. Altered serotonin metabolism in depressed patients with Parkinson's disease. Neurology 1984; 34:642–646.
2. Lebensohn ZM, Jenkins RB. Improvement of parkinsonism in depressed patients treated with ECT. Am J Psychiatr 1975; 132:283–284.
3. Jaffe ME. Clinical studies of carbidopa and L-dopa in the treatment of Parkinson's disease. In Yahr MD (ed). The Treatment of Parkinsonism; The Role of Dopadecarboxylase Inhibitors. New York: Raven Press, 1973.
4. Parkes JD. Domperidone and Parkinson's disease. Clin Neuropharmacol 1986; 9:517–532.
5. Nutt JG, Woodward W, Hammerstad JP, Carter JH, Anderson JL. The "on-off" phenomenon in Parkinson's disease: relation to levodopa absorption and transport. N Engl J Med 1984; 310:483–488.
6. Sechi GP, Tanda F, Motani R. Fatal hyperpyrexia after withdrawal of levodopa. Neurology 1984; 34:249–251.
7. Scholz E, Dichgans J. Treatment of drug-induced exogenous psychosis in parkinsonism with clozapine and fluperlapine. Eur Arch Psychiat Neurol Sci 1985; 235:60–64.
8. Lieberman AN. Treatment of Parkinson's disease. Mayo Clin Proc 1988; 63:1046–1049.
9. Rinne UK. Early combination of bromocriptine and levodopa in the treatment of Parkinson's disease: a 5-year follow-up. Neurology 1987; 37:826–828.
10. Barbeau A. High-level levodopa therapy in severely akinetic parkinsonian patients: twelve years later. In Rinne U, Klingler M, Stamm B (eds). Parkinson's Disease: Current Progress, Problems and Management. Amsterdam: Elsevier/North-Holland Biomedical Press, 1980:229–239.
11. Fahn S. Fluctuations in disability in Parkinson's disease: pathophysiology. In Marsden CD, Fahn S (eds). Movement Disorders. London: Butterworth Scientific, 1982:123–145.

12. Calne DB. Dopamine receptor agonists in treatment of basal ganglia disorders. Semin Neurol 1982; 2:359–364.

13. Eriksson T, Granerus AK, Linde A, Carlsson A. "On-off" phenomenon in Parkinson's disease: relation between dopa and other large neutral amino acids in plasma. Neurology 1988; 38:1245–1248.

14. Mayeux R, Stern Y, Mulvey K, Cote L. Reappraisal of temporary levodopa withdrawal ("drug holiday") in Parkinson's disease. N Engl J Med 1985; 313:724–728.

15. Muenter MD, Sharpless NS, Tyce GM, Darley FL. Patterns of dystonia ("D-I-D") in response to L-dopa therapy for Parkinson's disease. Mayo Clin Proc 1977; 52:163–174.

16. Fahn S, Bressman SB. Should levodopa therapy for parkinsonism be started early or late? Evidence against early treatment. Can J Neurol Sci 1984; 11:200–206.

17. Kelly PJ, Ahlskog JE, Goerss SJ, Daube JR, Duffy JR, Kall PA. Computer-assisted stereotactic ventralis lateralis thalamotomy with microelectrode recording control in patients with Parkinson's disease. Mayo Clin Proc 1987; 62:655–664.

18. Madrazo I, Drucker-Colin R, Diaz V, Martinez-Mata J, Torres C, Becerril JJ. Open microsurgical autograft of adrenal medulla to the right caudate nucleus in two patient with intractable Parkinson's disease. N Engl J Med 1987; 316:831–834.

19. Backlund E, Granberg P, Hamberger B, et al. Transplantation of adrenal medullary tissue to striatum in parkinsonism. J Neurosurg 1985; 62:169–173.

20. Langston JW, Irwin I. MPTP: current concepts and controversies. Clin Neuropharm 1986; 9:485–507.

Pelvic infections

D. Melessa Phillips ■ *Judith G. Gearhart*

■ Background

Pelvic infections, of which primary pelvic inflammatory disease (PID) is the prototype, constitute a major personal and public health hazard for women today. More then 1 million cases of PID are diagnosed yearly in the United States. It is estimated that the cost of management of PID and its sequelae will total over $3 billion per year in 1990.[1] Personal health risks for women diagnosed with PID are equally sobering: 17 per cent of patients are rendered infertile from post-PID tubal damage, and the risk of an ectopic pregnancy increases seven- to tenfold after PID.[2] Dyspareunia, chronic pelvic pain, recurrent PID, pelvic adhesions, and the need for surgery to correct pelvic structure damage are debilitating residua of PID for as many as one fourth of patients.

The most serious complication of sexually transmitted diseases, primary PID is the clinical syndrome of upper genital tract infection caused by ascending invasion of polymicrobes that originate in the vagina and cervix. Infection may be confined to the uterine cavity (endometritis), tubes (salpingitis), or ovaries (oophoritis). Extension of infection to adjacent intraperitoneal structures produces pyosalpinx, tubo-ovarian or broad ligament abscesses, and peritonitis. Women at the highest risk for primary PID are (1) those less than 25 years old, (2) those with multiple sexual partners, (3) those with a prior diagnosis of PID or a sexually transmitted disease, and (4) those who use an intrauterine device for contraception. Secondary pelvic infections are those unrelated to sexually transmitted causes, and they occur after invasive gynecologic procedures, pregnancy termination, spontaneous miscarriage, vaginal or cesarean delivery, and pelvic trauma, or in the presence of gynecologic malignancy. Secondary pelvic infections should be suspected whenever sepsis occurs in the postpartum or postoperative period.

Not all nonspecific pelvic pain is attributable to PID. Major and minor clinical criteria were established by Hager in 1983 to develop uniformity in accurately diagnosing the condition (Table 1). Physical examination criteria of pelvic and abdominal tenderness are highly subjective and may account for the popularity of the diagnosis in outpatient clinics and emergency departments. Clinicians must consider carefully the gy-

TABLE 1. Diagnostic Criteria for PID

All *three* required

- Direct abdominal tenderness with or without rebound tenderness
- Cervical and uterine tenderness to motion
- Adnexal tenderness

PLUS any *one* of the following:

- Temperature > 38° C (100.4° F)
- Pelvic mass or abscess on examination or sonography
- Peripheral WBC > 10,000/mm^3
- Endocervical gram-negative intracellular diplococci
- Peritoneal fluid leukocytosis (WBC > 15,000/mm^3) obtained by culdocentesis or laparoscopy

(From Hager WD, Eschenback DA, Spence MN, Sweet LR. Criteria for diagnosing and grading of salpingitis. Obstet Gynecol 1983; 61:113–114. Reprinted with permission from The American College of Obstetricians and Gynecologists.)

necologic history, risk factors present, the initial physical examination, and objective laboratory data before diagnosing a patient with PID.

Whenever the diagnosis of acute PID is considered, appropriate cultures must be taken at the time of the initial pelvic examination. If sexually transmitted PID is suspected, endocervical cultures for *N. gonorrhoeae* and probably *Chlamydia trachomatis* should be taken. Pharyngeal and rectal cultures should be obtained if the sexual history is relevant for infection at these sites. An endocervical specimen should be examined for the presence of gram-negative intracellular diplococci; a negative Gram stain does not exclude gonococcal disease. Aerobic and anaerobic blood cultures are probably most useful in establishing the etiologies of secondary pelvic infections, as multiple studies have documented poor correlation with lower genital tract microbiology in sexually transmitted PID. In women of childbearing age, a serum pregnancy test is recommended to exclude simultaneous intrauterine or ectopic pregnancy. Pelvic sonography is indicated whenever pain or peritoneal irritation is severe enough to preclude adequate pelvic examination[3] or if an adnexal mass is found. Whereas some centers routinely perform diagnostic laparoscopy for all suspected cases of primary PID, the procedure may not be available or practical in smaller communities. Patients should be referred for laparoscopy, however, if the diagnosis is in question, the pre-

senting symptoms are severe, or abscess formation or rupture is suspected.

Treatment of women with the clinical diagnosis of PID is difficult, because optimal therapy for the condition has yet to be defined. A major problem in establishing consistent treatment guidelines for PID arises from its changing polymicrobial nature. The pathogenesis of acute PID encompasses a broad spectrum of sexually transmitted, aerobic, and anaerobic micro-organisms (Table 2), any of which may be singly or in combination responsible for pelvic infections. Additionally, the number of available antibiotics is continually increasing in an attempt to deal with the emergence of bacterial resistance, drug-associated toxicity, new pharmacokinetics, and cost containment issues. Considerations in the therapy of secondary pelvic infections include the use of prophylactic antibiotics and the likelihood of specific pathogenic infections in the puerperal or postoperative period.

■ Management

The specific goal of treatment of all pelvic infections is complete eradication of the in-

TABLE 2. Microbiologic Causes of Pelvic Infections

Exogenous Agents
Sexually Transmitted Agents
Neisseria gonorrhoeae
Chlamydia trachomatis
Mycoplasma hominis
Ureaplasma urealyticum
Endogenous Agents
Aerobic Organisms
Gram-positive cocci: Streptococcus, Staphylococcus, Pneumococcus
Gram-positive bacilli: Diphtheroids, lactobacilli, *Listeria monocytogenes*
Gram-negative: Enterobacteriaceae: *Escherichia, Klebsiella, Proteus, Salmonella*
Gram-negative Other: *Pseudomonas, Gardnerella* (formerly *Haemophilus*)
Anaerobic Organisms
Gram-positive cocci: *Peptococcus, Peptostreptococcus*
Gram-positive bacilli: *Clostridium, Actinomyces, Bifidobacterium, Eubacterium, Propionibacterium*
Gram-negative cocci: Acidaminococcus, *Megasphaera, Veillonella*
Gram-negative rods: *Bacteroides, Fusobacterium*

(Reprinted with permission from Herbst AL, Mercer LJ: Overview of therapeutic and prophylactic antibiotics in obstetrics and gynecology. J Reprod Med 1988; 33:144–148.)

fectious process. Equally important goals in the therapy of primary PID are (1) preservation of fertility, and (2) prevention of the condition's chronic sequelae.

■ PRIMARY PELVIC INFLAMMATORY DISEASE

In 1986, Grimes and colleagues reviewed the prescribing habits of private physicians treating PID from 1966 to 1983.[4] The study noted that while most publications about PID treatment came from teaching hospitals, most women with PID actually were treated either as outpatients or as inpatients in community hospitals. Their survey of over 25 million antibiotic prescriptions, written predominantly by office-based primary care physicians, showed that (1) most patients with PID were treated as outpatients, with a single antibiotic, (2) cephalosporins became the most frequently prescribed drugs for inpatient therapy, replacing penicillin in combination regimens in the early 1980s, and (3) the rate of prescribing natural penicillins

declined dramatically while prescriptions for aminopenicillins more than doubled.

Clinicians traditionally have relied on the Centers for Disease Control (CDC) Sexually Transmitted Disease Treatment Guidelines for advice in the management of sexually transmitted diseases, including acute PID. In 1982, CDC guidelines for acute PID changed to reflect the availability of new antibiotics and the need to provide coverage for the condition's polymicrobial etiologies and for penicillinase-producing strains of *N. gonorrhoeae* (PPNG). The emergence in the 1970s of PPNG produced clinically significant bacterial resistance against three of the then most widely used antibiotics to treat gonorrhea: penicillins, tetracyclines, and aminoglycosides. In its latest guidelines, the CDC clearly states that "the treatment of choice for acute PID is not established."[5] It also emphasizes that no single drug is active against the entire spectrum of PID pathogens, and that despite in vivo studies, no antimicrobial combinations have been adequately evaluated for clinical efficacy in PID. Thus, practitioners must select an empiric regimen, based on the patient's history and initial

---

TABLE 3. CDC Recommendations for PID Management

Ambulatory Regimen

Cefoxitin (Mefoxin) 2 gm IM, plus probenecid, 1 gm PO

OR

Ceftriaxone (Rocephin), 250 mg IM, or equivalent cephalosporin

PLUS

Doxycycline (Vibramycin), 100 mg PO BID for 10–14 days

OR

Tetracycline, 500 mg PO QID for 10–14 days

Penicillin-allergic patients: Spectinomycin, 2 gm IM, followed by doxycycline or tetracycline for 10–14 days

Inpatient Regimen

Regimen A: Doxycycline (Vibramycin), 100 mg IV or PO BID

      PLUS

      Cefoxitin (Mefoxin), 2.0 gm IV every 6 hours

      OR

      Cefotetan* (Cefotan), 2.0 gm IV every 12 hours

Regimen B: Clindamycin (Cleocin), 900 mg IV every 8 hours

      PLUS

      Gentamicin (Garamycin), 2.0 mg/kg IV or IM followed by 1.5 mg/kg every 8 hours in patients with normal renal function

Continue drugs IV at least 4 days and at least 48 hours after patient improves. Follow Regimen A with doxycycline, 100 mg PO BID for 10–14 days, and Regimen B with doxycycline, 100 mg PO BID or clindamycin, 450 mg 5 times daily for 10–14 days

---

*Other cephalosporins such as ceftizoxime (Cefizox), cefotaxime (Claforan), and ceftriaxone (Rocephin), which provide adequate gonococcal, other facultative gram-negative aerobic, and anaerobic coverage, may be utilized in appropriate doses.

(From Centers for Disease Control. 1989 Sexually Transmitted Diseases Treatment Guidelines. Atlanta: Department of Health and Human Services, 1989.)

physical examination, while awaiting culture results that may not accurately reflect all etiologic pathogens.

Outpatient Therapy. The latest CDC regimens for the treatment of uncomplicated acute PID (salpingitis without peritonitis) are listed in Table 3. Conspicuously absent from the 1989 ambulatory treatment recommendations are ampicillin, amoxicillin, and aqueous procaine penicillin. Cephalosporins plus doxycycline/tetracycline provide activity against N. gonorrhoeae (including PPNG) and Chlamydia trachomatis. However, single doses of cephalosporin followed by oral tetracycline may not provide sustained activity against strains of nonbetalactamase–producing chromosomally mediated resistant N. gonorrhoeae (CMRNG) or the facultative or anaerobic organisms involved in PID. CDC recommendations for treatment of PPNG and CMRNG include spectinomycin, 2.0 gm IM, or ceftriaxone, 250 mg IM, followed by tetracycline, doxycycline, or erythromycin.[5] Women with PID should be monitored closely and seen again within 2 to 3 days after initiation of treatment to determine clinical improvement or worsening.

Inpatient Therapy. Hospitalization of patients with acute PID is indicated when (1) the diagnosis is uncertain, (2) surgical emergencies such as appendicitis or ectopic pregnancy cannot be excluded, (3) pelvic abscess is suspected, (4) the patient is pregnant, (5) the patient is a prepubertal child or adolescent, (6) the severity of the illness precludes outpatient management, (7) the patient is unable to follow or tolerate an outpatient regimen, (8) the patient has failed to respond to outpatient therapy, or (9) clinical follow-up within 72 hours of initial antibiotic treatment cannot be arranged.[5]

1989 CDC recommendations for inpatient management of PID are listed in Table 3 (Regimens A and B). Other parenteral treatment options of Regimen A include cefotaxime (Claforan), ceftriaxone (Rocephin), and ceftizoxime (Cefizox). Doxycycline may be given orally if the patient's condition warrants, as oral bioavailability of the drug is now known to be equal to that of parenteral administration. In Regimen B, the recommended dose of gentamicin for PID is higher than that used in other clinical situations; underdosing may occur if less than 1.5 mg/ kg every 8 hours is given. Patients with PID are generally young, with normal glomerular filtration rates, and can tolerate increased dosing without concomitant nephrotoxicity. Serum aminoglycoside levels should be monitored.

As new antibiotics and clinical trials emerge, a multiplicity of drug regimens has been studied in an attempt to find the "ideal" antibiotic. Mercer states that the ideal antibiotic for PID would possess the following characteristics: (1) broad-spectrum activity against gram-positive anaerobic organisms, PPNG, Chlamydia trachomatis, the full spectrum of Bacteroides species, gram-negative aerobic rods, and gram-positive aerobes, (2) a low incidence of side effects and toxicity, (3) a high degree of efficacy in an aerobic environment, (4) the ability to penetrate loculated pus at a high concentration, (5) a low propensity for the development of resistant strains, and (6) inexpensive to administer and monitor.[6]

Although no such perfect antibiotic exists, recent studies have shown several promising parenteral regimens, including an aztreonam (Azactam)-clindamycin combination,[7] a ceftizoxime (Cefizox)-doxycycline combination,[8] and single-drug regimens of ceftizoxime (Cefizox), imipenem (Primaxin), and ticarcillin–potassium clavulanate (Timetin).[9]

Despite the array of therapeutic possibilities, several general observations may help clarify the initial choice of therapy for patients with PID:

1. Antibiotics active against N. gonorrhoeae must always be included in the PID treatment regimen. PPNG should be considered in cases occurring in endemic urban areas and in cases of treatment failures.[10]
2. Two-drug therapy (initial therapy plus 10 to 14 days of follow-up antibiotic) is recommended for all cases of acute PID, whether managed as outpatient or inpatient. Antigonorrheal drugs alone do not provide adequate coverage for Chlamydia.
3. Anaerobic PID coverage is especially important for pregnant women, women with IUDs, and for women with severe or recurrent disease.
4. Treatment of Chlamydia trachomatis is essential in teenage women, since younger women are infected more frequently than women over 30 years of age.
5. Twenty to twenty-five per cent of women experience at least one recurrence of PID.[11] Repeated episodes of PID tend to be less often sexually transmitted,[2] and

treatment of recurrent PID should be selected accordingly.

The relationship of specific contraceptive methods and their association with PID deserves mention. Acute PID is very rare in women who are not sexually active. Women who use combined oral contraceptive pills have a lesser risk of developing PID than women who do not use a contraceptive method, and they tend to experience milder degrees of salpingitis than IUD users or women who use no contraception.[12] The IUD is generally considered to constitute a risk factor for the development of PID, particularly during the first few months of use.[2] Most authorities recommend removal of an IUD once PID is diagnosed and after antibiotics are instituted. Barrier contraceptives (diaphragm and condoms), when used with spermicides, afford excellent protection against sexually transmitted diseases (STDs) and PID, and their use probably should be encouraged in all sexually active women, even if another method is currently in use. Women who have had a tubal ligation have a minimal risk of contracting PID.[2]

■ SECONDARY PELVIC INFECTIONS

With the exception of sexually transmitted pathogens, organisms responsible for secondary pelvic infections are quite similar to those involved in primary PID. Bacteria endogenous to the female lower genital tract (see Table 2) may turn pathogenic following alterations of the pelvic anatomy. Examples of common secondary pelvic infections include Group B streptococcus, gram-negative anaerobes in postpartum endometritis, *Bacteroides* and *Enterococcus* in postcesarean endomyometritis, gram-positive streptococci and gram-negative anaerobes with penetrating abdominal trauma, and *Pseudomonas* in gynecologic malignancy.[13,14] *Clostridium* should be suspected in cases of non-sterile pregnancy termination or pelvic trauma. Group B streptococcus and *Listeria monocytogenes* are important obstetric pathogens that can cause serious maternal and neonatal infections. Chlamydial infection late in pregnancy has been associated with premature rupture of membranes, preterm delivery, delayed postpartum endometritis, and neonatal conjunctivitis and pneumonitis.[15]

Over the past decade, prophylactic antibiotics have been increasingly used prior to gynecologic and obstetric surgery to reduce the number of bacteria present at the operative site. Whether to use prophylaxis is perhaps best decided by considering the number of risk factors a patient has for potential infection (prolonged labor or rupture of membranes, presence of local pelvic infection or malignancy, postmenopausal patients undergoing hysterectomy, history of intravenous drug abuse) and the local hospital infection rate.

The recommendation for initial therapy of secondary pelvic infections is similar to that of PID—broad-spectrum anaerobic coverage (active against all *Bacteroides* species) and aerobic gram-positive and gram-negative organisms. First-generation cephalosporins are frequently used as prophylaxis prior to cesarean section but may not adequately cover for anaerobes in active infections. Second- and third-generation cephalosporins or a combination of ticarcillin–clavulanic acid may be effective, especially for *Enterococcus*, in the treatment of postoperative infections.

■ TUBO-OVARIAN ABSCESS

More than 50 per cent of women who develop tubo-ovarian abscesses have a history of pelvic inflammatory disease; in 70 per cent of the cases, the disease is unilateral.[16] Abscess rupture into the peritoneal cavity produces peritonitis, septicemia, and septic shock. Abscesses may be due to puerperal sepsis, an infected spontaneous or elective abortion, or a complication of pelvic surgery, or they may be associated with an IUD. Pathogens are usually endogenous bowel or vaginal flora secondarily invading pelvic tissues damaged by venereal disease, surgery, or delivery; anaerobes and gram-negative enteric bacilli are the most common pathogens.

Patients with tubo-ovarian abscesses are quite ill, with localized or diffuse abdominopelvic tenderness and an adnexal mass on pelvic examination. Sonography helps distinguish an inflammatory complex from other conditions (appendicitis, ectopic pregnancy, torsion of an ovarian cyst, septic abortion).

Initial management or unruptured tubo-ovarian abscesses remains controversial. Whereas some advocate immediate surgery, conservative therapy with broad-spectrum antibiotics is generally tried first. Commonly used parenteral regimens include (1) ampicillin or a first-generation cephalosporin in combination with an aminoglycoside and clindamycin, (2) ampicillin or a first-generation cephalosporin and metronidazol (Flagyl), with or without an aminoglycoside, (3) clindamycin and an aminoglycoside, or (4) cefoxitin and doxycycline.[16] If the patient fails to improve over the next 48 to 72 hours, or if intraperitoneal rupture is suspected, surgical intervention is indicated. Most surgeons currently prefer a conservative approach, utilizing unilateral adnexectomy rather than panhysterectomy, to preserve future fertility.

▪ Issues and Risks

▪ SIDE EFFECTS OF THERAPY

The three side effects most commonly associated with antibiotic therapy of PID are (1) nephrotoxicity, (2) bleeding abnormalities, and (3) diarrhea and pseudomembranous enterocolitis.[6]

Nephrotoxicity is most often an effect of aminoglycosides; however, abnormally high levels of any antibiotic can affect renal function and cause glomerular damage. Aminoglycoside levels should be monitored throughout therapy. Another factor contributing to renal dysfunction is retroperitoneal inflammation following the acute peritonitis caused by PID. The inflammatory reaction can result in functional obstruction of the ureters, which can increase susceptibility to antibiotic toxicity.

Another complication of antibiotic therapy is bleeding abnormalities. Two nonimmune mechanisms have been implicated: (1) cephalosporins that contain the N-methyl-thiotetrazole side chain are associated with an inhibition of vitamin K–dependent carboxylation and hypoprothrombinemia, and (2) alteration of binding proteins on the platelet surface leads to subsequent platelet dysfunction. Generally, the propensity for bleeding is not clinically significant but is enhanced by the use of other medications that interfere with clotting (such as nonsteroidal anti-inflammatory drugs), with impaired renal function, and with antibiotic administration to surgical patients. Other potential side effects of antibiotic administration are diarrhea and pseudomembra-

nous colitis. Oral ingestion or biliary excretion of an antibiotic alters normal gut flora and results in diarrhea, usually responsive to discontinuation of the antibiotic. This inconvenience may increase the expense of hydration, necessitate a change to another antibiotic, or delay discharge from the hospital, but it is seldom serious.

Pseudomembranous enterocolitis, on the other hand, may have more dramatic effects. It results from the antibiotic-induced overgrowth of *Clostridium difficile* in patients who harbor the organism asymptomatically. The enterotoxin-related diarrhea has been associated with all classes of antibiotics except the aminoglycosides. Selected overgrowth of *Clostridium difficile* is most often associated with drugs such as cefoxitin, which has a high biliary excretion rate and little gram-positive activity. Pseudomembranous colitis is treated with oral vancomycin or metronidazole.

To avoid diarrhea and *Clostridium difficile* overgrowth, the physician should select an antibiotic for PID treatment that has a broad spectrum but a low biliary excretion rate, thereby reducing the potential for accumulation of the antibiotic in the gastrointestinal tract. Antimicrobial resistance rates also must be considered in initial selection. Some new cephalosporins, though designed to resist enzyme degradation, have been recognized to induce beta-lactamase production.

▪ COSTS

As previously mentioned, STD and PID have a significant economic impact in the United States, annually costing more than $1 billion each. Hospitalization, antibiotics, nursing time, admixture fees, delivery systems (IV bags and tubing), monitoring of drug levels and resistance, and treatment of side effects contribute more than 80 per cent of the direct cost of management of PID, which results in 675 deaths per year. Ectopic pregnancy associated with PID results in an average of 24 deaths per year and accounts for 9 per cent of the direct costs. Fifty per cent of the morbidity and mortality associated with ectopic pregnancy is caused by PID.[1] Seventeen to twenty per cent of women with PID become infertile,[1,2] and the cost of infertility consultation and management accounts for 4.1 per cent of the direct costs.[1]

Indirect costs include lost workdays and wages, loss of household management for employed and unemployed women, and loss of lifetime earnings in the event of death. Annual indirect costs in the United States are currently estimated at over $1 billion.

■ PREVENTION

Primary prevention of PID includes counseling women about limiting the number of sexual contacts and choosing an appropriate contraceptive method. Barrier methods, including the diaphragm, enhance prevention when used with a spermicide. Oral contraceptive pills may discourage the development of PID, but not of vaginitis or cervicitis. IUDs may encourage development of PID secondary to STD and should be avoided in nulliparous patients for whom fertility is important. Treatment of patients to prevent PID and infertility and treatment of contacts of patients with known disease constitute secondary prevention. As with any STD, medical screening, treatment, and contact tracing should be carried out for the patient and partner with whom there has been sexual contact within the preceding 90 days.[6]

With either gonococcal or chlamydial infection, there is a 10 to 20 per cent risk of developing PID. Male partners of gonococcal PID patients are infected 40 to 50 per cent of the time; partners of nongonococcal PID patients are infected 15 per cent of the time. Many of these are asymptomatic and will reinfect their partner or infect new contacts if not screened. Therefore, all contacts of PID patients should be identified and screened for gonorrhea and chlamydia infection.[17] A priority situation for screening exists when PID is a result of a new PPNG infection in a previously uninfected community. Tertiary prevention (or preventing further sequelae in the patient with PID) involves testing for beta-lactamase production and sensitivity and using an anti-PPNG drug if patients are in an endemic area.[10]

■ PATIENT EDUCATION AND FOLLOW-UP

Each patient should be educated about the primary preventive measures mentioned

and should be cautioned to avoid sexual contact until noninfectious and asymptomatic. At the completion of treatment, a patient should have a test of cure. If the causative organism is a PPNG, reculture is recommended in 1 to 2 months.[10]

REFERENCES

1. Washington AE, Arno PS, Brooks MA. The economic cost of pelvic inflammatory disease. JAMA 1986; 255:1735–1738.
2. Westrom L. Pelvic inflammatory disease: bacteriology and sequelae. Contraception 1987; 36:111–128.
3. King LA. Pelvic inflammatory disease—its pathogenesis, diagnosis, and treatment. Postgrad Med 1987; 81:105–114.
4. Grimes DA, Blount JH, Patrick J, Washington AE. Antibiotic treatment of pelvic inflammatory disease—trends among private physicians in the United States, 1966 through 1983. JAMA 1986; 256:3223–3226.
5. Centers for Disease Control. 1985 STD Treatment Guidelines. Atlanta: US Department of Health and Human Services, reprinted Sept 1986.
6. Mercer LJ. Pelvic inflammatory disease—decision making in the pharmacy and therapeutics committee. J Reprod Med 1988; 33 (Suppl):135–141.
7. Dodson MG, Faro S, Gentry LO. Treatment of acute pelvic inflammatory disease with aztreonam, a new monocyclic β-lactam antibiotic, and clindamycin. Obstet Gynecol 1986; 67:657–662.
8. Hemsell DL. Acute pelvic inflammatory disease; etiologic and therapeutic considerations. J Reprod Med 1988; 33(Suppl):119–123.
9. Venezio FR, O'Keefe JP. Microbiologic considerations in the treatment of serious pelvic infections in women. J Reprod Med 1988; 33(Suppl):124–127.
10. Centers for Disease Control. Antibiotic-resistant strains of *Neisseria gonorrhoeae*; policy guidelines for detection, management and control. MMWR 1986; 36:15–145.
11. Bronham JC. Therapy for acute pelvic inflammatory disease: a critique of recent treatment trials. Am J Obstet Gynecol 1984; 148:235–240.
12. Rubin GL, Ory HW, Layde PM. Oral contraceptives and pelvic inflammatory disease. Am J Obstet Gynecol 1982; 144:630–638.
13. Herbst AL, Mercer LJ. Overview of therapeutic and prophylactic antibiotics in obstetrics and gynecology. J Reprod Med 1988; 33(Suppl):144–148.
14. Levine DP, Wilson RF. Treatment of penetrating abdominal trauma and gynecologic infections. J Reprod Med 1988; 33(Suppl):598–602.
15. Sweet RL, Landers DV, Walker C. *Chlamydia trachomatis* infection and pregnancy outcome. Am J Obstet Gynecol 1987; 156:824–833.
16. Lichtinger M. Emergency treatment of adnexal masses in a nonpregnant woman. Emerg Clin North Am 1987; 5:569–576.
17. McGregor JA, French JI, Spencer NE. Prevention of sexually transmitted diseases in women. J Reprod Med 1988; 33(Suppl):109–118.

Peptic ulcer disease in elderly patients

Alex H. Bruckstein

■ Background

■ CLINICAL FEATURES

Although the pathology of peptic ulcer disease in the elderly is similar to that in younger patients, the clinical features may vary considerably (Table 1) and confuse the physician. Many patients have classic postprandial epigastric discomfort relieved by food or antacids, but pain is less frequently the initial presentation in elderly patients. Melena is a relatively common presentation.[1] Some patients may present with mild abdominal discomfort, weight loss, anorexia, or vomiting, while in others the initial presentation is rather acute, when the ulcer perforates or bleeds. "Geriatric" ulcers (high in the cardia) cause misleading symptoms, such as substernal pain mimicking angina or dysphagia, suggestive of esophageal neoplasia. Chronic blood loss may lead to cerebral or cardiac symptoms that confuse the physician. Finally, with a giant duodenal or gastric ulcer, a patient may have weight loss and "failing health" that initially suggest neoplasia. The symptoms and signs of any complication of the disease may be masked, especially the peritoneal signs of perforation.

The incidence of elective peptic ulcer surgery is declining and the incidence of emergency operations remains the same, yet an age-adjusted analysis reveals that the incidence of both types of surgery are rising in elderly patients.[2] Even though the mortality rates of peptic ulcer disease show a consistent decrease in many countries, in patients over 60 years of age, especially women, a rising mortality rate is clear. In addition, the mortality rates are much higher in elderly than in young people, perhaps because of the occurrence of complications combined with the high mortality of abdominal sur-

gery in this age group. Also, many elderly patients are being treated with corticosteroids, anticoagulants, and nonsteroidal anti-inflammatory drugs (NSAIDs), which may increase the frequency and severity of ulcers in this age group. An additional factor is that gastric ulcers tend to heal more slowly than duodenal ulcers and to produce more complications in elderly patients.[3]

■ DIAGNOSIS

Elderly patients with suspected peptic ulcer disease should be evaluated if symptoms persist. The clinical features do not distinguish gastric from duodenal ulcer disease with certainty (Table 2) and present difficulty in distinguishing benign from malignant disease. Almost all elderly patients with peptic ulcer disease should undergo endoscopy, a safe procedure that is perhaps even easier than a barium study for elderly patients who may find it difficult to move around. In most cases, biopsy with histologic confirmation of the lesion is essential to exclude malignancy; endoscopy is thus the investigation of choice. Differentiating benign from malignant lesions is especially important in elderly patients because of the high incidence of gastrointestinal malignancy.[4]

■ Management

■ PHARMACOKINETICS

Aging does not alter the amount or rate of drug absorbed from the gastrointestinal tract,[5] but transit time in elderly ill patients is prolonged, which may result in increased absorption of medications. Once the medication is absorbed, two aspects of aging af-

TABLE 1. Common Features of Peptic Ulcer Disease in Elderly Patients

Heartburn	May be confused with cardiovascular disease or hiatus hernia with reflux
Anemia	May result from chronic blood loss. The patient occasionally may present with an acute gastrointestinal hemorrhage in the absence of a clear history of dyspepsia
Epigastric pain	Poor localization of pain common; pain may not be related to food
Nausea and vomiting	
Loss of appetite and weight	Symptoms are often confused with the diagnosis of neoplasm
Flatulence	
Regurgitation in mouth	A clear, tasteless fluid
Dysphagia	Results from an ulcer high in the cardia

fect the distribution of the absorbed drug: (1) a relative decrease in lean body mass, and (2) a relative increase in body fat. The decrease in lean body mass reduces the serum creatinine level, with the result that renal function appears better than it really is. The relative increase in body fat raises the steady-state level of drug after multiple doses, because lipid-soluble drugs may remain in the body longer before elimination.

Elderly patients may be at increased risk from relative overdosage of medication due to inefficient mechanisms for drug metabolism and elimination. Changes in the rate of drug elimination are most relevant for those

TABLE 2. Clinical Factors Differentiating Duodenal from Gastric Ulcer in Elderly Patients

	Duodenal Ulcer	Gastric Ulcer
Incidence	Decreases with age	Increases with age
Epigastric pain	Food relieves pain; maximal pain is 2–3 hr postprandial	Pain appears 1 hr post-prandial and lasts 2 hr
Weight	Stable	Weight loss
Eating habits	Frequent meals common in an attempt to relieve pain	Pain interferes with meals, so patient eats less

medications with a narrow therapeutic index, and defective elimination increases the tissue concentration and pharmacologic response of any given dose. This is a major cause of increased adverse drug reactions in the elderly. Hepatic drug metabolism changes with aging, and the response to the induction of microsomal enzymes declines with age.[6] Impaired renal elimination in elderly patients usually is a result of a reduction in glomerular filtration rate and tubular secretion of drugs, despite the lack of evidence of impaired renal function. Serum urea and creatinine values can be misleading because of the decrease in lean body mass; creatinine clearance is a better indicator of renal function.

■ DRUG THERAPY
(Table 3)

The trials for therapy of ulcer disease are usually conducted in younger patients. Although gastric secretion is reduced with age,[7] there is no evidence of any alteration in the relative efficacy of an agent, nor that reduced dosages of antisecretory agents are indicated in the elderly population. Relapses may be more common in elderly patients.[8] Thus, prolonged maintenance therapy is often indicated, together with early consideration of surgery in the patient who has a complication.

TABLE 3. Drug Therapy for Peptic Ulcers

Mechanism: Decrease Aggressive Forces

Antacids
  Many

H₂-receptor antagonists
  Cimetidine
  Ranitidine
  Famotidine
  Nizatidine

Prostaglandins*
  Misoprostol
  Enprostil

Antimuscarinics
  Telenzipine*
  Pirenzepine*

Proton-pump inhibitors
  Omeprazole*

Mechanism: Enhance Mucosal Defense

Sucralfate

Prostaglandins*

Colloidal bismuth subcitrate*

*Not currently available in the United States.

Recently, H_2-receptor antagonists have been widely used in the treatment and prevention of both gastric and duodenal ulcers. Although elderly patients have a higher incidence of frank achlorhydria, in clinical practice the gastric pH is not determined prior to initiation of therapy. A major advantage of these medications over antacid therapy is that compliance is somewhat better.

Compliance is affected by polypharmacy and by impairment of vision and memory. At a given level of noncompliance, elderly patients are at a greater risk of adverse drug reaction and therapeutic failure than are younger patients. Thus, the number of drugs prescribed should be limited, because the more drugs given, the greater the chance of a drug reaction or interaction, and the more likely it is that the patient will take the wrong medicine at the wrong time. To improve compliance, there must be an improved doctor-patient communication, recognition of the domestic situation, and easier access to medicines. Child-proof bottle tops and calendar bubble packs are difficult for the elderly patient to handle, which may reduce compliance.

Antacids

Care must be used when prescribing high-dose antacid therapy because of its potential complications. Magnesium-containing antacids have a cathartic effect, whereas the aluminum-containing antacids are constipating. Aluminum binds phosphate, which may result in hypophosphatemia. All antacids may lead to metabolic alkalosis, which may be a problem in an elderly patient with impaired renal function. Antacids may alter the rate of absorption, bioavailability, and renal excretion of many of the medications that elderly patients are taking. In the elderly patient who must take other medications in addition to antacids, they should be given one-half to one hour before or after the antacid medication, to avoid alteration in gastric absorption. All these factors argue against the long-term administration of antacids in elderly patients.

Anticholinergics

Anticholinergic therapy was once the therapy of choice for peptic ulcer disease, but it has lost favor because of the numerous side effects (e.g., gastric stasis, intestinal atony, obstructive uropathy, and acute glaucoma). The widespread distribution of muscarinic receptors has meant that the therapeutic effect of modulating the parietal cell is reduced by the additional effects of the drug on muscarinic receptors in other tissues. However, the recent discovery of subtypes of muscarinic receptors, M-1, has led to the development of drugs with selective actions, examples of which are telenzipine and pirenzepine. Pirenzepine has a selective action on M-1 receptors governing gastric acid and pepsinogen secretion. Thus, at levels sufficient to inhibit gastric acid and pepsinogen secretion, these drugs do not cause tachycardia, mydriasis, or impairment of gastric emptying. Pirenzepine has the additional advantage of being hydrophilic, thus not readily crossing the blood-brain barrier, avoiding central side effects. Despite this selectivity, dry mouth and blurred vision are commonly reported adverse effects.[9] Although glaucoma and prostatism—common diseases in the elderly—do not seem to be affected by pirenzepine, they are still considered a contraindication to its use.

Cimetidine

Although numerous side effects, such as diarrhea, skin rash, and pruritus, have been reported with this drug, considering the large number of patients treated worldwide for many years the incidence of side effects is quite rare.[10] Drug interactions may occur with cimetidine because of its inhibition of the cytochrome P-450 mixed-function enzyme system. Whether these interactions are clinically significant depends upon how narrow is the therapeutic range of the drug in question. Thus, adverse interactions are clinically significant in the patient who might be taking theophylline, warfarin, or phenytoin. If a patient has been on one of these medications, the addition of cimetidine may increase plasma levels of the drug, with resultant toxicity, but cimetidine may be safely administered if the dose of the index drug is reduced and plasma levels monitored.

Compared with the original dosing schedule of 300 mg four times daily, the nocturnal administration of cimetidine, 800 mg, may reduce adverse drug interactions.[11] In elderly patients with impaired renal function, a variety of neuropsychiatric effects have been reported, the most common of which is delirium in those in intensive care units. This may be a result of either a high plasma or a high cerebrospinal fluid level.

Ranitidine

Although ranitidine binds liver microsomal enzymes and the cytochrome P-450 enzyme system, the drug has only about one tenth of the binding affinity of cimetidine. Thus, the drug interactions demonstrated with cimetidine are seen much less commonly with ranitidine. The antiandrogenic effects that have been reported with cimetidine in patients who have taken it for a long period of time are not seen with ranitidine. In elderly ill patients, confusion has been associated with use of ranitidine.[12]

Famotidine

This new, highly specific, and potent H_2-receptor antagonist contains a thiazole ring structure, thus differing chemically from cimetidine and ranitidine. Pharmacologically, famotidine is 9 times more potent than ranitidine and 32 times more potent than cimetidine. It appears to be safe for elderly patients at therapeutic doses, has not yet been reported to cause antiandrogenic side effects, and is not yet known to interfere with hepatic oxidative metabolism. Further clinical experience will define famotidine's place in the clinical armamentarium against peptic ulcer disease in elderly patients.[13]

Nizatidine

Nizatidine is the newest of the H_2-antagonists that have been recently approved by the FDA. It is a structural analog of the other H_2-antagonists, consisting of the thiazole ring of famotidine and the ring side chains of ranitidine. Like the other H_2-antagonists, it is effective in a once-daily nocturnal dose. However, nizatidine may have an advantage over other drugs because of its bioavailability, resulting in more stable serum levels. Whether this is clinically significant in elderly patients remains to be proved.[14]

Sucralfate

The mechanisms by which sucralfate promotes ulcer healing is not completely understood. It appears to bind to proteins in the base of an ulcer, an effect that presumably protects the ulcer bed from acid-pepsin digestion. Sucralfate binds pepsin and bile acids and has been found to increase endogenous mucosal prostaglandin synthesis as well as to increase mucosal secretion of mucus and bicarbonate. The incidence of side effects is very low, with constipation being the most common. Because sucralfate has no effect on gastric acidity and because the drug is absorbed only minimally, interactions with other drugs are very rare. The major drawback to sucralfate therapy is that it is not yet available as a once daily dose.

Prostaglandin Analogs

The prostaglandins mediate a number of functions that are considered cytoprotective. These functions include maintenance of the gastric mucosal barrier, which is accomplished by synthesis of mucus and by stabilization of lysosomal enzymes so that mucus breakdown occurs less readily. Additionally, prostaglandins enhance gastric bicarbonate secretion and act to improve blood flow to the gastric mucosa, thus allowing for improved delivery of nutrients and tissue repair. Recent data suggest that surfactant activity is modulated by prostaglandins in the gastrointestinal tract in the same manner as in the lung, and that these surfactants may protect gastric mucosa. Prostaglandins seem to have a positive effect on the sodium-potassium-ATPase pump, a property that may trigger cellular processes that further improve mucosal resistance. Finally, prostaglandins increase the number of sulfhydryl molecules that act to protect against oxidative metabolism.

The major disadvantage of prostaglandin administration is that diarrhea and abdominal cramps can occur in about 20 per cent of patients. Of the clinically available prostaglandins, misoprostol and enprostil, there appears to be no significant advantage over currently available agents. Truly cytoprotective low-dose regimens of the prostaglandin analogs are inferior to currently available agents.[15]

Bismuth

Recent evidence suggests that factors other than acid play important roles in the genesis of acid-peptic diseases. Among these factors may be the presence of an infectious agent,

Helicobacter pylori. Much evidence suggests that *H. pylori* has a role in the development of gastritis, but its role in the pathogenesis of peptic ulcer remains less clear. Colloidal bismuth is undergoing a resurgence of interest because of its activity against this organism. Adverse effects are minimal, but compliance is limited by the blackening of the stool, darkening of the tongue, and the ammoniacal taste. Since absorbed bismuth is excreted by the kidneys, poor renal function in elderly patients may cause concern about toxicity with prolonged therapy.[16]

■ COST CONSIDERATIONS

There is not a significant cost difference among cimetidine, ranitidine, and sucralfate when recommended in usual doses.

■ Ulcer Healing

Differences between the pathophysiology of gastric and duodenal ulcer disease lead to different responses to ulcer therapy. In duodenal ulcer, healing rates for antisecretory agents depend on the degree of acid suppression. In contrast, in gastric ulcer patients the healing rate appears to depend more on the duration of treatment in elderly patients. A study of ulcers related to NSAIDs, which many elderly patients take, showed no apparent difference in healing achieved with the H_2-antagonist ranitidine, compared with the cytoprotective agent sucralfate.[17]

Because of drug interactions and toxicity in elderly patients, certain drugs should be excluded, even before considering their efficacy, especially when prolonged therapy is indicated. Thus, <u>ranitidine, famotidine, sucralfate, and bismuth appear to be among the first choices for ulcer therapy in the elderly.</u> Sucralfate's inconvenient dosing regimen, the side effect of constipation, and the occasional concern of aluminum toxicity make it less favored. Bismuth's drawback is its unpleasant taste and its four-times-daily regimen. Despite the fact that bismuth has healing rates comparable to those of H_2-receptor antagonists in the short-term, and despite its apparent advantage for the treatment of *H. pylori,* the question of possible toxicity with prolonged use remains. The H_2-receptor antagonists are equally effective in ulcer healing and appear to be equally safe, with the added advantage of being effective in a single nocturnal dose. The possibility of drug interactions, which were more likely with cimetidine, has been reduced with the nocturnal drug administration, provided that potentially interacting drugs are not given at the same time.

■ Summary and Conclusions

Therapy of peptic ulcer disease in elderly people has special problems. The efficacy and safety of the FDA-approved drugs are comparable. This allows for the personal preferences of patients and physicians. The nocturnal dosing regimen of the H_2-blockers is convenient, safe, and effective in the therapy of elderly patients. The clinician must be aware of the possibilities of adverse drug reactions or side effects in elderly patients because of prolonged therapy, polypharmacy, and altered pharmacokinetics. The simplest and most effective regimen should be chosen.

REFERENCES

1. Permutt RP, Cello JP. Duodenal ulcer disease in the hospitalized elderly patient. Dig Dis Sci 1982; 27:1–6.
2. Gustavsson S, Kelly KA, Melton LJ III, Zinsmeister AR. Trends in peptic ulcer surgery: a population-based study in Rochester, Minnesota, 1956–1985. Gastroenterology 1988; 94:688–694.
3. Somerville KW, Faulkner G, Langman MJS. Nonsteroidal anti-inflammatory drugs and bleeding peptic ulcer. Lancet 1986; 1:462–464.
4. Eshchar J, Pavlotzky MM, Cohen L, Tabac C. Gastrointestinal endoscopy in octogenarians. J Clin Gastroenterol 1986; 8:520–524.
5. Castelen CM, Volans CN, Raymond K. The effect of ageing on drug absorption from the gut. Age Ageing 1977; 6:138–143.
6. Salem SAM, Rajjayabun P, Shepherd AMM, Stevenson IH. Reduced induction of drug metabolism in the elderly. Age Ageing 1980; 7:68–73.
7. Kekki M, Samloff IM, Ihamaki T, Varis K, Sivrala M. Age- and sex-related behaviour of gastric acid secretion at the population level. Scand J Gastroenterol 1982; 17:737–743.
8. Van Deventer GM. Approaches to the long-term treatment of duodenal ulcer disease. Am J Med 1984; 77(Suppl 5B):15–22.
9. Giorgi-Conciato M, Daniotti S, Ferrari PA, et al. Efficacy and safety of pirenzepine in peptic ulcer and nonulcerous gastroduodenal diseases. Scand J Gastroenterol 1982; Suppl 81:1–41.

10. Colin Jones DG, Langman MJS, Lawson DH, Vessey MP. Post-marketing surveillance of the safety of cimetidine: twelve-month morbidity report. Q J Med 1985; 215:253–268.
11. Seaman JJ, Randolph WC, Peace KE, et al. Effects of two cimetidine dosage regimens on serum theophylline levels. Comparison of 800 mg hs and 300 mg qid. Postgrad Med 1985; 78(Nov Suppl):47–53.
12. Silverstone PH. Ranitidine and confusion. Lancet 1984; 1:1071.
13. Friedman G. GI Drug Column: Famotidine. Am J Gastroenterol 1987; 82:504–506.
14. Callaghan JT, Bergstrom RF, Rubin A, et al. A pharmacokinetic profile of nizatidine in man. Scand J Gastroenterol 1987; 22(Suppl 136):9–17.
15. Thomson AB. Treatment of duodenal ulcer with enprostil, a synthetic prostaglandin E_2 analogue. Am J Med 1986; 81(2A):59–63.
16. Coghlan JG, Gilligan D, Humphries H, et al. *Campylobacter pylori* and recurrence of duodenal ulcers: a 12-month follow-up study. Lancet 1987; 2:1109–1111.
17. Malchow-Moller A. Treatment of peptic ulcer disease induced by non-steroidal anti-inflammatory drugs. Scand J Gastroenterol 1987; 22(Suppl 127):87–91.

Peripheral neuropathy

Raymond A. Martin

Peripheral neuropathy (PN) is a disorder of peripheral nerves that has many causes. In most clinical settings, a cause can be determined approximately 50 per cent of the time on initial evaluation. Diagnostic accuracy may be as high as three fourths of patients in selected series at specially equipped centers.[1] In the absence of an initial diagnosis, longitudinal follow-up and later repetition of diagnostic studies may reveal a cause. Treatment of PN will be directed at the etiology, when known, or the symptoms, or both. Inability to cure or control rigidly the underlying disease process in many cases makes management of PN a challenging therapeutic endeavor.

■ Background

Symmetric distal involvement of sensory and motor nerves is the usual pattern in PN. This may be due to involvement of the myelin sheath and Schwann cells or of the axon itself. Clinical symptoms include proprioceptive loss, paresthesias, and numbness and weakness from involvement of large myelinated fibers. Pain, temperature loss, dysesthesias, and hyperpathia are seen when small unmyelinated fibers are affected. Axonal neuropathies are usually associated with sensory loss and weakness. The onset of these disorders may be acute, subacute, or chronic, usually depending on the underlying etiology.

Autonomic neuropathies affect bladder and anal sphincter control, sweating, pupillary responses, gastrointestinal motility, blood pressure, heart rate, and sexual function. Symptoms include orthostatism, impotence, delayed gastric emptying, and bladder and bowel incontinence.

Variations include neuropathies that are predominantly sensory, motor, autonomic, or mixed types with involvement of more than one subpopulation of nerve fibers. Mononeuropathies may occur singly or as multiple mononeuropathies, usually caused by pressure on nerves rendered more susceptible because of an underlying disease process. Mononeuritis multiplex implies multiple nerve involvement, often secondary to nerve infarction owing to disease of the vasa vasorum. Cranial nerves and spinal roots also may be involved, depending on the underlying disease process.

Etiologies of PN include diseases that are genetic, toxic, metabolic, inflammatory, infectious, postinfectious or immune, neoplastic, or due to dietary deficiencies. Many are idiopathic. Distinguishing among them often requires specialty training, application of nerve conduction and electromyographic

TABLE 1. Treatment of Hereditary Peripheral Neuropathy

Disease	Inheritance	Treatment
Hereditary sensory motor neuropathy (Charcot-Marie-Tooth; Déjérine-Sottas)	Autosomal dominant; occasionally recessive	Symptomatic
Refsum disease	Autosomal recessive	Plasmapheresis; restrict dietary phytol intake
Porphyria (acute intermittent, variegate, hereditary coproporphyria)	Autosomal dominant	Symptomatic; avoid triggering drugs, especially barbiturates

studies, and sometimes a peripheral nerve biopsy. For further discussion of this aspect, the interested reader is referred to the text by Dyck and associates.[2]

■ Management

The goal of therapy is treatment of the underlying disease process when known and alleviating the symptoms of neuropathy when possible. Often, treatment of disease only slows the progress of PN since disease cure is not possible, e.g., in diabetes mellitus. Commonly encountered peripheral neuropathies are listed in Tables 1 and 2, including specific therapies, if known.

Before discussing the symptomatic treatment of PN, some emphasis will be given to the latest recommendations for the treatment of Guillain-Barré syndrome and diabetic neuropathy.

Guillain-Barré Syndrome (GBS). Plasma-

TABLE 2. Treatment of Acquired Neuropathies

Disease	Etiology	Treatment
Diabetes mellitus	? abnormal polyol myoinositol metabolism; ? hypoxia	? aldose reductase inhibitors; strict diabetic control
Guillain-Barré syndrome	? autoimmune disease	Plasmapheresis
Uremia	Uremic toxin(s)	Dialysis; renal transplant
Myxedema	Thyroid hormone deficiency	Hormone replacement
Hepatic (cirrhosis)	Thiamine deficiency	Thiamine
Collagen vascular disease	Nerve infarction; nerve entrapment	Steroids, immunosuppressive drugs, plasmapheresis, surgical decompression
Infection		
Leprosy	*Mycobacterium leprae*	Dapsone, clofazimine, rifampin
Diphtheria	Neurotoxin	Antibiotics, specific antitoxin within 48 hr of infection
Herpes zoster	Direct viral invasion	Acyclovir
AIDS	Unknown	3'-Azido-2',3'-dideoxythymidine (AZT)
Sarcoid	Granuloma	Steroids
Deficiency states	Starvation; malabsorption	Beriberi (thiamine); pellagra (thiamine, B vitamins); B_{12} deficiency (Vitamin B_{12}); malabsorption (multiple vitamins, B complex, E, folate)
Toxins	Heavy metals	? chelation
	Drugs	Avoidance
	Solvents	Avoidance
Malignancy	Remote effect, circulating autoantibodies	Treatment of cancer; plasmapheresis in selected types

pheresis is now considered to be the only specific treatment for this syndrome. Steroids have no beneficial effects and may possibly be deleterious. If clinical criteria are met,[3] consideration is given to treating progressing patients in the first 2 to 3 weeks of illness. If patients approach inability to walk unassisted, develop bulbar weakness, or have significantly reduced respiratory capacity, plasmapheresis is started. Treatment aims at a total exchange of 200 to 250 ml of plasma per kg of body weight in 7 to 14 days. Three to five exchanges of 40 to 50 ml/kg are usually performed no oftener than every other day.[4] Exchange with albumin or artificial replacement fluids is recommended over fresh-frozen plasma to eliminate risk of infection with the hepatitis or AIDS viruses. Because of potential complications from plasmapheresis treatment, it should be performed in the ICU by physicians and personnel experienced in its use. With good supportive care and plasmapheresis, the clinical outcome can be improved, and the length and expense of illness can be reduced considerably.

Diabetic Peripheral Neuropathy (DPN). Hyperglycemia is currently believed to damage peripheral nerves through increased sorbitol levels, endoneurial hypoxia, and nonenzymatic glycolization of nerve proteins.[5] Although research studies are focusing on treatment with aldose reductase inhibitors (alrestatin, sorbinil, and tolrestat) and dietary myoinositol supplementation, lowering and normalizing blood glucose levels is considered to be the mainstay of treatment.[6] If rapid normalization leads to acute painful peripheral neuropathy, slower normalization in those patients is recommended. Pain in established DPN may improve with normoglycemia, since hyperglycemia enhances pain sensitivity, possibly through modulation of opioid receptors.[7] Until these experimental drugs and treatment regimens become available, maintenance of normoglycemia plus symptomatic treatment is the preferred approach.

■ **SYMPTOMATIC TREATMENT**

Chronic pain is often the most disabling symptom of sensory peripheral neuropathies. The pain may be lancinating in type or persistent with a burning dysesthetic quality. Lancinating pain often responds to anticonvulsant medications.[8] Therapy can

be initiated with carbamazepine (Tegretol), starting at an initial dose of 100 mg TID and increasing by 200 mg per week until a therapeutic blood level (8 to 12 μg/ml) or pain relief is obtained. Phenytoin (Dilantin) also may be effective and can be given in a once-daily dose of 300 mg to achieve a blood level of 10 to 20 μg/ml. A therapeutic trial of at least 1 month should be undertaken unless side effects or toxic manifestations occur. These may include allergic reactions, bone marrow suppression, hepatic dysfunction, and sedation. If the patient remains symptom-free for 3 months, an attempt to taper these medications may be undertaken.

Phenytoin should be used with caution in DPN, since high doses inhibit insulin secretion. Lancinating pains also may respond to treatment with baclofen (Lioresal), valproate (Depakote), and clonazepam (Klonopin).[8]

Persistent dysesthetic pain, especially if accompanied by depression and vegetative symptoms, may improve with tricyclic antidepressants (TCA), which enhance suppression of afferent pain impulses at the spinal cord entry level.[9] Amitriptyline (Amitril, Elavil, Endep), in doses of up to 150 mg/day,[10] and imipramine (Janimine, SK-Pramine, Tofranil), up to 100 mg/day,[11] have been beneficial in DPN. These drugs should be avoided when there is associated narrow angle glaucoma, cardiac arrhythmia, or symptomatic prostatic hypertrophy; they should be used judiciously in elderly patients or in patients with severe autonomic peripheral neuropathy (APN). Doses should begin at 10 to 25 mg in one nighttime dose and be increased slowly every 1 to 2 weeks until maximal dosage, side effects, or satisfactory results are obtained. They can be tried in PN of other etiologies if contraindications do not exist.

In more refractory cases, a short course of a TCA, such as amitriptyline or nortriptyline, combined with fluphenazine (Prolixin), can be tried. An effective combination is nortriptyline, 10 to 20 mg TID, and fluphenazine, 0.5 to 1 mg TID.[12] The same dose of fluphenazine can be used with one established daily dose of amitriptyline, as previously described. Short courses (3 to 6 months) of fluphenazine will lessen the incidence of tardive dyskinesia.

Susceptibility to peripheral nerve trauma in patients with PN may lead to painful deafferentation syndromes, such as causalgia and reflex sympathetic dystrophy (RSD). (Also see article on Reflex Sympathetic Dystrophy Syndromes.) These may improve with sympatholytic drugs such as oral phenoxybenzamine (Dibenzyline), 10 mg BID, and titrating upward to 20 to 40 mg BID or TID. The medication works by blocking alpha-adrenergic receptors and leaves beta-adrenergic receptors unopposed. Postural hypotension and tachycardia are limiting factors, and this drug should not be used in patients with APN. Oral nifedipine (Procardia), 10 to 30 mg TID, was reported to be beneficial in one recent study of pain treatment in RSD.[13] Hypotension may be a limiting factor.

Autonomic peripheral neuropathy is seen most frequently in diabetes, Guillain-Barré syndrome, and amyloidosis but may also occur in the PN of alcoholism, uremia, porphyria, and subacute combined degeneration due to vitamin B_{12} deficiency. Judicious use of pharmacotherapeutic agents is recommended, and avoidance is advocated when side effects are a risk to the patient.[14]

Orthostatism is a frequent and disabling symptom. Before medications are prescribed, practical therapeutic measures should include adequate hydration and avoidance of volume-depleting or hypotension-inducing drugs when possible. Elevation of the head of the patient's bed at night has been shown to lessen posture-induced salt and water loss.[15] Form-fitted elastic stockings and adequate salt ingestion are also beneficial. Initial drug therapy includes fludrocortisone (Florinef), 0.1 mg QD to QID, which enhances salt retention and arterial constriction.[16] If fludrocortisone is ineffective the sequence of medications shown in Table 3 can be considered.

Newer treatments include subcutaneous dihydroergotamine plus caffeine[20] and di-

Table 3. Medication Sequence for Treatment of Orthostatism

Drug	Dose	Effect
Indomethacin (Indocin, Indomed)	25–50 mg TID	Inhibition of prostaglandin-like substances[17]
Ephedrine	25–50 mg TID	Indirect alpha-agonist
Pindolol (Viskin)	5 mg BID–TID	Beta-blockade with intrinsic sympathomimetic activity[18]
Metoclopramide (Reglan, Octamide)	10 mg BID–QID	Dopamine vasodilation blockade[19]

phenylhydramine (Benadryl), 25 to 50 mg BID, combined with cimetidine (Tagamet), 300 mg BID or TID, which presumably work by combined H_1- and H_2-receptor blockade.[21] A detailed discussion of mechanisms and treatment is discussed by Low.[22]

Another manifestation of APN is cystopathy with insufficient bladder drainage. Frequent bladder emptying by voluntary voiding, Credé's maneuver, and intermittent self-catheterization should be accomplished to lessen the incidence of bladder infection. Bethanechol (Urecholine), 10 to 20 mg TID, may be of benefit. Diarrhea may respond to short-term treatment with tetracycline (Achromycin, Sumycin), 250 to 500 mg, at the onset of symptoms,[23] or to codeine phosphate or diphenoxylate (Lomotil), 2.5 mg TID.

Esophageal dysfunction producing dysphagia may improve with bethanechol. Bloating and abdominal fullness may be due to gastroparesis and delayed gastric emptying. Metoclopramide, 10 mg BID or QID before meals and at bedtime, is beneficial and may reduce concomitant nausea.

Male sexual dysfunction, if organic, responds poorly to drug therapy. A penile prosthesis may be the final resort of treatment.

Finally, motor disability and sensory loss may interfere with ambulation and use of the hands. There is increased susceptibility to poorly healing pressure sores and decubiti. Various orthotic and protective devices may improve considerably the comfort and functioning of patients impaired by PN. When significant impairment exists, referral to a physiatrist for evaluation and treatment is recommended. An adequate exercise program designed within the limits of patient capability is also recommended. Potential nerve compression sites, such as the elbows and knees, should be protected. Avoidance of alcohol consumption and smoking also should be strongly advised.

▪ Issues and Risks

The various diseases that cause PN often are not curable or identifiable, and progression frequently occurs. Periodic re-evaluation of patients is necessary to consider new therapies or to discontinue old ones that may now carry a risk because of disease progression. Polypharmacy is often part of the treatment regimen of patients with significant illness. Careful attention to drug interactions and side effects is of paramount importance to prevent iatrogenic symptoms or complications. The medications outlined here undoubtedly can benefit patients with symptoms of PN, but the best outcome will occur under the direction of the physician keenly aware of their indications, side effects, and interactions with other medications.

REFERENCES

1. Dyck PJ, Oviatt KF, Lambert EH. Intensive evaluation of referred unclassified neuropathies yields improved diagnosis. Ann Neurol 1981; 10:222–226.
2. Dyck PJ, Thomas PK, Lambert EH, Bunge R. Peripheral Neuropathy. 2nd ed. Philadelphia: WB Saunders, 1984.
3. Asbury AK, Arnason BG, Karp HR, McFarlin DE. Criteria for diagnosis of Guillain-Barré syndrome. Ann Neurol 1978; 3:565–566.
4. Guillain-Barré Study Group. Plasmapheresis and acute Guillain-Barré syndrome. Neurology 1985; 35:1096–1104.
5. Dyck PJ, Zimmerman BR, Vilen TH, et al. Nerve glucose, fructose, sorbitol, myo-inositol and fiber degeneration and regeneration in diabetic neuropathy. N Engl J Med 1988; 319:542–548.
6. American Neurological Association, Committee on Health Care Issues. Does improved control of glycemia prevent or ameliorate diabetic neuropathy? Ann Neurol 1986; 19(3):288–290.
7. Morley GK, Mooradian AD, Levine AS, Morley JE. Mechanism of pain in diabetic peripheral neuropathy. Effect of glucose on pain perception in humans. Am J Med 1984; 77:79–82.
8. Swerdlow M. Anticonvulsant drugs and chronic pain. Clin Neuropharmacol 1984; 7:51–82.
9. Basbaum AI, Fields HL. Endogenous pain control systems: brainstem spinal pathways and endorphin circuitry. Ann Rev Neurosci 1984; 7:309–338.
10. Max MB, Culnane M, Schafer SC, et al. Amitriptyline relieves diabetic neuropathy pain in patients with normal or depressed mood. Neurology 1987; 37:589–596.
11. Kvinesdal B, Molin J, Froland A, Gram LF. Imipramine treatment of painful diabetic neuropathy. JAMA 1984; 251:1727–1730.
12. Gomez-Perez FJ, Rull JA, Dies H, Rodriguez-Rivera JG, Gonzalez-Barranco J, Lozand-Castenada O. Nortriptyline and fluphenazine in the symptomatic treatment of diabetic neuropathy. A double blind cross-over study. Pain 1985; 23:395–400.
13. Prough DS, McLeskey CH, Borshy GC, et al. Efficacy of oral nifedipine in the treatment of reflex sympathetic dystrophy. Anesthesiology 1985; 62:796–799.
14. Portenoy RK. Drug treatment of pain syndromes. Semin Neurol 1987; 7:139–147.
15. Bannister R, Ardill L, Fentem P. An evaluation of different methods of treatment of idiopathic orthostatic hypotension. Q J Med 1969; 38:377–395.
16. Campbell IW, Ewing DJ, Clarke BF. 9-Alpha-fluorohydrocortisone in the treatment of postural hypotension in diabetic autonomic neuropathy. Diabetes 1975; 24:381–384.
17. Sutcliffe RL. Indomethacin treatment of postural hypotension (letter). Br Med J 1980; 280:1229.
18. Boesen F, Anderson EB, Kanstrup IL, et al. Treatment of diabetic orthostatic hypotension with pindolol. Acta Neurol Scand 1982; 66:386–391.
19. Kuchel O, Buu NT, Gutkowska J, Genest J. Treatment of severe orthostatic hypotension by metoclopramide. Ann Intern Med 1980; 93:841–843.
20. Hoeldtke RD, Cavanaugh ST, Hughes JD, Polansky M. Treatment of orthostatic hypotension with dihydroergotamine and caffeine. Ann Intern Med 1986; 105:168–173.
21. Stacpoole PW, Robertson D. Combination H_1 and H_2 receptor antagonist therapy in diabetic autonomic neuropathy. South Med J 1982; 75:634–635.
22. Low PA. Autonomic neuropathy. Semin Neurol 1987; 7:49–57.
23. Malins JM, French JJ. Diabetic diarrhea. Q J Med 1957; 26:467–480.

Pneumonia, nosocomial

Edward Tsou

A lung infection that develops in a hospitalized patient that is neither present nor incubating at the time of admission is a nosocomial pneumonia. A pneumonia acquired during hospitalization but not clinically recognized until after discharge may also be considered nosocomial. Hospital-acquired pneumonias are not usually apparent until at least 72 hours after admission.

Nosocomial infections develop in 5 to 10 per cent of all hospitalized patients. Although involvement of the lower respiratory tract accounts for only 15 per cent of these infections and ranks behind urinary tract (40 per cent) and surgical wound (25 per cent) infections, it is the most common lethal nosocomial infection, accounting for about 60 per cent of deaths causally related to nosocomial infection and 15 per cent of all hospital deaths.[1] About two thirds of deaths from nosocomial infection occur in critical, terminally ill patients.[1,2] In addition, nosocomial pneumonias lengthen hospital stays and increase hospital costs two to three times mean values for other hospital-acquired infections.[2,3] Rates of nosocomial pneumonia are highest in intensive care units, where as many as 15 to 70 per cent of patients may be affected; over half of patients who are mechanically ventilated, are immunocompromised, have significant underlying disease, or are infected with *Pseudomonas* will succumb.[2]

Nosocomial pneumonia is a difficult management problem because (1) it is most common in critically ill patients, who often lack specific signs and symptoms of pneumonia and have underlying lung disease that may mask infection (e.g., pulmonary edema, malignancy), (2) it can be caused by a myriad of organisms, (3) stains and cultures of respiratory secretions, fluids, and blood may not predict etiology or response to therapy reliably, (4) the role of invasive diagnostic procedures is not defined, (5) the physician must select empirically the most appropriate antibiotic among a bewildering array that will kill the probable causative microbes with the least toxicity and the lowest cost, and (6) prevention is the only recognized way to decrease the incidence, morbidity, and mortality of nosocomial pneumonia, but it remains an elusive goal.

■ Background

Nosocomial pneumonia may be acquired by bloodborne infection from intravenous lines, heart valves, veins, and remote sites, such as the urinary and gastrointestinal tracts, and by inhalation of aerosols from a contaminated environment or respiratory therapy equipment, but the majority of cases result from aspiration of oropharyngeal secretions. Aspiration occurs in most normal, healthy persons during sleep[4] but does not result in lower respiratory tract infection because of intact pulmonary defenses. Ill, hospitalized patients with depressed sensoriums; poor swallowing; nasogastric, endotracheal, and tracheostomy tubes; feeble cough mechanisms; neuromuscular weakness; and debilitated phagocytic, chemotactic, cellular/humoral immune, and inflammatory responses from disease and medication are more prone to aspirate and less able to fight off potential pathogens.

A diverse array of bacteria, fungi, viruses, mycobacteria, and parasites may cause nosocomial lower respiratory tract infections. The potential variety of pathogens and the potential severity of pneumonia increase in immunocompromised patients with organ transplants, hematologic malignancies, and AIDS and in those on antineoplastic, steroid, and immunosuppressive drugs.

Since the 1950s and early 1960s, when gram-negative bacilli accounted for only one third of hospital-acquired pneumonias, the role of these bacteria has increased and they now are responsible for 60 to 80 per cent of nosocomial lower respiratory tract infections.[2] A major reason appears to be the increased ability of gram-negative bacilli to colonize the upper respiratory tract as illness and debilitation progress. The oropharynx of a healthy individual is inhospitable to aerobic gram-negative bacilli, and only 2 per cent of normal persons transiently harbor these organisms. This prevalence rises to 30 to 40 per cent in hospitalized but not critically ill persons and to 73 per cent of moribund patients.[5] Over 40 per cent of patients may become colonized with aerobic gram-negative bacilli within 4 days of admission to an intensive care unit.[6]

Gram-negative bacilli adhere and bind to buccal and tracheobronchial cells of ill patients but not to the cells of healthy hosts. The reason for the increased cellular adherence of gram-negative bacteria is not precisely known, but it may be due to elevation of salivary proteases that deplete cell surface proteins, such as fibronectin, exposing receptor sites.[7] Loss of interbacterial inhibition and alterations in environmental pH also could play a role. The colonizing and infecting flora potentially arise from numerous exogenous sources, including sinks, water, aerosols, medical devices, hands of medical personnel, flowers, and food (especially salads). However, endogenous colonization from gastric sites also occurs, especially in patients on H$_2$-blockers, antacids, and enteral feedings.

The risk of colonization by aerobic gram-negative bacteria has been correlated with a host of risk factors (Table 1). The increased incidence of gram-negative nosocomial pneumonias in the 1970s and 1980s is presumably due to the increased number of hospitalized patients with these conditions.

The three most common aerobic gram-negative organisms causing lower respiratory nosocomial infection are *Klebsiella* sp, *Pseudomonas aeruginosa*, and *Escherichia coli*, but a variety of other gram-negatives may be involved, including *Haemophilus influenzae*. Although the majority of nosocomial bacterial pneumonias are the result of gram-negative bacilli, other pathogens occur at rates that vary with the institution and techniques of isolation. On cultures, up to 35 per cent of patients may show anaerobes, 10 to 15 per cent *Staphylococcus aureus*, 5 per cent *Streptococcus pneumoniae*, and 3 per cent coagulase-negative staphylococci, enterococci, or group B streptococci (Table 2). Polymicrobial infection is common, and multiple pathogens can be isolated in 50 to 60 per cent of nosocomial respiratory tract infections.[2] No pathogen may be detected on culture in one fourth or more of patients.[2] Approximately 20 per cent of hospital-acquired bacteremias with known sites of origin are due to pneumonia, and about 10 per

TABLE 1. Risk Factors Associated with Colonization of the Oropharynx by Gram-Negative Bacilli and Nosocomial Pneumonia

Advanced age
Increasing severity of illness
Long duration of hospitalization
Immunocompromised state
Intubation and mechanical ventilation
Major surgery, especially thoracic, thoracoabdominal, or upper abdominal
Tracheostomy
Nasogastric tubes
Poor nutrition
Enteral feedings
Use of antibiotics
Use of H$_2$-blockers and antacids
Alcoholism
Diabetes mellitus
Azotemia
Acidosis
Coma
Hypotension
White blood cell count less than 4000/mm^3 or greater than 15,000/mm^3

TABLE 2. Bacterial Etiologies of Nosocomial Pneumonia

Pathogen	Estimated Per Cent
Aerobic Gram-Negative Bacilli	
Klebsiella sp.	15
Pseudomonas aeruginosa	13
Escherichia coli	12
Enterobacter sp.	10
Proteus sp.	8
Serratia sp.	5
Haemophilus influenzae	4
Other *Pseudomonas* sp.	3
Other gram-negative aerobes	5
Gram-Positive Aerobes	
Staphylococcus aureus	13
Streptococcus pneumoniae	5
Other gram-positive cocci (enterococci, *Streptococcus* group B, coagulase-negative *Staphylococci*)	3
Anaerobes	
Only isolate	4
Total isolates	35
Mixed Infections	35
Bacteremic	10
No Pathogen Cultured or Isolated	25

Estimates are from multiple sources. Individual isolates total 100% and do not include those grown in mixed infections.

cent of nosocomial pneumonias are bacteremic.

Outbreaks of nosocomial lung infection caused by *Legionella* from contaminated water,[8] tuberculosis from uncontained aerosols,[9] and viruses (influenza, varicella) from infected persons[10] have been described. In immunocompromised patients, the spectrum of infective agents is extended to include fungi (*Aspergillus, Cryptococcus, Mucor, Candida*), viruses (cytomegalovirus, herpes), parasites (*Pneumocystis carinii, Toxoplasma gondii*), other bacteria (*Nocardia, Legionella micdadei*), and *Chlamydia*. It is the setting of critically ill patients with a variety of potential pathogens that makes management of nosocomial pneumonia extremely difficult.[11]

▪ Diagnosis

Clinical findings in patients with nosocomial pneumonia range from typical to subtle and concealed. Obvious cases present with fever, chills, cough productive of purulent sputum, leukocytosis, Gram stain and culture evidence of specific pathogens, and roentgen infiltrates. The most difficult patients to diagnose are critically ill or immunocompromised with underlying lung disease, who do not have typical signs and symptoms of pneumonia owing to coexisting illness or medication. The decision to perform basic laboratory studies, obtain stains and cultures, and treat empirically with antibiotics, or to pursue invasive diagnostic procedures to attempt isolation of specific pathogens, depends on the severity of illness and the presence of underlying conditions.

The initial step in the diagnosis of nosocomial pneumonias is to contemplate its presence. Although nosocomial pneumonia is a consideration in any hospitalized patient with new fever or increasing roentgenographic infiltrates, clinical signs and symptoms may be absent or misleading in elderly, debilitated patients on multiple drugs. Malignancy, vasculitis, pulmonary edema, lung hemorrhage, drug-induced lung disease, pulmonary thromboembolism, oxygen toxicity, the effects of radiation, and interstitial pneumonitis may all be mistaken for infection or mask its presence (Table 3).

After entertaining the possibility of nosocomial pneumonia, the probability of its presence is made by evaluation of risk factors, pulmonary symptoms, physical signs, chest roentgenograms, and laboratory findings.[11] Any hospitalized patient with depressed consciousness, esophageal disease,

TABLE 3. Etiology of Diseases That May Resemble Nosocomial Pneumonia

Alveolar cell carcinoma
Metastatic neoplasm
Lymphangitic spread of cancer
Radiation pneumonitis
Congestive heart failure
Adult respiratory distress syndrome
Re-expansion pulmonary edema (following rapid removal of air or fluid from the pleural space)
Pulmonary oxygen toxicity
Fat embolism
Pulmonary embolism and infarction
Sickle cell lung disease
Pulmonary vasculitis (e.g., systemic lupus erythematosus, Wegener's granulomatosis)
Pulmonary hemorrhage (e.g., bleeding secondary to invasive pulmonary procedure or coagulopathy)
Drug-induced lung disease (e.g., antineoplastic agents, nitrofurantoin)
Aspiration without infection (Mendelson's syndrome)
Bronchiolitis obliterans with organizing pneumonia
Bronchopulmonary aspergillosis (lung infiltrates appearing in a hospitalized asthmatic patient)

or neuromuscular weakness is at risk of aspiration. Up to 75 per cent of nosocomial pneumonias occur in surgical patients, depending on specific institutional populations. Risks for nosocomial pneumonia are highest in elderly men with underlying chronic obstructive pulmonary or cardiovascular disease who undergo lengthy thoracic, thoracoabdominal, or upper abdominal procedures. The risk of hospital-acquired lower respiratory tract infection may be 10 to 21 times greater in intubated, mechanically ventilated patients than in those not intubated.[12] One prospective study documented a 68 per cent incidence of nosocomial pneumonia in 108 patients with the adult respiratory distress syndrome.[13] Pneumonia in mechanically ventilated patients may be twice as high in patients on histamine H_2-receptor antagonists and antacids compared with those not treated with these drugs or on sucralfate.[14] An increased incidence of tracheal colonization and nosocomial pneumonia has been observed in mechanically ventilated patients receiving enteral nutrition.[15] One clinical postmortem study found that 36 per cent of patients thought to have only diffuse lung disease had pneumonia, and 20 per cent believed to have pneumonia had only diffuse lung disease. The overall misdiagnosis rate of 29 per cent suggests that errors in diagnosis based on clinical findings are common in the sickest patients.[16]

After the probability of nosocomial pneumonia is ascertained, a search should be made for a specific microbe. The likelihood of a bacterial etiology is greatly increased by the presence of purulent respiratory secretions. Malodorous sputums suggest anaerobic infection. Brick-red, gelatinous sputum resembling currant jelly, creamy or salmon-colored sputum, and rusty sputum are classic indications of *Klebsiella*, staphylococcus, and pneumococcus, respectively. *Legionella* pneumonia, however, is usually unaccompanied by sputum production. Less specific but common findings in bacterial pneumonias are true rigors and pleuritic chest pain. Risk factors should be assessed for the presence of mycobacteria (in-hospital exposure to infected persons), fungi (immunocompromised state, leukopenia), viruses (transplantation, immunocompromised state, exposure to persons with varicella, influenza), parasites (AIDS, immunocompromised state, foreign residence), and *Legionella* (in-hospital contaminated water or construction sites).

Although not sensitive for detection of causes of pneumonia, a careful physical examination may reveal specific clues to potential causes, such as mucocutaneous (ecthyma gangrenosum, infected intravenous sites or fistulas, rashes due to varicella, herpes simplex, or *Candida*), funduscopic (fluffy white fungal exudates, cytomegalovirus retinitis, choroidal tubercles), nasal *(Mucor, Aspergillus)*, oral (gingivitis, herpes labialis), or neurologic (*Cryptococcus, Nocardia*, anaerobes, *Staphylococcus*).[11]

The suspicion of nosocomial pneumonia usually results from the discovery of new infiltrates on the chest roentgenogram. However, the roentgenographic patterns are diverse and often nonspecific; in neutropenic patients, roentgen infiltrates may be absent in the presence of significant gram-negative pneumonia.[17]

A sputum Gram stain should be performed, as well as acid-fast, potassium hydroxide, *pneumocystis*, and direct immunofluorescent stains for *Legionella* if risk factors so indicate. Sputum examinations and blood cultures for bacteria are routinely obtained, and cultures for *Nocardia, Legionella*, funguses, mycobacteria, and viruses are performed when there is clinical suspicion for these entities. Despite the perceptual difficulty in distinguishing colonizing organisms from infecting ones, the main pathogenesis of nosocomial pneumonia is considered to be aspiration of colonizing flora. Supporting this concept is the ten times greater incidence of lower respiratory infection in colonized versus noncolonized patients, and the frequent correlation between colonizing organisms and those growing in the lower respiratory tract.[2,18] Pleural, pericardial, peritoneal, joint, cerebrospinal, or other clinically involved fluid or infected cutaneous sites also should be analyzed and cultured. If the diagnosis of nosocomial pneumonia and the probable infecting agent are sufficiently certain at this point, empiric antimicrobial therapy to cover the likely inciting agents can be started.

The decision to perform specific invasive diagnostic procedures is a clinical one. Rapid progression, the presence of immunosuppression, the increased likelihood of noninfectious disease, the absence of response to empiric therapy, and critical illness for which survival appears to demand specific diagnosis are situations that commonly prompt efforts to perform invasive diagnostic procedures to isolate distinctive pathogens or define noninfectious illness (Table 4). At present, however, there is no evidence that establishing a definite etiology alters outcome.[18-20]

Despite evidence supporting its diagnostic value, transtracheal aspiration has lost favor because of fear of complications and evidence that it samples colonizing upper respiratory tract flora. Percutaneous needle aspiration of pulmonary infiltrates can be performed in selected patients, especially those with pleural adhesions or with chest tubes in place, but the sickest patients can least afford the 9 to 26 per cent probability of pneumothorax despite its high yield of 55 to 76 per cent for specific etiologies.[18]

The initial procedure of choice is fiberoptic bronchoscopy with bronchoalveolar lavage, protected brush cultures, and transbronchial lung biopsy. Quantitative cultures should be performed, if available.[21] Specific diagnoses can be expected in over half of cases. Pneumothorax and minor hemorrhage occur in approximately 5 to 10 per cent of procedures.[18,19] When fiberoptic bronchoscopy fails to yield a diagnosis and

TABLE 4. Invasive Diagnostic Procedures in the Diagnosis of Nosocomial Pneumonia

| | | Estimated Per Cent | |
Procedure	*Yield Specific Diagnosis*	*Hemorrhage $>$ 25 ml*	*Pneumothorax*
Fiberoptic bronchoscopy with	30–84	0–26	0–19
bronchoalveolar lavage and	(52)	(7)	(7)
transbronchial biopsy			
Needle aspiration biopsy	55–76	3–18	9–26
Open lung biopsy	55–91	(1)	(8)
	(69)		

Mean percentages from several studies are given in parentheses.

(Adapted from Towes, GB. Nosocomial pneumonia. Clin Chest Med 1987; 8:467–479 and Matthay RA, Moritz ED. Invasive procedures for diagnosing pulmonary infection. Clin Chest Med 1981; 2:3–18.)

pulmonary disease does not improve on empiric therapy, open lung biopsy may establish a definitive diagnosis in about 70 per cent of patients (55 to 91 per cent) and may lead to a change in therapy in half of patients.[18,19] Performing open lung biopsy for diagnosis, especially in some immunocompromised patients, is a rational approach despite statistical evidence that it may not enhance survival.[18–20]

■ Management

The difficulty in managing nosocomial pneumonias has been compounded by the array of antimicrobial agents produced by the pharmaceutical industry in an attempt to match the diversity and pathogenicity of invading microbes. The number of agents is greatest and most effective against bacteria. For example, there are currently 27 cephalosporins, all but one of which begin with "cef-" (moxalactam), and 27 penicillins, all of which end in "-cillin."[22] Carbapenems (imipenem), monobactams (aztreonam, carumonam), quinolones (ciprofloxacin), and beta-lactamase inhibitors (clavulanic acid, sulbactam) are also relatively recent additions that have extended the spectrum and potency of antibacterial agents. There are currently no comprehensive comparative data about the clinical efficacy of each versus others or multiples of antibiotics; consequently, confusing relative differences in the in vitro spectrum of activity, minimum inhibitory concentrations (MICs) of antibiotics, comparative costs, and marketing techniques appear to determine in-hospital antimicrobial usage as much as true knowledge of outcome does. At present, no agent or combination of antibacterial agents can be considered drugs of choice in the treatment of nosocomial pneumonia, and only suggested therapy can be offered (Table 5). The armamentarium against viruses (acyclovir, ganciclovir, zidovudine, foscarnet, vidarabine), mycobacteria (rifabutin, clofazimine), *Pneumocystis carinii* (eflornithine, trimetrexate, dapsone/trimethoprim), *Toxoplasma* (spiramycin), and fungi (ketoconazole, fluconazole) has also increased, but with less success.

The initial antibiotic selection in treatment of nosocomial pneumonia is usually made empirically to cover the most likely

TABLE 5. Suggested Empiric Antibiotic Regimens for Treatment of Nosocomial Pneumonia

Mildly ill, non-neutropenic, nonimmunocompromised patient

Third-generation cephalosporin (e.g., cefoperazone, cefotaxime, ceftriaxone)

Alternatives: second-generation cephalosporin (e.g., cefuroxime), ticarcillin-clavulanate, ciprofloxacin

Moderately ill patient with or without underlying disease

Aminoglycoside plus antipseudomonal penicillin (e.g., piperacillin, azlocillin, mezlocillin, ticarcillin-clavulanate) or third-generation cephalosporin (e.g., ceftazidime)

Add vancomycin or nafcillin if staphylococcal infection is suspected. Substitute aztreonam for aminoglycoside in the presence of diminished renal function

Alternative: imipenem/cilastatin. Add vancomycin if methicillin-resistant or coagulase-negative staphylococci are isolated or suspected

Severely ill, immunocompromised, neutropenic patient

Vancomycin plus aminoglycoside plus antipseudomonal penicillin or third-generation cephalosporin plus erythromycin plus trimethoprim/sulfamethoxazole

Substitute aztreonam for aminoglycoside in the presence of diminished renal function

Alternative: imipenem/cilastatin plus erythromycin plus trimethoprim/sulfamethoxazole. Add vancomycin if methicillin-resistant or coagulase-negative staphylococci are isolated or suspected

Add amphotericin B if no response

pathogens, based on risk factors and clinical findings (Table 5). Antimicrobial therapy subsequently may be tailored by results of stains, cultures, biopsies, serology (rarely), and response to treatment. The more critically ill and immunocompromised the patient, the greater the pressure to use multiple agents to improve the spectrum and activity. Specific factors peculiar to each hospital, such as the incidence of methicillin-resistant staphylococci, aminoglycoside-resistant gram-negative bacilli, *Legionella*, tuberculosis (e.g., inner city general and Veterans Administration hospitals), and the prevalence of elderly, intensive care, surgical, and immunocompromised patients in the institution, also influence the number and types of antimicrobials used. When possible, comparative costs should be considered. When agents have similar potential efficacy, the least costly should be selected.

Patients who are not immunocompromised, are mildly ill, and have purulent sputum could be started on monotherapy with a third-generation cephalosporin, such as cefoperazone, which has been shown to be less expensive and as effective as clindamycin/gentamicin or cefazolin/gentamicin in the treatment of hospital-acquired pneumonia.[23] Many third-generation cephalosporins, such as cefoperazone, cefotaxime, and ceftriaxone, have poor activity against methacillin-resistant staphylococci, enterococci, and *Acinetobacter* and have variable activity against *Pseudomonas* and *Bacteroides fragilis*. In hospitals where methicillin-resistant *Staphylococcus aureus* is very common, where *Staphylococcus epidermidis* is suspected (e.g., infected intravenous sites), or where staphylococcal pneumonia is probable (creamy sputum, clusters of gram-positive cocci on sputum Gram stain), vancomycin should be added. If *Pseudomonas aeruginosa* is likely (e.g., chronic bronchiectasis, cystic fibrosis), the antipseudomonal cephalosporin ceftazidime is preferred, recognizing that it has a reduced gram-positive spectrum. The carboxypenicillins (carbenicillin, ticarcillin) and ureidopenicillins (azlocillin, mezlocillin, piperacillin) should not be used as single agents because of the rapid development of resistant gram-negative organisms. The comparative efficacy, toxicity, and costs of monotherapy with cephalosporins and beta-lactamase inhibitor–antibiotic combinations (ticarcillin-clavulanate, ampicillin-clavulanate, or sulbactam), quinolones (ciprofloxacin), and carbapenems (imipenem) have yet to be defined.

Antimicrobial therapy of nosocomial pneumonia in the critically ill patient has been performed mostly on patients with malignancy and granulocytopenia, using two- and three-drug regimens. Combination therapy with antipseudomonal aminoglycosides, plus either a third-generation cephalosporin with enhanced antipseudomonal activity (e.g., ceftazidime) or antipseudomonal penicillin, has been recommended.[18,22] The ureidopenicillins (azlocillin, mezlocillin, piperacillin) are preferred over the carboxypenicillins (carbenicillin, ticarcillin) because of their excellent activity against *Pseudomonas*; better *Klebsiella*, other gram-negative, and enterococcal coverage; lower sodium content; and lesser tendency to prolong bleeding time. With defective cell-mediated immunity or neutropenia, combinations of as many as five or more antibiotics have been recommended in critically ill patients, including vancomycin or nafcillin, aminoglycoside, third-generation cephalosporin or antipseudomonal penicillin, erythromycin, and trimethoprim-sulfamethoxazole.[22] Imipenem/cilastatin has the widest spectrum of the currently available antibiotics, and its use may eliminate the need for complex antibiotic regimens, but its role in the therapy of nosocomial pneumonia has not yet been fully evaluated. In some larger hospitals, amikacin has replaced gentamicin or tobramycin as the aminoglycoside of first choice, owing to the prevalence of gentamicin-resistant gram-negative organisms. The monobactam aztreonam has a spectrum of activity similar to that of the aminoglycosides but without nephrotoxicity, and it may be substituted in patients with diminished renal function. The addition of antifungal, antiviral, antituberculous, and antiparasitic agents to the regimen depends on the evidence or suspicion of coexisting infection or the absence of a response to antibacterials.

Although the duration of treatment is not known, most courses are given for a minimum of 10 days to 2 weeks or longer, depending on response. When no organism is isolated and the patient improves clinically, whether to continue a full course of antibiotics or stop therapy is debated, but recent evidence suggests that antibiotics may be discontinued safely in average cases after 4 days.[24] The finding of a specific pathogen usually indicates narrowing therapy for the particular organism. Optimizing the clearance of secretions, good nutrition, improving metabolic abnormalities, and enhancing host defenses appear to be obvious but may be difficult to achieve, and their effects on outcome remain largely unknown.

■ Prevention

The critical illness that brings patients to the hospital (partly due to the current strict criteria for hospital admission), the need for the airway to remain open for gas exchange, the difficulty of blocking aspiration, and the ability of pathogens to colonize the trachea despite bypassing the oropharynx with tracheostomy make prevention of nosocomial lower respiratory tract infection a desirable but nebulous goal. However, some logical measures may decrease the risk of hospital-acquired pneumonia:[12]

1. Handwashing prior to and following patient contact
2. Proper disinfection and changing of respiratory therapy equipment. This may include
   a. Proper disinfection of nebulization equipment, especially large volume, ultrasonic, and in-line nebulizers
   b. Filling of reservoirs with sterile, not tap water
   c. Preventing reflux back to the patient and proper disposal of contaminated tubing condensate
   d. Change of ventilator circuits every 48 hours
   e. Routine decontamination of bedside resuscitation bags and spirometers
   f. Use of unit dose medication and disposable equipment where feasible
3. Recognition that contaminated water, food, and environmental air may transmit infection, and avoidance when possible
4. Use of sucralfate instead of H_2-receptor antagonists and antacids possibly may decrease the incidence of nosocomial pneumonia

Although some encouraging data exist, the use of topical, aerosolized, or systemic prophylaxic antibiotics to prevent colonization and lung infection remains experimental.[25] There have been few clinically useful advances in enhancing pulmonary defenses or practical methods of preventing aspiration.

▪ Issues and Risks

Knowledge of risk factors for nosocomial pneumonia does not necessarily mean that they can be avoided (e.g., surgery, antibiotics, steroids, immunosuppressive drugs, antacids, tracheostomy, nasogastric suction, enteral feedings, mechanical ventilation).[12,14]

The need to perform invasive diagnostic procedures to confirm noninfectious illness or define specific pathogens is most logical in critically ill, immunocompromised, and neutropenic patients, but their value in terms of final outcome is uncertain. The decision to perform fiberoptic bronchoscopy,

needle aspiration, open lung, or other culture/biopsy techniques currently depends on risk factors, clinical status, and response to empiric therapy.

Based on current and rapidly changing data, no antibiotic or combination of antibiotics can be firmly recommended for nosocomial pneumonia. In general, the more critically ill and immunosuppressed the patient is, the greater the need for wider, potent antibiotic coverage.

Until development of ingenuous techniques to prevent colonization/aspiration and improve host defenses of critically ill patients, prevention of nosocomial pneumonia is largely limited to preventing transmission of pathogens from the environment to the patient. Until hospital-acquired respiratory infections can be truly prevented, a decrease in their incidence, morbidity, mortality, and cost cannot be expected.

REFERENCES

1. Gross PA, Neu HC, Aswapokee P, Antwerpen CV, Aswapokee N. Deaths from nosocomial infections: experience in a university hospital and a community hospital. Am J Med 1980; 68:219–223.
2. Jay SL. Nosocomial infections. Med Clin North Am 1984; 67:1251–1277.
3. Haley RW, Schaberg DR, Crossley KB, Von Allmen SD, McGowan JE. Extra charges and prolongation of stay attributable to nosocomial infections: a prospective interhospital comparison. Am J Med 1981; 70:51–58.
4. Huxley EJ, Viroslav J, Gray WR, Pierce AK. Pharyngeal aspiration in normal adults and patients with depressed consciousness. Am J Med 1978; 64:564–568.
5. Johanson WG Jr, Pierce AK, Sanford JP. Changing pharyngeal bacterial flora of hospitalized patients. Emergence of gram-negative bacilli. N Engl J Med 1969; 281:1137–1140.
6. Johanson WG Jr, Pierce AK, Sanford JP. Nosocomial respiratory infections with gram-negative bacilli. The significance of colonization of the respiratory tract. Ann Intern Med 1972; 77:701–706.
7. Dal Nogare AR, Towes GB, Pierce AK. Increased salivary elastase precedes gram-negative bacillary colonization in postoperative patients. Am Rev Resp Dis 1987; 135:671–675.
8. Stout J, Yu VL, Vickers RM, et al. Ubiquitousness of *Legionella pneumophila* in the water supply of a hospital with endemic Legionnaire's disease. N Engl J Med 1982; 306:466–468.
9. Kantor HS, Poblete R, Pusateri SL. Nosocomial transmission of tuberculosis from unsuspected disease. Am J Med 1988; 84:833–838.
10. Kapila R, Lintz DI, Tecson FT, Ziskin L, Louria DB. A nosocomial outbreak of influenza A. Chest 1977; 71:576–579.
11. Tsou E. Pneumonia, poorly resolved. *In* Taylor RB

(ed). Difficult Diagnosis. Philadelphia: WB Saunders, 1985:379–392.

12. Craven DE, Driks MR. Nosocomial pneumonia in the intubated patient. Semin Respir Infect 1987; 2:20–33.

13. Seidenfeld JJ, Pohl DF, Bell RC, Harris GD, Johanson WG Jr. Incidence, site, and outcome of infections in patients with the adult respiratory distress syndrome. Am Rev Resp Dis 1986; 134:12–16.

14. Driks MR, Craven DE, Celli BR, et al. Nosocomial pneumonia in intubated patients given sucralfate as compared with antacids or histamine type 2 blockers. The role of gastric colonization. N Engl J Med 1987; 317:1376–1382.

15. Pingleton SK, Hinthorn DR, Liu C. Enteral nutrition in a patient receiving mechanical ventilation. Multiple sources of tracheal colonization include the stomach. Am J Med 1986; 80:827–832.

16. Andrews CP, Coalson JJ, Smith JD, Johanson WG Jr. Diagnosis of nosocomial bacterial pneumonia in acute, diffuse lung injury. Chest 1981; 80:254–258.

17. Valdivieso M, Gil-Extremera B, Zornoza J, Rodriguez V, Bodey GP. Gram-negative bacillary pneumonia in the compromised host. Medicine 1977; 56:241–254.

18. Towes GB. Nosocomial pneumonia. Clin Chest Med 1987; 8:467–479.

19. Matthay RA, Moritz ED. Invasive procedures for diagnosing pulmonary infection. A critical review. Clin Chest Med 1981; 2:3–18.

20. Potter D, Pass HI, Brower S, et al. Prospective randomized study of open lung biopsy versus empirical antibiotic therapy for acute pneumonitis in nonneutropenic cancer patients. Ann Thorac Surg 1985; 40:422–428.

21. Chastre J, Fagon J, Soler P, et al. Diagnosis of nosocomial bacterial pneumonia in intubated patients undergoing ventilation: comparison of the usefulness of bronchoalveolar lavage and the protected specimen brush. Am J Med 1988; 85:499–506.

22. Sanford JP. Guide to antimicrobial therapy 1988. Bethesda, MD: Antimicrobial Therapy Inc, 1988: 23, 40.

23. Mangi RJ, Greco T, Ryan J, Thornton G, Andriole VT. Cefoperazone versus combination antibiotic therapy of hospital-acquired pneumonia. Am J Med 1988; 84:68–74.

24. McGehee JL, Podnos SD, Pierce AK, Weissler JC. Treatment of pneumonia in patients at risk of infection with gram-negative bacilli. Am J Med 1988; 84:597–602.

25. Pingleton SK. State of the art. Complications of acute respiratory failure. Am Rev Resp Dis 1988; 137:1463–1493.

Polycystic ovarian disease

David C. Cumming

■ Background

Polycystic ovarian disease (PCOD) is characterized by chronic anovulation accompanied by excess androgen production from the ovaries, the adrenal cortex, or both. While we generally discuss PCOD as if it were a single, well-defined clinical entity, it is probably a complex of disorders with a range of symptoms and signs. There are problems in determining the pathophysiologic mechanisms that lead to the clinical syndrome that is called PCOD. The relative contributions of abnormalities of adrenal and ovarian adrogenesis, hypothalamic function, and neurotransmitter control of the hypothalamic-pituitary-gonadal axis remain matters of conjecture. The use of a global term, *hyperandrogenic chronic anovulation*, might be more appropriate, but "polycystic ovarian disease" has become entrenched and is probably going to remain the generally accepted term.

Management of PCOD is management of the presenting reproductive need; this could include control of abnormal uterine bleeding, prevention of endometrial hyperplasia, treatment of hirsutism, induction of ovulation, reduction of obesity, or provision of contraceptive advice. The initial approach to the patient is to make the diagnosis and exclude other potentially more serious causes of the presenting symptom and then to deal with the patient's needs in a problem-solving fashion. Because symptomatology of PCOD is multifaceted, the various goals of the patient may be in conflict. It is difficult, for example, to seek pregnancy and treatment for hirsutism at the same time. Therefore, priorities must be set for the patient's goals. This article reviews polycystic ovarian disease, particularly emphasizing a goal-oriented approach for the patient.

■ Management

■ PROBLEMS IN MAKING THE DIAGNOSIS OF PCOD

The provisional diagnosis is usually fairly clear from the history and physical examination. The differential diagnosis is based on clinical and laboratory findings. Patients with PCOD usually have chronic anovulation associated with hyperandrogenism. The prevalence of symptoms and signs in a population of patients with anatomic (histologically proven) PCOD is summarized in Table 1.[1]

In practice, the clinical diagnosis of PCOD cannot be justified without the presence of amenorrhea or dysfunctional bleeding caused by chronic anovulation. Menstrual and other problems usually begin at puberty or soon after.[2] The time of menarche is usually normal, perhaps surprising, since obesity usually accelerates maturational processes. Obesity and even hirsutism often predate menarche. Hair growth tends to increase with increasing age; slight hair growth in a teenager may become substantially worse in later life. The manifestations of hyperandrogenism vary from slight to substantial and cannot be relied on for diagnosis.

Physical signs that should be sought include hair growth in inappropriate places (face, shoulders, suprapubic and midline abdominal and chest areas, fingers and toes), the distribution of obesity if present, clitorimegaly, and other signs of virilism including increased muscle mass, increased laryngeal size, frontal balding, or loss of breast tissue. Breast development and inspection of the vaginal lining, however, usually provide evidence of an estrogen effect. The amount of cervical mucus is often impressive.[3]

Although difficult in an obese patient, the pelvic examination may reveal bilaterally enlarged ovaries. It has been suggested that the demonstration of enlarged ovaries is crucial to the diagnosis of the clinical syndrome of polycystic ovarian disease. Therefore, emphasis has been placed at different times on careful bimanual examination, pneumoroentgenography, culdoscopy, and laparoscopy in the diagnosis of PCO. More recently, the increasing definition of ultrasound has led to suggestions that it should be considered essential in the diagnostic evaluation.[4] Although polycystic ovaries are commonly found in women with the clinical syndrome of PCO (over 50 per cent), the association is by no means invariable. Multicystic ovaries occur in about 3 per cent of women with regular menses. It is particularly emphasized that the incidental discovery of polycystic-appearing ovaries during surgery for an unrelated purpose in patients not seeking pregnancy should not lead to any surgical treatment of the ovaries.

Biochemical findings include a high luteinizing hormone (LH) to follicle-stimulating hormone (FSH) ratio (greater than 3:1), variable elevated androgen levels, and a high estrone to estradiol ratio. However, these results may be found in other forms of anovulation. Laboratory results, however, can be perplexing. A patient may appear to have clinical PCOD when her LH/FSH ratio is normal or, even more commonly, her androgens are normal. This can result from a recent spontaneous ovulation, which generally normalizes hormone levels for up to 6 weeks. Serum levels of biologically available testosterone—that is, free plus albumin-bound testosterone—can be increased without a change in serum total testosterone level because of an androgen-induced decrease in serum sex hormone–binding globulin (SHBG) levels. The measurement of free or bioavailable steroid has helped resolve this confusion.[5]

Minimal investigation of patients with possible PCOD should include measurement

TABLE 1. Clinical Symptoms and Signs in Women with Anatomic (Histologically Proved) Polycystic Ovaries

Symptom	Mean (%)	Range (%)
Obesity	41	16–49
Hirsutism	69	17–83
Virilization	21	0–28
Amenorrhea	51	15–77
Infertility	74	35–94
Dysfunctional bleeding	29	6–65
Biphasic temperature graph	15	12–40
Corpus luteum at surgery	22	0–71

(Data from Goldzieher JW, Axelrod LR: Clinical and biochemical features of polycystic ovarian disease. Fertil Steril 1963; 631–641.)

TABLE 2. Investigation of Patients with Suspected PCO

Minimal investigations:
  Luteinizing hormone
  Follicle-stimulating hormone
  Prolactin
  Testosterone
  DHEAS
  TSH, thyroid screen

"Optional" investigations:
  DHEA
  Androstenedione
  Biologically available testosterone
    Non-SHBG bound
    Free testosterone
  Estrone/estradiol ratio
  Ultrasound assessment of the ovaries

of LH, FSH, prolactin, androgens (testosterone and dehydropiandrosterone sulfate [DHEAS]), and thyroid-stimulating hormone (Table 2). More complete investigation could include assays of bioavailable testosterone, other androgens (e.g., DHEA and androstenedione), and the estrone/estradiol ratio. Ultrasound imaging can be used to assess the ovaries. However, this provides a restricted amount of information, since anatomic evidence of polycystic ovaries may occur without clinical problems and the clinical syndrome of PCOD may occur without ultrasound evidence of anatomic abnormalities in the ovaries. The presence or absence of anatomic abnormalities per se would do little to change the clinical management.

Specific testing may need to be performed to exclude other causes of hyperandrogenism with chronic anovulation (Table 3). Cushing's syndrome is usually suggested by its clinical features and can be confirmed by measurement of free cortisol levels in the 24-hour urine specimen or by a dexamethasone suppression test. The existence of acquired or late-onset heterozygote 21-hydroxylase deficiency is debated. Characteristically, there are increased circulating levels of 17-hydroxy progesterone and adrenal androgens (DHEA and DHEAS). It is suggested that an excessive 17-hydroxyprogesterone increment also may be observed in response to ACTH infusion when basal levels are normal, but a positive test is not consistent with evidence from genotyping.[6]

A sudden onset of masculinization suggests an androgen-producing tumor of the ovary or the adrenal gland. Androgen-producing tumors (Table 4) should be suspected in any patient with postpubertal onset of hirsutism with or without frontal balding or clitorimegaly. Virilization occurs only when testosterone levels approach the male range. Testosterone levels above 200 ng/dl or DHEAS levels above 700 μg/dl should prompt a search for a tumor.

Hyperthecosis is a histologic diagnosis generally found in patients resistant to conventional forms of therapy. Chronic anovulation may be related to weight in some women: they have regular menses when their weight is nearly normal, but they develop a biochemical and clinical profile resembling that of PCOD when they gain weight. Such patients tend to have a postmenarcheal onset of anovulation; diet often can lead to reproductive normality.[7]

TABLE 3. Differential Diagnosis of PCOD

Cushing's syndrome
Adrenal enzymatic deficiency
  Late-onset 21-hydroxylase deficiency
  3b-hydroxysteroid dehydrogenase-Δ4–5 isomerase
    deficiency
Functional tumors of ovary and adrenal
Hyperthecosis
Hyperprolactinemia
Thyroid deficiency
Simple hirsutism
Chronic anovulation asociated with obesity

■ TREATMENT OF PROBLEMS IN WOMEN WITH PCOD

After excluding potentially more serious causes for chronic anovulation with androgen excess, it is necessary to establish and set priorities for the reproductive needs and

TABLE 4. Androgen-Producing Tumors of the Ovary and Adrenal

Hilus cell tumor
Arrhenoblastoma (Sertoli-Leydig cell tumor)
Benign cystic teratoma
Luteinized thecoma
Adrenal rest tumor of the ovary
Adrenal adenoma
Adrenal carcinoma

other goals of the patient. The presenting problem(s) may include hirsutism, amenorrhea, irregular or excessive menstrual bleeding, obesity, infertility, and the need for contraception; there may be no specific complaint in patients who accept their physical and menstrual changes as being relatively normal.

■ OVULATION INDUCTION

Ovulation induction is generally necessary only in women who seek pregnancy. The medical approaches to the problem are fairly successful, so surgical approaches should be considered only when medical treatment has failed. A range of drugs has been used; clomiphene citrate has become the drug of first choice.

Clomiphene works well in PCOD patients seeking pregnancy. Up to 90 per cent of patients will ovulate with clomiphene citrate, 50 mg daily, for 5 days, beginning on the fifth day of a spontaneous period, with withdrawal bleeding induced by medroxyprogesterone acetate (10 mg daily for 7 to 10 days) or following a previous clomiphene cycle. Pregnancy occurs in about half the patients, but rates similar to those in normally ovulating women can be obtained.[8] Side effects are numerous but usually trivial. These include hot flashes, visual symptoms that are benign but troublesome, abdominal symptoms such as bloating or pain related to ovulation, nausea, vomiting, fatigue, headache, depression, dizziness, nervousness, changes in menstrual flow, reversible hair loss, and weight gain. Potentially serious problems include mild ovarian enlargement (in 15 per cent), hyperstimulation (dose-related and occurring in approximately 1 per cent), and multiple pregnancy, with twins being reported in 6 to 8 per cent of pregnancies. Miscarriage rates may be slightly higher than normal (perhaps because of the inadequate luteal phase) but

there is no evidence of an increase in fetal abnormalities. Failures are often associated with giving up treatment too soon[8] or other causes of infertility, including male and tubal problems. Clomiphene therapy may be unsuccessful because of a failure to induce ovulation or because pregnancy has not occurred despite an apparently successful ovulation induction. Reasons for failure on both counts remain obscure.

If the patient appears to ovulate normally but fails to achieve a pregnancy over four to six cycles, a fuller infertility investigation should be undertaken, including endometrial biopsy, hysterosalpingogram or laparoscopy, semen analysis, and a postcoital test (Table 5). The endometrial biopsy can indicate whether ovulation is adequate and suggest the need to alter the ovulation induction regime; there is no good evidence that the arbitrary increase of clomiphene has therapeutic benefit. The uses of hysterosal-

TABLE 5. Management of Clomiphene Failure

Failure to achieve pregnancy despite documented ovulation induction. *After three cycles:*
  1. Endometrial biopsy; exclude inadequate luteal phase
  2. Hysterosalpingogram (HSG) and/or laparoscopy; exclude tubal problems
  3. Postcoital test; exclude effects on cervix
  4. Semen analysis; exclude male factor in infertility

If results are normal, continue clomiphene for at least 12 months.

Failure to induce ovulation. *In succeeding cycles:*
  1. Increase dose by 50 mg per day to a maximum of 150 mg
  2. Increase duration of therapy to 7 days
  3. Consider high-dose regimen
  4. Consider addition of dexamethasone, 0.25–0.5 mg at night
  5. Consider addition of human chorionic gonadotropin (hCG) to stimulate ovulation and/or support the luteal phase
  6. If patient continues to be anovulatory, consider human menopausal gonadotropin (hMG)/hCG, pure FSH, or surgery to induce ovulation

pingography/laparoscopy and semen analysis are obvious. It is suggested that the antiestrogenic effect of clomiphene on the cervix may decrease sperm penetration. The significance of the cervical factor in infertility is very much debated, and its relevance in the treatment of PCOD is particularly difficult. The use of low doses of estrogen may improve the mucus but often at the expense of interfering with ovulation or its timing.

If the patient fails to ovulate with clomiphene or has a well-established inadquate luteal phase, the dose of clomiphene can be increased to a maximum of 150 mg per day for 5 days, or the duration of treatment can be increased up to 7 days (Table 5). Although ovulation may be induced with doses higher than 150 mg per day, pregnancy is less likely. Incremental regimens to much higher doses have been described,[9] but close patient supervision is essential.

Alternative forms of treatment have included the use of dexamethasone, pulsed gonadotropin-releasing hormone (GnRH), menopausal gonadotropins for follicular development with chorionic gonadotropin to trigger ovulation (hMG/hCG), "pure" FSH, and surgical techniques. Suppression of the hypothalamus has been attempted with birth control pills prior to ovulation induction and with GnRH analogs both prior to and during ovulation induction with hMG/hCG and with pure FSH.

Dexamethasone, 0.25 to 0.5 mg, may be added to clomiphene throughout the cycle at night; it dampens the adrenal contribution to the androgen pool and may inhibit ovarian androgenesis through glucocorticoid receptors in the ovary. The technique may be most appropriate in women with mild elevations of DHEAS or DHEA who fail to respond to the usual clomiphene regimes.[10] There appear to be few advantages in attempting to induce ovulation with glucocorticoids alone in PCOD, although it may be appropriate to do so when there is clear evidence of 21-hydroxylase deficiency. Other drugs have been used in combination with clomiphene, including hCG, progesterone, and bromocriptine. The hCG may be given as luteal phase support (1500 to 3000 units IM every 3 to 4 days once ovulation has occurred) or as an ovulating dose (e.g., 3000 to 6000 units IM just prior to ovulation), with 2000 units every 3 to 4 days as luteal phase support. Progesterone suppositories (25 mg twice daily or 50 mg daily per vagina) also can be used as luteal phase sup-

port; gestagens by mouth or injection should not be used for this purpose. Since the usual reason for failure to ovulate in response to clomiphene is a failure of follicular development, the use of hCG and progesterone is more appropriate for treatment of inadequate luteal phase than for failure of clomiphene to induce ovulation. In either event, there is little clear-cut evidence of their efficacy.

The use of pulsed GnRH in PCOD is frequently unsuccessful and should no longer be considered. Ovulation induction with hMG/hCG is difficult and should be undertaken only where monitoring facilities (same-day estradiol levels and accurate ultrasound measurement of follicular size) are available.[11] Ovulation induction rates approaching 100 per cent are reported, with pregnancies occurring in up to 70 per cent of cycles. Multiple pregnancies are a problem, with one third of patients achieving twins. Miscarriages occur in one quarter of patients. A particular problem in inducing ovulation with hMG/hCG in women with PCOD is the simultaneous partial development of several follicles that increase estradiol levels but do not mature to form an ovulatory follicle. The risk of hyperstimulation in PCOD patients is high, and if multiple follicular development does occur, the induction should be terminated. Other side effects of hMG/hCG treatment—pyrexia, joint pains, and tenderness at the site of injection—are rare.

"Pure" FSH, derived from postmenopausal urine in a manner similar to that of hMG but with LH removed, has been used to induce ovulation in women with PCOD.[12] The rationale behind such treatment is that follicular development is inadequate because of the low endogenous FSH levels. Careful monitoring remains essential. Ovulation has been reported in 57 of 68 attempted cycles, with pregnancies in 58.6 per cent of patients over time.[12] Clinical abortions occurred in 17.6 per cent of patients and multiple pregnancy in 5 patients. These and other similar figures from the studies that have been reported do not inspire confidence that the use of pure FSH is any better than use of hMG/hCG.

Suppression of the excessive pulsatile release of GnRH and LH has been attempted prior to other forms of ovulation induction. Birth control pills have been employed for this purpose, but success rates do not seem higher than without prior suppression.

GnRH agonists have been used to suppress the central axis prior to pulsed GnRH or, more recently, prior to and in conjunction with pure FSH. The results to date in the few published studies are promising but show no clear-cut advantage over the existing regimes.

If other forms of ovulation induction fail, surgical means can be employed. Failure of ovulation induction by nonsurgical means is now the only indication for wedge resection. The successful surgical induction of ovulation (up to 90 per cent) is accompanied by a relatively high immediate pregnancy rate, but the development of adhesions often prevents subsequent pregnancies.[13] A recently reported alternative is laparoscopic ovarian cautery using either the electrocautery[14] or, more recently, the laser.[15] Reported success rates are similar to those in wedge resection without the hospital stay or morbidity of the major surgery and perhaps with less risk of adhesions.[14]

In general, it seems fair to suggest that if clomiphene does not induce ovulation, other forms of therapy are much more hazardous and less successful. It should also be remembered that obesity can influence the success or failure of ovulation induction. Some patients can induce ovulation by dieting. Others can make the ovulation induction less difficult if they are prepared to lose weight. Successful dieting in women with PCOD is difficult and may result simply in a thin patient who still has PCOD. However, it is worthwhile both because of greater ease of ovulation induction and the benefits of good health.

■ HIRSUTISM

Opinions about what constitutes a socially acceptable amount of face and body hair in women are subsantially different around the world. The diagnosis of hirsutism is usually self-made, and patients will shop around for doctors who are prepared to offer treatment. Increased facial hair growth can distress women greatly because of doubts raised about their social acceptability and femininity. Treatment is worthwhile, although drugs used in the treatment have limited success in reversing the problem of hair growth induced by long-standing androgen excess. Physical methods (shaving, plucking, waxing, electrolysis, bleaching, depilatory creams) have a significant role to play in diminishing the cosmetic effects of hirsutism and should be discussed. They may augment the effects of medical treatment.

Response to medical treatment is slow, and patients and their doctors often become discouraged by the failure of an immediate response. Once undertaken, any specific therapy should continue for at least a year before being abandoned. Photographs or scoring systems can document the changes. Complete resolution of abnormal hair growth is an unrealistic goal; while considerable improvement may take place, there will always be some degree of problem to manage. Relapse will occur if therapy is discontinued and, therefore, at present management of hirsutism is a lifelong problem.

No drugs are approved for use in hirsutism in North America. Therefore, the advantages and disadvantages of any particular form of therapy should be carefully explained and a realistic estimate of the success provided. Available drugs include birth control pills, medroxyprogesterone acetate (MPA), glucocorticoids, spironolactone, and, in Europe and Canada, cyproterone acetate (CPA). The various forms of treatment work in several ways to reduce the increased androgen production and oppose its effects (Table 6).

TABLE 6. Mode of Action of Drugs Used in Hirsutism

Mode of Action	BCPs	Glucocorticoids	Spironolactone	MPA	CPA
Suppress LH levels	Yes	Yes	No	Yes	Yes
Suppress ovarian androgenesis	Yes	Yes	Yes	Yes	Yes
Suppress adrenal androgenesis	Yes	Yes	No	No	Yes
Increase SHBG	Yes	No	No	No	Yes
Block androgen receptor	Yes	No	Yes	No	Yes
Block conversion of testosterone to dihydrotestosterone	Yes	No	No	Yes	No

BCPs, birth control pills; CPA, cyproterone acetate; MPA, medroxyprogesterone acetate.

Low-androgen birth control pills (BCPs) are often recommended as initial therapy, but there is no good study suggesting significant differences among the various pills in treating hirsutism. Suggested pills are Brevicon/Modicon in the sub-50 μg estrogen dose pills and Demulen 50 in the 50 μg estrogen pills. BCPs generally will regulate menses and reduce androgen levels, but the degree of success in reducing hair growth is limited. Side effects are so well known that it would be redundant to mention them.

Glucocorticoids in physiologic doses (prednisone, 2.5 to 5 mg at night or dexamethasone, 0.25 to 0.5 mg at night) have little effect on hirsutism unless there is a very strong adrenal component. Concerns about adrenal suppression are not justified at this dosage, and side effects are unusual.

Spironolactone (50 to 200 mg per day in one or two doses) blocks binding to the androgen receptor in the cells and may reduce circulating testosterone levels in many women. This drug, originally formulated as a salt-wasting diuretic, may be the most powerful drug presently available in the United States to treat hirsutism.[16] Side effects include lethargy, nausea, and epigastric discomfort. Menstrual function may return to a more normal pattern, but there is also a tendency for dysfunctional bleeding to occur, which may be troublesome. Recently, the combination of spironolactone with either glucocorticoids or BCPs has provided better results, and this appears to be the method of choice at present. A good combination is spironolactone, 100 mg per day, with Demulen 50 or Modicon/Brevicon.[16] This prevents pregnancy and provides better cycle control than spironolactone alone. The possibility that spironolactone could block masculinization in the male fetus because of its effect on cellular androgen receptors has led to the general recommendation that some form of effective contraceptive be used when spironolactone is administered. In practice, no antiandrogenic effect has been reported. There is also anxiety that spironolactone may induce breast cancer, a concern similar to that with other drugs that have a progestational effect. Although breast tumors have been described in women taking spironolactone, there is no proof that the tumors were other than incidental, but unfortunately no proof that they

were not caused by the drug. This information should be shared with patients.

The use of cyproterone acetate is extensive in Europe, and its availability in Canada (where the drug is approved for treatment of prostatic cancer) has led to its use in hirsutism. A recent Canadian study has been published.[17] The usual regimen is the reverse sequential regimen in which ethinyl estradiol is given from cycle day 5 to day 25, and cyproterone acetate is given from day 5 to day 14 of the cycle. CPA has strong progestational effects and, unless combined with estrogen, tends to induce dysfunctional uterine bleeding. In Europe, CPA is available in a low-dose combined form as a birth control pill that seems to have a reasonable antiandrogenic potency without some of the side effects. It does not appear to have any significant advantage over spironolactone in treating hirsutism. There is also concern about the possibility of breast malignancy with CPA. Side effects include tiredness, lassitude, mood change, weight gain, breast discomfort, abnormal uterine bleeding, and thrombophlebitis. Although CPA is a significantly more potent androgen than spironolactone, it remains to be proved that it has any major advantages.

Medroxyprogesterone acetate (400 to 600 mg by IM injection, alternate weeks) has been reported to be effective in controlling hirsutism.[18] The side effects (complete disruption of menses, weight gain, headache, prolonged amenorrhea) together with a long delay in excretion make it a less than desirable choice, and it should perhaps be reserved for those patients who have problems with other forms of therapy.

GnRH analogs have been shown to reduce circulating androgens in women with PCOD,[19] but as yet no studies of their usefulness in hirsutism have appeared. Research into the topical use of drugs such as spironolactone has been carried out but without much success. A safe topical therapy would indeed be useful.

Present therapy for hirsutism remains unsatisfactory; removal of all unwanted hair is an unrealistic goal at present. However, the combination of medical therapy with physical removal of hair growth can make the majority of patients reasonably content with their appearance. Fuller understanding of the pathophysiology of hair growth will be required before complete success can be achieved in this area.

■ DYSFUNCTIONAL BLEEDING

Abnormal uterine bleeding can occur at intervals throughout the reproductive lifetime in women with PCOD as a result of the effects of unopposed estrogen on the endometrium. The continuing influence of unopposed estrogen can produce not only the lush but unstable proliferative endometrium of cystic hyperplasia but also adenomatous hyperplasia and endometrial carcinoma. Because of these possibilities, careful evaluation is necessary before considering therapy.

Endometrial sampling is essential in women over age 35 years with apparent dysfunctional bleeding, but it is unlikely that there would be unanimous agreement about the need for sampling of the endometrium in younger women, unless there is clear failure of a conservative treatment. Agreement over the sampling methodology is also unlikely.

Management of PCOD-related dysfunctional bleeding may involve arrest of the acute bleeding episode and the longer-term prevention of recurrent bleeding episodes and hyperplasia. Concurrent anemia may need to be treated either by oral iron therapy or occasionally by transfusion if the bleeding has been severe.

Although the endometrium is estrogen-dominated in PCOD, the use of progestational agents alone (e.g., medroxyprogesterone acetate or norethindrone, 10 mg daily for 21 days) is successful in stopping an acute bleeding episode in less than half of patients. Therefore these agents should not be used as primary therapy unless there is a strong contraindication to estrogen therapy. The arrest of the acute episode is best accomplished with combined birth control pill usage in doses of one pill four times daily until the bleeding is stopped, following which the dosage can be reduced gradually. Although a high estrogen dose is theoretically preferable, any combined BCPs can be used.[20] An alternative is to use conjugated estrogens, 2.5 mg four times daily (or the equivalent dose of another estrogen) for 3 weeks and combine this with medroxyprogesterone acetate, 10 mg daily for the last 10 days of treatment. Either regimen would be expected to stop 90 per cent of dysfunctional bleeding.[20] Nausea may be a major problem with the high doses of estrogen. Patients also should be warned that their periods following such a regimen may be heavy. Women who fail to respond to hormonal treatment require a fractional dilatation and curettage to exclude structural abormalities of the uterus (carcinoma, submucous fibroids, and so on).

Long-term prevention of dysfunctional bleeding usually can be obtained by means of withdrawal to medroxyprogesterone acetate, 10 mg daily for 10 to 14 days at 6- to 8-week intervals, or combined with birth control pills. Although the exact frequency of endometrial carcinoma in PCOD is not clearly known, the use of MPA as a safe and effective prophylaxis makes this the minimal therapy that should be applied to women with PCOD. Adenomatous hyperplasia may be treated by cyclic administration of medroxyprogesterone acetate, 10 mg daily for 21 days every 28 days over several months, then re-evaluated. Some evidence has supported this mode of therapy. It seems appropriate in women desiring to preserve their reproductive potential,[21] but it does require serial biopsies to ensure that the therapeutic goal has been achieved. If the adenomatous hyperplasia has reversed with the progestational treatment, it is logical to continue 10- to 14-day courses of medroxyprogesterone acetate, 10 mg daily at 6- to 8-week intervals until the patient wishes to attempt conception through ovulation induction.

Patients with endometrial carcinoma clearly require definitive therapy. Similarly, women with endometrial hyperplasia whose families are complete may reasonably opt for a definitive form of therapy for their problem. The role of hysterectomy in women with a history of adenomatous hyperplasia and indeed in PCOD patients in general when their families are complete remains controversial.

■ CONTRACEPTION IN WOMEN WITH PCOD

There is no reason why the birth control pill cannot be used in women with PCOD in the absence of a clear-cut contraindication. The choice would be a low-androgen pill, such as one containing 0.5 mg or less of norethindrone (Ovcon 35, Brevicon or Modicon) or ethynodiol diacetate (Demulen 50). The problem of breakthrough bleeding has frequently been addressed in normal women taking the birth control pill but rarely in women with PCOD using BCPs. There seems little problem in using a low-dose pill.

If it is elected to use another form of birth control (e.g., the barrier method or permanent sterilization of either partner), the minimal acceptable hormonal treatment (medroxyprogesterone acetate, 10 mg daily for 10 to 14 days at 4- to 8-week intervals) should be applied.

■ Issues and Risks

Management of patients with PCOD is clearly based on the reproductive needs of the patient, and these should be established from the first interview. The possibility of long-term sequelae from unopposed estrogen makes it important that patients should realize that PCOD is a lifetime diagnosis. Therefore, minimal treatment in women who are not sexually active is to prevent endometrial hyperplasia.

Polycystic ovarian disease is a relatively common problem, and the needs of the patients are usually clearly defined. The problem can be handled logically with a full understanding of the physiologic changes that are present. Ovulation induction is successful for most patients, and while the success of hirsutism treatment is more limited, the further development of drugs based on sound physiologic principles will enable us to control this aspect of PCOD. The long-term consequences of PCOD tend to be forgotten in trying to solve patients' immediate needs; the possibility that prolonged exposure to estrogen may have significant effects on the endometrium should not be overlooked. There is no consensus of optimal management of women with PCOD whose families are complete; for the present, cyclic gestagen therapy is the management of choice, although the possibility of hysterectomy with bilateral salpingo-oophorectomy can be discussed with individual patients.

REFERENCES

1. Goldzieher JW, Axelrod LR: Clinical and biochemical features of polycystic ovarian disease. Fertil Steril 1963; 14:631–641.

2. Yen SSC. The polycystic ovarian syndrome. Clin Endocrinol 1980; 12:177–208.

3. Cumming DC. Polycystic ovarian disease. Female Patient 1987; 12:19–64.

4. Franks S, Adams J, Mason H, Polson D. Ovulatory disorders in women with polycystic ovary syndrome. Clin Obstet Gynaecol 1985; 12:605–632.

5. Cumming DC, Wall SR. Non-SHBG bound testosterone as a marker for hyperandrogenism. J Clin Endocrinol Metab 1985; 61:873–876.

6. Dewailly D, Dufosse F, Vantyghem M-C, Racadot A, Lemaire C, Fossati P. Screening heterozygotes for 21-hydroxylase deficiency among hirsute women: lack of utility of the adrenocorticotropin hormone test. Fertil Steril 1988; 50:228–232.

7. Bates GW, Whitworth NS. Effect of body weight reduction on plasma androgens in obese infertile women. Fertil Steril 1982; 38:406–409.

8. Hull MGR, Savage PE, Jacobs HW. Investigation and treatment of amenorrhea resulting in normal fertility. Br Med J 1979; 1:1257–1261.

9. O'Herlihy C, Pepperall RJ, Brown JB, Smith MA, Sandri L, McBain JC. Incremental clomiphene therapy: a new method for treating persistent anovulation. Obstet Gynecol 1981; 58:535–542.

10. Lobo RA. The role of the adrenal in polycystic ovarian syndrome. Semin Reprod Endocrinol 1984; 2:251–262.

11. Wang CF, Gemzell C. The use of human gonadotropin for the induction of ovulation in women with the polycystic ovarian syndrome. Clin Endocrinol Metab 1980; 33:479–486.

12. Birkhauser MH, Huber PR, Neuenschwander E, Napflin S. Induction of follicle maturation with "pure" FSH in polycystic ovary syndrome. Geburts Frauend 1988; 48:220–227.

13. Adashi EY, Rock JA, Gizick D, Wentz A, Jones GS, Jones HW Jr. Fertility following bilateral ovarian wedge resection. A critical analysis of 90 consecutive cases of polycystic ovarian syndrome. Fertil Steril 1981; 36:320–325.

14. Gjonaess H. Polycystic ovarian syndrome treated by ovarian electrocautery through the laparoscope. Fertil Steril 1984; 41:20–25.

15. Huber J, Hosman J, Spona J. Polycystic ovarian syndrome treated by laser through the laparoscope (letter). Lancet 1988; 2:215.

16. Cumming DC. The use of spironolactone in treatment of hirsutism. Cleve Clin J Med, in press.

17. Belisle S, Love EJ. Clinical efficacy and safety of cyproterone acetate in severe hirsutism. Fertil Steril 1986; 46:1015–1020.

18. de Oliveira RFC, Novaes LP, Lima MB, Rodrigues J, France S, Khenaifes AI. A new treatment for hirsutism. Ann Intern Med 1975; 83:817–819.

19. Calogero AE, Macchi M, Montanini V, et al. Dynamics of plasma gonadotropin and sex steroid release in polycystic ovarian disease after pituitary-ovarian suppression with an analog of gonadotropin-releasing hormone. J Clin Endocrinol Metab 1987; 64:980–985.

20. Speroff L, Glass RH, Kase NG. Dysfunctional uterine bleeding. In Clinical Gynecological Endocrinology and Infertility. Baltimore: Williams and Wilkins, 1989:265–282.

21. Kistner RW. The treatment of hyperplasia and carcinoma in situ of the endometrium. Clin Obstet Gynecol 1982; 25:63–74.

Premenstrual syndromes

Anne D. Walling

■ Background

Few conditions can be more likely to cause the "heartsink" reaction[1] in physicians and bitter frustration in patients than premenstrual syndromes. This group of conditions has several different names, of which premenstrual tension (PMTS) and premenstrual syndrome (PMS) are the most widely used. Many authorities now prefer the term *premenstrual changes* to avoid negative stereotypes.[2] The interpretation of these terms is controversial, ranging from dismissal of the entire topic as a fad to belief in a classic disease model based on hormonal dysfunction.

Many definitions have been used for PMS, including a recent proposal to include late luteal dysphoric phase disorder (LLDPD) as a diagnostic category of the Diagnostic and Statistical Manual of the American Psychiatric Association (DSM-111).[3] Here, PMS is understood to consist of a clinical condition of recurrent physical and/or psychoemotional symptoms, sufficiently severe to interfere with normal functioning, which occur predictably and consistently in the luteal phase of the menstrual cycle and regress spontaneously during other phases of the cycle.

The essential feature of PMS is the *timing* of symptoms as opposed to the actual clinical presentation.[4] Over 200 symptoms have been described in PMS,[4] but each patient tends to have an individualized symptom pattern of a few specific symptoms that recur predictably every cycle.[5,6] The most common symptom clusters are summarized in Table 1. Surveys indicate that 20 to 90 per cent of women of childbearing age experience symptoms during the premenstrual phase, but only a small proportion, probably less than 10 per cent, have symptoms sufficiently severe to interfere with normal activities.[7,8]

Conversely, surveys have also identified an under-recognized group of women, also about 10 per cent of the total, who report positive premenstrual changes, such as high energy, well-being, and sexual arousal.[5,9]

PMS is characterized by controversy. Besides problems over definition, prevalence, and clinical features, there are multiple hypotheses of etiology and over 327 recommended treatments for this condition.[9] Scientific investigations have been hampered by the lack of an agreed definition, the subjective nature of many symptoms, and bias both in selecting patients and on the part of many investigators with strongly held beliefs concerning particular features of PMS.[10] Many recommendations have been made on the basis of uncontrolled trials or investigations of small numbers of patients.[10] There is no coherent literature to guide the physician in diagnosis, management, and prevention of PMS. On the other hand, over 30 books on PMS written for the general public are currently in print,[11] and the topic is regularly featured in magazines and radio or television programs targeted at women. This plethora of information and misinformation plays an important role in management.

■ Management

Because of the extensive public interest in PMS, the most common clinical scenario is for the patient to present seeking relief for her self-diagnosed PMS. However, physicians may consider the diagnosis in women presenting with a variety of symptoms if these symptoms can be linked to the menstrual cycle. A careful history clarifying the relationship of severe symptoms to the luteal phase of menstruation is the key factor in diagnosis.[4,12,13]

Patients present not just with a symptom complex but also with a set of beliefs and experiences.[13] Negative experiences and feelings of self-doubt, anger, isolation, and fear

TABLE 1. Premenstrual Syndromes: Clinical Features

Symptom Cluster	Reported Prevalance (%)	Suggested Treatment

Fluid Retention
  Weight gain
  Bloating
  Edema
	33–65	Spironolactone, 25 mg QID
		Other diuretics
		Low salt diet

Tension
  Irritability
  Anxiety
  Restlessness
  Mood swings
	66–90	Exercise
		Counseling
		Alprazolam, 0.25 mg TID
		Clonidine
		Verapamil (experimental)

Depression
  Depression
  Withdrawal
  Lethargy
	2–20	Exercise
		Counseling
		MAOI. Dosage:
		  individualized: lower than
		  for depression
		Lithium carbonate, 300 mg
		  BID or TID

Breast
  Mastalgia
  Breast engorgement
	20–38	Spironolactone
		Other diuretic
		Decrease caffeine
		Bromocriptine, 5 mg HS
		Danazol, 200 mg BID

Physical Symptoms
  Headache
  Backache
  Cramps
	20–36	Acetaminophen
		Mefenamic acid, 250 mg daily

Food Cravings
  Sweet ingestion
  Rebound hypoglycemia
	25–44	Education
		Low carbohydrate diet

Other
  Arousal
  Well-being
	10–15	

Exacerbation of:
  Asthma
  Epilepsy
  Migraines
  Violent behavior
	Unknown	Specific prophylactic therapy

of mental illness are common in PMS patients.[12,14] In addition, the patient may have read extensively on the subject and express strong loyalty to one particular definition, theory, and treatment plan for her condition. The situation may be complicated by overt or implied criticism of previous physicians, which poses a conflict of loyalties for the new physician and warns of the potential for manipulation of the physician-patient relationshp. The new PMS patient presents a clinical challenge involving both a caring response to the patient's distress and a suspicion of vulnerability to manipulation and failure.

The goal of treatment in PMS is control of symptoms to the extent that patients are able to function appropriately at all stages of the menstrual cycle. To achieve this "menstrual homeostasis"[4] requires a strong physician-patient relationship. Both patient and physician must acknowledge personal bias and the many unknowns and contradictions in suggested treatments for PMS. They must also be prepared to consider more than one strategy and to accept the long time scale involved in successful treatment. It is essential to set realistic goals that stress functional and subjective outcomes, including the alleviation, rather than the removal, of symptoms.

Without this cautious approach, there is a substantial risk of adding to the patient's problems without decreasing her symptoms. An oversolicitous approach, in which the physician undertakes the major responsibility to "cure" PMS, may encourage patient dependency and aggravate problems with self-esteem. Conversely, the physician who does not acknowledge the reality of the patient's symptoms is likely to create a hostile patient who may develop secondary symptoms and damage the physician's reputation in the community. Neither the dependent nor the angry patient gain in their ability to cope with PMS symptoms. The patient's role in developing and implementing the treatment plan is important but carries responsibilities. The patient is responsible for compliance with treatment and is the principal evaluator of its effectiveness. In addition, she has a responsibility to acknowledge the physician's role even when this involves areas of potential conflict, such as the duty of the physician to confront inappropriate behavior or refuse to prescribe an unproven treatment.

There are three stages in the management of PMS—evaluation, confirmation, and specific treatment (Fig. 1). Although the first two stages are primarily diagnostic, all three have therapeutic potential, and patients may experience considerable alleviation of symptoms before specific treatment with drugs or other modalities is instituted.[14]

■ MANAGEMENT STAGE 1. EVALUATION

History

It is important to gather information about the patient's beliefs and attitudes concerning PMS in addition to the conventional clinical history. Empathic listening to the patient's PMS story[14] provides both a description of the individual symptom complex and insight into the patient's goals, expectations, and previous experiences with health professionals. This may permit the physician to gauge the opportunities for patient education and participation in treatment.

The clinical history should pay special attention to family, social, gynecologic, and psychologic issues,[8] as these are believed to play a role in the etiology and expression of PMS. The relationshp of symptoms to the menstrual cycle is obviously critical but is

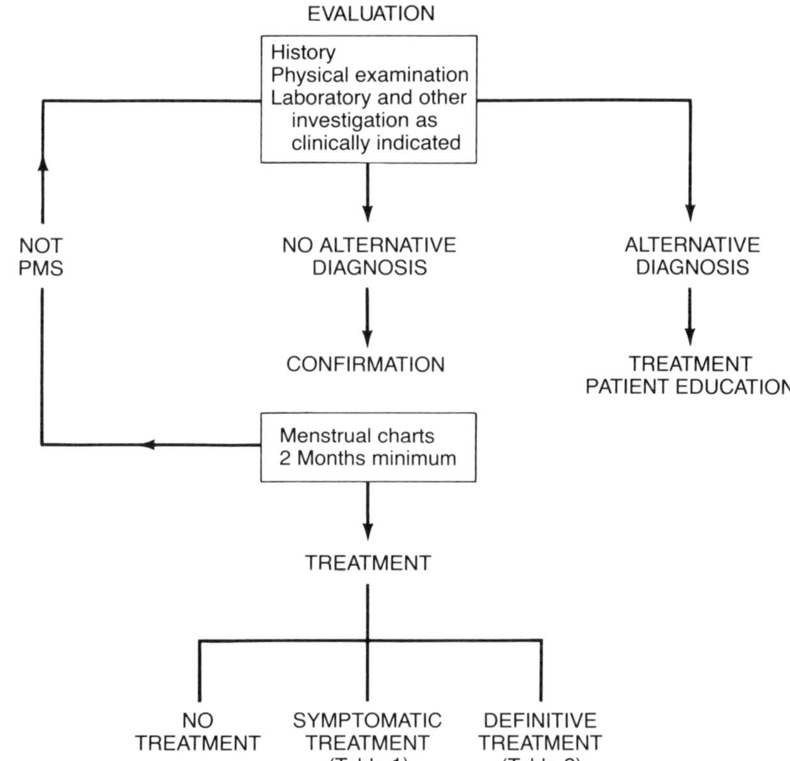

Figure 1. Investigation and management of PMS.

best documented by prospective charting, as described later.

Physical Examination

Each patient needs to be thoroughly evaluated by physical examination, including pelvic examination. With such a large potential spectrum of symptoms, the examination must be individualized for each patient to rule out significant other conditions that make up the differential diagnosis for each symptom cluster.

Other Assessments

Some investigators advocate elaborate protocols, which include blood chemistry, thyroid studies, prolactin levels, complete blood count, dexamethasone suppression test, and blood levels of estrogen, progesterone, magnesium, and pyridoxine, in addition to a battery of nutritional, psychologic, and neurometric tests.[15] A more pragmatic approach is to use an individualized program of laboratory and other diagnostic modalities to rule out coincidental and significant other disease that could explain the specific PMS symptom complex for each patient.[8] These investigations may well include psychologic tests or screens for depressive illness if emotional symptoms are a significant feature.

By the end of the evaluation stage, the physician should have a clear understanding of the specific symptom complex attributed to PMS and have ruled out other potential explanations for these symptoms. In addition, the evaluation should provide a comprehensive clinical data base on which to build appropriate treatment strategies.

■ MANAGEMENT STAGE 2. CONFIRMATION

It is essential to confirm the diagnosis by prospective documentation of symptoms during the luteal phase of the menstrual cycle for at least two and preferably more consecutive cycles.[8,10,12,14,15] Many symptom-reporting forms have been described, which range in sophistication from simple diaries[12] to visual analog scales.

Probably the best-known measurement devices are the Moos Menstrual Distress Questionnaire, the Premenstrual Assessment Form, and the Rubinow Visual Analogue Scale.[16] These commercially available forms have the advantage of being tested for validity and repeatability, but each has been criticized by those who do not share the designers' philosophy of PMS or specific area of expertise. Most forms require the patient to react to a large number of potential symptoms. This may cause problems, since each patient presents an individualized complex of a few symptoms. The questionnaires also may carry considerable powers of suggestion, which increase subjective bias. A simple approach is for the patient to record the presence of symptoms on a basal body temperature chart.[8] This confirms the historical description of the symptom complex and also relates it to the menstrual cycle (Fig. 2).

Because of the highly subjective nature of many symptoms, it may be useful also to gather data from a spouse or close associate of the patient.[12]

Failure to confirm the diagnosis of PMS by prospective charting is common in spite of the information widely available on the anticipated symptoms and subjective bias of all forms of charting. Several studies report that the diagnosis is confirmed in less than 50 per cent of PMS patients.[12,15] Charts from these patients show symptoms in other phases of the menstrual cycle. The patients require further investigation to explain their symptoms, and considerable patient education may be needed for them to accept that they do not suffer from PMS.

■ MANAGEMENT STAGE 3. TREATMENT

The many suggested treatments may be classified into four groups:

- general advice
- treatment for specific symptoms
- treatments based on theories of the etiology of PMS
- treatments that alter the menstrual cycle

A particular problem in evaluation of PMS treatment is the strong placebo response that occurs in 19 to 88 per cent of subjects.[9]

General Advice

Although there is overlap with therapies based on suggested etiologies, many inves-

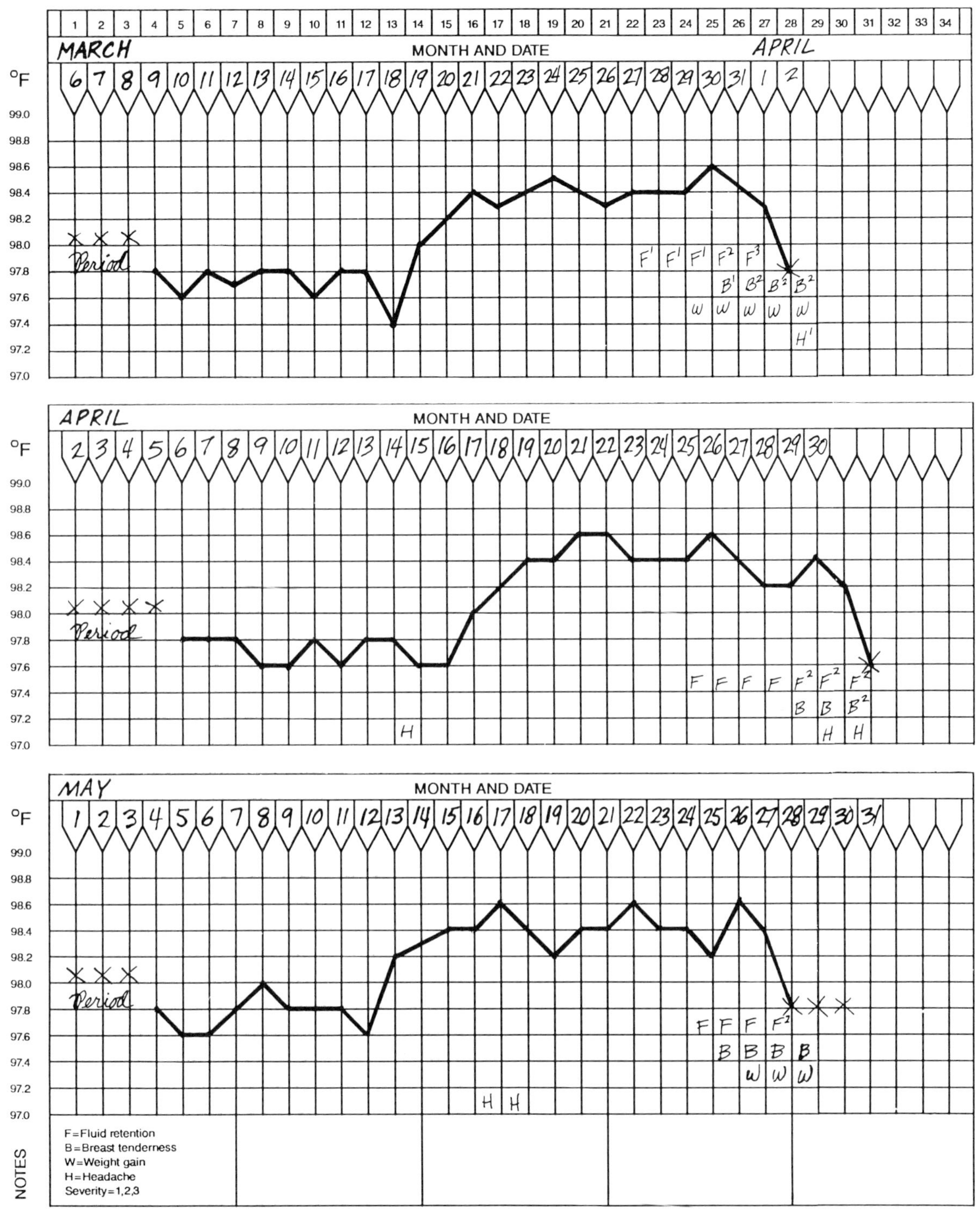

Figure 2. Basal body temperature and symptom charts in PMS.

tigators empirically recommend exercise, reassurance, avoidance of stress, reduction of smoking, moderation of caffeine and alcohol intake, and dietary modifications as a first line of treatment.[8,12,14,15] The general nature of this advice makes it suitable to begin such a program (individualized for each patient) for the long assessment period while the patient is charting symptoms and menstrual cycles. Besides direct health benefits, instituting such a program early emphasizes the patient's role in treatment and improves self-esteem.

Symptomatic Treatment

(See Table 1)

Fluid Retention. Diuretics have been used for many years to treat symptoms such as weight gain, edema, and bloating, which are commonly attributed to fluid retention in spite of the failure of physiologic studies to demonstrate true fluid retention or weight gain consistently in PMS.[17] The most widely studied diuretic has been spironolactone, perhaps because of its antiandrogenic and aldosterone-inhibiting properties. Spironolactone in dosages of 100 mg daily is widely recommended in spite of inconsistent study results.[8,14,15,17] Other diuretics and reduction of salt in the diet also have been advocated.[8,12]

Mood Swings/Irritability. Patient education, exercise, and counseling about techniques of stress reduction are particularly appropriate for this group of symptoms. For severe symptoms, the most widely used psychotropic medication is alprazolam (Xanax), which provided symptomatic relief in a small study of 22 patients.[18] The recommended dosage is 0.25 mg three times daily from day 20 until the second day of menstrual flow. The benefits of using alprazolam must be considered against unknown long-term safety and the concern about the potential of this drug for addiction.

Although not strictly psychotropic medications, clonidine and verapamil have been reported to alleviate symptoms in isolated case reports.[19,22] The mechanism may be through alpha-blockade, or it may be directly anxiolytic.

Depression. Although there is overlap with the preceding group, a smaller percentage of women have predominantly depressive features that may be severe enough to include suicidal ideation. The possibility of an underlying psychiatric condition, including alcohol or substance abuse, must be carefully excluded in all patients whose PMS symptoms are dominated by psychologic features. Another important consideration is the danger of reinforcing the idea to the patient that her symptoms are "all in her head" by the prescribing of psychotropic medications.

Monoamine oxidase inhibitors[12] and lithium carbonate have been recommended for patients with predominantly depressive symptoms.[8] Tricyclic drugs are considered inappropriate because of the 10- to 14-day delay before benefit is apparent.[12]

Breast Tenderness. Both bromocriptine (5 mg HS) and danazol (200 mg twice daily) have been reported to be effective in suppressing breast symptoms, but both are limited by side effects.[19-22] Diuretic therapy may also provide relief. Reduction of salt and caffeine intake is also recommended.

Headache and Other Pain Syndromes. Tension-type headaches and other pain syndromes may be relieved by simple analgesics such as aspirin and acetaminophen,[14] but particular attention has been paid to analgesics that block prostaglandin production. In a small study, mefenamic acid has been shown superior to placebo both in relieving pain and in improving mood swings.[20,22]

Other Symptoms. A craving for sweets, especially chocolate, has been reported to result in rebound hypoglycemia. This is best treated by patient education and the recommendation of small, carbohydrate-rich meals at frequent intervals. When other conditions, such as migraine, are triggered by premenstrual changes, it is important to avoid additional precipitants at that time and to use specific prophylactic therapy, such as beta-blockers or ergotamine preparations.

Etiology-Based Treatment

Progesterone. Progesterone treatment is the most controversial of all the issues in PMS. Uncontrolled studies have reported good results that have not been confirmed by carefully controlled double-blind studies.[4,8,10,15]

Particular problems in assessing the effectiveness of progesterone treatments are confusion about the substitution of synthetic progestins, which differ in physiologic action from natural progesterone, and the dosages necessry for therapeutic effect. Proponents advocate 25 to 100 mg of progesterone intramuscularly or 200 to 1600 mg daily by vaginal or rectal suppository from midcycle till the onset of menstrual flow.[12,15] Natural progesterone has a short half-life and is rapidly metabolized by the liver if given orally. This has led to the development of sublingual forms and gelatin capsules of micronized progesterone, which have been proved experimentally to provide adequate serum levels and were superior to placebo in one small study of PMS.[21] The dosage used was 100 mg in the morning and 200 mg at night for the 10 days of each cycle prior to menstruation. Although advocates claim that no adverse effects have been recorded with progesterone therapy even in prolonged treatment,[12] there is concern that this issue has not been adequately addressed.[10] The therapeutic dosages recommended—up to 1600 mg daily—are well in excess of physiologic rates of production, which are of the order of 40 mg daily in the midluteal phase and 210 mg per day in term pregnancy.[10]

Pyridoxine (B6). The B vitamins have been implicated in PMS either through a role in estrogen metabolism or as cofactors for neurotransmitters such as dopamine and serotonin.[4] Studies of pyridoxine supplementation have given inconsistent results[8,14,15] and are subject to all the problems of PMS research already described. Dosage is of particular concern in pyridoxine supplementation due to the danger of peripheral neuropathy. Advocates have given patients dosages of up to 6 gm daily. The daily dietary requirement is believed to be 2 to 4 mg, and the safety of a daily intake of over 200 mg has been seriously questioned.[15,19]

Others. Naltrexone, thyroid supplementation, bromocriptine, spironolactone, antifungal agents, and a bewildering array of nutritional interventions have been advocated in PMS[10,14,15,19] based on the many theories of etiology summarized in Table 2.

Treatment Altering the Menstrual Cycle

Depo-medroxyprogesterone (Depo-Provera) has been used to induce anovulation and amenorrhea in women with severe PMS. In addition to the long time-scale, this treatment has unpredictable effects and actually may exacerbate symptoms.[8,14,15,19]

This phenomenon of anovulation/amenorrhea also has been observed with oral contraceptives, which have been both advocated as a treatment and implicated as a cause of PMS.[8,12,14,15,19] Danazol has been used to disrupt the menstrual cycle through its depression of output of follicle-stimulating and luteinizing hormones, as well as competitive binding to gonadal hormones at target organs. It has been reported useful only for mastalgia[19] and has a significant incidence of side effects.[8]

Medical oophorectomy also has been attempted with gonadotropin-releasing hormone agonists that have been reported to be effective in small studies.[8,19] Surgical or radiation-induced menopause may not relieve PMS, although there may be a symptom-free gap of up to 1 year.[12] It has been suggested that PMS symptoms, particularly depression and psychologic problems, may be more severe following hysterectomy.[12] "Natural" menopause, however, is reported to terminate PMS, although an exacerbation of symptoms is common in the premenopausal period.[12]

■ Issues and Risks

Every aspect of PMS is surrounded by controversy. There is no agreed definition, etiology, diagnostic protocol, or treatment regimen, yet the condition is well-known to the general public. Patients may have considerably more "information" on the condition

---

TABLE 2. PMS Treatments Based on Theories of Etiology

Etiology	Daily Treatment	Comment
Progesterone deficiency	25–100 mg IM 200–1600 mg by vaginal or rectal suppository 300 mg oral micronized	Controversial; dosage individualized; treat from ovulation to menstruation
Pyridoxine	50–300 mg	Controversial; danger of neuropathy
Prolactin excess	Bromocriptine, 5 mg HS	
Prostaglandin deficiency	Diet supplement with zinc, magnesium, gamma-linoleic acid	Link with other theories; prostaglandin excess also postulated
Aldosteronism	Spironolactone, 25 mg QID	?Link to progesterone/prolactin
Hypothyroidism	As clinically indicated	
Endogenous opiates	Naltrexone, 25 mg BID	Experimental; links several other theories
Food allergies	PMS prevention diet	

than their physicians do, but this may be founded more on advocacy than on science. Many of the recommended treatments are based on flawed studies or empiric observations, and their usefulness is difficult to assess in view of the strong placebo effect. For some of these treatments, there is not only little proof of benefit, but also a danger of serious side effects. PMS is a strenuous challenge to the physician's skill in communication and empathy.

REFERENCES

1. O'Dowd TC. Five years of heartsink patients in general practice. Br Med J 1988; 297:528–530.
2. Endicott J, Halbreich U. Clinical significance of premenstrual dysphoric changes. J Clin Psychiatry 1988; 49:486–489.
3. American Psychiatric Association. Diagnostic and Statistical Manual of Mental Disorders. 3rd ed. Washington, DC: APA, 1987:367–369.
4. Halbreich U, Alt IH, Paul L. Premenstrual changes: impaired hormonal homeostasis. Endocrinol Metab Clin North Am 1988; 17:173–194.
5. Siegel JP, Myers BJ, Dineen MK. Premenstrual tension syndrome symptom clusters. J Reprod Med 1987; 32:395–399.
6. Widholm O. Epidemiology of premenstrual tension syndrome and primary dysmenorrhea. In Dawood MY, McGuire JL, Demers LM (eds). Premenstrual Syndrome and Dysmenorrhea. Baltimore: Urban & Schwarzenberg, 1985:3–12.
7. Woods NF, Most A, Derby GK. Prevalence of perimenstrual symptoms. Am J Public Health 1982; 72:1257–1264.
8. Wentz AC. Dysmenorrhea, premenstrual syndrome, and related disorders. In Jones HW III, Wentz AC, Burnett LS (eds). Novak's Textbook of Gynecology. 11th ed. Baltimore: Williams & Wilkins, 1988:251–259.
9. Blumenthal SJ, Nadelson CC. Mood changes associated with reproductive life events: an overview of research and treatment strategies. J Clin Psychiatry 1988; 49:466–468.
10. Dawood MY. Overview—consensus and controversy. In Dawood MY, McGuire JL, Demers LM (eds). Premenstrual Syndrome and Dysmenorrhea. Baltimore: Urban & Schwarzenberg, 1985:221–226.
11. Subject Guide to Books in Print 1986–1987. Vol. 3. New York: RR Bowker Co, 1986:5109–5110.
12. Dalton K. The premenstrual syndrome and progesterone therapy. 2nd ed. Chicago: William Heinemann, 1984:10–38.
13. Golub S. A developmental perspective. In Gise LH, Kase NG, Berkowitz RL (eds). The Premenstrual Syndromes. New York: Churchill Livingstone, 1988:7–19.
14. Keye WR. Premenstrual syndrome: seven steps in management. Postgrad Med 1988; 83:167–173.
15. Osofsky HJ, Keppel WH. Clinical evaluation and management. In Gise LH, Kase NG, Berkowitz RL (eds). The Premenstrual Syndromes. New York: Churchill Livingstone, 1988:97–108.
16. Rubinow DR, Roy-Byrne P, Hoban MC. Menstrually-related mood disorders: methodological and conceptual issues. In Dawood MY, McGuire JL, Demers LM (eds). Premenstrual Syndrome and Dysmenorrhea. Baltimore: Urban & Schwarzenberg, 1985:27–40.
17. Vellacott ID, O'Brien PMS. Effect of spironolactone on premenstrual syndrome symptoms. J. Reprod Med 1987; 32:429–434.
18. Smith S, Rinehart JS, Ruddock VE, Schiff R. Treatment of premenstrual syndrome with alprazolam. Obstet Gynecol 1987; 70:37–43.
19. Chuong CJ, Coulam CB. Current views and the beta-endorphin hypothesis. In Gise LH, Kase NG, Berkowitz RL (eds). The Premenstrual Syndromes. New York: Churchill Livingstone, 1988:75–96.
20. Mira M, McNeil D, Fraser IS, Vizzard J, Abraham S. Mefenamic acid in the treatment of premenstrual syndrome. Obstet Gynecol 1986; 68:395–398.
21. Dennerstein L, Spencer-Gardner C, Gotts G, Brown JB, Smith MA, Burrows GD. Progesterone and the premenstrual syndrome: a double-blind crossover trial. Br Med J 1985; 290:1617–1621.
22. Chihal HJ. Indications for drug therapy in premenstrual syndrome patients. J Reprod Med 1987; 32:449–52.

Pressure sores

Richard E. Melcher

Pressure sores (also referred to as decubitus ulcers) are a common but preventable clinical problem seen primarily in extended care facilities and acute care hospitals. It is estimated that 60 to 70 per cent of such lesions develop in elderly patients, occur most often during the first 2 weeks of hospital confinement, and add significantly to nursing time (up to 50 per cent) and cost per patient.[1] When preventive measures fail and a superficial sore develops, conservative treatment should effect healing. Deeper wounds may be life-threatening and require intensive and specialized care that employs a treatment plan familiar to nursing personnel to avoid confusion and speed recovery.

■ Background

The crucial factor in the formation of pressure sores is an uneven (shearing), excessive, repeated or prolonged application of pressure to high-risk tissue areas. Subcutaneous fat is extremely vulnerable to shearing forces that compromise blood supply by angular stretching of the vessels, leading to thrombosis. Skin padding over hard bony sites is equally vulnerable to direct pressure forces, with cellular ischemia occurring as a result of microvascular obstruction.

Pressures in excess of 30 mm Hg are sufficient to obstruct lymphatic, venous, and arteriolar circulation. Uninterrupted pressure in the range of 40 to 100 mm Hg is sufficient to produce irreversible ischemia and tissue necrosis. Although a sore may develop after one bout of sustained pressure, most sores result from repeated ischemic insults without adequate time for tissue recovery. Following the tissue insult, a number of destructive processes occur. Nutrient and oxygen transport as well as lymphatic drainage are compromised as tissue separation occurs. Vascular changes include platelet and red cell aggregation, microthrombi formation, and eventual intravascular fibrin deposition. The deposition of fibrin is primarily responsible for the delay in wound healing, and medications such as antibiotics and vasodilators are unable to reach the wound margin.[2]

Four major factors contribute to the development of pressure sores: pressure, time, shearing, and moisture. In the formation of pressure sores, there is a linear relation between skin integrity and age, and there is an inverse relation between time and pressure. Characteristics of patients prone to sores include bowel or bladder incontinence, excessive skin perspiration, altered nutritional status, and altered mental status. Patients with spinal cord injuries and stroke patients require special attention because of a decrease or loss of sensation and protective reflexes, and the presence of spasticity that interferes with proper positioning. Other patient-related risks include fractures, malignancy, diabetes, anemia, and cardiovascular and peripheral vascular disease. Overt environmental risk factors include oversedation, infrequent or incorrect turning techniques, neglect of hygienic skin care, misuse of electric beds (e.g., lack of footboards, food crumbs), and exfoliation of the skin with the removal of tape.[3]

More than 95 per cent of all pressure sores develop on the lower part of the body in five classic sites: the greater trochanter, sacrum, ischial tuberosity, lateral malleolus of the ankle, and the calcaneus. A useful classification system that is based upon the appearance of the lesion and the depth of invasion was introduced by J. D. Shea in 1975. A grade 1 sore is erythematous, warm, and indurated. It blanches with pressure and the skin is intact, and it is easily reversible with pressure relief. In grade 2, the lesion is often cool, and the skin break may extend down to, but not include, subcutaneous tissues. In grade 3, the tissue break penetrates the subcutaneous fat, demonstrates extensive undermining, is frequently necrotic and covered by a thick eschar, and when unroofed has a foul-smelling drainage. In grade 4, periosteum and bone may be involved or fistulas may be present. The risk for sepsis is high, and surgical repair and antibiotics are required.[4]

The complications of pressure sores are potentially life-threatening and often necessitate surgery. Typically, sepsis occurs with grade 3 or 4 sores and those colonized by certain gram-negative and anaerobic bacteria, including *Bacteroides fragilis*, *Proteus mirabilis*, and *Pseudomonas*.[5] Other infections include osteomyelitis (biopsy is necessary), cellulitis, and pyarthrosis. Systemic antibiotics are reserved for such complications, and choices are based on culture and sensitivity test results. Initial coverage includes an anaerobic agent (e.g., clindamycin) and an aminoglycoside (e.g., gentamicin). Wound colonization often results in poor correlation with infective organisms, thereby making swab cultures misleading. Systemic amyloidosis may occur as a consequence of chronic suppurative infection (such as osteomyelitis), and fistulas can penetrate to deep structures, including bowel and bladder.[6] Tetanus is another potential complication, and immunizations must be administered.

Risk assessment is vital to pressure sore prevention. A number of assessment scales may be employed to identify patients at greatest risk for developing a sore upon admission to a hospital or extended care facility. Any condition or agent that decreases spontaneous positional changes (e.g., sedatives), contributes to incontinence (diuretics, restraints), or reduces tissue perfusion (e.g., dehydration) can increase the risk.

Management

Countless techniques have been proposed for the prevention and management of pressure sores. Through the years, physicians have employed a variety of agents, including heavy metals, bismuth and bourbon paste, iodine and sugar paste, insulin, maggots, and more recently hyperbaric oxygen and fibrinolytic enhancement. Although it is difficult to assess and often duplicate the results of numerous techniques for prevention and treatment, most sores are superficial and will respond to conservative measures. The management of pressure sores can be improved in any facility by the implementation of a standardized approach based on four principles of care: (1) pressure relief, (2) debridement of necrotic tissue, (3) disinfection, and (4) support of granulation tissue growth. The use of an established skin care protocol should reduce confusion among nursing staff, contain costs, and achieve greater success in wound healing.[1]

■ PRESSURE RELIEF

Although it is well established that relief of pressure is the primary preventive and treatment measure, adequate steps often are not implemented, presumably due to limited personnel and materials. Regardless of a sore's classification, local wound pressure must be reduced to a level that allows for nutrient transport, oxygenation, and waste product removal. None of the currently available products is capable of 100 per cent pressure reduction. Their purpose is to reduce pressure and shear as much as possible.

Many wheelchairs have plastic or imitation leather surfaces, and the sling support does not allow for pressure distribution. Indeed, investigators have demonstrated pressures exceeding 300 mm Hg over the ischial tuberosities. A strong support such as plywood should be placed in the wheelchair to afford a flat, firm surface for equal weight distribution. This should be covered with a Jay cushion to further reduce ischial pressures and lessen the risk of shear. Every 20 to 30 minutes, patients should also perform pushups (lifts), or the staff should raise the patient, to allow for capillary recirculation.[7]

A number of bed devices are designed to redistribute or diminish pressure over bony prominences. Two classes of support systems exist—static and dynamic. The static devices are immobile, inexpensive, and somewhat effective for the redistribution of pressure and rely on material that cushions and molds to the body surface. Convoluted foam overlays (egg crates) are effective when thick enough so that the weight of the patient cannot completely compress the material. Gel, water, and air-filled devices are other static systems that are employed with success. (Sheepskins provide less pressure reduction but are somewhat effective in preventing shearing.) The siliconized hollow fiber mattress (e.g., Sierex) is a more expensive static support system that is also effective in minimizing pressure.

Dynamic devices employ an electrical pump to alternate currents of air to minimize pressure over bony prominences. One category of dynamic device is an air-fluidized bed (e.g., Clinitron), which utilizes an air column pumped through a bed of fine, medical-grade optical glass spheres to provide a form of levitation. This bed is employed after plastic surgical repair of deep sores, when multiple sores complicate positioning, and when wound deterioration occurs. It requires unique nursing care and is quite expensive.

A second type of dynamic device is the alternating pressure mattress, which consists of air cells arranged horizontally or vertically. Some provide for aeration of the patient's skin to reduce heat buildup and tissue maceration. Ideally, alternating pressure devices should remove pressure long enough to permit tissue perfusion; however, most systems do not achieve this goal and are not equal to air-fluidized beds. Therefore, it is essential that alternating pressure beds and static support systems be coupled with patient repositioning for successful pressure release.[8] Patients must be turned every 2 hours, and the 30-degree oblique positioning technique is employed in favor of 90-degree positioning. Rotational charts placed on the door should be maintained to verify treatments. Patient bridging with up to 6 pillows may be necessary to pad high-risk tissue surfaces.[9]

■ DEBRIDEMENT
(Table 1)

Necrotic tissue allows for bacterial growth, reduces oxygen tension, and prevents the formation of granulation tissue. Step-wise surgical debridement removes devitalized, nonviable tissue in grades 3 and 4 sores. The procedure is continued (usually three times a week) until healthy tissue is located, as evidenced by minimal bleeding. If pain control is needed, a systemic agent such as Vistaril, with or without an analgesic (e.g., Demerol), is administered 30 minutes prior to the procedure. Local wound infiltration is not satisfactory or desirable.

Enzymatic debridement may be employed during intervals between step-wise surgical debridement. Before application, loose necrotic debris should be irrigated from the wound with saline. A thin layer of agent is applied every 8 hours to the ulcer base not covered by eschar. Enzymatic debriding agents will not penetrate eschar or remove large amounts of necrotic tissue, and the simultaneous use of disinfectants will inactivate the enzyme agent. Wounds with excessive exudate can be effectively cleansed with dextranomers such as Debrisan. These agents absorb wound exudate, decrease inflammation, and are relatively easy to use.[10]

TABLE 1. Debridement: Modalities for Grades 3 and 4 Pressure Sores

Surgical
Employed two to three times per week. May be preceded by systemic analgesia
Mechanical
Wet-to-dry gauze dressings soaked in 0.9% sodium chloride or acetic acid
Enzyme
Applied thinly every 8 hours to supplement surgical debridement. Mesh gauze soaked in fibrinolysin-desoxyribonuclease solution may be used as adjunct to mechanical debridement
Hydrotherapy
Hubbard tank 3 to 5 days per week. Water Pik for bedridden or home-bound patients on daily basis with normal saline

Mesh gauze soaked with normal saline, acetic acid, or an enzyme system (e.g., Elase solution) can be applied to the sore as a wet-to-dry treatment for mechanical and combined mechanical-enzymatic debridement. The gauze must be packed into the sore to be successful. Hydrotherapy may achieve debridement as adjunctive therapy. Whirlpool or Hubbard tanks are commonly used in extended care facilities and hospitals (especially for lower extremity sores), but a Water Pik is effective and portable for bedside and home therapy.[7]

■ DISINFECTION

The wound's bacterial count must be kept low to effect healing. Studies suggest that wound closure is facilitated when bacterial counts are reduced to less than 10^5 bacteria per gram of wound tissue (or less than 10^6 bacteria per ml of exudate). Systemic antibiotics are ineffective because they do not penetrate the ulcer margin. Topical agents are effective against surface bacteria and do not penetrate deeper tissues. Once clean red granulation tissue develops, use of a disinfectant should be stopped. When enzyme systems are not being used, disinfection can be performed in conjunction with debridement to remove loosely adherent necrotic tissue and reduce bacterial contamination.[11]

Soaps, astringents, and antibacterial cleansers are of limited value in superficial sores, although they are useful in prevention. Topical antibiotics can sensitize the skin, have systemic toxic effects, lack efficacy against the bacterial moisture in the wound, and promote bacterial resistance. Their use is not recommended. Commonly used disinfectants include chlorhexidine gluconate (Hibiclens), povidone-iodine (Betadine), and acetic acid. Serious systemic toxicity and nephropathy can occur if an extremely large or deep sore is treated with povidone-iodine, and caution is advised.[12] When acetic acid is employed, the surrounding tissues can be protected with a thin rim of zinc oxide. Cleansing is carried out every 8 hours as a 2- to 5-minute wash with sterile gauze. A normal saline rinse should then be employed, followed by air drying. If the surrounding tissues become irritated, Granulex Spray may be applied and gently massaged into the skin to reduce epithelial desiccation and cornification.[13] All disinfection is discontinued when a clean red base is established.[14]

■ SUPPORT TISSUE GROWTH

Following the successful relief of pressure, debridement of all necrotic tissue, and adequate disinfection, the final step is to promote the growth of healthy granulation tissue. The newest forms of dressings—occlusive and semiocclusive materials—when properly applied, facilitate granulation by providing a clean, moist protective environment that permits fibroblast survival. Most synthetic dressings can be categorized into three groupings—hydrocolloid, polyurethane, and biodressings.

Hydrocolloid dressings are adhesive, gel-producing, water-impermeable membranes that can be left on for a maximum of 7 days. Advantages also include moderate fluid absorption, retention time, and wound-dressing interaction. Polyurethane film is an alternative dressing that is transparent-adherent. Although it is transparent and allows for wound inspection, exudate leakage is a problem, and absorption is minimal. Biodressings are hydrogels of water and polyethylene oxide reinforced with polyethylene film. The materials have a high water content and an adherence problem. All three synthetic dressings have efficacy in grade 2 and *superficial* grade 3 sores of limited size.[8] Occlusive dressings are not widely accepted for deeper grade 3 and grade 4 sores, because of the risk for re-emerging infection. In larger grade 3 and extensive grade 4 sores, linen gauze soaked with Ringer's solution (or normal saline) is applied wet and kept moist between dressing changes every 6 to 8 hours. The wound is inspected regularly for progress and infection. If infection re-emerges, disinfection is repeated.

To effect wound closure, the clinician must treat underlying conditions that retard the development of granulation tissue. Protein, carbohydrate, vitamin (especially C and A) and mineral (especially zinc) deficiencies must be corrected, and medical conditions such as diabetes and congestive heart failure must be controlled to achieve success.[14] If a pressure sore fails to improve or heal, or if infection recurs, the physician should investigate the need for further disinfection, debridement, and relief of pressure.

■ Issues and Risks

Pressure sores have frustrated physicians through the centuries and continue to pose a significant risk to institutionalized and debilitated patients. Although there is no consensus on the best method of treatment, clearly the cause is unrelieved pressure or shearing at critical hard sites. Prevention requires the identification of high-risk patients and maintenance of skin sanitation and pressure relief by nursing personnel.

In the absence of effective prevention, focus on a safe and standardized treatment approach that is familiar to the nursing staff. Pressure relief can be achieved with a number of devices that can reduce skin pressure below 40 mm Hg if coupled with frequent patient turning. The air-fluidized bed is the exception to this rule, but it is quite expensive and requires specialized nursing protocols. Debridement and disinfection clear the wound of necrotic material and excess bacteria, allowing oxygen tension to rise and the formation of granulation tissue.

Appropriate attention to underlying medical conditions is necessary to effect closure. Complications such as cellulitis, osteomyelitis, and sepsis require culturing and the institution of systemic antibiotics. Congestive heart failure, diabetes, and edematous states must be treated, or wound closure cannot be achieved.

Lastly, it is important to remember that most sores are superficial and require only conservative management.

REFERENCES

1. Melcher RE, Longe RL, Gelbart AO. Pressure sores in the elderly. Postgrad Med 1988; 83:299–307.
2. Seiler WO, Stahelin HB. Recent findings on decubitus ulcer pathology: implications for care. Geriatrics 1986; 41:47–50, 53–57, 60.
3. Staas WE, LaMantia JG. Decubitus ulcers and rehabilitation medicine. Int J Dermatol 1982; 21:437–444.
4. Shea JD. Pressure sore classification and management. Clin Orthop 1975; 112:89–100.
5. Bryan CS, Dew CE, Reynolds KL. Bacteria associated with decubitus ulcers. Arch Intern Med 1983; 143:2093–2095.
6. Sugarman B, Hawes S, Musher DM. Osteomyelitis beneath pressure sores. Arch Intern Med 1983; 143:683–688.

7. Rousseau P. Pressure sores in the elderly: part I. Geriatr Med Today 1988; 7:28–40.

8. Mulder GD, LaPan M. Decubitus ulcers: update on new approaches to treatment. Geriatrics 1988; 43:37–50.

9. Stewart P, Wharton GW. Bridging: an effective and practical method of preventive skin care for the immobilized person. South Med J 1976; 69:1469–1473.

10. Seiler W, Stahelin HB. Decubitus ulcers: treatment through five therapeutic principles. Geriatrics 1985; 409:30–44.

11. Krizek TJ, Robson MC. Evolution of quantitative bacteriology in wound management. Am J Surg 1975; 130:579–584.

12. Zamora JL. Chemical and microbiologic characteristics and toxicity of povidone-iodine solutions. Am J Surg 1986; 151:400–406.

13. Yucel VE, Basmajian JV. Decubitus ulcers: healing effects of an enzymatic spray. Arch Phys Med Rehab 1974; 55:517–519.

14. Bobel LM. Nutritional implications in the patient with pressure sores. Nurs Clin North Am 1987; 22:379–390.

Prostate cancer

Troy H. Guthrie, Jr.

▨ Background

Attitudes toward the management of prostate cancer have changed over the past two decades. As the number of men whose age exceeds 65 years has steadily increased, a realization has emerged that prostate cancer in an otherwise healthy elderly man will be the major limiting factor in his survival and requires therapy tailored to his other health factors and personal desires.

Adenocarcinoma of the prostate was diagnosed in approximately 90,000 men in 1989 and resulted in about 28,000 deaths. Approximately one half were diagnosed in a localized stage, and the other 50 per cent had metastatic disease. Prostate cancer has certain ethnic variations: it is less common in orientals and more aggressive in blacks.

The first factor that clearly influences aggressiveness of prostate cancer is *the histologic grade or degree of differentiation.* Numerous systems for grading prostate cancer exist, but probably best recognized is that proposed by Gleason.[1] Based on a retrospective analysis of a large series of patients with prostate cancer, Gleason's report indicated convincingly a relationship among tumor grade, the incidence of metastases, and long-term survival. A second factor that predicts the subsequent incidence of metastases and overall survival is *tumor volume of the pros-tate primary.*[2] The larger the tumor volume, the greater the incidence of local invasion and distant metastases. Of note is the fact that as the tumor volume increases, the degree of tumor anaplasia increases. Thus, large prostate primaries have higher tumor grades and a poorer overall prognosis.

A final factor influencing prognosis and management decisions is *the stage of the malignancy.* The system used by most physicians in this country is the American ABCD system. This clinical staging system is based on findings on digital rectal examination as well as the presence of either local invasion or distant metastases. *Stage A* is prostate cancer discovered incidentally on transurethral prostatectomy for obstructive uropathy symptoms. No lesion can be palpated by digital rectal examination. Stage A is usually divided into A_1, or cancer comprising less than 5 per cent of prostate removed and low grade on histologic review. Stage A_1 has a 5 per cent incidence of pelvic lymphadenopathy. In stage A_2, the cancer occupies more than 5 per cent of prostate removed and/or is of moderate to high grade. A 34 per cent incidence of pelvic lymph node metastases has been reported. *Stage B* is disease recognized by digital examination; it occupies more than 5 per cent of the prostate but does not extend through the prostate capsule or invade the seminal vesicles. Up to 40 per cent of patients with Stage B have pelvic adenopathy. *Stage C* is a cancer that invades periprostatic tissues or the seminal vesicles. The majority of patients with this stage ultimately give evidence of distant metastases. *Stage D* is a prostate primary of any size with detectable distant metastases. Survival curves show that stages A_2 through D have an increasing impact on survival when evaluated by an actuarial method.

■ PATTERNS OF PRESENTATION AND SUGGESTED DIAGNOSTIC EVALUATION

Prostate cancer has very predictable patterns of presentation that should prompt certain diagnostic studies to determine the stage of the disease prior to institution of therapy. These presentations include asymptomatic prostate nodules found incidentally on rectal examination; bone pain in elderly men; symptoms of bladder outlet obstruction or irritability, and asymptomatic azotemia. An important but uncommon pattern of presentation is that of carcinoma of unknown primaries in elderly men.

Asymptomatic prostate nodules, contrary to many physicians' beliefs, are usually malignant (60 per cent). When the rectal examination reveals a prostate nodule, the overall size, invasion, or fixation to other local tissues should be determined carefully. Blood for prostate acid phosphatase (PAP) and prostate-specific antigen (PSA) determination should be drawn no sooner than 2 days after the rectal examination. The patient's history should be reviewed for symptoms of bone pain and bladder outlet obstruction, and for constitutional symptoms such as weight loss. Any suggestion of metastatic disease, including nodules greater than 2 cm, invasion of periprostatic tissues upon rectal examination, or histories of bone pain or weight loss should be noted. A transrectal biopsy will confirm the diagnosis of malignancy. Once a tissue diagnosis is obtained, a bone scan should be done even if bone pain is absent, since 20 per cent of patients with bone involvement are initially asymptomatic. A computed tomography (CT) scan with contrast will better define periprostatic extension, bladder outlet invasion or obstruction, and regional lymph node metastases. Therapy then should be individualized based on stage, other health problems, and patient's preferences.

The second most common presentation is that of painful bone metastases in elderly men. Often this complaint is initially confused with complaints related to pre-existing osteoarthritis, rheumatoid arthritis, or low back syndrome. The pain of bone metastases, however, is relentlessly progressive, poorly relieved by nonsteroidal anti-inflammatory drugs, and primarily involves the lower axial skeleton. Plain films reveal the lytic-blastic lesions of prostate cancer, which preferentially involves the hips and lower spinal column. Rectal examination should reveal the primary lesion, which then can be biopsied for tissue diagnosis. Blood for determination of the tumor markers PAP and PSA should be drawn prior to palliative hormonal therapy to aid assessment of response.

Bladder outlet obstruction is another common initial manifestation of prostate cancer. This will be seen as symptoms of straining on voiding, dribbling, or frequency, or occasionally as asymptomatic azotemia. Many elderly men will not volunteer symptoms of bladder outlet obstruction so must be questioned carefully. Urinary tract infections and asymptomatic bacteriuria on routine urinalysis also should trigger an investigation for bladder outlet obstruction in older men. Likewise, plausible explanations for azotemia, including diabetes mellitus, hypertension, and nephrosclerosis may exist, but these are generally nonreversible; thus each elderly man with azotemia should have a careful evaluation to eliminate treatable bladder outlet obstruction as a cause of renal failure.

In patients found to have bladder outlet obstruction from prostatic pathology, a transrectal biopsy should be done for histologic diagnosis, followed by meaures to relieve the obstruction. If prostate cancer is documented, then staging should be undertaken as previously discussed.

Among the less common presentations of prostate cancer is that of carcinoma of unknown primary (CUP) syndrome. This syndrome accounts for 3 to 7 per cent of all diagnosed malignancies. The prognosis for most patients with CUP syndrome is bleak, with a median survival of 6 to 9 months and a 5-year survival rate of 3 per cent. Most of the CUP malignancies are found histologically to be adenocarcinomas. In elderly men, the only readily treatable metastatic adenocarcinoma is prostate cancer, which usually responds to hormonal maneuvers. Atypical presentations of prostate cancer include supraclavicular lymphadenopathy, pulmonary coin lesions, and primarily lytic bone metastases. If doubt exists about the site of origin of malignancies in elderly men, obtain serum PSA and PAP and review the case with the attending pathologist. If a prostate primary is possible, then immunoperoxidase stains of the biopsy specimen for PSA and PAP have a diagnostic accuracy approaching 100 per cent. Positive stains for PSA and PAP identify a prostate source of the CUP syndrome, and hormonal therapy likely will palliate the patient.

▪ Treatment

Therapy is stratified into modalities for patients with localized disease: stages A, B, and C, and those with metastatic disease stage D. In years past, many physicians were reluctant to treat elderly men with prostate cancer. The long natural history of prostate cancer, the coexistence of medical problems, combined with the fear of excessive toxicity, fostered a laissez-faire attitude toward prostate cancer. Improved survival of men in their 60s and 70s and a better understanding of how to use the treatment modalities available for prostate cancer has led to more aggressive approaches.

▪ LOCALIZED PROSTATE CANCER

Stages A_1, A_2, and B are treated with either surgery or radiation therapy. The selection of therapy is usually based on local health resources, the patient's physiologic state, and the sexual potency of the patient. Surgery is generally selected for patients who are physically able to tolerate a radical prostatectomy. Both the peritoneal and retropubic procedures are used, but neither has clear-cut superior results. The choice of procedure then becomes the surgeon's own preference, based on training and past experience. The ideal patient should have a small tumor and a projected long life expectancy. The major complications of radical prostatectomy are incontinence and loss of potency. All patients undergoing standard radical prostatectomy lose potency, and about 15 per cent have some degree of in-

continence.[3] Local recurrences develop in 10 per cent of patients, especially those with larger tumors or periprostatic invasion on histologic examination of the surgical specimen. Long-term disease-free survival for both stages A_2 and B disease is approximately 90 per cent at 5 years and 70 per cent at 10 years.[5] More recently, a potency-sparing operation has been developed. This spares the innervation of the corpus cavernosa on the side opposite the prostate primary. Approximately 70 per cent of men undergoing this operation retain potency one year later.[4] Whether the local recurrence rate and long-term disease-free survival equal a standard radical prostatectomy is unknown.

The development of high-energy radiation sources from linear accelerators, coupled with improvements in tumor localization and treatment planning techniques, has resulted in radiation therapy as an acceptable option for locoregional prostate cancer. Using tumoricidal doses of 7000 rads, radiation therapy obtains results comparable to surgery in stages A_2 and B prostate cancer. In addition, most patients with stage C prostate cancer currently are being treated with irradiation. Most series show an 80 per cent for 5-year and a 60 per cent for 10-year disease-specific survival for stage B. The comparable figures for stage C are 60 per cent and 40 per cent.[5]

Patients treated with radiation therapy tend to be older and physiologically more frail. Complications from radiation therapy include immediate tissue reactions requiring delays of radiation therapy, such as proctitis and desquamation of skin. Late side effects are relatively uncommon, and most patients retain potency.

▪ METASTATIC PROSTATE CANCER

The last decade has witnessed major advances in the understanding of the endocrinology of both normal and malignant prostate cells. Identification of testosterone receptors in prostate cancer has created a concept of hormonal maneuvers in prostate cancer similar to that of breast cancer. The concept of an interrelated hormonal axis involving the hypothalamus, pituitary, testes, adrenal, and prostate (Fig. 1) has led to better use of previously available hormonal

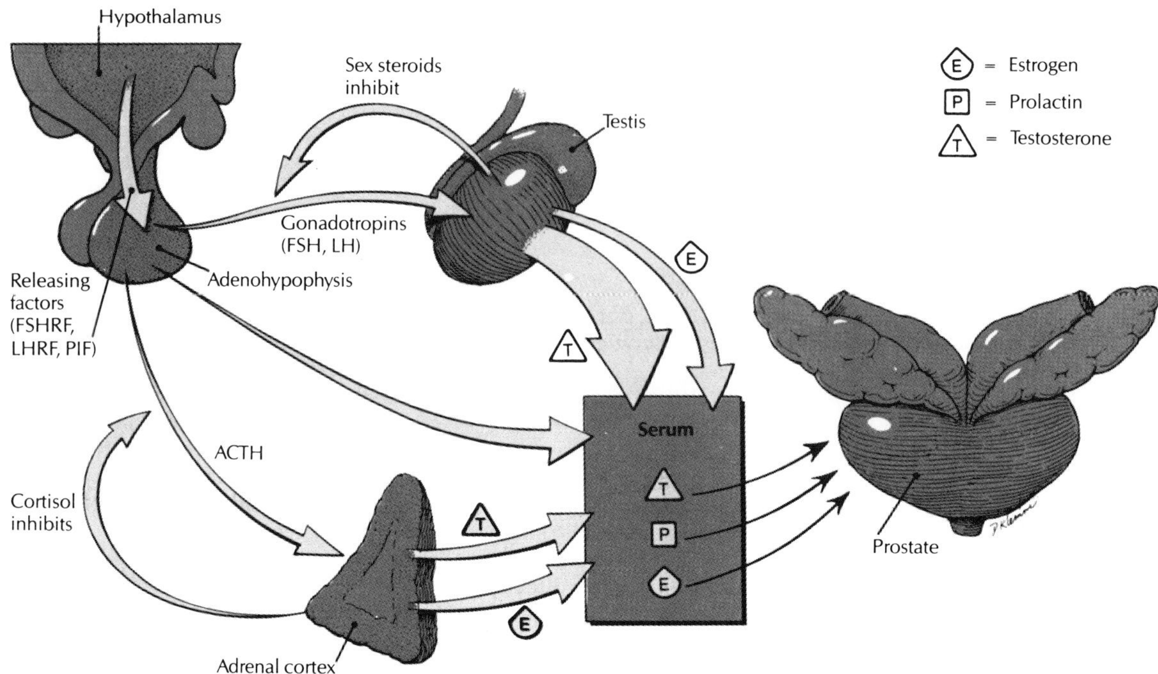

Figure 1. The prostate as an endocrine-responsive organ. Points to consider: (1) Testosterone receptors have been identified in normal and malignant prostate tissue. (2) There is evidence for the utility of testosterone receptor assay in predicting response to hormonal therapy. (3) A complex, interdependent hormonal pathway links the hypothalamus, the pituitary, the testes, and the prostate. Numerous areas exist in which hormonal maneuvers could affect prostatic tumor growth. ACTH, adrenocorticotropic hormone; FSH, follicle-stimulating hormone; FSHRF, follicle-stimulating hormone-releasing factor; LH, luteinizing hormone; LHRF, luteinizing hormone-releasing factor; PIF, prolactin-inhibiting factor. (Reprinted with permission from Guthrie TH Jr: Prostate cancer. Am Fam Physician 1987; 37:217–224, published by the American Academy of Family Physicians.)

maneuvers and development of new agents. Ten years ago only orchiectomy and diethylstilbestrol (DES) were commonly used forms of hormonal therapy. Today, gonadotropin-releasing hormone (GNRH) agonists and antiandrogens are commercially available and are having their role in treating metastatic prostate cancer better defined.

The current approach to metastatic disease is to treat symptomatic patients only. Some controversy exists about this approach, since retrospective analysis of the VA prostate cancer trials suggested some benefit in treating asymptomatic patients with adverse histologic features.[6] In addition, a nonrandomized trial at the Mayo Clinic also supported early therapy of asymptomatic patients.[7] Despite this information, until large-scale clinical trials lend further credence to this viewpoint, only symptomatic patients or patients judged at risk of impending symptoms should receive palliative radiation therapy or hormonal therapy.

Symptoms warranting therapy include bone pain, spinal cord compression, and obstructive uropathy. Less clear-cut indications include weight loss and malaise. Patients judged at risk for impending symptomatology include those with intensively positive bone scans or critical involvement of the spine and pelvis, those with rapidly enlarging tumor masses, and those with rapidly rising tumor markers (PAP and PSA).

Radiation Therapy. Patients with painful bone metastases not responsive to hormonal therapy or those with impending pathologic fractures in weight-bearing bones should receive palliative radiation therapy. In addition, patients with spinal cord compression should receive radiation therapy after institution of dexamethasone to prevent the initial inflammatory response of radiation. Radiation doses in the range of 3000 to 4000 rads given over 2 to 3 weeks are effective. Prophylactic or definitive orthopedic fixation of potential fractures of the hip joint or femur should be followed by regional irradiation with similar doses.

Estrogen Therapy. The most commonly employed hormonal therapy of metastatic prostate cancer is the use of estrogens, particularly DES. The most common dose of DES is 3 mg per day, given continuously until disease progression, with the usual duration of response being approximately 2 years. Growing evidence exists that doses of 3 mg per day increase the risk of thromboembolic disease and cardiovascular mortality.[8] Unfortunately, doses of DES of less than 3 mg per day erratically depress serum testosterone and give inferior control of prostate cancer in a substantial number of patients.

Orchiectomy. Castration rapidly drops serum testosterone to a baseline level of 15 μg/dl and produces control of prostate cancer in 60 to 80 per cent of patients. No increase in cardiovascular complications exists, but the loss of potency and the psychologic implication to the patient and his spouse often have an impact on treatment decisions.

GNRH Agonists. GNRH agonists that interfere with the release of pituitary luteinizing hormone (LH) and follicle-stimulating hormone (FSH) have become available. These agents result in an initial rise in the levels of LH, followed by subsequent cessation of secretion. This results in an initial rise in testicular production of testosterone that is often accompanied by disease flare; then testosterone levels drop to castrate levels, with disease control equal to that of DES or orchiectomy. The only commercially available GNRH agonist, leuprolide (Lupron), has the disadvantage of requiring daily subcutaneous injections and is thus suitable only for selected reliable patients. Another disadvantage of GNRH agonist is the expense, especially when compared with standard hormonal therapy.

Antiandrogens. In 1989, the first in a family of antiandrogens, flutamide, was released. Flutamide works by occupying the testosterone receptor at the cellular level. Serum testosterone levels remain normal, and many men retain potency.[9] No risk of thromboembolic or cardiovascular complications has been noted, and clinical trials suggest results equivalent to those of DES or orchiectomy. Minimal side effects have been observed. It is certain that flutamide and related drugs will see increasing use.

Other Hormonal Therapies. A number of other agents, including progesterones such as megestrol acetate, the antifungal drug ketoconazole, and the steroid inhibitor aminoglutethimide, have demonstrated activity in previously untreated patients, but have no advantage over the previously discussed drugs. All have had less critical evaluation.

Total Androgen Blockade. A concept developed by LaBrie and colleagues is that some patients' progression after the initial response is due to the presence of adrenal androgens.[10] In fact, sporadic reports of patients who failed DES or orchiectomy and responded to hypophysectomy, adrenalectomy, or medical adrenalectomy with aminoglutethimide exist. Unfortunately, these therapies carry considerable risks. As an alternative to these forms of therapy, controlled trials comparing GNRH agonists with placebo or flutamide have suggested a modest benefit for the combination of active drugs.[11] Both drugs are expensive, and until more mature information is available this should not be considered standard therapy.

Cytotoxic Chemotherapy

The role of cytotoxic chemotherapy in prostate cancer refractory to hormonal therapy is ill defined. Many problems exist in evaluating past clinical trials, including lack of specific response criteria, excessive morbidity in elderly patient populations, and, most importantly, failure to demonstrate survival benefit even in responding patients. Doxorubicin, cyclophosphamide, cisplatin, and others all have demonstrated some minimal activity. Combinations of agents have no proven superiority over single agents, and single agents have no proven superiority over supportive care.

This leads to the assessment that chemotherapy with cytotoxic drugs still belongs in the arena of clinical trials. If no appropriate clinical trial is available, then only selected physiologically vigorous patients should be offered chemotherapy. Response criteria should be well defined. If no response to initial therapy is obtained, a clear understanding should exist that only supportive care will be forthcoming.

■ Issues and Risks

Many issues still exist in the management of prostate cancer. Should prostate cancer be treated at all? What is the preferred therapy for localized disease? Which hormonal therapy is optimum? If DES is used, what is the preferred dose? Should hormonal therapy be combined? Finally, should cytotoxic chemotherapy be given outside the spectrum of a clinical trial?

All these questions can be answered by an honest assessment of your patient's physiologic, emotional, and pychosocial attributes; the risks of therapy; and your community's health resources.

Prostate cancer affects a wide spectrum of patients. On the one hand, there is the healthy 55 year old man who is still sexually active. Projected survival without prostate cancer would approach 20 years. He has teenaged children. Therapy should be aimed to retain potency in localized disease, which is probably best achieved with radiation therapy. Although potency-sparing operations exist, the long-term results are unknown, and few urologists have been trained in the procedure. If this same man has metastatic disease, he might be willing to undergo the added expense of flutamide to retain potency. In addition, with proper counseling, since modest survival benefits seem to accrue for total androgen blockade, he may be willing to forgo potency for a specific goal, such as seeing his children enter college.

Another characteristic patient is the man in his late 60s or 70s who has significant cardiovascular risk factors, is no longer potent, and is a widower. He does not want to drive 50 miles to the nearest radiation center. Localized disease in this man should be treated with prostatectomy and symptomatic metastatic disease with orchiectomy, flutamide, or GNRH agonists.

Finally, one is often faced with the frail, moderately demented, elderly man with severe medical problems. Survival of this patient is projected only for 1 to 2 years. In localized disease, if no significant obstruction exists, careful observation would be acceptable. If obstruction exists, then either radiation therapy or hormonal therapy is the best option. Only symptomatic metastatic disease should be treated, and since the patient is unreliable, orchiectomy would be the best form of therapy.

If an empathic approach and a careful review of the risks, benefits, and patients' goals are used, then the many controversies in the management of prostate cancer will fade away.

REFERENCES

1. Gleason DF: Histologic grading and clinical staging of prostate carcinoma. *In* Tannenbaum M (ed): Urologic Pathology: The Prostate. Philadelphia: Lea and Febiger, 1977: 171–192.
2. Byar DP, Mostof FK, and the VACURG: Carcinoma of the prostate; prognostic evaluation of certain pathologic features in 208 radical prostatectomies examined by the step section method. Cancer 1972; 30:5–13.
3. Gibbons RJ, Corea RJ, Brannen GE, et al: Total prostatectomy for localized prostate cancer. J Urol 1984; 131:73–76.
4. Walsh PC, Lopor H, Eggleston JC: Radical prostatectomy with preservation of sexual function. Anatomical and pathological considerations. Prostate 1983; 4:473–485.
5. Freiha FS, Bagashaw MA, Torti FM: Carcinoma of the prostate; pathology, staging, and treatment. Curr Probl Cancer 1989; 12:347–369.
6. Byar DP: VACURG studies on prostate carcinoma. *In* Tannenbaum M (ed): Urologic Pathology: The Prostate. Philadelphia; Lea and Febiger, 1977: 241.
7. Zincke K, Utz DC, Thiele FM, et al: Treatment options for patients with stage D adenocarcinoma of the prostate. Urology 1987; 30:307–315.
8. The Leuprolide Study Group: Leuprolide versus diethylstilbestrol for metastatic prostate cancer. N Engl J Med 1984; 311:1281.
9. Smith JA Jr: New methods of endocrine management of prostatic cancer. J Urol 1987; 137:1–30.
10. LaBrie F, Dupont A, Belanger A, et al: New approaches in the treatment of prostate cancer. Complete instead of partial withdrawal of androgens. Prostate 1983; 4:579–584.
11. Crawford E, Macleod D, Doana L: Treatment of newly diagnosed stage D_2 prostate cancer with leuprolide and flutamide or leuprolide alone. Phase III. Intergroup Study Proc ASCO 1988; 7:119A.

Pulmonary embolic disease

E. P. Trulock

The spectrum of venous thromboembolic disease includes deep venous thrombosis (DVT) and its complication, pulmonary embolism (PE). Both are common clinical problems that cause significant morbidity and mortality. The incidence of DVT and PE can be substantially reduced by appropriate prophylactic regimens. The management strategy of suspected DVT or PE is complex, because the diagnosis is difficult and the treatment modalities entail too many risks to be given empirically.

■ Background

■ INCIDENCE, MORTALITY, AND DIAGNOSTIC ACCURACY

The exact incidence of DVT and PE is uncertain. The frequency has usually been estimated from postmortem studies. The prevalence of significant or major PE (i.e., PE causing or contributing to death) at autopsy has varied among studies from 2 to 14 per cent,[1] but it is generally in the range of 7 to 9 per cent.[2] If such data are extrapolated to the mortality statistics of the United States, PE is a major factor in approximately 200,000 deaths annually. If another 300,000 nonfatal pulmonary embolism cases occur each year, as has been predicted, the annual incidence of PE would be around 500,000 cases.[2]

The incidence of DVT is more difficult to estimate. The deep venous system of the legs is not routinely dissected at autopsy; however, the frequency of DVT has been three to five times that of PE when this has been done. This extrapolates to 1.5 to 2.5 million cases of DVT per year, but the majority of these would not be detected. The incidence of clinically recognized DVT has been estimated to be around 250,000 cases yearly.[2]

Major PE is one of the most common unsuspected diagnoses discovered postmortem in hospitalized patients. The correct antemortem diagnostic rate for major PE is only around 30 per cent in autopsy series. Confounding factors that have been associated with diagnostic failure include pneumonia, congestive heart failure, and increasing age.[1] In addition, autopsy studies have revealed the inaccuracy of the "clinical" diagnosis of PE (i.e., diagnosis made by clinical features without a confirmatory imaging procedure). Only 30 to 60 per cent of pulmonary embolisms that were diagnosed "clinically" have been confirmed at autopsy.[1]

■ NATURAL HISTORY

Venous thrombosis develops in the lower extremities in the setting of venous stasis, endothelial injury, and/or hypercoagulability of the blood. The deep veins of the calf or the thigh may be involved, but proximal DVT is the most problematic. Superficial thrombosis poses no major threat unless the clot extends into the deep venous system. The three major complications of DVT are PE, recurrent DVT, and the postphlebitic syndrome. Whereas recurrent DVT and the postphlebitic syndrome are sources of considerable morbidity, PE is the most serious complication. Emboli occasionally arise from thrombi at other sites, such as the pelvic veins or the right heart chambers, but approximately 90 per cent of pulmonary embolisms originate from DVT. PE occurs in about 50 per cent of patients with documented DVT.[3]

The consequences of PE are determined by the extent of pulmonary vascular obstruction and the underlying cardiopulmonary status of the patient. In the absence of pre-existing cardiopulmonary disease, emboli must occlude more than 50 per cent of the pulmonary arterial circulation before the mean pulmonary arterial pressure rises. Occlusion of more than 75 per cent of the pulmonary arterial circulation raises the mean pulmonary arterial pressure to about 40 mm Hg; the previously normal right ventricle cannot sustain this degree of afterload, and right ventricular failure ensues. Massive PE (i.e., over 50 per cent obstruction of the pulmonary circulation) carries the worst prognosis. Approximately one half of all deaths from PE are due to massive embolism, and the majority of these fatalities occur during the first hour. The hospital mortality for patients with massive PE and hypotension may be as high as 32 per cent with conventional anticoagulant therapy,[3] and this subgroup of patients should be considered for more aggressive therapies, such as thrombolysis or embolectomy. In contrast, both massive and submassive pulmonary embolisms that do not cause hemodynamic compromise have only an 8 per cent mortality with anticoagulant treatment.[3]

The outcome of acute PE hinges on considering and confirming the diagnosis and on instituting proper treatment. Undiagnosed or untreated PE has a mortality rate of about 30 per cent, but the mortality rate of treated PE is only around 8 to 9 per cent. The long-term prognosis for survivors of acute PE depends primarily on their pre-embolic cardiac status. Pre-existing congestive heart failure is associated with a poor outcome during follow-up. In one study, only 19 per cent of the patients with left ventricular failure were alive 7 years after their PE, whereas 85 per cent of patients without cardiac disease were alive.[3] Deaths in both groups were not associated with recurrent PE.

The resolution of PE occurs principally by endogenous fibrinolysis. The dissolution begins within days, but it is rarely complete before 2 weeks in patients who are treated by anticoagulation. Therefore, diagnostic imaging procedures do not have to be performed on an emergency basis, and anticoagulant treatment can be started, if it is not contraindicated, without jeopardizing the yield of the tests. Ultimately, complete resolution of PE is the rule. Pulmonary hypertension secondary to unresolved or recurrent PE occurs in fewer than 2 per cent of patients after acute PE.[4]

■ RISK FACTORS

Venous thromboembolic disease is uncommon in the absence of a risk factor. Predisposing conditions include previous venous thromboembolism, cardiac disease, cancer, recent surgery, obesity, pregnancy and the puerperium, major trauma and burns, estrogen therapy, and prolonged immobility. The diagnosis should be considered in any patient with a risk factor who presents with suggestive signs or symptoms.

■ CLINICAL FEATURES

The symptoms and signs of PE are nonspecific and overlap with many other cardiopulmonary diseases. In patients suspected of having venous thromboembolism, the diagnosis is confirmed in only one half, or sometimes fewer, of the cases.[5] Routine tests, such as the chest radiograph and the electrocardiogram, are nondiagnostic, but they are helpful in ruling out other explanations of the symptoms and signs.

The arterial blood gas determination is an important test in any patient with cardiopulmonary signs or symptoms; however, it is not a reliable screening test in the evaluation of suspected PE. In the Pulmonary Embolism Trial and other studies, 11.5 to 13 per cent of patients with documented PE had a PO_2 above 80 mm Hg.[6] The alveolar-arterial (A-a) oxygen gradient may be normal, too.[7] Thus, neither the absence of hypoxia nor the presence of a normal A-a gradient excludes the diagnosis of PE. When hypoxia is present, it could be due to a variety of illnesses that mimic PE.

■ Management

■ DIAGNOSIS

A secure diagnosis is paramount in the management of PE and DVT. Clinical impression alone is unreliable, and objective imaging tests are essential to avoid serious diagnostic errors. Sensitive and specific noninvasive tests are widely available for both DVT and PE, and these should be employed liberally when the diagnosis is considered. The invasive contrast studies can be reserved for more selective indications.

Ventilation-Perfusion Lung Scintigraphy. The evaluation of suspected PE should begin with a ventilation-perfusion (V-P) radionuclide lung scintigram. Interpreted in conjunction with a concurrent chest radiograph, the V-P scintigraphic pattern is classified into one of four categories: normal, low probability, intermediate probability/ indeterminate, or high probability. Although there has been some controversy over the role of V-P scintigraphy in the diagnosis of PE, the preliminary results of the recently completed multicenter Prospective Investigation of Pulmonary Embolism Diagnosis (PIOPED) validate its utility.[8]

A "normal" V-P scan effectively excludes PE, and a "low probability" interpretation implies that the likelihood of PE is small (10 per cent or less). A "high probability" scan carries a reasonable assurance (about 90 per cent) of a correct diagnosis of PE. Results in these two categories are usually adequate to exclude or confirm PE in most circumstances; however, if a "high" or "low probability" result is discordant with the clinical impression, it should be confirmed angiographically.

Most "intermediate probability" or "indeterminate" scans deserve further investigation. PE is found by angiography in 20 to 35 per cent of patients with such scans. Finally, even if the V-P scan is expected to be inconclusive, it generally should be done anyway as the initial step. V-P scan results are not always predictable, and an abnormal, yet nondiagnostic, scan may guide selective pulmonary angiography.

Pulmonary Angiography. This is the gold standard for the diagnosis of PE. The indications for angiography are "intermediate probability" or "indeterminate" V-P scan, discordance between the V-P scan interpretation and the clinical impression, high risk of bleeding with anticoagulation, and anticipation of inferior vena cava interruption or thrombolytic therapy. Although an angiogram is not mandatory for the third or fourth indication, it should be done if there is any uncertainty. Pulmonary angiography is a safe procedure, even in the setting of severe chronic pulmonary hypertension.[9] The risks of the procedure are less than the risk of complications from empiric treatment with anticoagulants,[10] and it should not be underutilized.

Noninvasive Venous Tests. The evaluation of suspected DVT usually should begin with noninvasive venous studies. Noninvasive techniques include impedance plethysmography (IPG), Doppler ultrasonography, and duplex scanning. The results of all three modalities have a strong correlation with venographic findings. The respective sensitivity and specificity in the diagnosis of proximal DVT are 93 and 94 per cent for IPG, 84 and 88 per cent for Doppler ultrasonography, and 90 and 95 per cent for duplex scanning.[11,12] Neither IPG nor Doppler ultrasonography is sensitive in the detection of isolated calf vein thrombosis; however, duplex scanning is extremely useful. IPG and Doppler ultrasonography depend on venous outflow, and these techniques cannot distinguish between thrombotic and nonthrombotic causes of venous obstruction. False-positive tests for DVT may be obtained with extraluminal compression or elevated central venous pressure. Duplex scanning is a useful adjunct because it directly images the echogenic material of an intravascular thrombus. All these tests are portable and can be done at the bedside.

Venography. This is the gold standard for the diagnosis of DVT. Considerable expertise is required to perform and interpret a venogram accurately. Incomplete venous filling with contrast and other technical artifacts may lead to a false-positive interpretation. The most reliable criterion for the diagnosis of DVT is a constant intraluminal filling defect that is visible in several projections. Venography should be done if reliable noninvasive techniques are not available, if there is a discrepancy between the clinical impression and the noninvasive test results, or if the noninvasive tests give either equivocal or potentially false-positive results.

Diagnostic Strategy. DVT and PE often occur together, and this concurrence may be helpful in the diagnostic approach to suspected PE. For example, if the ventilation-perfusion lung scan results in indeterminate or intermediate probability, noninvasive venous tests of the legs might reveal DVT. Since the therapy is usually the same for DVT and PE, angiography might be avoided by this strategy. On the other hand, negative studies for DVT cannot be used to exclude PE. PE has been found by angiography in 35 per cent of patients with simultaneously negative bilateral venograms[5] and in 47 per cent of patients with negative noninvasive venous examinations.[13]

■ TREATMENT

Several treatment options are available for venous thromboembolism. The therapeutic approaches include conventional anticoagulation, inferior vena cava interruption, thrombolysis, and embolectomy. The choice of therapy should be governed primarily by the hemodynamic status of the patient and the presence or absence of contraindications to anticoagulation or thrombolysis.

Anticoagulation

Conventional anticoagulation with heparin followed by warfarin is the standard treatment for uncomplicated first episodes of DVT and PE in patients without hemodynamic compromise and without a contraindication. Adequate anticoagulation with heparin in the acute phase and warfarin in the chronic phase is effective in preventing recurrent DVT and PE.[14-16] Prior to initiation of treatment, a careful history, physical examination, chart review, and laboratory evaluation should be conducted to identify risk factors for bleeding.

If there are no contraindications and the bleeding risk is not high, heparin may be started while diagnostic tests are planned and carried out. No diagnostic sensitivity will be sacrificed, and the risk of a complication is low if the patient has been carefully screened. However, the diagnosis must be pursued by an appropriate imaging procedure as soon as practical, and therapy should not be continued without confirmation. If there is a contraindication to heparin or if the patient's bleeding risk is high, heparin should be withheld and the diagnostic studies undertaken without delay.

Heparin should be given by continuous intravenous infusion rather than by intermittent intravenous bolus injection; however, an adjusted subcutaneous regimen may be an effective alternative.[17] A protocol for the initiation and maintenance of heparin is outlined in Table 1. Heparin therapy should be monitored by the partial thromboplastin time (PTT), and the dose should be adjusted to maintain the PTT between 1.5 and 2.5 times control value. PTT values of less than 1.5 times control are associated with higher recurrence rates. The correlation between PTT values and bleeding complications has been inconsistent among studies, but there may be an increased risk at PTT values greater than 2.5 to 3.0 times control. The optimal duration of heparin treatment has not been determined; however, a minimum of 7 days is customary.

Subtherapeutic anticoagulation is a common problem during the first few days of heparin administration. In a recent survey, 60 per cent of patients did not have a single therapeutic PTT during the first 24 hours of treatment.[18] Practices that contributed to the delay in achieving a therapeutic PTT included insufficient doses of heparin initially, delays in obtaining the first PTT on heparin, inadequate dose change in response to a subtherapeutic PTT, and excessive and prolonged reductions in dose in response to a PTT greater than 3.0 times control. The early emphasis during heparinization should be on achieving a therapeutic dose. There should be less concern initially about overdosing with heparin; this is uncommon with the usual doses, and bleeding complications correlate poorly, if at all, with the PTT.

After the acute phase of heparin treatment, the chronic phase of treatment should continue for 3 months for an uncomplicated first episode of venous thromboembolism. For a recurrence or for a persistent major risk factor, the duration of anticoagulation should be extended. Chronic anticoagulation may be accomplished with oral warfarin or adjusted-dose subcutaneous heparin. Warfarin is usually chosen, but subcutaneous heparin is the method of choice during pregnancy.

Warfarin should be started after a few days of heparin therapy and overlap with the completion of the heparin course. Dose requirements of warfarin vary substantially among patients because of differences in drug elimination and interactions with other medications. An initial warfarin dose of 5 to 15 mg daily is reasonable. The maintenance dose should be regulated subsequently by monitoring the prothrombin time (PT). Using the rabbit brain thromboplastin assay, a PT ratio (patient PT/control

TABLE 1. Protocol for Heparin Anticoagulation

Obtain pretreatment coagulation profile (PT, PTT platelet count).

Begin heparin with 5000 units IV bolus followed by continuous infusion of about 1000 units/hr.

Monitor PTT q 4–6 hr until stable in the therapeutic range (1.5–2.5 × mean control or pretreatment value).

Re-bolus and/or adjust infusion rate as indicated by the PTT.

Monitor PTT daily once stable, monitor complete blood count (with platelets) every second or third day.

Continue heparin for at least 7 days and until oral anticoagulation is adequate.

PT) of 1.2 to 1.5 is recommended as the therapeutic range.[19]

Subcutaneous heparin must be given in a dose-adjusted fashion for maintenance anticoagulation. Fixed-dose subcutaneous heparin at 5000 units every 12 hours has been shown to be ineffective.[15,20] Subcutaneous heparin is given every 12 hours and is monitored by the mid-interval PTT. The dose is adjusted initially to achieve a mid-interval PTT 1.5 times control; thereafter, no monitoring is usually needed.

Thrombolysis

Although three effective thrombolytic drugs—streptokinase (SK), urokinase (UK), and tissue plasminogen activator (tPA)—are available, the precise role of thrombolysis in the management of venous thromboembolism is controversial. Thrombolysis has several theoretic advantages over conventional anticoagulation. Unlike anticoagulation, which merely prevents propagation of thrombi, thrombolysis actively promotes dissolution of emboli and thrombi. Hemodynamic alterations secondary to PE can be reversed more rapidly, and venous valvular damage and its sequelae, chronic venous insufficiency and the postphlebitic syndrome, may be avoided or minimized. In spite of its theoretic superiority, thrombolysis did not prove more effective than conventional anticoagulation in reducing mortality from PE in the Pulmonary Embolism Trial.[21] Furthermore, the lytic activity of the available drugs is not specific for venous thrombi or pulmonary emboli; fresh clots at any site are subject to dissolution, and bleeding complication rates have generally been higher with thrombolysis than with anticoagulation. For these reasons, the use of thrombolytic agents in routine management has remained relatively restricted.

The primary indication for thrombolytic therapy is PE with circulatory compromise that does not respond readily to supportive measures. This group of patients has a poor prognosis, and the opportunity for rapid hemodynamic improvement justifies the risks of thrombolysis if there are no contraindications. Reversal of hemodynamic alterations has been demonstrated with SK, UK, and tPA.[21-23] Other proposed indications for thrombolysis include submassive PE in patients who might not tolerate further cardiopulmonary compromise, massive PE without hemodynamic compromise, heparin treatment failure, and extensive proximal DVT; all these are less compelling than the primary indication.

Patients selected for thrombolytic therapy should have a well-documented diagnosis, and the thromboemboli should be recent, preferably less than 7 days old. Absolute contraindications to thrombolytic therapy are active internal bleeding and recent (less than 2 months) cerebrovascular accident or other active intracranial process. Relative major contraindications are recent (less than 10 days) major surgery, obstetric delivery, organ biopsy, or previous puncture of a noncompressible vessel; recent serious gastrointestinal bleeding; recent serious trauma; and severe arterial hypertension (over 200 mm Hg systolic or over 110 mm Hg diastolic). Consideration must also be given to a host of relatively minor contraindications.[24]

The best choice of a thrombolytic agent is unclear. All three drugs—SK, UK and tPA—appear equally suitable, but UK and tPA are more expensive than SK. Although only SK and UK have been approved by the Food and Drug Administration for this indication, there is ample published experience with tPA in PE.[23,25-27] UK and tPA have been compared directly.[28] With the regimens of tPA and UK employed, tPA appeared to act more rapidly and to have fewer bleeding complications than UK; however, a number of methodologic criticisms have questioned the validity of the comparison.

All the agents should be given by peripheral intravenous infusion; there is no advantage to intrapulmonary administration. A protocol for treatment is presented in Table 2. The role of laboratory monitoring is limited to establishing the presence of a lytic state, and this is necessary only with SK and UK. Once a lytic state is verified, no dose adjustment is made. A lytic state may be documented by several laboratory parameters, including a prolonged thrombin time, elevated fibrin degradation products, or prolonged PT or PTT. When the lytic infusion is completed, a maintenance infusion of heparin should be resumed when the PTT is approximately two times control. Heparin and warfarin are then given as previously described.

Inferior Vena Cava Interruption

Interruption of the inferior vena cava (IVC) prevents PE from DVT. The indications for IVC interruption are a contraindication to

TABLE 2. Protocols for Thrombolytic Therapy

Discontinue heparin and allow anticoagulant effect to dissipate. Minimize invasive procedures.

Infuse thrombolytic agent by peripheral vein.

SK: 250,000 IU loading dose over 30 min
100,000 IU/hr maintenance dose for 24 hr

UK: 4000 IU/kg loading dose over 10 min
4000 IU/kg/hr maintenance dose for 12 hr

tPA: Optimal regimen undetermined
Loading dose not necessary
Consider: 100 mg over 2 hr or 50 mg over 2 hr followed by an additional 50 mg over next 4–5 hr if not improved

Confirm lytic state with SK or UK by monitoring the thrombin time or fibrin degradation products approximately 4 hr into infusion. This is not necessary for tPA.

Discontinue thrombolytic drug. Resume maintenance heparin infusion when PTT is approximately 2.0 × control.

anticoagulation, a complication of anticoagulation that requires its premature discontinuation, recurrent PE during adequate anticoagulation, embolectomy, and prophylaxis against potentially life-threatening PE. The latter indication pertains to patients who have suffered a massive PE and could not tolerate an early recurrence and to patients who have a tenuous cardiopulmonary status due to another heart or lung disease and might succumb to a submassive PE.

Several techniques have been described, but the Greenfield vena caval filter is currently preferred by most surgeons and invasive radiologists. This cone-shaped device is inserted percutaneously through the internal jugular or femoral vein and is placed in the inferior vena cava under fluoroscopic guidance. The recurrence rate of PE after a filter is about 5 per cent, and the long-term patency rate is around 98 per cent.[28] Anticoagulation may be resumed or started after filter placement if it is not contraindicated.

Embolectomy

Surgical extraction of emboli is rarely indicated. If the resources are available, embolectomy should be considered in the otherwise healthy patient with a life-threatening PE who cannot be treated with, or who fails to respond to, thrombolysis. Since the majority of deaths due to massive PE occur within the first hour, and most of the patients who survive longer will respond to nonoperative therapy, surgical skill and experience with embolectomy are limited.

Two techniques may be used, transvenous catheter embolectomy and open embolectomy. Transvenous catheter embolectomy is performed with a ballon-tipped suction catheter that is floated into position in a pulmonary artery by fluoroscopic guidance. The position of the catheter at the site of an embolus is confirmed by injection of a small amount of a contrast agent. Suction is applied to the catheter, and the embolus is extracted as the catheter is withdrawn. Multiple retrievals are usually necessary before hemodynamic improvement is seen. In experienced hands, emboli have been extracted successfully in up to 85 per cent of patients; however, the acute mortality rate in patients treated with this approach was 32 per cent.[28]

Open embolectomy may be done with or without cardiopulmonary bypass. The overall mortality rate with cardiopulmonary bypass is around 30 per cent,[29] and without bypass it is about 38 per cent.[30] With or without bypass, patients who have suffered cardiac arrest prior to the embolectomy have a mortality rate near 70 per cent. In contrast, patients who have not suffered cardiac arrest before the embolectomy have only a 10 to 20 per cent mortality rate.

■ Issues and Risks

■ COMPLICATIONS

The major complication of the treatment with anticoagulation or thrombolysis is bleeding. In the Pulmonary Embolism Trial, the incidence of bleeding was 27 per cent in the heparin group and 45 per cent in the urokinase group, but in only 4 per cent of the heparin group and 10 per cent of the urokinase group was the bleeding severe enough to stop treatment or to require blood transfusion.[21] These rates are probably excessive for both modalities because of the invasive procedures mandated by the protocol, and lower rates may be expected by carefully selecting patients and by avoiding unnecessary invasive procedures. Nonetheless, the risk of bleeding is probably greater with thrombolysis than with anticoagulation, and thrombolytic therapy should be reserved for those situations in which the benefits justify the risks.

The approach to bleeding during heparin therapy depends on the site and severity of hemorrhage and on the PTT. If the PTT is excessively prolonged and the bleeding is not major, it may be managed by a temporary cessation of heparin with subsequent resumption at an adjusted dose. If significant bleeding occurs with a therapeutic PTT, heparin must be discontinued. The PTT will usually return to normal in a few hours, but the reversal can be expedited in emergencies by the administration of protamine sulfate. An alternative therapy, such as vena cava interruption, will have to be considered.

Minor bleeding from puncture sites is common during thrombolytic therapy and usually can be managed by local compression. Major bleeding will require cessation of thrombolytic therapy. With UK and SK, the lytic state will reverse relatively quickly because of the short half-life of these drugs, but the lytic action of tPA outlasts its apparent half-life. Fresh-frozen plasma can be used to replete coagulation factors, and epsilon-aminocaproic acid can be given in more urgent situations.

Long-term anticoagulation with warfarin is also associated with a significant incidence of hemorrhagic complications. The risk of bleeding may be reduced by adjusting the PT ratio to 1.2 to 1.5 X control without a significant increase in the risk of recurrent venous thromboembolism.[31] The approach to bleeding during warfarin treatment depends on the site and severity of hemorrhage and the PT. If the bleeding is minor and the PT is excessively prolonged, a dose adjustment to return the PT to the therapeutic range may be sufficient. If the bleeding is more significant and the PT is in or near the therapeutic range, warfarin must be stopped and anticoagulation reversed. The PT can be returned to normal by infusion of fresh-frozen plasma or by administration of vitamin K. The decision regarding alternative therapy for venous thromboembolism after discontinuation of warfarin will depend primarily on the risk of recurrence. If the risk is high, vena cava interruption should be considered. If the risk is low, it may be acceptable to monitor carefully for recurrence of DVT using serial noninvasive studies. Bleeding that occurs with a therapeutic PT should be investigated further to determine the cause.

■ RISK-BENEFIT CONSIDERATIONS IN DIAGNOSIS AND TREATMENT

The clinical diagnosis of DVT and PE is notoriously inaccurate, and reliance on clinical impression alone will lead to serious errors in management. Both underdiagnosis and overdiagnosis will result in unnecessary morbidity and mortality. The diagnosis of DVT and PE can be confirmed or refuted by an appropriate diagnostic strategy utilizing invasive and/or noninvasive imaging procedures. The risks of these procedures, including pulmonary angiography, are quite low—much lower, in fact, than the risk of

TABLE 3. Risk and Prevention of DVT and PE

Patient Group	Incidence of Venous Thrombosis* (%)	Incidence of Fatal PE (%)	Prophylaxis
Orthopedic surgery (major hip or knee)	40–70	7–10	Adjusted dose heparin; low-dose warfarin; pneumatic compression (knee only)
General abdominal, thoracic, and gynecologic surgery	10–20	1	Low-dose heparin
Urologic surgery	15–20	<5	Pneumatic compression
Neurosurgery	15–20	<1	Pneumatic compression
Medical patients	<15	<1	Low-dose heparin

*Risk is increased by advancing age, malignancy, heart failure, and prolonged immobility.
(Data from National Institutes of Health Consensus Conference. Prevention of venous thrombosis and pulmonary embolism. JAMA 1986; 256:744–749 and Hull RD, Raskob GE, Hirsh J. Prophylaxis of venous thromboembolism: an overview. Chest 1986; 89:374S–383S.

death from underdiagnosis and undertreatment or the risk of hemorrhage from overdiagnosis and overtreatment. Hence, when there is diagnostic uncertainty, a pulmonary angiogram or venogram is usually safer than the alternative strategy of treating or not treating on the basis of clinical impression or empiricism.

■ PREVENTION

One key to reducing the morbidity and mortality of venous thromboembolism is prevention of DVT. The risk of DVT, as well as the efficacy and safety of prophylaxis, are different in various patient groups. A guide to risk assessment and prophylaxis is presented in Table 3.

The most widely applicable and best-studied method of prophylaxis is low-dose heparin. Beneficial results have been shown in both surgical and medical patients, using a regimen of subcutaneous heparin, 5000 units, given 2 hours preoperatively (surgical) or within 12 hours of admission (medical) and continued every 8 to 12 hours thereafter.[32,33]

The low-dose heparin regimen is not suitable for all patients. Contraindications to this regimen include coagulopathy, active or recent gastrointestinal bleeding or peptic ulcer disease, advanced renal or hepatic disease, pericardial effusion, or acute cerebrovascular event (until hemorrhage has been excluded). If low-dose heparin is contraindicated or if any bleeding risk is unacceptable, external pneumatic compression is the best alternative. The low-dose heparin regimen is relatively ineffective in preventing DVT in high-risk orthopedic patients, and more intense approaches are advised.[34,35]

Although prophylaxis substantially lowers the incidence of venous thromboembolism, it does not guarantee protection.[36] If a clinical suspicion of acute DVT or PE arises, it should be evaluated even though prophylaxis has been given.

REFERENCES

1. Goldhaber SZ. Strategies for diagnosis. *In* Goldhaber SZ (ed). Pulmonary Embolism and Deep Venous Thrombosis. Philadelphia: WB Saunders, 1985:79–97.
2. Coon WW. Venous thromboembolism. Prevalence, risk factors, and prevention. Clin Chest Med 1984; 5(3):391–401.
3. Dalen JE, Paraskos JA, Ockene IS, Alpert JS, Hirsh J. Venous thromboembolism. Scope of the problem. Chest 1986; 89(5):370S–373S.
4. Benotti JR, Dalen JE. The natural history of pulmonary embolism. Clin Chest Med 1984; 5(3):403–410.
5. Hull RD, Hirsh J, Carter CJ, et al. Pulmonary angiography, ventilation lung scanning, and venography for clinically suspected pulmonary embolism with abnormal perfusion lung scan. Ann Intern Med 1983; 98:891–899.
6. D'Alonzo GE, Dantzker DR. Gas exchange alterations following pulmonary thromboembolism. Clin Chest Med 1984; 5(3):411–419.
7. Overton DT, Bocka JJ. The alveolar-arterial oxygen gradient in patients with documented pulmonary embolism. Arch Intern Med 1988; 148:1617–1619.
8. Highlights: ATS Symposia. Recent advances in diagnosis of pulmonary embolism and deep venous thrombosis. Am Rev Resp Dis 1988; 138:1046–1047.
9. Nicod P, Peterson K, Levine M, et al. Pulmonary angiography in severe chronic pulmonary hypertension. Ann Intern Med 1987; 107:565–568.
10. Cheely R, McCartney WH, Perry JR, et al. The role of noninvasive tests versus pulmonary angiography in the diagnosis of pulmonary embolism. Am J Med 1981; 70:17–22.
11. Wheeler HB, Anderson FA. Diagnostic approaches for deep vein thrombosis. Chest 1986; 89(5):407S–412S.
12. Oliver MA. Duplex scanning in venous disease. Bruit 1985; 9:206–209.
13. Schiff MJ, Feinberg AW, Naidich JB. Noninvasive venous examinations as a screening test for pulmonary embolism. Arch Intern Med 1987; 147:505–507.
14. Barritt DW, Jordan SD. Anticoagulant drugs in the treatment of pulmonary embolism. Lancet 1960; 1:1309.
15. Hull R, Delmore T, Genton E, et al. Warfarin sodium versus low-dose heparin in the long-term treatment of venous thrombosis. N Engl J Med 1979; 301:855–858.
16. Hull RD, Raskob GE, Hirsh J, et al. Continuous intravenous heparin compared with intermittent subcutaneous heparin in the initial treatment of proximal-vein thrombosis. N Engl J Med 1986; 325:1109–1114.
17. Doyle DJ, Turpie AGG, Hirsh J, et al. Adjusted subcutaneous heparin or continuous intravenous heparin in patients with acute deep vein thrombosis. Ann Intern Med 1987; 107:441–445.
18. Wheeler AP, Jaquiss RDB, Newman JH. Physician practices in the treatment of pulmonary embolism and deep venous thrombosis. Arch Intern Med 1988; 148:1321–1325.
19. Hirsh J, Deykin D, Poller L. "Therapeutic range" for oral anticoagulant therapy. Chest 1986; 89:11S–15S.
20. Hull R, Delmore T, Carter C, et al. Adjusted subcutaneous heparin versus warfarin sodium in the long-term treatment of venous thrombosis. N Engl J Med 1982; 306:189–194.
21. The Urokinase-Pulmonary Embolism Trial. A national cooperative study. Circulation 1973; 47(suppl II):1–108.
22. Urokinase-Streptokinase Embolism Trial. Phase 2 results. A cooperative study. JAMA 1974; 229:1606–1613.
23. Come PC, Kim D, Parker A, et al. Early reversal of right ventricular dysfunction in patients with acute

pulmonary embolism after treatment with intravenous tissue plasminogen activator. J Am Coll Cardiol 1987; 10:971–978.

24. National Institutes of Health Consensus Development Conference. Thrombolytic therapy in thrombosis. Ann Intern Med 1980; 93:141–144.

25. Goldhaber SZ, Markis JE, Meyerovitz MF, et al. Acute pulmonary embolism treated with tissue plasminogen activator. Lancet 1986; 2:886–889.

26. Goldhaber SZ, Heit J, Sharma GVRK, et al. Randomised controlled trial of recombinant tissue plasminogen activator versus urokinase in the treatment of acute pulmonary embolism. Lancet 1988; 2:293–298.

27. Verstraete M, Miller GAH, Bounameaux H, et al. Intravenous and intrapulmonary recombinant tissue-type plasminogen activator in the treatment of acute massive pulmonary embolism. Circulation 1988; 77:353–360.

28. Greenfield LJ. Vena caval interruption and pulmonary embolectomy. Clin Chest Med 1984; 5(3):495–505.

29. Gray H, Morgan J, Paneth M, Miller GAH. Pulmonary embolectomy for acute massive pulmonary embolism: an analysis of 71 cases. Br Heart J 1988; 60:196–200.

30. Clarke DB, Abrams LD. Pulmonary embolectomy: a 25 year experience. J Thorac Cardiovasc Surg 1986; 92:442–445.

31. Hull R, Hirsh J, Jay R, et al. Different intensities of oral anticoagulant therapy in the treatment of proximal-vein thrombosis. N Engl J Med 1982; 307:1676–1681.

32. Collins R, Scrimgeour A, Yusuf S, Peto R. Reduction in fatal pulmonary embolism and venous thrombosis by perioperative administration of subcutaneous heparin. Overview of results of randomized trials in general, orthopedic, and urologic surgery. N Engl J Med 1988; 318:1162–1173.

33. Halkin H, et al. Reduction of mortality in general medical in-patients by low-dose heparin prophylaxis. Ann Intern Med 1982; 96:561–565.

34. National Institutes of Health Consensus Conference. Prevention of venous thrombosis and pulmonary embolism. JAMA 1986; 256:744–749.

35. Hyers TM, Hull RD, Weg JG. Antithrombotic therapy for venous thromboembolic disease. ACCP-NHLBI National Conference on Antithrombotic Therapy. Chest 1986; 89:26S–35S.

36. Hull RD, Raskob GE, Hirsh J. Prophylaxis of venous thromboembolism: an overview. Chest 1986; 89:374S–383S.

Recreational athlete, medical care of the

William L. Toffler

■ Background

There has been a dramatic change over the past several years in the way that Americans view exercise. The Harvard Alumni study has increased our understanding of activity and exercise by showing that physical activity is not only associated with better health, but also with increased longevity.[1] The study found that routine activities, including walking and stair climbing, relate inversely to mortality—primarily from cardiovascular and respiratory causes. Similarly, the Multiple Risk Factor Intervention Trial supports this conclusion and indicates that gardening for 45 minutes is as good as running for 2 hours in preventing death from coronary artery disease.[2] Millions of Americans who previously might not have considered participation in any sort of recreational athletic endeavor can be assured of some significant health benefit even from relatively low-level (in terms of frequency and intensity) activity. A growing awareness of these issues may explain, at least in part, why the number of people participating in regular physical activity is increasing. Over 40 million Americans participate in exercise walking and more than 25 million jog or run.[3] This represents a significant increase over sampling taken just a few years previously.

Among these millions of Americans are people with known ailments such as coronary artery disease, diabetes, and asthma. At the same time, some of these individuals have as yet undetected abnormalities. For example, when the basketball star Pete Maravich died, he was found to lack a major coronary artery. These and other related issues require special consideration in the overall medical care of the recreational athlete.

■ Management

■ CORONARY ARTERY DISEASE

The treatment of individuals with coronary artery disease (CAD) has changed markedly in the past few decades. Not only have drug therapy and surgical options improved outcome, but the recommendations for activity and exercise for such patients have become much more liberal. Patients previously had been confined to bed for as long as 3 to 6 weeks after a myocardial infarction. In contrast, exercise now has a definite place in the treatment of the patient with CAD through all phases of illness. In fact, a recent report suggests that early exercise following coronary artery bypass grafting may improve subsequent graft patency.[4] Physical training probably should be started as early as possible after bypass surgery to improve both graft patency and cardiac function. Unfortunately, the precise details of how cardiac rehabilitation is best carried out and the optimal duration of medically supervised exercise are still not clearly defined.

Although the use of routine exercise testing among healthy adults to screen for cardiovascular complications has been questioned, exercise testing clearly helps identify cardiac patients who are at increased risk for exercise-related cardiovascular complications.[6] Patients with increased risk include those with previous heart attacks, impaired left ventricular function, exercise angina, and ventricular dysrhythmia. Coronary angiography should be considered for all patients with marked ST segment depression. Family members and friends should be trained in cardiopulmonary resuscitation, and the individual with heart disease should engage in activity with companions who have this skill. Patients should be encouraged to take their own pulses and to obtain an electrocardiogram when heart rate and rhythm irregularities are detected. Appropriate warm-up and cool-down procedures should be emphasized. The initial period of activity and the

cool-down periods are times of higher risk. An appropriate warm-up may decrease the occurrence of the ischemic ST segment depression. The cool-down may reduce the possibility of postexercise hypertension and the detrimental effect of the rise of plasma catecholamines following exercise.[6] Patients who disregard appropriate warm-up and cool-down are at risk, as are those who consistently exceed prescribed training heart rates.

It is imperative that individuals with CAD know their recommended heart range for training and how to stay in this range. One can learn to correlate heart rate with perceived level of exertion in the absence of interfering medications such as beta-blockers. The level of exercise at which a person becomes short of breath but is still able to carry on a conversation correlates well with the heart rate that approximates the desired range for exercise. Checking the heart rate to assure accurate correlation is essential, along with strict adherence to prescribed training rates. High-risk patients should be encouraged to engage in activities at lower levels of intensity and under more controlled situations. They should avoid competitive recreational games. One can compensate for the reduced intensity of training, in part, by more frequent training sessions. Individuals with CAD who are on beta-blockers are limited with respect to improvements in maximal oxygen uptake. Switching to calcium channel blockers may offer an alternative to control angina or hypertension without limiting either the training effect or the beneficial effect of exercise on the lipid profile.

Hypothermic and hyperthermic conditions are important aspects to emphasize as a part of patient education. Despite appropriate dress, exposure to cold air may cause angina pectoris. Patients exercising in cold weather should wear a mask or scarf over the nose and mouth, be aware of extreme wind chill factors, change wet clothing, wear several layers of light clothing that can be shed or replaced as needed, keep moving to increase body heat production, and protect body surface areas that have a large surface area to mass ratio, such as the hands and cheeks.[6] Hyperthermic conditions can cause increases in body temperature and metabolism that result in a disproportionate increase in myocardial oxygen demand. Those who exercise in hot weather should decrease exercise intensity, exercise during the cooler parts of the day, and adjust to porous, light-colored clothing to facilitate cooling by evaporation.

■ ASTHMA

In the past, many patients with asthma have been advised to restrict their participation in exercise because of the concerns about triggering exercise-induced asthma (EIA). Such limitations are generally ill-founded and unnecessary. To illustrate this point, 67 athletes at the 1984 Olympic Games had EIA, and 41 of them won medals.[7] Swimming is an excellent exercise for most people with asthma. In addition, athletes with EIA generally perform with less difficulty in sports that require short bursts of energy, such as gymnastics, baseball, football, and short-distance track and field events. Factors that determine the severity of airway response to exercising include duration, intensity, and type of exercise as well as the ambient air conditions. The precise mechanisms underlying EIA are not fully established but are related to many factors, including respiratory heat and water loss, airway rewarming, intensity of exercise, and possibly mast cell–driven mediator release. In addition, there are clear data indicating that the severity of EIA depends not only on airway cooling but also upon the rapidity and magnitude of air-

way rewarming postexercise.[8] Appreciation of these underlying mechanisms provides a basis for strategies to minimize the triggering of EIA. An athlete may be able to reduce or prevent an episode entirely by avoiding abrupt changes in work intensity before, during, and after exercise. A gradual warm-up over 10 to 15 minutes and a gradual cooldown over 10 to 30 minutes can be very helpful to some athletes with EIA.

Many people with EIA do not realize that their symptoms of exercise intolerance actually may be asthma. In an evaluation of over 300 athletes, only 2.6 per cent gave a history of or knew that they had asthma, yet an additional 17 per cent demonstrated airway hyperreactivity when they were tested by methacholine inhalation.[7] On re-evaluation of these athletes with more specific questioning, almost one-third of them had symptoms of coughing, wheezing, or chest tightness during exercise, compatible with previously undiagnosed EIA.

Once a diagnosis of EIA has been confirmed, medication treatment options must be considered (Table 1). Aerosol medications have distinctive advantages, including shorter onset of action and fewer side effects. Beta-adrenergic agonists are first-line treatment options, including drugs such metaproterenol, albuterol, terbutaline, and bitolterol. Treatment can be administered either by metered dose inhaler (MDI) or self-administered nebulizer. Oral beta-agonists

TABLE 1. Suggested Approach to Medication Management for EIA

Medications		*Dosing & Frequency**
Initiate Therapy:		
Aerosol β-2 adrenergic agonist	metaproterenol sulfate (Alupent, Metaprel)	q 4 hr
	terbutaline sulfate (Brethaire, Brethine)	q 4–6 hr
	bitolterol mesylate (Tornalate)	q 4–6 hr
	albuterol (Proventil, Ventolin)	q 4–6 hr
Alternative to Initiate Therapy or Use Concomitantly:		
Mast cell stabilizer	cromolyn sodium (Intal)	10–15 minutes before exercise or up to QID
In Difficult Cases:		
Anticholinergic agent	ipratropium bromide (Atrovent)	q 4 hr
Inhaled corticosteroids	tramcinolone acetonide (Azmacort)	q 6–12 hr
	beclomethasone (Beclovent, Vanceril)	q 6–12 hr
	flunisolide (AeroBid)	q 6–12 hr
Calcium channel blockers (controversial)	nifedine (Procardia, Adalat)	10–20 mg, PO or SL ½–1 hr before exercise or may be given TID

*Aerosol: two inhalations.

are available but offer little protection from EIA and are associated with a higher incidence of adverse effects. In addition, although the aerosol forms of metaproterenol and albuterol are allowed in competition, the oral formulations of these drugs (and many other antiasthmatic agents) are prohibited by the United States Olympic Committee. For most patients with mild EIA, use of a metered-dose inhaler 10 to 15 minutes before exercise will prevent bronchospasm. The appropriate technique with use of an MDI is extremely important to assure maximum delivery of medication to the airways of the lung. Athletes should exhale partially and then begin a very slow inhalation, establishing a laminar inflow of air prior to releasing medication from the MDI. The inhalation should continue after medication release for 6 or more seconds. Persons not able to cooperate with this technique may benefit from any one of a number of inhalation assist devices that improve delivery of the medication to the lung.

Cromolyn sodium is an alternative treatment for EIA. Cromolyn also can be given by MDI or by nebulizer before exercising. Cromolyn is usually free of adverse effects and blocks not only the immediate asthmatic response, but also the late-phase reaction in those persons with dual responses to exercise. This late-phase reaction usually occurs approximately 4 to 6 hours after exercise and is usually less intense than the immediate asthmatic response. Theophylline has limited effectiveness as a single agent but at times can be tried in combination with the aforementioned agents in difficult cases. Similarly, anticholinergic agents have limited usefulnes alone but sometimes can be used in combination treatment with a beta-agonist and cromolyn. Inhaled corticosteroids also should be considered for use in those patients whose EIA is unresponsive to other medications. Use of calcium channel antagonists in the management of patients with EIA has a theoretic basis and may directly effect the relaxation of bronchial smooth muscle or may indirectly inhibit mast cell secretion. Although their use is still somewhat experimental, nifedipine can be tried before exercise in patients when other measures are unsuccessful.[9] Unfortunately, most studies have demonstrated that calcium antagonists have only modest and highly variable effects on airway smooth muscle contraction.[10]

In addition to the appropriate utilization of medications, athletes with EIA need to be aware of the respiratory irritants and allergens that may also contribute to the frequency or severity of episodes. Exercising in an area with elevated levels of particulates and other pollutants or at a track adjacent to a freshly mown football field may undermine medical measures that otherwise would have resulted in successful control of an athlete's EIA.

■ DIABETES MELLITUS

Exercise results in improved control of diabetes as well as better weight control, higher self-esteem, and an improved high-to-low density lipoprotein cholesterol ratio. The glycemic response to exercise is significantly related to the duration of activity, and even low-intensity activity produces a significant, but modest, decrease in glucose levels.[11] In addition, the physically conditioned athlete with diabetes usually requires lower doses of insulin. Exercise in diabetes can be harmful if the individual is pushed into a volume-depleted ketotic or ketoacidotic state. If insulin dosages are inadequate, glucose is not used efficiently as an energy source and fatty acids become used as an energy source, resulting in the production of ketone bodies. This situation usually does not occur unless diabetic control is inadequate, placing the athlete at risk of ketoacidosis as a result of exercise. On the other hand, an individual with tightly controlled diabetes may become hypoglycemic in the early phases of exercise, during the workout, or after prolonged exertion.[12] This hypoglycemia is in part caused by an increased rate of insulin absorption from the injection site, resulting in increased uptake of sugar by muscle tissue.

It is essential that glucose control be reasonable before an athlete begins an exercise program. Athletes with repeated blood glucose levels greater than 300 mg/dl should have improved glucose control prior to exercise. Athletes with tight control should consider "relaxing" insulin doses prior to any contemplated change in activity level. To minimize difficulties with blood sugar control, exercise should be done regularly each day or every other day, preferably at approximately the same time of the day. Drugs that increase the risk of hypoglycemia, such as beta-blockers and alcohol, should be avoided. The timing of exercise and the peak effect of insulin administered before exercise are of paramount importance. Blood glucose should be monitored more closely during the first week of activity—both before and after approximately 30 minutes of exercise. If exercise is performed near the peak effect of insulin given, a snack can be utilized prior to exercise to minimize the tendency to hypoglycemia. A source of glucose to treat mild hypoglycemia should be available during and after exercise, including juice, fruit, or a commercial glucose-rich prepartaion. More severe hypoglycemia resulting in vomiting or an altered state of consciousness can be treated with glucagon intramuscularly. Although glucagon has a gluconeogenic effect initially, it is a potent direct stimulus to insulin secretion, which can result in rebound hypoglycemia, so that attention must be given to other measures to raise blood glucose levels (Table 2). Subsequent adjustments in the insulin dose preceding exercise should be reduced by 10 to 20 per cent, depending on the severity of the hypoglycemia.

Athletes with diabetes should wear Alert bracelets identifying their condition and should strive always to exercise with companions who are knowledgeable with respect to the symptoms, signs, and treatment of hypoglycemia. Sports that place the diabetic patient at risk for injury to the eye or head, such as football, should be discouraged. Sports, such as gymnastics and diving, that place the diabetic patient at risk for injury-producing falls should be avoided.[12] Ultimately, after consideration of the risks and alternatives, the athlete must decide and is responsible. (See further discussion in "Issues and Risks.")

TABLE 2. An Approach to Symptomatic Hypoglycemia

Mild
Juice, fruit, or commercial glucose preparation
Assure glucose control prior to return to exercise

Moderate to Severe
Glucagon, 0.5 – 1.0 mg SC, IM, or IV (may repeat every 15–20 minutes prn)
If available, dextrose 50% in water, 1 ml/kg up to 50 ml, IV (may repeat if needed)
Give oral carbohydrate when fully conscious to assure sustained effect
Adjust insulin to assure glucose control

■ HEAT INJURY

Vigorous physical activity results in significant energy expenditure and generation of heat. Energy expenditure per hour can range from 400 kilocalories for the novice runner to as much as 1200 kilocalories for the elite runner, resulting in a change in core body termperature from 37°C to 39 to 41° C.[13] Dissipation of generated heat occurs by conduction, radiation, convection, and evaporation of sweat. A variety of environmental factors can greatly alter these mechanisms, including the ambient temperature, humidity, direct exposure to the sun's radiation, and the types and amounts of clothing worn. In addition, medications that interfere with the sympathetic nervous system, such as anticholinergic agents and beta-blockers, also may be implicated in alteration of an athlete's ability to sweat. Lack of attention to any one or more of these factors can result in heat injury. During prolonged-endurance exercise, such as running a marathon, hyperthermia is one of the primary factors limiting athletic performance.[14]

Heat injuries are easier to prevent than to treat. The American College of Sports Medicine recommends that distance races should not be conducted when the wet bulb temperature exceeds 28°C.[15] The cooler periods of the day and the early morning or late evening hours are usually best for sports. Adequate fluid replacement is an essential factor in preventing heat injury and should be initiated prior to exercise. Use of water is quite appropriate, and an electrolyte solution is rarely needed except under extremely severe climatic conditions in an individual not yet acclimatized. Athletes should be encouraged to drink 8 ounces of fluid 10 to 15 minutes before competition and to pause and drink more fluid at regular intervals during exercise. Excessive glucose concentrations in electrolyte solutions can impair gastric emptying and absorption of free water, thereby defeating the purpose of fluid replacement.[13] Awareness of these issues and recommendations should help minimize the incidence of thermal injury during periods of high temperature and humidity.

Attempts have been made to reduce core temperature by artificial skin wetting, as with a water sprinkler, but these have not proved to be effective. Although spraying produces a significant reduction in mean skin temperature, this is offset by an overall reduction in skin conductance, presumably as a result of cutaneous vasoconstriction resulting in no net heat transfer from the core.[14]

Heat injuries range from heat exhaustion to heatstroke. Heatstroke is a serious, life-threatening disease caused when the body's thermoregulatory system fails and the core temperature rises to extreme levels. Rectal temperature can range from 40.6°C to as high as 42.5°C. Mild cases of heat-related illness can be treated with rest and water replacement. Heatstroke is a medical emergency requiring rapid cooling and intravenous fluid and electrolyte replacement. An icewater bath is an ideal measure, but in less extreme cases, a cooling mattress and ice packs may suffice. When core temperature declines to about 39°C, cooling should be modified becasue of the danger of excessive cooling and overshoot. In serious cases, monitoring of fluid and electrolyte balance, acid-base balance, and cardiac rhythm must be accomplished. Unfortunately, even with maximal therapy, mortality from heatstroke is high.

■ PREGNANCY

There has been a significant cultural shift in our society's view of exercise and activity during pregnancy. Not so many years ago, a woman might have been advised to cease working or even might have been asked to leave the workplace simply because she had become pregnant. Now exercise is often a part of a woman's lifestyle, and a woman who chooses to continue to exercise can do so throughout pregnancy. The effects of pregnancy and exercise combine to influence heart rate, cardiac output, blood pressure, and blood flow. Physiologic changes that normally occur during pregnancy are affected by exercise, usually to the woman's benefit.[16] At the same time, several anatomic and physiologic changes occur during pregnancy that make exercise difficult. These include an increase in maternal weight, the presence of exaggerated lordosis, increased joint laxity, and increased fluid retention. There is also a shift in the center of gravity that can decrease coordination, balance, and agility. Exercise actually can be helpful and can offset some of these changes by causing a strengthening of bones, ligaments, and

muscle. In addition, exercise directly helps improve coordination and joint mobility and reduce water retention and leg swelling, with improved venous circulation of the legs. Exercise also can minimize low backache and improve posture.

Animal studies have shown that with prolonged exhaustive exercise, cardiac output is redistributed, with increased blood flow to exercising muscle and decreased blood flow to the uterus.[16] There is considerable controversy as to whether uteroplacental blood flow is autoregulated, which might offset this phenomenon. Even if autoregulation occurs, there is concern that this mechanism may be overwhelmed with increasing intensity and duration of exercise. Therefore it seems prudent to avoid initiating training during pregnancy and to limit intensity to no more than prepregnancy levels. With increasing gestational age, pulmonary reserve is reduced, and even women with a high level of physical fitness will fatigue more quickly. At the same time, a fit pregnant woman can maintain more strenuous activity and delay the possible occurrence of oxygen debt during the later stages of pregnancy.

No amount of exercise is appropriate when conditions are already present that compromise placental blood flow. These include toxemia, hypertension, or intrauterine growth retardation. In addition, any sign of bleeding, premature labor, or incompetent cervix, suspected or documented fetal disease, and infection are contraindications to exercise. Activity levels and exercise should be highly individualized in mothers with multiple gestation and diabetes.

■ Issues and Risks

■ SUDDEN DEATH DURING EXERCISE

In spite of the many benefits associated with exercise, lingering concerns remain regarding the possibility of sudden death while exercising. In individuals without any previously identified heart disease, the risk of sudden death during exercise is seven times the death rate during sedentary activities.[6] Siskovich reported that the relative risk of cardiac arrest during exercise, compared with other times, is 56 times greater among men with a low level of habitual activity and only five times greater among men with high levels.[17] However, the total risk of cardiac arrest among habitually vigorous men is only 40 per cent of that for sedentary men. Therefore, physical activity protects against sudden death overall, even though the risk of death during the activity itself is higher.

The incidence of cardiovascular complications during exercise among persons with cardiac diseases is extremely variable but is considerably greater than among healthy individuals. Even so, current cardiac rehabilitation practice allows for prescribed supervised exercise to be performed at a low risk of complications. In a review of 167 rehabilitation programs, the incidence rates per million patient hours were 8.9 for cardiac arrest, 3.4 for myocardial infarction, and 1.3 for fatalities.[18] The two most frequent complications are cardiac arrest and myocardial infarction; the former occurs seven times more often than the latter.[6]

The sudden death of a well-known individual such as Jim Fixx, runner and author, focuses tremendous public attention on this problem. Despite the pressure of liability concerns to detect abnormalities prospectively, screening exercise testing is not generally useful in predicting significant cardiovascular complications in asymptomatic persons.[19]

■ PARTICIPATION ISSUES

Many student athletes are required to have a yearly physical examination before they may participate in school-sponsored sports. Individual guidelines vary widely from state to state, and even within a particular state the local guidelines may vary.[20] Guidelines are often incomplete, so the completeness and appropriateness of the examination depend chiefly on the sports medicine knowledge and interest of the examining physician.[21] The Committee on Sports Medicine for the American Academy of Pediatrics published the recommendations for participation in competitive sports in 1988.[22] Previous guidelines have become obsolete because of changes not only in safety equipment but also in societal attitudes toward the rights of athletes to compete despite a medical condition that may increase the risk of sustaining an injury or aggravat-

ing a pre-existing medical condition.[22,23] The decision often brings the physician's concern for an athlete's safety into conflict with the athlete's right to pursue an interest in sports. The Committee considered that the physician, the athlete, and the parents must weigh whether the advantages of participation in athletics are worth whatever risks are involved.[22] The risks appear to be different for a young adolescent going out for a sport than for an adult whose sport is a central part of his or her life. The concept of "assumption of risk" covers a legally competent adult who wishes to subject himself or herself to an increased risk.[23] The delivery of medical care to the athlete appears to be following the evolving norms in other areas of medicine and in our society in general. The controversial decision by Sugar Ray Leonard to continue to box after experiencing a retinal detachment is an example of this evolution. An athlete has the right to all the available information concerning alternatives and risks to participation in a given activity or sport.[16] Only with this information can an informed choice, appropriate to the individual, be made.

REFERENCES

1. Paffenbarger RS, Jr, Hyde RT, Wing AL, et al. Physical activity, all-cause mortality, and longevity of college alumni. N Engl J Med 1986; 314:605–613.
2. Leon AS, Connett H, Jacobs DR Jr, et al. Leisure time physical activity levels and risk of coronary heart disease and death: the multiple risk factor intervention trial. JAMA 1987; 258:2388–2395.
3. Cinque C. Are Americans fit? Survey data conflict. Phys Sportsmed 1986; 14(11):24.
4. Nakai Y, Katoaka Y, Bando M, et al. Effects of physical exercise training on cardiac function and graft patency after coronary bypass grafting. J Thorac Cardiovasc Surg 1987; 93:65–72.
5. Winslow EBJ. Cardiac rehabilitation. JAMA 1987; 258(14):1937–1938.
6. Franklin BA. Safety of outpatient cardiac exercise therapy: reducing the incidence of complications. Phys Sportsmed 1986; 14(9):235–248.
7. Schroeckenstein DC, Busse W. Exercise and asthma: not incompatible. J Resp Dis 1988; 9(6):29–45.
8. McFadden ER Jr, Lenner KAM, Strohl VP. Postexertional airway rewarming and thermally induced asthma: new insights into pathophysiology and possible pathogenesis. J Clin Invest 1986; 788:18–25.
9. Corris PA, Nariman S, Gibson GJ. Nifedipine in the prevention of asthma induced by exercise and histamine. Am Rev Resp Dis 1983; 128:991–992
10. Massey KL, Hendeles L. Calcium antagonists in the management of asthma: breakthrough or ballyhoo? Drug Intell Clin Pharm 1987; 21(6):505–509.

11. Paternostro-Bayles M, Wing RR, Robertston RJ. Effect of life-style activity of varying duration on glycemic control in type II diabetic women. Diabetes Care 1989; 12:34–37.
12. Stephens P, Hoffman WH, Karlson K, et al: Exercise for children with chronic disease: what is allowable? J Musculo Skel Med 1988; 5(2):13–29.
13. Puffer JC. Sports medicine. In Taylor RB (ed). Family Medicine: Principles and Practice. New York: Springer Verlag, 1988:703–720.
14. Basset DR Jr, Nagle FG, Mookerjee S, et al. Thermoregulatory responses to skin wetting during prolonged treadmill running. Med Sci Sports Exerc 1907; 19(1):28–32.
15. American College of Sports Medicine. Position stand on the prevention of thermal injury during distance running. Sports Med Bull 1984; 19(3):8.
16. Kulpa PJ. Exercise during pregnancy. Fam Pract Recert 1989; 11(1):35–56.
17. Siskovich DS, Weiss NS, Fletcher RH, et al. The incidence of primary cardiac arrest during vigorous exercise. N Engl J Med 1984; 311:874–877.
18. Van Camp SP, Peterson RA. Cardiovascular complications of outpatient cardiac rehabilitation programs. JAMA 1986; 256(9):1160–1163.
19. Malinow MR, McGarry DL, Kuehl KS. Is exercise testing indicated for asymptomatic people? J Cardiac Rehabil 1984; 4:376–380.
20. Feinstein RA, Soileau EJ, Daniel WA. A national survey of preparticipation physical examination requirements. Phys Sportsmed 1988; 16(5):51–59.
21. Samples P. Preparticipation exams: are they worth the time and trouble? Phys Sportsmed 1986; 14(10)180–187.
22. Committee on Sports Medicine. Recommendations for participation in competitive sports. Pediatrics 1988; 81(5):737–740.
23. Dorsen PJ. Should athletes with one eye, kidney, or testicle play contact sports? Phys Sportsmed 1986; 14(7):130–138.

Reflex sympathetic dystrophy syndrome

David L. Smith ■ *Stephen M. Campbell*

In the classic form, reflex sympathetic dystrophy syndrome (RSDS) is characterized by distal extremity pain, swelling, and dystrophic skin changes, coupled with episodic vasodilatation or vasoconstriction (vasomotor instability). Other associated features of RSDS include limitation of shoulder motion, finger flexion deformities, sweat gland stimulation, and hair or nail changes. Not all these clinical features are always apparent at presentation, and they may vary with time. Although unilateral upper extremity involvement is most common, lower extremity or bilateral involvement can occur.

■ Background

Since its initial description in the Civil War era,[1] other terms, such as causalgia, shoulder-hand syndrome, Sudeck's atrophy, and postinfarction sclerodactyly, have been employed to depict the same symptom complex. The term *reflex sympathetic dystrophy* syndrome was introduced in 1947 by Evans[2] in an attempt to unite overlapping terminology. Frozen shoulder syndrome[3] or adhesive shoulder capsulitis is felt by many investigators to be a variant of RSDS;[3,4] transient regional osteoporosis[5] also has coexisting features (Fig. 1).

RSDS is a diagnostic challenge, since there is a wide variety of underlying or associated conditions that potentially could go unrecognized and trigger the symptom complex, lack of uniform clinical diagnostic criteria, and perhaps an underappreciation of radiographic or scintigraphic abnormalities that can support the diagnosis. Also, RSDS remains a therapeutic challenge since management of the patients can be difficult despite a wide variety of effective modalities reported. Although spontaneous recovery may occur in adults, patients may develop chronic symptoms, and end-stage disease may become irreversible, resulting in a poor functional outcome.[6] RSDS also has been described in children.[7,8] In contrast to the adult form, RSDS in children tends to be self-lim-

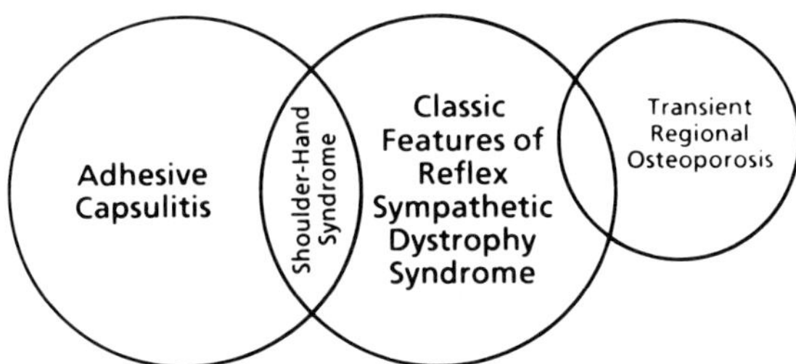

Figure 1. Overlapping features of adhesive shoulder capsulitis, RSDS, and transient regional osteoporosis (TRO). Adhesive shoulder capsulitis (frozen shoulder syndrome) without coexisting features of RSDS is felt to be a variant of RSDS. Shoulder-hand syndrome is a term applied to RSDS when adhesive capsulitis and signs of hand vasomotor instability and dystrophic skin changes exist. Features that distinguish TRO from RSDS include absence of vasomotor and skin signs with TRO. On the other hand, radiographic evidence of migratory osteopenia with RSDS is usually absent. In general, TRO is felt to be a variant of RSDS.

iting, and less aggressive therapeutic modalities are most often employed.[9,10]

■ TRIGGERING EVENTS AND PATHOGENESIS

RSDS has been associated with many underlying traumatic, surgical, and medical conditions (Table 1). The precise pathopsychology of RSDS remains unknown.[11] Medical and surgical conditions or traumatic events can trigger the sympathetic autonomic nerve supply to the involved extremity. Although earlier investigators focused on peripheral mechanisms[12] (e.g., artificial synapse theory), central spinal cord dysfunction has gained attention more recently.[13] A leading model suggests that tissue damage or disruption evokes chronic afferent nociceptic pain fiber excitation. Accentuated spinal cord internuncial or wide dynamic-range neuronal activity develops. Spinal cord internuncial neurons become sensitized to any further stimulation induced from A-fiber mechanoreceptors. This leads to touch-evoked pain (allodynia). Sympathetic efferents are stimulated, and cross-stimulation to blood vessels, sweat glands, muscles, bone, skin, or synovium can result[14] (Fig. 2).

■ CLINICAL SIGNS AND SYMPTOMS

Signs and symptoms have been divided into early, middle, and late phases. Since these

TABLE 1. Triggering Events of Conditions Associated with RSDS

Precipitant	Interval Preceding Features of RSDS	Per Cent of All Cases*
TRAUMA		
Wrist/hand fractures	2–4 wks.	30
Ankle/foot fractures		
Crush injuries		
Contusions and sprains of neck, shoulder, or arm		
Lacerations		
Spinal cord injuries		
Electrical or thermal burns		
POSTOPERATIVE		
Carpal tunnel decompression	2–4 wks.	10
Dupuytren's contracture repair		
Ganglion excision		
Hip surgery		
Knee arthroscopy		
NEUROLOGIC		
Cerebrovascular accident	2–6 wks.	20
Peripheral nerve entrapment or injury (i.e., median or ulnar nerve)		
Head trauma		
INTRATHORACIC		
Myocardial infarction	1 day–6 wks.	10
Thoracic or cardiac surgery		
Infection		
OTHER		
Neoplasm	?	20
Cervical osteoarthritis		
Herpes zoster		
Metabolic bone disease		
Drugs		
IDIOPATHIC	?	10
TOTAL		100

*Since multiple descriptions and terminology have been used for RSDS, the "per cent of all cases" should be viewed as an approximation rather than an absolute.

(Adapted with permission from Smith DL, Campbell SM. Reflex sympathetic dystrophy syndrome. Diagnosis and management. West J Med 1987; 147:342–345.)

designations are arbitrary, symptoms or findings can overlap or coexist between phases.

Early. In this phase, findings from vasodilation are evident. The distal aspect of the arm or leg is red, warm, and edematous. Erythema may be enhanced in the dependent position. Nondermatomal sharp or burning pain is pronounced, often with minimal touch (allodynia or hyperpathia). Accelerated hair and nail growth or smooth and sweaty skin may also be present. The hand

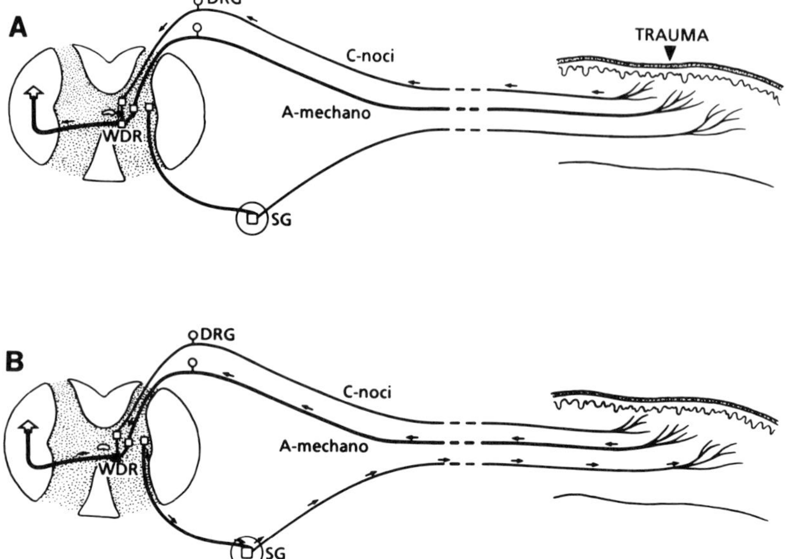

Figure 2. *A,* Trauma or other triggering event (e.g., myocardial infarction) can trigger afferent nociceptive pain fibers. Wide dynamic range (WDR) spinal cord neuron activity develops. *B,* Further WDR stimulation can be induced by A-fiber mechanoreceptors such as touching the skin. Sympathetic efferent neurons are excited and may augment skin mechanical or pain receptor activity. An abnormal cycle of nerve fiber stimulation activity occurs without further triggering events. This model on the pathogenesis is supported in part by animal studies. The precise pathophysiology remains unknown. DRG, dorsal root ganglia; SG, sympathetic ganglia. (Adapted with permission from Roberts WJ: A hypothesis on the physiologic basis for causalgia and related pains. Pain 1986; 24:297–311.)

is held in a flexed and guarded position. Finger stiffness or early joint contractures may be present. Shoulder stiffness with a mild, painful loss of range of motion may occur. This phase may last up to 6 months.

Middle. In this phase, findings from distal vasoconstriction are apparent. The hand or foot is cool and blanched or even cyanotic. Atrophy of subcutaneous tissue and intrinsic hand or foot muscles is present. Digit flexion contractures occur while hypersensitivity and/or burning pain persists. Usually, shoulder mobility becomes markedly impaired with upper extremity involvement. The skin of the hand or foot is smooth or even glazed in appearance. Hair and nail growth abates. This phase lasts several months; however, 20 per cent of cases become chronic and some degree of impairment persists.[14]

Late. Late-phase symptoms and findings are characterized by advanced skin, subcutaneous, and intrinsic hand or foot muscle atrophy. Digit flexion contractures frequently become fixed. Abnormal vasomotor activity and hyperpathia diminish while shoulder immobility persists. Dupuytren's-type contractures may be visible. This stage may last up to 12 months, and 30 per cent of the patients have a chronic or irreversible course, despite aggressive treatment.

■ DIAGNOSIS

Although firm clinical or laboratory diagnostic criteria have not been established for RSDS, preliminary criteria have been proposed.[15] These should help the clinician make a diagnosis (Table 2). Heightened awareness of the cardinal clinical features (Table 3) and knowledge of the phases and progression of RSDS, coupled with a joint imaging study[16] should facilitate diagnostic efforts (Fig. 3). Radiographic abnormalities, consisting of patchy or diffuse osteopenia in the involved distal extremity, are present in approximately 70 per cent of cases.[17] Unfortunately, these abnormalities are not present until symptoms have been present for at least 6 weeks.[18] Moreover, these radiographic findings are not pathognomonic for RSDS. Similar radiographic findings can be seen in patients with disuse osteoporosis or in those who have inflammatory arthritis.[19] On the other hand, three-phase scintigraphy using technetium-99m diphosphonate appears to have good diagnostic utility for classic or definite cases of RSDS (based on clinical criteria). An abnormal scintigram has a sensitivity of 96 per cent and a specificity of 97 per cent in classic or definite cases.[16] These are abnormal prior to radiographic changes and may also help predict response to therapy.[15] In addition, at least in children,

TABLE 2. Diagnostic Clinical Features and Supportive Criteria for the Reflex Sympathetic Dystrophy Syndrome (RSDS)

Definite RSDS
Pain, swelling, and tenderness in an extremity
Symptoms and signs of vasoconstriction or
   vasodilation
Dystrophic skin or nail changes usually present

Probable RSDS
Pain and tenderness in an extremity and
   EITHER
      symptoms and signs of vasoconstriction or
        vasodilations
   OR
   swelling
Dystrophic skin or nail changes often are present

Possible RSDS
Symptoms or signs of vasoconstriction or vasodilation and
   EITHER
   swelling
   OR
   tenderness
Dystrophic skin or nail changes are occasionally
   present

Doubtful RSDS
Unexplained pain and tenderness in an extremity
   without history or evidence of vasoconstriction
   or vasodilation
Dystrophic skin or nail changes are not present

Supportive Criteria
Abnormal delayed-image radionuclide bone scans
   show increased periarticular activity in multiple
   joints
Radiographs of the affected distal extremity show
   localized patchy osteopenia

(With permission, from Smith DL, Campbell SM. Reflex sympathetic dystrophy syndrome. Diagnosis and management. West J Med 1987; 147:342–345. These proposed criteria are modified from Kozin F. Reflex sympathetic dystrophy syndrome. Bull Rheum Dis 1986; 36:1–8.)

thermography may be useful as an aid in establishing the correct diagnosis.[20]

■ Management

No one knows what constitutes optimal therapy for RSDS. The many presentations of the syndrome, its variable course, and the lack of easily reproducible objective criteria for response have made the study of therapy difficult.

At least two generalizations are widely accepted:

1. Spontaneous recovery. Many patients with RSDS will recover spontaneously. If patients with strokes or injuries are followed carefully, many will develop scintigraphic, radiographic, or subtle clinical findings of RSDS; most of these patients eventually will return to normal without therapy and never develop the full-blown clinical syndrome.[16,21]
2. Early treatment. Successful therapy of RSDS depends on its early institution.[22] Therapy instituted in the first few weeks or months of the syndrome is far more likely to result in improvement; therapy delayed for months or years, when RSDS has entered its chronic form, often results in little or no benefit.

The clinical dilemma is obvious. Many patients seen early in the course of RSDS are likely to get better on their own, but if therapy is going to be used it must be instituted early. How can we treat those patients who need to be treated, yet avoid possibly toxic therapy in those who will recover spontaneously? The answer is unknown. Given the potential for chronic pain and disability, it seems better to err on the side of treating. Thus, patients who have definite findings of RSDS (particularly early in the course or shortly after a precipitating event) and those

TABLE 3. Clinical Findings in the Reflex Sympathetic Dystrophy Syndrome*

Clinical Finding	Per Cent with Finding (Range)
Pain	
Distal pain	98 (96–100)†
Tenderness	72 (55–88)†
Hyperesthesia	79 (69–88)†
Swelling	62 (46–69)†
Vasomotor changes	
Erythema	47 (36–60)†
Cyanosis	8 (5–16)
Warmth	15 (6–21)†
Raynaud's phenomenon	12 (2–20)
Dystrophic changes	
Hypertrichosis, nail changes, atrophy	47 (21–60)
Hyperhidrosis	32 (21–40)†
Decreased hand/finger movement	77 (37–88)†
Bilateral (clinical findings)	22 (10–25)

*This table represents a compilation of four studies encompassing 714 patients. Not all findings were noted in each study. Patients at all stages of disease were described. Those changes usually seen in early disease are marked with a dagger(†).

(Reprinted with permission from Smith DL, Campbell SM. Reflex sympathetic dystrophy syndrome. Diagnosis and management. West J Med 1987; 147:342–345).

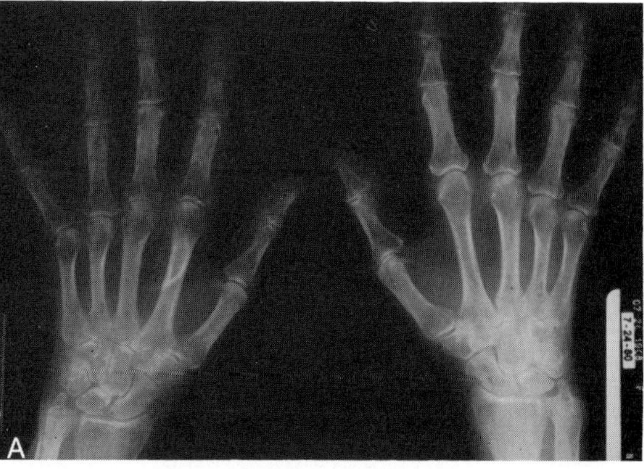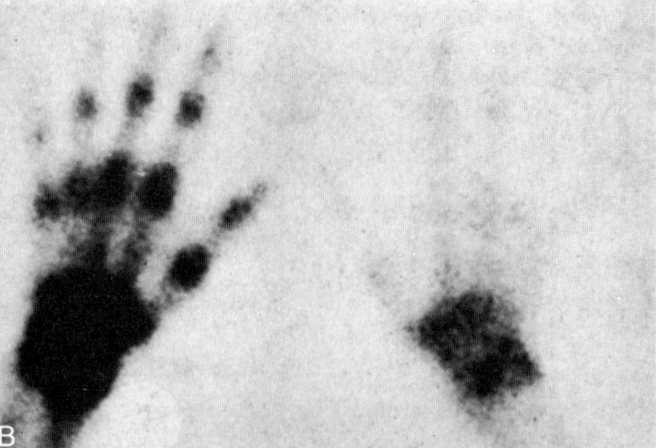

Figure 3. *A*, Bilateral hand radiograph. In the left hand, pronounced periarticular osteopenia is present about multiple metacarpal phalangeal joints, while patchy osteopenia is present in the radial carpal joint area. The uninvolved right hand demonstrates normal bone caliber. *B*, Bilateral hand joint imaging study using 99m technetium diphosphonate. On the left side, an abnormal, markedly increased uptake in multiple joints is present (delayed image scan). These abnormalities were seen in the patient shown in *A* who had an abnormal radiograph. Minimal activity is present in the right wrist area (uninvolved side). In the setting of lefthand vasomotor instability and cutaneous abnormalities, an abnormal delayed scintigram such as this is virtually pathognomonic for RSDS.

whose symptoms or signs progress certainly should receive therapy; those patients with less definite RSDS or with chronic stable findings (many months or years) should be approached more cautiously.

■ GENERAL RULES

Given a decision to treat a patient with RSDS, there are at least three widely accepted general rules:

1. Treat early. If you decide to treat, go ahead and do it; further delay in therapy yields less successful results.
2. Expect slow or partial improvement. The patients do not improve quickly: signs of improvement may take weeks or even months to develop and may be incomplete. Partial improvement does not mean that treatment was unsuccessful.
3. Try several modes of therapy. Failure or only partial improvement with one type of therapy does not mean that other therapy will not work. This is not surprising, given the uncertainty surrounding the pathogenesis of RSDS.

■ SPECIFIC THERAPY

The therapies proposed for RSDS are depicted in Figure 4 and listed in Table 4. Sup-

port in the literature for many of these is sparse.

■ PHYSICAL THERAPY

Physical therapy (PT) plays an important role in the treatment of RSDS. The rationale is partly empiric (based on apparent clinical improvement in patients with therapy) and partly theoretic (altering the balance of nociceptive somatic inflow and sympathetic outflow, thus breaking the reflex arc underlying RSDS).

Most investigators agree that *mobilization of the extremity* is important in the treatment of RSDS.[23-25] In part this may be traced to the perception that immobilization may cause or worsen RSDS. Patients should be encouraged to use passive and active range of motion aggressively. This may not be well tolerated when the pain and stiffness are severe. In fact, therapy that causes significant or prolonged worsening of the pain actually may worsen the entire syndrome, perhaps by potentiating the central reflexes or afferent sympathetic outflow underlying RSDS.

Many other types of PT have been suggested as being valuable. Few objective data support their use, but some patients seem to benefit. PT in RSDS often uses some kind of sensory stimulus, such as alternating hot and cold treatments, ultrasound,[26] or transcutaneous nerve stimulation,[27,28] in an attempt to alter somatic nociceptive influx

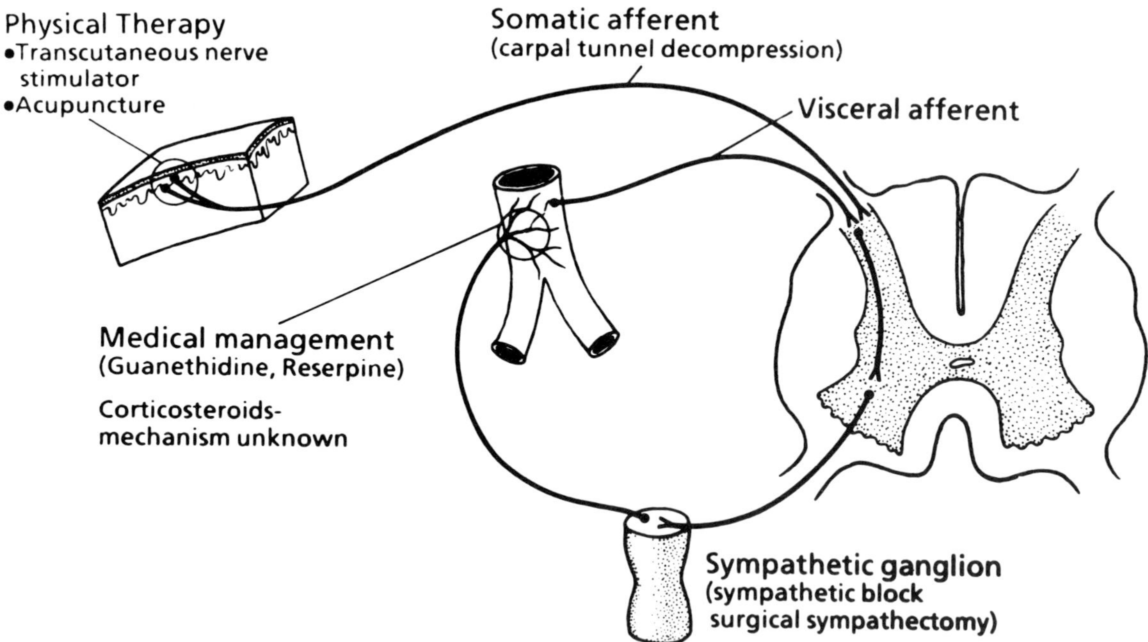

Figure 4. Various therapeutic modalities and their sites of action. Surgically correcting a peripheral nerve entrapment (e.g., carpal tunnel decompression) should improve abnormal diminished afferent nociceptive activity. Abnormal efferent activity can be modified or corrected by both surgical and medical modalities.

and thus break the reflex arc perpetuating RSDS.

In summary, the best PT for RSDS is mobilization of an extremity, preferably immediately after an injury to pre-empt the development of the syndrome, or early in the course of the disease. Mobilization should be aggressive, but not to the point of markedly increasing the patient's pain. Other types of PT may help by diminishing

or masking the pain, or by increasing the efficacy of mobilization.

■ SYMPATHETIC BLOCKADE

Sympathetic blockade is the standard therapy for RSDS. Blocking sympathetic activity in the periphery not only decreases the trophic and vasomotor changes seen in the skin and subcutaneous tissue, but also diminishes pain perception and hyperpathia. This allows more vigorous use of the extremity, with the aforementioned benefits.

Some form of sympathetic blockade has been available for 50 years. Though many studies attest to clinical benefits in many, if not most, patients, few studies compare sympathetic blockade with placebo or with other medical therapy, or compare different regimens of sympathetic blockade. Given the frequency of spontaneous recovery in RSDS, this is unfortunate. However, since many patients with advanced RSDS (who would not be expected to recover spontaneously) do respond to sympathetic blockade, it seems clear that these techniques do indeed work with some frequency.

Regional Sympathetic Blockade. These techniques involve exposing the sympa-

---

TABLE 4. Therapy of Reflex Sympathetic Dystrophy Syndrome

Physical Therapy
  Mobilization*
  Transcutaneous nerve stimulation*
  Contrast temperature therapy
  Acupuncture/electroacupuncture
  Ultrasound
Sympathetic Blockade
  Regional sympathetic blockade*
  Paravertebral ganglion blockade*
  Surgical sympathectomy*
Medical Therapy
  Corticosteroids*
  Propranolol
  Phenoxybenzamine
  Nifedipine
  Calcitonin

*Therapies most commonly used, or those with extensive support in the literature.

thetic nerves of an involved extremity to some kind of sympathetic blockade given intravenously.[29,30] A *Bier block* is usually used to achieve high concentrations of sympathetic blocker while avoiding systemic toxicity. In essence, an intravenous catheter is placed in the affected arm or leg, the extremity is exsanguinated using elastic bandages, and a blood pressure cuff is placed and inflated to above systolic pressure. The sympathetic blocking agent is then infused through the IV catheter and allowed to bind to tissue receptors for 10 to 15 minutes; the blood pressure cuff is then deflated.

Active substances used with this technique have included lidocaine, reserpine, guanethedine, and methylprednisolone (which is thought to decrease postinfusion edema).[29-35] Benefit has been observed in 25 to 75 per cent of patients treated, sometimes lasting for a day or two to several months. Most studies suggest that repeated infusions (e.g., every other day for a total of 4 infusions) are often necessary. Only a few studies have compared regional sympathetic blockade with paravertebral sympathetic blockade, with uncertain results. Overall, the two techniques probably afford similar results.[36,37]

Paravertebral Sympathetic Blockade. The most widely used form of sympathetic blockade is paravertebral sympathetic blockade, and specifically stellate ganglion blockade. In these techniques, an anesthetic (e.g., lidocaine or bupivicaine) is injected into the prevertebral fascia along which the sympathetic ganglia run: the stellate and thoracic ganglia for the arm, and the lumbar ganglia for the leg. Achievement of a successful stellate ganglion block is demonstrated, for example, by rapid relief of pain, a cool dry hand, and development of an ipsilateral Horner's syndrome.

Good-to-excellent results can be achieved in 25 to 75 per cent of patients: these effects may be temporary (days) or permanent.[38-40] As with other therapy of RSDS, the earlier the therapy the better. Best results are seen in the first 6 months of disease. Most patients require several paravertebral sympathetic blocks; lack of significant response to daily or every other day blocks after 5 to 7 days should be considered a failure of the therapy. Several reports have described placing an indwelling catheter into the prevertebral fascia and infusing anesthetic constantly for several days.[41] Ganglionic block-

ade of the leg is more difficult; it may be necessary to try to localize the levels involved, using sensory epidural anesthesia, before attempting paravertebral ganglionic blockade.[42]

Surgical Sympathectomy. Permanent sympathetic blockade can be obtained by surgically removing the sympathetic ganglia.[39-45] Generally speaking, this therapy is reserved for those patients who respond fairly well but only temporarily to paravertebral sympathetic blockade. These patients appear to have a good likelihood of responding permanently to surgical sympathectomy. Patients who do not benefit from paravertebral sympathetic blockade are unlikely to respond to surgical therapy.

■ MEDICAL THERAPY

At this time there is little evidence, with a few exceptions, to suggest that medical therapy helps RSDS. Many drugs have been tried, usually with no benefit. The strongest data available concern corticosteroid therapy.

Corticosteroids. Although the mechanism of action is unknown, corticosteroids have been used since the early 1950s to treat shoulder-hand syndrome and, hence, RSDS. Several controlled and uncontrolled trials have shown that patients with RSDS benefit from corticosteroid therapy.[22,46] In a randomized controlled study of 23 patients, 13 patients were treated with prednisone, 10 mg three times a day, to recovery or to a maximum of 12 weeks; all 13 had more than 75 per cent improvement in their symptoms. In contrast, only 2 of 10 patients given placebo had similar improvement.[47] In another study, more than 60 per cent of patients treated with higher doses of prednisone (initially, 40 to 60 mg per day with a rapid taper) for 2 to 4 weeks had good-to-excellent responses to treatment; many of these patients had previously not responded to stellate ganglion blockade.[15] It appeared that abnormal scintigraphy predicted steroid responsiveness, but that otherwise the duration of symptoms did not seem to be related to a likelihood of response.

Other Medical Therapy. Propranolol, which produces nonselective beta-blockade, has been described as having some benefit in a few patients.[48,49] In another series of patients, oral phenoxybenzamine (40 to 120 mg a day for 6 to 8 weeks) was used to try to achieve systemic sympathetic blockade; a large number of these patients, and nearly all of those with acute RSDS, had excellent and prolonged responses.[50] In an uncontrolled study, nifedipine, which may affect vascular tone and hence blood supply in an extremity, was given in doses of 10 to 30 mg three times a day. Seven of thirteen patients had complete relief of their symptoms.[51] Finally, there is some interest in the European literature on the use of calcitonin as an adjunct to PT.[52,53]

■ Issues and Risks

■ DIAGNOSIS

The diagnosis of RSDS may be difficult in some cases. In some patients, RSDS symptoms may mimic those of Raynaud's disease, transient regional osteoporosis, thromboembolic disease, or connective tissue diseases such as systemic sclerosis or an asymmetric inflammatory arthritis. A detailed history and examination combined with a three-phase nuclear scintigram should lead to the correct diagnosis (see Fig. 3B).

■ TREATMENT

A variety of modalities, from PT alone to surgical sympathectomy or corticosteroid use in conjunction with PT, have been advocated for RSDS. Although clinical studies have attested to the usefulness of each of these, the optimal treatment of RSDS is unknown. In adult patients, the issues or controversies about treatment are whether a surgical approach, regional sympathetic blockade, or a trial of corticosteroids should be used initially. A logical approach consists of considering the following salient points.

Avoid the development of RSDS by promptly diagnosing any associated conditions or correcting or modifying precipitating causes. In general, early mobilization after injury should be encouraged. If the syndrome develops, treat it early in order to optimize results. Mobilization of the affected extremity is important, but not to the extreme that increased pain or other symptoms occur. Use of other modalities of physical therapy, such as transcutaneous nerve

stimulation, may afford increased mobilization without enhancing pain perception. If severity of symptoms and progression of disease become apparent, consider whether more aggressive therapy is warranted. In adults, choose between sympathetic blockade (regional or paravertebral ganglion blocks) or systemic corticosteroid therapy, based on the availability of consultants with experience in these techniques, the patient's other medical problems, and the patient's own wishes. Failure of one form of therapy does not mean other therapy will fail; try other modalities.

Although long-term steroid use has the inherent risk of causing bony compression fractures or cataracts, a short course (4 weeks) of a tapering prednisone dose should minimize these untoward effects. Alternatively, regional or paravertebral sympathetic blockade can be performed and may be successful, especially when used early in the course of RSDS with a sympathetic blocker or local anesthetic. It is our view that surgical sympathectomy should be reserved for patients in whom a trial of steroids was unsuccessful and paravertebral sympathetic blockade afforded good but only temporary results.

In children, corticosteroids, sympathetic blockade, and sympathectomy are usually not necessary. Typically, PT, transcutaneous nerve stimulation, and analgesics will allow recovery, since a self-limited form of RSDS is the rule.[10]

REFERENCES

1. Mitchell SW, Morehouse GR, Keen WW. Gunshot Wounds and Other Injuries to Nerves. Philadelphia: JB Lippincott, 1864:1–164.
2. Evans JA. Reflex sympathetic dystrophy; report on 57 cases. Ann Intern Med 1947; 26:417–426.
3. Risk TE, Pinals RS. Frozen shoulder. Semin Arthritis Rheum 1982; 11:440–452.
4. Steinbrocker O, Spitzer N, Friedman HH. The shoulder-hand syndrome in reflex dystrophy of the upper extremity. Ann Intern Med 1947; 29:22–52.
5. Lakhanpal S, Ginsburg WW, Luthra HS, Hunder GG. Transient regional osteoporosis. A study of 56 cases and review of the literature. Ann Intern Med 1987; 106:444–450.
6. Steinbrocker O, Argyros TG. The shoulder-hand syndrome: present status as a diagnostic and therapeutic entity. Med Clin North Am 1958; 42:1533–1553.
7. Fermaglich DR: Reflex sympathetic dystrophy in childhood. J Pediatr 1977; 60:881–883.
8. Bernstein BH, Singsen BH, Kent JT, et al. Reflex neu-

rovascular dystrophy in childhood. J Pediatr 1978; 93:211–215.

9. Forster RS, Fu FH. Reflex sympathetic dystrophy in children. A case report and review of the literature. Orthopedics 1985; 8:475–477.

10. Ruggeri SB, Athreya BH, Doughty R, Gregg JR. Das MM. Reflex sympathetic dystrophy in children. Clin-Orthop 1982; 163:225–230.

11. Folkerts JF, Wiertz-Hoessels MJ, Krediet P, Snee AJ. Reflex sympathetic dystrophy. A clinical, histological and experimental study. Confin Neurol 1969; 31:145–175.

12. Granit R, Leksell L, Skoglund CR. Fibre interaction in injured or compressed region of nerve. Brain 1944; 67:125–140.

13. Roberts WJ. A hypothesis on the physiologic basis for causalgia and related pains. Pain 1986; 24:297–311.

14. Smith DL, Campbell SM. Reflex sympathetic dystrophy syndrome. Diagnosis and management. West J Med 1987; 147:342–345.

15. Kozin F, Ryan LM, Carerra GF, Soin JS, Wortmann RL. The reflex sympathetic dystrophy syndrome. III. Scintigraphic studies, further evidence for the therapeutic efficacy of systemic corticosteroids and proposed diagnostic criteria. Am J Med 1981; 70:23–30.

16. Holder LE, MacKinnon SE. Reflex sympathetic dystrophy in the hands: clinical and scintigraphic criteria. Radiology 1984; 152:517–522.

17. Kozin F, Soin JS, Ryan LM, Carrera GF, Wortmann RL. Bone scintigraphy in the reflex sympathetic dystrophy syndrome. Radiology 1981; 138:437–443.

18. Kozin F, Genant HK, Bekerman C, McCarty D. The reflex sympathetic dystrophy syndrome. II. Roentgenographic and scintigraphic evidence of bilaterality and of periarticular accentuation. Am J Med 1976; 60:332–338.

19. Kozin F. Reflex sympathetic dystrophy syndrome. Bull Rheum Dis 1986; 36:1–8.

20. Lightman HI, Pochaczevsky R, Aprin H, Iiowite NT. Thermography in childhood reflex sympathetic dystrophy. J Pediatr 1987; 111:551–555.

21. Tepperman PS, Greyson ND, Hilbert L, Jiminez J, Williams HI. Reflex sympathetic dystrophy in hemiplegia. Arch Phys Med Rehabil 1984; 65:442–447.

22. Rosen PS, Graham W. The shoulder-hand syndrome: historical review with observations on 73 patients. Can Med Assoc J 1957; 77:86–93.

23. Goldsmith JL. Causes and prevention of reflex sympathetic dystrophy. J Hand Surg 1980; 5:295–296.

24. Goodman CR. Therapy of shoulder-hand syndrome. NY State J Med 1971; 71:559–562.

25. Subbarao J, Stillwell GK. Reflex sympathetic dystrophy syndrome of the upper extremity: analysis of total outcome of management of 125 cases. Arch Phys Med Rehabil 1981; 62:549–554.

26. Portwood MM, Lieberman JS, Taylor RG. Ultrasound treatment of reflex sympathetic dystrophy. Arch Phys Med Rehabil 1987; 68:116–118.

27. Richlin DM, Carron H, Rowlington JC, Sussman MD, Baugher WH, Goldner RD. Reflex sympathetic dystrophy: successful treatment with transcutaneous nerve stimulation. J Pediatr 1978; 93:84–86.

28. Meyer GA, Fields HL. Causalgia treated by selective large fibre stimulation of peripheral nerve. Brain 1972; 95:163–168.

29. Hannington-Kiff JG. Intravenous regional sympathetic blockade with guanethidine. Lancet 1974; 1:1019–1020.

30. Hannington-Kiff JG. Relief of Sudeck's atrophy with regional intravenous guanethidine. Lancet 1977; 1:1132–1133.

31. Glynn CJ, Basedow RW, Walsh JA. Pain relief following post-ganglionic sympathetic blockade with IV guanethidine. Br J Anaesth 1981; 1297–1301.

32. Chuinard RG, Dabezies EJ, Gould JS. Murphy GA, Matthews RE. Intravenous reserpine for reflex sympathetic dystrophy. South Med J 1981; 74:1481–1484.

33. Driesen J, Weikers CVD, Nicolai JPA, Cral JF. Clinical effects of regional intravenous guanethidine in reflex sympathetic dystrophy. Acta Anaesthesiol Scand 1983; 27:505–509.

34. Duncan KH, Lewis RD, Racz G, Nordyke MD. Treatment of upper extremity reflex sympathetic dystrophy with joint stiffness using sympatholytic Bier blocks and manipulation. Orthopedics 1988; 11:883–886.

35. Poplawski ZJ, Wiley AM, Murray JF. Post-traumatic dystrophy of the extremities; a clinical review and trial of treatment. J Bone Joint Surg 1983; 65A:642–655.

36. McKain CW, Urban BJ, Goldner JL. The effects of intravenous regional guanethidine and reserpine. J Bone Joint Surg 1983; 65A:808–811.

37. Bonelli S, Conoscente F, Movilia PG, Restelli L, Francucci B, Grossi E. Regional intravenous guanethidine vs. stellate ganglion block in reflex sympathetic dystrophies: a randomized trial. Pain 1983; 16:297–307.

38. Steinbrocker O, Neustadt D, Lapin L. Shoulder-hand syndrome—sympathetic blockade compared with corticotropin and cortisone therapy. JAMA 1946; 153:788–791.

39. Rasmussen TB, Freedman H. Treatment of causalgia. An analysis of 100 cases. J Neurosurg 1946; 3:165–173.

40. Wang JK, Johnson KA, Ilstrup DM. Sympathetic blocks for reflex sympathetic dystrophy. Pain 1985; 23:13–17.

41. Linson MA, Leffert P, Todd DD. Treatment of upper extremity reflex sympathetic blockade with prolonged continuous stellate ganglion block. J Hand Surg 1983; 8:153–159.

42. Erdemir H, Gelman S, Galbraith JG. Prediction of the needed level of sympathectomy for post traumatic reflex sympathetic dystrophy. Surg Neurol 1982; 17:353–354.

43. Kleinert HE, Cook FW, Kritz JE. Neurovascular disorders of the upper extremity treated by transaxillary sympathectomy. Arch Surg 1965; 90:612–616.

44. Patman RD, Thomson JE, Persson AV. Management of post traumatic pain syndrome: report of 113 cases. Ann Surg 1973; 177:780–787.

45. Schumacher HB, Abramson DI. Posttraumatic vasomotor disorders: with particular reference to late manifestations and therapy. Surg Gynecol Obstet 1949; 88:417–434.

46. Glick RN. Reflex dystrophy (algoneurodystrophy): results of therapy by corticosteroids. Rheumatol Rehabil 1973; 12:84–88.

47. Christensen K, Jensen EM, Noer I. The reflex dystrophy syndrome: response to treatment with systemic corticosteroids. Acta Chir Scand 1982; 148:653–655.

48. Simson G. Propranolol for causalgia and Sudeck's atrophy. JAMA 1974; 227:327.

49. Vistsunthorn U, Prete P. Reflex sympathetic dystrophy of the lower extremity. A complication of herpes zoster with dramatic response to propranolol. West J Med 1981; 135:62–66.

50. Ghostine SY, Comair YG, Turner DM, et al. Phenoxybenzamine in the treatment of causalgia. Report of 40 cases. J Neurosurg 1984; 60:1263–1268.
51. Prough DS, McLeskey CH, Poehling GG, et al. Efficacy of oral nifedipine in the treatment of reflex sympathetic dystrophy. Anesthesiology 1985; 62:796–799.
52. McKay NNS. Post-traumatic reflex sympathetic dystrophy syndrome (Sudeck's atrophy)—effect of regional guanethidine infusion and salmon calcitonin. Br Med J 1977; 1:1575–1576.
53. Gobelet C, Meier JL, Schaffner W, Bischof-Delaloye A, Gerster JC, Berckhardt P. Calcitonin and reflex sympathetic dystrophy syndrome. Clin Rheumatol 1986; 5:382–388.

Renal failure, acute

Randy L. Howard ■ *John D. Conger* ■ *Robert W. Schrier*

■ Background

Acute renal failure is an abrupt decline in renal function sufficient to result in retention of nitrogenous waste products in the body. The classic clinical feature of acute renal failure for years was felt to be oliguria. It is now clear that a nonoliguric form of acute renal failure exists and that this entity carries a better prognosis.[1] Acute renal failure is often referred to as acute tubular necrosis although frequently only minimal detectable morphologic changes of the renal tubules are observed. Acute tubular necrosis has become a term commonly used in clinical practice to describe tubular damage resulting from ischemia or various nephrotoxins (Table 1). This article will be directed primarily toward management of the acute renal failure associated with tubular damage. The detailed management of acute renal failure resulting from prerenal factors, postrenal factors, or intrinsic renal diseases, such as glomerulonephritis, vasculitis, and interstitial nephritis, will not be discussed.

Estimates of the frequency of acute renal failure were first obtained during World War II. One of ten patients with severe trauma developed acute renal failure, and the mortality rate was 90 per cent. During the Korean War, the incidence decreased to 1 in 200 severely traumatized patients, and the mortality rate decreased to approximately 60 per cent with the use of hemodialysis treatment. In the Vietnam War, the incidence of acute renal failure was further decreased to 1 in approximately 2000 casualties, but the mortality rate remained in the 50 to 60 per cent range. Acute renal failure is commonly encountered in contemporary medical practice. Approximately 4 to 5 per cent of all admissions to a general medical hospital develop acute renal failure. A higher incidence of acute renal failure is seen in intensive care units, in patients with rhabdomyolysis or severe burns, and in patients receiving aminoglycoside therapy.

In spite of improved dialysis techniques and regimens, the mortality rate of patients with acute renal failure who require dialysis has not changed significantly over the past 40 years.[2] The mortality rate for surgically related acute renal failure is in the range of 50 to 70 per cent, whereas acute renal failure in the medical setting is associated with mortality rates of 20 to 50 per cent.

Acute renal failure can result from three major processes: (1) a decrease in renal perfusion with a resultant decrease in glomerular filtration rate (prerenal azotemia), (2) intrinsic renal parenchymal disease (renal-azotemia), and (3) obstruction to urine flow (postrenal azotemia). Common causes of the three types of acute azotemia can be found in standard nephrology textbooks. Prerenal azotemia accounts for 40 to 80 per cent of acute renal failure, whereas postrenal azotemia accounts for 2 to 5 per cent.[3,4] The remainder of the cases of acute renal failure are due to renal azotemia. Prerenal and

TABLE 1. Causes of Acute Renal Failure Association with Tubular Damage

Hemodynamic	Nephrotoxic	
	Exogenous	*Endogenous*
Intravascular volume depletion	Aminoglycosides	Hyperuricemia
Hemorrhage	Sulfonamides	Myoglobinuria
GI fluid loss	NSAIDs	Hemoglobinuria
Third-space loss (e.g.,	Contrast media	Hypercalcemia
peritonitis, pancreatitis,	Heavy metals	
burns)	Methotrexate	
Reduced cardiac output	Cis-platinum	
Myocardial infarction	Acetaminophen	
Arrhythmias	Ethylene glycol	
Cardiomyopathy		
Valvular heart disease		
Pericardial tamponade		
Reduced vascular resistance		
Sepsis		
Antihypertensive agents		
Major surgery		

postrenal azotemia are usually reversible but in a prolonged state can lead to acute tubular necrosis.

▪ Management

In this section, we will discuss the initial conservative management of acute renal failure, complications associated with acute renal failure and their management, and dialysis therapy for acute renal failure. We will also briefly discuss management of specific nephrotoxins and the role of renal biopsy in acute renal failure.

Initial management of the patient with acute renal failure is outlined in Table 2. Correction of prerenal factors and provision for adequate drainage of the urinary system are essential. If the patient has obstruction of the urinary system, a Foley catheter or nephrostomies are necessary, depending on

TABLE 2. Initial Management of Acute Renal Failure

1. Exclude any reversible etiology
    Correct prerenal factors
    Provide for adequate drainage of urinary system
2. Attempt to induce a nonoliguric state if patient remains oliguric after correction of prerenal factors
    Mannitol
    Furosemide
    Dopamine
    Combination of furosemide and dopamine

the location of obstruction. The presence of injury to the renal vasculature and interstitial processes must be considered.

Little specific therapy is available once the diagnosis of acute renal failure is established. No specific therapy has been proved to improve glomerular filtration rate in established acute renal failure. If the patient remains oliguric after correction of prerenal factors, either mannitol, furosemide (Lasix),[5] or dopamine[6] can be administered in an attempt to induce a nonoliguric state. Furosemide can be administered at an initial dose of 1 mg/kg. The dose can be progressively increased at 2-hour intervals to a maximum of 5 mg/kg, administered intravenously over 20 to 30 minutes, if a diuresis is not established. Mannitol may be administered at a dose of 0.25 to 0.50 gm/kg. Hyperosmolarity may occur if a diruesis is not established and repeated doses of mannitol are administered. Dopamine can be administered as a continuous intravenous infusion at a rate of 1 to 3 μg/kg/min. Although the existence of a renal vasodilatory dose of dopamine remains controversial, some patients seem to benefit from the combination of dopamine and furosemide. Prospective studies have demonstrated that nonoliguric acute renal failure is a less severe form of acute renal failure.[1] Following these maneuvers, the patient is managed conservatively until dialysis becomes necessary.

Conservative management includes the following principles (Table 3): The intake of nitrogen, water, and electrolytes is decreased to match output. Adequate calories

TABLE 3. Conservative Management of Acute Renal Failure

1. Decrease intake of nitrogen, water, and electrolytes to match output
2. Provide adequate calories
3. Adjust medication dosage
4. Clinical monitoring
    Daily physical examination
    Intake and output
    Daily weights
5. Biochemical monitoring
    Complete blood count
    Electrolytes
    Blood urea nitrogen and creatinine
    Calcium and phosphorus
    Magnesium

are provided in an attempt to decrease tissue catabolism. Medication doses are adjusted for the degree of renal failure. Physical examination is performed daily to assess the patient for complications that will be discussed in the next section. Daily weights, along with intake and output, require close monitoring. Biochemical monitoring of complete blood count, electrolytes, blood urea nitrogen, and serum creatinine will be required at least daily. Calcium, phosphorus, and magnesium can be followed less frequently.

■ **COMPLICATIONS**

Table 4 outlines the complications associated with acute renal failure.

Fluid and Electrolytes. Renal elimination of nitrogenous wastes, water, electrolytes, and acids is impaired during acute renal failure. Three factors that determine the magnitude of biochemical abnormalities are urine volume (oliguric or nonoliguric), catabolic state of the patient, and severity of the reduction in glomerular filtration rate. Oliguric, catabolic patients have the most profound biochemical abnormalities.

The blood urea nitrogen and serum creatinine can be expected to increase daily 10 to 20 and 0.5 to 1.0 mg/dl, respectively, in oliguric, noncatabolic patients. Rhabdomyolysis, fever, sepsis, surgery, and trauma will result in greater increases in blood urea nitrogen and serum creatinine. Attempts to limit catabolism by treating fever and infection while providing adequate nutrition may decrease increments in nitrogenous

wastes. The optimal method for achieving nutrition remains controversial. To minimize endogenous tissue breakdown and prevent starvation ketoacidosis, at least 100 grams of carbohydrate should be provided daily. Hyperalimentation, a form of nutrition often used in critically ill patients, may lead to fluid overload and electrolyte disturbances.

With the development of acute renal failure, the kidney becomes less capable of excreting salt and water. Salt and water retention resulting in peripheral edema, pulmonary edema, and hyponatremia is an ever-present concern. The potential for development of fluid overload is greatest in oliguric patients and is usually due to excessive volume administration. In patients with acute renal failure, fluid intake should be limited to urine output plus insensible losses plus any extrarenal losses (gastrointestinal, wound drainage). Insensible losses occur from the respiratory tract and through the skin and increase with fever and tachypnea. Patients who require mechanical ventilation have minimal respiratory losses owing to the use of humidified oxygen.

Hyponatremia occurs frequently in acute renal failure. Patients are unable to excrete solute-free water and their free water intake should be limited as determined by the

TABLE 4. Complications of Acute Renal Failure

1. Fluid and electrolytes
    Azotemia
    Volume overload
    Hyponatremia
    Hyperkalemia
2. Divalent ion metabolism
    Hyperphosphatemia
    Hypocalcemia
    Hypermagnesemia
3. Acid-base disturbances
    Anion gap metabolic acidosis
4. Hematologic complications
    Normochromic, normocytic anemia
    Bleeding tendencies
5. Infectious
6. Cardiovascular
    Hypertension
    Volume overload
7. Neurologic
    Lethargy, somnolence, confusion, agitation
    Seizures
8. Gastrointestinal
    Nausea and vomiting
    Ileus
    Hemorrhage

serum sodium concentration. Hyponatremia indicates excess and hypernatremia denotes deficient solute-free water.

Hyperkalemia occurs frequently in acute renal failure because of decreased renal excretion of potassium. Other factors contributing to hyperkalemia include catabolism, which increases release of potassium from tissues, and acidemia, which shifts potassium out of cells. The major clinical effects of hyperkalemia are related to the cardiovascular and peripheral neuromuscular systems. Progressive effects of hyperkalemia on the cardiac conduction system include peaked T waves, prolongation of the P-R interval, depression of S-T segments, lengthening of the QRS interval, loss of P waves, and finally coarse ventricular fibrillation. Neuromuscular effects of hyperkalemia include weakness and paralysis. Treatment of hyperkalemia depends on the plasma potassium concentration and the extent of cardiovascular and neuromuscular symptoms. The principles of treatment of hyperkalemia involve counteracting the effect of potassium on muscle cell membrane potential, redistribution of potassium from the extracellular to the intracellular space, and finally removal of potassium from the body (Table 5). Increasing the extracellular calcium with calcium gluconate (10 to 20 ml of a 10 per cent solution) counteracts the effect of hyperkalemia on muscle cell membrane potential. Redistribution of potassium from the extracellular to the intracellular space can be accomplished with administration of sodium bicarbonate (50 to 100 mEq) or infusion of glucose and insulin (50 ml of 50 per cent dextrose with 10 units of regular insulin). Removal of potassium from the body can be accomplished with exchange resins such as sodium polystyrene (Kayexalate, 25 to 50 gm with sorbitol orally or without sorbitol as a retention enema) and with dialysis.

Phosphorus and Calcium. Hyperphosphatemia occurs with acute renal failure, owing to decreased renal elimination. Phosphorus levels are higher in catabolic patients and in those patients with extensive tissue damage. Treatment of hyperphosphatemia consists of administration of 30 to 60 ml of aluminum hydroxide orally four to six times per day.

Hypocalcemia is frequently encountered in acute renal failure. Causes include tissue deposition of calcium phosphate in the presence of hyperphosphatemia, skeletal resistance to the calcemic effect of parathyroid hormone, and decreased renal production of 1,25-dihydroxyvitamin D. The hypocalcemia associated with acute renal failure rarely requires specific therapy because the ionized component of total calcium is increased because of acidemia and frequent hypoalbuminemia. Acute administration of alkali to correct acidosis may result in increased protein binding of calcium and can lead to tetany or seizures owing to decreased ionized calcium.

Acid-Base. Metabolic acidosis occurs in all patients with acute renal failure because of an inability of the kidney to excrete the daily acid production of approximately 1 mEq/kg. The mild acidosis generally does not require treatment until the serum bicarbonate concentration falls to less than 15 mEq/liter. If treatment becomes necessary, then bicarbonate or citrate solutions can be given. Citrate is metabolized to bicarbonate by the liver. Administration of citrate to raise the bicarbonate concentration, together with aluminum in the form of aluminum hydroxide to control hyperphosphatemia, can increase aluminum absorption and lead to aluminum intoxication.

Hematologic. A normocytic, normochromic anemia usually develops in acute renal failure because of decreased erythropoiesis, extracorpuscular hemolysis, hemodilution, and gastrointestinal blood loss. The hematocrit usually stabilizes at between 20 and 30 per cent. Bleeding tendencies, although not common, may occur owing to qualitative platelet defects, poorly defined coagulation

TABLE 5. Management of Hyperkalemia

Therapy	Mechanism	Onset	Duration
Calcium chloride	Antagonism	Immediate	Brief
Glucose plus insulin	Redistribution	Minutes	Hours
Intravenous NaHCO$_3$	Redistribution	Minutes	Hours
Kayexalate	Removal	Hours	Hours
Dialysis	Removal	Hours	Hours

defects, anemia, and changes in blood vessels. Bleeding is more common if the hematocrit is less than 30 per cent.[7] The best clinical parameters to follow are the platelet count and bleeding time. Therapies to improve the bleeding tendency include correction of anemia, platelet transfusions, infusion of cryoprecipitate (10 units), infusion of deamino-arginine vasopressin (0.3 μg/kg), and administration of conjugated estrogens (10 to 30 mg daily).[8,9] Decreasing the blood urea nitrogen concentration with dialysis will also improve the bleeding tendency. Correction of bleeding tendencies should be accomplished in all patients with acute renal failure prior to surgery.

Infectious. Infections are commonly associated with and constitute the leading cause of death in patients with acute renal failure. Not only are infections commonly associated with the development of acute renal failure, but also infections involving surgical wounds, the respiratory tract, and the urinary tract frequently complicate acute renal failure. Thirty to seventy per cent of deaths in patients with acute tubular necrosis are due to infectious complications. A majority of patients with acute renal failure require treatment with antibiotics. Early removal of invasive devices (endotracheal tube, Foley catheter, central venous lines) can help decrease infections in patients with acute renal failure.

Cardiovascular. Cardiovascular complications associated with acute renal failure include circulatory congestion and hypertension. As noted, fluid overload is usually due to excessive volume administration in combination with a decreased ability to excrete salt and water. Hypertension usually occurs in the setting of fluid overload. Pericarditis rarely occurs now in patients with acute renal failure.

Other. Neurologic and gastrointestinal complications are common in acute renal failure. The neurologic symptoms include lethargy, somnolence, confusion, agitation, and seizures. These symptoms are more common in elderly patients. Gastrointestinal complications include anorexia, nausea, vomiting, ileus, and abdominal pains. The coagulopathy, along with the stress of acute renal failure, may lead to gastrointestinal hemorrhage in 10 to 30 per cent of patients. Conservative management with antacids that do not contain magnesium and with histamine-2 blockers is usually adequate.

The neurologic and gastrointestinal symptoms usually respond well to initiation of dialysis.

Renal failure affects bioavailability, distribution, metabolism, and renal elimination of many medications. Therefore, appropriate adjustments in the dosing of most medications must be made in renal failure. Some medications should be avoided because of marked changes in pharmacokinetics.[10]

■ DIALYSIS

When conservative measures fail to control biochemical alterations and other complications of acute renal failure, then institution of dialysis may become necessary. Indications for dialytic therapy are shown in Table 6. Earlier initiation of dialysis has been shown to decrease mortality, and most centers now begin dialysis when the BUN reaches the 100 to 120 mg/dl range. Early dialysis can simplify patient management by allowing more liberal sodium, potassium, and fluid intake. "Intensive" dialysis, in which the serum creatinine was kept below 5.1 mg/dl had no effect on mortality when compared with "less intensive" dialysis, in which the mean predialysis serum creatinine level was 9.1 mg/dl.[11]

Several options that exist when dialytic therapy is necessary in acute renal failure[12] are listed in Table 7. The two familiar modalities of dialysis are hemodialysis and peritoneal dialysis. Two other options that can be quite useful in critically ill patients are continuous arteriovenous hemofiltration and continuous arteriovenous hemodialysis.

Hemodialysis is a commonly used process in which the solute and water composition of blood is altered by exposing the blood to dialysate solution. A semipermeable membrane or artificial kidney separates the blood from the dialysate. Solutes can pass through the membrane by diffusion and ultrafiltration (convection). Water movement can be adjusted by controlling the pressures in the

TABLE 6. Indications for Dialysis

Volume overload
Hyperkalemia refractory to medical management
Severe metabolic acidosis refractory to medical
   management
Central nervous system symptoms of uremia
Pericarditis

TABLE 7. Dialysis Management of Acute Renal Failure

Modality	Indication
Peritoneal dialysis	Low catabolic rates Intact peritoneum Lack of trained personnel
Hemodialysis	Increased catabolic rate Hemodynamic stability Trained personnel
CAVH (continuous arteriovenous hemofiltration)	Moderate catabolic rate Hemodynamic instability Ultrafiltration as major goal Partially trained personnel
CAVHD (continuous arteriovenous hemodialysis)	Moderate-to-high catabolic rate Hemodynamic instability Ultrafiltration and dialysis needed Partially trained personnel

blood and dialysate compartments. To perform hemodialysis, access to the vascular space must be obtained. In the acute setting this is usually accomplished by insertion of a flexible double-lumen dialysis catheter into the subclavian, internal jugular, or femoral vein. These catheters can be used immediately after placement. Another option for vascular access is operative insertion of a Quinton-Scribner Teflon arteriovenous shunt. Common complications of hemodialysis include hypotension, headache, nausea, vomiting, cramps, bleeding from heparin used to prevent clotting in the dialyzer, and hypoxemia from pulmonary vascular white blood cell and platelet sequestration along with alveolar hypoventilation. Factors favoring the use of hemodialysis are availability of machinery and personnel, hemodynamic stability, and a catabolic patient.

In peritoneal dialysis, a catheter is placed into the peritoneal cavity, either surgically or percutaneously. Dialysate solution is infused into the peritoneum, and toxic materials move from the blood and surrounding tissues by diffusion and osmotic drive into the dialysate solution. Removal of these substances from the body occurs when the dialysate solution is drained. Disadvantages of peritoneal dialysis include the risk of peritonitis, inability to use this method in patients with large disruptions of the peritoneal space or perforations of the diaphragm, and inadequate clearance of nitrogenous wastes in catabolic patients. Advantages include technical simplicity and no need for

anticoagulation or development of disequilibrium symptoms. The disequilibrium syndrome is a set of systemic and neurologic symptoms that can occur during or soon after hemodialysis. The etiology is controversial but may be related to changes in brain water content associated with dialysis. Symptoms can include nausea, vomiting, restlessness, headache, seizures, obtundation, and coma. Situations favoring the use of peritoneal dialysis are lack of technical support, absolute contraindication to heparin, and a hemodynamically unstable, noncatabolic patient.

Continuous arteriovenous hemofiltration (CAVH) is an extracorporeal process that utilizes the patient's arterial to venous hydraulic pressure gradient to generate and remove an ultrafiltrate.[13,14] A small filtration cell containing a membrane highly permeable to water and small molecular weight solutes is used. When blood pressure falls, the ultrafiltration rate decreases and there is less risk of hemodynamic instability. Low blood flow rates (20 to 50 ml/min) can result in high ultrafiltration rates (300 to 500 ml/hr) and removal of excess fluids. Solute removal occurs via the process of convection. In patients who produce less than 10 grams per day of urea nitrogen, the BUN can be maintained at less than 90 mg/dl with an exchange volume of 10 to 12 liters in 24 hours. In catabolic patients, CAVH can be used to remove excess fluids and allow use of hyperalimentation. Arterial and venous access is usually obtained using the femoral artery and vein, although in this situation too the Quinton-Scribner shunt can be employed. Common complications include vascular compromise, infection, and hemorrhagic complications associated with anticoagulation of the extracorporeal circuit. CAVH is most beneficial in hemodynamically unstable patients in whom volume status is the major concern.

If solute removal in addition to fluid removal is a major concern, then continuous arteriovenous hemodialysis (CAVHD) can be performed. The circuit is similar to that used in CAVH except that dialysate now flows through the ultrafiltration cartridge, and the cartridge becomes a dialyzer. Diffusion of solutes from the blood into the dialysate occurs along with ultrafiltration. Ultrafiltration rates with CAVHD can be quite low. As in CAVH, the arterial to venous hydraulic pressure gradient generates the ultrafiltrate, and hemodynamic stability is maintained.

■ MANAGEMENT OF SPECIFIC NEPHROTOXINS

The various nephrotoxins that can cause acute renal failure associated with tubular damage are shown in Table 1. Once acute renal failure due to nephrotoxins becomes established, the management follows the principles previously outlined. Nephrotoxic injury to the kidney can be prevented in many circumstances. The major therapy in the prevention of nephrotoxic injury involves adequate hydration and a brisk urine flow rate. Urine alkalinization may be beneficial in circumstances involving methotrexate, hyperuricemia, myoglobinuria, or hemoglobinuria. Hydration along with mannitol can prevent the acute renal failure caused by radiocontrast agents.[15] Other specific therapies include leucovorin with methotrexate infusions, allopurinol to prevent hyperuricemia, and N-acetylcysteine (Mucomyst) to treat acetaminophen toxicity.

The ingestion of ethylene glycol is toxic to the neurologic, cardiovascular, and renal systems. Acute renal failure is a common occurrence. A metabolic acidosis with an elevated anion gap and osmolal gap should raise the suspicion of ethylene glycol ingestion. Ethylene glycol itself is not a toxic substance, but the various metabolites produced by the enzyme alcohol dehydrogenase are toxic. Therefore, treatment consists of ethanol to competitively inhibit alcohol dehydrogenase and hemodialysis to remove ethylene glycol and metabolites from the body. A serum ethanol level of 100 mg/dl is the goal, and it can be obtained with a loading dose of 0.6 gm/kg and a maintenance dose of 109 mg/kg/hr. During dialysis, the maintenance dose will have to be increased to account for removal of ethanol by the dialysis membrane. Hemodialysis should be performed until the anion and osmolal gaps have normalized.

■ RENAL BIOPSY IN ACUTE RENAL FAILURE

The indication for renal biopsy in acute renal failure varies considerably among clinicians. The biopsy may help determine the nature of the pathologic process, the prognosis, and the potential reversibility of the renal disease and suggest whether specific therapy is indicated. The renal biopsy may be useful when acute glomerular, vascular, or tubulointerstitial disease is suspected.

■ Issues and Risks

■ PROPHYLAXIS OF ACUTE RENAL FAILURE

Prevention has become a cornerstone of medical therapy in the 1980s. In patients at high risk to develop acute renal failure, prophylactic treatment can attenuate or prevent deterioration of renal function. These high-risk patients include diabetics, elderly patients, septic patients, and patients undergoing major surgery.

Prophylactic therapy consists of administration of saline to prevent volume depletion. Administration of either mannitol or furosemide may prevent contrast-induced acute renal failure.[15] In the absence of volume depletion, saline is much inferior as a prophylactic measure compared with the higher solute excretion achieved with mannitol or furosemide with replacement of urinary losses.

■ AUTOREGULATION

The normal kidney has mechanisms that maintain renal blood flow and glomerular filtration rate within a narrow range, despite wide variations in blood pressure. This process is referred to as autoregulation. In ischemic acute renal failure, autoregulation becomes disrupted,[16] and the renal vasculature responds excessively to vasoconstrictor stimuli, such as hypotension and renal nerve stimulation.[17] This loss of autoregulation may have significant clinical implications in acute renal failure. A fall in blood pressure that normally would not be considered significant may cause recurrent ischemic damage because of the loss of autoregulation in acute renal failure. Likewise, hemodialysis that is frequently complicated by hypotension may prolong acute renal failure by inducing recurrent ischemic damage.

REFERENCES

1. Anderson RJ, Linas SL, Berns AS, et al. Nonoliguric acute renal failure. N Engl J Med 1977; 296:1134–1138.
2. Kjellstrand CM, Gornick C, Davin T. Recovery from acute renal failure. Clin Exp Dial Apheresis 1981; 5:143–161.
3. Hou SH, Bushinsky DA, Wish JB, Cohen JJ, Harrington JT. Hospital-acquired renal insufficiency: a prospective study. Am J Med 1983; 74:243–248.
4. Norman RW, Mack FG, Awad SA, Belitsky P, Schwarz RD, Lannon SG. Renal failure secondary to bilateral ureteric obstruction: review of 50 cases. Can Med Assoc J 1982; 127:601–604.
5. Brown CB, Ogg CS, Cameron JS. High dose furosemide in acute renal failure: a controlled trial. Clin Nephrol 1981; 15:90–96.
6. Graziani G, Cantaluppi A, Casati S, et al. Dopamine and furosemide in oliguric acute renal failure. Nephron 1984; 37:39–42.
7. Livio M, Marchesi D, Remuzzi G, Gotti E, Mecca G, de Gaetano G. Uraemic bleeding: role of anaemia and beneficial effect of red cell transfusions. Lancet 1982; 2:1013–1015.
8. Remuzzi G. Bleeding in renal failure. Lancet 1988; 1:1205–1207.
9. Deykin D. Uremic bleeding. Kidney Int 1983; 24:698–705.
10. Bennett WM, Aronoff GR, Golper TA, Morrison G, Singer I, Brater DC. Drug Prescribing in Renal Failure: Dosing Guidelines for Adults. Philadelphia: American College of Physicians, 1987.
11. Gillum DM, Dixon BS, Yanover MJ, et al. The role of intensive dialysis in acute renal failure. Clin Nephrol 1986; 25:149–155.
12. Alfred HJ, Cohen AJ. Use of dialytic procedures in the intensive care unit. In Rippe JM, Irwin RS, Alpert JS, Dalen JE (eds). Intensive Care Medicine. Boston: Little, Brown, 1985:562–582.
13. Lauer A, Saccaggi A, Ronco C, Belledonne M, Glabman S, Bosch JP. Continuous arteriovenous hemofiltration in the critically ill patient. Ann Intern Med 1983; 99:455–460.
14. Kaplan AA, Longnecker RE, Folkert VW. Continuous arteriovenous hemofiltration. Ann Intern Med 1984; 100:358–367.
15. Old CW, Lehner LM. Prevention of radiocontrast-induced acute renal failure with mannitol. Lancet 1980; 1:885.
16. Matthys E, Patton MK, Osgood, RW, Venkatachalam MA, Stein JH. Alterations in vascular function and morphology in acute ischemic renal failure. Kidney Int 1983; 23:717–724.
17. Kelleher SP, Robinette JB, Conger JD. Sympathetic nervous system in the loss of autoregulation in acute renal failure. Am J Phys 1984; 246:F379–386.

Rheumatoid arthritis

Sanford H. Roth ■ *Paul H. Caldron* ■ *Ralph E. Bennett*

■ Background

In medical writing, the struggle to describe the clinical appearance of rheumatoid arthritis (RA) appears to have begun with a case report by Hippocrates, and difficulty persists through the most recent revision (1987) of the American College of Rheumatology criteria for the diagnosis of RA.[1] These new criteria (Table 1) are more streamlined, and appear to recognize that longer lists of features and exclusions cannot supplant the clinician's gestalt. RA remains a systemic disorder of unknown etiology, with prominent, peculiarly symmetric synovitis. The variable presentation expands the differential diagnosis and heightens the challenge of early accuracy, since the evolution of therapy in the 1980s has reversed our former attitude about waiting for erosive joint damage before initiating aggressive immunomodulatory therapy.

Whereas certain gene products, such as HLA-DR4, and certain DNA fragments found on gene probing can identify populations at increased risk, the community practitioner can find solace in the fact that RA remains a clinical diagnosis that is common to approximately 1 per cent of the population, and little sophisticated laboratory investigation is needed before embarking upon therapy. As with most rheumatic diseases, there is a strong female preponderance and an increasing prevalence through the third to seventh decades.

TABLE 1. The 1987 Criteria for Classification of Rheumatoid Arthritis (Traditional Format)*

Criterion	Definition
1. Morning stiffness	Morning stiffness in and around the joints, lasting at least 1 hour before maximal improvement
2. Arthritis of 3 or more joint areas	At least 3 joint areas simultaneously have had soft tissue swelling or fluid (not bony overgrowth alone) observed by a physician. The 14 possible areas are right or left PIP, MCP, wrist, elbow, knee, ankle, and MTP joint
3. Arthritis of hand joints	At least one area swollen (as defined above) in a wrist, MCP, or PIP joint
4. Symmetric arthritis	Simultaneous involvement of the same joint areas (as defined in No. 2) on both sides of the body (bilateral involvement of PIPs, MCPs, or MTPs is acceptable without absolute symmetry)
5. Rheumatoid nodules	Subcutaneous nodules over bony prominences or extensor surfaces, or in juxta-articular regions, observed by a physician
6. Serum rheumatoid factor	Demonstration of abnormal amounts of serum rheumatoid factor by any method for which the result has been positive in $<5\%$ of normal control subjects
7. Radiographic changes	Radiographic changes typical of rheumatoid arthritis on posteroanterior hand and wrist radiographs, which must include erosions of unequivocal bony decalcification localized in or most marked adjacent to the involved joints (osteoarthritis changes alone do not qualify)

*For classification purposes, a patient shall be said to have rheumatoid arthritis if he or she has satisfied at least four of these seven criteria. Criteria 1 through 4 must have been present for at least 6 weeks. Patients with two clinical diagnoses are not excluded. Designation as classic, definite, or probable rheumatoid arthritis is *not* to be made.

PIP, proximal interphalangeal; MCP, metacarpophalangeal; MTP, metatarsophalangeal.

(From Arnett FC, Edworthy SM, Block DA, et al: The American Rheumatism Association 1987 revised criteria for the classification of rheumatoid arthritis. Arthritis Rheum 1988; 31:315–324. © 1988. Used by permission of the American College of Rheumatology).

■ CLINICAL PRESENTATION

About two thirds of patients will have an insidious onset with varying systemic symptoms, including malaise, fatigue, diffuse body aches, and morning stiffness, gradually congealing to a rather symmetric, clinically apparent synovitis. Others may have one or a few peripheral joints involved initially, which over a period of weeks to months become additive with other joints to create the more typical distribution of rheumatoid polysynovitis (Fig. 1). Low-grade fever, anemia, and weight loss are common. High fever and chills with a dramatically acute onset of intense polysynovitis must always suggest endovascular infection, but it is not a rare picture of new rheumatoid disease. Likewise, whereas systemic infection is a major cause of death in well-established RA, flares of the primary disease may have impressive constitutional features.

More unusual is palindromic rheumatism, in which approximately one third of patients eventually develop symmetric synovitis, yet for weeks to many months beforehand they will have episodic monarthritis lasting hours to days with intercritical peri-

ods. This pattern is distinguished from gout and other crystalline arthropathies by lack of crystals in joint aspirates.

The juvenile onset of RA is distinguished in the child from other forms of juvenile chronic arthritis by its adherence to a symmetric peripheral pattern typical of adult RA, and in the adult by the age of onset, the presence of postinflammatory micrognathia, and growth retardation. In general, medical management does not differ in RA on the basis of age of onset, although concerns about child-bearing potential may influence the selection of some immunosuppressive agents.

As with virtually all rheumatic diseases, evaluation of the efficacy of selected treatments is confounded by the known variability in the course of RA. Many individuals who meet the criteria for RA early turn out to have other self-limiting disease or treatable infection and get better, whereas some evolve to manifest other chronic rheumatic diseases or malignancies. One fourth to one third of patients will have a course of active disease punctuated by brief periods of remission; up to 14 per cent may have prolonged remissions in the absence of ther-

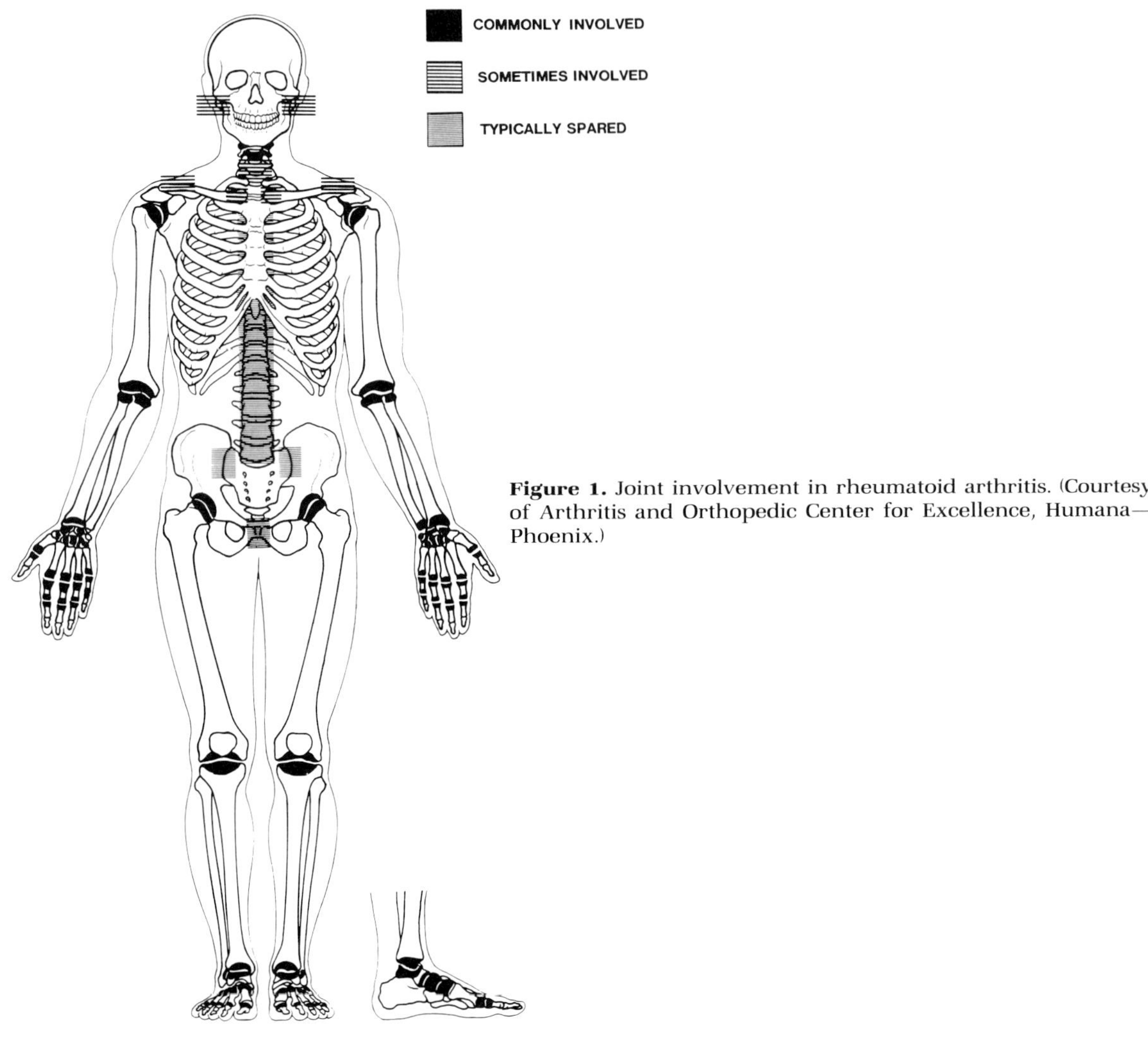

Figure 1. Joint involvement in rheumatoid arthritis. (Courtesy of Arthritis and Orthopedic Center for Excellence, Humana—Phoenix.)

apy.[2] A small portion seem to have a relentless destructive course that leads to loss of independent living within a decade or less. The goal of medical management in the absence of recognized cause or cure for RA is to induce and maintain remission states as much as possible and thus limit permanent joint damage and maximize the quality of life.

EXTRA-ARTICULAR MANIFESTATIONS

Along with the constitutional attendants mentioned, this systemic disease of immune disregulation and immune complexes may involve most organ systems in one or more ways (Fig. 2). In large measure, these features are managed on whole with the synovitis by anti-inflammatory and immunomodulatory therapies. Specific adjunctive treatment, such as artificial tears during the day and ophthalmic gels at night, as well as sugar-free mints, a tote of water, and conspicuous attention to dental hygiene, are enormously useful for the sicca complex of Sjögren's syndrome. Rheumatoid nodules are rarely more than a cosmetic problem, although excision may be required if local interference with dexterity or post-traumatic infection occurs. Rheumatoid pleural and pericardial effusions need to be aspirated only for diagnostic exclusions or for symptomatic cardiopulmonary compromise. Felty's syndrome in RA, with neutropenia and splenic enlargement, is an uncommon scenario encountered in long-established disease. Massive, painful splenomegaly and severe neutropenia with recurrent pyogenic

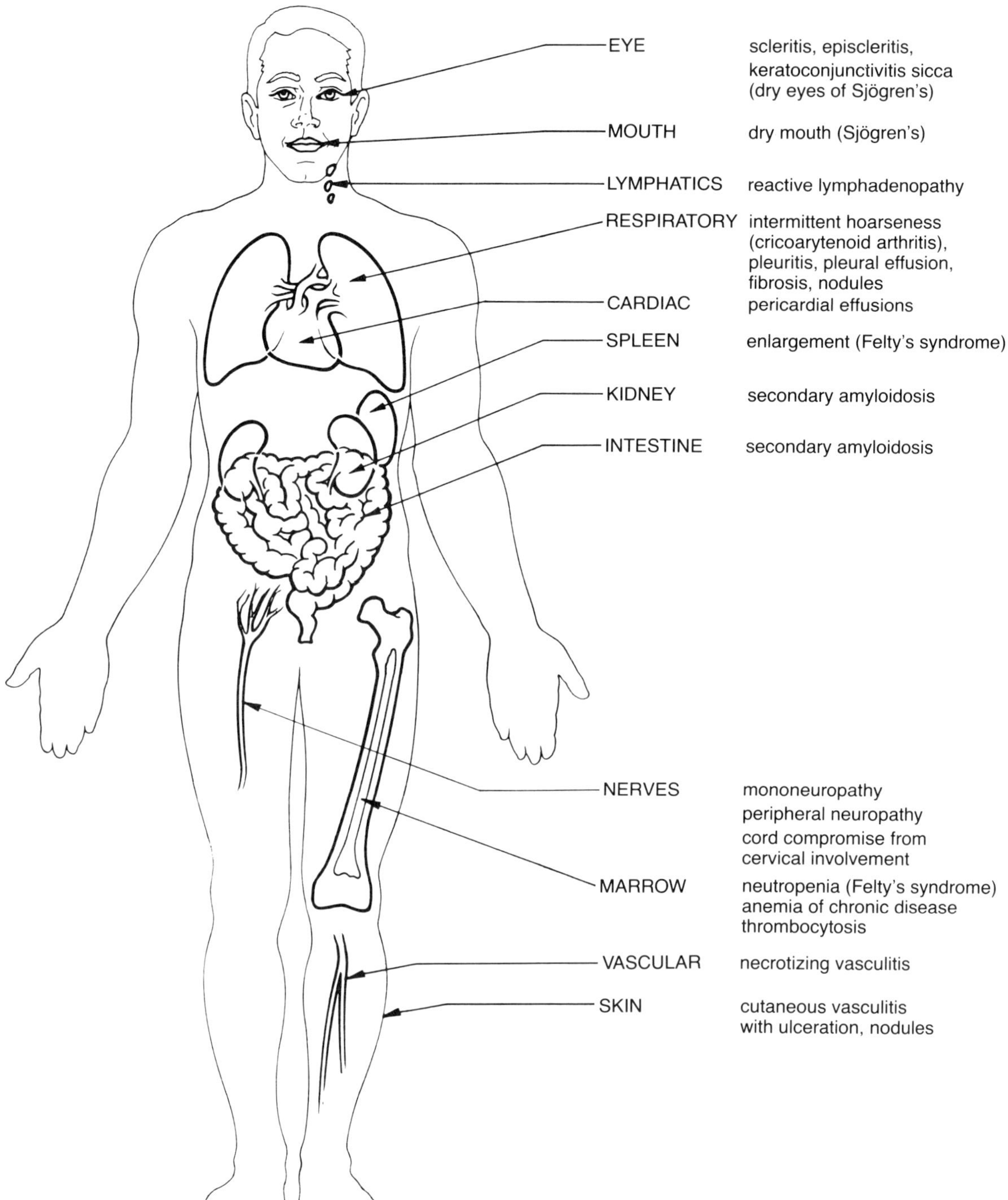

Figure 2. Extra-articular manifestations of rheumatoid arthritis. (Courtesy of Arthritis and Orthopedic Center for Excellence, Humana—Phoenix.)

infections are indications for splenectomy.[3] Systemic vasculitis with skin ulceration, mononeuropathies, digital infarction, pericarditis, or evidence of arteritis of visceral organs calls for acute inpatient support with cytotoxic therapy, possibly apheresis, and medical management of the organ systems involved.[4] Rheumatoid synovitis and instability of the atlantoaxial articulation are usually manageable with cervical collars and precautions regarding travel, but surgical stabilization, often with odontoidectomy, may be required if long tract symptoms occur. Special care always should be afforded during transfers and intubation of such patients undergoing anesthesia.[5]

■ DIAGNOSIS AND ASSESSMENT

The diagnostic criteria are listed in Table 1, and further elaboration of diagnostic procedures is not within the scope of this text. However, the clinician should bear in mind that joint aspiration should be performed in acute presentations or flares when an effusion is present, to rule out joint sepsis, or when gout or pseudogout may mimic or coexist with RA.

The utility of rheumatoid factor deserves comment. Although this antiglobulin immune complex occurs in 80 per cent of RA patients, it should not be construed as diagnostic; other diseases in which nonspecific immunoglobulin activation and joint swelling occur together should be considered. Under appropriate circumstances, these may include other rheumatic diseases; viral infections such as mononucleosis, hepatitis, rubella, influenza and others; vaccinations; parasitic infections; subacute bacterial endocarditis; mycobacterial infections; postirradiation or chemotherapy for neoplasms; sarcoidosis; chronic liver disease; and paraproteinemias.

A plethora of laboratory, radiographic, physical, functional, and psychologic measurements are available to assess clinical status and response to therapy, but most decisions for usual therapy are based on the clinician's global assessment. This is usually heavily weighted upon the duration of morning stiffness, the "energy level," the presence of active synovitis or extra-articular disease, and evidence of adverse effects of current therapy. The erythrocyte sedimentation rate (ESR) and the hemoglobin determination are the numerical data points used most commonly to corroborate the en face impression of disease control or deterioration.

A comprehensive differential list may include any entity that causes arthralgias or synovitis, yet a few common clinical circumstances bear further mention here. What presents as classic polymyalgia rheumatica (PMR) in elderly patients sometimes evolves into typical RA, replete with rheumatoid factor that may have been previously undetectable. Benign hypermobility syndrome in adolescents and younger adults, with prolonged postactivity arthralgias and frequently concomitant fibrositis, may sound much like RA until the examination is performed. Previously undiagnosed late tophaceous gout may require joint aspiration to distinguish its sometimes identical appearance from nodular RA. When subluxed joints fall back into alignment upon flattening of the hands on a firm surface, Jaccoud's arthropathy of recurrent rheumatic fever or systemic lupus erythematosus is a more likely diagnosis. Chronic Lyme disease arthropathy may mimic RA, if earlier stage manifestations are overlooked.

■ Management

The long-range goal of the management of chronic RA is the prevention of disability and the maintenance of independent functioning. These long-term goals must be balanced against the patient's short-term goal of pain relief and the short-term (and often short-sighted) goal of the physician who attempts to react to laboratory values alone.

Education must be a primary function of the physician caring for the patient with RA. Chronic fatigue and inability to continue some activities lead to a loss of self-esteem. Patients who do not have a strong support system will suffer the most. The concept of pacing and frequent rest periods must be explained early in the onset of the disease course and reinforced regularly. Patients who have realistic expectations of their treatment program will be more compliant. Psychologic counseling, physical therapy,[6] and reconstructive surgery are complements to the traditional "pyramid" approach to the medical treatment of RA (Fig. 3).

■ NONSTEROIDAL ANTI-INFLAMMATORY DRUGS (NSAIDs)

Anti-inflammatories have long been used as the foundation of RA treatment. These drugs are relatively fast acting, and their discontinuation is quickly followed by a recrudescence of symptoms. When effective, NSAIDs can reduce the swelling and erythema of an

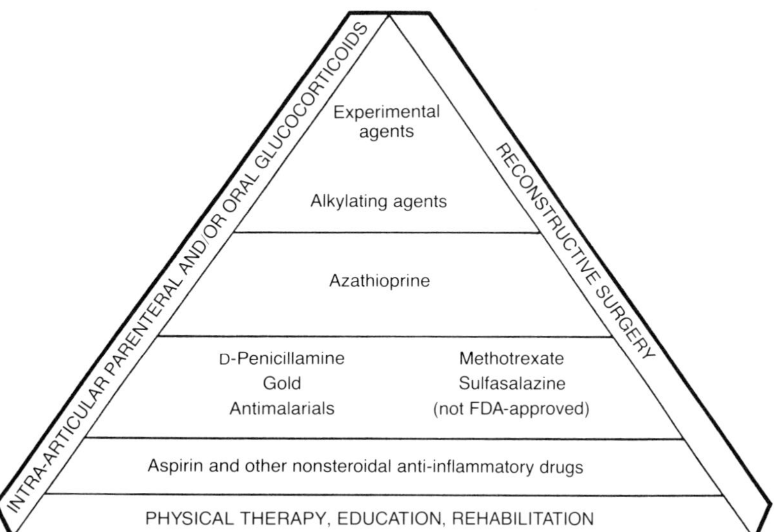

Figure 3. Therapy of rheumatoid arthritis. (Courtesy of Arthritis and Orthopedic Center for Excellence, Humana—Phoenix.)

arthritic joint. They also have analgesic and antipyretic activity. They do not affect or modify disease progression, nor have they been shown consistently to reduce laboratory indices of disease progression.

Though they appear different from each other chemically, most NSAIDs fall within several chemical groups (Table 2). All are

TABLE 2. Classification of NSAIDs

Class	Generic Name
Salicylates	Aspirin
	Choline magnesium
	trisalicylate
	Diflunisal
	Salsalate
Carboxylic Acids	
Proprionic acids	Carprofen
	Fenoprofen
	Flurbiprofen
	Ibuprofen
	Ketoprofen
	Naproxen
	Suprofen
Indoleacetic and	Indomethacin
indeneacetic	Sulindac
acids	
Pyrrole alkanoic	Tolmetin
acid	
Pyrazalone	Oxyphenbutazone
Derivatives	Phenylbutazone
Fenamates	Meclofenamate sodium
	Mefanamic acid
Oxicams	Piroxicam
	Isoxicam
Acetic Acid	Diclofenac sodium
Derivative	

believed to produce their anti-inflammatory actions through inhibition of the cyclo-oxygenase pathway. Since clinical efficacy does not always correlate with cyclo-oxygenase inhibition, other mechanisms of action have been investigated, including inhibition of lipoxygenase production, granulocyte and monocyte regulation, and bradykinin production. It is possible that these various effects vary in importance from NSAID to NSAID, which may explain why one medication may be more effective in a given patient than another. There is no hierarchy in terms of potency of these medications, and a 1- to 2-week trial of several medications may be worthwhile if a satisfactory response is not obtained.

Tolerability. Prostaglandin inhibition results in toxicities that must always be considered in certain populations at risk. In patients with liver disease and ascites, congestive heart failure (CHF), diuretic treatment, and hypotension, glomerular function may be dependent on prostaglandins. NSAID inhibition of prostaglandin production may result in increasing renal insufficiency and toxicity from concurrent reduction secondary to reduced renal clearance.

Gastropathy resulting from NSAID usage is now being recognized as the most serious common problem associated with medical therapy. A strategy for circumventing this problem is discussed in detail later.

Some patients do not respond to any NSAID or, more commonly, are unable to tolerate any NSAID, usually because of NSAID gastropathy or because of a history of severe allergic reactions. Using an NSAID as baseline therapy in RA should not be considered as absolutely essential, for low-dose glucocorticoid therapy, remittive agents, and intra-articular glucocorticoids are available as therapy.

■ GLUCOCORTICOIDS

Because of the catastrophic side effects that occur at higher dosages of glucocorticoids, most rheumatologists presently attempt to limit daily dosage to the equivalent of 7.5 mg or less of prednisone. Even at these dosages, institution of treatment should be started with careful informed consent, as it may be difficult to taper the glucocorticoids and side effects are very common. Weight gain, cushingoid facies, osteopenia, and ecchymoses still may occur in a high percentage of patients. Posterior subcapsular cataracts, hyperglycemia, myopathy, avascular necrosis, and psychiatric reactions are possible even with these low doses.

With these caveats aside, glucocorticoid treatment still has a mainstream role in the treatment of RA. When used in a daily dosage of 7.5 mg prednisone equivalent, glucocorticoids can provide relief of constitutional symptoms, and they have a potent anti-inflammatory action. Because of their quick onset of action, they may be used to bridge therapy between the fast-acting and less potent NSAIDs and slower-acting remittive treatment. Once relief is obtained, tapering of the prednisone can be started. If treatment has been maintained for more than several months, then a tapering schedule of no faster than 0.5 mg every 2 weeks will provide a steady reduction in dosage while minimizing the risk of flare.

Because of their potent anti-inflammatory and immunosuppressive effects, glucocorticoids may be needed in moderately high doses in such potentially life-threatening associated situations as a necrotizing arteritis, mononeuritis multiplex, active interstitial pulmonary disease, acute and hemodynamically significant pericarditis, or pleural effusion. They usually are not appropriate in the treatment of the granulocytopenia of Felty's syndrome.

Intra-articular (IA) local glucocorticoid injections are most useful for those whose disease is controlled except for one or a few actively inflamed joints. The less soluble and microcrystalline suspensions may provide a longer duration of action, though there is a small risk of a crystal-induced arthropathy with the latter.

Relief from IA injections may be dramatic in 85 to 95 per cent of patients in most series, with relief lasting several weeks to months. The same joint should not be injected multiple times in a short time frame. Though it is not always feasible, it is best to wait at least 6 months before reinjecting a given joint. Animal studies have demonstrated multiple cartilage abnormalities, such as decreased luster, fissuring, fibrillation, loss of metachromasia, and degeneration with repeated injections.

Other side effects include tendon rupture, depigmentation of the skin at the injection site, subcutaneous fat atrophy, and septic arthritis. If there is any doubt as to whether an isolated, severely inflamed joint is infected, the fluid should be aspirated and infection ruled out prior to injection of any glucocorticoid.

■ DISEASE-MODIFYING ANTIRHEUMATIC DRUGS (DMARDs)

In a significant portion of patients with RA, treatment with NSAIDs or low-dose glucocorticoids will not sufficiently suppress disease activity. In these patients, slow-acting (and potentially disease-modifying) antirheumatic drugs may be beneficial. These drugs, when effective, can control disease symptoms and provide a steroid-sparing effect. In certain instances, they have been shown radiologically to alter the progression of the disease. The DMARDs presently available for the treatment of RA are listed in Table 3.

Chrysotherapy. Injection of gold salts for use in RA is a relatively old treatment. Jacques Forestier first developed it in the early 1930s. Its efficacy was best proved by the classic Empire Rheumatism Council study,[7,8] which demonstrated that a 6-month course of the drug has a beneficial effect lasting 12 to 18 months.

Gold is available for intramuscular injection with either the water-based preparation gold sodium thiomalate (Myochrysine) or the oil-based preparation aurothioglucose (Solganal). The oil-based preparation does not have a nitrotoid reaction as a possible

TABLE 3. Disease-Modifying Antirheumatic Drugs (DMARDs)

Drug	Serious Toxicities	Monitoring Schedule
Gold	Proteinuria, cytopenias, mucocutaneous	CBC, urinalysis every week for first 4 weeks then every other injection (not less than 1 per month); chemistries every 3rd month
D-Penicillamine	Proteinuria, cytopenias, mucocutaneous, autoimmune diseases	CBC, urinalysis, every 2 weeks first month, then every 4–6 weeks; chemistries every 4–6 weeks
Antimalarials	Retinal toxicity	Biannual ophthalmologic examination
Sulfasalazine	Gastrointestinal toxicities, hepatitis, rash, hemolytic anemia, toxic nephrosis with crystalluria	Periodic chemistries, frequent CBC and urinalysis (guidelines not established)
Immunosuppressives		
Alkylating agents	Cytopenias, infections, neoplasia, hemorrhagic cystitis	CBC every 1–2 weeks the first month, then every month; chemistries every 3 months; urinalysis every month
Antimetabolites	Cytopenias, hepatitis cirrhosis (methotrexate), pneumonitis, neoplasia (possibly azathioprine)	CBC every 1–2 weeks first month, then every 1–2 months; chemistries every 1–3 months; chest radiograph yearly

side effect as does the water-based preparation. This annoying vasomotor symptom may prompt switching to aurothioglucose.

Gold is first given as a test dose of 10 mg. It is advisable to have the patient remain in the office for 20 minutes following the injection to monitor for ill effects. If tolerated, 25 mg and then 50 mg may be given as weekly doses. The typical drop-out rate due to ill effects in most studies is approximately one third.

An adequate trial consists of administration once weekly for 6 months. If no benefit is obtained, this therapy should be discontinued. Once a therapeutic effect is obtained, the frequency of injections can be decreased to every other, then every third, then every fourth week.

An oral preparation in the form of auranofin (Ridaura) has also recently become available. This has a lesser frequency of severe dermatologic and renal symptoms, though the frequency of some gastrointestinal disturbance ranges from 30 to 45 per cent, with approximately 10 per cent of patients experiencing diarrhea so severe that treatment must be discontinued. Though injectable gold may achieve its effect in an average of 3 to 4 months, oral gold usually will take as long as 6 months to achieve a comparable effect.

D-Penicillamine. Penicillamine has been approved for use by the Food and Drug Administration (FDA) since 1978. Early studies that used dosages as high as 1.5 gm daily showed a high incidence of side effects, though more recent studies limiting daily dosage to between 750 mg and 1 gm show a lesser frequency. Some side effects are idiosyncratic and include induction of such life-threatening autoimmune illnesses as myasthenia gravis, Goodpasture's syndrome, obliterating bronchiolitis, systemic lupus erythematosus, hemolytic anemia, and pemphigus. Because of these and other unpredictable ill effects, penicillamine may be the least attractive DMARD to use for the nonspecialist.

D-Penicillamine should be started at a dose of 125 mg daily, given either 1 to 2 hours prior to or 2 to 3 hours after meals. The dosage may be increased in 125- to 250-mg increments every 8 weeks until the desired therapeutic effect is achieved.

Antimalarials. Quinacrine was the first antimalarial drug used in the treatment of inflammatory arthritis, in 1951. The 4-aminoquinolones now used most commonly are chloroquine and particularly hydroxychloroquine. These are the slowest-acting of the antirheumatic drugs. Though some patients achieve an early response in 1 to 2 months, studies demonstrating clinical efficacy have had to last at least 6 months. Though fears of retinal toxicity related to cumulative usage have limited their popularity, the incidence of this side effect can be minimized by restricting dosage to 4 to 6 mg/kg of lean body weight.[9]

Chloroquine is available only in 250- and 500-mg tablets. Because its ocular toxicity is minimized if a dosage of 4 mg/kg is not exceeded, this one tablet daily is rarely exceeded and indeed may be excessive for many patients. The maximum dosage of hydroxychloroquine is 6 mg/lean body weight expressed in kg, or 400 mg daily. Exceeding these dosages may result in retinal accumulation and toxicity, with edema and a bull's eye appearance of the macula. The definitive tests for ophthalmologic monitoring have not been established, but biannual monitoring with a red Amsler grid is one commonly accepted method. If retinal abnormality attributable to these medications develops, immediate cessation of treatment is required.

Other side effects include nausea, bloating, gastrointestinal distress (though not ulcers), ototoxicity, a diffuse maculopapular or urticarial rash occurring within 2 to 4 weeks of initiation of treatment, hemolytic anemia, and, rarely, a neuromyopathy. In addition to the aforementioned retinal toxicity, a transient difficulty in visual accommodation may occur.

At proper dosages, these drugs may be maintained indefinitely. With the vicissitudes in general health associated with other medical illnesses, care should be taken to adjust the dosage to changes in renal function and weight.

Sulfasalazine. This azo compound of sulfapyridine and 5-aminosalicylic acid was initially used in the 1940s as treatment in arthritis, but only recently has it gained popularity in the United States as a second-line agent in RA.[10] Though there are some studies showing efficacy, long-term studies are not available.

Common side effects include gastrointestinal toxicity, which is dose related and is often the dose-limiting toxicity, hemolytic anemia, myelosuppression, rash, hepatotoxicity, and pneumonitis. Enteric-coated preparations may allow a higher dosage to be tolerated.

◼ IMMUNOREGULATORY DRUGS

The most commonly used drugs of this class fall into three major groups: purine analogs, folic acid antagonists, and alkylating agents. Although these agents are also looked upon as DMARDs, they are considered separately here because their use has been derived from chemotherapy for neoplasia, and they are recognized to be immunomodulatory.

Purine Analogs. Azathioprine was the first chemotherapeutic agent approved for use by the FDA. Like other antimetabolites, its cellular toxicity is cycle specific. It is commonly used in the treatment of aggressive refractory rheumatoid arthritis, vasculitis, and other nonarticular complications.

Azathioprine is metabolized to 6-mercaptopurine, which is then incorporated into RNA and can therefore affect DNA synthesis. Its mechanism of action is unclear. The main toxicities include a severe gastrointestinal disturbance, bone marrow suppression, allergic hepatitis, herpes zoster, and a susceptibility to infections that does not always relate directly to the leukopenia. The increased risk of development of malignancies in RA patients remains a difficult epidemiologic problem to sort out.

Azathioprine has been shown to be effective in doses of 0.75 to 2.5 mg/kg in both short- and long-term studies. Adjustment of the dosage should be made for patients with a creatinine clearance of less than 15 ml/min and for patients taking allopurinol.

Methotrexate (MTX). MTX is a folate antagonist that has been used widely in a variety of rheumatic diseases since the late 1940s, but only in the past year was it approved by the FDA for use in RA. This analog of folic acid interferes with the enzyme dihydrofolate reductase, thus preventing the reduction of folic to folinic acid, a step necessary in the assembly of thymidine and purine.

MTX is given as a once-weekly pulse therapy, usually in a dosage range of 5 to 15 mg, though some rheumatologists exceed this. Common toxicities include gastrointestinal disturbances, stomatitis, and mild alopecia. These are usually manageable without discontinuing the medicine. A transient elevation in transaminase levels is common and, if less than twofold, may warrant only observation or cessation of treatment for a brief period. More serious toxicities include cirrhosis that may not relate to transaminase levels and a hypersensitivity pneumonitis. Because cirrhosis rarely reaches clinical significance[11,12] in a properly selected patient population, many rheumatologists advise against routine liver biopsies. Alcoholism and impaired hepatic function are risk factors for cirrhosis. It is also said that diabetes and obesity are risk factors, though the evidence for this is less clear. Impaired renal function is a major risk factor for other toxicities. No study has shown MTX to be carcinogenic.

MTX has a relatively rapid rate of onset, with the average onset being about 6 weeks. The average time from cessation of treatment to flare is only about 3 weeks, which has caused some to wonder whether its efficacy is related more to an anti-inflammatory than an immunosuppressive action.

Alkylating Agents. Alkylating agents act by directly binding to DNA at guanidyl residues and causing chain breakage or miscoding at these sites. The prototype of this class of drugs is mechlorethamine (nitrogen mustard), which is administered intravenously. Though not commonly used, it has been shown to be useful in the treatment of the acute RA flare. Its principal toxicities include nausea and vomiting, phlebitis, and hematologic suppression. A total of 0.3 mg/kg or 17 mg (whichever is less) may be given over 5 to 6 days with careful administration by a physician or oncologic nurse to prevent any extravasation and resulting tissue damage.

Cyclophosphamide is more commonly used in the treatment of RA. It has a much slower onset of action and a longer half-life. It has been clearly shown to be effective in RA in doses of 1 to 2 mg/kg/day and has also been demonstrated to suppress erosive disease. However, its long list of side effects includes gastrointestinal toxicity, alopecia, infertility, myelosuppression, hemorrhagic cystitis, and even the induction of neoplasia. Because of these problems, it is rarely warranted for use in articular disease alone, though its use in necrotizing vasculitis and other life- and limb-threatening complications may be warranted. Its administration by monthly pulses may limit these side effects, but efficacy has yet to be demonstrated in articular disease.

■ INVESTIGATIONAL TREATMENT

Cyclosporin A, an antifungal agent with immunoregulatory properties, may prove to be useful in the treatment of RA. However, its multiple toxicities, including development of lymphoma and frequent nephrotoxicity, limit its use at present. Several other drugs are currently under investigation and have not yet been approved for use by the FDA.

In addition to these slow-acting drugs, several methods, including plasmapheresis and total lymph node irradiation, have been investigated. The expense and risk of these procedures and their questionable efficacy have limited their usefulness in clinical medicine.

■ Issues and Risks

Effective drug therapy remains the key to successful rheumatoid arthritis management for, without control of pain and inflammation, rehabilitative efforts have been shown to deteriorate ultimately; compliance fails, and reactive depression often results with its attendant impact on general health and nutrition. The key to arthritis therapy is not often a single agent, but rather an NSAID/DMARD combination; the NSAID targets analgesia and local inflammation, and the DMARD aims at immunomodulation of the proliferative destructive process, which commonly persists for decades. Corticosteroids, at times, can form a useful bridge to the time when the DMARD becomes effective.

Rheumatoid disease is unique to host response. Clinicians agree that infection and trauma may trigger acute flares. It has also been recognized that difficulties with stress adaptation can trigger undesirable neurohormonal responses and hence, precipitate rheumatoid exacerbations.[13] Whereas synovitis may be persistently destructive over many years, recent data suggest that the establishment of granulomatous proliferative synovitis and hence the destructive changes in joints are most accelerated during the first few years of the disease.[14] It is likely that a narrow time window—the first year or two—is when our medical therapy may have its best long-term beneficial impact. This appears true even when the disease has its onset late in life. Some epidemiologic data suggest that RA may have the mortality potential of treated Hodgkin's disease.[15]

Since recognizing these important points about the natural history of RA, two major issues have emerged, leading us to re-evaluate the philosophy of our traditional rheumatoid therapy pyramid.

■ EVOLVING DMARD USE

First, for decades the various DMARDs traditionally have been used later in the rheumatoid disease, probably after the "window of opportunity" to significantly alter the proliferative destructive process has been closed. A consensus is emerging that DMARDs should be instituted at the time of diagnosis.

In addition to this general point on use of DMARDs, a changing gestalt with respect to the individual DMARDs has taken place. Although gold salt therapy and penicillamine were the most traditional DMARDs used in the United States, it has been appreciated that a relatively small percentage of patients actually achieve major disease suppression, compared with the high percentage who experience significant adverse drug reactions.[2,16] Consequently, the emerging role of methotrexate as the most used DMARD in rheumatoid arthritis therapy in the late 1980s, even prior to FDA approval for this indication, is based upon its increasingly recognized superior risk/benefit ratio over other DMARDS.

Whichever DMARD is used, those who treat rheumatoid arthritis, while still concerned about side effects, are equally concerned about "no effects" of therapy. Spending many months or years on slower-acting DMARDs like gold and penicillamine during those very important early months and years of the disease is becoming a less acceptable option. Approximately 80 per cent of patients on methotrexate will experience benefit within the first 8 weeks. Some have a similar experience with azathioprine. In addition, there is increaseing interest in combined remittive therapy, such as combinations of oral gold with methotrexate or azathioprine, or low doses of methotrexate and azathioprine or other agents at appropriately adjusted doses. It is likely that this sort of combination chemotherapy will evolve rapidly over the coming decade. In sum, a less rigid posture has led the rheumatology community to consider the advantages of introducing more aggressive DMARD therapy before destructive granulomatous disease has become entrenched.

■ EVOLVING NSAID USE

The second major issue of therapy that has evolved recently concerns our recognition that NSAIDs are not simple, safe agents for casual use at anti-inflammatory doses. Just recently, the FDA has required new class labeling for all NSAIDs for serious complications of ulcers, bleeding, and perforation that may occur at any time in therapy. Such complications now account for more side effects than from all other drugs used in medicine today and probably account for more than 10,000 deaths annually. The economic costs of gastropathy by way of hospitalization, lost work time, and also treatment are staggering. Largely for this reason the role of NSAIDs as primary therapy has come under scrutiny and encouraged us to look harder at our choices of NSAIDs, our dosing schemes, particularly in elderly patients, and the evaluation of other methodologies to improve the risk/benefit ratio of these agents.[17] Our appropriately increasing discomfort with this group of drugs is another major reason why we look at earlier DMARD therapy in the rational management of rheumatoid arthritis.

More than other exotic experimental therapies, such as apheresis, radiation therapy, and selective diets, all of which appear to be decreasing in promise, these two convergent issues of NSAID gastrotoxicity and earlier immunomodulation with newer DMARDs have held the lion's share of attention recently in the evolution of treatment of rheumatoid arthritis.

In the long road of arthritis therapy, there are ups and downs and turns. There is no simplistic algorithm for individual case management, which will continue to depend upon the attention, experience, and skilled monitoring by the clinician. Optimal long-term management will usually be predicated upon use of a team approach, including health care workers in rehabilitation, behavioral medicine, and nutrition, and, where necessary, reconstructive orthopedic surgeons. Although primary care physicians still see the majority of rheumatoid arthritis patients, the increasing sophistication in the treatment of rheumatoid arthritis calls for early involvement of the rheumatologist as the pivotal point in networking this system of care for the RA patient. Attention to these issues should allow us to return the majority of patients to a more normal, productive life.

REFERENCES

1. Arnett FC, Edworthy SM, Block DA, et al. The American Rheumatism Association 1987 revised criteria for the classification of rheumatoid arthritis. Arthritis Rheum 1988; 31(3):315–324.
2. Wolfe F, Hawley DJ. Remission in rheumatoid arthritis. J Rheumatol 1985; 12:245–252.
3. Blumfelder TM, Logue GL, Shimm DS. Felty's syndrome: effects of splenectomy upon granulocyte count and granulocyte-associated IgG. Ann Intern Med 1981; 94:623–628.
4. Cupps TR, Fauci AS. Systemic necrotizing vasculitis of the polyarteritis nodosa group. In Smith LD (ed). The Vasculitides, Philadelphia, WB Saunders, 1981:26–49.
5. Raskin RJ, Schnapf DJ, Wolf CR, et al. Computerized tomography in evaluation of atlantoaxial subluxation in rheumatoid arthritis. J Rheumatol 1983; 10(1):33–41.
6. Spiegel JS, Spiegel TM. Are rehabilitation programs for rheumatoid arthritis patients effective? Semin Arthritis Rheum 1987; 260–270.
7. Empire Rheumatism Council. Gold therapy in rheumatoid arthritis. Report of a multicentre controlled trial. Ann Rheum Dis 1960; 19:95–119.
8. Empire Rheumatism Council. Gold therapy in rheumatoid arthritis. Final report of a multicentre controlled trial. Ann Rheum Dis 1961; 20:315–334.
9. Mackenzie AH. Dose refinements in long-term therapy of rheumatoid arthritis with antimalarials. Proceedings of a Symposium. Am J Med 1983; 75(1a):40–45.
10. Pinals RS, Kaplan SB, Lawson JG, Hepburn B. Sulfasalazine in rheumatoid arthritis. A double-blind, placebo-controlled trial. Arthritis Rheum 1986; 29:1427–1434.
11. Kremer JM, Lee RG, Tolman KG. Liver histology in rheumatoid arthritis reviewing long-term methotrexate therapy. Arthritis Rheum 1989; 20:121–127.
12. Aponto J, Petrelli M. Histopathologic findings in the liver of rheumatoid arthritis patients treated with methotrexate. Arthritis Rheum 1988; 31:1457–1464.
13. Zautra A, Okun M, Robinson S, Lee D, Roth S, Jansen E. Life stress and lymphocyte alterations among patients with rheumatoid arthritis. Health Psychol 1989; 8(1):1–14.
14. Scot DL, Symmons DPM, Popert AJ. Long-term outcome of treating rheumatoid arthritis; results after twenty years. Lancet 1987; 2:1108–1111.
15. Pincus T, Callahan LF. Taking mortality in rheumatoid arthritis seriously—predictive markers, social economic status and comorbidity. J Rheumatol 1986; 14:841–845.
16. Wilske KR, Healey LA. Remodelling the pyramid—a concept whose time has come (editorial). J Rheumatol. Publication pending.
17. Roth SH: NSAID and gastropathy: a rheumatologist's review. J Rheumatol 1988; 15:912–919.

Seizures during childhood

John T. MacDonald

Seizures are common during childhood, with 3 to 4 per cent of all children experiencing a febrile seizure and 0.5 per cent a nonfebrile convulsion. Management of these disorders has undergone major changes in the last 2 decades: febrile seizures are no longer routinely treated, and most patients who need medication are managed with a single drug if possible. Childhood epilepsy is hard to treat since there is such a wide spectrum of epileptic syndromes, and often one child will experience many different types of seizures. In addition, the psychologic impact upon the child and family frequently complicates medical management, and the monitoring of drug side effects is often quite difficult in the younger age groups.

■ Background

Effective medical management depends upon proper diagnosis. Childhood epilepsy presents with many different clinical signs and symptoms. The International Classification of Epileptic Seizures attempts to utilize clinical symptoms to separate seizures into two main categories: partial (focal) and generalized (bilateral brain involvement).[1] Partial seizures may or may not be associated with loss of consciousness whereas, in the generalized type, there is an early loss of awareness. The older terminology for common seizure types is compared with the newer classification system in Table 1. The newer system, based upon clinical signs and

TABLE 1. Classification of Seizures

International Seizure Classification	*Prior Terminology*
Partial seizures	Focal seizures
Simple partial seizures	
with motor symptoms	Jacksonian seizures
with sensory symptoms	Focal sensory
with autonomic/ psychic symptoms	
Complex partial seizures	Temporal lobe Psychomotor seizures
Partial with secondary generalization	Grand mal with focal onset
Generalized seizures	Grand mal
Absence	Petit mal
simple absence	
atypical absence	
Myoclonic	Minor motor infantile spasms
Atonic	Drop attacks
Tonic-clonic	Grand mal
Clonic-tonic	Grand mal

symptoms, is useful in formulating a diagnosis, prognosis, and treatment plan. The choice of the initial anticonvulsant drug depends upon correct classification of the seizure disorder, and child neurologists now favor treatment with a single drug (monotherapy) for most types of childhood epilepsies.[2]

Other systems attempt to combine electroencephalographic (EEG) and clinical data into identifiable childhood epileptic syndromes.[3] Several of these syndromes have an age-related onset. In the neonate, for example, the disorder benign familial neonatal convulsions has a favorable outcome, whereas myoclonic seizures in the first year of life carry a poor prognosis. A self-limited disorder, benign childhood epilepsy with centrotemporal spikes (rolandic seizures), with onset in late childhood presenting as partial nocturnal seizures with temporal lobe spikes on the EEG, must be differentiated from complex partial seizures that are more difficult to treat successfully and have a more guarded long-term prognosis.

▪ Management

Not every child with a seizure is epileptic, and anticonvulsant drugs may not be indicated.[4] In the child with a nonfebrile seizure, a correct classification of the disorder will help determine whether immediate treatment is necessary and what drugs are most likely to control the convulsions. Those who present in status epilepticus obviously will need chronic anticonvulsants. When more than one drug has been given intravenously to stop the status, it is generally possible later to taper all but one medication for chronic use.

In neonates, phenobarbital is preferred following status epilepticus since phenytoin (Dilantin) levels are difficult to maintain in the first months of life. In older children, one may choose phenytoin as the chronic medication, since it produces fewer behavioral side effects than does phenobarbital. Infants with infantile myoclonic spasms, older children with Lennox Gastaut syndrome, and patients with absence and complex partial seizures tend to have recurrent attacks and must be treated aggressively. Those children who have a single unprovoked generalized tonic-clonic seizure, however, may not need to be started on chronic anticonvulsant drugs, since the recurrence rate may not be greater than 30 per cent.[5,6]

A common problem are those small children who experience a brief febrile convulsion; no longer are they routinely placed on phenobarbital. Only 9 to 15 per cent of children with a single febrile seizure will have recurrences.[7] When febrile convulsions recur, become more prolonged, or produce focal deficits, especially in a neurologically abnormal child, then that patient may need continuous phenobarbital prophylaxis.[8] Intermittent phenobarbital during an illness is not effective. Phenytoin and carbamazepine (Tegretol) have not proved effective in preventing recurrent febrile seizures. Valproate (Depakene), although an effective prophylactic agent, should be avoided, if possible, in children under 2 years of age owing to the increased risk of liver toxicity.[9] In most cases, when parents are informed of the generally benign nature of the condition, no medications will be required. When used, phenobarbital can be given once a day at 4 to 5 mg/kg/day to maintain a therapeutic level; the child must be watched closely for side effects (hyperactivity, irritability, sleep problems). Usually the drug is discontinued when the child is seizure free for 1 to 2 years or aged 3 years.[10] In Europe, rectal diazepam, given every 8 to 12 hours during a febrile illness, is prescribed, but this treatment has not been widely accepted in the United States.[11]

Two epileptic syndromes that occur in early childhood, infantile myoclonic spasms (West's syndrome) and the Lennox Gastaut syndrome, present difficult management problems. Infantile spasms usually occurs in the first year of life, with sudden onset of bilateral flexion of the neck and trunk, which occurs in a repetitive pattern for short intervals each day. The attacks increase in frequency over time, and infants show neurologic regressions.[12] Some infants have had a prior central nervous system (CNS) injury at birth, but many are normal at the onset of the spasms. The prognosis is poor; most patients develop epilepsy and mental retardation despite control of the seizure disorder. Valproate (Depakene, Depakote), at 15 to 60 mg/kg/day, may control the spasms in some patients, but most are also treated with oral steroids or ACTH injections. The Lennox Gastaut syndrome (LGS) may evolve from infantile spasms with a mixed seizure disorder, including absence, atonic head drops, and generalized tonic-clonic seizures all present in the same child. LGS is associated with mental retardation and a typical EEG pattern. Treatment with valproate or clonazepam (Klonopin) for the myoclonic and absence seizures is combined with phenytoin or carbamazepine for generalized attacks, but the results are poor. The child with LGS also may be treated with oral steroids or ACTH if standard anticonvulsant therapy fails. The dose of ACTH varies in the literature but typically is in the range of 40 to 160 units/day, given intramuscularly. A dramatic improvement is expected within the first week, and then the drug is slowly tapered over many weeks; if no major change occurs within the first week of ACTH treatment, many neurologists quickly discontinue the drug.[12]

The child with a newly diagnosed seizure disorder should be followed closely, and certain commonsense precautions around water and heights are appropriate. In some older children and adolescents, if may be necessary to restrict certain contact sports temporarily until the seizures are well controlled. Parents and the school must be cautioned against overprotection. The family and school should be presented correct information regarding the child's disorder, and, when old enough, the child deserves a simple age-appropriate explanation of what has happened and why and for how long medication will be necessary. Particularly in teenagers, compliance with medical treatment improves when the family and patient are fully informed.

The choice of a specific medication should be based upon the classification of the seizure (Table 2). The tendency now is to avoid using multiple agents and to manage most epileptics with one drug (monotherapy).[13] For example, the hepatic toxicity of valproate is minimized when it is used as a single agent. Compliance is also much improved on one drug, and it is easier to monitor side effects (Table 3). It should be noted that adverse behavioral effects may occur even when the child is on relatively low doses of medication. In some studies, there is not only less toxicity but also an improvement

TABLE 2. Choice of Anticonvulsant Medication

| | Medication | |
Type of Seizure	*First Choice*	*Second Choice*
Partial seizures		
Simple	Phenytoin	Phenobarbital
	Carbamazepine	Primidone
Complex partial	Carbamazepine	Valproate
	Phenytoin	Primidone
Generalized seizures		
Simple absence	Ethosuximide	Valproate
Atypical absence	Valproate	Ethosuximide
Myoclonic	Valproate	Clonazepam
		Phenobarbital
		Phenytoin
		ACTH
Atonic	Valproate	Clonazepam
		Phenytoin
Tonic-clonic	Carbamazepine	Phenobarbital
	Phenytoin	Valproate

TABLE 3. Side Effects of Anticonvulsants

Drug	Dose-Related	Nondose-Related	Idiosyncratic
Carbamazepine	Diplopia Blurred vision Lethargy	Stomach upset Diarrhea Fluid retention	Allergic dermatitis Aplastic anemia Granulocytopenia
Clonazepam	Drowsiness Ataxia Congestion	Behavior problems Confusion	Anemia
Ethosuximide	Nausea Dizziness Headache Anorexia	Stomach upset Fatigue	Allergic dermatitis Pancytopenia
Phenytoin	Nystagmus Ataxia Cognitive	Gum hyperplasia Hair growth Lymphadenopathy Coarse face Folate deficiency Neuropathy	Allergic dermatitis Aplastic anemia Lupus reaction Fetal syndrome Hepatic failure Granulocytopenia
Phenobarbital	Cognitive Sleep disorder Hyperactivity Ataxia	Lethargy Hyperactivity Sleep disorder Osteopenia	Allergic dermatitis Granulocytopenia
Valproate	Stomach upset Tremor Cognitive	Nausea Weight gain Hair loss	Hepatic failure Pancreatitis Fetal syndrome

in seizure control when multiple drugs are replaced by monotherapy.[14]

To initiate treatment, a single drug is chosen appropriate for the type of seizure, and the dose is adjusted over time to attain a therapeutic level (Table 4). Phenytoin and phenobarbital are started at a maintenance dose, but carbamazepine, valproate, and others must be slowly increased to a maintenance level to avoid initial side effects. Doses should be changed only if the last dose change has resulted in a steady state (five half-lives of the drug) and the seizures continue. It is important to obtain blood levels of drug at steady state to document a therapeutic level; however, if the child is well controlled and tolerates the drug, it may not always be necessary to increase dosage to attain a "normal" blood level. When seizures persist despite high therapeutic blood levels or signs of toxicity occur, then a second drug should be substituted for the first medication, which is slowly tapered after the new medication is within the low therapeutic range. If a severe toxicity occurs, it may be necessary to discontinue the anticonvulsant abruptly.

Generalized tonic-clonic seizures in children are frequently treated with carbamazepine or phenytoin as first-line drugs. In the infant with generalized seizures, especially if some are provoked by fever, one may wish to consider phenobarbital first. With older children who do not respond to the initial medications, valproate may prove useful.

Absence seizures commonly present as "staring spells." In children with behavioral problems, one must first determine whether

TABLE 4. Anticonvulsant Pharmacokinetic Data

Drug	Starting Dose (mg/kg/day)	Therapeutic Serum Level (µg/ml)	Days Required to Reach Steady State
Carbamazepine	10	4–12	3–4
Clonazepam	0.03	0.02–0.08	6
Ethosuximide	10	40–100	7–10
Phenobarbital	5	15–40	21
Phenytoin	5	10–20	7–8
Primidone	3–5	5–12	4–7
Valproate	15	50–120	2–4

the symptom is secondary to a short attention span, boredom, or daydreaming. A true absence usually presents as an abrupt halting of activity that occurs "out of context," lasts 5 to 20 seconds, and may be associated with eye blinking, and the child does not remember the event. The physician may be able to provoke a typical attack in the office by hyperventilating the child for 3 minutes.[15] The differential diagnosis of staring spells must also include a more common seizure disorder, complex partial convulsions. Children with these attacks generally have longer spells followed by a postictal state of confusion or lethargy. Complex partial seizures may include "forced thoughts," memory distortions, brief but intense affectual changes, and automatisms, such as repetitive hand movements or purposeless walking about. The treatment of absence is with ethosuximide (Zarontin) or valproate; children with complex partial seizures are started initially on carbamazepine or phenytoin, with valproate or primidone beneficial in some cases. The child with typical absence usually responds to ethosuximide slowly increased into a range of 20 to 30 mg/kg/day. If unsuccessful or other seizures develop (myoclonic, generalized tonic-clonic), then valproate may be effective at a dose of 15 to 60 mg/kg/day. In smaller children, valproate is usually given in three to four doses during the day. With refractory cases, one may add acetazolamide (Diamox) at 20 mg/kg/day to either initial drug, or try clonazepam (Klonopin)[16] at a dose of 0.05 to 0.2 mg/kg/day.

Complex partial seizures are frequently difficult to control fully. Carbamazepine is a first-line drug and usually is well tolerated in children.[17] Younger patients can be started at 10 mg/kg/day in three divided doses, with the dose increased weekly; a complete blood count and platelets should be monitored on a regular basis, even though hematologic side effects are very rare. If carbamazepine fails, phenytoin may be added with a slow taper off the carbamazepine. The 50-mg phenytoin chewable tablet is well accepted, and the child is started at 5 to 6 mg/kg/day in three divided doses. Valproate and primidone also can be tried in refractory cases. Many of these children eventually will need a combination of medications, and then they must be closely monitored for side effects by way of frequent blood level checks for drug, owing to the

TABLE 5. Antiepileptic Drug Interactions

Drug	Drug Level Decreased By	Drug Level Increased By
Carbamazepine	Phenobarbital Phenytoin Primidone Clonazepam	Valproate
Phenytoin	Carbamazepine Valproate (rare)	Carbamazepine (rare)
Valproate	Carbamazepine Phenytoin Phenobarbital Primidone	
Phenobarbital		Valproate
Ethosuximide	Carbamazepine	Valproate

complicated drug interactions[18] (Table 5). Blood levels should be obtained at a consistent time in relation to the dose, with trough levels (before a dose) to determine whether the patient is undertreated or peak levels (after a dose) to evaluate for toxicity.

When seizures persist despite multiple changes in anticonvulsants, one may wish to try a ketogenic diet.[19] This diet consists of a very high fat intake to produce daily urine ketosis. It is primarily useful in poorly controlled atypical absence, atonic, and myoclonic disorders; strict compliance is essential and a dietitian must be involved to help the family and child adhere to the diet. Multivitamins are rarely helpful except in rare cases of B_6-dependent seizures, usually presenting in early infancy or the neonatal period; in the infant with poorly controlled seizures a trial of vitamin B_6, 50 to 100 mg/day, may be considered.

■ Issues and Risks

Children with convulsions may do better than the family and physician initially expect. Although the underlying etiology is important in these patients, the longer a child remains seizure-free after initial treatment, the more likely the outcome will be favorable when anticonvulsants are discontinued. The duration of drug treatment depends somewhat upon the type of convulsive syndrome and the age of the child. The child with infantile spasms is usually treated for many years, whereas those with simple febrile seizures, if treated, are typically taken off medication within 1 to 2 years or by age 3 years. In patients with generalized tonic-clonic or complex partial seizures, it may be possible to stop medication after 2 seizure-free years, with a 75 per cent long-term success rate reported in one study.[20] However, some neurologists continue anticonvulsant drugs for 4 to 5 years, particularly if the EEG remains paroxysmal, the child is entering puberty, or the seizures were difficult to stop initially. These clinical decisions must be individualized and discussed openly with the family and child, so that everyone involved is well informed and comfortable with the duration of treatment. When a drug is to be stopped, it should be decreased slowly. Most recurrences occur within the first year after discontinuation of the anticovulsant.

A small number of children with intractable epilepsy unresponsive to multiple medications may benefit from neurosurgery. Patient selection is critical; these patients need a full evaluation at a medical center with expertise in this area. Surgical resection of abnormal cortex or section of the corpus callosum may be beneficial in certain children.[21]

REFERENCES

1. Commission on Classification and Terminology of the International League Against Epilepsy. Proposal for revised clinical and EEG classification of epileptic seizures. Epilepsia 1981; 22:489–501.
2. Penry JK (ed). Epilepsy: Diagnosis, Management, Quality of Life. New York, Raven Press, 1986:1–20.
3. Commission on Classification and Terminology of the International League Against Epilepsy. Proposal for the classification of the epilepsies and epileptic syndromes. Epilepsia 1985; 26:268–278.
4. Vining EPG, Freeman JM. Management of non-febrile seizures. Pediatr Rev 1986; 8:185–190.
5. Hauser WA, Anderson VE, Lowenson RB. Seizure recurrence after a first unprovoked seizure. N Engl J Med 1982; 307:522–528.
6. Camfield PR, Camfield CS, Dooley JM. Epilepsy after a first unprovoked seizure in childhood. Neurology 1985; 35:1657–1660.
7. Nelson KB, Ellenberg JH. Predictors of epilepsy in children who have experienced febrile seizures. N Engl J Med 1976; 295:1029–1033.
8. NIH Consensus Development Conference Summary. Febrile seizures—long-term management of children with fever-associated seizures. Pediatrics 1980; 66:1009–1012.
9. Driefuss FE, Santilli N, Langer DH, Sweeney KP, Moline KA, Menander KB. Valproic acid hepatic fatalities: a retrospective review. Neurology 1987; 37:379–385.
10. Camfield PR, Camfield C, Shapiro S. The first febrile seizure—antipyretic instruction plus either phenobarbital or placebo to prevent a recurrence. J Pediatr 1980; 97:16–21.
11. Knudsen FV, Vestermark S. Prophylactic diazepam or phenobarbitone in febrile convulsions: a prospective, controlled study. Arch Dis Child 1978; 53:660–663.
12. Snead OC, Benton JW, Myers GJ. ACTH and prednisone in childhood seizure disorders. Neurology 1983; 33:966–970.
13. Collaborative Group for Epidemiology of Epilepsy: Adverse reactions to antiepileptic drugs: a multicenter study of clinical practice. Epilepsia 1986; 27:323–330.
14. Covanis A, Gupta AK, Jeavons PM. Sodium valproate: monotherapy and polypharmacy. Epilepsia 1982; 23:693–720.
15. Drury I, Driefuss FE. Pyknoleptic petit mal. Acta Neurol Scand 1985; 72;353–362.
16. Sato S, Penry JK, Driefuss FE, Dyken PR. Clonazepam in the treatment of absence seizures. A double blind clinical trial. Neurology 1977; 27:371.
17. Mattson RH, Cramer JA, Collins JF. Comparison of carbamazepine, phenobarbital, phenytoin and primidone in partial and secondary generalized tonic-clonic seizures. N Engl J Med 1985; 313:145–151.
18. Levy R: Drug interactions in epileptic children. In Morselli PL, Pippenger CE, Penry JK (eds). Antiepileptic Drug Therapy in Pediatrics. New York, Raven Press, 1983:75–84.
19. Livingston S, Pauli LL, Pruce I. Ketogenic diet in the treatment of childhood epilepsy. Dev Med Child Neurol 1977; 19:833–834.
20. Shinnar S, Vining EPG, Mellitis J. Discontinuing antiepileptic medication in children with epilepsy after two years without seizures: a prospective study. N Engl J Med 1985; 313:976–989.
21. Green RC, Adler JR, Erba G. Epilepsy surgery in children. J Child Neurol 1988; 3:155–166.

Sickle cell disease

Alan E. Lichtin

The oxygen-carrying protein in red blood cells, hemoglobin, is composed of four globin chains: two alpha (α) and two beta (β) chains. Sickle cell diseases occur when there is an amino acid substitution at the sixth position (valine for glutamic acid) of β-globin. When blood passes through capillaries and enters venules, deoxygenation occurs. Normally, deoxygenated hemoglobin retains approximately the same shape as oxygenated hemoglobin. However, in sickle cell disease, the deoxygenated hemoglobin assumes a conformational change that causes the red blood cell to alter its shape. The normal biconcave disc shape of the red blood cell changes into a sickled, rigid, comma-shaped cell. It is this shape change that leads to the morbidity and mortality of the sickle cell diseases.

There are many excellent reviews of sickle cell disease.[1,2] The references cited and the text will be useful for the reader interested in pursuing this topic further.

■ Background

Sickle cell disease refers to many different syndromes. Depending upon the genetics of the family tree, patients may have combinations of a sickle cell gene and other genes related to α- or β-globin gene abnormalities. Individuals inheriting a sickle β-globin gene from one parent and a normal β-globin gene from another parent have the condition called sickle cell trait. Sickle cell trait is probably not associated with increased mortality.[3] Some patients with sickle cell trait may experience hematuria, an inability to concentrate the urine, splenic infarctions at high altitudes, or bacteriuria and pyelonephritis during pregnancy. There are isolated case reports of patients with sickle cell trait dying suddenly after extreme exertion at high altitudes; this point is controversial.[4]

When one parent transmits a sickle β-globin gene and the other transmits another structural variant of the β-globin gene, for example hemoglobin C, the patient has a condition called hemoglobin sickle C disease. When one parent transmits a sickle β-globin gene and the other parent transmits a β-thalassemic gene, the condition is called sickle β-thalassemia. In general, the variants of sickle cell disease (sickle C, sickle β-thalassemia) are milder than the homozygous abnormality, in which both parents transmit a sickle β-globin gene to the offspring. This latter condition is called sickle cell anemia.

Eight per cent of black Americans carry the sickle cell trait. Based on chance pairings among these individuals, the incidence of sickle cell anemia in the United States is 1 in every 650 black Americans. Approximately 1 in every 1120 blacks has sickle C disease, and 1 in every 3200 blacks has sickle β-thalassemia.

Patients with sickle cell disease have chronic hemolysis, with anemia, compensatory reticulocytosis, indirect hyperbilirubinemia, sickled red blood cells on peripheral smear, elevated lactate dehydrogenase (LDH), and erythroid hyperplasia on bone marrow examination.

Sickle cell disease can manifest itself in many clinical presentations. The most common is the vaso-occlusive or "painful" crisis. In this setting, sickled red cells "log jam" in the microcirculation, causing distal infarction. This infarction leads to tissue ischemia and death, which causes the patient to have pain. As the crisis resolves, the area with ischemia either develops collateral circulation or becomes oxygenated in some fashion (the log jam resolves), or the infarcted tissue dies and there is a reparative process. The painful crisis can last from a few days to several weeks. It is usually the painful crisis that causes the most interactions with the health care system for the sickle cell patient.

Patients will present with pain, usually in the long bones or axial skeleton. The affected part will be tender to palpation. Patients may have fever and tachycardia. The pain may migrate from area to area or remain localized. The pain is usually constant, or it may be mild and brief. The pain may be excruciating, requiring weeks of hospitalization. Various factors are thought to precipitate sickle cell crises, including emotional stress, cold or hot weather, infection, and pregnancy. Laboratory findings may or may not be different from baseline values for patients. Some investigators feel an elevated LDH over the baseline value may help discriminate those patients actually having crisis from those who are not.

There have been reports of changes in the number of irreversibly sickled cells, decreased deformability, and decline in the dense cell fraction during painful crises, but how these observations relate to the clinical management of patients is yet to be delineated.

Part of the evaluation of patients with sickle cell disease who present with pain includes asking the question, "Is this pain typical of your previous crises or is it different?" If a patient usually presents with leg and back pain but then presents with abdominal pain and vomiting, a search for a cause other than vaso-occlusive crisis should be undertaken. The minimum evaluation includes a urinalysis and culture, if pyuria is seen, a complete blood count with differential and platelet count, reticulocyte count, and an LDH value.

Obviously, a white blood cell count higher than usual for the patient, in association with fever, should lead the clinician to seek an infectious source. Patients with sickle cell disease do not deal well with encapsulated bacterial infections. Patients may appear stable but decompensate rapidly in the setting of pneumococcal or gram-negative sepsis.

Other abnormalities that may cause morbidity or mortality for the patient include the following (where applicable, a brief description of treatment is added):

Cardiopulmonary System. When an infarctive crisis occurs in the lungs, the patients may present with fever, dyspnea, radiographic findings of an infiltrate, and even hemoptysis. It is difficult to discriminate whether these patients have pneumonia or the "acute chest syndrome." Most clinicians will treat these patients with antibiotics until blood and sputum cultures return neg-

ative.[5] Some patients who are predisposed to this type of sickling in the lung may develop pulmonary hypertension and cor pulmonale.

Liver and Biliary System. Patients with sickle cell disease have a hemolytic anemia and can be jaundiced on that basis alone, without invoking a hepatic etiology. There can be infarctive crises in the liver, causing right upper quadrant pain. This can be confused with biliary tract pain or cholelithiasis. Because of the lifelong hemolysis, sickle cell disease patients are prone to develop bilirubin gallstones as early as adolescence. Prophylactic cholecystectomies are recommended for patients with sickle cell disease in their early 20s.[6]

Spleen. The majority of patients with sickle cell anemia undergo a process of multiple infarctions of the spleen and over time have "autosplenectomy." Because of the loss of splenic function, Howell-Jolly bodies are seen on the peripheral smear. These patients also are predisposed to infections with encapsulated bacteria. Fulminant pneumococcal sepsis has been recorded not infrequently in patients with sickle cell disease. For that reason, the prophylactic use of penicillin has been tested and shown to be of proven benefit to prevent infections with encapsulated bacteria, especially pneumococcus, in the early age groups of sickle cell patients.[7]

Genitourinary System. The renal medulla, because of its function in forming a concentrated urine, tends to be a location where red blood cells sickle. Papillary necrosis, hematuria, difficulty concentrating the urine, and predisposition to infection in the renal pelvis occur.

Priapism. Young men with sickle cell disease may develop a painful constant erection of the penis, which is termed *priapism*. The onset of this condition may be unrelated to sexual activity. There is vaso-occlusion within the erectile tissue of the corpora cavernosae and corpus spongiosum. If medical attention is sought quickly, this may be relieved by the use of vasodilators and sedatives. Exchange transfusions do have a role in resolving priapism, if the patient seeks attention within the first 3 to 6 hours. Once the priapism is allowed to persist beyond 24 hours, the ability lowers to resolve this medically. Surgical decompression of the corpora cavernosae by the Winter's procedure or a cavernospongiosum shunt is sometimes necessary.[8] Priapism, left untreated beyond 24 hours and requiring surgical decompression, may lead to a permanent erectile dysfunction.

Problems with Pregnancy. Because of the increased burdens of pregnancy on the cardiovascular and hematopoietic systems, female patients with sickle cell disease who become pregnant may have several problems. They may develop an increased incidence of vaso-occlusive crises or worsening anemia and heart failure. Pyelonephritis is common in this setting. There is increased risk for premature birth and fetal death; placental infarctions are a likely cause for this. It used to be standard practice to give prophylactic red blood cell transfusions to pregnant sickle cell patients in the second and third trimesters. A recent study has demonstrated a reduction in painful crises in pregnant women with sickle cell disease who receive prophylactic red cell transfusions; however, there were no significant differences in the perinatal outcome between the offspring of mothers with sickle cell disease who were receiving prophylactic transfusions and those who were not.[9]

Central Nervous System. Approximately 8 to 10 per cent of patients with sickle cell disease will develop a stroke, often in childhood. This can lead to unfortunate neurologic morbidity. The patients who do suffer one stroke often have further strokes. Strokes are one of the few indications for exchange transfusion in the emergent setting, as well as for at least 1 year beyond the time of the stroke, to prevent second strokes.

Eye. Sickle cell patients may have obstruction of small peripheral, retinal vessels, leading to neovascularization and arteriovenous aneurysms. Patients may develop retinal detachment and blindness over time.

Bony Abnormalities. Patients with sickle cell disease have widened bone marrow spaces and thin cortices. The "codfish spine" is a condition in which the vertebral bodies have a biconcavity on the upper and lower plates. The infarctive crises in bone can lead to necrosis of the femoral head. Patients may require hip replacements if the degeneration of the femoral head leads to severe difficulty with ambulation. The marrow that is infarcted during a crisis may be an area for infection to develop. Osteomyelitis with anaerobic organisms, *Salmonella*, or other bacteria has been described.

Leg Ulcers. As with other hemoglobinop-athies, e.g., thalassemia major, patients with sickle cell disease may develop ulceration over the medial or lateral malleoli. The reason for this is infarction of the small subdermal and dermal vessels in the thinned skin overlying these bony prominences. Careful avoidance of trauma to these bony areas is important. When ulceration occurs, the use of whirlpools, dressing changes, keeping the areas clean, and the use of Unna boots have been shown to lead to relief of this problem. Unfortunately, once one ulcer occurs, the skin may never quite become normal again, and further ulceration may occur.

Sequestration Crisis. Sequestration occurs primarily in infants and children. There is pooling of red blood cells in the spleen, leading to a sudden increase in the size of the spleen. Patients may become markedly more anemic than their baseline and die of hypotension and cardiac arrest.

▪ Management

In the care of a patient with sickle cell disease, it is important to establish a strong bond between treating physicians, nurses, social workers, other therapists, and the patient. This is best done in the setting of a sickle cell clinic. The dedicated team can best serve the patient by providing educational materials and emotional support to families and developing communication with the patient when he or she is in steady state as well as when ill. This leads to uniformity of treatment. Patients with sickle cell disease often are treated in emergency rooms by different physicians and may develop narcotic addiction because of the variable attempts by physicians to control the pain of the vaso-occlusive crisis. When one physician is the prescriber for narcotics, the patient and the doctor can better assess exactly what is wrong with the patient, which may obviate the need for narcotics at certain times.

▪ EPISODIC TREATMENT

In the paragraphs above, some episodic treatments are described for various abnormalities, e.g., the use of exchange transfusions for stroke or priapism. The most frequent interaction patients with sickle cell disease have with their physicians revolves around the "painful" crisis. Patients who have sickle cell crisis pain should be given analgesic medicine. Initial attempts at non-narcotic analgesics may be successful. Usually, however, morphine or some other narcotic is needed, given subcutaneously or intramuscularly every 2 to 3 hours. Meperidine causes an increased incidence of seizures and should be avoided, especially in patients with renal or neurologic disease. Oxycodone should be avoided in young children. Methadone should never be used routinely. It may be possible to switch a patient who has previously been on meperidine to a methadone program and keep the patient on oral medicine, which, it is hoped, might avoid hospitalization. For milder pain, codeine, aspirin, acetaminophen, or ibuprofen may be useful. It is best to avoid the chronic use of outpatient narcotics, because of the potential for addiction. The use of other narcotics, for example butorphanol, has been studied and may be of benefit.[10] Transcutaneous electrical nerve stimulation for the treatment of sickle cell pain may be used as an adjunctive maneuver.[11] Behavioral modification, acupuncture, and patient-controlled analgesia have been attempted; however, they have not yet become standards of care.

In the first 24 hours, it is advisable to give morphine on a fixed schedule, approximately every 2 to 3 hours at a dose of 0.15 mg/kg, not to exceed 10 mg/dose. Acetaminophen, aspirin, or ibuprofen is given concomitantly. Oxygen and intravenous fluids also have a role in treating the pain crisis. After the first 1 to 2 days at the initial morphine dose, if the pain begins to subside a tapering of the dose by approximately one fifth every day may be attempted, but there should be no change in the dosage interval. Over 3 to 4 days of gradual tapering, with the patient being part of the decision making, it is possible to have most patients switch to oral medication by about the fourth through seventh day. Some patients do not require such a gradual tapering and can be switched to oral medicine sooner.

The most remarkable aspect of sickle cell disease is its variability—that some patients have multiple crises and are in the hospital frequently, whereas others may hardly ever interact with the health care system, because they "handle their crises" by themselves or simply seldom have a crisis. Nur-

turing home environments and stable psychosocial backgrounds may play a role.

Recently, elevated hemoglobin F levels, low MCV levels, concurrent alpha-thalassemia, and certain profiles of patients' DNA, using restriction endonucleases, have been associated with milder courses.[12] Hydroxyurea, 5-azacytidine, and cytarabine have been administered to patients with sickle cell diseases to elevate the hemoglobin F levels.[13,14] These patients have shown sustained elevations of their hemoglobin F level with decreased frequency of vaso-occlusive crises; however, such therapy may be leukemogenic and may be associated with decreases in white blood cell count and platelet count. Bone marrow transplantation has been performed for patients with thalassemia and, in rare instance, sickle cell anemia.[15] This should be reserved for young children whose sickle cell anemia has not caused end-organ damage. Bone marrow transplantation has a defined morbidity and mortality that has to be weighed against a positive outcome. These individuals would have to receive allogeneic transplants from HLA-histocompatible donors, so there is the risk of graft vs. host disease. Recombinant DNA techniques can yield erythropoietin in pharmacologic quantities. Its role in sickle cell anemia is unclear at this time. All these manipulations are highly experimental.

■ PROPHYLACTIC TREATMENT

It has been shown clearly that the prophylactic use of penicillin decreases the risk of infection in children with sickle cell anemia.[7] Identifying as early as possible that a child has sickle cell disease is important for the reduction of morbidity in these patients. Neonatal screening of hemoglobin is widely recognized as a cost-effective method of decreasing the morbidity and mortality of sickle cell disease.[16] Chorionic villous sampling and amniocentesis can yield cellular DNA that can be analyzed by restriction endonucleases[17] or gene amplification.[18] Thus, the in utero detection of fetuses with sickle cell anemia may give parents the option of terminating a pregnancy in which the fetus carries sickle cell disease. Obviously, the ethical issues pertinent to such a decision have to be thoroughly discussed, and the couples need to be counseled. Couples in whom both members have sickle cell trait or variants of the β-globin gene abnormality associated with sickle cell diseases need to be educated about their risks of having a child with sickle cell disease. Unfortunately, usually a woman is already pregnant when she has a hemoglobin electrophoresis that determines the chance of carrying a fetus with sickle cell disease.

The other forms of prophylactic treatment that may be of benefit include, as stated, the use of transfusions during the later stages of pregnancy; however, there is recent controversy in this area.[9] Patients with sickle cell disease who are about to undergo general anesthesia should have some manipulation of their blood to decrease the hemoglobin S concentration. It is not clear whether simple transfusion to a hemoglobin of 10 gm/dl or exchange transfusion to decrease the hemoglobin S level below 30 to 60 per cent avoids the increased risks sickle cell patients have with general anesthesia.[19] This includes the occurrence of severe vaso-occlusive crisis on awakening from anesthesia, strokes, myocardial infarctions, and so on. A nationwide study is currently being conducted randomizing patients to these two procedures (simple transfusion vs. exchange transfusion) in sickle cell patients about to undergo elective surgery.

Annual ophthalmologic examinations by ophthalmologists acquainted with sickle retinopathy help prevent visual impairment. The avoidance of smoking and severe extremes of exercise, especially on hot days, also may decrease morbidity for the sickle cell patient. Avoidance of known precipitating factors, for example, emotional stresses, strenuous exercise, and extremes of cold and heat, may reduce the number of vaso-occlusive crises.

■ Issues and Risks

As in any chronic illness, sickle cell disease patients may have problems coping with their illness. Sickle cell disease patients have significant psychosocial distress in the areas of employment and finances, sleeping and eating, and performance of normal daily activities; fear and anxiety regarding deterioration of physical function, lack of assertiveness in social relationships, and depression are also found.[20] Antidepressants have

been used to help as an adjunct in pain control and may help in the area of depression in sickle cell patients.

It is emphasized that close, long-term relationships of staff members (physicians, nurses, social workers) with patients are important to make them feel that their health status is being monitored carefully. Through community and patient education, genetic counseling, and newborn screening programs, the medical community can do much to decrease the incidence and morbidity of this illness.[21]

REFERENCES

1. Beutler E. The sickle cell diseases and related disorders. *In* Williams WJ, Beutler E, Erslev AJ, Lichtman MA (eds). Hematology. New York: McGraw-Hill, 1990:613–644.
2. Serjeant GR. Sickle Cell Disease. New York: Oxford University Press, 1985.
3. Sears DA. The morbidity of sickle cell trait. Am J Med 1978; 64:1021–1036.
4. Kark JA, Posey DM, Schumacher HR, Ruehle CJ. Sickle cell trait as a risk factor for sudden death in physical training. N Engl J Med 1987; 317:781–787.
5. Poncz M, Kane E, Gill FM. Acute chest syndrome in sickle cell disease: etiology and clinical correlates. J Pediatr 1985; 107:861–866.
6. Schubert TT. Hepatobiliary system in sickle cell disease. Gastroenterology 1986; 90:2013–2021.
7. Gaston MH, Verter JI, Woods G, et al. Prophylaxis with oral penicillin in children with sickle cell anemia. N Engl J Med 1986; 314:1593–1599.
8. Ercole CJJ, Pontes JE, Pierce JM Jr. Changing surgical concepts in the treatment of priapism. J Urol 1981; 125:210–211.
9. Koshy M, Burd L, Wallace D, Moawad A, Baron J. Prophylactic red cell transfusions in pregnant patients with sickle cell disease. N Engl J Med 1988; 319:1447–1452.
10. Gonzalez ER, Ornato JP, Ware D, Bull D, Evens RP. Comparison of intramuscular analgesic activity of butorphanol and morphine in patients with sickle cell disease. Ann Emerg Med 1988; 17:788–791.
11. Wang WC, George SL, Wilimas JA. Transcutaneous electrical nerve stimulation treatment of sickle cell pain crises. Acta Haematol 1988; 80:99–102.
12. Embury SH, Dozy AM, Miller J, et al. Concurrent sickle cell anemia and alpha thalassemia. N Engl J Med 1982; 306:270–274.
13. Dover GJ, Charache S, Boyer SH, Vogelsang G, Moyer M. 5-Azacytidine increases HbF production and reduces anemia in sickle cell disease: dose-response analysis of subcutaneous and oral dosage regimens. Blood 1985; 66:527–532.
14. Veith R, Galanello R, Papyannopoulou T, Stamatoyannopoulous G. Stimulation of F-cell production in patients with sickle cell anemia treated with cytarabine or hydroxyurea. N Engl J Med 1985; 313:1571–1575.
15. Johnson FL, Look AT, Gockerman J, Ruggiero MR, Dalla-Pozza L, Billings FT. Bone marrow transplan-

tation in a patient with sickle cell anemia. N Engl J Med 1984; 311:780–783.

16. Vichinsky E, Hurst D, Earles A, Kleman K, Lubin B. Newborn screening for sickle cell disease: effect on mortality. Pediatrics 1988; 81:749–755.

17. Boehm CD, Antonarakis SE, Phillips JA III, Stetten G, Kazazian HH Jr. Prenatal diagnosis using DNA polymorphisms: report on 95 pregnancies at risk for sickle cell disease or β-thalassemia. N Engl J Med 1983; 308:1054–1058.

18. Embury SH, Scharf SJ, Saiki RK, et al. Rapid prenatal diagnosis of sickle cell anemia by a new method of DNA analysis. N Engl J Med 1987; 316:656–661.

19. Roizen MF. Anesthetic implications of concurrent diseases. *In* Miller RD (ed). Anesthesia. New York: Churchill Livingstone, 1986:320–321.

20. Barrett DH, Wisotzek IE, Abel GG, et al. Assessment of psychosocial functioning of patients with sickle cell disease. South Med J 1988; 81:745–750.

21. Nash KB. Overview of humanistic progress in sickle cell anemia during the past ten years. Am J Pediatr Hematol Oncol 1983; 5:352–359.

Sleep apnea

Michael Donahoe ■ *Mark H. Sanders*

■ Background

Recent years have seen a dramatic increase in the study of ventilatory control and mechanics during sleep. Sleep apnea is now recognized as a substantial cause of significant morbidity and possibly mortality. Despite recent advances in this field, major knowledge gaps remain that prohibit definitive conclusions regarding the indications for therapy of sleep-disordered breathing. The level and frequency of nocturnal arterial desaturation and the frequency of sleep-disordered breathing events that demand intervention are unclear.[1,2] A significant proportion of asymptomatic and otherwise healthy subjects, particularly elderly people, have evidence of sleep apnea.[3] A major unresolved issue is whether sleep apnea can represent a normal variant in the absence of cardiovascular or cognitive disturbance or whether all sleep apnea is associated with disorders of function, which at times may be subclinical.

The majority of investigators agree on the need to treat patients with marked abnormalities on polysomnographic evaluation and well-defined measures of morbidity, including cor pulmonale, pulmonary hypertension, excessive daytime hypersomnolence, and altered alertness or mental function. However, along with increased public awareness, physicians are faced with a growing population of patients with less definitive symptoms and polysomnographic test results. Before the appropriate indications and type of therapy for sleep apnea can be established, long-term multicenter studies of this disorder are badly needed.[4] The uncertainty of diagnosis is paralleled by a similar uncertainty regarding the indications and efficacy of the therapeutic approaches. A single therapeutic option applicable for all patients presenting with sleep apnea does not exist. The clinical disorder of "sleep apnea" most likely represents a final common pathway of a heterogeneous list of pathophysiologic abnormalities, similar to the clinical disorder of "congestive heart failure." Until more detailed information regarding the pathophysiology of this disorder is available, the best treatment alternative is an individualized approach based upon the patient's symptoms, preferences, polysomnographic findings, and tolerance of the available therapeutic measures. This approach must be supplemented by subsequent confirmation of therapeutic efficacy on follow-up evaluation.

■ Management

The therapeutic options to be discussed are directed primarily toward the patient suffering from mixed and obstructive apneas. Patients with predominantly central sleep apnea are relatively uncommon (less than 10 per cent). As will be discussed, many patients with evidence of mixed or central apneas respond to the conventional measures employed for the treatment of obstructive sleep apnea. The therapeutic approach to sleep apnea is summarized in Figure 1.

■ RISK FACTOR MANAGEMENT

Attention to factors that may either precipitate sleep apnea or aggravate an underlying tendency toward the disorder provides the foundation for effective treatment. In a small percentage of patients, attending to these factors alone may be successful and obviate the need for aggressive intervention.

Weight Reduction. Obesity is a common, although not universal, accompaniment of sleep apnea. This problem may be either lifelong or of recent development and related to the onset of symptoms. Weight reduction may result in marked relief from, if not elimination of, the symptoms and clinical manifestations of sleep apnea.[5,6] Even modest weight reduction may result in improvement in clinical signs and symptoms.[5-7] Smith and associates documented a significant decrease in apnea frequency and desaturation in 15 patients with obstructive sleep apnea following a mean weight reduction of only 9 per cent.[5] This knowledge, combined with the recognized benefits to overall general medical health of weight reduction, makes this a cornerstone of therapy

for a large portion of patients evaluated for sleep apnea. Unfortunately, obesity is often poorly responsive to the conventional therapies, and patients who successfully lose weight may relapse.

Patients with more urgent medical indications for treatment of sleep apnea, who receive more aggressive therapies, still require counseling regarding the importance of weight reduction. If weight reduction is successful, they may then require re-evaluation with polysomnography to determine the need for continued treatment. Likewise, patients who regain lost weight may experience the return of sleep apnea symptoms that had resolved during the previous period of weight loss.

Sleeping Position. Investigators have suggested that the lateral decubitus position is associated with a decreased frequency of sleep apnea.[8] Interviews with the patient and bed partner frequently will disclose an increase in the patient's snoring and apnea in the supine position, which is confirmed by monitoring sleep position during polysomnography. Theoretically, the gravitational effects of the supine position cause apposition of the tongue with the posterior pharyngeal wall, leading to upper airway obstruction. If supine-dependent apnea is documented, the "sleep-ball" technique can be employed to maintain the patient in the lateral decubitus position during sleep. A ball is sewn into the back of the patient's sleeping garments, which "alerts" the patient of the need to change position when supine.

Manipulation of sleep position represents

Figure 1. The therapeutic approach and options for sleep apnea.

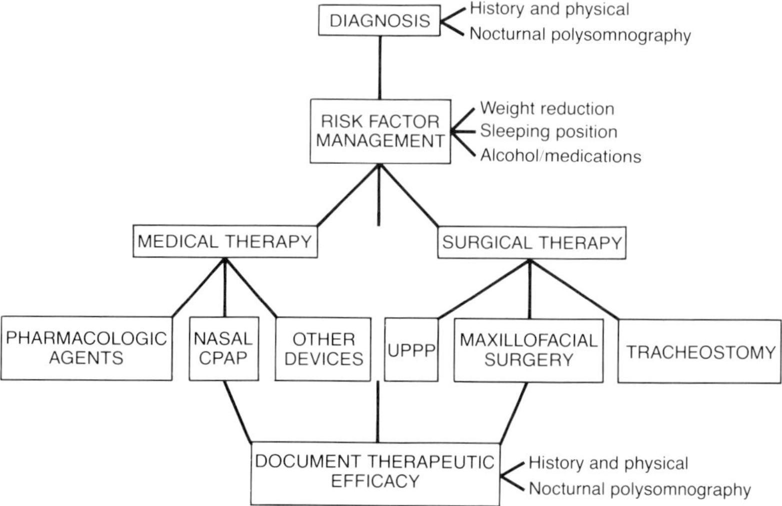

the sole therapeutic option required in a minority of patients. George and associates have suggested that the lateral decubitus sleeping position reduces apnea events only in nonrapid eye movement (non-REM) sleep, as compared with REM sleep, and does not reduce the frequency of patient arousals.[8] Despite these findings, manipulation of the sleeping position may represent an effective therapeutic option for patients with minimal REM apnea, and it also can be used to increase the likelihood for success of other therapies.

Alcohol/Medications. The adverse effect of alcohol on sleep apnea frequently can be appreciated from the patient interview. The patient or bed partner will relate that the snoring is louder, the apneas are longer, and the daytime hypersomnolence is greater following the ingestion of alcohol. These changes result from alcohol's interference with the normal neuromuscular tone of the upper airway, resulting in decreased airway diameter and an increased likelihood of sleep apnea.[9] In addition, alcohol reduces the arousal response to hypoxia and hypercapnia, which could prolong underlying apnea events.[10] This combination of effects makes alcohol a "forbidden vice" for patients with sleep apnea, and all patients need to be instructed repeatedly in this regard.

In addition to questions regarding alcohol consumption, the evaluation of patients with suspected sleep apnea requires a detailed drug history. The list is growing of medications recognized to precipitate or aggravate sleep apnea. Any medication with known sedative properties should be avoided if possible. Benzodiazepines, commonly used as sedatives, are included in this list. Flurazepam is recognized to augment the frequency of sleep apnea events.[11] Although the mechanism and extent of alteration in sleep ventilation associated with the benzodiazepines remain controversial, these medications are best avoided in patients with suspected sleep apnea.

In a similar fashion, the barbiturate and narcotics classes of pharmacologic agents are believed to have undesirable effects on upper airway muscle tone and ventilatory chemosensitivity. This knowledge is especially important in sleep apnea patients who must undergo surgery. Recognition of the effects of commonly employed sedatives on upper airway diameter and ventilatory control demands careful monitoring in the perioperative period.

Endocrine Disorders. The administration of exogenous androgenic hormones appears to aggravate sleep apnea.[12] Certainly, the disorder is more prevalent in men and postmenopausal women, which supports a hormonal influence. Although the mechanism remains controversial, these agents should be avoided by this patient population.

Recent work has confirmed the previously suspected association of hypothyroidism with sleep apnea. In one series, nine of eleven patients with hypothyroidism demonstrated obstructive sleep apnea, which resolved with thyroid replacement.[13] The clinical manifestations of sleep apnea often are more apparent than those of hypothyroidism, especially in elderly people. Therefore, all patients evaluated for sleep apnea also should undergo the necessary evaluation to exclude hypothyroidism.

Anatomic Abnormalities. Anatomic abnormalities of the upper airway may predispose patients to the development of sleep apnea. These structural lesions may include nasal deformities, nasal polyps, hypertrophic tonsils or adenoids, tumors in the oro- or hypopharynx, macroglossia, or craniofacial disproportions. Adults with hypertrophied tonsils may benefit from tonsillectomy, although the likelihood of a surgical cure of the apnea is much less than in younger patients.[14] Similarly, patients with nasal obstruction are unlikely to be cured completely from nasal surgery alone.[14] Nevertheless, all patients should undergo a detailed evaluation of the upper airway, with decisions regarding the need for surgical intervention made on an individual basis with surgical consultation.

■ MEDICAL THERAPY FOR SLEEP APNEA

Pharmacologic Agents. Oxygen administration during sleep is a therapeutic option that can be employed successfully in certain patients with sleep apnea. Recurrent hypoxemia in association with periods of apnea or hypopnea is believed to play a major pathophysiologic role in the signs and symptoms of sleep apnea, including pulmonary hypertension, arrhythmias, polycythemia, sleep arousal and fragmentation, and possibly disturbances of cognition. Administration of oxygen alone has been shown to reduce apnea time and frequency in patients with eucapnic sleep apnea.[15] However, isolated oxygen administration to this patient population is not without risk. Following the acute administration of oxygen to patients with sleep apnea, initial prolongation of apnea time may be noted.[15] All patients treated with oxygen therapy should undergo polysomnography during the initial trial of oxygen to determine oxygen requirements and to document the safety of oxygen administration, especially with respect to its effect on apnea time and frequency.

Protriptyline is a nonsedating tricyclic antidepressant that is beneficial in some patients with sleep apnea. It suppresses REM sleep,[16] that stage of sleep generally characterized by the most prolonged and frequent apneas. This medication has also been reported to convert non-REM apnea events to hypopneas.[17] Regardless of its mechanism of action, most investigations have suggested that protriptyline does not result in the complete elimination of sleep apnea except for those patients with mild disease. Polysomnography is required to document the therapeutic response to this therapy, as some patients report subjective improvement in daytime hypersomnolence without documented improvement in the severity of their sleep apnea. A limiting factor to the use of protriptyline is often the side effects of the medication, which are related primarily to its anticholinergic properties.

Progesterone, a known ventilatory stimulant, has been proposed for the treatment of sleep apnea. Medroxyprogesterone improves awake ventilatory chemosensitivity; however, its effectiveness during sleep for patients with obstructive sleep apnea has been less convincing.[18] In the absence of adequate studies, this therapeutic agent cannot be recommended as a first-line agent for the treatment of either obstructive or central sleep apnea.

Theophylline, another medication recognized to augment ventilatory chemosensitivity, has been employed to treat apneas during infancy and therefore has been investigated for the treatment of sleep apnea in adults. Espinoza and associates concluded that theophylline appeared to reduce central apneas and the central component of mixed apneas, while simultaneously increasing sleep fragmentation.[19] No effect was seen on the frequency or duration of obstructive apneas. Theophylline does not appear to offer a major therapeutic advantage for patients with sleep apnea, although it may have a role in the treatment of patients with predominantly central apneas.

Nicotine may affect upper airway dilator muscle activity, making it an appropriate therapeutic intervention for patients with sleep apnea. Gothe and associates reported a reduction in obstructive and mixed apneas over a short interval following the administration of nicotine chewing gum.[20] This small study requires confirmation, as well as investigation into methods of nicotine delivery that would allow the sustained action necessary for sleep.

Metabolic acidosis is a known respiratory stimulant. In this regard, medications such as acetazolamide, which can induce a metabolic acidosis, have been employed for the treatment of sleep apnea. The numbers of patients investigated with this medication to date are small and preclude any firm recommendations regarding its use in either obstructive or central sleep apnea. Of concern is a report by Sharp and colleagues that suggests that the augmented ventilatory stimulus associated with this medication produces an increase in the severity of obstructive apneas.[21]

Additional agents investigated as therapeutic modalities for this disorder include naloxone, bromocriptine, baclofen, atropine, almitrine, L-tryptophan, chlorimipramine, prochlorperazine, and strychnine. These medications cannot be recommended at this time in the absence of evidence to support their safety and efficacy.

Nasal Continuous Positive Airway Pressure (Nasal CPAP). The application of nasal continuous airway pressure as a method to "splint" open the upper airway during sleep has become an important therapeutic alternative for patients with sleep apnea. A variety of commercial and custom-built devices are now in use. The most common CPAP system consists of a silicone mask that fits snugly at the nose (Figure 2). The mask is attached to an air blower able to generate high airflows. The expiratory limb of this device contains an adjustable or fixed valve that provides the necessary resistance to airflow to generate the required positive airway pressure.

As might be expected, nasal CPAP results in significant improvement in apnea and oxygen desaturation in patients with obstruc-

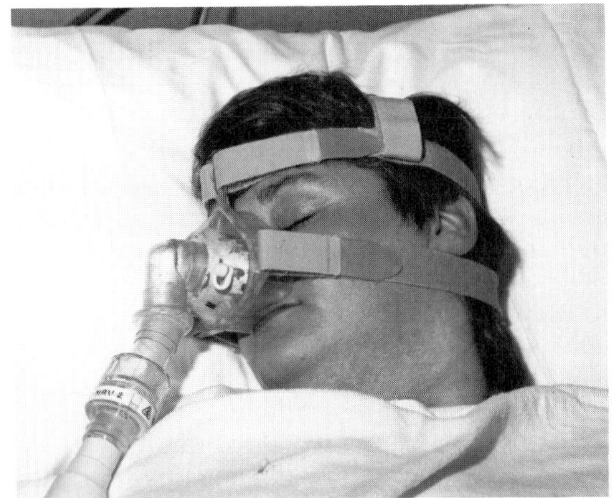

Figure 2. Sleeping with a standard nasal CPAP mask and the associated head straps, which are designed to maintain the position of the mask during sleep.

tive apnea.[22] An additional finding was the report by Sanders that CPAP also effectively reduced or eliminated mixed apneas, including both the obstructive and central components, and tended to reduce central apnea frequency.[23] Issa and Sullivan subsequently confirmed these findings.[24] Subsequent work has suggested that some central apneas actually may result from an obstructing event in the ventilatory cycle.[25] This knowledge would support a trial of nasal CPAP in all patients with sleep apnea, even those with evidence of predominantly central apneas. The heterogeneous pathophysiology of central apneas suggests that nasal CPAP will not be uniformly successful for all patients, but it will represent a viable alternative for some.

When patients are evaluated whose clinical symptoms do not correspond to findings obtained during a polysomnographic evaluation, the low-risk, high–patient-compliance nature of nasal CPAP allows it to be used as a diagnostic tool. A therapeutic trial of nasal CPAP can be employed in patients whose complaints are in excess of documented abnormalities on polysomnography, to assess the effect of eliminating sleep apnea on the patients' complaints. Likewise, patients who have minimal daytime complaints but marked abnormalities on polysomnography may notice a dramatic clinical improvement in previously unrecognized symptoms following the initiation of nasal CPAP.

Approximately 75 to 85 per cent of patients deemed acceptable for the therapeutic administration of nasal CPAP are able to comply with home therapy.[26] The majority of patients require between 5 and 15 cm H_2O of continuous nasal CPAP for effective treatment. The high rate of patient compliance depends on a strong patient support system. This support system is structured at three levels:

- *Patient Education.* This aspect of treatment begins during the initial patient evaluation and continues with follow-up by the patient's physician or the sleep laboratory personnel or both.
- *Equipment Maintenance and Repair.* The patient must have ready access to qualified personnel able to deal with technical problems related to the home use of the equipment.
- *Peer Support.* Patient organizations provide much-needed peer support to allay the fears and anxieties of patients initially beginning therapy with CPAP. In addition, these groups assist this patient population in dealing with the social isolation that is frequently a significant problem in their pretreatment lifestyle.

Nasal CPAP has proved to be remarkably benign in terms of significant side effects. Pneumomediastinum or pneumothorax has not occurred to our knowledge, nor has impairment of cardiac function been reported. The majority of complications with nasal CPAP are related to local effects of the high-pressure airflow or nasal mask. These include dry eyes, dry mouth, nasal congestion and rhinorrhea, conjunctivitis, and nose and mouth irritation from the mask. An occasional patient may complain of chest heaviness or discomfort following the use of nasal CPAP, which usually has no apparent cardiopulmonary origin and is most frequently attributed to musculoskeletal pain. Despite the relative safety of this therapeutic maneuver, nasal CPAP should not be prescribed for any patient without a complete evaluation by polysomnography. This should include evaluation of a sleep interval during the administration of the nasal CPAP. This testing will allow determination of the optimal level of nasal CPAP required to control the patient's sleep apnea; it will document the safety of this form of therapeutic intervention; and it allows exposure of the patient to this unique form of nocturnal ventilation under controlled laboratory conditions with experienced personnel.

The introduction of nasal CPAP has provided an effective therapeutic option for the majority of patients with sleep apnea. In addition to its documented efficacy, a major advantage is the high level of patient acceptance and the low level of patient risk.

Other Devices. Other devices proposed to maintain the patency of the upper airway during sleep include the nasopharyngeal airway and the tongue-retaining device. Although a nasopharyngeal airway theoretically would be an effective means of preventing upper airway obstruction during sleep, this technique has not been useful in our experience. The device is poorly tolerated by the majority of patients because of the associated nasal discomfort and occasional activation of the gag reflex.

The tongue-retaining device, as described by Cartwright,[27] attaches to the tongue by suction and maintains the tongue in a forward position during sleep. Preliminary investigation suggests that this device may be most effective in patients who have lesser degrees of obesity and predominantly supine position–dependent apnea. Approximately 60 per cent of patients are able to tolerate the device, although only a small number of patients have been evaluated in the literature to date. An oral appliance, using principles similar to the tongue-retaining device, also has been described;[28] however, this apparatus has not been evaluated in significant patient numbers to allow conclusions about its efficacy.

■ SURGICAL THERAPY FOR SLEEP APNEA

The surgical therapy of sleep apnea is designed to modify the characteristics of the airway to bypass or reduce the area of obstruction. As discussed, all patients should undergo otolaryngologic examination to eliminate the possibility of upper airway abnormalities that can precipitate or aggravate sleep apnea. This section will deal primarily with surgical options for patients with normal anatomy of the upper airway.

Uvulopalatopharyngoplasty. Uvulopalatopharyngoplasty (UPPP) is a procedure designed to reduce upper airway obstruction through resection of the uvula, bilateral tonsils, a variable portion of the free margin of the soft palate, and lateral pharyngeal wall. Based on the reported series, this procedure is effective in approximately 50 per cent of patients.[29,30] At present, criteria to identify those patients who will benefit from UPPP have not been established. Up to 80 per cent of patients may report symptomatic improvement following this procedure.[30] As with all other therapies discussed, the subjective improvements described by the patients do not always correlate with the more objective determination of changes in sleep breathing patterns, raising the possibility of a placebo effect. Follow-up polysomnography is indicated approximately 6 to 8 weeks following the procedure, when the healing is complete, to document a physiologic improvement.

UPPP can be complicated by chronic nasal regurgitation in up to 5 per cent of patients, although this problem may be seen acutely in up to 50 per cent of patients.[29] Of concern in the acute postoperative period is the report of early postoperative UPPP deaths.[31] The potential complication of swelling, with airway compromise, has led some surgical specialists to advocate prophylactic tracheostomy with this procedure. Sanders et al and Johnson et al have recently reported their experience with polysomnography in the immediate post-operative period following UPPP.[32,33] This evaluation, confined to patients who were normocapnic in the awake preoperative period, suggested that in the study population the combined apnea/hypopnea index and the level of oxyhemoglobin desaturation were not different in the postoperative period. However, some patients were clearly worse in the early postoperative period. Further, patients who required oxygen in the postoperative period were allowed to use the oxygen during the postoperative polysomnographic evaluation. These patients likely would have been at risk for significant desaturation if supplemental oxygen had not been provided.

In summary, UPPP is a surgical option that appears to be effective in approximately 50 per cent of patients with obstructive sleep apnea. Unfortunately, patients' responses to the procedure cannot be predicted preoperatively, and this has been the major limitation in widespread application of this operation. The procedure can generally be done without tracheostomy in experienced hands, but postoperative monitoring with attention to patients' potential supplemental oxygen needs is essential. The procedure is almost uniformly successful in the elimination of unacceptable snoring, although this problem may improve without significant changes in patients' sleep apnea.

Maxillofacial Surgery. Cephalometric radiographs of patients with sleep apnea have suggested that a significant portion of the patients have maxillofacial abnormalities that cannot be determined by routine physical examination. Techniques to normalize the bony relationships are being evaluated. These techniques require highly skilled surgical intervention, combined with detailed experience in the management of the upper airway during this type of surgery through both the intraoperative and postoperative periods. Until long-term studies of adequate sample size have been completed, the potential risks associated with these procedures, as well as the significant patient morbidity, prohibit their widespread application to the population of patients with sleep apnea.

Tracheostomy. Although tracheostomy provides an immediate bypass of upper airway obstruction during sleep, it has obvious disadvantages. In addition to the psychologic effects on the patient that might result from the surgically produced cosmetic changes, the surgical procedure and postoperative care can be technically difficult. Many obese patients have short necks, anterior adipose tissue, and posteriorly displaced tracheas, which can make placement and general care of the tracheostomy difficult. Postoperative problems can include bleeding, infection, strictures, aspiration, and stomal or tracheal granulation tissue. Fortunately, the development of nasal CPAP has made the need for tracheostomy to manage patients with sleep apnea relatively rare. This procedure can now be reserved exclusively for those patients who cannot be controlled with other, less invasive, therapies.

■ Issues and Risks

The primary issue facing the physician who encounters the patient with signs and symptoms consistent with sleep apnea is determining which patients require therapy, and how urgently that therapy is needed. Certainly, patients with marked daytime hypersomnolence, often associated with falling asleep while driving, have significant morbidity that should be treated promptly. Polysomnographic findings of frequent noc-

turnal arrhythmias, including bradycardia, or marked arterial desaturation during sleep necessitate immediate intervention. Less clear is the management of patients with intermediate symptoms and objective findings. Each case must be approached on an individual basis until more information is available regarding the pathophysiology of sleep apnea. It is hoped that further investigation of this disorder will allow the selection of treatment based on analysis of the associated pathophysiologic abnormality.

As a foundation to all therapeutic options, an attempt should be made by the patient and physician to modify those risk factors known to precipitate or aggravate the sleep apnea syndrome. Nasal CPAP appears to be an appropriate therapeutic modality for the majority of patients. It offers a low risk:benefit ratio but still acceptable patient compliance. Nasal CPAP is evaluated as an initial trial before other, more invasive techniques with unpredictable outcomes, such as UPPP, are attempted. Regardless of the therapy selected, the care of the patient with sleep apnea requires follow-up documentation, by both patient history and polysomnography.

REFERENCES

1. Berry DTR, Webb WB, Block AJ. Sleep apnea syndrome: a critical review of the apnea index as a diagnostic criterion. Chest 1984; 86:529–531.
2. Sanders MH, Rogers RM. Sleep apnea: when does better become benefit? Chest 1985; 88:320–321.
3. Knight H, Millman RP, Gur RC, Saykin AJ, Doherty JU, Pack AI. Clinical significance of sleep apnea in the elderly. Am Rev Resp Dis 1987; 136:845–850.
4. Weil JV, Cherniack NS, Dempsey JA, Edelman NH, Phillipson EA, Remmers JA, Kiley JP. Respiratory disorders of sleep; NHLBI Workshop Summary. Am Rev Resp Dis 1987; 136:755–761.
5. Smith PL, Gold AR, Meyers DA, Haponik EF, Bleecker ER. Weight loss in mildly to moderately obese patients with obstructive sleep apnea. Ann Intern Med 1985; 103:850–855.
6. Harman EM, Wynne JW, Block AJ. The effect of weight loss on sleep-disordered breathing and oxygen desaturation in morbidly obese men. Chest 1982; 82:291–294.
7. Sugarman HJ, Fairman RP, Baron PL, Kwentus JA. Gastric surgery for respiratory insufficiency of obesity. Chest 1986; 90:81–86.
8. George CF, Millar TW, Kryger MH. Sleep apnea and body position during sleep. Sleep 1988; 11:90–99.
9. Krol RC, Knuth SL, Bartlett D Jr. Selective reduction of genioglossal muscle activity by alcohol in normal human subjects. Am Rev Resp Dis 1984; 129:247–251.
10. Anthonisen NR, Kryger M. Ventilatory and arousal

responses to hypoxemia in sleep. Am Rev Resp Dis 1982; 126:1–2.

11. Dolly FR, Block AJ. Effect of flurazepam on sleep-disordered breathing and nocturnal oxygen desaturation in asymptomatic subjects. Am J Med 1982; 73:239–243.

12. Sandblom RE, Matsumoto AM, Schoene RB, Lee KA, Giblin EC, Bremner WJ, Pierson DJ. Obstructive sleep apnea syndrome induced by testosterone administration. N Engl J Med 1983; 308:508–510.

13. Rajagopal KR, Abbrecht PH, Derderian SS, Pickett C, Hofeldt F, Tellis CJ, Zwillich CW. Obstructive sleep apnea in hypothyroidism. Ann Intern Med 1984; 101:491–494.

14. Rubin AH, Eliaschar I, Joachim Z, Alroy G, Lavie P. Effects of nasal surgery and tonsillectomy on sleep apnea. Bull Eur Physiopathol Resp 1983; 19:612–615.

15. Martin RJ, Sanders MH, Gray BA, Pennock BE. Acute and long-term ventilatory effects of hyperoxia in the adult sleep apnea syndrome. Am Rev Resp Dis 1982; 125:175–180.

16. Brownell LG, West P, Sweatman P, Acres JC, Kryger MH. Protriptyline in obstructive sleep apnea. A double-bind trial. N Engl J Med 1982; 307:1037–1042.

17. Smith PL, Haponik EF, Allen RP, Bleecker ER. The effects of protriptyline in sleep-disordered breathing. Am Rev Resp Dis 1983; 127:8–13.

18. Rajagopal KR, Abbrecht PH, Jabbari B. Effects of medroxyprogesterone acetate in obstructive sleep apnea. Chest 1986; 90:815–821.

19. Espinoza II, Antic R, Thornton AT, McEvoy RD. The effects of aminophylline on sleep and sleep-disordered breathing in patients with obstructive sleep apnea syndrome. Am Rev Resp Dis 1987; 136:80–84.

20. Gothe B, Strohl KP, Levin S, Cherniack NS. Nicotine:a different approach to treatment of obstructive sleep apnea. Chest 1985; 87:11–17.

21. Sharp JT, Druz WS, D'Souza V, Diamond E. Effect of metabolic acidosis upon sleep apnea. Chest 1985; 87:619–624.

22. Sanders MH, Moore SE, Eveslage J. CPAP via nasal mask: a treatment for occlusive sleep apnea. Chest 1983; 83:144–145.

23. Sanders MH. Nasal CPAP effect on patterns of sleep apnea. Chest 1984; 86:839–844.

24. Issa FG, Sullivan CE. Reversal of central sleep apnea using nasal CPAP. Chest 1986; 90:165–171.

25. Sanders MH, Rogers RM, Pennock BE. Prolonged expiratory phase in sleep apnea. A unifying hypothesis. Am Rev Resp Dis 1985; 131:401–408.

26. Sanders MH, Gruendl CA, Rogers RM. Compliance of patients with nasal CPAP therapy for sleep apnea. Chest 1986; 90:330–333.

27. Cartwright RD. Predicting response to the tongue-retaining device for sleep apnea syndrome. Arch Otolaryngol 1985; 111:385–388.

28. George PT. A modified functional appliance for treatment of obstructive sleep apnea. J Clin Orthodont 1987; 21:171–175.

29. Simmons FB, Guilleminault C, Miles LE. The palatopharyngoplasty operation for snoring and sleep apnea: an interim report. Otolaryngol Head Neck Surg 1984; 92:375–380.

30. Conway W, Fujita S, Zorick F, Sicklesteel J, Roehrs T, Wittig R, Roth T. Uvulopalatopharyngoplasty. One year follow-up. Chest 1985; 88:385–387.

31. Kramer M, Anand VK, Schoen L, Draper E. Death associated with uvulopalatopharyngoplasty: a case report. Sleep Res 1985: 14:180.

32. Sanders MH, Johnson JT, Keller FA, Segar L. The acute effects of uvulopalatopharyngoplasty on breathing during sleep in sleep apnea patients. Sleep 1988; 11:75–89.

33. Johnson JT, Sanders MH. Breathing during sleep immediately after uvulopalatopharyngoplasty. Laryngoscope 1986; 96:1236–1238.

Smoke inhalation

Thomas J. Iberti ■ *Peter J. Papadakos*

Smoke inhalation commonly produces respiratory dysfunction with or without significant surface burns. Despite the advent of improved treatment modalities for burns and burn-shock, inhalation-related pulmonary injuries, especially when combined with severe burns, remain a leading cause of morbidity and mortality. The mortality rate associated with patients suffering isolated severe inhalation injuries is 5 to 8 per cent, whereas the mortality rate may exceed 50 per cent in patients with both burns and inhalation injuries.[1–3]

■ Background

■ PATHOPHYSIOLOGY

Smoke inhalation produces pulmonary dysfunction and systemic injury by thermal, hypoxic, and chemical mechanisms. Although they will be discussed individually, these mechanisms of injury commonly are all present in the smoke-injured patient.

Thermal Injuries. Thermal-induced respiratory injury usually results in damage to the upper airway (pharynx, vocal cords) and produces mucosal and laryngeal edema. This may produce marked increases in the work of breathing.[1] Severe injury may progress to upper airway obstruction. These injuries usually become manifest within the first 24 hours and resolve within 3 to 5 days. Thermal injury below the vocal cords is uncommon, due to the efficient cooling of the upper airway, but it may occur when superheated steam is inhaled.[2]

Hypoxic Injuries. Hypoxia results from upper airway obstruction, ventilation-perfusion mismatching, carbon monoxide poisoning, and, occasionally, cyanide gas. With severe hypoxia, arterial hypoxemia develops, resulting in a markedly decreased tissue oxygenation. In such cases, a metabolic acidosis secondary to increased lactic acid production results.[1]

Chemical Injuries. Chemical injuries occur from the inhalation of toxic particles contained in smoke and from the irritant effects of these compounds on the airways. These products consist of a suspension of small particles in hot air, and gases that contain both particulate and gaseous components. The components of smoke include carbon dioxide, carbon monoxide, oxides of sulfur, oxides of nitrogen, chlorine, phosgene, ammonia, and hydrogen cyanide. Phosgene is produced by burning plastic and may react with water in the airway to produce hydrochloric acid.[1] The exact composition of smoke depends upon the material burning, but all fires contain carbon monoxide and carbon dioxide. The byproducts of combustion may adhere to the mucosal layer of the airway and, in the presence of water, form corrosive acids and alkalis that produce further damage.[1,5]

Initial symptoms of chemical injuries are variable and can range from no early symptoms to severe bronchoconstriction, with evidence of decreased compliance, obstructive atelectasis, ventilation-perfusion mismatching, and increased shunt.[1,3] Later, mucosal airway edema impairs normal mucociliary function.

In severe injuries, noncardiogenic pulmonary edema may result. Within 3 to 4 days following the serious injury, the mucosa may slough, producing infection and obstruction in the distal airways. This produces a cascade of decreasing lung compliance, increased work of breathing, increases in airway resistance, hypoxemia, and increases in the pulmonary shunt days after the initial inhalation injury.[1-3]

■ Diagnosis

The diagnosis of smoke inhalation often requires a high index of suspicion, as the initial patient presentation may be extremely variable. Injury to the lungs most commonly occurs in closed-space accidents, such as house fires and explosions.[4] Close attention to the neurologic examination is important, since mental status changes may be early indicators of hypoxemia or carbon monoxide poisoning, both requiring emergency therapy. Early neurologic findings, such as lethargy, confusion, and obtundation, should be considered a result of carbon monoxide or cyanide toxicity and treated prior to confirmatory tests. Of note is the fact that cyanosis frequently is not present in early carbon monoxide poisoning.

Symptoms such as hoarseness, wheezing, or carbonaceous sputum production occur in less than 50 per cent of smoke inhalation victims.[4] Although the incidence of pulmonary complications in burn patients usually correlates with the severity of the burn, a significant percentage of burn patients may present with respiratory injury and no evidence of oropharyngeal or facial burns. The pulmonary examination may be helpful if abnormal, but, again, a normal examination does not exclude this diagnosis. Close attention to changes in the pulmonary examination over time is indicated, because both thermal and chemical injuries may demonstrate a progressive worsening of symptoms.

Essential laboratory evaluation consists of an arterial blood gas determination with carbon monoxide and oxygen saturation and a chest roentgenogram. Except for elevated carbon monoxide levels (to be discussed), these tests are neither specific nor sensitive indicators of pulmonary injury. Newer modalities, such as fiberoptic bronchoscopy, [133]xenon lung scanning, and pulmonary function tests, can be helpful in diagnosing the patient with suspected inhalation injury.[2,3,5]

Fiberoptic bronchoscopy is especially useful because it can be done in the emergency room or at the patient's bedside.[2] Endoscopic criteria for the diagnosis of inhalational injury include laryngeal or tracheal-bronchial inflammation, airway edema, necrosis of ulceration of the trachea, and the presence of soot in or charring of the airway. In addition, directed suctioning may be performed through the bronchoscope. The efficacy of bronchial lavage is unknown. Initial evaluation of the upper airway, either by bronchoscopy or direct laryngoscopy, will demonstrate the extent of injury but does not have prognostic value. Pulmonary function tests and [133]xenon scans may add to a more accurate determination of the extent of the lung damage and can be followed over time.[1-3,6]

If any doubt remains regarding the severity of inhalation injury, even in the asymptomatic patient, the patient should be admitted for continued observation.

■ Management

The mainstay of treatment in inhalation injuries is adequate ventilation and oxygenation, maintenance of a patent airway, and adequate oxygen delivery to the tissues. Since burn patients often have other injuries, individualization of therapy and an organized approach to the emergency treatment of such patients are of critical importance.

Early complications of smoke inhalation include airway obstruction and carbon monoxide poisoning. Patients with impending upper airway obstruction often present with hoarseness, difficulty in speaking, and stridor. If edema is present upon evaluation of the upper airway via bronchoscopy or direct laryngoscopy, the airway should be secured by either an endotracheal tube or a tracheostomy.[1,2,7] Direct endotracheal intubation via bronchoscopic guidance may prove helpful with difficult intubations. With severe upper airway obstruction, physicians skilled at emergency tracheostomy/cricothyroidotomy should be consulted immediately. Tracheostomy through an area of burn tissue is relatively contraindicated due to the high infection risk.[1] Other criteria for intubation are smoke inhalation associated with coma and respiratory depression, posterior pharyngeal edema, and circumferential neck burns.

Smoke inhalation also may trigger bronchospasm and produce lower airway obstruction. Therapy in this instance again includes close attention to the airway, in addition to humidified air and bronchodilators. Sloughing of the airway mucosa may occur in severe injury and produce obstruction and infection in the distal airways.[1-3,8] In this setting, lung compliance is reduced and the work of breathing markedly increased. It is important to remember that bronchospasm occasionally may be caused by the aspiration of a foreign body present in the smoke. Noncardiogenic pulmonary edema also may be seen in a minority of cases and can be exacerbated by the large volume requirements found in patients with surface burns.[1]

Carbon monoxide poisoning is the most frequent immediate cause of death from fire. Carbon monoxide is an odorless, colorless, nonirritating gas that is produced by the incomplete combustion of carbonaceous material. The burning of wood and furniture in closed spaces frequently produces toxic concentrations of carbon monoxide. Carbon monoxide has an affinity for hemoglobin 210 times that of oxygen. Thus, small amounts have profound effects on the oxygen hemoglobin saturation curve to the left. This results in a diminished ability to unload oxygen to the tissues.[1-3]

The overall net effect of carbon monoxide poisoning is severe tissue hypoxia. Carbon monoxide levels should be obtained on all patients suspected of smoke inhalation. The signs and symptoms of carbon monoxide poisoning are related to the carboxyhemoglobin concentration. Levels below 20 to 40 per cent frequently cause headache, nausea, and dizziness. Levels greater than 40 per cent frequently produce irreversible neurologic damage and death.[1-3]

Tachypnea is often not present in carbon monoxide poisoning. This is because the carotid body sees a normal partial pressure of oxygen.[1] Carbon monoxide does not affect the partial pressure of oxygen in arterial blood but rather binds tightly to hemoglobin. This reduces oxygen-carrying capacity.

In the severely intoxicated patients, minute ventilation will increase only when lactic acidosis secondary to tissue hypoxia occurs.[1]

All patients with altered mental status and a history of smoke inhalation should be suspected of carbon monoxide poisoning.[1] Successful management of carbon monoxide poisoning requires early diagnosis based upon a high level of suspicion and appropriate laboratory tests. Therapy is 100 per cent oxygen, which will reduce the half-life of carbon monoxide in the body from 250 minutes to 50 minutes. Endotracheal intubation will insure 100 per cent oxygen delivery. Hyperbaric oxygen, when readily available, will reduce elimination time further and may help provide more dissolved oxygen to the tissues. At 3 atmospheres, the half-life may be reduced to 25 minutes.

Recent data suggest that neither steroids nor prophylactic antibiotics are indicated in the treatment of inhalational injuries.[9] In patients who develop subsequent pneumonia, antibiotics should be directed at the typical nosocomial flora in the hospital until positive identification can be made. Strict attention to pulmonary toilet and adequate suctioning are the mainstays of therapy. Follow-up on survivors of the smoke inhalation syndrome reveals variable airway obstruc-tion that usually resolves. Persistence of an obstructive impairment may be secondary to the development of large airway stenosis, bronchiectasis, or bronchiolitis obliterans.

REFERENCES:

1. Cahalane M, Demling RH. Early respiratory abnormalities from smoke inhalation. JAMA 1984; 251:771–773.
2. Herndon DN, Thompson PB, Traber DL. Pulmonary injury in burned patients. Crit Care Clin 1985; 1:79–96.
3. Robinson L, Miller RH. Smoke inhalation injuries. Am J Otolaryngol 1986; 7:375–380.
4. Papadakos PJ, Iberti TJ. Smoke inhalation injuries. Emerg Decisions 1988; 4:30–34.
5. Moylan JA Jr, Wilmore DW, Mouton DE, et al. Early diagnosis of inhalation injury using ^{133}xenon lung scan. Ann Surg 1972; 176:477–484.
6. Robinson L, Miller RH. Smoke inhalation injuries. Am J Otolaryngol 1986; 7:375–380.
7. Robinson NB, Hudson LD, Robertson HT, Thorning DR, Carrico CJ, Heimbach DM. Ventilation and perfusion alterations after smoke inhalation injury. Surgery 1981; 90:352–363.
8. Venus B, Matsuda T, Copiozo JB, Mathru M. Prophylactic intubation and continuous positive airway pressure in the management of inhalation injury in burn victims. Crit Care Med 1981; 9:519–523.
9. Burns TR, Greenberg SD, Cartwright J, Jachimczyk JA. Smoke inhalation: an ultrastructural study of reaction to injury in the human alveolar wall. Environ Res 1986; 41:447–457.

Snakebite

Clifford C. Snyder

▪ Background

Among difficult medical management problems, the treatment for the bite of a snake appears to be one of universal perplexity. Very few physicians encounter even one snake-bitten patient in a lifetime of practice, and those who unexpectedly do are usually unfamiliar with bites of snakes. In reality, even the experts differ regarding the correct mode of snake bite therapy, and therefore the inexperienced therapist may be led to confusion and dread complications. The rate of mortality is not disastrously high, but the morbidity is frequently prolonged, with severe physical disability. The therapeutic rationale of envenomation will never be determined by treating an occasional victim, because there are deceptive gradients of response. Unlike patients with acute appendicitis or renal stone colic, snake bite patients do *not* all react in the same manner. There are more reports and books concerning serpentine envenomation than most physicians have the time to peruse; many of these offer personal opinions in good faith that actually are of little value and sometimes include harmful advice.

The amounts of snake venom per bite are exceedingly divergent. There are reports that snakes may govern the amount of venom they inject into their prey—that is, either an infinitesimal quantity or a deadly dose, decided by the serpent's physical and emotional circumstance.[1] The fangs of a venomous snake may penetrate the victim's skin without depositing detectable venom or leaving clinical findings of envenomation.[2] Such a patient could be treated in any manner and pronounced "cured," which would mislead not only the therapist but also the readers of the report into future erroneous prognoses.

Other variables that must be considered are the potency of the snake venoms of different species, the anatomic site of the bite, the depth of the venom deposit, the victim's blood volume, and the victim's sensitivity to the venom. Venom potency depends upon its pharmacologic complexity and its influence upon the tissue being attacked. The meerkat, mongoose, and hedgehog are typical examples of tissue resistance to venoms, whereas the human being and the rabbit display poor tolerance to snake venoms. The envenomation of a thigh muscle is more detrimental than antigen-injected scalp, because the moving leg muscles disperse the poison into muscle mass, vessels, and nerves and create difficulty in retrieving the poison spread. In contrast, the scalp is thin and the musculature is adherent to the skull, thus prohibiting deep penetration or spread yet easy retrieval of the antigen. Therefore, the site of the bite is an important variable. The limited blood volume of children is responsible for venom hemoconcentration and severe envenomation, necessitating more antivenin therapy than in an adult, whose large blood volume acts as a diluent to the venom. Because venom is an allergen and about one-third of the world population is allergy-prone, physicians must be alert to this possible sensitivity.[3]

■ CARDINAL FINDINGS

The cardinal findings of serpentine envenomation are (1) fang puncture wound(s), (2) pain, and (3) swelling.

Fang Puncture Wounds. Physicians must search carefully for fang punctures. When the patient has been struck on the fingers or toes, there may be one puncture on one digit, two punctures on one digit, or punctures on each of two digits. There may be one, two, or more fang inflictions, and even six punctures have been detected. Numerous punctures are from more than one bite, or from snakes that have multiple fangs.[4]

Pain. The victim's first reaction to the bite is fright, which is immediately followed by excruciating pain. I can verify this subjective symptom from personal experience. The pain may be eased by direct digital pressure at the bite site, and also by the application of an ice pack. But these therapies are only temporary. Many times the initial pain is accompanied by nausea, weakness, sweating, and vomiting.[5]

Swelling. Within minutes of the bite, the venom initiates a histamine-like phenomenon locally, accompanied by extravasation of blood and resulting edema and hematoma. The swelling progresses both proximally and distally and becomes brawny and pitting. The increase or the abatement of the edema may act as a gauge of the victim's progress.

■ ANCILLARY FINDINGS

Accompanying the fang penetration are a local capillary congestion (erythema) and blood vessel fragility with extravasation (ecchymosis) caused by the venom vasculotoxicity. Petechiae are concurrent with the erythrocytic diapedesis. The appearance of serum or hemorrhagic transudate (bullae) into the integument denotes the severity of the envenomation. Nausea and emesis are common vagal annoyances. Hyperesthesia in the bite area is experienced immediately, which subsides and yields to numbness and later paresthesias. These paresthesias simulate formications, prickings, tinglings, and the like, epidermally and subdermally. They may continue long after the emergency has ended and terminate as causalgia, a lasting sequela. Muscle-dermal twitchings, called fasciculations, are fine spontaneous spasmodic contractions of integumentary muscle fibers innervated by motor nerve filaments; these are prominently observed periorally. Progressive pitting edema ensues which is due to lymphatic and vascular compression, resulting in cyanosis, necrosis, and tissue slough. Rapid feeble pulse, dyspnea, vertigo, dimmed vision, pinpoint pupils, and malaise are prodromes to shock, coma, and possibly death.

■ Management

The management of one who has been bitten by a snake must be considered a formidable emergency until it is known that the offender was nonpoisonous or that the person did not receive a significant amount of venom. The first step in treatment is to identify the snake and, if possible, ascertain whether it was poisonous. The second step is to assess the severity and progress of the envenomation. The third step is to establish the patient's sensitivity to horse serum. And the fourth step is to treat the envenomation aggressively, once it is graded, to save limb and life, with the assistance of colleagues experienced with this type of emergency.

Factors that influence snake bite therapy include:

1. Age and size of victim. Children are affected more seriously.
2. Species and size of snake. Species, not size, is important.
3. Time elapsed after the snake bite. The earlier treated, the better.
4. Location, depth, and number of bites. Superficial versus subfascial.
5. Amount of venom injected. Numerous pharmacologic effects.
6. Sensitivity of victim to venom. Allergy is common and is serious.
7. Efficacy of first-aid treatment. Correct history is essential.

Because of the numerous variables involved with envenomation, snake bites need classifying so the practitioner may plan a course of therapy. An easily understood and applicable method of classification for pit viper bites is:

1. *No envenomation.* Although fang puncture(s) is present, the patient is free of pain and there is the bare minimum of swelling. The only treatment is to cleanse the wound.

2. *Mild envenomation.* Fang puncture(s) or fang scratches are visible, the patient is apprehensive, minimal local swelling is evident, there is some complaint of pain, and

the laboratory findings are irrelevant. Observe this patient.

3. *Moderate envenomation.* Puncture wounds are conspicuous, with oozing of blood, local cyanosis, ecchymosis, progressive regional edema, and moderate pain. The patient is excited and nauseated and may experience transient syncope. The laboratory findings include a decrease in red blood cells, hematocrit, platelets, and fibrinogen level, and a prolonged bleeding time. Hospitalize this patient and monitor hourly. Use one vial of polyvalent crotalid antivenin (Wyeth) intravenously, and excise the puncture wounds under local anesthesia. Repeat the blood studies and, if there is no increase in the findings, stabilize the bite site, elevate the area, and keep it cool to inhibit pain and decrease local metabolic processes.

4. *Severe envenomation.* Fang penetration is associated with immediate excruciating pain locally and regionally, and rapid progression of edema both distally and proximally to the infliction. There is usually subcutaneous emphysema with crepitation. Cyanosis is prevalent and is host to petechiae, bullae, and ichor. Neurologic sequelae include nausea, vomiting diaphoresis, weakness, dyspnea, hemoptysis, hypotension, and vertigo. The signs and symptoms may increase and include eyelid ptosis, interval hemorrhaging, hematuria, and coma. The laboratory findings are correlative. All patients with severe envenomations are hospitalized, monitored continuously, and treated aggressively. The patient's family must be advised promptly about changing conditions, and discussion with medical colleagues about alarming alterations is necessary.

The classification for elapid envenomation is comparable to that of the pit viper (Crotalid). The coral snakes and the cobras are responsible for most of the elapid bites in the United States.

1. *No envenomation.* Because the fangs of the coral snake are small, these may leave minute puncture wounds that are difficult to locate. Scratches are common. A history of being bitten may be the only positive indication of the incident.

2. *Mild envenomation.* Fang punctures are definite, with edema, streaky cyanosis, bullae, petechiae, moderate pain, miosis, eyelid ptosis, and muscle weakness. Hospitalization is necessary because many of the signs and symptoms are delayed. The bite site

should be excised as soon as possible, and, in the case of coral snake bite, North American coral snake antivenin (Wyeth) instituted intravenously.

3. *Moderate-severe envenomation.* The findings are as observed in the previous two classifications, plus neurologic symptoms such as severe muscle paralysis, dyspnea, aphasia, dysphagia, and coma. Immediate airway clearance is mandatory and oxygen therapy necessary. The bite site is excised while antivenin is administered. Because the patient is paralyzed and unable to breathe or move, conversation may be carried on with eyelid signals of "yes" and "no."

■ PROPHYLACTIC THERAPY

- Avoid hiking and camping in known snake-infested areas.
- Do not explore concealed caves, dens, lairs, and rock crevices.
- Be on the alert for snakes sunning on warm days.
- Watch where you sit, stretch, and step in unknown terrain.
- When mountain climbing, avoid reaching over hidden ledges.
- Wear protective gear such as trousers, slacks, and long-sleeved shirts.
- Hike with a friend; it may be life-saving.
- Keep your horse or vehicle near.
- Do not molest a snake; they have more fangs than you do.
- Zoos are better qualified to keep snakes as pets.
- Carry a snakebite kit and read the instructions at the time of purchase instead of at the time of the accident.

■ EMERGENCY FIELD THERAPY

There are no absolute rules, only practical ones.

- Avoid exciting or exerting the victim, which will increase circulation and spread venom.
- Kill the offender and keep for identification.
- Apply a flat tourniquet (belt, neckerchief) between bite site and heart, and only loosen it if swelling increases.
- Cleanse and incise fang puncture(s) lin-

early through skin only. No cruciate incisions.
- Digitally express or suction venom through linear incisions.
- Rest bitten leg or arm horizontally with level of the heart.
- Administer antivenin intravenously if the patient is not allergic.
- Arrange transport of patient to medical facility.

■ EMERGENCY DEPARTMENT THERAPY

- Identify the injury as envenomous (fang marks, swelling, pain).
- Obtain patient history, including allergies and concomitant diseases.
- Administer antivenin intravenously. If the patient is allergic to antivenin, titrate with 100 ml of normal saline plus 100 mg of hydrocortisone sodium succinate (Solu-Cortef).
- Elliptically excise fang punctures.
- Administer medications as needed (antibiotics, analgesics, tetanus toxoid).
- Hospitalize patient for observation and laboratory analysis (CBC, fibrinogen, platelet count, hematocrit, prothrombin time).

■ Issues and Risks

■ THE ENVENOMERS

Poisonous snakes of North America stem from the family of Crotalidae (pit vipers) and the family of Elapidae (coral snakes and cobras). The pit vipers are so named because of the sensory pit organ located between the eye and nostril. The poisonous coral snake may be identified by its black head ("black head means dead"), and body bands of red, yellow and black ("red bands on yellow can kill a fellow").[6]

■ THE VENOM

Poisonous snake venoms comprise some of the world's most powerful enzymes, proteins, and polypeptides, The enzyme L-arginine esterase releases bradykinin, which probably causes the pain, hypotension, nausea, vomiting, and sweating in snake-bitten victims. The protease, phospholipase A, destroys red blood cell membranes, and hyaluronidase breaks down connective tissue. Amino acid esterase exhibits a bipartite function: it prevents clotting by partially splitting fibrinogen to fibrin, or if present in sufficient quantity it may persuade clotting, producing the classic syndrome of disseminated intravascular coagulation. This dual mechanism is puzzling to the inexperienced physician and may lead to improper therapy.

■ THE TOURNIQUET

This device was designed to compress blood vessels and stop bleeding, but it is not to be used in this manner in snake bite therapy. It is used to occlude superficial venous and lymphatic flow *only* and not impede the deep venous or arterial circulation. Complications ensue when the band is applied too tightly and too long. The tourniquet should be flat, to inhibit cutting into the soft tissues. A snugly applied tourniquet, compared with a wrist watch band, will permit a finger beneath it as a test and will function properly.

■ ICE PACKS

Cooling the bite area decreases the metabolic reaction and relieves the pain. Ice packs should be used only over the bite site, with a small towel in place between the ice and the skin of the host tissue. The bite area should never be placed in ice water in a pail or bucket for continuous soaking. A snake bite is serious; when superimposed with frostbite, it is disastrous.[7]

■ CORTICOSTEROIDS

This controversial medical therapy is used to dissociate the antigen-antibody reaction, and it is beneficial when administered in combination with antivenin to reduce reactions in allergic patients. It is also used in serum sickness complications.

■ FASCIOTOMY

Fasciotomy is a heatedly debated subject.[8] It is proposed as a diagnostic as well as a therapeutic procedure.[9] Proponents of fasciotomy use it to differentiate between a subfascial snake envenomation and a subdermal deposit of venom, and it is the basis of their therapeutic approach. The opponents of fasciotomy condemn the severity of the surgical procedure in comparison with antivenin therapy.[10]

■ ANTIVENIN THERAPY

Antivenin is a horse serum product that is capable of generating severe idiosyncrasies. Although antivenin administration is unequivocally a necessity in the treatment of snake bite, it must not be given injudiciously for every envenomation problem. It is best given early, because tissue destruction is rapid and antivenin does not correct the loss of vital structures.[11] Antivenin should never be administered by inexperienced lay personnel. It is to be given intravenously or intra-arterially by a physician, nurse, dentist, veterinarian, or physician's assistant.

■ EXCISION OF FANG PUNCTURE WOUNDS

Excision of the envenomated area by a knowledgeable family physician or surgical specialist is the course of choice. Excision of the fang punctures and surrounding tissue is accomplished immediately postbite under local anesthesia. The line of excision is 1 to 2 cm equidistant from the puncture wounds. Digital bites do not necessitate wide excisions, as the venom is deposited superficially. The tourniquet placed proximal to the bitten area prevents hemorrhaging. Because the direction of the fang tips is difficult to verify, inclusive excision will remove most of the venom and devitalized tissue. This technique is particularly helpful in elapid (neurotoxic) envenomations, but must be achieved early postbite. The resultant wound is treated as are comparable surgical wounds. Because the excision is elliptic, the skin margins later approximate easily. If tension is found in closing the wound, a split thickness skin graft for coverage is remarkably aesthetic. If the snake-bitten area is neglected, the result is necrosis, slough, infection, and loss of vital tissues.

It is interesting that through the years the commonest therapy for snake bite has been to use cross-hatch (cruciate) incisions and suction, and such an approach is accepted as a proven technique by both the medical profession and lay technicians. This method of retrieving the injected venom harms the victim, who must tolerate the results of "scar face," hypertrophic cicatrices, keloids, and traumatic neuromas. There is very little retrieval of incarcerated venom by this method, and infection is common due to the poor blood supply to the skin tips of the cross-hatches. A crust or eschar forms over the wound, producing an anaerobic environment that is at risk for clostridial invasion.

REFERENCES

1. Allon N, Kochva E. The quantities of venom injected into prey of different size by Vipera palaestinae in a single bite. J Exp Zool 1974; 188(1):71–75.
2. Van Mierop LH. Poisonous snakebite: a review: 1. Snakes and their venom. 2. Symptomatology and treatment. J Fla Med Assoc 1976; 63(3):191–210.
3. Snyder CC, Mayer TA. Animal, snake, and insect bites. In Mayer TA (ed). Emergency Management of Trauma. Philadelphia: WB Saunders, 1985:466–483.
4. Snyder CC, Hunter GR, Browne EZ. Malevolent inflictions: bites and stings. In Shires GT (ed). Care of the Trauma Patient. New York: McGraw-Hill, 1979:176–206.
5. Snyder CC, Knowles RP. Snake bites: guidelines for practical management. Postgrad Med 1988; 83(6):52–75.
6. Ditmars RL. The Reptiles of North America. New York: Doubleday, 1951:306–314.
7. Frey C, Minton SA, Snyder CC, et al. National Research Council, Committee on Emergency Medical Service. Meeting of National Academy of Science. Bethesda, MD, 1977.
8. Glass TG Jr. More on snakebite. Texas Med 1982; 78:13–18.
9. Lockhart WE. Treatment of snakebite. JAMA 1965; 193:36–38.
10. Garfin SR, Castilonia RR, Mubarak SJ, et al. An evaluation of the role of surgical decompression in the treatment of the rattlesnake bites. In Russell FE (ed). Snake Venom Poisoning. Philadelphia: JB Lippincott, 1980:319.
11. Tu AT. Local tissue damaging (hemorrhage and myonecrosis) toxins from rattlesnake and pit viper venoms. J Toxicol 1983; 2:205–207.

Thyroid disease in the elderly patient

Frank M. Price ■ *James V. Felicetta*

■ Primary Hypothyroidism

Hypothyroidism, as diagnosed by low T4 and elevated TSH levels, occurs in from 1 to 5 per cent of elderly people.[1–5] Based on pathologic examinations and population surveys for antithyroidal antibodies, Hashimoto's autoimmune thyroiditis is recognized as the most common cause of hypothyroidism in older patients. However, many cases are also seen in patients with a remote history of radioactive iodine therapy or thyroid surgery.[6] Several researchers have recommended routine screening for hypothyroidism in geriatric populations, such as those admitted to hospital inpatient units or geriatric evaluation units.[3,4]

Even if routine screening is not done, a number of findings on history and physical examination may suggest a possible diagnosis of hypothyroidism. The patient may mention cold intolerance, fatigue, or weight gain during a routine office visit. More advanced disease will cause dry skin, hoarse voice, memory loss, or depression. On physical examination, the thyroid gland is rarely palpable. Skin may be doughy. The tongue may be thick and the hair, coarse. The heart size may be increased, and heart tones are muffled. Bowel sounds may be decreased, and fecal impaction may be noted on rectal examination. Ankle or sacral edema is mild to moderate. Deep tendon reflexes are normal initially, but the relaxation phase is prolonged. The chest radiograph may show cardiomegaly. Laboratory tests often show anemia, hyponatremia, hypercholesterolemia, and hypertriglyceridemia.[6]

There is much debate over whether clinically euthyroid patients with a normal T4 level but a mildly elevated thyroid-stimulating hormone (TSH) level should be treated. Some investigators have used the term *subclinical hypothyroidism* for this set of laboratory findings. It is clear that patients with elevated TSH levels are at increased risk of developing clinical hypothyroidism in the future, and treatment at the subclinical stage will obviate some of the extremely close follow-up needed for untreated patients. On the other hand, it is not clear whether the as-yet-undetermined metabolic abnormalities associated with an elevated TSH level are truly detrimental. Some clinicians, therefore, prefer to check serum T4 and TSH levels as often as every 3 to 6 months, and to treat with replacement therapy only when the T4 level falls to subnormal levels. We prefer a more proactive approach to prevent any complications that might develop. We therefore recommend administering low doses of thyroid hormone as soon as an elevated TSH level is demonstrated. We start with a daily dose of 0.05 mg of levothyroxine and increase by 0.025 mg every 2 months until both TSH and T4 levels are within normal limits. It is important to note that it may take the pituitary up to 2 months to adapt to a higher ambient thyroid hormone level by reducing TSH secretion.

For those patients with clinical hypothyroidism, as documented by low serum T4 and elevated TSH levels, the usual maintenance replacement dose of levothyroxine (T4) will be between 0.1 and 0.2 mg per day. Most elderly patients require a dose closer to 0.1 mg. Any elderly patient who is not rendered clinically and chemically euthyroid on 0.2 mg per day should be re-evaluated in terms of the diagnosis and compliance. Increasing the daily dose beyond this level probably will not improve the thyroid status but may well lead to headaches, palpitations, nervousness, confusion, disorientation, and angina pectoris, as well as significant worsening of other coexisting problems. Likewise, the relatively common practice of prescribing dried (desiccated) bovine thyroid extract, which contains unpredictable amounts of both T4 and T3, should be avoided. Only synthetic preparations of pure hormone should be used.

In the elderly patient without a history or physical findings suggestive of coronary artery disease, replacement therapy should begin with a daily dose of 0.05 mg of levothyroxine. The dose can be increased by 0.025 mg every 2 weeks, up to a daily dose of 0.1 mg. Maintain the patient at this dose for 6 weeks, then recheck levels of T4 and TSH. If the patient is euthyroid both chemically and clinically at this point, continue with a daily dose of 0.1 mg. If thyroid function tests still indicate hypothyroidism, increase the daily dose by 0.025 mg and recheck levels in another 8 weeks, making the appropriate adjustments at that time based on the laboratory values. If the patient is chemically hyperthyroid, reduce the daily dose by 0.025 mg and carefully review the medication history.

When patients are treated with the usual replacement doses of T4, the euthyroid state is achieved in 4 to 8 weeks. Symptomatic improvement occurs in as little as 7 days. In the elderly patient who is using reduced doses of thyroid hormone initially, the time to noticeable improvement may be longer. The trade-off for this slower recovery is a decreased risk of causing dangerous manifestations of coronary artery disease. If the T4 level is in the low normal range and the patient still complains of hypothyroid symptoms, it may be reasonable to increase the daily dose by 0.025 mg. If the high normal range of T4 concentration is achieved and the elderly patient still feels hypothyroid, a re-evaluation of the patient's symptoms may be in order. It is also worthwhile rechecking the TSH level. Whereas a normal T4 level confirms only recent compliance, a normal TSH level indicates daily compliance for several weeks. With the "supersensitive" TSH assay, a level below 0.5 μU/ml may indicate excessive levothyroxine replacement.

Replacement with triiodothyronine (T3), instead of thyroxine (T4), has been discussed for as long as the preparation has been available. A dose of 25 μg of T3 is equivalent to 100 μg of T4. In addition, when given orally, T3 works more rapidly to reverse clinical manifestations of hypothyroidism, presumably because of a lesser degree of protein binding. However, for the noncomatose patient, there is no need to replace with T3. Replacement with T4 will provide adequate levels of T3 in the serum, through the peripheral (extrathyroidal) conversion of T4 to T3. Because of its short serum half-life, T3 must be given two or three times a day. Also, if replaced solely with T3, the serum T3 level will fluctuate widely, whereas on T4 the T3 level will gradually reach a plateau and remain there. This stability makes it easier to follow thyroid hormone levels serially.

■ Hypothyroidism with Coronary Artery Disease

It is well-known that hypothyroidism is associated with hypercholesterolemia and hypertriglyceridemia.[6] Clinically, a wide range of manifestations of coronary artery disease is seen in patients with hypothyroidism.[7,8] In a large series reported by the Mayo Clinic, less than 7 per cent of hypothyroid patients reported angina pectoris prior to replacement therapy.[9] Likewise, myocardial infarction in this setting is rare,[7] but when it does occur, it is often complicated by congestive heart failure and lethal arrhythmias. In all probability, the dearth of clinical manifestations of coronary artery disease results from the markedly decreased basal metabolic demands and inactive lifestyle of most patients with hypothyroidism.

Coronary disease manifestations are infrequent during thyroid replacement therapy, but they can be disastrous. One can see angina pectoris, myocardial infarction, and congestive heart failure. In the large Mayo Clinic series, 35 of 1503 hypothyroid patients developed angina pectoris for the first time during replacement therapy.[9] There was a previous history of angina pectoris in another 55 patients. The frequency and severity of angina improved during therapy in 21 patients, remained unchanged in 25, and worsened significantly in 9 patients. Six in the latter group suffered myocardial infarctions during replacement therapy. Because of increased release, decreased catabolism, and decreased renal excretion, creatine phosphokinase (CPK) and lactate dehydrogenase (LDH) levels can be elevated in uncomplicated hypothyroidism. The pattern of LDH isoenzyme elevations seen in hypothyroidism may be identical to that associated with myocardial infarction.[10] The most reliable guidelines in diagnosing acute myocardial infarction in the hypothyroid patient are the characteristic pattern of rise and fall of the various enzymes, and an increase in the MB fraction of CPK. This isoenzyme is not routinely elevated in uncomplicated hypothyroidism.

Before beginning replacement therapy, it is important to determine whether the patient has significant coronary artery disease. This knowledge may prompt closer follow-up of these high-risk patients. Hypothyroidism alone can cause various forms of atrioventricular block, extrasystoles, and T wave abnormalities. During exercise treadmill testing, there is a significant incidence of S-T segment and T wave abnormalities in hypothyroid patients without coronary artery disease. Large studies of the value of radionuclide testing have not yet been performed in hypothyroid patients. In patients who are otherwise healthy and experiencing angina, cardiac catheterization remains the gold standard in determining the extent of coronary artery disease.

In patients with chest pain who undergo cardiac catheterization and have little or no coronary artery disease, it is safe to begin a usual course of thyroid hormone replacement therapy. In fact, chest pain, dyspnea on exertion, dizziness, and syncope actually may resolve with administration of thyroid hormone. In this small group of hypothyroid patients, these "coronary" symptoms may be due to pericardial fluid, interstitial lung edema, or impaired myocardial pump function secondary to the hypothyroidism. It has been shown that hypothyroidism causes reversible echocardiographic abnormalities consistent with a cardiomyopathy similar to that seen in idiopathic hypertrophic subaortic stenosis (IHSS).[11]

In hypothyroid patients with coronary artery disease who cannot undergo coronary artery bypass graft (CABG) surgery, one should begin replacement therapy with an extremely low dose of levothyroxine, in the range of 0.0125 to 0.025 mg per day, and very gradually increase the daily dose by 0.025 every 2 to 3 weeks.

Should angina occur or worsen as the dose is increased, the dose should be decreased to the previous level for 2 to 3 weeks and then increased by a smaller amount every month. Bearing in mind the potential side effects of beta-blockers in hypothyroid patients (symptomatic bradycardia and atrioventricular block), one of these agents or a calcium channel blocker should be administered. The ultimate goal is the standard replacement dose of 0.1 to 0.15 mg per day. However, due to worsening angina, some patients with significant coronary artery disease are intolerant of these doses. In these patients it may be necessary to maintain replacement doses at an inadequate level and trade a small degree of hypothyroidism for a lifestyle less encumbered by chest pain.

Myxedema Coma

In the most severe form of hypothyroidism, myxedema coma, multiple metabolic changes make the treatment of hypothyroidism more challenging and dangerous. This entity will continue to increase in incidence primarily because of the introduction of radioiodine therapy for hyperthyroidism, with the subsequent predisposition to hypothyroidism.[12] The diagnosis is typically made in an elderly woman, usually in the seventh or eighth decade of life.[13] Physical examination reveals hypothermia, a low-pitched, hoarse voice, hearing loss, dry skin, large tongue, obesity, alopecia, eyelid edema, bradycardia, abdominal distention, urinary retention,[14] and fecal impaction. Most patients present during the winter months.[12,15] It is not uncommon for myxedema coma to develop after the patient has been admitted to the hospital. In this setting, there is usually a recent history of surgery or the administration of narcotics, anesthetics, or phenothiazines.[12]

Hypoventilation and CO_2 narcosis in myxedema coma are due primarily to a decrease in the hypoxic respiratory drive and less importantly, to a minor alteration in the normal response to hypercapnia.[13] Pleural effusions and ascites can further compromise respiratory function. The swollen tongue due to mucopolysaccharide infiltrates also can cause partial airway obstruction. Lastly, superimposed infection, especially in the pulmonary system, can cause further decreases in the arterial Po_2. Thyroid hormone therapy will improve the respiratory response to hypoxemia, but it will not affect mechanical ventilatory function. Treatment of hypoventilation consists of mechanical

ventilatory support when indicated, usually for the first 2 to 3 days of therapy. More severe cases may require up to 1 month of assisted ventilation. The frequent recurrence of ventilatory failure after extubation may be avoided mainly by continuing mechanical ventilatory support until the patient is fully conscious and breathing independently.[12]

Hyponatremia is caused primarily by impaired free water excretion, resulting from inadequate delivery of free water to the distal tubule.[13] Most myxedematous patients have decreased plasma volume and a decreased glomerular filtration rate. Therapy is directed toward reducing the excessive volume of total body water while maintaining a normal or slightly increased total body sodium content. Although free water restriction alone is adequate in milder cases, many patients with a serum sodium concentration of less than 120 mEq/L require more aggressive therapy. One method is to administer 50 to 100 ml of 3 per cent NaCl cautiously and follow that up with 40 mg of intravenous furosemide to promote a free water diuresis. In patients with a history or examination suggestive of congestive heart failure, monitoring with a CVP catheter or Swan-Ganz catheter may be necessary.

Hypothermia, sometimes to temperatures less than 80°F, is seen in 75 per cent of patients presenting in myxedema coma. Conversely, the diagnosis of myxedema also should be considered in an elderly patient who presents with an infection but no fever. Core body temperatures of less than 32.5° (90°F) is a predictor of a stormy hospital course and increased mortality. Concurrent hypoglycemia can worsen the hypothermic problem. Therapy consists of passive warming with blankets and administration of thyroid hormone. Active rewarming can cause vasodilation, which can lead to hypotension.

Abnormal gastrointestinal motility, including paralytic ileus, is another common problem in myxedema. Motility disorders result from a neuropathy and from a mucopolysaccharide infiltrate in the muscularis layer. Such a patient presents with a history of increased abdominal gas and constipation.[13] It is often difficult to rule out mechanical bowel obstruction. The distinction is crucial, for patients who undergo abdominal exploratory surgery while in myxedema coma do extremely poorly. Likewise, although the motility problems respond to thyroid hormone replacement, the hormone cannot be given orally because GI absorption is so poor.[12]

Myxedematous patients become hypotensive because of inadequate intravascular fluid volume.[10] This occurs despite an increased extracellular fluid volume. Basic therapy consists of dextrose in saline, along with hydrocortisone, 100 mg, every 8 hours. Constant surveillance is necessary to prevent overt congestive heart failure. For severe hypotension and shock, pressors may be required for the first few days of therapy. However, pressors often have little effect on blood pressure unless the patient is also given thyroid hormone replacement.

Cardiomegaly, caused primarily by accumulation of pericardial fluid rich in mucopolysaccharide, is extremely common in severe cases of myxedema.[10] The pericardial fluid accumulates over a long period of time; acute pericardial tamponade is rare.[16] In some cases, there is a mild degree of coexistent left ventricular dilation. Heart tones are muffled. Electrocardiographic changes include bradycardia, atrioventricular block, low voltage, prolonged Q-T intervals, and T wave abnormalities. Despite significantly decreased stroke volume and cardiac output, myxedematous patients rarely present in congestive heart failure. Heart failure is usually due to underlying coronary artery disease or hypertension, combined with iatrogenic saline administration. Therapy for all cardiovascular problems consists of prompt administration of thyroid hormone replacement and, when hypotension is severe, pressor agents such as dopamine.[17]

Because of the stuporous condition of most patients in myxedema coma and concurrent hyponatremia, which itself can cause confusion and cranial nerve dysfunction, seizures and aspiration are common. Occult aspiration pneumonias, without fever, cough, or sputum production, greatly increase short-term mortality, especially if not detected and treated promptly. Whereas the role of prophylactic antibiotics for the first 24 to 48 hours is unclear, measures to prevent aspiration are essential.[12]

Myxedematous patients with hypotension, hypothermia, hypoglycemia, hyponatremia, and hyperkalemia should be evaluated for coexisting adrenal insufficiency. A significant decrease in adrenal reserve is seen in 5 to 10 per cent of patients with hypothyroidism.[13] It is usually due to hypopi-tuitarism or to primary autoimmune adrenal failure coexisting with Hashimoto's autoimmune thyroiditis. Whereas baseline cortisol levels and the response to exogenous ACTH are normal, adrenal and pituitary reserves may be limited. In addition, although the pituitary-adrenal axis response time is slowed in myxedema, thyroid hormone replacement therapy causes a marked increase in cortisol metabolism. This can lead to an insufficient supply of corticosteroids. Before administering steroids, a 1-hour ACTH stimulation test is a good idea. The patient can be given 10 mg of dexamethasone empirically during the test, providing glucocorticoid and mineralocorticoid protection without affecting test results. The usual recommended dose of steroids is 100 mg of hydrocortisone intravenously every 6 to 8 hours for the first 10 days of therapy. This dose can be gradually tapered thereafter, based on the patient's blood pressure, level of consciousness, and general response to therapy.

Thyroid hormone replacement is the mainstay of treatment of myxedema coma.[17] An ongoing controversy is whether to give T4, T3, or both. Concerns center on achieving adequate replacement in a timely manner without inducing significant cardiovascular complications. Undoubtedly, T4 replacement provides a steady onset of action, gradual increase in levels, and fewer side effects. Parenteral preparations of T3 are difficult to obtain. Administration of replacement hormone via nasogastric tube is unlikely to succeed, owing to impaired gastrointestinal absorption; in the worst-case scenario, it can provide a route and substrate for aspiration.

When levothyroxine is given intravenously in a bolus of 500 μg, almost complete replacement of the extrathyroidal pool of T4 is achieved (the usual pool is 300 to 600 μg). T4 levels normalize within 24 hours. A daily maintenance dose of 50 to 100 μg will normalize TSH levels in about 2 to 4 weeks. Larger doses of T4 are unnecessary and potentially dangerous. Nonthyroidal illness inhibits peripheral conversion of T4 to T3, and T3 levels may remain depressed despite adequate T4 replacement. For this reason, some experts recommend giving small doses of T3 for the first few days. Likewise, in the severely hypothermic patient, T3 will cause a significant rise in core body temperature in 2 to 3 hours, whereas the effect of T4 on temperature may take as long as 12 to 14 hours. In the elderly patient who has a statistically increased likelihood of coronary artery disease, daily electrocardiograms and 24-hour monitoring for ischemic changes and arrhythmias are mandatory for the first few days of therapy.

The mortality rate of myxedema coma can be as high as 60 per cent.[15] Treatment is essential, but one must be cautious with replacement therapy so as not to cause T3-related side effects. A reasonable approach to thyroid hormone replacement therapy includes a loading bolus of T4 of 200 to 300 μg intravenously (4 μg/kg lean body weight), followed by 100 μg 24 hours later. Beginning on the third day of therapy, the daily dose should be 50 μg of T4. Some would advocate giving T3 in a dose of 25 μg intravenously every 12 hours, right from the beginning. If T3 is used, it can be continued until the patient is fully awake and capable of taking T4 orally.

■ Hyperthyroidism

Although hyperthyroidism is not as common as hypothyroidism, large surveys have detected it in 0.5 to 1 per cent of individuals over the age of 60 years.[1,2,4,18] Conversely, 15 to 20 per cent of cases of hyperthyroidism occur in patients over the age of 60 years. Graves' disease is not uncommon in elderly people, but, with increasing age, patients with toxic multinodular goiter and autonomously functioning thyroid nodules comprise a larger portion of the hyperthyroid population than do younger cohorts. Rather than the classic manifestations of thyrotoxicosis, presentation in elderly patients often consists of subtle weight loss, syncope, cardiac or gastrointestinal complaints, or psychiatric changes ranging from lassitude to violent psychosis.[19] The term *apathetic hyperthyroidism* has been used to describe the passive, flat affect of many elderly hyperthyroid patients, in sharp contrast to the presentation of younger hyperthyroid patients.[20] Because of the difficulty in diagnosing hyperthyroidism in elderly people solely on the basis of history and physical examination, many investigators recommend thyroid function tests for all elderly hospitalized patients.[18,21] In the outpatient setting, all patients with significant new complaints, es-

pecially of the cardiovascular, gastrointestinal, or central nervous systems, or chronic wasting of unknown etiology should be tested for hyperthyroidism. Although treatment goals and methods are generally similar, distinct differences in etiology, natural history, and prognosis favor an individualized approach to each hyperthyroid patient. Therapy for hyperthyroidism in elderly patients consists of thionamides, beta-blockers, radioactive iodine, or surgery, alone or in combination, to be described.

■ THIONAMIDES

The thionamides, propylthiouracil and methimazole, inhibit thyroid hormone production by blocking the oxidative iodination step and the coupling step in the intrathyroidal synthesis of thyroid hormone. In addition, propylthiouracil (PTU) blocks the peripheral conversion of T4 to T3, although methimazole (MMI) does not. T4 levels will usually normalize within 14 to 60 days of the start of therapy. PTU is typically started at a dose of 300 to 450 mg per day, in three divided doses. Once euthyroidism is achieved, the maintenance dose is 50 to 200 mg per day, given in one to three divided doses. MMI, with a slower onset of action and a longer half-life, is started at 30 mg per day until the patient is euthyroid, then decreased to 5 to 20 mg per day. It is given only once daily. If the dose of thionamide is cut too soon or by too large an increment, hyperthyroidism usually returns. Failure of therapy is usually due to noncompliance, except in the case of a large, toxic multinodular goiter in a patient who has received large doses of stable iodine recently. Concurrent treatment with T4 supplements, thought by some to protect against the development of hypothyroidism, is unwarranted.

As definitive therapy for hyperthyroidism, thionamides work best in mild cases of short duration. They are also excellent agents for attaining euthyroid status prior to radioactive iodine (RAI) treatment or surgery and may be continued after surgery to control thyrotoxicosis. However, it is important to withdraw PTU for at least 3 days prior to RAI uptakes, scans, or ablative therapy and not to restart it for 5 days after RAI has been given. Otherwise the PTU will interfere with the uptake of the radioactive iodine by the thyroid gland. Most patients who are going to relapse upon cessation of thionamide therapy do so within 6 months.[22] The small increases in T4 and T3 levels seen immediately after stopping thionamide therapy are usually transient and have no bearing on the likelihood of eventual relapse.

Adverse effects of the thionamides include hypersensitivity reactions, manifested by pruritus, rash, and fever. These often resolve despite continuation of the medication, but it is usually wise to switch to another thionamide. Arthralgias and serum sickness are rarely encountered. Granulocytopenia occurs in less than 1 per cent of patients, usually at 4 to 8 weeks of therapy. After the thionamide is stopped, the bone marrow usually recovers within 2 weeks. However, rare cases of fatal granulocytopenia have been described. Fatal hepatic necrosis also has been reported in several patients.

■ STABLE IODINE

Stable iodine usage in elderly patients should be limited to the rare case of true thyroid storm, in which it can be employed in conjunction with PTU and beta-blockers. In physiologic doses of less than 1.0 μg/day, stable iodine causes a dose-related increase in thyroid hormone synthesis. In high doses, a critical level of intrathyroidal iodine is achieved acutely, causing a dramatic drop in the rate of hormone synthesis. This is known as the Wolff-Chaikoff effect. Usually this effect is transient, because the thyroid will adapt to increased iodine levels by decreasing the rate of iodide transport into the thyroid, and the intrathyroidal iodide concentration will gradually fall. This adaptation is known as escape. Iodine in pharmacologic doses also causes an increase in colloid stores, with a marked drop in the rate of hormone release. Symptoms usually improve within 3 to 4 days, owing to a combination of both effects. The increase in colloid content results in increased firmness of the gland and decreased vascularity. Stable iodine is available in two commonly used forms: Lugol's solution, which contains 6 mg of iodide per drop, is given in doses of 3 drops thrice daily. Saturated solution of potassium iodide (SSKI), which contains 50 mg of iodide per drop, is given in doses of 1 drop thrice daily.

■ BETA-BLOCKERS

Although beta-blockers are known to inhibit the peripheral conversion of T4 to T3, much larger doses of these medications are required to actually block the conversion than are needed to ameliorate the symptoms of hyperthyroidism. Theoretically, an excess of thyroid hormone causes an increase in the number of beta-adrenergic receptors on the cell. Beta-blockers block the attachment of hormone to the receptors. The major use for propranolol and the other beta-blockers in the treatment of hyperthyroidism is to minimize symptoms while other more definitive therapy is being instituted.[23] Beta-blockers ameliorate the cardiovascular effects of hyperthyroidism, but they leave the patient hyperthyroid. The usual starting dose is 40 mg of propranolol orally every 6 hours. The goal is titration to a resting heart rate of 70 to 80 beats per minute.

■ RADIOACTIVE IODINE

Radioactive iodine is currently the therapy of choice for most elderly patients with hyperthyroidism. The goal of radioactive iodine (RAI) therapy is the production of sufficient radiation thyroiditis to reduce thyroid function to normal without causing hypothyroidism. The response to RAI is a two-stage phenomenon. Initially, in 3 to 7 days, there is an acute radiation response. Afterwards there is a chronic, gradual atrophy of the thyroid. The acute onset of hypothyroidism is clearly dose related. What remains unclear is whether the late onset of hypothyroidism is dose related.[24,25]

There are two schools of thought concerning treatment of hyperthyroidism with RAI. The first, rarely encountered in the United States, is to give a dose high enough to produce hypothyroidism in all patients and to treat everyone with T4 replacement.[26] To achieve this ablative effect, the usual total dose is in the range of 20 to 30 mCi. The other school of thought aims for cure without hypothyroidism. Here the dose is 3 to 10 mCi of ^{131}I, which provides about 50 to 80 μCi per gram of thyroid tissue. Estimates of early-onset hypothyroidism within the first year run to about 10 per cent with low-dose RAI, with late-onset hypothyroidism occurring at about 1 to 2 per cent per year.[27,28] If the low-dose regimen is used, one should check thyroid function tests every 2 to 3 months for the first year. If the patient is euthyroid at 1 year, as shown by T4 and TSH levels, there is a smaller chance of eventual hypothyroidism. However, if the TSH level is elevated, new hypothyroidism occurs in about 5 per cent.[29] It is important to note that early hypothyroidism, especially with low doses, is often transient, whereas hypothyroidism after 1 year is almost always permanent. If a patient is still hyperthyroid 6 months after RAI therapy, it is usually necessary to re-treat. Second doses in Graves' disease may have to be higher, because the remaining cells are partially radiation-resistant. Although chemical evidence of worsened thyrotoxicosis about 3 to 14 days after RAI ablation is common, patients rarely report clinical evidence of worsened hyperthyroidism. Likewise, radiation thyroiditis rarely causes symptoms.

RAI therapy causes subclinical hypoparathyroidism in 10 to 40 per cent of patients, but symptomatic disease is very rare. There is a slightly increased risk of lymphoma in patients with Graves' disease, but this risk is not altered by surgery or RAI treatment.[30] It is known that very low-dose RAI, below what is recommended, may indeed damage thyroid cells and lead to an increased risk of cancer. Recommendations for RAI therapy include a minimum dose of 200 rads to the thyroid, the usual dose being 400 to 500 rads. This dose is well above the cancer-inducing range, and no increased risk of malignancy is seen with this dose. Concern over possible teratogenic effects of RAI is not a consideration in elderly patients.

■ THYROIDECTOMY

Surgery for hyperthyroidism is largely a therapy of the past, especially in the elderly. However, if surgery is contemplated, the recommended procedure is usually a subtotal thyroidectomy, which involves the removal of all but the posterior capsule and small portions of the inferior poles of one or both lobes.[31] This procedure reduces the risk of damage to the recurrent laryngeal nerve, hypoparathyroidism, and permanent hypothyroidism. Propranolol, either alone or in combination with PTU, will prepare the patient for surgery adequately.[23] Long-term studies show that about 65 to 70 per cent of

patients remain euthyroid postoperatively. After 6 months, elevated TSH levels indicate inadequate thyroid reserve, with a high risk of hypothyroidism.[23] Here regular follow-up is mandatory. Late-onset hypothyroidism occurs in about 1 per cent per year. Persistent hyperthyroidism means removal of insufficient amounts of thyroid tissue.[23] Almost half of the cases of recurrent hyperthyroidism present at least 5 years after surgery; a significant percentage of cases presents more than 30 years later. [131]I is recommended for recurrent hyperthyroidism; hypothyroidism is often the end result.

Mortality from surgery is virtually nonexistent. Thyroid storm is rare. About 20 per cent of patients experience hypocalcemia owing to ischemia, trauma, or recovery of the system from hyperthyroid bone disease.[32] Permanent hypoparathyroidism occurs in less than 1 per cent of cases, but decreased parathyroid reserve is seen in up to 25 per cent of cases. Bilateral vocal cord paralysis is rare, but unilateral cord paralysis is seen in 1 in 200 patients.[33]

■ Graves' Disease

Graves' disease is the most common cause of hyperthyroidism in elderly people. It is caused by stimulation of the thyroid gland's TSH receptors by thyroid-stimulating immunoglobulins (TSI). Common systemic manifestations include tachycardia, tremor, nervousness, weight loss, and occasionally angina or high-output congestive heart failure. Diarrhea may be a prominent complaint. The thyroid is diffusely enlarged. Fine, smooth skin, tachycardia, cachexia, nervousness, cardiac gallop, pretibial edema, and tremor may be striking or absent. Hyperactive deep tendon reflexes and muscle weakness are common. Generally, elderly people with Graves' disease have very modest eye findings, often limited to a dry or itchy sensation. The serum T4 is almost uniformly elevated, and supersensitive TSH assays are below 0.5 μU/ml.

The elderly patient with Graves' disease responds best to ablative therapy with radioactive iodine. Thionamide therapy occasionally may produce long-term euthyroidism, but most patients will return to a hyperthyroid state within 6 months of cessation of therapy. Beta-blockers will ameliorate symptoms, especially in those patients suffering from angina or high-output heart failure. Surgery is virtually never recommended for this disease in elderly people.

■ Toxic Multinodular Goiter (TMNG)

This form of hyperthyroidism is much more common in elderly patients than in younger patients. This disparity in frequency is probably due to the slow rate of growth of hot nodules. When TSH secretion is suppressed, the normal thyroid will still display a low level of autonomous function distributed evenly throughout all of the follicles. In the TMNG, follicles with a high degree of autonomous function coexist with normal and cold follicles. Hot follicles can be distributed either in a random fashion throughout the gland or in discrete clusters. If the cluster is large enough, it will show up as hot on isotope scans.[34] Whenever the hormonal output of the hot follicles exceeds the requirements of the body, thyrotoxicosis results.

In euthyroid patients with MNG, one finds that T4 and T3 levels are normal, TSH is low, and the TSH response to thyroid-releasing hormone (TRH) administration is blunted. In the normal thyroid gland, an increase in the iodine load causes a small increase in the production of thyroid hormone. This inhibits secretion of TSH; the function of the thyroid follicle is reset at a lower level. In TMNG, however, in which TSH is already suppressed, a small increase in iodine load can lead to a significant increase in thyroid hormone production. The incidence of iodine-induced hyperthyroidism is unknown, but certainly exposure to excessive doses of iodine may accelerate the appearance of hyperthyroidism in patients with nodular goiter.

Clinically, TMNG is typically seen in an elderly woman who has had a goiter for years. Mild symptoms of hyperthyroidism are superimposed on those resulting from coexisting nonthyroidal disease. Typical findings include tachycardia, atrial fibrillation, weight loss, depression, anxiety, and insomnia. Angina pectoris or high-output congestive heart failure often may be the major presenting complaint. In many cases, these clues appear months to years before the onset of classic hyperthyroidism. It is important to rule out thyroid disease in any presentation of acute or chronic disease in an elderly patient with MNG. This is most easily done with assays of T4 and TSH levels. In those patients with normal thyroid hormone levels, a subnormal value for the recently introduced supersensitive TSH assay may be helpful. If all are normal, a normal TRH stimulation test rules out thyroid disease. A blunted TSH response curve is consistent with subclinical hyperthyroidism, but it also can result from nonthyroidal illness.

Therapy in TMNG should be undertaken soon after the diagnosis is made, especially in elderly patients who may have coronary artery disease. The use of PTU in the same doses as for treatment of Graves' disease is recommended until the patient is euthyroid. Propranolol is helpful if the patient is tremulous or tachycardic or experiencing chest pain. In TMNG, stopping PTU almost always will result in a return to the hyperthyroid state. RAI is the preferred therapy for TMNG in an elderly patient. Since the isotope is preferentially taken up by the hot nodules, they will receive most of the effects of the radiation. Because the hot follicles are relatively radioresistant, a larger dose of RAI is needed than is used with Graves' patients. A typical treatment dose for Graves' patients is 5 to 10 mCi, but the usual dose of RAI in TMNG is 15 to 20 mCi. Occasionally, when there is enough autonomous activity in other follicles, RAI will be taken up by all follicles, and hypothyroidism will result.

■ Autonomously Functioning Thyroid Nodule

The autonomously functioning thyroid nodule (AFTN) is a discrete thyroid nodule that functions independently of TSH. Radioisotope scans demonstrate increased uptake of isotope only by the nodule, with minimal evidence of any activity in the rest of the gland. The nodule cannot be suppressed by the administration of oral T3, but the rest of the thyroid gland can be stimulated by the administration of exogenous TSH. The natural history of this type of nodule is not clearly understood. The end result is a highly active nodule producing enough thyroid hormone to suppress TSH secretion and thus suppress the metabolic activity of the rest of the thyroid gland. If the nodule is big enough, usually greater than 4 cm in diameter, the patient will eventually become hyperthyroid.[35]

Clinically, the ratio of female to male patients is about 6 to 1. In patients older than 60 years, about 50 per cent of AFTN will cause hyperthyroidism, whereas in patients younger than 60 years, the frequency is only about 10 per cent. Diagnosis is made in the appropriate clinical setting by an elevated serum T4 and/or T3 level. Most commonly, the overall radioactive uptake is in the high-normal range, which is in contrast to the usual marked elevation seen in Graves' disease. Thyroid scans should show that most or all of the uptake of tracer isotope is occurring in the nodule.[36]

Therapy for a toxic hyperfunctioning nodule consists of either radioactive iodine or surgery. Radioactive iodine is the treatment of choice in elderly patients. A large dose of isotope is usually recommended, as the colloid-packed nodule is often less sensitive to radiation than is the goiter of Graves' disease. If there is any uptake in other parts of the thyroid on scans, the patient should be pretreated with T3, 25 μg daily by mouth for 5 days, to prevent RAI uptake by the rest of the gland. Likewise, for the same reason, it is important to delay RAI therapy for at least 7 days after any injections of TSH. Some thyroidologists routinely administer iodine for 4 to 6 weeks after RAI is given in the event that TSH secretion recovers. For most nodules, 20 to 25 mCi should do the job. However, for nodules with a diameter of more than 3 cm, 50 to 75 mCi may be needed.[37] Because of Nuclear Regulatory Commission regulations, any dose of 30 mCi or greater must be administered on an inpatient basis, because of the radioactive hazard posed to others by such a patient. Surgery is recommended only for extremely large nodules that would require exceedingly high doses of RAI. If an elderly patient with an autonomous nodule presents with cardiovascular manifestations, therapy with RAI should be undertaken as quickly as possible, along with the administration of beta-blockers.

REFERENCES

1. Atkinson RL, Dahms WT, Fisher DA, Nichols AL. Occult thyroid disease in an elderly hospitalized population. J Gerontol 1978; 33:372–376.
2. Jefferys PM. The prevalence of thyroid disease in patients admitted to a geriatric department. Age Ageing 1972; 1:33–37.
3. Bahemuka M, Hodkinson HM. Screening for hypothyroidism in elderly inpatients. Br Med J 1975; 1:601–603.
4. Livingston EH, Hershman JM, Sawin CT, Yoshikawa TT. Prevalance of thyroid disease and abnormal thyroid tests in older hospitalized and ambulatory persons. J Am Geriatr Soc 1987; 35:109–114.
5. Lloyd WH, Goldberg IJ. Incidence of hypothyroidism in the elderly. Br Med J 1961; 2:1256–1259.
6. Watanakunakorn C, Hodges RE, Evans TC. Myxedema. A study of 400 cases. Arch Intern Med 1965; 116:183–190.
7. Vanhaelst L, Neve P, Chailly P, Bastenie PA. Coronary-artery disease in hypothyroidism. Lancet 1967; 2:800–802.
8. Steinberg AD. Myxedema and coronary artery disease—a comparative autopsy study. Ann Intern Med 1968; 68:338–344.
9. Keating FR, Parkin TW, Selby JB, Dickinson LS. Treatment of heart disease associated with myxedema. Prog Cardiovasc Dis 1960; 3:364–381.
10. Aber CP, Thompson GS. The heart in hypothyroidism. Am Heart J 1964; 68:428–430.
11. Santos AD, Miller RP, Mathew PK, Wallace WA, Cave WT, Hinojosa L. Echocardiographic characterization of the reversible cardiomyopathy of hypothyroidism. Am J Med 1980; 68:675–682.
12. Senior RM, Birge SJ, Wessler S, Avioli LV. The recognition and management of myxedema coma. J Am Med Assoc 1971; 217:61–65.
13. Blum M. Myxedema coma. Am J Med Sci 1972; 264:432–443.
14. Evans W. A case of myxedema with ascites and atony of the urinary bladder. Endocrinology 1932; 17:409–416.
15. Le Marquand HS, Hausmann W, Hemsted EH. Myxoedema as a cause of death. Report of two cases. Br Med J 1953; 1:704–706.
16. Kerber RE, Sherman B. Echocardiographic evaluation of pericardial effusion in myxedema. Circulation 1975; 52:823–827.
17. Crowley WF, Ridgway EC, Bough EW, et al. Noninvasive evaluation of cardiac function in hypothyroidism. N Engl J Med 1977; 296:1–6.
18. Tibaldi JM, Barzel US, Albin J, Sirks M. Thyrotoxicosis in the very old. Am J Med 1986; 81:619–622.
19. Davis PJ, Davis FB. Hyperthyroidism in patients over the age of 60 years. Medicine 1974; 53:161–181.
20. Caplan RH, Glasser JE, Davis K, Foster K, Wickus G. Thyroid function tests in elderly hyperthyroid patients. J Am Geriatr Soc 1978; 26:116–120.
21. Griffin MA, Solomon DH. Hyperthyroidism in the elderly. J Am Geriatr Soc 1986; 34:887–892.
22. Greer MA, Kammer H. Bouma DJ. Short-term antithyroid drug therapy for the thyrotoxicosis of Graves' disease. N Engl J Med 1977; 297:173–176.
23. Toft AD, Irvine WJ, Sinclair I, McIntosh D, Seth J, Cameron EH. Thyroid function after surgical treatment of thyrotoxicosis. A report of 100 cases treated with propranolol before operation. N Engl J Med 1978; 298:643–647.

24. Roudebush CP, Hoye KE, DeGroot LJ. Compensated low-dose ^{131}I therapy of Graves' disease. Ann Intern Med 1977; 87:441–443.
25. Smith RN, Wilson GM. Clinical trial of different doses of ^{131}I in treatment of thyrotoxicosis. Br Med J 1967; 1:129–132.
26. Safa AM, Skillern PG. Treatment of hyperthyroidism with a large initial dose of sodium iodide I-131. Arch Intern Med 1975; 135:673–675.
27. Nofal MM, Beierwaltes WH, Patno ME. Treatment of hyperthyroidism with sodium iodide I^{131}: a 16-year experience. JAMA 1966; 197:605–610.
28. Dunn JT, Chapman EM. Rising incidence of hypothyroidism after radioactive-iodine therapy in thyrotoxicosis. N Engl J Med 1964; 271:1037–1042.
29. Toft AD, Seth J, Irvine WJ, Hunter WM, Cameron EH. Thyroid function in the long-term follow-up of patients treated with iodine-131 for thyrotoxicosis. Lancet 1975; 2:576–578.
30. Saenger EL, Thoma GE, Tompkins EA. Incidence of leukemia following treatment of hyperthyroidism. Preliminary report of the Cooperative Thyrotoxicosis Therapy Follow-Up Study. JAMA 1968; 205:855–862.
31. Klementschitsch P, Shen K. Kaplan EL. Reemergence of thyroidectomy as treatment for Graves' disease. Surg Clin North Am 1979; 59:35–44.
32. Rude RK, Oldham SB, Singer FR, Nicoloff JT. Treatment of thyrotoxic hypercalcemia with propranolol. N Engl J Med 1976; 294:431–433.
33. Farrar WB. Complications of thyroidectomy. Surg Clin North Am 1983; 63:1353–1361.
34. Miller JM, Block MA. Functional autonomy in multinodular goiter. JAMA 1970; 214:535–539.
35. Blum M, Shenkman L, Hollander CS. The autonomous nodule of the thyroid: correlation of patient age, nodule size and functional status. Am J Med Sci 1975; 269:43–50.
36. Silverstein GE, Burke G, Cogan R. The natural history of the autonomous hyperfunctioning thyroid nodule. Ann Intern Med 1967; 67:539–548.
37. Gorman CA, Robertson JS. Radiation dose in the selection of ^{131}I or surgical treatment for toxic thyroid adenoma. Ann Intern Med 1978; 89:85–90.

Tourette's syndrome

Ruth Dowling Bruun

Tourette's syndrome (TS) is a neuropsychiatric disorder manifested primarily by multiple motor and vocal tics. The diagnostic criteria set forth by the Diagnostic and Statistical Manual of Mental Disorders-III-R (1987) are the presence of sudden, rapid, recurrent, nonrhythmic, stereotyped motor movements (tics) and one or more vocal tics; the tics are experienced as irresistible, but they can be suppressed for varying periods of time; they vary in location, number, frequency, complexity, and severity with time; onset occurs before the age of 21 years; and duration is of more than 1 year.

These criteria, however, are not precisely accurate (e.g., a few cases have been reported with onsets after age 21 years, and some of the movements may be slower and more dystonic in nature), nor do they adequately convey a picture of the multiple problems experienced by many patients with Tourette's syndrome.

■ Background

Tourette's syndrome has been termed "a model neuropsychiatric disorder" because, in addition to involuntary movements, many patients suffer from behavioral difficulties, such as obsessive-compulsive disorder, attention deficit hyperactivity disorder, poor impulse control, and emotional lability.[1-3] Thus, control of the involuntary movements, which are the hallmark of TS, may not be sufficient for adequate treatment of a TS patient. In fact, behavioral problems may far outshadow tics in impairing the patient.

■ TIC SYMPTOMS

The motor tics of Tourette's syndrome vary from simple ones such as eye blinking, nose twitching, facial grimacing, head tossing, and jerky movements of the extremities to complex ones that may give the patient a bizarre appearance. Some of the more common complex motor tics are touching people or things, twirling around, smelling objects, dancing movements, and obscene gesturing.

Vocal tics are also divided into simple and complex types. Simple vocal tics include barking, snorting, throat clearing, clucking, whistling, spitting, and vocalizing parts of words (syllables such as uh, fu, eeh, and so on). Complex vocal tics consist of words or phrases such as "bull," "fat," "you know," "I'm okay," and so on. Additionally, there may be coprolalic utterances consisting of a variety of obscene or otherwise socially objectionable words or phrases.

Other symptoms that seem related to tics are palilalia, echolalia, speech irregularities (unusual, meaningless accentuations, stammering and rapid speech, for example), echopraxia, and copropraxia.

■ OBSESSIVE-COMPULSIVE BEHAVIOR

Obsessive-compulsive behavior is present in many TS patients. The incidence has been reported to be as high as 90 per cent.[4] Also, recent genetic research has indicated that obsessive-compulsive symptomatology actually may be an alternative or additional expression of the TS gene.[5,6] Sometimes obsessive-compulsive symptoms, because of their severity, will have a greater priority for treatment than tics.

Often the distinction between a tic and a compulsive action may be hard to make. Many TS patients will feel a need to "even up" (e.g., touch something with one hand and then with the other), to perform an act a certain number of times, or to perform it over and over until it "feels right." These behaviors are quite clearly compulsive in nature. However, many patients will also describe an unpleasant sensation, or urge, which immediately precedes or actually causes a tic. Thus some tics are carried out in order to relieve a sensation whereas others seem to arise spontaneously with little or no premonitory sensation. To the physician these tics appear the same, but are some tics actually compulsions and other tics just plain tics? Although this may seem to be purely an academic dilemma, the distinc-

tion becomes more relevant when one realizes that medications that are effective for tic diminution are not the same medications that are effective for obsessive-compulsive symptoms.

■ ATTENTION DEFICIT HYPERACTIVITY DISORDER

Up to 50 per cent of TS patients have attention deficit hyperactivity disorder (ADHD). (Also see the article on this disorder.) This is often present before the onset of TS symptoms. As with obsessive-compulsive disorders, some genetic research suggests that ADHD is an integral part of TS.[7] However, there is considerable dispute over this.[8] The symptoms of ADHD—poor attention span, easy distractibility, impulsivity, and motor hyperactivity—frequently worsen as tics develop and may cause severe problems with schooling. Children with the combination of TS and ADHD are often the ones who have the most difficulty in coping with educational demands and in dealing with life in general. Attention deficits may persist into adulthood and, together with a tic disorder, will often seriously impair the TS patient's ability to maintain employment appropriate for his or her intelligence. Unfortunately, treatment with stimulant medications that may control ADHD symptoms is generally contraindicated for the TS patient, since these medications may provoke a worsening of tics. (Treatment of ADHD is discussed later.)

■ EMOTIONAL LABILITY, IMPULSIVITY, AND AGGRESSIVITY

Although there is much disagreement as to what percentage of TS patients are affected by emotional lability, aggressivity, and impulsivity, most researchers agree that the number is significant.[3,9] Many TS patients, even those without attention problems, will describe a sense of inner tension that will wax and wane along with the tics. Irritability, emotional incontinence, and explosive temper outbursts are not uncommon in such patients. Management of these behaviors can be the most difficult part of the treatment of the TS patient, particularly because they cause so much distress to the patient's family as well as to the patient.

■ COGNITIVE DISABILITIES

Along with behavioral problems, many TS patients also suffer from a variety of learning problems.[10] In addition to specific learning disabilities, many patients have difficulties in reading because they will "get stuck" on a certain word or line, or their tics will cause them constantly to lose their place on a page. Others will simply be too distracted by the need to inhibit their tics to concentrate on anything else. Additionally, patients who are being medicated may suffer from a variety of side effects that impair their concentration (see under Specific Medications).

■ Management

Since there has been a growing awareness of Tourette's syndrome in the United States, the diagnosis is more frequently being made in cases whose symptoms are not so severe. These milder cases often do not require treatment with medication. It may be sufficient for these patients to understand the nature of their condition and to know that they are not alone in having it. Many adult Tourette patients have been concealing their symptoms for years in the belief that they would be considered "weird" by their friends and even by their families. Others have turned to self-analysis or to religion for answers that they could not obtain from doctors. In such cases there is often a tremendous sense of relief when the condition can be officially named and recognized as a known disorder. Younger patients with mild symptoms are also usually better treated with reassurance and education. Both the patient and the family will need this sort of advice. The Tourette Syndrome Association (42-40 Bell Boulevard, Bayside, NY 11361) can provide pamphlets and other literature as well as some excellent videotapes that will be helpful.

School personnel also should be informed, and certain adjustments in the school routine may be made when deemed appropriate. If, for example, children are allowed to leave the classroom for a few minutes when tics are bothersome, they may be able to handle their symptoms without being disruptive to the class. Supportive counseling may be helpful if the counselor is well versed in the symptomatology of TS and does not try to make psychologic interpretations when they are not appropriate. Counseling should be directed toward coping with a chronic physically, socially, and sometimes emotionally disabling condition. It is also helpful for the child to know that many TS patients spontaneously improve in the later teen years and that it is unusual, in any case, for a patient to get worse after this age.[11]

Since the clinical manifestations of Tourette's syndrome may be so variable, it is of the utmost importance that a complete picture of the patient be obtained before undertaking treatment. Although the presence of tics is essential for the diagnosis, this may not be the most disabling symptom. Therefore, a clear understanding of the "target symptoms" is the first step in treatment.

■ MEDICATION

The decision to give medication should be made when TS symptoms are preventing patients from functioning at the level which they should reasonably be expected to achieve, or when the social consequences of appearing strange to others become a significant deterrent to normal social development. At this point, there are a number of different medications to consider.

Although haloperidol has been considered the drug of choice for Tourette's syndrome in the past, it is a potent medication with a host of potential side effects. Therefore, many physicians with experience in the treatment of TS will prefer to try other medications with lower potential for side effects first. One such medication is clonidine.

Clonidine

Clonidine (Catapres) is an imidazoline derivative long established as an effective antihypertensive medication. Since 1979, it has been considered to be useful in the treatment of TS.[12] As an alpha-adrenergic agonist, clondine acts directly on the adrenergic system and indirectly on a number of other neurotransmitter systems, including serotonin and dopamine.

Although clonidine originally was felt to be more effective against tics than later studies have indicated, it has been widely accepted as a medication that is useful for the treatment of TS, since it is also considered helpful for many of the associated behavioral manifestations of the disorder.[13]

Clonidine is initiated at a dose of 0.025 to 0.05 mg, once or twice daily, and the dosage is very gradually raised over a period of weeks until an effective level is reached or the medication is deemed unsatisfactory. Many patients do well at low levels such as 0.1 to 0.15 mg per day. Others require total daily doses as high as 0.5 or 0.6 mg (the latter is unusual). Clonidine is best given in small doses three to four time daily, since it has a relatively short half-life (about 6 hours). An alternative dosing method is the transdermal patch (Catapres-TTS), which delivers a total daily dosage continuously and needs to be changed only every week. While this is at least theoretically an ideal method of administering the drug, my experience has been that active children have a great deal of trouble keeping these patches on for more than a day or two at a time.

When clonidine is working effectively, the TS patient will experience a relief of inner tension, a decreased drive to produce tics, less obsessional thinking and irritability, and an increased ability to concentrate and to control impulses. The onset of these beneficial effects may be quite delayed, however, and it may be necessary to take the medication for a period of months (at least 3) before the fullest effect is experienced.

Most common side effects are dry mouth, sedation, easy fatigue, headache, and lightheadedness. These may often be avoided by a very slow increase of dosage. Others, such as increased irritability, nightmares, and insomnia are rarer but may be an indication that clonidine is less likely to work for that patient. Nevertheless, some patients experience these side effects transiently only after every increase of dosage and find that they disappear after a short while. As a rule, hypotension is not a concern. Tolerance to the beneficial effects of clonidine does not seem to develop, and no dangerous effects of long-term use have been described.

If it becomes necessary to discontinue clonidine treatment, the dosage should be reduced gradually. Abrupt withdrawal may cause a rebound hypertension in rare patients or, more commonly, has been known to cause motoric hyperactivity, anxiety, and insomnia.[14]

Haloperidol

Haloperidol (Haldol) was the first medication to be documented as effective against the tics of TS. This recognition came in the early 1960s and reopened an interest in Tourette's syndrome, which had been almost forgotten for several decades. The fact that a dopamine-blocking neuroleptic was able to control both motor and vocal tics, including that most mysterious symptom, coprolalia, led to the recognition that TS was an organic syndrome and that many patients, once considered hopeless, might now be helped. Furthermore, the discovery advanced research in the area of dopamine-mediated disorders and spurred much new research that still continues on the role of neurotransmitters on motor control and behavior.[15,16]

Although haloperidol remains the medication most commonly prescribed for TS, there is now a growing awareness of its many side effects that, it is hoped, will lead the enlightened physician to gauge carefully the need for such medication before prescribing it. Assuming, however, that the physician is aware of the potential complications of treatment with haloperidol and is willing to monitor the patient for them, this may be a most effective medication. It has been estimated that up to 80 per cent of patients will benefit from the judicious use of this neuroleptic with significant suppression of tics. Its effects on hyperactivity, impulse control, and aggressive behaviors also may be beneficial, although this has been less well documented. It does not seem particularly effective in controlling or ameliorating obsessive-compulsive behavior.

Haloperidol is best given initially at a dose of 0.25 to 0.5 mg at bedtime. The daily bedtime dosage will avoid initial sedation in the daytime and is quite satisfactory. The dose is then raised as needed every 5 to 7 days by 0.25- or 0.5-mg increments. During this time, frequent telephone calls to the patient (or parents) will greatly facilitate the treatment and avoid the development of debilitating side effects. Since tics are often suppressed in the doctor's office, it is of little use to examine the patient each time a change of medication is contemplated. A self-report or a parent's report on the changes noted during the past few days will be much more useful for these purposes.

Parkinsonian symptoms (tremor, muscular rigidity, slowed movement, drooling, and so on) may occur during the first few weeks of treatment. If so, anticholinergic medications such as benztropine (Cogentin) or trihexyphenidyl (Artane) may be used. However, if the haloperidol is raised slowly, these side effects do not often occur. Akathisia is somewhat more common. It is characterized by a motor restlessness that may be mistaken for an increase in hyperactivity, or for anxiety. This particular side effect may be hard to treat. Diazepam (Valium) may be effective but should be avoided for long-term use because of its addictive potential. There have been some reports that clonidine may be effective against akathisia, and this has been suggested as an indication for combined haloperidol and clonidine treatment.[17] However, it is certainly preferable to try diminishing doses of haloperidol before resorting to treatment with two pharmacologic agents. Drowsiness may be handled by consumption of coffee or caffeine-containing soft drinks. However, some patients find that caffeine will cause a tic increase. Behavioral changes that are, in fact, side effects may be insidious and may easily be mistaken for psychiatric disorders unrelated to medication effect.[18,19] These include depressions (which may become severe), increased irritability, or school and social phobias. These do not respond to anticholinergics and are best treated by decreasing or discontinuing haloperidol.

One imperative reason to discontinue haloperidol is the development of symptoms of tardive dyskinesia. Although reports of this complication are relatively rare in TS patients, this is a potentially permanent, disabling condition. The movements of tardive dyskinesia are distinguishable from those of TS in that they are usually choreoathetoid in nature and more constant than tics. They occur most commonly in the facial muscles, consisting typically of chewing movements and fine, wormlike movements of the tongue. Mild choreoathetoid movements of the extremities also may be an early sign. Since the movements of tardive dyskinesia may be temporarily relieved by an increase of haloperidol, there is a real danger of starting a morbid cycle of dosage increases that

eventually only worsen the underlying dyskinesia.

The desired end-point in dosage adjustment is reached when the greatest symptom control is achieved without side effects or with minimal side effects. Thus, the lowest effective dosage is the optimum. Most patients will respond to doses of under 5 mg/day. Many will do well on doses as low as 1 mg/day or even less. A few patients seem to need much higher doses, in the range of 10 to 30 mg/day. However, there is considerable disagreement as to the merits of continuing to increase the dose at such high levels.

Patients who have been taking haloperidol for a period of time may experience withdrawal symptoms when the dose is decreased. These will be manifested by a heightened restlessness, insomnia, irritability, and an increase in tic activity. Such reactions may last for several weeks. Therefore, it is most important to decrease the dose slowly and to be aware that one is working with a withdrawal syndrome rather than with the "real" status of the patient.

Pimozide

Pimozide (Orap) is a relatively new neuroleptic that has been marketed in the United States (since 1984) solely for the treatment of Tourette's syndrome. It is considered to be equally as effective as haloperidol for suppression of tics and is often better tolerated. In several studies it has been shown to have a lower incidence of side effects than haloperidol.[20] It should be understood, however, that it does have the potential to cause any or all of the side effects already discussed in relation to haloperidol. In addition, it has been found to cause a prolongation of the electrocardiographic Q-T interval; flattening, notching, and inversion of T waves; and the appearance of U waves in some patients. Therefore, it is recommended by the manufacturer that an electrocardiogram (ECG) be obtained prior to treatment and at regular intervals during treatment. If the Q-T interval is increased beyond 0.47 sec (children) or 0.52 sec (adults), or 25 per cent over the normal level for that patient, pimozide should be discontinued. Because of these ECG changes, it is recommended that pimozide not be tried unless a patient has failed to respond to haloperidol. However, many physicians who treat large numbers of TS patients feel that the potentially low side effect spectrum makes this drug a very attractive alternative to haloperidol.

Pimozide is started at a dose of 1 to 2 mg at bedtime and raised slowly, as needed, by 1-mg increments until the optimal dose level is attained. Titration to the proper dose is done in the same manner as that of haloperidol (i.e., slowly and only up to the minimum effective dose). Withdrawal effects may occur just as they do for haloperidol.

Fluphenazine

Although fluphenazine (Prolixin) has not received the attention that haloperidol and pimozide have, studies show that it has equal capacity to suppress tics.[21] While it has approximately the same spectrum of side effects, it may be better tolerated by some patients and should, therefore, be given equal weight when the use of a neuroleptic is being considered. Fluphenazine may be started at a dose of 0.5 to 1 mg per day at bedtime and increased in the same fashion as haloperidol until the lowest effective daily dosage has been reached. As with haloperidol and pimozide, it should be withdrawn slowly to avoid withdrawal symptoms.

Other Neuroleptics

There are a few reports of successful tic suppression with other neuroleptics, such as thiothixene (Navane), chlorpromazine (Thorazine), and trifluoperazine (Stelazine).[21,22] These do not appear to be as effective for most patients, but occasional patients will respond well to one or another of them.

Clonazepam

Clonazepam (Klonopin) is a benzodiazepine used for the treatment of certain forms of epilepsy. It is also considered helpful for a variety of movement disorders. It appears to have a mild tic-suppressing effect and may be useful for mild tic symptoms, or it may be given in combination with another more potent medication.[21] The most common side effects are sedation, memory lapses, confusion, and depression. It is an addictive substance and has all the potential hazards associated with other benzodiazepines.

Miscellaneous Other Tic-Suppressing Medications

The recent literature on TS includes reports of successful tic suppression through the use of calcium channel blockers and reserpine. Three other medications that are available only experimentally in the United States at this time but have been shown to be effective for TS are tetrabenazine, clozapine, penfluridol, and Ro22-1319.[21]

■ TREATMENT OF OBSESSIVE-COMPULSIVE SYMPTOMS

With the possible exception of clonidine, the drugs just discussed are not helpful for obsessive-compulsive (OC) symptoms. Recently, however, a bicyclic antidepressant, fluoxetine (Prozac), has become available in the United States and has been shown to be effective in controlling obsessions and compulsions in at least 50 per cent of patients tested.[23] Fluoxetine has a long half-life (3 days) and, therefore, may be given once daily or even once every other day without loss of potency. It may be effective in very low dosages (10 to 20 mg/day) after a few weeks of administration, but some patients will require as much as 80 mg daily for maximum control of OC symptoms. Side effects most commonly encountered are nausea, anorexia, anxiety, nervousness, headache, insomnia, or drowsiness.

Clomipramine (Anafranil) has also been proved effective as treatment for OC symptoms.[24] It is a tricyclic antidepressant given in dosages similar to those of amitriptyline or imipramine. The daily dosage effective for treatment of OCD varies between 75 and 300 mg/day. Side effects are similar to those encountered with other tricyclic antidepressants.

Behavior therapy may be helpful for the treatment of OC symptoms associated with TS, but this has not yet been established by any scientific study.

■ TREATMENT OF ATTENTION DEFICIT HYPERACTIVITY DISORDER/

Although many TS patients also have ADHD, it is important for the treating physician to know that stimulant medications have been reported to produce tics in tic-prone individuals or to exacerbate tics in those who already manifest them. Thus, it is advisable to avoid prescribing stimulant medications in TS patients or in their family members if at all possible.[25] In such cases clonidine, haloperidol, or another neuroleptic or imipramine may be helpful for ADHD symptoms. If these medications are not sufficient to control the symptoms of hyperactivity, careful administration of methylphenidate (Ritalin) or another stimulant may be necessary. The patient (and family) always should be carefully advised of the risks before undertaking such treatment. In some cases a combination of neuroleptic and methylphenidate or clonidine and methylphenidate may be effective.

■ TREATMENT OF OTHER ASSOCIATED BEHAVIORAL SYMPTOMS

A small handful of TS patients, particularly in the late adolescent years, will have severely disruptive behavioral symptoms in addition to the more conventional TS symptomatology. Irritability, anger, and explosive outbursts of temper, as well as emotional immaturity with extreme lability of mood, are characteristics of this type of TS patient. Bouts of temper will be followed by periods of remorse and depression. Although there is no standard formula for the treatment of such cases, medication may be helpful. Some patients have responded positively to a combination of a neuroleptic with lithium, carbamazepine (Tegretol), or an antidepressant such as trazodone (Desyrel). These cases are difficult to treat and require very careful monitoring, as well as support and encouragement for the patient and the whole family. Behavioral therapy or family therapy may be required in addition to, or instead of, medicine. There is very little evidence that behavioral therapy will be of help for tic suppression, yet it may be an essential part of treatment for such associated behavioral problems and possibly for obsessive-compulsive symptoms as well.

REFERENCES

1. Gilles de la Tourette G. Étude sur une affection nerveuse caractérisée par de l'incoordination motrice accompagné d'echolalie et de coprolalie. Arch Neurol 1885; 9:19-42, 158-200.
2. Cohen DJ, Bruun RD, Leckman JF (eds). Tourette's Syndrome and Tic Disorders: Clinical Understanding and Treatment. New York: John Wiley and Sons, 1988.
3. Singer HS, Rosenberg LA. Development of behavioral and emotional problems in Tourette syndrome. Pediatr Neurol 1989; 5:41-44.
4. Nee LE, Polinsky RJ, Ebert MH. Tourette syndrome: clinical and family studies. In Friedhoff AJ, Chase TN (eds). Gilles de la Tourette Syndrome. New York: Raven Press, 1982:291-296.
5. Pauls DL, Leckman JF. The inheritance of Gilles de la Tourette's syndrome and associated behaviors: evidence for autosomal dominant transmission. N Engl J Med 1986; 315:993-997.
6. Pauls DL, Towbin KE, Leckman JF, Zahner GEP, Cohen DJ. Gilles de la Tourette syndrome and obsessive compulsive disorder: evidence supporting an etiological relationship. Arch Gen Psychiatr 1986; 43:1180-1182.
7. Comings DE, Comings BG. Tourette's syndrome and attention deficit disorder. In Cohen DJ, Bruun RD, Leckman JF (eds). Tourette's Syndrome and Tic Disorders: Clinical Understanding and Treatment. New York: John Wiley and Sons, 1988:120-135.
8. Pauls DL, Hurst CR, Kruger SD, Leckman JF, Kidd KK, Cohen DJ. Gilles de la Tourette's syndrome and attention deficit disorder with hyperactivity: evidence against a genetic relationship. Arch Gen Psychiatr 1986; 43:1177-1179.
9. Riddle MA, Hardin MT, Ort SI, Leckman JF, Cohen DJ. Behavioral symptoms in Tourette's syndrome. In Cohen DJ, Bruun RD, Leckman JF (eds). Tourette's Syndrome and Tic Disorders: Clinical Understanding and Treatment. New York: John Wiley and Sons, 1988:152-162.
10. Hagin RA, Kugler J. School problems associated with Tourette's syndrome. In Cohen DJ, Bruun RD, Leckman JF (eds). Tourette's Syndrome and Tic Disorders: Clinical Understanding and Treatment. New York: John Wiley and Sons, 1988:224-236.
11. Bruun RD. The natural history of Tourette's syndrome. In Cohen DJ, Bruun RD, Leckman JF (eds). Tourette's Syndrome and Tic Disorders: Clinical Understanding and Treatment. New York: John Wiley and Sons, 1988:22-39.
12. Cohen DJ, Young JG, Nathanson JA, Shaywitz BA. Clonidine in Tourette's syndrome. Lancet 1979; 2:551-553.
13. Leckman JF, Walkup JT, Cohen DJ. Clonidine treatment of Tourette's syndrome. In Cohen DJ, Bruun RD, Leckman JF (eds). Tourette's Syndrome and Tic Disorders: Clinical Understanding and Treatment. New York: John Wiley and Sons, 1988:292-301.
14. Leckman JF, Ort S, Cohen DJ, Caruso KA, Anderson GM, Riddle MA. Rebound phenomena in Tourette's syndrome after abrupt withdrawal of clonidine: behavioral cardiovascular and neurochemical effects. Arch Gen Psychiatr 1986; 43:1168–1176.
15. Shapiro AK, Shapiro E. Treatment of tic disorders with haloperidol. In Cohen DJ, Bruun RD, Leckman JF (eds). Tourette's Syndrome and Tic Disorders: Clinical Understanding and Treatment. New York: John Wiley and Sons, 1988:268-280.
16. Leckman JF, Riddle MA, Cohen DJ. Pathobiology of Tourette's syndrome. In Cohen DJ, Bruun RD, Leckman JF (eds). Tourette's Syndrome and Tic Disor-

ders: Clinical Understanding and Treatment. New York: John Wiley and Sons, 1988:104-116.

17. Zubenko GS, Cohen BM, Lipinski JF, Jonas JM. Use of clonidine in treatment of akathisia. Psychiatry Res 1984; 13:253–259.

18. Bruun RD. Subtle and underrecognized side effects of neuroleptic treatment in children with Tourette's disorder. Am J Psychiatry 1988; 145:621-624.

19. Bruun RD. Dysphoric phenomena associated with haloperidol treatment of Tourette syndrome. In Friedhoff AJ, Chase TN (eds). Gilles de la Tourette Syndrome. New York: Raven Press, 1982:433-436.

20. Moldofsky H, Sandor P. Pimozide in the treatment of Tourette's syndrome. In Cohen DJ, Bruun RD, Leckman JF (eds). Tourette's Syndrome and Tic Disorders: Clinical Understanding and Treatment. New York: John Wiley and Sons, 1988:282-289.

21. Singer HS, Trifiletti R, Gammon K. The role of "other" neuroleptic drugs in the treatment of Tourette's syndrome. In Cohen DJ, Bruun RD, Leckman JF (eds). Tourette's Syndrome and Tic Disorders: Clinical Understanding and Treatment. New York: John Wiley and Sons, 1988:304-316.

22. Bruun RD. Gilles de la Tourette's syndrome: an overview of clinical experience. J Am Acad Child Psychiatr 1984; 23:126-133.

23. Fontaine R, Chownard G. An open clinical trial of fluoxetine in the treatment of obsessive-compulsive disorder. J Clin Psychopharmacol 1986; 6:98-101.

24. Zohar J, Insel TR. Diagnosis and treatment of obsessive-compulsive disorder. Psychiatr Ann 1988; 18:168-171.

25. Golden GS. The use of stimulants in the treatment of Tourette's syndrome. In Cohen DJ, Bruun RD, Leckman JF (eds). Tourette's Syndrome and Tic Disorders: Clinical Understanding and Treatment. New York: John Wiley and Sons, 1988:318-325.

Toxic megacolon in inflammatory bowel disease

Janet Ruth Todorczuk ■ *Richard W. McCallum*

■ Background

Toxic dilatation of the colon complicating severe inflammatory bowel disease was described as early as the 1930s. The term *toxic megacolon* was introduced in 1950 by Marshak and associates to describe this acute, fulminating, often lethal complication of ulcerative colitis.[1]

It was once assumed that toxic megacolon occurred only in association with ulcerative colitis; however, this entity has also been reported to complicate other diseases, such as ischemic colitis, amebic colitis, bacillary dysentery, pseudomembranous colitis, and Crohn's colitis.[2-6] The incidence of toxic dilatation of the colon has been decreasing in recent years.[5,6] This is attributed to better medical management of inflammatory bowel disease in general and earlier recognition of toxic megacolon by physicians. The incidence in ulcerative colitis has been reported to be from 1.6 to 8 per cent of all cases of ulcerative colitis,[4,6,8] although some older reports still quote an incidence of up to 13 per cent.[7] In Crohn's colitis, the incidence is approximately 6 per cent.[4,5]

Toxic megacolon is characterized by dilatation of the colon and full-thickness inflammation. The involvement of the colon may be either total or segmental. Generally total colonic involvement is the rule, although toxic megacolon also has been reported in disease of the left colon only.[6]

Toxic megacolon usually occurs with a severe attack of previously diagnosed ulcerative colitis; however, in 25 to 40 per cent of the cases, it occurs as an initial manifestation of the disease.[9,10] Toxic megacolon in Crohn's colitis may occur as an early manifestation of the disease, before extensive transmural fibrosis has developed.[4] Because of this, toxic dilatation of the colon is rare in late Crohn's colitis.

■ PATHOGENESIS

The basic pathologic process in the production of toxic megacolon is the same, no matter what type of colitis is involved. Inflammation of the colonic mucosa penetrates to involve all layers of the colonic wall, including the circular and longitudinal muscle layers as well as the serosa. Ultimately, this transmural inflammation results in almost complete paralysis of the involved area of the colon. The colon loses its ability to contract and promote propulsion, and it becomes dilated.

Certain factors have been implicated as contributing to the development of toxic megacolon, and these factors have been incriminated in as many as 70 per cent of the cases.[6,9,11] Excessive use of narcotics, anticholinergics, and antidiarrheals can worsen colonic dilatation by inhibiting normal motility.[9,11–13] Toxic megacolon has been described following proctoscopic and barium enema examinations of patients with acute exacerbations.[14–16] These procedures require air insufflation, and excessive use of air may lead to rapid distention of the colon. Electrolyte deficiencies may also be triggering factors, although some investigators believe that hypokalemia is the result of, and not the cause of, toxic dilatation of the colon.[4]

■ DIAGNOSIS

Clinical Findings (Table 1). Toxic megacolon is found in all age groups and its occurrence during pregnancy has been described.[17–19] One group of workers has suggested that younger age groups are more likely to develop toxic megacolon, based on the fact that 69 per cent of patients studied were under the age of 30 years.[8] In the setting of an acute exacerbation of colitis, toxic megacolon may be difficult to recognize. This is particularly true in patients on long-term steroids, in whom the clinical picture

TABLE 1. Clinical Findings in Toxic Megacolon

Abdominal pain
Bloody diarrhea
Fever: temperature $> 38.5°$ C (101.5° F)
Tachycardia: pulse > 120 beats/min
Leukocytosis: WBC $> 12,000/mm^3$
Anemia: hemoglobin < 10 gm/dl
Hypoalbuminemia: albumin < 3.0 gm/dl
Electrolyte disturbances (i.e., low K, Na, Cl)
Radiographic evidence of colonic dilatation:
   maximum diameter > 6 cm

may be masked by the steroids. A change in the pattern of the patient's abdominal pain is usually the initial complaint. The pain may change from crampy and intermittent pain to steady and diffuse pain, not relieved by bowel movements.

Bowel movements may vary. Diarrhea may be persistent, although some patients will experience a reduction or cessation of bowel movements, particularly those patients being treated with motility-reducing antidiarrheal agents. A cessation of bowel movements in acute fulminant colitis should not give a false sense of security to the treating physician, as this change does not necessarily signify clinical improvement; rather it may signify worsening of the colitis or development of toxic dilatation of the colon.[6]

The patient will usually appear acutely ill, with a fever, tachycardia, hypotension, and signs of volume depletion. Some patients may manifest mental status changes ranging from profound anxiety and hysteria to disorientation and listlessness.

A thorough and careful abdominal examination is very important. The abdomen is usually distended and tympanitic. Bowel sounds are diminished or absent due to the markedly reduced peristaltic activity of the colon. The examining physician should be aware that an inconsistency may exist between the physical finding of abdominal distention and the degree of dilatation of the colon. There may be only mild distention of the abdomen despite extreme dilatation found on an abdominal radiograph.

Abdominal tenderness is usually diffuse, but it may be localized to the left lower quadrant or periumbilical area. Rebound tenderness, guarding, and other signs of peritoneal irritation suggest impending perforation. An early sign of perforation in a clinically well-appearing patient is loss of hepatic dullness.[12] Systemic complications such as thrombophlebitis also may be present.[6]

Laboratory Findings. Laboratory studies reflect acute inflammation of the colon. The most common finding is marked leukocytosis and a leftward shift. Toxic granulations may be seen on the blood smear. The sedimentation rate is usually over 50 mm per hour. Anemia is common and is due to colonic bleeding. Electrolyte abnormalities include low potassium, sodium, chloride, magnesium, and calcium levels. A low, serum albumin level may also be seen, and this is secondary to excessive colonic loss of protein.[6,12,13,20]

Radiologic Findings. Classically, a plain abdominal x-ray film will reveal dilatation of the transverse colon early in the course of the disease. Segments of the right or left colon also may be dilated, but the rectum is usually not involved in toxic dilatation. There is often distention of the small bowel as well. The dilated transverse colon usually exceeds 6 cm in diameter[6,11,12] (Fig. 1). Other radiographic features also will be present, and they are equally important in the diagnosis[6] (Table 2). Normal haustral markings are lost in the involved segment of the colon. Less involved portions of bowel will show thickened haustra. Numerous broad-based pseudopolyps may be seen extending into the lumen from the bowel wall. The bowel lumen may appear scalloped and have toothlike projections, representing deep ulcers (Fig. 2). Submucosal leakage of air occasionally is seen, producing a subserosal radiolucent line in the wall of the colon.[8,21] A more ominous radiographic sign is free air, visible on an erect or lateral decubitus view

TABLE 2. Radiographic Features of Toxic Megacolon

Marked distention of the colon (>6 cm)
Loss of normal haustral and mucosal markings
Nodular, polypoid, intraluminal projections: pseudopolyps
Irregular contours of the bowel lumen: deep ulcers
Relative shortening of the colon

of the abdomen. This indicates free perforation. Other radiologic examinations (e.g., barium enema films) are not indicated in the diagnosis of this disease because of the potential of contributing to perforation.

■ Management

The patient with toxic dilatation of the colon due to the various types of colitis requires constant observation, preferably in an intensive care unit. A surgeon who is familiar with inflammatory bowel disease and skilled in gastrointestinal surgery should see the patient on admission and should follow

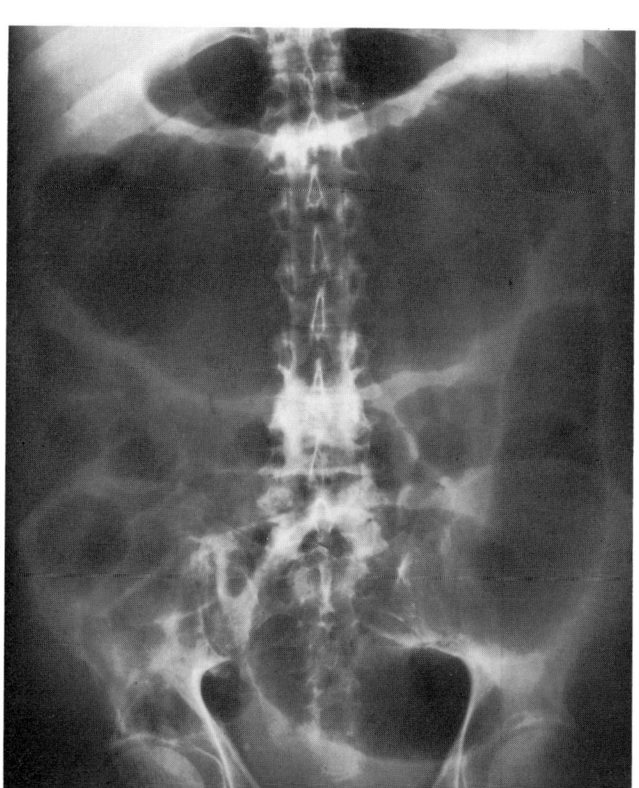

Figure 1. Abdominal radiograph in a patient with toxic megacolon, illustrating a markedly dilated transverse colon, over 6 cm in diameter.

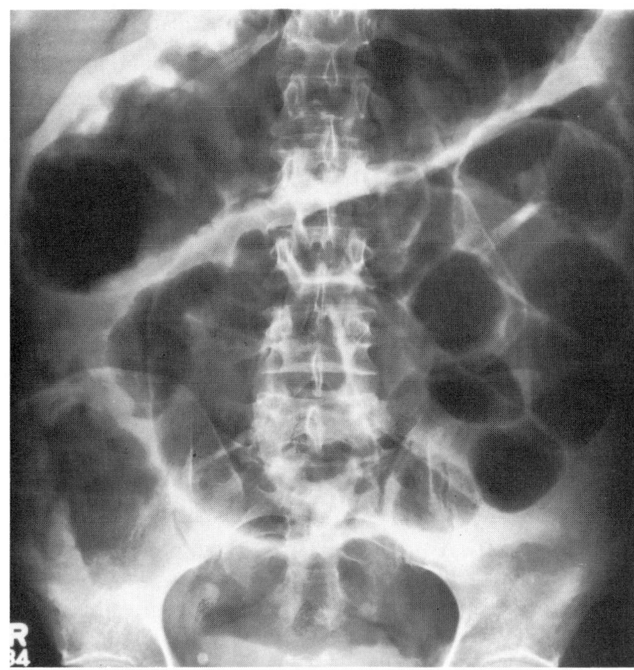

Figure 2. Abdominal radiograph in a patient with toxic megacolon, illustrating intraluminal projections (pseudopolyps) and irregular contours of the bowel lumen, representing ulcerations in the transverse colon.

the patient closely with the primary physician. The patient should be assessed frequently, at least three times daily in the early stages, for any change in physical findings or symptoms. Hourly monitoring of vital signs in the course of the disease is prudent. Worsening of the disease will be suggested by persistent tachycardia and hypotension. Persistent fever in a patient on high-dose steroids for over 48 hours is particularly worrisome, as this would suggest a perforation or abscess.

Blood studies—a complete blood count, sedimentation rate, electrolytes, blood urea nitrogen, and creatinine—should be monitored daily. Some authorities recommend documenting stool frequency, consistency, and amount of blood loss to help in monitoring the progress of the patient.

Blood cultures and stool cultures for *Salmonella*, *Shigella*, *Yersinia*, and *Campylobacter*, as well as stool examination for amebiasis, should be obtained on admission. A stool sample for *Clostridium difficile* culture and toxin is also warranted. A limited, rigid proctoscopy to about 5 cm (without air insufflation) is probably safe despite the severe illness. This procedure enables the physician to evaluate the rectal mucosa for evidence of active disease and to obtain a biopsy, stool cultures, and stool samples for ova and parasites. This examination may

give information about the extent of the disease and possible etiology of the colitis.

An admission and daily chest radiograph and an abdominal film are necessary to look for signs of free perforation and to assess resolution of the colonic dilatation.

■ SUPPORTIVE THERAPY

Initial medical management includes bowel rest and decompression of the colon. The patient should have nothing by mouth (NPO). Decompression of the dilated colon with the use of a nasogastric tube is probably sufficient, although some authorities favor the use of a long tube, such as a Cantor or Miller-Abbott tube.[6,12,13,20] This tube should be passed into the duodenum under the guidance of fluoroscopy to facilitate passage into the distal small bowel. Continuous suction on this tube reduces small bowel gas and thereby reduces the amount of gas entering the already dilated colon.[6] A rectal tube may also aid in colonic decompression.[6]

Other methods to decompress the colon have been mentioned in the literature. The most successful method involves rolling the patient to a prone position for 10 to 15 minutes to redistribute the colonic gas from the transverse colon to the descending colon.[12,13,20] Colonic gas preferentially accumulates in the transverse colon, particularly when the patient is supine in bed, because it is the most anterior part of the colon. The prone position facilitates the passage of colonic gas to the rectum for eventual expulsion. The patient's position should be changed every 2 hours. Decreasing colonic distention may allow more time for the healing of colitis with the other measures outlined subsequently.

Fluid and electrolyte replacement is equally important to correct dehydration and electrolyte imbalances. Careful monitoring of electrolytes and of calcium and magnesium levels is needed, because a deficiency may contribute to the continuing colonic dilation.

If the patient is anemic from colonic bleeding, blood transfusions may be required to maintain a hematocrit about 25 per cent. Hypoalbuminemia may benefit from intravenous administration of salt-free albumin to raise the serum albumin level to at least 3 gm/dl.

Narcotic pain medications, anticholinergics, and antidiarrheals should not be used early in the course of toxic megacolon. These agents can worsen the toxic dilatation of the colon because of their motility-reducing properties. Pain requiring frequent narcotic analgesics should signal the physician that an abscess or perforation exists. Severe pain should not persist in toxic megacolon once the patient has been adequately decompressed.[12,13]

■ SPECIFIC THERAPY

Steroids. The therapeutic value of corticosteroids in toxic megacolon is a controversial point,[10,22] but most investigators recommend their use.[6,12,13,20,22] Steroid use in toxic megacolon is particularly important if the patient had received steroid treatment prior to the flare of colitis. In such patients steroids are needed to prevent an adrenal crisis precipitated by the added stress of the acute toxicity.

If the patient with toxic megacolon has previously received steroids, then intravenous hydrocortisone (Solu-Cortef), 100 mg every 8 hours, is recommended.[12,13,20,23] Higher dosages may not be needed, but some physicians have used up to 1 gram daily.[13] Some workers advocate the use of a continuous infusion of steroids rather than bolus administration.[12,13,20]

The decision to use hydrocortisone versus adrenocorticotropic hormone (ACTH—Cortrosyn, Cortrophin ACTH) in the treatment of the fulminant colitis is quite controversial. Some believe that ACTH, at a dosage of 40 units every 8 hours, is more effective than hydrocortisone in patients not previously receiving steroids for the colitis.[23] It should be noted that the use of ACTH in this manner is not universally accepted by all gastroenterologists.

Since both ACTH and hydrocortisone can produce hypokalemia, the serum potassium level should be monitored regularly. This is particularly important with the use of ACTH because the hypokalemia is more severe.

Rectal steroids are not effective in this disease. Parenteral steroids should be avoided in patients with toxic megacolon who have clinical evidence on admission of a free perforation or a sealed-off perforation.[12,13,20] The exception to this is the patient who has recently received steroid treatment prior to the development of the toxic megacolon. Again, in this situation, steroids are needed to prevent an adrenal crisis.

Although there is no evidence that steroids contribute to an increased risk of colonic perforation,[22] they do mask the clinical signs of perforation, and extra attention is needed in following these patients.

Antibiotics. Antibiotics are usually employed in toxic megacolon because of the danger of fecal spillage should the colon perforate, and because of secondary bacterial invasion of the bowel wall. Antibiotic agents must be active against the anaerobic and aerobic organisms commonly present in the colon. The combination of metronidazole (Flagyl), an aminoglycoside, and ampicillin (for enterococci coverage) is recommended.[12,13,20] A third-generation cephalosporin plus metronidazole is also a reasonable choice. Antibiotics should be continued for 7 to 10 days through the course of the acute illness.[12,13,20]

Parenteral Nutrition. Intravenous hyperalimentation may be required in patients with toxic megacolon who are likely to remain NPO for prolonged periods of time. (See article, "Nutritional support of the acutely and chronically ill patient.") However, there is no evidence that parenteral alimentation helps heal the colon in toxic megacolon or that it helps avoid surgery.[5,12,13,20] Parenteral nutrition is usually not necessary if the patient improves after a few days of medical treatment. Likewise, it is not prudent to delay what may be life-saving surgery and prolong medical therapy in order to "improve the patient's nutritional status before surgery" with parenteral alimentation.

Sulfasalazine, 5-ASA, and Immunosuppressives. Sulfasalazine (Azulfidine) and the new 5-ASA enemas (Rowasa) should not be used in the treatment of toxic megacolon. Likewise, there is no role for immunosuppressives in the acute management of this entity.[13,20] These drugs have a very long response time (over 4 weeks).

■ Issues and Risks

■ ASSESSING THE RESPONSE TO MEDICAL THERAPY

Early recognition and treatment of toxic megacolon is crucial to successful medical management. The first 48 to 72 hours of medical therapy are the most important and will decide the outcome of toxic megacolon.[5,6,11,24] Monitoring vital signs, bowel movements, daily flat and upright abdominal radiographs, clinical signs, and laboratory parameters is necessary in assessing response to therapy. Some patients will experience a dramatic improvement with medical management. This is manifested by a decrease in abdominal distention, a return of bowel sounds, defervescence of fever, and normalization of laboratory parameters. The plain film of the abdomen will show colonic decompression. This will correlate with the clinical improvement of the patient. Patients who respond to medical management should be maintained on high-dose steroids for 10 to 14 days. Oral steroids, such as prednisone, 40 to 60 mg daily, can be instituted when the patient is tolerating liquids. The nasogastric tube can be removed when an abdominal film documents persistent colonic decompression even with the tube clamped for 24 hours. Antibiotic coverage should be continued for a full 10- to 14-day course. With adequate colonic decompression and reversal of the signs of toxicity, the patient should be able to tolerate oral intake and gradual advancement of diet.

Unfortunately, medical treatment of toxic megacolon may reverse the process in less than 50 per cent of the cases.[8–10] Patients not responding to the treatment just outlined will continue to show distention of the abdomen and dilation of the colon, as well as evidence of toxicity. Signs of perforation in these patients should be closely monitored. These include persistent tachycardia, hypotension, a new fever in a previously afebrile patient, or leukocytosis with a previously normal white blood cell count. Because the rate of perforation in these patients can be as high as 50 per cent, intensive medical management of toxic megacolon should not continue beyond 3 days in the patient who is not showing signs of improvement.

■ TIMING OF SURGERY

Some surgeons argue that toxic megacolon is a surgical emergency and that medical management should be limited to preoperative correction of fluid and electrolyte deficiencies in preparation for surgery.[7,21] A great number of patients in whom toxic megacolon develops will require surgery eventually for control of their colitis. Nevertheless, a trial of maximal medical management is warranted, with surgery reserved for the cases of unsuccessful medical management. Aggressive medical therapy is recommended particularly in the patient who presents with toxic megacolon as the first manifestation of the colitis.[6,12,20] Certain conditions are strong indications for immediate surgery. These include (1) persistent or progressive dilatation of the colon despite supportive therapy, even though the clinical signs of toxicity have abated, (2) signs of perforation of the colon, and (3) uncontrollable hemorrhage from the colon.[8,11,24]

■ SURGICAL TREATMENT

The choice of operation depends on the severity of the clinical illness. In general, a cecostomy or a completely diverting ileostomy alone is probably inadequate surgical treatment.[4] A single-stage proctocolectomy is too extensive an operation for a critically ill patient, carrying a mortality rate of 14 to 30 per cent.[4] The best procedure is a total or subtotal colectomy with an end ileostomy and mucous fistula, the Hartman procedure.[4,6] This procedure will enable the surgeon to reoperate at a later date and perform an ileoanal anastomosis. In deciding to perform surgery for toxic megacolon not responsive to medical management, the etiology of the colitis is not necessarily important. The various procedures are the same for toxic megacolon due to Crohn's colitis or ulcerative colitis. However, long-term results and prognosis are not the same, as ulcerative colitis will be cured by total proctocolectomy but Crohn's colitis may not.

■ PROGNOSIS

The outcome of therapy may be affected by certain factors. These include the age of the patient, the timing of surgery, and the incidence of perforation.[25] Patients under 40 years of age do better. Likewise, elective colectomy after stabilization of the disease carries a mortality rate of 5 to 10 per cent, whereas emergency surgery performed within the first few days of medical treatment carries a mortality of 20 to 50 per cent.[9,19] This is particularly true when surgery is performed because of perforation. Patients who are successfully treated medically and who do not require surgery during the initial hospitalization have a low mortality rate, about 2 per cent.[9,12,19] Death in these patients frequently is due to pulmonary emboli.[12]

About 50 per cent of patients with toxic megacolon will respond to the initial medical treatment; the remainder will require surgical intervention during the hospitalization because of a perforation or the inability to control the colitis. It is therefore extremely important for the physician to identify those patients who will require emergency surgery. The physician should realize that patients with toxic megacolon have a more severe form of colitis, and that 60 per cent of the patients who avoid surgery with the initial episode of toxic megacolon will require hospitalization for fulminant colitis or toxic megacolon with 1 year and may require surgery at that time.[21,24]

REFERENCES

1. Marshak RH, Lester LJ, Friedman Al. Megacolon: a complication of ulcerative colitis. Gastroenterology 1950; 16:768-772.
2. Brown CH, Ferrante WA, Davis WD. Toxic dilatation of the colon complicating pseudomembranous enterocolitis. Am J Dig Dis 1968; 13:813-821.
3. Burke GW, Wilson ME, Mehrez IO. Absence of diarrhea in toxic megacolon complicating *Clostridium difficile* pseudomembranous colitis. Am J Gastroenterol 1988; 83:304-307.
4. Grieco MB, Bordan DL, Geiss AC, Beil AR. Toxic megacolon complicating Crohn's colitis. Ann Surg 1980; 191:75-80.
5. Cunsolo A, Bragaglia RB, Arena N, et al. Toxic megacolon complicating ulcerative colitis and Crohn's disease. Int Surg 1985; 70:339-343.
6. Huizenga KA, Schroeder KW. Gastrointestinal complications of ulcerative colitis and Crohn's. In Kirsner JB, Shorter RG (eds). Inflammatory Bowel Disease. Philadelphia: Lea & Febiger, 1988: 269-275.
7. Grant CS, Dozois RR. Toxic megacolon: ultimate fate of patients after successful medical management. Am J Surg 1984; 147:106-110.
8. Harlong WA, Arvanitakis C, Skibba RM, Klotz AP. Treatment of toxic megacolon. A comparative review of 29 patients. Am J Dig Dis 1977; 22:195-200.
9. Roys G, Kaplan MS, Juler GL. Surgical management of toxic megacolon. Am J Gastroenterol 1977; 68:161-163.
10. Chare MJB, Aubrey DA. Management of toxic megacolon. Br J Clin Prac 1982; 36:175-180.
11. Heppell J, Farkouh E, Dube S, et al. Toxic megacolon. An analysis of 70 cases. Dis Colon Rectum 1986; 29:789-792.
12. Present DH. Management of toxic megacolon. In Korelitz BI, Sohn N (eds). Inflammatory Bowel Disease: Experience and Controversy. New York: Grune & Stratton, 1985:217-222.
13. Present DH. Fulminant colitis and toxic megacolon. In Bayless TM (ed). Current Therapy in Gastroenterology and Liver Disease-2. Toronto, Philadelphia: BC Decker, 1986:284-291.
14. Reddy KR, Thomas E. Toxic megacolon after proctosigmoidoscopy in ulcerative colitis. South Med J 1983; 76:1072-1073.
15. Goldberg HI. The barium enema and toxic megacolon: cause-effect relationship (correspondence)? Gastroenterology 1975; 68:617-618.
16. Wruble LD, Bronstein MW. Toxic dilatation of the colon following barium enema examination during the quiescent stage of chronic ulcerative colitis. Am J Dig Dis 1968; 13:918-923.
17. Becker IM. Pregnancy and toxic dilatation of the colon. Am J Dig Dis 1972; 17:79-84.
18. Cooksey G, Gunn A, Witherspoon WC. Surgery for acute ulcerative colitis and toxic megacolon during pregnancy. Br J Surg 1985; 72:547.
19. Thomford NR. Toxic megacolon. Surg Annu 1980; 12:341-350.
20. Present DH. Fulminant colitis. In Bayless TM (ed). Current Management of Inflammatory Bowel Disease. Toronto, Philadelphia: BC Decker, 1989:82-86.
21. Adams JT. Toxic dilatation of the colon. A surgical disease. Arch Surg 1973; 106:673-682.
22. Meyer S, Janowitz HD. The place of steroids in the therapy of toxic megacolon. Gastroenterology 1978; 75:729-731.
23. Meyers S, Sachar DB, Goldberg JD, Janowitz HD. Corticotropin versus hydrocortisone in the intravenous treatment of ulcerative colitis. Gastroenterology 1983; 85:351-357.
24. Soyer MT, Aldrete JS. Surgical treatment of toxic megacolon and proposal for a program of therapy. Am J Surg 1980; 140:421-425.
25. Greenstein AJ, Sachar DB, Gibas A, et al. Outcome of toxic dilatation in ulcerative and Crohn's colitis. J Clin Gastroenterol 1985; 7:137-144.

Transient ischemic attacks

John B. Chawluk

The major challenge to physicians treating transient ischemic attacks (TIAs) is to select therapies with *proven* efficacy in improving the natural history of the disease process. Difficulties in management stem from the dearth of rigorous therapeutic trials and the relatively high risks of some therapeutic alternatives. Aspirin has been shown to reduce the risk of stroke and death after TIA, although this effect is less apparent in women than in men. Other pharmacologic measures for stroke prevention after TIA have been less well studied. Even more controversial is the role of carotid endarterectomy in the treatment of TIA. Though intuitively logical, this procedure has never been proved to alter natural history in a carefully designed randomized study and is associated at times with unacceptably high morbidity and mortality rates.

Stroke is the third leading cause of death in the United States.[1] TIAs precede at least 10 per cent of all strokes and over 50 per cent of carotid territory strokes associated with carotid artery stenosis.[2] These statistics emphasize the need for an informed and rational approach to TIA management *now*, despite the current paucity of sound clinical research data.

■ Background

A TIA is, by definition, temporary (less than 24 hours) focal neurologic dysfunction resulting from a reduction in cerebral blood flow so that metabolic demands in a given brain region are not met. This definition of TIA was established before the modern era of x-ray computed tomographic (CT) and magnetic resonance (MR) scanning. A time window of 24 hours was therefore imposed, based on expectations of histopathologic infarction if ischemia were to persist longer than a day. A typical TIA lasts most commonly for minutes, although in some cases symptoms may last for hours. Sensitive neuroimaging techniques may demonstrate permanent tissue damage (infarction) in individuals who otherwise meet clinical criteria for TIA. This subgroup has not been separately considered in treatment studies and will be considered here to be representative of the more typical TIA population (no neuroimaging evidence for completed infarction).

■ TYPES OF TIA

An understanding of the several subtypes of TIA and various etiologic factors is essential to rational management. Amaurosis fugax is a form of TIA in which the retina is ischemic, as opposed to ischemia of actual brain tissue. Its recognition as a form of TIA is important for several reasons. Since the ophthalmic artery is an end-vessel from the internal carotid artery, thromboembolic events affecting the retina may also affect the ipsilateral cerebral hemisphere. The incidence of internal carotid artery disease and subsequent stroke is higher in patients with amaurosis fugax compared with a matched population without it. However, the risk of subsequent stroke in amaurosis fugax patients is lower than in individuals with transient cerebral ischemia.

Anterior circulation TIA refers to cerebral ischemia in the distributions of the anterior and middle cerebral arteries. These vessels are supplied by the internal carotid artery. Posterior circulation TIA is due to occlusive phenomena in the distribution of the vertebral and basilar arteries, which feed vessels supplying flow to the brain stem, cerebellum, occipital lobes, thalamus, and mesial temporal lobes. Because of differences in bulk flow patterns, vessel caliber, surgical accessibility, and the nature of the TIA symptoms, approaches to management may differ. For instance, one may be reluctant to administer anticoagulant drugs to a patient whose posterior circulation TIAs are manifested by vertigo and drop attacks that could expose the patient to risks from serious falls. Surgical approaches to vertebrobasilar disease are limited and experimental, whereas carotid endarterectomy is a widely practiced procedure. Posterior circulation events may be more commonly related to sluggish flow in small caliber perforating vessels, suggesting a possible theoretic advantage to hemorrheologic agents (e.g., pentoxifylline [Trental]).

Crescendo TIA, analogous to crescendo angina, is defined as episodes of stereotypical TIA increasing in frequency, severity, and duration. The implication is that these patients may be at particularly high risk of imminent stroke and should be managed differently from ordinary TIA sufferers.

■ CAUSES OF TIA

A useful etiologic classification of TIA from a therapeutic vantage considers TIA due to (1) cardiac embolization; (2) medium caliber artery (e.g., internal carotid artery or vertebrobasilar) atherosclerotic changes, with embolization to the brain or downstream hypoperfusion related to hemodynamic factors; and (3) arteriosclerotic disease in smaller, penetrating intracranial vessels. Consideration of these mechanisms helps the physician decide among surgical, antiplatelet, anticoagulant, and hemorrheologic modalities.

■ Management

■ DIAGNOSTIC CONSIDERATIONS

Diagnostic studies should (1) help determine the cause for the TIA (brain CT or MR scan, carotid duplex Doppler ultrasound, electrocardiogram); (2) identify risk factors for vascular disease (fasting lipids and glucose, sedimentation rate, syphilis serology, prothrombin time [PT], and partial thromboplastin time [PTT]); (3) identify factors that could predispose to prolonged ischemia and subsequent infarction (serum glucose, hematocrit determination, platelet count); and (4) provide baseline data for monitoring therapies (CT/MR scan, duplex ultrasound, PT/PTT, hematocrit, platelet count). These basic investigations will be obtained in most

TIA patients and offer very little risk. Other studies may be performed based upon results from the initial tests. These include Holter monitor, echocardiogram with or without cardiac Doppler examination, cerebrospinal fluid examination, tests for coagulopathies, transcranial Doppler examination, and angiography. A search for less common causes of cerebral ischemia (e.g., vasculitis, hyperviscosity syndromes) may be warranted in unusual cases, especially in young patients with no apparent cerebrovascular risk factors.

■ GENERAL PRINCIPLES

Physicians treating TIA patients often overreact to elevations in systemic blood pressure (BP).[3] Hypertension accelerates atherosclerosis and arteriosclerosis, but this is a long-term effect and not relevant to the acute management of cerebral ischemia. Hypertensive encephalopathy is a rare cerebrovascular disorder manifested by focal neurologic symptoms and signs, seizures, mental status changes, funduscopic abnormalities, ischemic electrocardiogram (ECG) changes, and renal abnormalities (BUN, creatinine, urinary sediment). This is usually easily distinguished from an ordinary TIA. There are no other neurologic reasons to lower the blood pressure acutely in a TIA patient (unless the patient is to be fully anticoagulated; see later discussion). Acute elevation of BP during and after a TIA is a homeostatic response to focal cerebral hypoperfusion. Measures taken to counteract this protective mechanism may cause a stroke rather than prevent it. In general, one should not treat hypertension in the setting of acute cerebral ischemia if the BP is less than 200/120. This depends, however, on the prior hypertensive history and evidence for other significant acute end-organ dysfunction (heart, kidney). A blood pressure of over 200/120 may also be treated safely with bed rest alone, although cautious use of short-acting antihypertensive agents may be considered, initially lowering the mean BP by no more than 20 per cent.

TIA and carotid artery disease are being recognized increasingly as important harbingers of coronary artery disease. The cardiac morbidity and mortality after TIA are at least as great as the risk of fatal and nonfatal stroke. A TIA, therefore, should provoke the same evaluation for coronary artery disease that would be called for if the patient presented with angina pectoris.

Other general management principles concern the prompt correction of medical conditions made apparent by the initial diagnostic evaluation. The TIA patient should be kept well-hydrated; if diuretics are leading to volume depletion, they should be discontinued temporarily when possible, until specific TIA therapy has been established. There is evidence to suggest that the presence of hyperglycemia at the time of cerebral ischemia may predispose to more severe tissue damage.[4] Therefore, attempts should be made to maintain a normoglycemic state as strictly as possible. Polycythemia should be promptly treated with isovolemic phlebotomy. Hypercoagulable or thrombocytotic states should be corrected. Appropriate steps should be taken to ameliorate hyperviscosity states (e.g., plasmapheresis), depending on the underlying cause. Vasculitis due to collagen vascular disorders should be identified and treated with high-dose corticosteroids (60 mg or more of prednisone a day or dose equivalent). Central nervous system syphilis should be treated with high-dose intravenous penicillin G, 2 to 4 million units every 4 hours, for 14 to 21 days, followed by intramuscular benzathine penicillin G, 2.4 million units weekly for three doses.

Cerebral ischemia in young adults needs brief mention. The possibility of drug abuse should be thoroughly investigated, especially use of sympathomimetic agents (e.g., cocaine, amphetamines, phenylpropranolamine in diet pills or cold preparations). In general, women taking oral contraceptives should discontinue these medications. Although the thromboembolic risks are small, especially with lower estrogen–containing preparations, a warning TIA in an oral contraceptive user without other cause for cerebral ischemia may implicate the contraceptives etiologically. Somewhat paradoxically, there is no evidence to suggest increased thromboembolism in middle-aged or older women using conjugated estrogen preparations.

 THERAPEUTIC OPTIONS

Antiplatelet Therapy. Aspirin (ASA) has been the best studied and most convincingly effective therapy for TIA to date. The optimal antiplatelet dose of ASA in vivo has not been determined. A recent large multicenter trial of ASA in TIA reported no difference in benefits between 325 mg daily and 650 mg BID.[5] Adverse effects were significantly reduced at the lower dosage. Since even lower dosages have not been adequately evaluated, the current recommended ASA dose for stroke prophylaxis is 325 mg daily. For patients with gastric intolerance to this dose of ordinary ASA, enteric-coated products can be used.

The effectiveness of ASA therapy in women is not as apparent as in men, most likely due to the lower morbidity (stroke) and mortality rates in female patients at risk for stroke. Clinical trials, therefore, require very large numbers of female patients in order to demonstrate statistically significant benefits. Nevertheless, studies such as those of Bousser and colleagues have demonstrated such benefits of ASA in women at risk for stroke. Based on current data, a dose for women of 325 mg daily is also reasonable.

Dipyridamole (Persantine) has been tested in combination with ASA for stroke prevention after TIA and has never been shown to enhance significantly the salutary effects of ASA alone.[6] A possible remaining role for dipyridamole in treating cerebral ischemia may be for the small group of patients with nontissue prosthetic heart valves who continue to have cerebral embolic events while receiving ASA and warfarin sodium (Coumadin).

Brief mention should be made of ticlopidine hydrochloride, a drug that may soon be available for stroke prophylaxis in the United States. A very recent multicenter trial indicates that ticlopidine is more effective than ASA in lowering mortality and subsequent stroke rates in patients with TIA or minor stroke.[7] This effect, most likely from inhibition of fibrinogen binding and platelet aggregation, appears to extend equally to men and women, suggesting a further advantage over ASA. Gastric complications are substantially less with ticlopidine. An important adverse effect with ticlopidine, however, is reversible neutropenia, occurring in close to 1 per cent of treated patients.

Anticoagulant Therapy. The use of anticoagulant therapy in ischemic cerebrovascular disease has long been a subject of controversy, related to the limitations of early studies (high anticoagulant dosages, CT technology not yet available) and the potential risk of anticoagulant drugs. An excellent review of this literature to 1977 concluded that the values of anticoagulants in TIA remained unproved.[8] Several studies since 1979 have examined the benefit of anticoagulants versus ASA in TIAs.[9] Although various aspects of these studies are open to criticism, the conclusions are worth citing: (1) both ASA and anticoagulants appear to reduce the risk of cerebral infarction after TIA (although the evidence is stronger in support of ASA); (2) the risk of *serious* hemorrhagic complications is greater with anticoagulants; and (3) the incidence of other side effects, especially gastrointestinal intolerance, is greater with ASA. Most neurologists and other physicians treating TIA (*except* TIA due to cardiac embolization) would therefore use ASA rather than Coumadin.

There appears to be a distinct role, however, for anticoagulants in the treatment of TIA caused by embolus from the heart. This is most commonly seen with atrial fibrillation and until 10 to 20 years ago was frequently in association with rheumatic heart disease. There is very little controversy regarding the use of chronic anticoagulation in patients with cerebral ischemia, rheumatic heart disease, and atrial fibrillation. The risk of recurrent cerebral ischemia in rheumatic heart disease and atrial fibrillation is approximately 10 per cent a year and appears to be independent of other clinical factors, such as left atrial size, presence of atrial thrombus, chronicity of the atrial fibrillation, and so on.[10] An oft-cited complication rate from chronic anticoagulation is 5 per cent per year, with serious or fatal complications at 1 per cent per year.[11] Even these data are not secure, however. A recent review suggests a complication range of 2 to 22 per cent per year of major bleeding and 2 to 9 per cent per year of fatal bleeding.[12] This same review also emphasizes another important point. Confusion over reagents used to measure prothrombin time (PT) (rabbit brain thromboplastin verus human brain thromboplastin) has led to confusion over the appropriate therapeutic range for the PT. Initial attempts at stroke prophylaxis with Coumadin should aim at a PT of 1.3 to 1.5 times the control value, rather than the traditional goal of 2 to 2.5 times baseline PT. Using these guidelines, the potential benefit of chronic Coumadin therapy in rheumatic heart disease and atrial fibrillation (a stroke reduction rate of at least 50 per cent[13]) uld outweigh the risks. The risk of cere-

bral hemorrhage is increased in the presence of extreme hypertension, and care should be taken to lower the blood pressure to at least 190/110 before beginning anticoagulants.

Less certain is the risk:benefit ratio of chronic anticoagulation after TIA in patients with nonrheumatic atrial fibrillation. (Also see article on pages 100–106.) This is the most common cardiac cause of cerebral embolism. Considerable data suggest that these patients are at greater risk for stroke compared with the general population. No data are available, however, that define an optimal therapy. A preliminary comparison of nonrheumatic atrial fibrillation patients with and without anticoagulant treatment showed no differences in morbidity or mortality between the two groups.[14] Until a well-designed prospective study of anticoagulation in nonrheumatic atrial fibrillation has been performed, a reasonable approach to management of TIAs in these patients would be to use ASA (325 mg daily) initially and consider low-dose Coumadin (PT of 1.3 to 1.5 times baseline) if recurrent cerebral ischemia occurs. Although theoretically one might not expect antiplatelet drugs to be effective against atrial clot, they are empirically effective in venous thrombosis, in which similar mechanisms are operative.

TIA after a recent myocardial infarction (MI) may very well be due to ventricular (mural) thrombus, even when not demonstrable by echocardiography. In this instance only a short course of anticoagulation should be necessary, since the incidence of stroke more than 3 months post-MI drops off precipitously. Pending the diagnostic evaluation outlined earlier, a recent MI patient with a TIA should be started on intravenous heparin (bolus of 5000 units, followed by infusion pump administration of 800 to 1200 units/hr, depending on patient size), aiming for a partial thromboplastin time (PTT) of 1.5 to 2.0 times baseline. Coumadin therapy can be initiated simultaneously and the heparin discontinued when the PT is in the desired range (1.3 to 1.5 times control value). After 3 months of full anticoagulant therapy, the patient can be switched to ASA, 325 mg daily.

The management of TIA in patients with dilated cardiomyopathy is similarly empiric, with a probable role for full anticoagulation. (Also see article on pages 132–137.) The risk of chronic anticoagulation in such individuals may be quite high, given the possibility of global cerebral hypoperfusion, syncope, falls, and so on. Nevertheless, the risk of stroke after TIA is also high, especially in the presence of demonstrable ventricular thrombus by echocardiography. Although no controlled studies have been performed, the high risk of recurrent embolization has led to the general use of chronic anticoagulation in these patients.[10] Again, caution must be exercised in monitoring for bleeding and avoiding overanticoagulation.

The one cardiac source for cerebral emboli in which antiplatelet drugs are the logical first choice is mitral valve prolapse. The etiology of cerebral ischemia (most commonly TIA) in patients with mitral valve prolapse appears to be related to platelet-fibrin deposition on myxomatously degenerated valves. The percentage of individuals with mitral valve prolapse and cerebral ischemic events is relatively small, and no large studies of stroke prophylaxis in these patients have been performed. Several small series have indicated a possible benefit of ASA in reducing stroke risk from mitral valve prolapse.[15] On this basis, patients with TIA found to have mitral valve prolapse should be treated with ASA, 325 mg daily.

Another possible role for anticoagulant therapy is in the treatment of *crescendo TIA*. The use of anticoagulation in this setting is empiric, since no adequate studies are available. A recent report suggests a high incidence of carotid stenosis of greater than 75 per cent, with or without deep plaque ulceration, in a select group of patients with frequent anterior circulation TIAs.[16] Very little harm is likely to occur with well-monitored short-term heparin therapy in patients without contraindications, although they must be observed closely for the development of heparin-induced thrombocytopenia (see later discussion). Immediate anticoagulation in this setting may buy time while antiplatelet drugs are taking effect and the diagnostic evaluation is underway. If the patient is already on antiplatelet agents when the flurry of TIAs takes place, full heparinization may provide additional benefit while a more permanent course of action is developed.

Physicians treating cerebrovascular ischemia with heparin must not forget the risk of iatrogenic thrombosis caused by heparin-induced thrombocytopenia.[17] A baseline platelet count should be obtained before initiating heparin therapy, and the platelet count should be followed on a daily basis. If the platelet count drops by 30 per cent, heparin should be discontinued.

Hemorrheologic Agents. Viscosity is one of the three major factors affecting flow through vessels (in addition to pulse pressure and vessel caliber). Modification of blood viscosity to improve flow through arterial stenoses, thus improving cerebral circulation, makes intuitive sense. The only currently available oral agent in the United States for lowering blood viscosity is pentoxifylline (PTX) (Trental). No large controlled studies of use of this drug after TIA have been performed. Preliminary data indicate a reduction in stroke and TIA with pentoxifylline compared with ASA.[18] Since dipyridamole *has* been well studied and shown not to be effective in preventing recurrent cerebral ischemia, pentoxifylline 400 mg orally TID, should be considered instead, as an adjunct to antiplatelet therapy with ASA. In theory, this agent might be particularly useful in posterior circulation TIAs, especially those involving the brainstem, where smaller caliber perforating vessels may be affected; and in patients with diabetes or hypertension, in whom small vessel arteriosclerosis appears to underlie the cerebral ischemic event. The major side effects of pentoxifylline are gastrointestinal (nausea, eructation, heartburn), and can be reduced by lowering the dose to 400 mg once or twice daily as necessary.

Carotid Endarterectomy (CEA). Thirty-five years after the procedure was first performed, the role for endarterectomy in stroke prophylaxis has yet to be defined. The apparent logic, elegance, and value of this procedure in TIA patients who subsequently never suffer another cerebral ischemic event cannot be denied. One must temper these instincts, however, recalling that over a 5-year period the risk of stroke in unselected *untreated* TIA patients is less than 50 per cent! The variability of natural history in subgroups of TIA patients and the wide range of reported surgical outcomes lead to considerable uncertainty about the true efficacy of carotid endarterectomy. A full discussion of these issues is well beyond the scope of this article.[19,20] Several national and international multicenter trials of carotid endarterectomy in TIA and asymptomatic carotid stenosis are ongoing. Pending results from these studies, certain general guidelines regarding the use of carotid endarterectomy can be proposed:

- It should be performed only on arteries supplying the ischemic vascular territory.

TABLE 1. Current Treatments for TIA

Treatment	Status	Indication	Major Risks	Comments	Dose
aspirin (ASA)	P	Noncardiogenic TIA, mitral valve prolapse	Gastrointestinal (GI) hemorrhage, allergic reactions	Enteric-coated preparations may be better tolerated	325 mg QD
pentoxifylline (PTX) (Trental)	U	Adjunct to ASA; small vessel disease	None (GI intolerance)	Lower dose (QD, BID) if TID not tolerated	400 mg TID
ticlopidine HCl	E	Noncardiogenic TIA, ? other TIA	Neutropenia (reversible)	As opposed to ASA, equally effective in women and men; expensive ($1–2 QD)	250 mg BID
heparin	U	Initial treatment of cardiogenic TIA,* crescendo TIA	Major hemorrhage, thrombocytopenia with thrombosis	5–7 day course; infusion pump; daily platelet counts	PTT 1.5–2.0 times control
sodium warfarin (Coumadin)	U	Cardiogenic TIA,* ? other TIA	Major hemorrhage (>4 per cent per yr risk)	Well-tolerated	PT 1.3–1.5 times control
carotid endarterectomy	S	TIA in territory of stenosed artery	Arteriographic and surgical (stroke, death, myocardial infarction)	Certain TIA subgroups likely to benefit most	—

*Except mitral valve prolapse.
P = proved effective in large, well-controlled trials.
U = uncertain; data support efficacy but further studies needed.
E = experimental; promising preliminary data, US availability likely soon.
S = under study; multicenter trials ongoing.

This can be determined clinically, angiographically, or by Doppler studies.

- With stenoses of less than 80 per cent diameter reduction, it should be reserved for TIA patients who fail medical therapy (ASA with or without pentoxifylline).
- In patients with TIA and carotid stenosis of 80 to 90 per cent, it can be reserved for those patients who demonstrate progressive stenosis on noninvasive testing repeated at 3- to 6-month intervals. Transcranial Doppler testing is a new, noninvasive technique that can provide valuable information regarding adequacy of collateral channels.[21] This may aid in identifying patients at increased risk of stroke (abnormal intracranial hemodynamics, insufficient collateral flow) who may benefit from it.
- The combined short-term (under 3 months) risk of arteriography and carotid endarterectomy (based upon institutional audit) should be 5 per cent or less.
- Special caution should be exercised when considering it in TIA patients with poorly controlled medical conditions (diabetes, hypertension, coronary artery disease), with multiple cerebral vessel involvement (carotid artery plus disease in any of the following arteries: intracranial vessels, contralateral carotid, vertebral, basilar, subclavian), or with crescendo TIAs.

Table 1 summarizes current available therapies for TIA. Treatment of TIA remains a frustrating challenge. We search diligently for more effective and less harmful interventions, while today's patient faces death or severe functional handicap. The uncertain physician at the bedside is well-advised to recall the fractured adage and "not just do something, but stand there," think, and remain informed!

REFERENCES

1. Wolf PA, Kannel WB, McGee DL. Epidemiology of strokes in North America. In Barnett HJM, Mohr JP, Stein BM, Yatsu FM (eds). Stroke: Pathophysiology, Diagnosis, and Management. New York: Churchill Livingstone, 1986:19-29.
2. Mohr JP, Pessin MS. Extracranial carotid artery dis-

ease. *In* Barnett HJM, Mohr JP, Stein BM, Yatsu FM (eds). Stroke: Pathophysiology, Diagnosis, and Management. New York: Churchill Livingstone, 1986:293-336.

3. Lavin P. Management of hypertension in patients with acute stroke. Arch Intern Med 1986; 146:66-68.

4. Helgason CM. Blood glucose and stroke. Stroke 1988; 19:1049-1053.

5. UK-TIA Study Group. United Kingdom transient ischaemic attack (UK-TIA) aspirin trial: interim results. Br Med J 1988; 296:316-320.

6. Bousser MG, Eschwege E, Haguenau M, LeFaucconnier JM, Thibult N, Touboul D, Touboul PJ. "AICLA" controlled trial of aspirin and dipyridamole in the secondary prevention of athero-thrombotic cerebral ischemia. Stroke 1983; 14:5-14.

7. Hass WK, Easton JD, Adams HP Jr, Pryse-Phillips W, Molony BA, Anderson S, Kamm B. A randomized trial comparing ticlopidine hydrochloride with aspirin for the prevention of stroke in high-risk patients. N Engl J Med 1989; 321:501–507.

8. Brust JCM. Transient ischemic attacks: natural history and anticoagulation. Neurology 1977; 27:701-707.

9. Garde A, Samuelsson K, Fahlgren H, Hedberg E, Hjerne L-G, Ostman J. Treatment after transient ischemic attacks: a comparison between anticoagulant drug and inhibition of platelet aggregation. Stroke 1983; 14:677-681.

10. Cerebral Embolism Task Force. Cardiogenic brain embolism. Arch Neurol 1986; 43:71-84.

11. Scheinberg P. Controversies in the management of cerebral vascular disease. Neurology 1988; 38:1609-1616.

12. Levine M, Hirsh J. Hemorrhagic complications of long-term anticoagulant therapy for ischemic cerebral vascular disease. Stroke 1986; 17:111-116.

13. Szekely P. Systemic embolism and anticoagulant prophylaxis in rheumatic heart disease. Br Med J 1964; 1:1209-1212.

14. Lodder J, Dennis MS, Van Raak L, Jones LN, Warlow CP. Cooperative study on the value of long-term anticoagulation in patients with stroke and non-rheumatic atrial fibrillation. Br Med J 1988; 296:1435-1438.

15. Watson RT. TIA, stroke, and mitral valve prolapse. Neurology 1979; 886–889.

16. Rothrock JF, Lyden PD, Yee J, Wiederholt WC. "Crescendo" transient ischemic attacks: clinical and angiographic correlations. Neurology 1988; 38:198-201.

17. Ramirez-Lassepas M, Cipolle RJ, Rodvold KA, Seifert RD, Strand L, Taddeini L, Cusulos M. Heparin-induced thrombocytopenia in patients with cerebrovascular ischemic disease. Neurology 1984; 34:736-740.

18. Herskovits E, Famulari A, Tamaroff L, Gonzalez AM, Vasquez A, Dominguez R, Fraiman H, Vila J. Preventive treatment of cerebral transient ischemia: comparative randomized trial of pentoxifylline versus conventional antiaggregants. Eur Neurol 1985; 24:73-81.

19. Barnett HJM, Plum F, Walton JN. Carotid endarterectomy—an expression of concern. Stroke 1984; 15:941-943.

20. Patterson RH, Jonas S, Hachinski V. Can carotid endarterectomy be justified? Arch Neurol 1987; 44:651-654.

21. DeWitt LD, Wechsler LR. Transcranial doppler. Stroke 1988; 19:915-921.

Transplantation patient, medical care of the

Morris A. Flaum ■ *Hector O. Ventura* ■ *Daniel H. Hayes* ■ *Luis A. Balart* ■ *Clifford H. Van Meter, Jr.* ■ *John L. Hussey* ■ *Julio E. Figueroa*

Organ and bone marrow transplantation have become widely accepted modes of management for a number of severe and life-threatening disorders. This article summarizes the indications and management of patients who are to undergo bone marrow, cardiac, liver, pulmonary, and renal transplantation.

■ Bone Marrow Transplantation

Bone marrow transplantation has been utilized in several broad categories of disease: bone marrow failure, immune deficiency states, storage diseases, and malignant disorders. Bone marrow for transplantation may be obtained from identical twins (syngeneic transplant), human leukocyte antigen (HLA)-identical siblings (allogeneic transplant), or the patient concerned (autologous transplant).

■ ALLOGENEIC TRANSPLANTATION

Allogeneic bone marrow transplantation has been most extensively studied in aplastic anemia, acute myelocytic anemia, acute lymphocytic leukemia, and chronic myelogenous leukemia (Table 1). Bone marrow transplantation has been demonstrated to be effective in hematologic reconstitution of patients with aplastic anemia. Bone marrow transplantation has been shown to compare favorably to androgens or supportive care, with a long-term survival rate of 57 per cent in the transplanted group.[1] Subsequent trials have indicated that immunosuppressive therapy with either antilymphocyte globulin or antithymocyte globulin may result in equivalent response and survival.[2] Alloge-

TABLE 1. Indications for Allogeneic Bone Marrow Transplantation

Bone Marrow Failure
Aplastic anemia
Fanconi's anemia
Myelodysplastic disorders
Diamond-Blackfan syndrome

Congenital Disorders
Chronic granulomatous disease
Severe combined immune deficiency disorder
Wiskott-Aldrich syndrome
Chediak-Higashi syndrome
Infantile osteopetrosis
Thalassemia
Sickle cell anemia
Storage diseases
  Gaucher's disease
  Fabry's disease
  Hurler's disease
  Hunter's disease
  Metachromatic leukodystrophy
  Sanfilippo's syndrome
  Maroteaux-Lamy syndrome
  Morquio's syndrome
  Adrenoleukodystrophy

Malignant Diseases
Acute myelogenous leukemia
Acute lymphocytic leukemia
Chronic myelogenous leukemia
Hodgkin's disease
Non-Hodgkin's lymphoma

TABLE 2. Representative Survival Results of Allogeneic Bone Marrow Transplantation Versus Chemotherapy in AML (Actual Survival at 3–5 Years)

	BMT (%)	Chemotherapy (%)
1st CR		
age < 30 yr	50–70	20–40
age > 30 yr	30–45	10–35
Initial relapse or 2nd CR	30	<10
Advanced	10–20	0

AML = acute myelogenous leukemia; BMT = bone marrow transplantation; CR = complete remission.
(Reprinted with permission from Champlin R: Acute myeologenous leukemia; biology and treatment. Mediguide Oncol 1988;8:1–9.

neic bone marrow transplantation also has been utilized extensively in patients with acute myelogenous leukemia. The optimal timing and selection criteria remain controversial. Disease-free survival has been estimated to range between 50 and 70 per cent, with a relapse rate ranging from 10 to 40 per cent. Age is a significant prognostic criterion; patients older than 30 years of age have decreased survival. In patients undergoing bone marrow transplant, superior long-term disease-free survival at 5 years (48 per cent) has been demonstrated when compared with survival of patients treated with chemotherapy alone (21 per cent).[3] A graft-versus-leukemia effect has been demonstrated by the decreased relapse rate and increased survival of patients manifesting graft-versus-host disease when compared with patients without graft-versus-host disease.[4] In patients who are not optimal candidates for bone marrow transplantation in first remission, such as patients older than age 30 years, bone marrow transplantation has been suggested in early relapse or in second complete remission (Table 2).[5]

In acute lymphocytic leukemia (ALL), the optimal benefit of allogeneic bone marrow transplantation has not been clearly defined. In children, allogeneic transplant is recommended in second or subsequent remissions, with a disease-free survival rate of 40 to 64 per cent.[6] In adult ALL, the prognosis of standard therapy remains unsatisfactory, and transplantation in first remission may be considered for adults with poor prognostic signs, such as an elevated white blood cell or blast count, B or null cell disease, presence of the Philadelphia chromosome, or prolonged period to attain remission.

Transplantation in chronic myelocytic leukemia may be curative. Disease-free survival in the chronic phase is 50 to 60 per cent, with a relapse rate of 10 to 20 per cent. Data from Seattle indicate an improved prognosis when transplantation is performed within 1 year of diagnosis.[7] Patients undergoing transplantation in more advanced stages of disease, such as blast crisis or accelerated phase, exhibit a high incidence of relapse and diminished disease-free survival.

In patients with acute leukemia or chronic myelocytic leukemia in whom an HLA-identical match is unavailable, partially mismatched or unrelated donors may be considered.

■ AUTOLOGOUS TRANSPLANTATION

Infusion of the patient's own previously stored bone marrow serves to repopulate the bone marrow after the application of myeloablative doses of radiation, chemotherapy, or both. It has found application in disorders in which there is a steep dose-response curve to chemotherapy (Table 3). This has been evaluated particularly in patients in whom the malignant disease is sensitive to the modality employed. Autologous transplantation has been extensively evaluated in the hematologic malignancies. In Hodgkin's disease, a 79 to 87 per cent response rate has been noted in patients treated with either single-agent or combination chemotherapy. Similar satisfactory responses have been noted in patients with non-Hodgkin's lymphomas.[8] Patients with minimal or responsive disease fare better than patients with extensive or refractory disease.

Autologous transplantation has been utilized in acute myelocytic leukemia with both untreated and treated bone marrow. Bone marrow may be treated with monoclonal antibodies or 4-hydroperoxycyclophosphamide. Positive responses with the use of both purged and unpurged bone marrow, especially the latter, have been noted. Eleven of 25 patients in second or third complete remission remained in complete remission after therapy with busulfan and cyclophosphamide or cyclophosphamide, total body irradiation, and infusion of bone marrow treated with 4-hydroperoxycyclophosphamide.[9]

Bone marrow from patients with acute lymphoblastic leukemia has also been reinfused either in the purged or unpurged state. Agents utilized to treat bone marrow include monoclonal antibodies, 4-hydroperoxycyclophosphamide, or mafosfamide. These trials are not conclusive but suggest a role for autologous transplantation in this disease entity.

Solid tumors demonstrate less responsiveness to chemotherapeutic agents, and therefore results with autologous transplantation have been less promising. However, children with advanced neuroblastoma have been shown to have a significantly improved survival and an overall response rate of 44 to 46 per cent when treated with autologous transplantation.[8]

Autologous bone marrow transplantation may be of benefit in the treatment of other solid tumors, including breast carcinoma, small cell lung carcinoma, glioma, testicular carcinoma, and melanoma. However, the role of this modality of therapy remains undefined. Although responses have been noted, these tend to be short-lived, and impact on survival has not been demonstrated definitively.

TABLE 3. Indications for Autologous Bone Marrow Transplantation

Effective
Acute myelogenous leukemia
Acute lymphocytic leukemia
Hodgkin's disease
Non-Hodgkin's lymphoma
Neuroblastoma

Possibly Effective
Breast carcinoma
Melanoma
Small cell lung cancer
Testicular carcinoma

■ MANAGEMENT

Graft-Versus-Host Disease (GVHD).

GVHD occurs in 25 to 70 per cent of patients undergoing allogeneic bone marrow transplantation, as a consequence of the infusion of immunocompetent T lymphocytes that recognize host antigens. Acute GVHD occurs within the first 100 days of bone marrow transplant and results in skin, liver, and gastrointestinal damage. The disease is graded according to the extent and severity of involvement of these organs (Grades I through IV). Development of GVHD results in an increased risk of fatality. Major efforts have been expended in attempts to prevent acute GVHD. The agents commonly used in its prevention are methotrexate, cyclosporine, antithymocyte globulin, and corticosteroids.

Patients with acute nonlymphoblastic leukemia in first remission or chronic myelocytic leukemia in the chronic phase who underwent allogeneic bone marrow transplantation were treated with either cyclosporine alone or a combination of cyclosporine and methotrexate. Combination therapy resulted in a decrease in the incidence and severity of GVHD and an improved actuarial survival rate.[10] Cyclosporine has also been used in combination with corticosteroids, with similar beneficial results.

An alternative method of decreasing the incidence of graft-versus-host disease has been the use of monoclonal antibody techniques to remove the immunocompetent lymphocytes. However, studies have indicated an increased incidence of graft failure and relapse of leukemia.[11]

The mainstay of therapy for graft-versus-host disease has been corticosteroids. Other agents utilized for therapy of GVHD include antithymocyte globulin, cyclosporine, thalidomide, and a monoclonal antibody linked to ricin (Xomazyme). However, therapy remains unsatisfactory, and acute GVHD continues to be a major cause of mortality in patients undergoing allogeneic transplantation.

Chronic GVHD occurs after day 100 of allogeneic transplant. The target organs are those that may be involved in acute GVHD. Skin involvement may result in the development of a scleroderma-like or lichen planus–like skin lesion. Other manifestations of chronic GVHD include hepatic, oral, ocular, and esophageal involvement. A major complication of chronic GVHD is immunoincompetence and the development of infectious complications. The mainstay of therapy for chronic GVHD has been corticosteroids with or without the addition of azathioprine. Cyclosporine and thalidomide have also shown promise in its therapy.

Infection

Infection is a common occurrence in bone marrow transplant recipients. It occurs as a consequence of profound leukopenia, disruption of skin and mucous membrane barriers, and immunosuppression. The period of aplasia may last for 3 to 4 weeks. The interruption of integrity of the skin and mucous membranes due to chemotherapy side effects and indwelling catheters provides a portal of entry for skin and enteric organisms. The organisms seen during this phase of transplantation include *Escherichia coli*, *Klebsiella pneumoniae*, *Pseudomonas aeruginosa*, *Staphylococcus aureus*, *Staphylococcus epidermidis*, and streptococci. The patient is also at risk for developing fungal infections from *Candida* and *Aspergillus* species. Attempts at decreasing the incidence of infection include the use of protective isolation, sterile or low-bacterial diets, and decontamination with oral nonabsorbable antibiotics. Prophylaxis with trimethoprim-sulfamethoxazole has been effective in decreasing the incidence of *Pneumocystis carinii* infections. Because of profound immunosuppression, fever during the granulocytopenic stage must be investigated aggressively, and broad-spectrum antibiotics should be begun empirically. A common regimen utilizes the combination of ticarcillin and clavulanate with gentamicin or tobramycin. Vancomycin is also frequently added to improve coverage for *S. epidermidis*. If the patient remains febrile and no organism is clearly identified, empiric therapy with the antifungal agent amphotericin B is recommended. Antibiotics are usually continued until granulocytopenia has resolved.

Herpes simplex may be a common cause of morbidity in patients undergoing transplant. Intravenous acyclovir (Zovirax), either prophylactically in seropositive patients or therapeutically, is effective in reducing this complication. Varicella zoster infections occur later in the post-transplant period and also should be treated with acyclovir.

Interstitial pneumonitis is a feared complication that may occur during the recovery phase. The etiologic factors implicated in the development of interstitial pneumonitis include chemotherapy, radiation therapy, and cytomegalovirus (CMV). Efforts to prevent the development of CMV interstitial pneumonitis have included the use of high-titer anti-CMV immune globulin and the use of CMV antibody-negative blood products in patients who are CMV antibody-negative. Therapy for CMV interstitial pneumonitis is suboptimal; gancyclovir is currently being investigated.

Patients with chronic GVHD remain immunocompromised and are at risk for developing infection with encapsulated organisms (*S. pneumoniae* and *H. influenzae*). The risk of infection is decreased by the continuation of prophylaxis with trimethoprim-sulfamethoxazole or penicillin.

■ SUPPORTIVE CARE

Nutritional Support. As a consequence of multiple physiologic abnormalities that result from bone marrow transplantation, nutrition is adversely affected. It is therefore critical to provide the transplant recipient with adequate nutrition to prevent superimposed morbidity and mortality due to malnutrition. Total parenteral nutrition is needed to meet the requirements of a patient undergoing transplant. Amino acid solutions provide nitrogen and result in a positive nitrogen balance. Fluids and electrolytes are required to provide adequate hydration and repletion of electrolyte losses. Dextrose and fat solutions are utilized to provide enhanced caloric intake. Fat solutions also prevent essential fatty acid deficiency. The delivery of total parenteral nutrition, as well as other intravenous fluids, has been simplified by the use of double-lumen right atrial catheters.

Blood Bank Support. Bone marrow transplant recipients require intensive transfusion support. The blood bank is called upon to provide red blood cells, platelets, and granulocytes. Blood products should be irradiated to prevent transfusion of immunocompetent lymphocytes, which may result in GVHD. To prevent hemorrhage, platelets are transfused prophylactically when the count falls below 20,000/microliter.

Optimal supportive care of a transplant patient requires the coordinated efforts of an integrated team of physicians from a number of subspecialty departments, including Infectious Disease, Gastroenterology, Pathology, Surgery, and the Blood Bank, as well as a dedicated nursing staff and a psychosocial supportive system.

■ Cardiac Transplantation

Since the report by Lower and Shumway[12] of the orthotopic heart transplantation technique and the first human-to-human heart transplant performed by Barnard in 1967,[13] major developments in cardiac transplantation have made this procedure very suitable for the treatment of end-stage cardiomyopathy.

The improvement in patient survival has been associated with improvements in the diagnosis and management of infections and the introduction of endomyocardial biopsy for the diagnosis of allograft rejection and of cyclosporine as an immunosuppressive agent.[14]

■ RECIPIENT CRITERIA

The primary reasons for referring patients for heart transplantation include very limited prognosis (life expectancy of less than 12 months) and inability to lead a satisfactory life due to physical limitations secondary to heart failure. Most of these patients are New York Heart Association functional class III or IV. Transplantation should be considered when the patient's prognosis with medical therapy is unlikely to exceed the expected survival with cardiac transplantation of approximately 80 to 90 per cent at 1 year. Recipient criteria as well as contraindications for transplantation are seen in Table 4.

■ DONOR CRITERIA

The diagnosis of brain death must be confirmed prior to donor preparation (Table 5). Because of donor shortages, the age limit for acceptability as a donor has been increased to 40 years for men and 50 years for women. In certain cases, coronary arteriography must be performed in the donor heart to rule out coronary artery disease, especially in donors who are older than 40 years of age. Of

TABLE 4. Cardiac Transplantation Recipient Criteria

1. Severe NHA Class III or IV cardiac dysfunction not controlled by medical or surgical treatment
2. Limited life expectancy, with 1-year mortality estimated to be more than 50%
3. Physiologic age less than 60 years, absolute upper limit for chronologic age 65 years
4. No systemic illness other than abnormalities related to heart failure
5. Emotional stability
6. Strong family support system.
7. Absence of the following exclusion criteria:
   a. Severe pulmonary hypertension (paraventricular nuclear stratum [PVR] more than 8 Wood units, or PVR more than 6 Wood units with failure of nitroprusside infusion to reduce PVR to below 3 or to reduce PA systolic pressure below 50 mm Hg) or transpulmonary gradient greater than 15 mm Hg
   b. Severe, irreversible hepatic, renal, or pulmonary disease
   c. Active systemic or pulmonary infection
   d. Recent pulmonary infarction
   e. Insulin-dependent diabetes
   f. History of uncontrollable hypertension
   g. Systemic vascular or cerebrovascular disease
   h. Active peptic ulcer disease
   i. History of substance abuse (including alcohol) or behavior problem

importance is the patient's history of a "significant" period of severe hypotension, high-dose inotropic requirements, or cardiac arrest.

■ DONOR-RECIPIENT MATCHING

The weight of the donor should be within 25 per cent of the body weight of the recipient. Larger donor hearts are used for patients with elevated pulmonary vascular resistance. ABO blood group compatibility is also very important, since no case of survival of an ABO-incompatible donor heart has been reported. Moreover, a donor-specific cross-

TABLE 5. Brain Death Criteria

No spontaneous respiration
Deep coma
No voluntary movement (except deep tendon reflexes)
Absence of brain stem reflexes
No depressant drugs in blood or urine
Absence of profound metabolic disorder

(Drawn from Copeland TG, Stinson EB. Human heart transplantation. Curr Prob Cardiol 1979;4:12–15.)

match is required if recipient serum is more than 5 per cent reactive to a random lymphocyte panel.

■ MANAGEMENT

Rejection. *Hyperacute rejection* of a donor heart is very uncommon, but it is likely if the recipient is found to be positive in a screening for cytotoxic antibodies. To minimize the chance of hyperacute rejection, all potential recipients with cytotoxic antibodies must have a negative lymphocyte cross-match with any potential donor heart before its acceptance.

Acute rejection remains one of the major challenges in cardiac transplantation. This type of rejection is cell mediated and can be categorized as mild, moderate, or severe. Mild acute rejection represents cellular changes associated with the appearance of perivascular and endocardial monocyte infiltrate but without myocyte necrosis. Moderate rejection poses a more extensive threat to viability of the graft. Histologically, more extensive lymphocyte infiltrate extends to all areas and is also associated with focal myocyte necrosis. However, this process is reversible if treatment is instituted immediately.

Major acute rejection episodes occur within the first 6 months of transplantation; despite improvements in immunosuppressive therapy, acute rejection remains a major cause of death within the first year of cardiac transplantation.

The development of accelerated graft atherosclerosis has been called *chronic rejection*. This process is one of the primary factors limiting survival in cardiac transplantation, and it occurs in 44 per cent of transplant recipients. The coronary disease is diffuse, with distal obliteration of the vessels.

Chronic rejection can result in congestive heart failure, myocardial infarction, or sudden death. Moreover, it can be associated with higher levels of cholesterol and low-density lipoproteins. The treatment of choice for patients with advanced transplant coronary artery disease is retransplantation, but the incidence of recurrent coronary artery disease in the second graft is very high. Since the clinical manifestations of accelerated coronary disease are not very prominent because the transplanted heart is de-

TABLE 6. Oschner Medical Institutions Immunosuppressive Protocol

Preoperative
Cyclosporine, 10 mg/kg PO 2 hr before surgery
Azathioprine, 4 mg/kg IV 2hr before surgery

Intraoperative
Methylprednisolone IV, 500 mg

Postoperative
1. Methylprednisolone, 125 mg IV 8 hr × 3 doses
   Prednisone, 1 mg/kg/day PO in 2 divided doses;
      taper 0.1 mg/kg every 48 hr until 0.3 mg/kg/day;
      0.1 mg/kg/day by 6 weeks
2. Cyclosporine
   Postoperative day 1: Initial dose: 4 mg/kg
   Postoperative day 2:
   If creatinine level is < 1.5 mg/dl: 8 mg/kg/day PO
      in 2 divided doses
   If creatinine level is 1.5–2.0 mg/dl: 5 mg/kg/day PO
      in 2 divided doses
   If creatinine level is > 2.0 mg/dl: hold cyclosporine
   Maintenance dose: 4 mg/kg/day
   Check serum levels: 200–300 units first 6 wk post-
      transplant, 100-200 units thereafter
3. Azathioprine
   Give 2 mg/kg PO once daily
   Adjust dose according to WBC/mm³; aim for WBC
      of approximately 5000

nervated and therefore chest pain is not present, annual cardiac catheterization is indicated to facilitate the diagnosis.

Immunosuppression. The immunosuppressive protocol utilized at the Ochsner Medical Institutions, which consists of a combination of cyclosporine, azathioprine, and methylprednisolone, is shown in Tables 6 and 7. The introduction of OKT 3, a monoclonal antibody directed against the T_3 receptor of T cells, is a significant advance in the treatment of allograft rejection.[15] It can be used to treat refractory cardiac allograft

TABLE 7. Ochsner Medical Institutions Treatment of Acute Rejection

Mild Acute Rejection
Methylprednisolone, 1 gm IV daily × 3 days
Prednisone, 1 mg/kg/day PO in 2 divided doses × 2
   days and then tapered to 0.1 mg/kg/day
Biopsy: 48 hours after methylprednisolone completed

Moderate Acute Rejection
Hospitalize
Methylprednisolone, 1 gm IV daily × 3 days
Rebiopsy before tapering methylprednisolone
If biopsy reveals ongoing rejection, begin OKT 3, 5
   mg IV daily × 10–14 days

Severe Acute Rejection
Methylprednisolone, 1 gm IV daily × 3 days or/and
   OKT 3, 5 mg IV daily × 10–14 days

rejection and, in some institutions, has replaced antithymocyte globulin (ATG) in the early post-transplant period. The adverse reactions associated with OKT 3 are self-limited and do not require discontinuation of the drug.

Diagnosis of Graft Rejection. The use of routine endomyocardial biopsy to diagnose allograft rejection has changed the survival rates in cardiac transplant patients, since the histologic changes of acute rejection appear before the patient develops clinical signs of rejection. This procedure usually is performed early in the course of heart transplantation, when the likelihood of rejection is greatest. Clinical findings associated with acute graft rejection are those of congestive heart failure (dyspnea on exertion, decline in exercise tolerance, jugular venous distention, and S3 gallop).

Infection. Mediastinitis may occur. The cause is usually bacterial (*S. aureus* or *S. epidermidis*) or fungal.

Infection with *Toxoplasma* should be considered in patients with fever of unknown origin. Toxoplasmosis can be a primary disease that is reactivated, or it may be transferred from the donor heart. Treatment with sulfadiazine and pyrimethamine is usually successful. Coccidioidomycosis usually can be treated successfully with amphotericin B. Infections with *Nocardia* and *P. carinii* are associated with fever and pulmonary infiltrates; lung biopsy is often required for diagnosis. *Nocardia* infection is treated with sulfadiazine or minocycline, whereas *Pneumocystis* infection is treated with pentamidine or trimethoprim-sulfamethoxazole.

Cytomegalovirus is the most common infection occurring in heart transplant recipients today. Clinically, it can be associated with fever, epigastric discomfort, sepsis, pulmonary infiltrates, or hepatitis. Biopsy of pulmonary infiltrates or liver biopsy confirms the diagnosis. The standard treatment is gancyclovir.[16]

■ Liver Transplantation

The management of a patient who has undergone liver transplantation has evolved extensively since the first liver transplant was done by Dr. Thomas Starzl in 1963.[17] The ensuing decades have seen a steady rise in survival figures, from a 1-year survival of

TABLE 8. Indications for Liver Transplantation

Chronic active hepatitis
Sclerosing cholangitis
Primary biliary cirrhosis
Fulminant and subacute hepatic necrosis
Primary hepatic neoplasms
Metabolic disorders
Hepatic veno-occlusive disease (Budd-Chiari syndrome)
Laennec cirrhosis (inactive)
Biliary atresia
Polycystic disease
Failed prior liver transplant

20 per cent to a 1-year survival of 80 per cent today.

This improvement in patient survival is due to many factors: refinement of the surgical technique, particularly with the use of the veno-venous bypass pump; development of newer and better immunosuppresive drugs, such as cyclosporine; better anesthetic and critical care management; the aggressive use of percutaneous biopsy for the diagnosis of rejection; and better understanding and control of infectious processes that invade these patients.

Proper patient selection equates to successful postoperative outcome. The indications for liver transplantation have been expanding rapidly over the past decade. The accepted indications for liver transplantation are found in Table 8. The contraindications and relative contraindications to liver transplantation can be found in Table 9. Many controversial indications for liver transplantation must be evaluated individually by the transplant team. One of these

TABLE 9. Contraindications to Liver Transplantation

Absolute Contraindications
Systemic sepsis
Extrahepatic malignancy
Acute drug or alcohol abuse
Advanced cardiopulmonary disease
Uncorrectable congenital anomalies
HIV positivity

Relative Contraindications
Age greater than 60 years
Irreversible renal failure
Prior extensive biliary or right upper quadrant surgery
Portal vein thrombosis
Hepatitis B surface antigen, positive state
Major psychosocial disorders
Diabetes mellitus

TABLE 10. Surgical Complications of Liver Transplantation

Postoperative hemorrhage
Biliary complications
   Early bile leak and late bile duct stricture (intrahepatic and anastomotic)
Hepatic artery thrombosis
Portal vein stenosis

controversial indications is metastatic hepatic malignancy.[18] Postoperative management of a liver transplant recipient is medically oriented. Surgical intervention in the postoperative period is related to specific surgical complications, the most common of which are found in Table 10.

■ MANAGEMENT

Nutrition. Essentially all patients with chronic end-stage liver disease are malnourished. Malnutrition leads to delayed wound healing and metabolic derangements in the postoperative period. Early in the postoperative period, all patients are placed on enteral or parenteral nutrition. This regimen is used also in patients who were in a normal nutritional state preoperatively (those with acute hepatic failure). Specific metabolic problems that are commonly seen are hypernatremia, hyperkalemia (secondary to blood tranfusion), and metabolic alkalosis (blood transfusion). Other metabolic derangements can be seen as the result of specific complications.

Renal Function. All patients are on low-dose dopamine (2 to 5 μg/kg/min) to maximize renal function. Close scrutiny is paid to renal dysfunction, which can be secondary to multiple potential nephrotoxic events and drugs. Common causes of renal dysfunction include aminoglycoside antibiotics, cyclosporine, and intraoperative events such as venovenous bypass, clamping of the inferior vena cava, and hemodynamic instability.

Immunosuppression. The immunosuppression regimen consists of triple-drug maintenance therapy. Steroids are given intravenously for the first week and are then tapered. The rapidity of the steroid taper depends upon the immunologic acceptance of the allograft. Patients who experience early rejection episodes will receive higher-dose steroids for longer periods, whereas patients who have no evidence of graft rejection or minimal rejection can be tapered more rapidly.

Azathioprine is given in a dose of 1.5 to 2 mg/kg/day, depending upon bone marrow response. The most common side effects of azathioprine, which require either discontinuance of the medication or a reduced dose, are leukopenia, thrombocytopenia, and infection

Cyclosporine is given intravenously in the early postoperative period until intestinal bile concentrations are sufficient for the adequate absorption and maintenance of cyclosporine levels. Cyclosporine is a liquid in an oil-based carrier; therefore, intraluminal bile is necessary for gastrointestinal absorption. Intravenous cyclosporine is used for approximately 1 to 2 weeks postoperatively. Intravenous cyclosporine can be given by continuous infusion, starting at 2 mg/hr and increasing to 5 to 7 mg/hr, to maintain a random whole blood cyclosporine level of 200 ng/dl.

The side effects of cyclosporine are multiple. The most common and problematic are nephrotoxicity and hypertension. Table 11 lists the various side effects of cyclosporine.[19,20]

Triple immunosuppressive therapy allows for the use of lower cyclosporine doses than combination cyclosporine with steroids only. As a result of the lower dose of cyclosporine, the complications of this drug are reduced and are more easily manageable.

Rejection. The timing of rejection has been the most important advance of liver transplantation. The use of percutaneous liver biopsy in the post-transplant period is essential. Most transplant centers have adopted the use of routine protocol biopsy, which is usually done on a weekly basis for the first 3 to 4 weeks following transplantation. Thereafter, biopsies are performed at select intervals and during times of suspected rejection or to evaluate significant biochemical abnormalities.

Protocol biopsy allows for the histologic examination of the allograft. Obtaining specimens of the hepatic parenchyma, central veins, and portal tracts allows one to determine the overall function of liver and detect subclinical rejection.

The hallmark of the treatment of rejection is bolus steroid therapy. Steroid-resistant rejection is treated by monoclonal antibody therapy (OKT 3).

Infection. Infectious complications in hepatic allograft recipients are multiple. Bacterial infections arise from the same sources as would be expected in any critically ill patient postoperatively. The use of gut decontamination significantly reduces the rate of postoperative bacterial infection, not only of blood-borne sepsis but also of intra-abdominal abcesses. Gut decontamination is begun prior to transplantation and continued for several weeks after transplantation.

Prophylactic broad-spectrum antibiotics are used for the first 48 hours. They usually include an aminoglycoside and a third-generation cephalosporin or semisynthetic penicillin. Empiric therapy is then used for specific indications. The most common postoperative sources are from indwelling venous catheters.

Viral infections are most commonly caused by herpes simplex and cytomegalovirus (CMV). Prophylactic acyclovir is used in the postoperative period initially, intravenously and then orally. The oral dose is given for several months during the postoperative period, until the immunosuppression doses are at a maintenance level. The Mayo Clinic group has shown the significance of CMV in transplant recipients. A CMV seronegative recipient who receives a CMV seropositive organ is at risk for developing a clinically significant infection in the postoperative period.[21] CMV infections commonly cause high-spiking fevers, arthralgia, and myalgia. However, CMV pneumonitis and hepatitis can be life-threatening complications in this patient population. An experimental drug, gancyclovir, an analog of acyclovir, has been very successful in treating CMV infections in the liver transplant population.

The opportunistic infection caused by *Pneumocystis carinii* is rare but often fatal. In a heavily immunosuppressed patient, particularly one being treated for graft rejec-

TABLE 11. Side Effects of Cyclosporine

Nephrotoxicity
Hypertension
Hepatotoxicity
Neurologic reactions
    seizures
    intracranial hemorrhage
    confusion
    cortical blindness
    quadriplegia
Malignancy

tion, prophylaxis against *Pneumocystis* consists of oral trimethoprim-sulfamethoxazole. The treatment of an active *Pneumocystis* infection should consist of intravenous trimethoprim-sulfamethoxazole and/or pentamidine, either intravenously or in the aerosolized form.

The *Candida* species represents the most common fungal infection in this patient population. Candidemia is unusual and is more frequently found in patients who receive repeated treatments for rejection or long-term broad-spectrum antibiotics. Other fungal infections are seen infrequently. The mainstay of the treatment of fungal infections is amphotericin B. Ketoconazole and its newer derivatives are difficult drugs to use because of their competition for cyclosporine metabolism in the liver.

Malignancy. The incidence of malignancy in liver transplant patients is increased over the general population. The most common is a lymphoproliferative disorder; however, all malignancies, including adenocarcinomas, are increased.[22]

The long-term care of the recipient of a liver transplant is a coordinated effort between the transplant center and the local or referring physician. Patients require continuous biochemical monitoring for liver function, cyclosporine levels, bone marrow suppression, and renal function. The longest surviving liver transplant recipient underwent transplantation surgery in 1967. This patient gives us hope that indefinite survival after liver transplant can be accomplished with intensive management and follow-up.

■ Pulmonary Transplantation

The success of numerous heart transplantation programs has led to expansion of the principles and techniques of transplantation to include the pulmonary system. Early attempts at pulmonary transplantation were anecdotal and generally unsuccessful, but the pioneering work of Cooper and others with the Toronto Lung Transplant Group have set the standard for the modern era.[23] The hallmark of this group's contribution is the use of a vascularized omental pedicle to surround and reinforce the bronchial or tracheal anastomosis, which historically had been the limiting factor in the success of pulmonary transplantation in the cyclosporine era. With adherence to rigid recipient criteria, careful donor selection, use of proper surgical technique, and meticulous postoperative acute and chronic patient management, long-term survival rates with single- or double-lung transplantation can exceed 65 per cent.

■ INDICATIONS

Initially, patients considered potential recipients for single-lung transplantation included only those with idiopathic pulmonary fibrosis. In isolated instances, patients with emphysema and primary pulmonary hypertension have also received single-lung transplants, but these operations are few in number and will require further investigation. Double-lung transplantation has been performed successfully in patients with emphysema, cystic fibrosis, and pulmonary hypertension.[24,25] With the current survival rate in patients receiving double-lung transplantation and the scarcity of all donor organs relative to the number of potential recipients, it is believed by many that single- or double-lung transplantation may replace heart-lung transplantation for patients with primary or secondary end-stage lung disease.

■ MANAGEMENT

Immunosuppression. As with all transplant patients, the obstacle in postoperative management is to maintain adequate immunosuppression to prevent acute or chronic rejection of the transplanted organ while avoiding the hazards of opportunistic infection. In the immediate postoperative period, cyclosporine and azathioprine are administered. Corticosteroids are then begun 1 month after transplant or with the first rejection episode and are then tapered and discontinued within 1 year. Transbronchial biopsy[26] and bronchoalveolar lavage are used, often simultaneously, to maintain surveillance for infection and rejection. Varying degrees of benefit from these techniques have been observed in the early postoperative period.

Infection. Appropriate antiviral, antifungal, and antibiotic regimens are required for the management of infection in these severely compromised patients. The need for monitoring for infection and rapid intervention cannot be overemphasized. In 21 patients undergoing single-lung transplantation by the Toronto Lung Transplant Group, four patients had early death; two were caused by pneumonia—one of viral and the other of bacterial origin. Of the four late deaths, two were due to infection. The only long-term antibiotic prophylaxis used in these patients was trimethoprim-sulfamethoxazole (Bactrim, Septra), 800 mg tablets taken twice daily to prevent *P. carinii* infection. Therefore, it is apparent that long-term survival of these patients depends upon the early recognition and prompt, appropriate treatment of any infections that develop. Infection is often manifested early by deterioration in pulmonary function. It is therefore suggested that these patients monitor their pulmonary function daily with a hand-held device. If a deterioration of function is observed for 3 consecutive days, they should undergo biopsy and bronchoalveolar lavage. Obviously, any other systemic or constitutional signs of infection also should be investigated. The cooperation of infectious disease specialists and pathologists in an institutional effort is vital to the success of long-term management.

■ COMPLICATIONS

The long-term complications seen in patients undergoing cardiac transplantation continue to be hypertension and the development of obliterative arteritis, but patients who have undergone pulmonary transplantation also may develop bronchiolitis obliterans. Investigators believe this may be a result of the loss of direct vascular supply to the bronchioli, with subsequent dependence on retrograde flow from the pulmonary arteries. At the First International Symposium on Transplantation for End-Stage Lung Disease, no more than a handful of cases of obliterative bronchiolitis were reported. This is compared with the significant incidence of obliterative bronchiolitis, 33 per cent, in the 55 per cent of heart/lung transplant patients who are 2-year survivors. Although this statistic is encouraging, these patients nonetheless should be observed for evidence of delayed chronic re-

jection and bronchial or tracheal anastomotic narrowing.

In patients with pulmonary fibrosis or cystic fibrosis, recurrence of the primary disease in the transplanted lung has not been observed. Only one patient with sarcoidosis had a recurrence in the transplanted lung, and in patients undergoing lung transplantation for pulmonary hypertension the results are as yet unconfirmed. There is also an approximate 2 per cent incidence of lymphoproliferative disease in patients at risk. However, this may be reversible with manipulation of the immunosuppressive regimen.

Patients must maintain rigid compliance with their immunosuppressive medications and be attentive to unassociated illnesses, such as gastrointestinal disturbances, that might lead to poor absorption of medications and subsequent alteration in serum levels. Pulmonary function must be monitored daily and any sustained abnormalities or deviations in clinical status reported to the transplant physicians so that appropriate investigational steps may be taken.

■ Renal Transplantation

■ BACKGROUND

Since the first successful renal transplant performed in Boston in 1955,[27] renal transplantation has become the treatment of choice for end-stage renal disease. Nearly a decade later, chronic dialysis was developed to sustain life in end-stage renal failure.[28] Over the next 25 years, a series of breakthroughs have brought transplantation to its current enviable therapeutic status:

1. The identification of histocompatibility loci important in matching grafts with patients.[29]
2. Identification of more specific immunosuppressive drugs targeted toward cellular (acute) rejection. For nearly 20 years, the standard immunosuppressive therapy was azathioprine and corticosteroids. Antilymphocyte globulin (ALG) and antithymocyte globulin (ATG) were identified and refined to take a place in current quadruple therapy (ALG/ATG, steroids, azathioprine and cyclosporine). One of the most important advances was the de-

velopment of an anti-T cell immunosuppressant, cyclosporine-A, allowing a 20 to 30 per cent increase in short-term (5-year) graft survival.[30]
3. Recognition that pretransplant blood transfusions improved cadaver graft survival and permitted better living donor selection through donor-specific transfusions.[31]
4. Advancement of organ preservation with the introduction of UW (Belzer) solution, which kept kidneys viable for at least 72 hours.
5. Development of a national organ-sharing agency and certified regional procurement agencies, which increased kidney utilization and decreased wastage of this precious resource.
6. Recent development of mono-specific antibodies to target-specific T cells causing an acute rejection, i.e., OKT 3.[32]
7. Advances in the development of more effective agents against viruses (i.e., gancyclovir, acyclovir), which have reduced infectious complications in immunocompromised hosts.
8. The most recent work involves antibodies against interleukin II receptors,[33] and an interleukin II diphtheria toxin hybrid is being developed that will be tested clinically in the near future.[34]

All these advances have made renal transplantation the most successful therapeutic approach for treatment of end-stage renal failure, with a 1-year graft survival exceeding 90 per cent in living donors[35] and 80 per cent in cadaver donors.[36]

■ MANAGEMENT

Recipient Selection and Preparation

Most patients with end-stage renal disease who are younger than 60 years of age and have no other serious complicating illness are considered good candidates for kidney transplantation. Uncontrolled malignancies, severe cardiovascular and peripheral vascular disease, lack of compliance with medical advice, and intercurrent chronic infection are all relative contraindications to renal transplantation. Most (but not all) patients receive chronic maintenance dialysis prior to transplantation.

Prior to transplantation, evaluation of cardiac function, particularly directed toward the detection of coronary artery disease, is important. Also, evaluation of the urinary bladder and lower urinary tract is necessary. ABO blood group determination, HLA tissue typing, and determination of cytotoxic antibody sensitivity are required. In most centers, blood transfusions to the recipient, whether they are random third-party transfusions or donor-specific, are used in pretransplant conditioning and screening.

In living donor transplantation, donor-specific transfusion (DST) under cover of low-dose azathioprine (1 to 1.5 mg/kg/day) to prevent sensitization is associated with increased graft survival (85 to 95 per cent at 1 yr). Before cadaver donor transplantation, the recipient is given five or more transfusions from random blood bank donors.

All patients receive basic immunosuppressive therapy (methylprednisolone and azathioprine) hours before the transplant procedure. Cyclosporine is not given until urinary output and renal function are adequate (usually 1 to 7 days). Renal transplant function is monitored by measurements of blood urea nitrogen (BUN), serum creatinine, and urinary output. Renal scintigrams and color flow Doppler ultrasound examinations of the kidney are performed to monitor blood flow and renal function and help detect evidence of rejection. Fine-needle aspiration biopsies of the transplanted kidneys are often performed. This technique is safe and can help differentiate rejection from cyclosporine toxicity. When the diagnosis of acute rejection is made, the patient is first treated with high-dose intravenous corticosteroids, then with oral prednisone that is gradually tapered.

OKT 3 (monoclonal antibody) is used in steroid-resistant acute rejection. Recurrent episodes of rejection can be treated with either therapy. Steroids are preferred, although the cumulative dose can have serious side effects. The presence of anti-OKT 3 antibodies should be determined prior to repeated retreatment. High levels of anti-OKT 3 antibodies preclude retreatment. Absent or low levels of OKT 3 antibodies suggest that retreatment could be successful.

Use of prophylactic antibiotic and antiviral agents is arbitrary. Some transplant centers use trimethoprim-sulfamethoxazole and acyclovir in combination as prophylaxis for *P. carinii* and opportunistic viral infections.

Donor Preparation and Evaluation

Because of the growing shortage of cadaver organs and the improved success of living transplantation, identification of potential living donors and their preparation are important. Evaluation for kidney donors includes donor ABO testing, tissue typing (HLA, DR, and mixed leukocyte culture), and direct cytotoxic cross-matching between the potential donor/recipient pairs. Living donors are usually direct family members (brother, sister, father, mother, son, or daughter).

Unrelated living donors are occasionally suitable. After the selection of the best donor, the potential donor is evaluated physically and emotionally. A donor who is acceptable then undergoes renal function studies and arteriography to assess donor renal anatomy.

Potential cadaver donors are screened by organ procurement agencies. Most donors are between the ages of 5 and 55 years. Screening for infection (pyogenic, viral, HIV, and so on) is routinely performed prior to transplant. Improved organ preservation has made cadaver transplantation a nearly elective procedure, and hence evaluation of the recipient and donor can be more thoroughly accomplished prior to the transplant. Despite efforts to increase cadaver organ availability, the number of patients awaiting kidney transplants increases yearly. Further innovative approaches to this problem are necessary if we are to increase the precious resource of available organs for transplantation.

■ ISSUES AND RISKS

Renal Transplant Recipient Follow-Up. The recipient is followed postoperatively by members of the transplant team, including the transplant surgeon, the nephrologist, social workers, clinical nurse specialists, and renal dietitians. Signs suggestive of decreased renal function or infection are among the parameters followed during regular visits. Blood levels of cyclosporine-A are also monitored, and the doses adjusted appropriately.

Antihypertensive therapy is necessary in many patients after renal transplantation. Hypertension is a significant side effect of cyclosporine therapy and is usually managed with diuretics, beta-blockers, and calcium channel blockers. Angiotensin-converting enzyme (ACE) inhibitors should be avoided because of their potential to decrease renal blood flow and glomerular filtration rate, resulting in worsening renal function and hyperkalemia.

Diabetes mellitus can develop after transplantation, especially in patients who have latent diabetes, are overweight, and abuse carbohydrates. It can be aggravated by corticosteroids, especially when rejection is treated repetitively, but it can also be found in patients receiving maintenance prednisone. Patients who develop diabetes can be treated with diet, oral hypoglycemics, or insulin. Most diabetics who are insulin dependent prior to transplantation require increased insulin to control diabetes. Often the combination of intermediate and regular insulin several times daily is necessary. Renal transplant patients are immunocompromised and more susceptible to infection. Infection can be serious, particularly if the patient has borderline renal function and requires significant immunosuppression to maintain viability of the organ. Frequent treatment for rejection must be carefully weighed in view of borderline function because the risk of life-threatening infection may outweigh graft maintenance. Bacterial infections should be treated aggressively with conventional antibiotic therapy. Viral infections, including CMV, herpes simplex (either localized or systemic), and herpes zoster, are difficult to treat. Newer antiviral agents such as acyclovir or gancyclovir have markedly improved the therapy of these infections. Epidemic outbreaks of *Pneumocystis* infection have occurred in some transplant centers, and trimethoprim-sulfamethoxazole has been used prophylactically.

■ POST-TRANSPLANT COMPLICATIONS

Renal function can remain relatively stable for years but can decrease gradually with time. This occurrence is probably the result of chronic rejection characterized by vascular wall thickening, reduction in blood flow, and gradual loss of glomerular filtration. Acute decreases in renal function in long-term survivors usually indicate an acute rejection episode and require therapy. Acute rejection episodes may be the result of intentional or inadvertent discontinuation of immunosuppressive therapy.

Transplant renal arterial stenosis has been reported. Narrowing of the artery commonly occurs at the anastamotic site and occasionally occurs in the proximal donor artery. When stenosis is present, hypertension worsens and renal function may decrease rapidly. A bruit may appear in the transplant site, or a previously present bruit may increase. Surgical correction of the renal arterial stenosis or, when appropriate, balloon angioplasty can return the blood pressure to normal and improve renal function.

Stenosis of the transplanted ureter can occur acutely or chronically. Signs and symptoms of obstructive uropathy may develop. The diagnosis is usually made by ultrasonography, renal scintigraphy, or intravenous pyelography.

The incidence of malignancy in long-term survivors with renal transplants is slightly increased over the incidence in the general population. Cutaneous malignancies and lymphoproliferative disorders are the most common types. Among the latter, it is peculiar and characteristic of renal transplant recipients to develop central nervous system lymphomas. Awareness of this characteristic presentation makes early diagnosis possible and more effective therapy applicable.

REFERENCES

1. Camitta BM, Thomas ED, Nathan GL, et al. Prospective study of androgens and bone marrow transplantation for treatment of severe aplastic anemia. Blood 1979; 53:504–514.
2. Gluckman E, Marmont A, Speck B, Gordon-Smith EC for the Working Party on Severe Aplastic Anemia of the European Group for Bone Marrow Transplantation. Immunosuppressive treatment of aplastic anemia as an alternative for bone marrow transplantation. Semin Hematol 1984; 21:11–19.
3. Appelbaum FR, Fisher LD, Thomas ED, The Seattle Marrow Transplant Team. Chemotherapy v marrow transplantation for adults with acute nonlymphocytic leukemia: a five-year follow-up. Blood 1988; 72:179–184.
4. Weiden PL, Fluornoy N, Sanders JE, Sullivan KM, Thomas ED. Antileukemic effect of graft-versus-host disease contributes to improved survival after allogeneic marrow transplantation. Transplant Proc 1981; 13:248–251.
5. Wiernik PH (ed). Mediguide to Oncology. Wayne, NJ: Lederle Laboratories, 1988; 8:1–6.
6. Appelbaum RF. Marrow transplantation for hematologic malignancies: Brief review of current status and future prospects. Sem Hematol 1988; 25(Suppl 3):16–22.
7. Storb R. Bone marrow transplantation for the treatment of chronic myelogenous leukemia. Am J Med Sci 1988; 31:87–94.
8. Cheson BD, Lacerna L, Leyland-Jones B, Sarosy C, Wittes RE. Autologous bone marrow transplantation. Ann Intern Med 1989; 110:51–64.
9. Yeager AM, Kaizer H, Santos GW, et al. Autologous bone marrow transplantation in patients with acute nonlymphocytic leukemia using ex vivo marrow treatment with 4-hydroperoxycyclophosphamide. N Engl J Med 1986; 315:141–147.
10. Storb R, Deeg HJ, Whitehead J, et al. Methotrexate and cyclosporine compared with cyclosporine alone for prophylaxis of acute graft versus host disease after marrow transplantation for leukemia. N Engl J Med 1986; 314:729–735.
11. Apperley JF, Jones L, Hill G, et al. Bone marrow transplantation for patients with chronic myeloid leukemia; T-cell depletion with Campath I reduces the incidence of graft-versus-host disease, but may increase the risk of leukemic relapse. Bone Marrow Transplant 1986; 1:53–56.
12. Lower RR, Shumway NE. Studies on orthotopic homotransplantation of the canine heart. Surg Forum 1960; 11:18–19.
13. Barnard CN: A human cardiac transplant: an interim report of a successful operation performed at Groote Schuer Hospital, Cape Town. S Afr Med J 1967; 41:1272–1274.
14. Copeland TG. Cardiac Transplantation. Curr Prob Cardiol 1988; 13:163–224.
15. Costanzo-Nordin MR, Silver MA, O'Connell JB, et al. Successful reversal of acute cardiac allograft rejection with OKT3 monoclonal antibody. Circulation 1987; 76:V71–80.
16. Watson FS, O'Connell JB, Amber IJ, et al. Treatment of cytomegalovirus pneumonia in heart transplant recipients with 9(1,3-dihydroxy-2-proproxymethyl)-guanine (DHPG). Heart Transplant 1988; 7:102–105.
17. Starzl TE, Groth CG, Brettschneider L, et al. Orthotopic homotransplantation of the human liver. Ann Surg 1988; 168:392–415.
18. Jenkins RL, Fairchild RB. Role of transplantation in liver disease. Surg Clin North Am 1989; 69:371–382.
19. De Groen PC, Aksamit AJ, Rakela J, Forbes GS, Krom RAF. Central nervous system toxicity after liver transplantation: the role of cyclosporine and cholesterol. N Engl J Med 1987; 317:861–866.
20. Ptachcinski RJ, Burckart GJ, Venkataramanan R. Cyclosporine. Drug Intell Clin Pharm 1985; 19:90–100.
21. Rakela J, Weisner R, Taswell PE, et al. Increased CMV infections and relation to donor/recipient serology status in liver transplantation. Transplant Proc 1987; 19:2399–2402.
22. Penn I. Cancers following cyclosporine therapy. Transplantation 1987; 43:32–35.
23. The Toronto Lung Transplant Group. Experience with single-lung transplantation for pulmonary fibrosis. JAMA 1988; 259:2258–2262.
24. Cooper JD, Patterson GA, Grossman R, Maurer J, Toronto Lung Transplant Group. Double-lung transplant for advanced chronic obstructive lung disease. Am Rev Respir Dis 1989; 139:303–307.

25. Patterson GA, Cooper JD, Goldman B, et al. Technique of successful clinical double-lung transplantation. Ann Thorac Surg 1988; 45:626–633.
26. Hutter JA, Stewart S, Higenbottam T, Scott JP, Wallwork J. Histologic changes in heart-lung transplant recipients during rejection episodes and at routine biopsy. J Heart Transplant 1988; 7:440–444.
27. Merrill JP, Murray JE, Harrison JH, Guild WR. Successful homotransplantation of human kidney between identical twins. JAMA 1956; 160:277–282.
28. Scribner BH, Buri R, Caner J, Hegstrom R, Burnell JM. Treatment of chronic uremia by means of intermittent hemodialysis: a preliminary report. Trans Am Soc Artif Int Organs 1960; 6:114–122.
29. Opelz G, for The Collaborative Transplant Study. Effect of HLA matching in 10,000 cyclosporine-treated cadaver kidney transplants. Transplant Proc 1987; 19:641–646.
30. Rolles K, Friend PJ, Calve RY. Seven years' experience of cyclosporine in renal transplantation. Transplant Proc 1986; 18:1242–1243.
31. Tiwari JL. Blood transfusion and kidney graft survival: a review. In Terasaki PL (ed). Clinical Transplants, 1986. Los Angeles: UCLA Tissue Typing Laboratory, 1986:341–343.
32. Goldstein G (ed). Therapeutic use of the monoclonal antibody orthoclone OKT-3. Transplant Proc 1987; 19(Suppl 1):1–57.
33. Soulillou JP, Le Mauff B, Olive D, et al. Prevention of rejection of kidney transplants by monoclonal antibody directed against interleukin 2. Lancet 1987; 1:1339–1342.
34. Stromm TB, Kelley VE. Toward more selective therapies to block undesired immune responses. Kidney Int 1989; 35:1026–1033.
35. Salvatierra O Jr, Melzer J, Vincenti F, et al. Donor-specific blood transfusions versus cyclosporine—the DST story. Transplant Proc 1987; 19:160–166.
36. Tiwari JL. Cyclosporine and kidney graft survival: a review. In Terasaki PL (ed). Clinical Transplants, 1986. Los Angeles: UCLA Tissue Typing Laboratory, 1986:345–366.

Urinary incontinence

L. Keith Lloyd

■ Background

Urinary incontinence, the involuntary loss of urine, is often treated as a diagnostic entity but in reality is a sign or symptom that has a multiplicity of causes. Although urinary incontinence is seen in all age groups, it reaches its highest incidence among elderly people. Community-based studies have shown a prevalence of between 10 and 20 per cent among persons 65 years or older.[1] The incidence among institutionalized elderly patients reaches nearly 50 per cent and, along with bowel incontinence, is a major reason for admission to a nursing facility.[2] Adult urinary incontinence is far more common in women but becomes somewhat more evenly distributed between the sexes with advancing age.

Urinary incontinence does not result in serious disease but may be associated with skin rash or even decubitus sores, particularly in debilitated or hospitalized patients. Urinary incontinence may result in depression and withdrawn or reclusive behavior. It has been estimated, however, that as many as half the patients with urinary incontinence have not consulted a physician about treatment. Conservative estimates place the cost of managing urinary incontinence at greater than 10 billion dollars annually. Approximately 70 per cent of this figure is spent on community dwellers and 30 per cent on nursing home residents.[2] With the current and anticipated increase in numbers of elderly persons, it must be anticipated that the numbers of incontinent patients will increase, and the cost of care for these patients will increase. Cost-effective strategies for evaluation and care of patients, therefore, will be increasingly in demand in the future.

Urinary incontinence may be caused by a variety of disturbances, but this article focuses on clinical evaluation and treatment of the most commonly encountered forms of urinary incontinence in adults. These include genuine stress incontinence, urgency incontinence, overflow incontinence, and

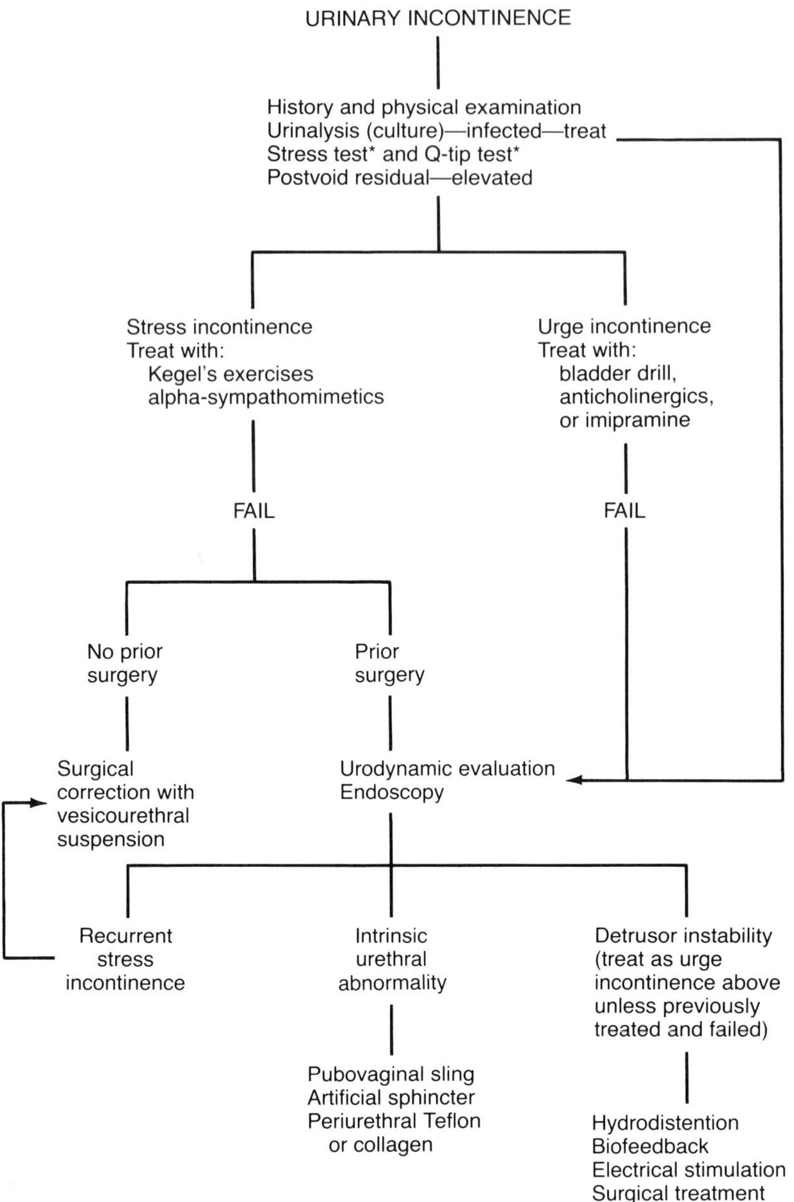

Figure 1. Algorithm depicting staged management of urinary incontinence. Initial evaluation consists of simple in-office procedures. Residuals elevated greater than 100 ml require urodynamic evaluation and endoscopy. Other patients are then treated according to the protocol, with additional evaluation and management of patients who fail to respond to initial measures.

mixed incontinence.[2] Figure 1 is an algorithm showing how many patients can be managed at least initially with simple office evaluation.

---

*In the stress test, the patient is asked to cough. If leakage is observed, then the anterior bladder wall is elevated slightly and the patient is asked to cough again. If this maneuver prevents leakage, this is suggestive of stress incontinence. The Q-tip test is performed by placing a cotton applicator into the urethra so that the cotton tip is at the bladder neck. The patient is then asked to cough. If the opposite end of the Q-tip moves anteriorly, this also is suggestive of stress incontinence.

■ Management

As with most conditions, proper management is predicated upon accurate diagnosis and use of the least invasive and least costly therapies as initial treatment. Management of urinary incontinence does not have to be an all-or-none phenomenon. Many patients, because of social conditioning or associated medical problems, will be quite content simply with reduction in frequency and severity of incontinence as a result of simple and noninvasive treatments. Utilizing this approach, treatment is staged, and patients advance to higher stages of treatment depending upon response and willingness to accept specific treatment modalities. Initial testing via the algorithm will separate patients who have urinary tract infection as an initiating or aggravating factor from patients who have large residuals combined with incontinence (overflow incontinence).

■ URINARY INFECTION

Urinary infection alone is not generally an initiating factor for incontinence but may be a significant aggravating factor. Urinary infection, particularly in older patients, may not be associated with the usual symptomatology. When urinary tract infection is detected, it should be treated appropriately with antibiotic therapy for a period of 7 to 10 days and the incontinence reassessed before proceeding to additional evaluation and therapies.

■ OVERFLOW INCONTINENCE

In our experience, overflow incontinence is a relatively uncommon cause of urinary incontinence and one that is generally detected easily by physical examination and confirmed with the postvoid residual urine determination. It occurs usually on the basis of significant neurologic disease or urinary tract obstruction. In either case, intermittent catheterization can be used either as a definitive or temporary therapy. Overflow incontinence due to bladder outlet obstruction is treated surgically by endoscopic or open removal of the obstructive tissue.

■ STRESS INCONTINENCE

Stress urinary incontinence is defined as the involuntary loss of urine when intravesical pressure exceeds urethral pressure in the absence of detrusor activity.[3] This diagnosis is suggested by the history and can be confirmed by simple observation in the office. It is, perhaps, the most common cause of incontinence in adult women. As seen in the algorithm, a tentative diagnosis of stress urinary incontinence may be made and treatment instituted with pelvic floor–strengthening exercises and pharmacologic therapy.

Kegel reported significant improvement in urinary incontinence among patients treated with pelvic floor–strengthening exercises.[4] He used a form of biofeedback, since patients were instructed to contract the vaginal muscles on a balloon device, the perineometer, which gave a visual display of the effect of the muscle contraction. These exercises have largely fallen into disuse, however, because of perceived less effective results.[5] Most patients are not taught strengthening exercises with the use of a perineometer and often are told simply to interrupt the urinary stream during voiding.

Many women do not understand which muscle to contract when told to contract the pelvic floor or to interrupt urinary flow. Contraction of the pelvic floor muscles should be taught by placing a finger in the rectum and asking the patient to contract the external anal sphincter. The external anal sphincter, urinary sphincter, and levator sling muscles will contract in concert. It often takes a few moments to demonstrate to the patient which muscles should be contracted. Once the patient is certain of the muscles to be contracted, then isometric exercises are done, with sustained contraction for 3 seconds and relaxation for 3 seconds, with repetition of this exercise 30 times. The set of exercises is then repeated three times a day. The patient should be cautioned that progress with this activity will be slow and that the strengthening exercises should be continued indefinitely. Weight loss and general body exercise through walking are also beneficial.

Klarskov and colleagues randomly divided patients either to surgery or to a pelvic floor–training program for treatment of stress urinary incontinence.[6] Whereas surgical therapy clearly proved superior, 42 per cent of the patients were satisfied with the outcome of pelvic floor–strengthening exercises and did not wish to have surgical correction. Furthermore, the surgical outcome in patients who had received pelvic floor training was especially good, and patients with residual symptoms after surgery benefited from the training program. Their program was intensively guided by a physiotherapist, and the importance of muscle consciousness and education about the pelvic floor was stressed.

Pharmacologic therapy may be utilized separately, in place of, or in our opinion ideally in conjunction with pelvic floor exercises. Phenylpropanolamine (Propadrine),

50 mg two to four times per day,[7] or pseudoephedrine (Sudafed), 30 to 60 mg two to four times per day, may produce some increase in maximum urethral closure pressure and subjective improvement in symptomatology. These drugs must be used with caution in patients with hypertension or cardiovascular disease. Imipramine (Tofranil), in an uncontrolled study, also has been shown to be beneficial for stress urinary incontinence.[8] The dose of imipramine is 25 mg, two to three times per day. Again, caution is required in patients with vascular disease, and central nervous system side effects, including excessive drowsiness, may be experienced with this medication.

Electrostimulation, using either an intravaginal device or an anal plug, has been reported to reduce symptoms in stress and urge incontinence.[9,10] These devices have not been used to any great extent in this country, however, and currently are not generally available. Surgical treatment has been the mainstay of treating stress urinary incontinence in this country and the aforementioned methods are not widely used, except in patients with the very mildest degrees of incontinence.

Surgical Treatment

Numerous surgical procedures have been described for the correction of stress urinary incontinence. No series of patients of significant size, however, has achieved the elusive goal of perfect results. Many procedures report success rates as high as 90 to 95 per cent in well-selected patients. Surgical procedures broadly fall into two categories: vaginal/needle suspension procedures or suprapubic suspension procedures. The goal of these operations is to restore the vesical neck and urethra to a proper, or even exaggerated, anterior position, so that increases in intra-abdominal pressure are transmitted equally to the bladder and urethra. Although results with the two types of procedures are similar, there has been increasing use of the vaginal/needle suspension procedures in recent years because of decreased perioperative morbidity and shorter hospitalization.

Needle suspension procedures were first described by Pereyra in 1959,[11] and, although results were good, the procedure never gained wide popularity until modifications introduced by Stamey and separately by Boyd and Raz were developed and advocated in recent years.[12,13] The addition of endoscopic examination to be certain that the needles do not perforate the bladder or urethra has been a significant advance in the effectiveness and safety of these procedures. More recently, Gittes and Loughlin have simplified the procedure even further by eliminating any vaginal incision.[14,15]

In the procedure described by Gittes, the needles are passed through two small suprapubic incisions behind the pubis and through the anterior vaginal wall lateral to the bladder neck. A helical suture is then formed by taking two sutures through the anterior vaginal wall and then passing the vaginal end of the suture back up to the suprapubic incision where it is tied. Postoperatively, the sutures cut through the vaginal mucosa and become buried in scar tissue in the vaginal wall. This procedure can be done quickly and even under local anesthesia in patients who may require that. It is ideally suited for patients with primary stress incontinence or older patients who are suboptimal surgical candidates. Urinary retention following this procedure is relatively common, and a short period of suprapubic catheter drainage or intermittent catheterization is often required.

Early results with this procedure appear to be quite good, but long-term follow-up is needed to determine whether the repair will stand the test of time. This procedure can be performed in patients who have had previous operations, provided the appropriate physical findings are present.

Suprapubic bladder suspension procedures were first described by Marshall, Marchetti, and Krantz in 1948.[16] Currently, most of the suprapubic procedures are either a classic Marshall-Marchetti-Krantz procedure, modifications thereof, or modifications of the Burch colposuspension.[17] These procedures all involve dissection of the retropubic space and suspension of the anterior vaginal wall, either to the periosteum of the pubis, Cooper's ligament, or the anterior abdominal fascia. These procedures are indicated when other open suprapubic surgery is being performed, in patients who have failed needle suspension procedures with recurrent loss of bladder base support, and perhaps in younger patients in whom the long-term results of suprapubic procedures might be slightly superior to the needle suspension operations. However, overall results of both suprapubic procedures and needle suspension procedures are quite similar; patient selection, surgeon preference, and local practice patterns probably play the major roles in decision for a surgical procedure.[18]

Treatment of Surgical Failures

As stated, no operative procedure for correcting stress urinary incontinence has proved 100 per cent successful. Patients who have failed previous surgical correction for stress urinary incontinence should undergo comprehensive urodynamic evaluation. In some of these patients, technical failures will be demonstrated, and repeat bladder neck suspension procedures are indicated. In others, however, the incontinence is more severe, physical examination will demonstrate the urethra and bladder neck to be positioned well anteriorly, and videourodynamic studies often show an open bladder neck at resting detrusor pressures. In this situation, the defect is usually intrinsic urethral weakness and not simply anatomic incontinence. Simple surgical resuspension in these patients frequently will fail, and a procedure that provides compression or coaptation of the proximal urethra will have a greater chance of success. We prefer the pubovaginal sling procedure for these patients and prefer to use a strip of anterior abdominal fascia since it allows the operation to be performed through one incision.[19] Overall surgical results of this procedure are quite good, but there is a significant postoperative incidence of detrusor instability or urge urinary incontinence.

Artificial urinary sphincters have been utilized for treating patients with intrinsic urethral defects. Initial surgical results were not good, but improved patient selection has made this a viable surgical alternative.[20] Ideal candidates generally are younger patients who have good tissue integrity and have not undergone multiple surgical procedures.

Patients with intrinsic urethral abnormalities have been treated in recent years with periurethral injections of polytetrafluoroethylene paste, as described by Politano.[21] This is a simple outpatient surgical procedure that can be performed under local anesthesia. It produces compression of the proximal urethra/bladder neck area by a bolus of injected Teflon paste. Collagen recently has been used in a similar manner for periurethral injection with good short-term results.[22]

■ URGE INCONTINENCE

Urgency incontinence is perhaps the most common type of incontinence encountered in the older population. It is defined simply as loss of urine when the patient senses a desire to void but is unable to inhibit voiding long enough for proper toileting.[3] Recently it has been shown that as many as half of elderly patients with urge incontinence also have impaired bladder contractions and elevated residual urines.[23] Often a specific cause is not identified, but this type of incontinence can be associated with a variety of central nervous system diseases and with local irritating factors such as urinary infection or bladder outlet obstruction.

As seen from the algorithm, patients clinically diagnosed with urge incontinence may be treated initially with bladder training or bladder drill with or without added pharmacologic therapy. Currently in the United States, simple pharmacologic treatment is probably the most common form of therapy for these patients.

Bladder Training

Adequate cognitive function and motivation are essential components for a successful bladder training program. The key to bladder training is use of the voiding chart or voiding diary. In its simplest form, this is a record the patient keeps, over several 24-hour periods, of the times voided, volumes voided, and incontinence episodes. The voiding chart is then examined and the average interval between voiding episodes determined. If voiding is frequent and volumes are low, as would be expected with urge incontinence, the patient is asked to increase progressively the interval between voidings. For example, the patient who is voiding at hourly intervals might be asked to increase the interval by 15 minutes the first week; when that goal is achieved, a new goal is established to lengthen further the interval between voiding episodes. Frewen first described this procedure in 1978 and achieved high success rates in curing or improving symptoms of urgency and urge incontinence.[24] His program, however, included a

2-week stay in the hospital with fairly intense training and supportive therapy. This approach is not practical in this country, but good results with the modified program have been described.[25]

This is an easy form of treatment to institute. It is particularly suitable for older patients, since it does not involve surgical treatment or pharmacologic therapy, which might have significant side effects. It also gives the patient a sense of control over the problem, with specific steps to take to achieve improvement in urinary incontinence.

Pharmacologic Therapy

This has probably been the mainstay of treatment of urge incontinence in this country. Anticholinergics and smooth muscle relaxants are the most commonly used agents.[26] They inhibit detrusor contractility and may improve bladder capacity with subsequent increase in the intervoid interval, as well as improvement or control of urinary incontinence. Propantheline (Pro-Banthine) inhibits the action of acetylcholine at postganglionic nerve endings in the bladder. It may be used at a dose of 7.5 to 30 mg three to four times per day. We start with lower doses, particularly in elderly patients, and gradually increase the dose until the desired therapeutic effect is achieved. Significant side effects of dry mouth and constipation may occur at higher doses. Propantheline should not be given to patients with glaucoma and should be used cautiously in elderly people or patients with significant cardiac disease.

Oxybutynin hydrochloride (Ditropan), which has both anticholinergic and antispasmodic effects on bladder smooth muscle, also has been an extremely useful agent in controlling symptoms of urgency and urge incontinence. The usual dose is 2.5 to 10 mg three to four times per day, depending on severity of symptoms and response. Side effects and precautions are similar to those of propantheline.

Imipramine has been a very useful drug in treating urgency incontinence. We have seen many patients respond to imipramine when earlier trials of anticholinergics have not been successful. This agent is the original tricyclic antidepressant, but all its mechanisms of action are still not clearly understood. It appears to have both anticholinergic and direct smooth muscle relaxant effects on the bladder, as well as enhancement of alpha-sympathetic activity in the bladder neck and proximal urethra, the combined effects of which promote urinary continence. It also appears to have an effect in the basal ganglia, which may in reality be its most important effect in controlling urge incontinence in elderly patients as well as childhood enuresis. We prefer to start initially with a bedtime dose of 25 to 50 mg and increase progressively to a maximum dose of 150 mg per day. The drug may be given in divided doses if necessary for improved control of daytime symptomatology. The most pronounced side effect of the drug is sedation, and treatment at night helps circumvent this in most patients. Anticholinergic side effects, such as dryness of the mouth and constipation, are frequently seen. Again, the drug should be used with caution in elderly patients and in those with significant cardiac disease. It may also be given in combination with anticholinergics, with improved results in some patients.

Women who display postmenopausal changes in the vaginal mucosa (atrophic vaginitis) should also be treated with topical estrogens. Low doses of 0.5 to 1.5 mg of conjugated estrogens may be given in vaginal creams two to three times per week. Such low doses provide beneficial effects for the vaginal and urethral mucosa and minimize the risk of any systemic ill effects. This agent should not be used in women with known breast or genital cancer or past history of thromboembolic disorder. It should be used cyclically and discontinued at 3- to 6-month intervals, depending on patient response.

Other Management Methods

Patients who show apparent improvement or cure with pharmacologic treatment should be followed for the possibility of developing increasing residual urines or urinary tract infection. Patients who fail to respond to the aforementioned methods need further investigation with urodynamic studies and possibly endoscopy. Alternative treatments may then be considered.

Hydrodistention. Overstretching the bladder causes disruption of myoneural junctions and some ischemic atrophy of the smooth muscle.[26] This can be performed under spinal or epidural anesthesial; the bladder is left distended to a pressure of about 100 cm H_2O for two hours. This may produce beneficial effects in a significant number of patients. Bladder rupture is a possibility with this procedure, but it is generally extravesical and can be treated with Foley catheter drainage.

Biofeedback. This is simply a form of behavioral training that attempts to alter physiologic responses by providing demonstrative evidence of the response (feedback) to the patient, so that the response can be altered. A system utilizing visual information of intravesical pressure, pelvic floor muscle activity, and intra-abdominal pressure was devised by investigators at the National Institute on Aging.[5] In a small sample of patients, they achieved significant improvement in urinary incontinence. This methodology has not been used widely to date because of the complexity of the system and the time involved in training individual patients.

Electrical Stimulation. Electrical stimulation with intravaginal or intrarectal devices has been shown to improve urgency incontinence in significant numbers of patients.[9,10] These devices are not widely available, nor have significant trials been done comparing them with other methods of controlling urge incontinence.

Surgical Treatment. Surgical treatment is really a treatment of last resort in a sense and has not been used to a great extent in this country. Surgical ablation of the S-3 roots has been shown effective in abolishing uninhibited contractions but has the side effects of perineal anesthesia and alterations in bowel and sexual function. A variety of surgical incisions within the bladder have been used, predominantly in England, with satisfactory results.[27]

Subtrigonal injections of ethanol, while not strictly a surgical procedure, can ablate parasympathetic nerves as they enter the bladder base. This has been reported to have beneficial effects in at least one small series of patients and can be applied relatively easily.[28] There was significant risk of vesicovaginal fistula in this study. Very careful patient selection and attention to technique are important aspects of this procedure.

■ Issues and Risks

Urinary incontinence is a socially and psychologically disabling condition that causes depressive and withdrawn behavior. It has been accepted as a normal consequence of aging to a large degree, and many patients do not seek medical evaluation or treatment. Recent studies have shown that elderly or even institutionalized patients can be evaluated and effectively treated. This, at least, has the potential for improving or curing urinary incontinence in many, possibly avoiding institutionalization, and certainly easing the burden of aging for both the patient and family. Patients with advanced medical diseases or severe cognitive impairment are not good candidates for evaluation and treatment and may be best served by judicious use of catheters or external devices for controlling incontinence.

Patients with severe alterations in bladder/urethral anatomy and physiology may sometimes best be treated by supravesical urinary diversion. Continent diversions that provide, in a sense, a substitute bladder constructed from ileum or large bowel may provide a satisfactory method of urinary management in patients with severe bladder disability. These types of appliance-free diversions require commitment by both the surgeon and the patient. Catheterization of the reservoir several times per day is required, however, and the reoperation rate is significant. For appropriately selected patients, continent diversion appears to provide an acceptable form of urinary management in patients whose bladders are lost to malignancy or when the severity of the condition precludes use of the modalities discussed to control incontinence.

Urinary incontinence can be improved or controlled in most patients. A logical and staged treatment approach, as described here, should provide the maximum amount of benefit with the minimum amount of intervention and cost.

REFERENCES

1. Vetter N, Joner D, Victor C. Urinary incontinence in the elderly at home. Lancet 1981; 2:1275–1277.
2. National Institutes of Health Consensus Development Conference. Urinary incontinence in adults. National Institutes of Health Consensus Development Conference Statement 1988; 7(5)1–11.
3. International Continence Society. First report on the standardization of terminology of lower urinary tract function. Br J Urol 1976; 48:39–42.
4. Kegel AH. Stress incontinence of urine in women: physiologic treatment. J Int Coll Surg 1956; 25:487–499.
5. Burgio KL, Burgio LD. Behavior therapies for urinary incontinence in the elderly. Clin Geriat Med 1986; 2:809–827.
6. Klarskov P, Belving D, Bischoff N. Pelvic floor ex-

ercises versus surgery for female urinary stress incontinence. Urol Int 1986; 41:129–132.
7. Lehtonen T, Rannikko S, Lindell O, Talja M, Wuokko E, Lindskog M. The effect of phenylpropanolamine on female stress urinary incontinence. Ann Chir Gynecol 1986; 75:236–241.
8. Gilja I, Radej M, Kovacic M, Parazajder J. Conservative treatment of female stress incontinence with imipramine. J Urol 1984; 132:909–911.
9. Eriksen BC, Bergmann S, Mjøinerød OK. Effect of anal electrostimulation with the "INCONTAN" device in women with urinary incontinence. Br J Obstet Gynaecol 1987; 94:147–156.
10. Fall M. Does electro-stimulation cure urinary incontinence? J Urol 1984; 131:664–667.
11. Pereyra AJ. A simplified surgical procedure for the correction of stress incontinence in women. West J Surg Obstet Gynecol 1959; 67:223–226.
12. Stamey TA. Endoscopic suspension of the vesical neck for urinary incontinence in females: report on 203 consecutive patients. Ann Surg 1980; 192:465–471.
13. Boyd SD, Raz S. Needle bladder neck suspension for female stress incontinence. Urol Clin North Am 1984; 11:357–366.
14. Gittes RF, Loughlin KR. No-incision pubovaginal suspension for stress incontinence. J Urol 1987; 138:568–570.
15. Morales A, VanCott GF. The Gittes procedure as an improved simplification of current techniques for vesical neck suspensions. Surg Gynecol Obstet 1988; 167:243–245.
16. Marshall VF, Marchetti AA, Krantz KE. The correction of stress incontinence by simple vesico-urethral suspension. Surg Gynecol Obstet 1949; 88:509–518.
17. Burch JC. Cooper's ligament urethrovesical suspension for stress incontinence. Am J Obstet Gynecol 1968; 100:764–772.
18. Green DF, McGuire EJ, Lytton B. A comparison of endoscopic suspension of the vesical neck versus anterior urethropexy for the treatment of stress urinary incontinence. J Urol 1986; 136:1205–1207.
19. McGuire EJ, Bennett CJ, Konnak JA, et al. Experience with pubovaginal slings for urinary incontinence at the University of Michigan. J Urol 1987; 138:525–526.
20. Diokno AC, Hollander JB, Alderson TP. Artificial urinary sphincter for recurrent female urinary incontinence: indications and results. J Urol 1987; 138:778–780.
21. Politano VA. Periurethral Teflon injection for urinary incontinence. Urol Clin North Am 1978; 5:415–422.
22. Appell RA, Goodman JR, McGuire EJ, et al. Multicenter study of peri- and transurethral GAX-collagen injection for urinary incontinence (abstract). J Urol 1989; 141:359A.
23. Resnick NM, Yalla SV, Laurino E. The pathophysiology of urinary incontinence among institutionalized elderly persons. N Engl J Med 1989; 320:1–7.
24. Frewen WK. The management of urgency and frequency of micturition. Br J Urol 1980; 52:367–369.
25. Ouslander JG, Sier HC. Drug therapy for geriatric urinary incontinence. Clin Geriat Med 1986; 2:789–807.
26. Korda A, Krieger M, Hunter P. The use of prolonged bladder distension in the treatment of intractable urinary incontinence in females with detrusor instability. Aust NZ J Obstet Gynecol 1987; 27:155–157.
27. Mundy AR. The surgical treatment of urge incontinence of urine. J Urol 1982; 128:481–483.
28. Harris RG, Constantinou CE, Stamey TA. Extravesical subtrigonal injection of fifty per cent ethanol for detrusor instability. J Urol 1988; 140:111–116.

Urinary tract infections, recurrent

Douglas R. Smucker ■ ***Larry W. Johnson***

Urinary tract infections (UTI) in adult patients are encountered frequently in clinical practice. Most uncomplicated lower UTIs are easily recognized and respond promptly to appropriate antibiotic therapy. However, a small percentage of patients will develop patterns of recurrent infections that may pose more difficult diagnostic and therapeutic dilemmas. Armed with an understanding of the pathophysiology of recurrent infections of the urinary tract and knowledge of prophylactic antimicrobial regimens, primary care physicians can diagnose accurately and control successfully most recurrent infections.

■ Background

Urinary tract infections include a variety of syndromes defined by the presence of significant numbers of bacteria in the urine. Infections can be described as symptomatic or asymptomatic and hospital or community-acquired, and they range in severity from acute, uncomplicated cystitis in a young woman to life-threatening pyelonephritis and sepsis in an elderly one. Symptomatic UTIs can be placed in the following simple classification:[1,2]

1. First or occasional infection
2. Frequent infection
   a. Reinfection
   b. Persistent infection

The distinction between "occasional" and "frequent" infections is subjective in patients who experience more than one UTI. However, studies of nonpregnant women with recurrent UTI show a bimodal distribution of infection frequency.[3] Approximately 85 per cent of women with recurrent UTI average about one infection every 3 years and might best be characterized as having "occasional" infections. The remaining 15 per cent experience two or more infections each year, perhaps best described as "frequent" UTIs.

Frequent infections in men or women can be the result of reinfection from organisms originating outside the urinary tract or from persistent infection by the same organism, usually from a focus within the urinary tract. Between episodes of reinfection, the urinary tract is free of bacteria. Organisms that cause reinfections gain entrance to the urinary tract most often from colonization of the vaginal or perianal areas. Reinfections may be occasional or frequent.

Persistent infections occur when the source of infection within the urinary tract continues to inoculate the urine despite antimicrobial therapy. Persistent infections are always frequent and occur promptly after discontinuing therapy, since infected calculi or other foci of infection cannot be successfully sterilized by antimicrobial agents. The same organism, identified by sensitivity patterns or serotype, grows from urine culture during each infection in a cluster of UTIs from bacterial persistence.

Distinguishing between reinfection and persistent infection helps guide diagnostic investigation and therapeutic planning. Consideration of differences in pathogenesis and natural history of bacteriuria in women, men, and elderly patients is also important when planning management of recurrent infections.

■ RECURRENT INFECTIONS IN WOMEN

Uncomplicated lower urinary tract infections in women are the most common UTIs seen by physicians. Approximately one of five women will have a UTI during their lifetime, and 3 per cent of those will have recurrent infections.[4] Bacteriuria is more common in women that in men in all age groups except during infancy. The higher rate of infection is primarily because of easier entrance of bacteria through the shorter female urethra and bacterial colonization of the vagina and perineum.

The most common bacterial pathogen for all UTIs in women is *Escherichia coli*. Of the 150 different serotypes of *E. coli*, only 6 are responsible for most UTIs.[5] Approximately 80 to 85 per cent of recurrent infections in women are due to *E. coli*. *Proteus mirabilis*, *Klebsiella* spp., and *Streptococcus faecalis* are responsible for most other recurrent infections.[6]

The great majority (99 per cent) of recurrent UTIs in women are reinfections. Occasional infections that occur less than once per year are always reinfections.[1] Women who have frequent reinfections often have clusters of two or more UTIs in close succession, followed by a 6-month or longer infection-free period.[6] Reinfections that occur in close succession are often caused by serotypically identical organisms. In contrast to persistent infection, however, each occurrence within a cluster of reinfections is followed by a negative urine culture while the woman is not taking antimicrobial therapy.

Persistent infection, marked by the inability to sterilize the urinary tract for even short periods, is relatively rare in women. The most common causes of bacterial persistence in women are infected urinary calculi, congenital abnormalities that have become secondarily infected, foreign bodies, and papillary necrosis.[7] Frequent infection with organisms other than *E. coli*, particulary *Proteus mirabilis*, *Klebsiella* spp., or

Pseudomonas spp., are more common in persistent infections and should prompt an investigation for infection stones or structural urinary tract abnormalities.[1] The kidney is never the source of bacterial persistence in the absence of stones, necrotic papillae, congenital abnormalities, or azotemia.[7]

A patient's susceptibility to frequent reinfection of the urinary tract is an interplay between host defenses and characteristics of infecting organisms. Colonization of the vagina, perineum, and urethra with pathogenic bacteria is more common in women with frequent infections than in those who remain infection-free.[8] The best explanation for differing rates of colonization and subsequent infection is related to increased adherence of gram-negative bacteria to vaginal and bladder epithelial cells in susceptible women.[4,9] Bacterial "adhesins" in the form of fimbriae or pili attach to receptors on host epithelial cells. In some women, the bacterial adherence that results is strong enough to withstand the usual cleansing effect of urine flow through the urethra, allowing bacteria to gain access more easily to and multiply in the lower urinary tract.

Other risk factors for frequent reinfection of the female urinary tract include sexual activity, use of a diaphragm, and increasing age. After intercourse, a woman is 60 times more likely to develop a UTI within 48 hours than a woman who has not had intercourse.[10] Diaphragm use alters normal vaginal flora, can obstruct the urethra, and acts as a foreign body that can introduce pathogenic bacteria into the vagina. The prevalence of bacteriuria, both symptomatic and asymptomatic, increases with age in both men and women.[11]

■ RECURRENT INFECTIONS IN MEN

Men experience fewer recurrent UTIs than women. When they do occur, however, persistent bacterial infection from a focus within the urinary tract is much more common in men. The most frequent cause of persistent bacteriuria in men, both symptomatic and asymptomatic, is chronic bacterial prostatitis.[12] Mild-to-moderate symptoms of irritative voiding dysfunction, urinary frequency or hesitancy, or discomfort in the perineum, lower abdomen, lower back, or genitalia may be experienced. Pain

with ejaculation and hemospermia also may occur. Chills and fever are uncommon with chronic infection.[13]

The hallmark of chronic bacterial prostatitis is the occurrence of relapsing urinary tract infection by the same pathogenic bacteria, with inability to sterilize the urinary tract following short courses of antimicrobial therapy. Laboratory diagnosis of chronic prostatitis can be difficult. Microscopic examination of prostatic fluid expressed during digital rectal examination may show leukocytes and macrophages. The diagnosis is best confirmed by bacteriologic cultures that localize the pathogen to the prostatic secretions.[14]

The incidence of small prostatic calculi increases with advancing age.[12] These calculi can sometimes be seen on pelvic x-ray films. Careful autopsy examinations have shown that tiny prostatic stones, often invisble on x-ray films, occur in almost every adult prostate.[15] Prostatic calculi can become infected and act as a source of bacterial persistence and recurring urinary tract infections.

Although the prostate gland is the most common source of recurrent infection, radiologic studies should be obtained in any man with persistent bacteriuria to rule out other foci of infection. Urologic consultation should be considered if bladder outlet obstruction from an enlarged prostate gland is suspected.

■ Management

■ RECURRENT INFECTIONS IN WOMEN

The cornerstone of management of frequent reinfections of the female urinary tract is oral antibiotic therapy. The goals of treatment are to minimize the discomfort and disability of frequent infections, treat symptomatic occurrences promptly, and avoid induction of bacterial resistance or other adverse effects of frequent antibiotic administration.

The frequency and pattern of recurrent infections and the level of discomfort from symptomatic episodes are the primary factors influencing management decisions for women with frequent reinfections (Fig. 1).

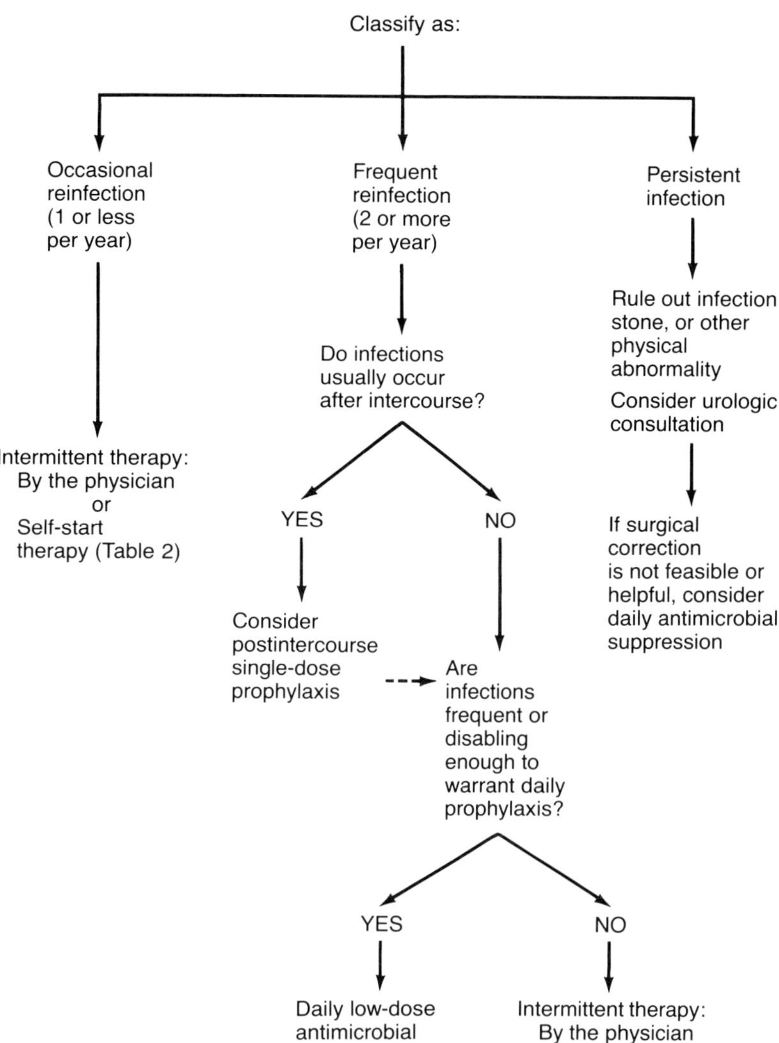

Figure 1. Treatment decisions for women with recurrent, uncomplicated lower urinary tract infections.

Patients can be reassured that recurrent, uncomplicated urinary tract infections do not lead to other problems, such as cancer or infertility, and that they are not sexually transmissable. In the absence of pregnancy, diabetes mellitus, immunosuppression, or obstruction of the urinary tract, serious morbidity from frequent reinfections is rare.[1] With these facts in mind, the physician can decide with the patient whether the frequency or level of discomfort from symptomatic infections warrants a prophylactic antibiotic regimen to minimize the number of infections, or whether prompt intermittent antibiotic therapy for symptomatic infections is sufficient.

Daily low-dose oral antibiotic prophylaxis is often the best choice of treatment for women who experience very frequent, symptomatic, or disabling infections. The goals of daily prophylaxis are to prevent reinfections, either by decreasing the number of bacteria colonizing the vagina and perineum or by clearing bacteria from the urine before symptomatic infection occurs. Ideally, these goals should be achieved with an antibiotic that causes few adverse side effects, is safely taken over a long period of time, and does not encourage bacterial resistance in the rectal or vaginal flora. Daily antibiotic regimens that meet these requirements and successfully prevent recurrent

TABLE 1. Oral Antimicrobial Regimens for Daily Prophylaxis of Recurrent UTIs in Women

Trimethoprim/sulfamethoxazole (Bactrim, Septra) (one-half single-strength tablet)	40 mg/200 mg
Nitrofurantoin (Furadantin)	100 mg q HS
Cinoxacin (Cinobac)	250 mg q HS
Trimethoprim (Proloprim, Trimpex)	50 mg q HS

infections in women are listed in Table 1. Some antimicrobials, such as ampicillin, tetracycline, and cephalexin, may promote bacterial resistance in fecal flora and should not be used for long-term prophylaxis.[4,16]

The daily antibiotic dose is best given at bedtime. This allows the highest levels of antimicrobial in the urine to remain in the bladder overnight during sleep and may enchance effectiveness. Most studies of women who average two to four reinfections per year show a decrease to 0.1 to 0.4 infection per year with once-a-day antibiotic therapy.[1]

If symptoms of a lower urinary tract infection occur during prophylactic therapy, the daily antibiotic should be discontinued and a midstream urine sample obtained for urinalysis, culture, and sensitivity testing. Since the organism that caused the symptomatic infection is likely to be resistant to the antibiotic being used for prophylaxis, a different oral antibiotic regimen at full treatment doses should be started promptly, after urine has been obtained for culture. Any necessary changes in antibiotic choice can be made once sensitivity results are available. Sterilization of the urine should be confirmed by a repeat culture 1 week later, before daily antibiotic prophylaxis is restarted.

Initial treatment with daily antibiotic prophylaxis should continue for at least 6 months. Women who continue to have frequent reinfections following 6 months of daily therapy can safely remain on low-dose prophylactic antibiotics for a much longer period of time. One study has shown the safety and efficacy of 5 years of continuous, low-dose prophylaxis with trimethoprim-sulfamethoxazole.[17]

If reinfections tend to occur within 48 hours of intercourse, a single-dose prophylactic regimen following intercourse may be indicated.[4] If a single-dose antibiotic is used more frequently than once a week, the intermittent effect on bowel and vaginal flora is more likely to induce bacterial resistance than a daily antibiotic dosage. Therefore, this regimen is best for women who have intercourse only occasionally. Women with recurrent infections who use a diaphragm should be counseled to switch to another form of contraception. Voiding soon after intercourse also may reduce the risk of a reinfection.[10]

Women who experience reinfections fewer than once a year, or those who would prefer not to take daily prophylactic antibiotics, may be instructed in the use of intermittent self-start antibiotic therapy for symptomatic infections (Table 2).[16,18] To enchance the accuracy of self-diagnosis, patients should be instructed to collect a clean-catch, midstream urine sample for culture before starting antibiotics. Instructing the patient in the use of a dip-slide device for urine culture may be more efficient and less expensive than relying on standard culture techniques.[16]

Once symptoms have been recognized by the patient and a urine culture has been obtained, a single-dose or 3-day antibiotic course is started promptly (Table 2). If symptoms of UTI recur or persist within 2 to 3 days following self-start therapy, sensitivities of the infective organism should be assessed and a full seven- to ten-day course of appropriate oral antibiotics prescribed promptly. Self-start intermittent therapy is not appropriate if pregnancy, diabetes mellitus, or other complicating conditions are present.

Some treatments or advice traditionally given to women with recurrent infections have not been shown to be helpful in clinical trials. Treatment of an apparent stenotic urethra by repeated dilatation is not useful in the treatment of reinfections.[16] Behavioral aspects, including perianal hygiene, the direction of wiping after bowel movements, frequency of voiding, and the type of material worn as undergarments, also do not appear to be related to the recurrence of UTIs in adult women.[10]

Any suspicion of persistent bacterial infection in a female patient requires investigation of possible anatomic or structural abnormalities of the urinary tract. Urologic consultation should be sought for most

TABLE 2. Protocol for Self-Start Intermittent Antimicrobial Therapy

1. The patient is instructed on recognition of symptoms of lower UTI. She should contact her physician if fever, chills, flank pain or hematuria occurs.
2. When symptoms occur, the patient obtains a clean-catch, midstream urine sample in a sterile container and either
    a. Refrigerates it until the specimen can be taken to a laboratory for culture and sensitivity within 24 hours.
    or
    b. Performs a dip slide culture and takes it to the physician's office for interpretation within 48 hours.
3. The patient then takes one of the following single-dose or 3-day regimens:
    Trimethoprim/sulfamethoxazole, two DS tablets (single dose)
    Trimethoprim/sulfamethoxazole, one DS tablet BID for 3 days
    Norfloxacin, 400 mg BID for 3 days
    Ciprofloxacin, 500 mg BID for 3 days
    Nitrofurantoin, 100 mg QID for 3 days
4. If the initial culture is positive, a repeat urine culture is obtianed 1 week later to ensure adequate treatment.
5. The patient should contact her physican if symptoms recur after single-dose or 3-day therapy.

women with suspected bacterial persistence. If no surgically correctable abnormalities are found or if surgical correction is not possible or indicated, antibiotic suppression of persistent bacterial infection may be necessary.[1] Although sterilization of the infected focus within the urinary system is usually not possible, a daily single-dose antimicrobial agent to which the infecting organism is susceptible will prevent recurring symptomatic infections. The induction of bacterial resistance in bowel flora is a less important consideration when suppressing persistent infections. The choice of treatment should be dictated primarily by culture and sensitivity data and the side effect profile of antibiotics chosen.[1]

■ RECURRENT INFECTIONS IN MEN

Recurrent UTIs caused by bacterial persistence from chronic bacterial prostatitis are best managed initially by long-term oral antibiotic therapy. Most antimicrobial agents do not penetrate into prostatic secretions in high levels, particularly when the prostate is not acutely inflamed. However, a few antibiotics have been shown to be effective in the treatment of chronic infection (Table 3). Trimethoprim-sulfamethoxazole is the most commonly used antimicrobial. Patients who receive trimethoprim-sulfamethoxazole as a double-strength tablet twice a day for 4 to 16 weeks show a rate of cure in various studies of from 30 to 40 per cent.[12] At least 4 to 6 weeks of continuous daily treatment is necessary, although the optimal duration of therapy has not yet been established.

Recent studies have shown the efficacy of norfloxicin in the treatment of recurring urinary tract infections. Norfloxicin has a wide spectrum of activity against bacteria isolated from men with recurrent urinary tract infections. A dose of 400 mg twice a day is tolerated well over a long term of treatment and may be more effective than trimethoprim-sulfamethoxazole in eradicating organisms from the prostate gland.[19]

Patients who are not cured by at least 6 weeks of full-dose oral antibiotics can be managed with low-dose antimicrobial suppression. Trimethoprim-sulfamethoxazole in a dose of one single-strength tablet each day or nitrofurantoin, 100 mg once or twice daily, are reasonable choices since neither is prone to produce resistant fecal bacteria and both are well tolerated in long-term use.[12]

Surgical treatment should also be considered for men who fail 6 or more weeks of oral antibiotic therapy. As many as one third of patients with chronic prostatitis may be helped by transurethral resection of the prostate gland.[20] Success of a transurethral

TABLE 3. Oral Antimicrobial Regimens for Treatment of Chronic Bacterial Prostatitis

Full dose, daily dosing for 4 to 16 weeks:	
Norfloxacin (Noroxin)	400 mg BID
Trimethoprim/sulfamethoxazole (Bactrim, Septra)	160 mg/800 mg BID
Carbenicillin indanyl sodium (Geocillin)	2 tablets QID
Erythromycin (Erythrocin, others)	500 mg QID
Doxycycline (Vibramycin)	100 mg BID

resection depends on the removal of all infected prostatic calculi. This may be difficult, since the peripheral areas of the prostate gland often are the most prominent for prostatic calculi and infection.[12]

■ SPECIAL CONSIDERATIONS IN ELDERLY PATIENTS

Asymptomatic bacteriuria increases in incidence with advancing age in both men and women. It is particularly common in elderly people.[11] Although most physicians agree that asymptomatic bacteriuria in an elderly patient with an otherwise normal urinary tract does not require antibiotic treatment, controversy still exists. In a study of institutionalized elderly men who were not catheterized, antibiotic therapy for asymptomatic bacteria was found to be neither necessary nor effective.[21] However, in ambulatory elderly women who experience recurrent symptomatic UTIs, treatment of asymptomatic bacteriuria may decrease the frequency of symptomatic infection.[22] There is no evidence that treatment of asymptomatic bacteriuria improves mortality rates among elderly people.

In postmenopausal women with recurrent UTIs, a common physiologic cause is decreased natural defenses caused by atrophic vaginitis. Estrogen in the form of topical vaginal cream or oral therapy may decrease the frequency of recurrent infections in women with atrophic vaginitis.[23]

Elderly persons who are in long-term care facilities often have indwelling urinary bladder catheters in place for a variety of reasons. Although rates of urinary tract infection from a single bladder catheterization are less than 1 per cent, colonization and infection develop in nearly all patients with indwelling catheters. By the end of 2 weeks, at least 50 per cent of catheterized patients have significant bacteriuria, and after 30 days nearly all patients are colonized with bacteria.[11] Intermittent antimicrobial treatment of asymptomatic colonization in a catheterized patient will lead to reinfection with increasingly resistant organisms. Antibiotic treatment of recurrent bacteriuria in a catheterized patient is indicated only if signs and symptoms of UTI occur.

■ Issues and Risks

Recurrent urinary tract infections account for millions of visits to physicians' offices each year in the United States. The cost of diagnosis, treatment, and lost time at work due to disability is significant, particularly for patients who experience frequent infections. The safety and efficacy of low-dose daily antibiotic prophylaxis or self-start intermittent antibiotic therapy for frequent reinfections have been clearly established. Use of these techniques can significantly decrease the impact of recurrent infections, either by preventing their occurrence or diminishing their effect with prompt treatment.

The most important risk involved with daily administration of antibiotics is the development of resistant bacterial strains. Careful choice of antibiotics minimizes the dangers of bacterial resistance and reinfection.[1,4] The physician must work closely with the patient to insure adherence to daily or self-start intermittent protocols in order to minimize the chance of bacterial resistance.

The major risk of long-term morbidity from uncomplicated recurrent infections comes with persistent bacteriuria from a focus within the urinary tract. A major diagnostic task of the primary care physician is to rule out peristent bacteriuria caused by obstructive uropathy, stone formation, or congenital abnormalities. Prompt treatment of acute infections, careful follow-up to insure sterilization of urine, and urologic referral when indicated decrease the risk of renal scarring and other serious morbidity from recurrent infections.

Future approaches to the management of recurrent urinary tract infections focus on lessening the adherence of bacteria to mucosal surfaces in the lower urinary tract. Such efforts include replacement of the mucin layer on bladder epithelium, competitive exclusion of pathogenic bacteria with nonpathogenic *Lactobacillus* strains, developing substances that block the adherence of bacteria to receptors on epithelial cells, and immunization against the most common urologic pathogens.[24] Although these techniques are still in early stages of development, initial studies show some promise for eventual clinical application to patients with recurrent urinary tract infections.

REFERENCES

1. Fowler JE. Urinary tract infections in women. Urol Clin North Am 1986; 13:673–683.
2. Stamey TA. A clinical classification of urinary tract infections. South Med J 1975; 68:934–939.
3. Mabeck CE. Treatment of uncomplicated urinary tract infection in nonpregnant women. Postgrad Med 1972; 48:69–75.
4. Shortliffe LMD, Stamey TA. Urinary infections in adult women. *In* Walsh PC, Gittes RF, Perlmutter AD, Stamey TA (eds). Campbell's Urology. Philadelphia: WB Saunders, 1986:797–830.
5. Rantz LA. Serologic grouping of *Escherichia coli*. Arch Intern Med 1962; 129:1153–1157.
6. Kraft JK, Stamey TA. The natural history of symptomatic recurrent bacteriuria in women. Medicine 1977; 56:55–60.
7. Shortliffe LMD, Stamey TA. Infections of the urinary tract: introductions and general principles. *In* Walsh PC, Gittes RF, Perlmutter AD, Stamey TA (eds). Campbell's Urology. Philadelphia: WB Saunders; 1986:738–796.
8. Stamey TA, Sexton CC. The role of vaginal colonization with Enterobacteriaceae in recurrent urinary infections. J Urol 1975; 113:214–217.
9. Fowler JE, Stamey TA. Studies of introital colonization in women with recurrent urinary infections; the role of bacterial adherence. J Urol 1977; 117:472–476.
10. Fihn SD. Behavioral aspects of urinary tract infection. Urology 1988; 32(Suppl 3):16–18.
11. Zilkoski MW, Smucker DR, Mayhew HE. Urinary tract infections in the elderly. Postgrad Med 1988; 84:191–206.
12. Meares EM. Prostatitis and related disorders. *In* Walsh PC, Gittes RF, Perlmutter AD, Stamey TA (eds). Campbell's Urology. Philadelphia: WB Saunders, 1986:868–887.
13. Meares EM. Urinary tract infections in the male patient. Urology 1988; 32(Suppl 3):19–20.
14. Meares EM. Acute and chronic prostatitis: diagnosis and treatment. Infect Dis Clin North Am 1987; 1:855–873.
15. Fox M. The natural history and significance of stone formation in the prostatic gland. J Urol 1963; 89:716–727.
16. Schaeffer AJ. Recurrent urinary tract infections in women. Postgrad Med 1987; 81:51–58.
17. Nicolle LE, Harding GKM, Thomson M, Kennedy J, Urias B, Ronald AR. Efficacy of five years of continuous, low-dose trimethoprim-sulfamethoxazole prophylaxis for urinary tract infection. J Infect Dis 1988; 157:1239–1242.
18. Wong ES, McKevitt M, Running K, Counts GW, Turck M, Stamm WE. Management of recurrent urinary tract infections with patient-administered single-dose therapy. Ann Intern Med 1985; 102:302–307.
19. Sabbaj J, Hoagland VL, Cook T. Norfloxacin versus co-trimoxazole in the treatment of recurring urinary tract infection in men. Scand J Infect Dis 1986; 48(Suppl 1):48–53.
20. Kaye D. Urinary tract infections in the elderly. Bull NY Acad Med 1980; 56:209–220.
21. Nicolle LE, Bjornson J, Harding GK, et al. Bacteriuria in elderly institutionalized men. N Engl J Med 1983; 309:1420–1425.
22. Boscia JA, Kobasa WD, Knight RA, Abrutyn E, Levison ME, Kaye D. Therapy versus no therapy for bacteriuria in elderly, ambulatory, non-hospitalized women. JAMA 1987; 257:1067–1071.
23. Privette M, Cade R, Peterson J, Mars D. Prevention of recurrent urinary tract infections in postmenopausal women. Nephron 1988; 50:24–27.
24. Uehling DT. Future approaches to the management of urinary tract infections. Urol Clin North Am 1986; 13:749–758.

Urticaria and angioedema

William Wagner

■ Background

Hives may be nearly as frustrating for the physician as they are for the patient experiencing them. If the hives are of very recent onset, the cause may be identified. If the hives are chronic, the cause may never be established definitely. Fortunately, control of the urticaria is frequently possible. In addition to pharmacologic measures, management includes avoidance of identifiable trigger factors, investigation and treatment of concurrent illnesses, and resolution of inevitable questions of allergic reactions.

In a study of 554 cases of urticaria and angioedema, the etiology was unknown in 79 per cent of the cases.[1] Cases that were thought to be due to drug eruption other than aspirin were not included in the survey. Aspirin-sensitive patients and patients with psychologic factors were included in the unknown etiology category, since the aspirin and psychologic factors were usually contributory but not the sole cause of urticaria. Cholinergic urticaria accounted for 5.1 per cent of the cases. Physical urticarias, including cold, light, and pressure urticaria, together comprised 3.4 per cent. Dermographism was found in 8.5 per cent. After elimination of drug reactions, 3.1 per cent of the patients were believed to be allergically triggered. Urticaria occurred without angioedema in 40 per cent; urticaria and angioedema occurred together in 49 per cent; and angioedema occurred alone in 11 per cent. The median duration of activity was the longest for patients having combined urticaria and angioedema. Fifty per cent of the cases were still active after 5 years. The median duration of urticaria alone was 6 months, and the median duration of angioedema was 1 year.

CLINICAL APPEARANCE

Typical hives are pruritic papules that develop quickly and resolve in less than 48 hours, leaving normal-appearing skin. The diameter varies from a few millimeters to several centimeters. There may be large areas of confluent dermal swelling. Tiny hives occurring in response to heat suggest cholinergic urticaria. The distribution of hives may suggest one of the physical urticarias (cold, heat, solar, pressure, or vibratory) or contact urticarias (chemicals, foods, or cosmetics). The urticarial papule is principally due to the accumulation of intradermal edema. In a histopathologic study of 45 patients with chronic urticaria, Monroe and associates described 9 cases (20 per cent) with leukocytoclastic vasculitis.[2] The sedimentation rate was elevated in 56 per cent of the vasculitis group, compared with 29 per cent for the sparse infiltrate group. Arthralgias occurred in 44 per cent of the vasculitis group and 29 per cent of the sparse infiltrate group. In a study of 16 urticaria patients with cutaneous necrotizing venulitis, an elevated erythrocyte sedimentation rate was the most common laboratory abnormality.[3] Pain and stiffness of the joints occurred in 15 of the 16 patients. Sedimentation rate should be included in the initial evaluation of urticaria to assess the degree of inflammation.

Angioedema frequently accompanies urticaria. The vascular fluid leakage of angioedema is in the subcutaneous tissue, producing a diffuse swelling. Typical areas of involvement are eyelids, lips, tongue, throat, hands, feet, and genitalia. Pruritus is mild or absent. Angioedema may be associated with chest discomfort, dysphagia, and abdominal pain. Angioedema occurring without hives, even in the absence of a family history of angioedema, should be evaluated for the complement abnormalities (low C4 and absent or nonfunctioning C1 esterase inhibitor) associated with hereditary angioedema, since the management is unique.

ACUTE URTICARIA

Urticaria is often assumed to represent an allergic reaction. This is more often true in acute urticaria than in chronic urticaria. If an external allergen can be identified, the optimal management is avoidance. Drug reactions are a common cause of acute urticaria. A prior history of tolerance of the drug does not rule out allergic reaction; in fact, prior exposure is needed to generate the antibodies participating in the reaction. The clinical history may be complicated by multiple drug administration, concurrent infection, and the possibility of delayed immune reactions to drugs. In the effort to identify a drug contributing to urticaria, first consider the last drug started prior to the onset of hives. Also review the patient's medications for known offenders, such as beta-lactam antibiotics, sulfonamides, narcotic analgesics, radiographic dyes, aspirin, and other nonsteroidal anti-inflammatory drugs. Allergy skin testing is helpful in selected cases, such as penicillin, insulin, and local anesthetic reactions.[4] When the suspected drug cannot be eliminated, desensitization may be needed. Desensitization facilitates continued administration of the allergenic drug while symptoms are treated.

Food allergies may also trigger urticaria. Consistently associated symptoms such as itching of the mouth, vomiting, abdominal cramps, or diarrhea improve the likelihood that a food reaction is occurring. Positive food allergy skin tests with a negative control skin test identify potential clinical food allergies but do not establish the diagnosis. Negative food skin tests with an appropriate positive control are helpful in reducing the likelihood of food allergy. Blind oral challenge may be needed to establish a cause and effect relationship firmly. Food and drug additives, such as tartrazine and sulfites, need to be considered, but reactions confirmed by blind challenge are rare.[5,6] In chronic urticaria, the patient may have accumulated a long list of "red herrings." Elimination of concern over food allergy may greatly facilitate management of the urticaria and protect the patient from unnecessary alteration of lifestyle.

Acute urticaria also may occur after allergy shots. Urticaria distant from the injection site indicates a systemic reaction. In addition to pharmacologic control of the acute symptoms, the injection record should be reviewed for possible errors in extract concentration, time interval, or dosage. Allergists are cautious to avoid administration of allergy shots to patients taking beta-blocker drugs. Calcium channel blockers often may be used in place of beta-blockers in patients on allergy injections. For hypertension, the angiotensin-converting enzyme inhibitors are widely used; however, angioedema has been associated with these drugs.

Allergic contact urticaria commonly occurs among animal dander–sensitive patients after contact with the animal's fur or saliva. Angioedema of the eyelids may occur after petting an animal even though no hives appear on the hands. Contact with foods such as fish, shrimp, beef, chicken, potatoes, nuts, and eggs may cause urticaria on the hands, even though the same foods may be tolerated when ingested.[7] Wearing gloves to handle the food controls the problem.

Some cases of acute urticaria are associated with infection. In evaluating 76 cases of acute urticaria in children and young adults, Schuller found 60 per cent of the cases associated with infections (pharyngitis, viral rhinitis, otitis media, sinusitis, pneumonitis, and urinary tract infection).[8] Urticaria also has been associated with hepatitis, mononucleosis, and helminthic infestations.[9]

In most cases of allergic urticaria, the food or drug allergen will be recognized and avoided, resulting in resolution of the hives. Urticaria secondary to infections may be expected to resolve once the infection is eliminated.

■ CHRONIC URTICARIA

The physical urticarias are a subset of chronic urticaria that should be recognized.

Identification of a physical trigger factor assists in prevention of recurrent urticaria when avoidance is possible.

Cholinergic urticaria is induced by elevation of the body temperature. Typical lesions are 2- to 4-mm pruritic papules on the upper trunk and arms, but systemic manifestations may include hypotension, wheezing, and gastrointestinal complaints.[10] Cholinergic urticaria may be induced by exercise or by passive heat exposure. The lesions usually clear with cooling of the skin. The H_1 blocker hydroxyzine (Atarax, Vistaril) may be effective in preventing cholinergic urticaria.[11] A temporary refractory period may be induced by a cautious hot bath.[12]

Essential acquired cold urticaria is another common physical urticaria. Cold air exposure may induce hives of the face and extremities, and handling frozen food may cause swelling of the hands. The most serious risk comes from cold water immersion, which may result in generalized hives and hypotension. Cold beverages also represent a special risk. In addition to avoidance of cold exposure, antihistamines such as cyproheptadine (Periactin), 2 to 4 mg orally two or three times per day, or doxepin (Adapin, Sinequan), 10 to 25 mg orally two or three times per day, help prevent cold-induced urticaria.[13] The ice cube test, the induction of a hive on the forearm after 3 to 5 minutes' contact with an ice cube, may be used to confirm the diagnosis and to check the adequacy of therapy. Fortunately, the cold urticaria tendency may spontaneously remit after a few months to 1 or 2 years.[10]

Solar urticaria occurs in light-exposed areas. Onset is within 1 to 30 minutes of exposure, and lesions persist for 15 minutes to 3 hours.[10] Management involves avoidance, use of sun blockers, and antihistamines. Temporary tolerance may be induced by controlled light exposure.

Hives often develop in areas of physical pressure. A rare form of delayed pressure urticaria has an atypical presentation. The test pressure stimulus for identification of this condition is 15 pounds applied to the skin for 15 minutes. In this condition, painful indurated lesions develop at the pressure site several hours after the pressure stimulus. Chills, fever, and arthralgias usually accompany the skin lesions. Patients also have typical chronic urticaria. The delayed pressure lesions do not respond to antihistamines but improve with nonsteroidal anti-inflammatory drugs and with corticosteroids.[14]

■ Management

Systemic urticaria developing acutely in the doctor's office or presenting in the emergency room should be treated as a form of anaphylaxis. Initial treatment includes epinephrine 1:1000, 0.3 to 0.5 ml subcutaneously for adults, and 0.01 ml/kg of body weight up to 0.3 ml for children. Diphenhydramine (Benadryl and others) is the second drug used. Intramuscular (IM) administration is usually appropriate in the emergency room. For adults, use 25 to 50 mg IM. For children, use 1 mg/kg weight up to 25 mg. Corticosteroids are rarely needed for acutely developing urticaria. Keep in mind that corticosteroids begin to have pharmacologic effect after approximately 4 hours. If the acute reaction follows a subcutaneous injection in the arm, a tourniquet should be applied briefly above the injection site. If hypotensive, the patient should be placed in the supine position. Intravenous saline may be needed to restore intravascular volume.

In the emergency situation, an external triggering factor is often apparent. Allergens, infections, or physical factors may be identified, leading to specific intervention in patients presenting after a few days or weeks of hives. The difficult management cases are the patients presenting after months and years of hives or angioedema or both, without consistent external cause.

Antihistamines are currently the first line of management. The goal is prevention of hives. Once a hive is present, it will resolve spontaneously within 24 to 48 hours. Failure of an individual lesion to resolve within this time frame casts doubt on the diagnosis of simple urticaria. Antihistamines work by competing with histamine for the tissue receptor sites (H_1 and H_2). The antihistamine works best when it is in the tissue before the histamine is released. Patients with chronic urticaria developing hives at least 2 or 3 days per week will have the best chance of prevention of hives if the drug is taken daily. Diphenhydramine is used in the acute treatment situation but is often too sedating for chronic therapy. Numerous H_1 antihistamines are available. With the exception of terfenadine (Seldane) and astemizole (Hismanal), sedation is a common side effect.

Among the H_1 antihistamines, hydroxyzine (Atarax, Vistaril, and others) is favored because of a long duration of action. Hydroxyzine has been shown to suppress histamine-induced wheal and flare for 36 to 60 hours, respectively.[15] In responsive patients, a single bedtime dose of 20 mg will prevent hives. In resistant cases, the dose may be divided and vary up to 200 mg per day.[9]

Terfenadine (Seldane) and astemizole (Hismanal) are the H_1 antihistamines available for patients intolerant of the more sedating antihistamines. In a double-blind comparison of terfenadine, 60 mg PO BID, with chlorpheniramine, 4 mg PO TID, and with placebo in treatment of chronic idiopathic urticaria, terfenadine was statistically superior to placebo in all 6 weeks of the study.[16] Terfenadine caused less drowsiness and fatigue than chlorpheniramine. In an 8-week double-blind placebo-controlled study of the treatment of chronic idiopathic urticaria, astemizole-treated patients reported significant improvement compared with placebo in control of pruritus, erythema, and extent of wheals.[17] Mild sedative effects were observed in only 2 of 27 patients receiving astemizole. Five of the astemizole-treated patients reported increased appetite. The astemizole dose used was 30 mg PO on the first day, 20 mg PO on the second day, and 10 mg PO on subsequent days. Astemizole has a very long terminal elimination half-life. In repeated administration trials, this value ranged from 18 to 30 days.[18] Any desired allergy skin testing would need to be completed prior to starting astemizole.

Unfortunately, not all patients will achieve satisfactory control of their hives with H_1 blockers alone. Although H_2 blockers are not effective alone in chronic urticaria, the addition of an H_2 blocker to an H_1 blocker improves control of urticaria. In a controlled trial of therapy in chronic urticaria, hydroxyzine, 25 mg PO QID, plus cimetidine (Tagamet), 300 mg PO QID, was compared with hydroxyzine plus each of the following: placebo, terbutaline, cyproheptadine, and chlorpheniramine. The hydroxyzine-cimetidine combination was favored by 58 per cent of the patients and produced the lowest symptom scores and greatest histamine wheal suppression.[19] A double-blind cross-over study of 18 patients showed a statistically significant improvement in itching and in the frequency, number, and size of hives when cimetidine, 300 mg PO QID, was added to the baseline regimen of hydroxyzine, 20 mg PO QID.[20]

Because of the antiandrogen side effects and influence on the hepatic metabolism of other drugs associated with cimetidine, newer H_2 blockers are being tried in combination with H_1 blockers in refractory urticaria. The addition of the H_2 blocker ranitidine (Zantac) to the H_1 blocker clemastine (Tavist) enhanced suppression of allergen-induced cutaneous wheal and flare reactions.[21] Use of the tricyclic antidepressant doxepin (Adapin, Sinequan) in the treatment of chronic urticaria has been proposed because this drug has potent H_1 and H_2 blocker activity. In a double-blind crossover study of doxepin, 25 mg PO TID, in chronic idiopathic urticaria, the doxepin-treated patients experienced fewer lesions, less itching, and less swelling or angioedema.[22] Lethargy, dry mouth, and constipation were commonly observed.

It is recognized that histamine is not the only mediator involved in urticaria. Control of urticaria with antihistamines is often not complete. When severe chronic urticaria interferes with daily living despite antihistamine therapy, corticosteroids are considered. The natural history of chronic urticaria often spans years; if corticosteroids were used for years, adverse effects would be inevitable. In the management of common urticaria, corticosteroid use is kept to a minimum. Doses are decreased and alternate-day therapy is attempted. Antihistamines should be continued to help minimize the duration of therapy with corticosteroids. In certain cases of urticarial vasculitis, the use of prednisone is justified. In some cases of hypocomplementemic urticarial vasculitis, the response has been better to hydroxychloroquine.[23]

■ HEREDITARY ANGIOEDEMA

Hereditary angioedema, associated with deficiency or impaired function of C1 esterase inhibitor, is rare in contrast to the common type of angioedema associated with urticaria. During an acute attack of angioedema in a C1 esterase–deficient patient, the first priority is to be sure the airway is maintained. The unique aspect of management is in the prevention of attacks using attenu-

ated androgens. In a study of 27 patients with hereditary angioedema, the minimal effective dose of stanozolol (Winstrol) needed to reduce the signs and symptoms of angioedema in the presence of minimal side effects ranged from 0.5 to 2.0 mg per day.[24] Stanozolol was started at 2 mg per day. After signs and symptoms of angioedema were controlled on 1 or 2 mg per day for 2 months, the drug dose was individually minimized. Therapy did not have to be interrupted, but while the minimum dose was being attained, 18 patients experienced adverse reactions. The most common was biochemical evidence of hepatic dysfunction. At the minimal effective dose, the hepatic enzymes were in normal range. On minimum dose treatment, the angioedema attack frequency was reduced, even though the C4 and C1 esterase inhibitor levels did not return to normal.

■ Issues and Risks

One of the most common issues for the patient is determining the cause of the urticaria and angioedema. In some cases, an allergic or physical basis can be established. In a few cases, an underlying illness such as an infection can be eradicated with resolution of the urticaria. In the majority of chronic urticaria cases, the intellectual satisfaction of finding the cause of the hives will be absent. Patients should return for periodic follow-up appointments, especially when there is a change in the hives or when new symptoms appear.

Although H_1 antihistamines are usually safe medication, sedation may be hazardous depending on the occupation of the patient. Confusion or other mental status changes are not rare in geriatric patients on antihistamines. Urinary retention is not rare in older men on antihistamines. The H_2 antihistamines are not yet approved for use in management of urticaria, but some patients will benefit from combined use of H_1 and H_2 antihistamines. Use of H_2 blockers alone in urticaria has not been helpful. Corticosteroid therapy is the third line of pharmacologic management. The duration of corticosteroid use is kept to a minimum. The corticosteroid should be the first drug discontinued as severe hives improve. The patient should not expect to be hive-free at the expense of the long-term side effects of corticosteroid treatment.

The role of allergy evaluation for urticaria has two sides. In some cases, an allergic etiology will be established, and the hives can be prevented by avoidance of further exposure. More commonly, patients with chronic urticaria are faced with the bewildering assumption that a food or other environmental allergen is responsible for their hives. Allergy skin tests or RAST tests for specific IgE can be of great help in assessing the probability of allergic reaction to specific foods and environmental allergens. The urticaria patient may be saved from years of unnecessary dietary limitation. In some cases it may be necessary to do blind oral challenges to establish whether a certain food is causing urticaria.

Research efforts into the mechanisms of allergic reactions, the effects of mast cell mediators, and methods to intervene in these events are leading us to greater understanding and more effective treatment for the mystery of urticaria.

REFERENCES

1. Champion RH, Roberts SOB, Carpenter RG, Roger JH. Urticaria and angioedema. Br J Dermatol 1969; 81:588–597.
2. Monroe EW, Schulz CI, Maize JC, Jordon RE. Vasculitis in chronic urticaria: an immunopathologic study. J Invest Dermatol 1981; 76:103–107.
3. Soter NA. Chronic urticaria as a manifestation of necrotizing venulitis. N Engl J Med 1977; 296:1440–1442.
4. Patterson R, DeSwarte RD, Greenberger PA, Grammer LC. Drug allergy and protocols for management of drug allergies. NER Allergy Proc 1986; 7:325–342.
5. Stevenson DD, Simon RA, Lumry WR, Mathison DA. Adverse reactions to tartrazine. J Allergy Clin Immunol 1986; 78:182–191.
6. Bush RK, Taylor SL, Busse W. A critical evaluation of clinical trials of reactions to sulfites. J Allergy Clin Immunol 1986; 78:191–202.
7. Burdick AE, Mathias CGT. The contact urticaria syndrome. Dermatol Clinics 1985; 3:71–84.
8. Schuller DE. Acute urticaria in children. Postgrad Med 1982; 72:179–185.
9. Kaplan AP. Chronic urticaria. Postgrad Med 1983; 74:209–222.
10. Casale TB, Sampson HA, Hanifin J, et al. Guide to physical urticarias. J Allergy Clin Immunol 1988; 82:758–763.
11. Jorizzo JL, Smith EB. The physical urticarias. Arch Dermatol 1982; 118:194–201.
12. Moore-Robinson M, Warin RP. Some clinical aspects of cholinergic urticaria. Br J Dermatol 1968; 80:794–799.
13. Wanderer AA, Grandel KE, Wasserman SI, Farr RS. Clinical characteristics of cold-induced systemic reactions in acquired cold urticaria syndromes: recommendations for prevention of this complication and a proposal for a diagnostic classification of cold urticaria. J Allergy Clin Immunol 1986; 78:417–423.
14. Sussman GL, Harvey RP, Schocket AL. Delayed pressure urticaria. J Allergy Clin Immunol 1982; 70:337–342.
15. Simons FE, Simons KJ, Frith EM. The pharmacokinetics and antihistaminic properties of the H_1 receptor antagonist hydroxyzine. J Allergy Clin Immunol 1984; 73:69–75.
16. Grant JA, Bernstein DI, Buckley CE, et al. Double-blind comparison of terfenadine, chlorpheniramine, and placebo in the treatment of chronic idiopathic urticaria. J Allergy Clin Immunol 1988; 81:574–579.
17. Bernstein IL, Bernstein DI. Efficacy and safety of astemizole, a long-acting and nonsedating H_1 antagonist for the treatment of chronic idiopathic urticaria. J Allergy Clin Immunol 1986; 77:37–42.
18. Woodard JK. Pharmacology and toxicology of nonclassical antihistamine. Cutis 1988; 42:5–9.
19. Harvey RP, Wegs J, Schocket AL. A controlled trial of therapy in chronic urticaria. J Allergy Clin Immunol 1981; 68:262–266.
20. Monroe EW, Cohen SH, Kalbfleisch J, Schulz CI. Combined H_1 and H_2 antihistamine therapy in chronic urticaria. Arch Dermatol 1981; 117:404–407.
21. Thomas RHM, Browne PD, Kirby JDT. The effect of ranitidine, alone and in combination with clemastine, on allergen-induced cutaneous wheal-and-flare reactions in human skin. J Allergy Clin Immunol 1985; 76:864–869.
22. Goldsobel AB, Rohr AS, Siegel SC, et al. Efficacy of doxepin in the treatment of chronic idiopathic urticaria. J Allergy Clin Immunol 1986; 78:867–873.
23. Lopez LR, Davis KC, Kohler PF, Schocket AL. The hypocomplementemic urticarial-vasculitis syndrome: therapeutic response to hydroxychloroquine. J Allergy Clin Immunol 1984; 73:600–603.
24. Sheffer AL, Fearon DT, Austen KF. Hereditary angioedema: a decade of management with stanozolol. J Allergy Clin Immunol 1987; 80:855–860.

Vaginitis, recurrent

Sebastian Faro

■ Background

■ SYMPTOMS

Vaginitis, a term often misused, describes a clinical condition causing symptoms thought to originate from the vagina. The term *vaginitis* signifies the existence of an inflammatory state, detected by the presence of white blood cells. The patient usually complains of one of the following symptoms: pain, itching, soreness, burning, nondescript discomfort, sensation of sandpaper, or dyspareunia. The discharge is usually foul smelling and has changed from a white or slate gray, the normal color, to dirty gray, cream, yellow, or green.[1,2] The term *bacterial vaginosis* has been coined to describe a condition characterized by polymicrobial overgrowth, particularly anaerobes, a noticeable absence of white blood cells, and a thin watery discharge. The lack of white blood cells indicates that inflammation is not associated with this condition, thus the term *vaginosis*. Another cause of bacterial vaginitis, although controversial, is *Gardnerella vaginalis*; this organism can be found in association with anaerobes (bacterial vaginosis) or can be the predominant organism in vaginitis. *G. vaginalis* vaginitis is characterized by a foul-smelling, dirty gray discharge and the patient often complains of a nondescript discomfort or burning.

The two most common nonbacterial causes of vaginitis are *Trichomonas vaginalis* and *Candida albicans*. *T. vaginalis*, a flagellated protozoan, is responsible for 180 million cases of vaginitis worldwide each year. Many women infected with this organism are asymptomatic. Approximately 50 to 75 per cent of the female patients have a discharge that varies from dirty gray to yellow or cream colored. Twenty-five to fifty per cent of patients complain of vulvovaginal irritation. It is interesting that 5 to 10 per cent of the patients complain of lower abdominal pain.[3] Examination of the vaginal walls and cervix may reveal the presence of petechial hemorrhages, the so-called "strawberry cervix." Since *T. vaginalis* is one of the most common sexually transmitted organisms, coexisting sexually transmitted organisms, such as *Neisseria gonorrhoeae*, *Chlamydia trachomatis*, and *herpes simplex* are often found.

Fungal infection of the vagina is most frequently due to *Candida albicans*, although other species of *Candida* have been identified as causes of vaginitis. Typically, the symptomatic patient has pruritus of the vulva and vagina; erythema is prominent, and edema may also be present. Excoriations are often present and may be severe. The discharge is usually thick and adherent to the vaginal walls, but may be thin and liquid.

■ PHYSICAL EXAMINATION

The pelvic examination begins with a thorough inspection of the vulva for signs of infection: inflammation, ulcers, papules, areas of raised epithelium, or a cobblestone appearance of the epithelium. The folds between the labia should be examined for ulcers, which are likely to go unnoticed. The prepuce of the clitoris should be drawn back to expose the clitoris and surrounding tissue. If any lesions are found, appropriate specimens should be obtained for the detection of specific organisms, e.g., *Treponema pallidum*, *Haemophilus ducreyi*, *Chlamydia trachomatis*, and *herpes simplex*. Areas suspicious for human papilloma virus (HPV) infection appear as discrete zones of erythema or small papules or blisters. The virus, when found in this subtle presentation as differentiated from frank condyloma, appears to have a preference for the inferomedial aspect of the labia minora. These areas are usually tender or painful to gentle palpation.

Application of 5 per cent acetic acid to these areas results in the development of aceto-white epithelium, which is characteristic but not pathognomonic of HPV cellular infection.[4] Areas suspicious for malignant changes should be painted with toluidine blue. The dye should remain on the tissue for 5 minutes, followed by washing with 5 per cent acetic acid. Those areas that retained the toluidine dye should be biopsied and specimens sent for histologic study.

The vestibule should be examined to determine whether the urethral meatus is inflamed, there is purulent discharge, or Skene's or Bartholin's glands are infected. Specimens obtained from the urethra and Skene's and Bartholin's glands should be cultured for *Neisseria gonorrhoeae*, *Chlamydia trachomatis*, *Mycoplasma hominis*, and *Ureaplasma urealyticum*. If Skene's or Bartholin's glands are abscessed, the specimens also should be cultured for aerobic bacteria such as *Streptococcus agalactiae*, members of the Enterobacteriaceae, and anaerobes, such as *Bacteroides*, *Fusobacterium* and *Peptostreptococcus*.

A speculum should be gently inserted into the vagina, taking care to avoid traumatizing the cervix to prevent bleeding that would interfere with the evaluation of the vagina. The vaginal walls should be examined for ulcerated lesions, petechial hemorrhages, cobblestoning of the epithelium, areas of raised white epithelium, and abnormal vascular pattern. The vaginal discharge should be characterized as to quantity, consistency, color, and odor.

■ LABORATORY

The laboratory investigation of recurrent vaginitis can be divided into immediate application of simple laboratory procedures versus more involved tests. Significant information can be obtained by performing inexpensive tests in the office.

One or two drops of vaginal discharge are mixed with one or two drops of concentrated potassium hydroxide (KOH) to determine whether a fishy odor is emitted (whiff test). The presence of amines (fishy odor) is associated with an overgrowth of *Gardnerella vaginalis* or anaerobes or both. This specimen also should be examined microscopically for the presence of yeast. Pseudohyphae of *C. albicans*, which contain chitin, are resistant to concentrated alkali. The alkaline solution will dissolve and disrupt the squamous epithelial cells, white blood cells, and bacteria, which facilitates the identification and recognition of yeast forms.

The pH of the vaginal fluid is normally 3.8 to 4.2 and can be easily determined by immersing litmus paper in the vaginal discharge. The color change can be compared with the chart provided on the container housing the litmus paper to determine the pH value. A pH of 4.5 or more indicates abnormal bacterial growth.[2] When a yeast infection is present, the pH may be less than 4.5, since fungi typically prefer a more acidic environment than do bacteria. However, a pH above 4.5 does not rule out the presence of *C. albicans*.

One or two drops of vaginal discharge are mixed with 1 to 2 ml of normal saline, and a drop of this diluted discharge is examined microscopically. Normal vaginal discharge contains mature squamous epithelial cells, if there is adequate estrogen. If estrogen is deficient, a large number of immature squamous cells will be seen. These are circular to elliptical with a large central nucleus, and are referred to as parabasal cells. Mature squamous cells, in the healthy or normal state, are not covered by debris and bacteria. The nucleus is easily identified, the cells' membrane is sharply delineated, and cytoplasm is neither densely granulated nor obliterated. White blood cells are rare, and the free-floating bacteria are not clumped together. The predominant bacteria are *Lactobacillus*, which are rod-shaped and appear blue to violet when Gram-stained. (Fig. 1A).

When the bacterial flora is abnormal, different presentations are possible on microscopic examination after discharge.[5] The one common finding is the presence of "clue cells," which are squamous epithelial cells densely covered with adherent bacteria (Fig. 1B) that stain red (gram-negative). These gram-negative bacilli are usually *Gardnerella vaginalis*. Gram-positive and gram-negative bacilli, as well as cocci, are usually present in the vaginal fluid. If the patient has *Gardnerella vaginalis* vaginitis, clue cells are present, the bacteria in the surrounding medium are clumped together, and there is a noticeable absence of white blood cells. Patients with bacterial vaginosis have a vaginal discharge similar to that seen with *G. vaginalis* vaginitis. The difference is that

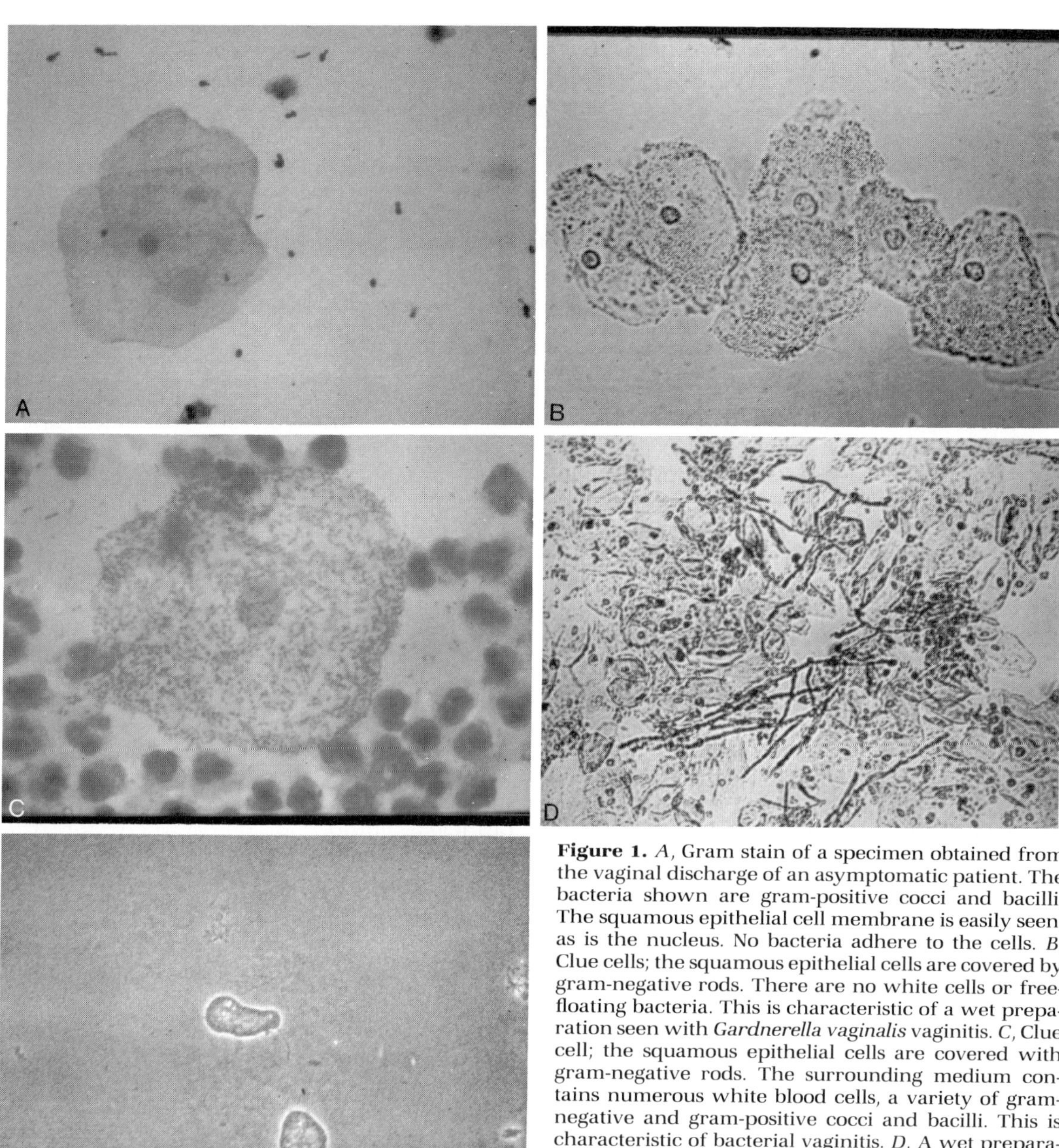

Figure 1. *A*, Gram stain of a specimen obtained from the vaginal discharge of an asymptomatic patient. The bacteria shown are gram-positive cocci and bacilli. The squamous epithelial cell membrane is easily seen, as is the nucleus. No bacteria adhere to the cells. *B*, Clue cells; the squamous epithelial cells are covered by gram-negative rods. There are no white cells or free-floating bacteria. This is characteristic of a wet preparation seen with *Gardnerella vaginalis* vaginitis. *C*, Clue cell; the squamous epithelial cells are covered with gram-negative rods. The surrounding medium contains numerous white blood cells, a variety of gram-negative and gram-positive cocci and bacilli. This is characteristic of bacterial vaginitis. *D*, A wet preparation of vaginal discharge from a patient with *C. albicans* vaginitis. Note the presence of hyphal structures (dark filaments). Numerous squamous epithelial cells are present. *E*, Wet preparation of vaginal discharge containing *Trichomonas vaginalis*.

bacteria in the vaginal fluid are not clumped together but retain their individuality. Patients with bacterial vaginitis will have clue cells, many different free-floating bacteria that are not clumped together, and numerous white blood cells (Fig. 1C). If the preparation is Gram stained, there are numerous gram-positive and gram-negative bacteria (Table 1).

Patients with *C. albicans* vaginitis usually have a pH of 4.2 or less; the discharge characteristically is white and pasty, described as cottage cheese-like. A pH greater than 4.2 does not rule out the presence of *Candida*. *C. albicans* may coexist with bacterial vaginitis. If it is difficult to see yeast cells, budding yeast cells or pseudohyphae, the discharge should be mixed with concentrated

TABLE 1. Characteristics of Vaginal Discharge

Characteristic	Normal	*G. vaginalis*	Bacterial vaginosis	Bacterial vaginitis
pH	3.8–4.2	≥4.5	≥4.5	≥4.5
Amines	—	+	+	+
Clue cells	—	+	+	+
WBC	±	—	—	+
Bacteria	bacilli	clumped bacilli, cocci	free-floating bacilli, cocci	free-floating bacilli, cocci

KOH as described earlier (Fig. 1*D*). If the patient's symptoms suggest a yeast infection but it cannot be substantiated by examining the vaginal discharge microscopically, a specimen should be obtained for the culture of *Candida* by inoculating a specimen on one of the commercially available media.

If the vaginal discharge has a pH of 4.5 or more and appears frothy, then the presence of *T. vaginalis* should be suspected. *T. vaginalis* can be easily identified by its motility and beating flagella (Fig. 1*E*). Patients with a history of recurrent infection in which no protozoa can be seen should have a vaginal specimen for the culture of *T. vaginalis*. Commercial media, e.g., Diamond's or Feinberg-Whittington media—can increase the accuracy of the diagnosis. Approximately 95 per cent of the cases can be confirmed by culturing the organism. When resistance is suspected, antibiotic sensitivities can be conducted on the isolated protozoan.

The patient with recurrent bacterial vaginitis or vaginosis who has been treated with various antimicrobial agents should have a vaginal specimen obtained for the isolation of aerobes and anaerobes. Some authorities would not recommend obtaining a specimen for culture. However, these patients often have been treated with several courses of metronidazole, cephalosporins, ampicillin, clindamycin, and sulfonamide preparations but continue to be symptomatic. Therefore, it seems appropriate to determine the types of bacteria present and which organisms dominate. The specimen should be transported in an anaerobic vial since the vagina contains many different bacteria (Table 2), especially anaerobes, which are usually fastidious. Knowing the concentration of bacteria per milliliter of vaginal fluid will establish which organisms are dominant. Antibiotic sensitivities (specifically, oral antibiotics) should be determined for the dominant organisms.

■ Management

The management of patients with a recurrent vaginal infection is difficult because the patient is often frustrated, may be angry, and has spent a considerable amount of

TABLE 2. Indigenous Bacteria of the Vagina

Aerobes	Anaerobes
Lactobacillus	*Bacteroides bivius*
Diphtheroids	*Bacteroides disiens*
Corynebacterium	*Bacteroides distasonis*
beta-hemolytic streptococcus	*Bacteroides fragilis*
Escherichia coli	*Bacteroides melaninogenicus*
Enterobacter cloacae	*Fusobacterium*
Enterobacter aerogenes	
Enterobacter agglomerans	
Proteus mirabilis	
Klebsiella pneumoniae	
Staphylococcus epidermidis	
Staphylococcus aureus	
non-group D streptococcus	
group D streptococcus	
Streptococcus agalactiae	
Streptococcus faecalis	

TABLE 3. Treatment Regimens for Bacterial Vaginitis

Disease	Antibiotic	Dosage
Gardnerella vaginalis	Cefuroxime axetil (Ceftin)	250 mg, BID × 7 days
	Cephalexin (Keflex)	
Bacterial vaginitis	Amoxicillin/clavulanic acid (Augmentin)	500 mg, TID × 7 days
Bacterial vaginosis	Metronidazole (Flagyl)	500 mg, TID × 7 days

money for both doctors' fees and treatment regimens. These patients have usually seen many different physicians, seeking someone to cure their condition. It is important to establish good communication with the patient and attempt to educate her about the characteristics of a normal vagina. Explain that the goal is to restore the normal microflora and discharge to the vagina. The treatment of vaginitis depends upon determining the specific etiology, because inappropriate treatment will result in significant alteration of the vaginal flora (Table 3). Empiric or "shot-gun" treatment results in complicating the identification of the specific cause of vaginitis.

Controversy exists over whether or not bacterial infections are sexually transmitted, and whether or not the partner should be treated. Since these patients have recurrent infection and it is more than likely that the man was offered treatment, both should be counseled. The man should be advised to wear a condom during the treatment and follow-up period. This will eliminate the possibility of re-infection. If the patient and her partner participate in oral-genital or anal intercourse, they should be encouraged to discontinue these practices during the treatment and follow-up period. These activities may result in the introduction of large numbers of bacteria into the vagina.

Many individuals find it difficult to take medication three or four times a day for 10 days. Since compliance is often incomplete, it is important to impress upon the patient that she must complete the course of medication as prescribed.

■ BACTERIAL VAGINOSIS, VAGINITIS, AND *G. VAGINALIS* VAGINITIS

These forms of abnormal bacterial vaginal flora are all characterized by the presence of a dominant flora that may or may not be anaerobes. Bacterial vaginosis and *G. vaginalis* vaginitis are both characterized by the presence of clue cells and *G. vaginalis*. Treatment with metronidazole appears to be illogical since *G. vaginalis* tends to be resistant to this antibiotic. In addition, patients with recurrent bacterial vaginitis have more likely received repeated courses of metronidazole, and the bacteria that are now present may be resistant. Therefore, a culture establishing the dominant bacteria and determination of their antibiotic sensitivities should be carried out. Recurrent bacterial vaginitis is frequently polymicrobial, involving anaerobes as well as members of the Enterobacteriaceae. Therefore, it would be wise to use an agent such as amoxicillin/clavulanic acid (Augmentin), 500 mg orally, three times a day for 10 days, which can be initiated before knowing the identity of the bacteria and the antibiotic sensitivities. Augmentin has a spectrum of activity that includes aerobes and facultative and obligate anaerobes. The presence of clavulanic acid will inhibit the beta-lactamase enzymes produced by many of these bacteria. Thus, a single antibiotic can treat these complex conditions.

When *G. vaginalis* is present with a predominance of anaerobes, it is usually not found in a concentration exceeding 10^3 colony-forming units (cfu)/ml. This is characteristic of bacterial vaginosis. Clindamycin, 300 mg orally three times daily for 10 days, is suitable. This agent has excellent anaerobic activity as well as activity against *G. vaginalis*.

Patients in whom *G. vaginalis* is present in a concentration greater than 10^5 cfu/ml usually do not have a significant number of other bacteria. It is not unusual for these other bacteria to be members of the Enterobacteriaceae family. Augmentin, 500 mg orally three times daily, or cefuroxime (Ceftin), 250 mg orally twice daily for 10 days may be used in therapy.

■ TRICHOMONIASIS

Treatment of *T. vaginalis* vaginitis must include the male partner. *T. vaginalis*, a sexually transmitted organism, has been recovered from 70 per cent of men whose female partners were infected and 85 per cent of women who had infected male partners. Since this is a frequently occurring sexually transmitted organism, it is not uncommon to find other coexisting sexually transmitted organisms.[6] Two situations make it difficult to eradicate this organism from the vagina; one is pregnancy and the other is the so-called metronidazole-resistant infection.

Although transmission is principally via sexual intercourse, nonvenereal transmission is possible. Urine, semen, vaginal exudates, and towels have been shown to act as vectors. Neonatal trichomoniasis has been reported in approximately 5 per cent of female infants born to infected women.[7] Thus, it is extremely important to point out to the patient the need for meticulous hygiene.

Treatment can be initated by administering metronidazole, 2 gm as a single oral dose. However, this is not suitable for the patient with recurrent disease. Initially, 500 mg of oral metronidazole three times daily for 7 days can be used for patients with recurrent disease. The male partner, although treated simultaneously, should wear a condom during sexual intercourse. This allows the physician to determine whether the patient responds to metronidazole in the prescribed dosage. If the patient's vagina has not been cleared of the protozoan, the dosage can be increased by administering 500 mg orally three times daily in conjunction with 500-mg vaginal suppositories twice a day. If this regimen is unsuccessful, then the presence of resistance must be considered and the physician must obtain material for antibiotic sensitivity testing. Strains of *T. vaginalis* resistant to metronidazole are rare.[8,9] However, even if the organism is resistant, metronidazole is the primary agent for the treatment of *T. vaginalis* and can be administered in higher dosages. The dosage can be increased to 3 or even 4 grams per day, which will usually cause nausea that may require the use of antiemetics. The patient may have to be hospitalized to allow

for the administration of high doses of metronidazole because of the possible toxicity. The dosage may be divided between oral, rectal, vaginal, or intravenous routes, which may reduce the incidence and severity of the nausea, metallic taste, and perhaps neurotoxicity.

■ YEAST VAGINITIS

The two most common species of *Candida* are *C. albicans* and *C. glabrata*; the former is the most frequent cause of yeast vaginitis. *C. glabrata* differs from *C. albicans* in that it is a smaller organism and grows as a budding yeast. *C. glabrata* is not inhibited by the usual concentration of miconazole, nystatin, enconazole, and butaconazole. This species develops resistance to the azole antifungal agents rapidly.[10] *C. glabrata* is sensitive to clotrimazole, ketoconazole, and amphotericin B.

The patient who has been treated with several courses of antifungals, such as miconazole, but continues to be infected should have the fungus isolated and identified as to species. Species other than *C. albicans* may be responsible. It is also possible that the patient is being reinfected from her own gastrointestinal (GI) tract or her sexual partner. It is extremely difficult to clear the rectum of microorganisms, but an attempt at controlling the GI population is possible with an agent such as ketoconazole. Prior to instituting long-term therapy, the patient should be instructed not to wear tight-fitting synthetic garments and to avoid perfumed douches. The physican should determine whether she is taking antibiotics (even maintenance doses) or corticosteroids, and she should be screened for diabetes and acquired immunodeficiency disease.

Several different regimens have been advocated for the treatment of recurrent candidiasis. Thus far, in all studies, when the maintenance antifungal agent was discontinued, the disease recurred within 3 months.[11–13]

One approach is to treat the symptomatic patient with an antifungal agent for a period of 7 to 10 days, then re-examine to determine whether the yeast has been eradicated or the problem has been reduced to an asymptomatic state. The patient can be advised to use the agent for two to three days prior to and after the menses. Another approach is to treat the patient with ketoconazole, 400 mg, given orally for 14 days. This is followed with 100 mg of ketoconazole daily for 6 months.[13] Patients on ketoconazole must be monitored for nausea, rash, headaches, and anaphylaxis. They must also be advised that ketoconazole can cause liver toxicity, and, therefore, liver function tests must be performed regularly.

Issues and Risks

BACTERIAL VAGINITIS

Bacterial vaginal infections, including vaginosis, may be precursors to postoperative infection, chorioamnionitis, premature rupture of membranes, premature labor, and premature delivery.[14] The spectrum of bacterial vaginitis may represent a continuum that is influenced by the treatment. This is specifically seen when antimicrobial therapy is prescribed without examining and evaluating the patient. Inappropriate therapy will result in selection of resistant bacteria, resulting in further alteration of the vaginal microflora. The presence of an abnormal bacterial flora can be determined upon examination and office laboratory testing, as discussed earlier. The difficulty arises in treating these conditions, since they are polymicrobial infections. Treatment must also consider outside influences such as the sexual partner, although his role has not been elucidated.

TRICHOMONIASIS

The pregnant patient with *T. vaginalis* poses an interesting challenge. The safety of metronidazole has not been firmly established, and animal data suggest that the drug may be teratogenic and carcinogenic. The antibiotic has been shown to induce tumors in laboratory animals receiving high doses over a prolonged period of time.[15,16] However, recent studies in humans have not confirmed these concerns. A possible alternative to the use of metronidazole for the treatment of *T. vaginalis* vaginitis in the pregnant patient is clotrimazole. A dose of 100 mg, administered intravaginally daily for 6 days, has been effective.

The association between *T. vaginalis* and vaginal bacteria needs to be studied. Since *T. vaginalis* is a motile organism, does it serve as a source of transportation for bacteria? Does the presence of *T. vaginalis* indicate that the vaginal bacterial flora is abnormal; that is, is there a predominance of anaerobes and other potentially pathogenic bacteria?

YEAST VAGINITIS

Treatment of recurrent *C. albicans* vaginitis has been unsatisfactory. The best that can be hoped for is to suppress the organism to numbers that do not cause symptoms. Infection is dependent upon inoculum size; thus, if the number of yeast cells can be kept below a threshold number, then symptomatic infection may be prevented. It does not appear that vaginal medication will be successful in curing the patient with recurrent yeast vaginitis. Recent studies have proposed that there is a local immunologic defect in the lower genital tract of individuals with recurrent disease. There appears to be a transient inhibition of cell-mediated immunity in the vagina, manifested by the inability of vaginal lymphocytes to mount a proliferative response to *Candida albicans*. This impairment allows *C. albicans* to proliferate, adhere to the vaginal epithelium, and cause symptoms.[17]

REFERENCES

1. Faro S, Phillips, LE. Non-specific vaginitis or vaginitis of undetermined aetiology. Int J Tiss Reac 1987; IX(2):173–177.
2. Amsel R, Totten PA, Spiegel CA, Chenk CS. Non-specific vaginitis: diagnostic criteria and microbial and epidemiological associations. Am J Med 1983; 74:14–22.
3. Honigberg B. Trichomonads of importance to human medicine. *In* Krier JP (ed). Parasitic Protozoa. Vol 2. New York: Academic Press, 1978: 275.
4. Champion MJ. Clinical manifestations and natural history of genital human papillomavirus infection. Obstet Gynecol Clin North Am 1987; 14:363–388.
5. Larsen B, Galask RP. Vaginal microbial flora: composition and influences of host physiology. Ann Intern Med 1982; 96:926–930.
6. Judson FN. The importance of co-existing syphilitic, chlamydia, mycoplasmal, and trichomonal infections in the treatment of gonorrhea. Sex Trans Dis 1979; 6:112–114.
7. Al-Salihi FL, et al. Neonatal *Trichomonas vaginalis:* report of three cases and review of the literature. Pediatrics 1974; 53:196–198.
8. Ralph ED, Darwish R, Austin TW, et al. Susceptibil-

ity of *T. vaginalis* strains to metronidazole: response to treatment. Sex Trans Dis 1983; 10:119–122.

9. Muller M, Lossick JG, Gorrell TE. In vitro suscepti-bility of *T. vaginalis* to metronidazole and treatment outcome in vaginal trichomoniasis. Sex Trans Dis 1988; 15:17–24.

10. Segal E. Pathogenesis of human mycoses: role of adhesion to host surfaces. Microbiol Sci 1987; 4(11):344–347.

11. Warnoch DW, Burke J, Cope NJ, Johnson EM, et al. Fluconazole resistance in *Candida glabrata*. Lancet 1984; 2:1310.

12. Sobel JD. Management of recurrent vulvovaginal candidiasis with intermittent ketoconazole prophy-laxis. Obstet Gynecol 1985; 65:435–440.

13. Sobel JD. Recurrent vulvovaginal candidiasis. A

prospective study of the efficacy of maintenance ketoconazole therapy. N Engl J Med 1986; 315:1455–1458.

14. Faro S, Phillips LE, Martens MG. Perspectives on the bacteriology of postoperative obstetric-gynecologic infections. AM J Obstet Gynecol 1988; 158:694–700.

15. Beard CM, Noller KO, O'Fallan WM, et al. Cancer after exposure to metronidazole. Mayo Clin Proc 1988; 63:147–153.

16. Roe JFC. A critical appraisal of the toxicology of metronidazole. *In* Phillips I, Collier J (eds). Metronidazole: Proceedings of the Second International Symposium on Anaerobic Infections. London: Academic Press, 1979:215–222.

17. Witkin SS. Immunology of recurrent vaginitis. Am J Reproduc Med 1987; 15:34–37.

Ventricular arrhythmias

Steven P. Kutalek ■ *Joel Morganroth*

Ventricular arrhythmias comprise a group of commonly occurring cardiac rhythm disorders originating distal to the AV node, of varying complexity and severity. The clinical spectrum ranges from asymptomatic ventricular premature complexes (VPCs) and nonsustained ventricular tachycardia (NSVT) to life-threatening, often fatal, sustained ventricular tachycardia (VT) and ventricular fibrillation (VF). Ventricular arrhythmias represent a difficult medical management problem because of their variable prognosis, the need for risk stratification to identify patients prone to fatal arrhythmia, the inadequacy and toxicity of many forms of medical therapy, the overall poor prognosis in patients with sustained arrhythmias, and the uncertainty as to whether antiarrhythmic therapy improves long-term prognosis in many patients with asymptomatic, potentially malignant arrhythmias in the absence of sustained ventricular tachycardia.

■ Background

The presentation of ventricular arrhythmias is acute or chronic. Selection of modes of therapy follows stratification of risk into be-

nign, potentially lethal, or lethal forms. Identification and differential diagnosis are accomplished by 12-lead electrocardiography and ambulatory monitoring for benign or potentially lethal arrhythmias, or by clinical cardiac electrophysiologic testing for paroxysmal sustained ventricular tachycardia or ventricular fibrillation. These methods also provide parameters to measure efficacy of therapy and electropharmacologic toxicity of medical agents.[1-3]

Acute sustained ventricular tachycardia or ventricular fibrillation occurs in association with acute myocardial infarction or cardiac ischemia; in the presence of severe electrolyte, pH, or metabolic disturbances; secondary to proarrhythmic (arrhythmia-exacerbating) effects of antiarrhythmic drugs; or spontaneously in patients with ischemic or nonischemic cardiomyopathy and the long QT syndrome. These lethal rhythm disorders often result in syncope and hemodynamic collapse, accounting for the majority (80 per cent) of episodes of sudden cardiac death.[4-6] Acute nonsustained, hemodynamically compromising ventricular tachycardia that results in lightheadedness or syncope must also be considered life threatening.

Benign chronic ventricular premature complexes or nonsustained ventricular tachycardia, asymptomatic or producing palpitations, occurs in structurally normal hearts and carries minimal sudden death risk.[7,8] In association with organic myocardial disease, however, 10 or more VPCs per hour on ambulatory monitor or NSVT significantly increases sudden death risk, and thus may be classified as potentially lethal.[9–11] Structural cardiac disease includes regional wall motion abnormalities caused by myocardial infarction, cardiomyopathy with left ventricular ejection fraction less than 40 per cent, or hypertrophic cardiomyopathy.

The acute onset of benign or potentially lethal arrhythmias may be marked by palpitations or remain asymptomatic, being detected only by electrocardiographic monitoring. Sustained lethal arrhythmias may present as lightheadedness, syncope, sudden death, progressive angina, congestive heart failure, or palpitations. Catecholamines and a variety of stimulant medications can exacerbate or precipitate acute ventricular arrhythmias.

Ventricular arrhythmias may be automatic, due to enhanced rates of phase 4 depolarization; this resting phase of the ventricular action potential normally manifests only slow spontaneous depolarization. More frequently, ventricular arrhythmias result from re-entry caused by microcircuits in the subendocardium or, less frequently, macrore-entry. These arrhythmias are most often left ventricular in origin. The re-entrant form frequently can be terminated by programmed electrical stimulation or overdrive pacing, whereas definitive correction of automatic arrhythmias requires removal of the inciting stimulus.

■ Management

Therapeutic goals are the prevention of sudden cardiac death, or relief of symptomatic palpitations and lightheadedness when the risk of treatment is warranted. Chronic, prolonged suppressive antiarrhythmic therapy is indicated for patients with lethal arrhythmias.

■ ACUTE THERAPY

Acute sustained ventricular tachycardia or ventricular fibrillation requires immediate therapy. In the presence of hemodynamic compromise (which may result in heart failure, uncontrolled angina, hypotension, or signs of acute hypoperfusion, including lightheadedness or syncope), direct current electrical cardioversion is the treatment of choice. VF requires transthoracic defibrillation with 200 joules, followed by an additional 200–360 joules if the initial shock is unsuccessful.[12] Acute sustained monomorphic VT often can be cardioverted with lower energies, starting at 50 joules, but increasing rapidly as required. With organized VT, cardioversion *synchronized* with the QRS complex will minimize the potential for acceleration to VF. Concomitant acute therapy with intravenous lidocaine (Xylocaine) should be initiated unless there is allergy to the medication. Correction of electrolyte abnormalities, pH, oxygenation, congestive heart failure, and ischemia plays an important role in the acute control of malignant VT or VF, as does withdrawal of medications that may exacerbate the arrhythmia. Table 1 lists some potentially proarrhythmic drugs.

Upon failure of lidocaine and metabolic correction, intravenous bretylium (Bretylol) may be useful for acute control, especially for VF,[12] but prolonged use (greater than 48 hours) is not recommended, since the drug may deplete catecholamine stores. Intravenous procainamide (Pronestyl) also provides an effective second-line defense for breakthrough arrhythmias after lidocaine; however, the administration rate must be controlled at a maximum of 50 mg/min to avoid severe vasodilatory hypotension, and thus the drug takes longer to load than does lidocaine. Procainamide-induced hypotension may be treated by decreasing the rate of drug infusion and cautiously administering IV fluids. Since catecholamine stimulants may exacerbate acute ventricular arrhythmias, they should be avoided if possible unless required to maintain blood pressure.

Especially in proarrhythmic patients or

TABLE 1. Examples of Potentially Proarrhythmic Drugs

Catecholamines
Theophylline derivatives
Antiarrhythmic medications, including digitalis
Diuretics causing hypokalemia
Tricyclic antidepressants
Alcohol and caffeine

those with the prolonged QT syndrome, continuous pacing of the atrium or ventricle at rates greater than the sinus rate may suppress VT or torsade de pointes by decreasing ventricular refractory period disparity. Ventricular pacing has the advantage of lead stability and avoids potential irregularities in R-R intervals due to AV Wenckebach. Pacing also remains the therapy of choice for bradycardia-induced VT or VF. Intravenous isoproterenol (Isuprel) increases sinus rate and can be used to treat torsade de pointes, but catecholamines may stimulate the arrhythmogenic focus in some patients.

Subsequent to acute control of sustained VT or VF, unless a distinct etiology can be defined that precipitated the event, electrophysiologic testing may be indicated with the patient off antiarrhythmic medications, to guide chronic antiarrhythmic therapy[2,3,13] (Table 2).

Infrequently, the acute onset of palpitations and lightheadedness may be associated with VPCs or NSVT. If hemodynamic compromise is suspected, the arrhythmia should be approached aggressively with the patient in hospital. Otherwise, chronic therapy defined on the basis of risk stratification is indicated.

■ CHRONIC THERAPY

Chronic management of ventricular arrhythmias involves therapy with antiarrhythmic medications or devices. Table 3 delineates commonly used drugs and dosages for long-term control of these arrhythmias. Decisions to treat are based on stratification of sudden death risk and an understanding of potential toxicities and adverse effects of antiarrhythmic therapy (Table 4).

TABLE 2. Sequence for Electrophysiologic Testing Using Programmed Ventricular Stimulation (PVS)

1. Stop antiarrhythmic medications that affect ventricular arrhythmias and let drugs wash out
2. Baseline PVS off antiarrhythmic medications; induce arrhythmia
3. Acute IV administration of antiarrhythmic drug and repeat PVS
4. Oral administration of antiarrhythmic drug and achieve steady rate
5. Repeat PVS on oral drug
6. Repeat steps 4 and 5 as required

TABLE 3. Antiarrhythmic Medications for Ventricular Arrhythmias

Class	Generic Name	Common Dosages† (mg)
IA	Procainamide*	250–1000 QID
	Quinidine*	200–400 QID
	Disopyramide*	100–300 QID
IB	Tocainide	300–600 TID
	Mexiletine	150–400 TID
	Lidocaine	IV infusion at 1–4 mg/min
IC	Flecainide	100–200 BID
	Encainide	25–50 TID
	Propafenone	150–300 TID
II	Propranolol*	10–100 TID
III	Amiodarone	200–600 OD
	Bretylium	IV infusion at 1–4 mg/min

*Sustained-release preparations available.
†Dosages for individual patients may vary outside the ranges indicated.

Benign nuisance palpitations due to VPCs or NSVT in patients with intrinsically normal myocardium and no echocardiographic or exercise-testing abnormalities should first be approached with reassurance and anxiolytics as required. Beta-blockers remain the

TABLE 4. Representative Adverse Effects of Antiarrhythmic Drugs

Drug	Adverse Effect*
Procainamide	GI effects, lupus syndrome, fever
Quinidine	GI effects, cinchonism, thrombocytopenia
Disopyramide	Anticholinergic effects (including dry mouth, blurred vision, urinary retention), negative inotropy
Tocainide	GI and CNS effects, paresthesias, thrombocytopenia
Mexiletine	GI and CNS effects, tremor, hepatic dysfunction
Lidocaine	GI and CNS effects
Flecainide	Blurred vision, IVCD, negative inotropy
Encainide	Blurred vision, paresthesias, IVCD, negative inotropy
Propafenone	GI and CNS effects, IVCD, negative inotropy
Propranolol	Lethargy, bradyarrhythmia, heart block, bronchospasm, negative inotropy
Amiodarone	GI effects, pulmonary toxicity, hypo- or hyperthyroidism, hepatitis, corneal microdeposits, sun sensitivity
Bretylium	GI effects, hypotension, catecholamine sensitivity

*Any antiarrhythmic drug can cause proarrhythmia.
IVCD, Intraventricular conduction delay.

antiarrhythmic therapy of choice for patients with persistent arrhythmia-related symptoms in this group and often will suppress ectopy sufficiently to provide comfort to the patient. Any of the beta-blocking, membrane-stabilizing agents in low-to-moderate dosages may prove effective in individual patients. The utility of drugs with intrinsic sympathomimetic activity for ventricular arrhythmias has not been clearly defined. Some advantage may be obtained with nonselective, i.e., beta$_1$-beta$_2$ blockers that diminish the tendency to peripheral hypokalemia, especially in patients receiving potassium-wasting diuretic therapy. For patients whose symptoms remain significant despite therapeutic trials with beta-blocking agents, Class I antiarrhythmic drugs may prove effective; however, each of these drugs has the potential for significant adverse, toxic, and potentially fatal effects with prolonged use. The risk/benefit ratio of therapy with antiarrhythmic drugs must be cautiously balanced when one considers therapy for arrhythmias that are not life threatening. The highly toxic agent amiodarone (Cordarone) should be avoided in this group.

Patients with NSVT or frequent VPCs or both in association with structural cardiac disease possess an increased risk for sustained VT or sudden death.[9–11] Precise delineation of individuals at greatest risk is not yet possible. The efficacy of therapy for these patients with *potentially lethal* arrhythmias must be weighed against the risks of antiarrhythmic drugs. Further, with the exception of beta-blockers in post-MI patients,[14,15] it is unclear whether suppression of ventricular arrhythmias in this patient population reduces sudden death risk; risk is increased by Class IC drugs in post-MI patients with chronic ventricular arrhythmias.[16] At present, the only antiarrhythmic drug appropriate for use in this group is one that has been clearly shown not to increase mortality. Thus, for now, only beta-blockers are indicated for suppression of ventricular ectopy in this group, and we would avoid all Class I antiarrhythmic agents until further data are forthcoming.

Since empiric or noninvasive ambulatory monitor-guided therapy for VPC suppression in patients with *lethal* ventricular arrhythmias is not as effective in predicting survival as directed therapy with serial electrophysiologic (EP) studies, invasive testing is indicated in patients with a history of sustained VT, VF, or cardiac arrest.[17] Drugs are selected based on efficacy, with allowance for a greater degree of risk from the medications themselves owing to the malignant nature of the underlying rhythm disorder. Individual drug efficacy rates range from 10 to 40 per cent for these arrhythmias (Table 5).

Class IA medications such as procainamide (Pronestyl, Procan SR) and quinidine (Quinidex, Quinaglute) provide first-line defense for sustained arrhythmias if proven effective for the patient at electrophysiologic testing. Higher dosages may be required than are used for less severe arrhythmias. Despite being moderately effective and familiar drugs, each of these agents carries toxic potential with prolonged use (see Table 4). Disopyramide (Norpace, Norpace CR), with negative inotropic effects, often is not tolerated because of the depressed left ventricular contractility present in the majority of patients with sustained ventricular arrhythmias.

The oral Class IB drugs, tocainide (Tonocard) and mexiletine (Mexitil), possess relatively low efficacy for suppression of sustained arrhythmias when used alone, but they may be synergistic when used together with Class IA drugs. Drugs used in combination may be administered at reduced dosage, decreasing the potential for intolerable side effects and dose-related electropharmacologic toxicities. The possibility for irreversible agranulocytosis in some patients treated with tocainide reserves its use only for patients with lethal ventricular arrhythmias. Despite side effects and toxicities on other organs, the Class IB agents possess lit-

TABLE 5. Efficacy Rates for Arrhythmia Suppression by Oral Antiarrhythmic Drugs

	% Effective	
Drug	***VPCs & NSVT***	***Sustained VT & VF***
Procainamide	60	25
Quinidine	65	25
Disopyramide	50	25*
Tocainide	40–50	10
Mexiletine	50	10
Encainide	80–85	25
Flecainide	80–85	25*
Propafenone	65–75	20*
Propranolol	50	5*
Amiodarone	N/A	20–40

*Increased likelihood of exacerbating heart failure.
N/A, Not applicable.

tle in the way of cardiac toxic manifestations (i.e., conduction slowing or negative inotropy). They may also be useful in combination with Class IC drugs and with amiodarone. IB/IC and IB/amiodarone combinations should be used only in patients with lethal arrhythmias.

Whereas Class IC drugs—encainide (Enkaid), flecainide (Tambocor), and propafenone (Rhythmol)—have greatest efficacy for nonsustained ventricular arrhythmias,[13,18] Class IC agents may increase sudden death rates in the potentially lethal arrhythmia population.[16,19,20] Thus, their use in patients with ventricular arrhythmias is limited to those with lethal forms, i.e., sustained ventricular tachycardia or ventricular fibrillation, albeit as a second- or third-line choice. These drugs are most proarrhythmic, however, in patients with severely depressed left ventricular ejection and the most hemodynamically compromising rapid ventricular tachycardias, [21] namely in those patients at greatest risk for arrhythmia recurrence and sudden cardiac death. After initiating therapy, dosage should be increased no more frequently than every 48 to 72 hours to decrease the potential for adverse hemodynamic or proarrhythmic effects. Each agent carries negative inotropic potential, and propafenone has concomitant beta-blocking effects. Efficacy rates for sustained ventricular tachycardia are moderate-to-low when these agents are used alone.

Suppression of sustained ventricular tachyarrhythmias with beta-blockers (Class II drugs) alone is uncommon, and the drugs have negative inotropic effects. They have greater efficacy for isolated VPCs and NSVT; they can be used in combination with other agents.

Amiodarone is the most effective single medication for sustained ventricular tachycardia but also is significantly toxic.[22] In-hospital loading requires 1 to 2 weeks, with the full loading duration extending several months. When compared with other agents, a lower percentage of patients with inducible VT on amiodarone will have clinical recurrence, but the tachycardia rate of induced VT correlates well with the rate of spontaneous VT, if it occurs. Major toxic manifestations involving pulmonary fibrosis or severe hepatic dysfunction require discontinuation of therapy. Hypo- or hyperthyroidism, owing to the iodine content of the drug, can be treated in the usual manner.

Device therapy is appropriate for patients with lethal ventricular arrhythmias in that it avoids drug toxicity and provides improved overall survival.[23] The automatic implantable cardioverter defibrillator (AICD) can be placed via sternotomy or thoracotomy in patients not suppressed with conventional medical therapy, who are intolerant to antiarrhythmic drugs, or in patients with cardiac arrest whose arrhythmia cannot be initiated in the electrophysiologic laboratory, i.e., with no marker of efficacy for antiarrhythmic medication. Antitachycardia pacing is useful in patients with sustained VT with moderate rates but may cause acceleration to VF. Thus, if used in the automatic mode, concomitant AICD implantation is recommended. Device interaction between pacemaker and AICD can be significant.

Antitachycardia pacing also can be used in the manual magnet-activated mode in the emergency department under monitored conditions. Demonstrated efficacy requires extensive electrophysiologic testing both intraoperatively and after surgery. Catheter ablation of the re-entrant circuit initiating sustained ventricular tachycardia requires extensive ventricular catheter mapping in the EP laboratory during VT; this can be performed only in patients with a hemodynamically tolerated arrhythmia. VT recurrence rates within 1 to 2 years after ablation are significant, up to 50 per cent.

Surgical endocardial resection and cryoablation may be performed in conjunction with aneurysmectomy to interrupt the re-entrant pathway initiating VT.[24] Intraoperative mapping proves useful in guiding resection for VT that does not originate in an obvious endocardial scar, but blind resection often proves successful. Surgical mortality remains as high as 15 per cent, even at centers where there are experienced staff. Follow-up inpatient EP testing demonstrates efficacy. The procedure is useful in patients with intractable VT or in those who require concomitant cardiac surgery. It does provide definitive cure in up to 90 per cent of those who survive the procedure. Concomitant AICD implantation or drug therapy may be necessary in some patients.

Patients with intractable, recurrent, sustained ventricular tachycardia in association with severe coronary artery disease or congestive heart failure may require cardiac transplantation. Antiarrhythmic drugs or devices may be used as a bridge to transplant.

■ Issues and Risks

Because of uncertainty about the long-term benefits of medical treatment with respect to improved survival in patients with potentially lethal arrhythmias, caution is necessary to avoid harmful effects of antiarrhythmic therapy in that population. Proarrhythmia occurs with any antiarrhythmic drug in 2 to 15 per cent of patients treated.[19-21] This may involve a new onset of asymptomatic or hemodynamically compromising atrial or ventricular arrhythmias, sustained VT, or sudden death. Initiation of medical therapy requires follow-up with ambulatory monitoring or EP testing, as well as regular examinations for signs or laboratory abnormalities consistent with organ toxicity. Combined intolerance and cardiac/noncardiac toxic effects lead to discontinuation of therapy with oral antiarrhythmic drugs in about 30 per cent of patients.

Despite medical therapy for sustained ventricular arrhythmias, recurrence rates remain significant in those with severely reduced myocardial contractility. This, together with the toxic potential of antiarrhythmic medications, has led to increased acceptance of device therapy, which may significantly prolong survival. Operative mortality limits the use of endocardial resection to selected patients with aneurysm or intractable ventricular tachycardia, whereas implantation of defibrillators carries less operative risk. However, use of devices entails considerable expense.

Combined transvenous antitachycardia pacing/defibrillation units hold promise.

REFERENCES

1. Morganroth J. Ambulatory "Holter" electrocardiography: choice of technologies and clinical uses. Ann Intern Med 1985; 102:73–82.
2. Horowitz LN, Josephson ME, Farshidi A, Spielman SR, Michelson EL, Greenspan AM. Recurrent sustained ventricular tachycardia. III. Role of the electrophysiologic study in selection of antiarrhythmic regimens. Circulation 1978; 58:986–997.
3. Ruskin JN, DiMarco JP, Garan H. Out-of-hospital cardiac arrest. Electrophysiologic observations and selection of long-term antiarrhythmic therapy. N Engl J Med 1980; 303:607–613.
4. Lown B. Sudden cardiac death. The major challenge confronting contemporary cardiology. Am J Cardiol 1979; 43:313–328.
5. Panidis IP, Morganroth J. Sudden death in hospitalized patients: cardiac rhythm disturbances detected by ambulatory electrocardiographic monitoring. J Am Coll Cardiol 1983; 2:798–805.
6. Savage DD, Castelli WP, Anderson SJ, Kannel WB. Sudden unexpected death during ambulatory electrocardiographic monitoring: the Framingham study. Am J Med 1983; 74:148–152.
7. Brodsky M, Wu D, Denes P, Kanakis C, Rosen KM. Arrhythmias documented by 24-hour continuous electrocardiographic monitoring in 50 male medical students without apparent heart disease. Am J Cardiol 1977; 39:390–395.
8. Kostis JB, McCrone K, Moreyra AE, Gotzoyannis S, Aglitz NM, Natarajan N, Kuo PT. Premature ventricular complexes in the absence of identifiable heart disease. Circulation 1981; 63:1351–1356.
9. Kotler MN, Tabatznik B, Mower MM, Tominaga S. Prognostic significance of ventricular ectopic beats with respect to sudden death in the late postinfarction period. Circulation 1973; 47:959–966.
10. Bigger JT, Weld FM, Rolnitzky LM. Prevalence, characteristics and significance of ventricular tachycardia (three or more complexes) detected with ambulatory electrocardiographic recording in the late hospital phase of acute myocardial infarction. Am J Cardiol 1981; 48:815–823.
11. The Multicenter Postinfarction Research Group. Risk stratification and survival after myocardial infarction. N Engl J Med 1983; 309:331–336.
12. American Heart Association Textbook of Advanced Cardiac Life Support. 1987:238–239.
13. DiBianco R, Fletcher RD, Cohen RI, Gottdiener JS. Treatment of frequent ventricular arrhythmia with encainide: assessment using serial ambulatory electrocardiograms, intracardiac electrophysiologic studies, treadmill exercise tests, and radionuclide cineangiographic studies. Circulation 1982; 65:1134–1137.
14. Beta-Blocker Heart Attack Trial Research Group. A randomized trial of propranolol in patients with acute myocardial infarction. I. Mortality results. JAMA 1982; 247:1707–1713.
15. Lichstein E, Morganroth J, Harrist R, Hubble E. Effect of propranolol on ventricular arrhythmia. The Beta Blocker Heart Attack Trial experience. Circulation 1983; 67(Suppl II):II1–II5.
16. The Cardiac Arrhythmia Suppression Trial (CAST) investigators. Increased mortality due to encainide or flecainide in a randomized trial of arrhythmia suppression after myocardial infarction. N Engl J Med 1989; 31:406–412.
17. Platia EV, Reid PR. Comparison of programmed electrical stimulation and ambulatory electrocardiographic (Holter) monitoring in the management of ventricular tachycardia and ventricular fibrillation. J Am Coll Cardiol 1984; 4:493–500.
18. The Flecainide-Quinidine Research Group. Flecainide versus quinidine for treatment of chronic ventricular arrhythmias: a multicenter clinical trial. Circulation 1983; 67:1117–1123.
19. Velebit V, Podrid P, Lown B, Cohen BH, Graboys TB. Aggravation and provocation of ventricular arrhymias by antiarrhythmic drugs. Circulation 1982; 65:886–894.
20. Morganroth J, Borland M, Chao G. Application of a

frequency definition of ventricular proarrhythmia. Am J Cardiol 1987; 59:97–99.

21. Morganroth J, Anderson JL, Gentzkow GD. Classification by type of ventricular arrhythmia predicts frequency of adverse cardiac effects from flecainide. J Am Coll Cardiol 1986; 8:607–615.

22. Mason JW. Amiodarone. N Engl J Med 1987; 316:455–466.

23. Marchlinski FE, Flores BT, Buxton AE, Hargrove WC III, Addonizio VP, Stephenson LW, Harken AH, Doherty JU, Grogan EW Jr, Josephson ME. The automatic implantable cardioverter-defibrillator: efficacy, complications, and device failures. Ann Intern Med 1986; 104:481–488.

24. Horowitz LN, Harken AH, Kastor JA, Josephson ME. Ventricular resection guided by epicardial mapping for the treatment of recurrent ventricular tachycardia. N Engl J Med 1980; 302:591–593.

Index